Get started with your **Connected Casebook**

Redeem your code below to access the **e-book** with search, highlighting, and note-taking capabilities; **case briefing** and **outlining** tools to support efficient learning; and more.

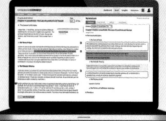

1. Go to www.casebookconnect.com
2. Enter your access code in the box and click **Register**
3. Follow the steps to complete your registration and verify your email address

If you have already registered at CasebookConnect.com, simply log into your account and redeem additional access codes from your Dashboard.

ACCESS CODE:
Scratch off with care.

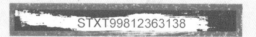

STXT99812363138

Is this a used casebook? Access code already redeemed? Purchase a digital version at **CasebookConnect.com/catalog**.

If you purchased a digital bundle with additional components, your additional access codes will appear below.

"I liked being able to search quickly while in class."

"Being able to highlight and easily create case briefs was a fantastic resource and time saver for me!"

D1716331

"I loved it! I was able to ~~ on the go and create a more effective outline."

For technical support, please visit http://support.wklegaledu.com.

ASPEN COURSEBOOK SERIES

LAW AND NEUROSCIENCE

Second Edition

OWEN D. JONES

*Glenn M. Weaver, M.D. and Mary Ellen Weaver Chair
in Law, Brain, and Behavior
Professor of Law & Professor of Biological Sciences
Vanderbilt University
Director, MacArthur Foundation Research Network
on Law and Neuroscience*

JEFFREY D. SCHALL

*E. Bronson Ingram Professor of Neuroscience
Vanderbilt University*

FRANCIS X. SHEN

*Professor, University of Minnesota Law School
Executive Director, MGH Center for Law, Brain & Behavior
Instructor in Psychology, Harvard Medical School*

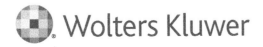

Published by Wolters Kluwer in New York.

Wolters Kluwer Legal & Regulatory U.S. serves customers worldwide with CCH, Aspen Publishers, and Kluwer Law International products. (www.WKLegaledu.com)

Cover image: iStock.com/metamorworks

To contact Customer Service, e-mail customer.service@wolterskluwer.com, call 1-800-234-1660, fax 1-800-901-9075, or mail correspondence to:

Wolters Kluwer
Attn: Order Department
PO Box 990
Frederick, MD 21705

Printed in the United States of America.

1 2 3 4 5 6 7 8 9 0

ISBN 978-1-5438-0109-5

Library of Congress Cataloging-in-Publication Data

Names: Jones, Owen D., author. | Schall, Jeffrey D., author. | Shen,
    Francis X. (Professor) author.
Title: Law and neuroscience / Owen D. Jones, Glenn M. Weaver, M.D. and
    Mary Ellen Weaver Chair in Law, Brain, and Behavior,
    Professor of Law & Professor of Biological Sciences,
    Vanderbilt University, Director, MacArthur Foundation Research
    Network on Law and Neuroscience; Jeffrey D. Schall, E. Bronson Ingram Professor of
    Neuroscience, Vanderbilt University; Francis X. Shen, Professor,
    University of Minnesota Law School, Executive Director, MGH Center for Law,
    Brain & Behavior, Instructor in Psychology, Harvard Medical School.
Description: Second edition. | New York : Wolters Kluwer, [2021] | Series:
    Aspen coursebook series | Includes bibliographical references and index. |
    Summary: "Coursebook on law and neuroscience, including the bearing of
    neuroscience on criminal law, criminal procedure, and evidence" —
    Provided by publisher.
Identifiers: LCCN 2020030500 (print) | LCCN 2020030501 (ebook) | ISBN
    9781543801095 (paperback) | ISBN 9781543823318 (ebook)
Subjects: LCSH: Practice of law — Psychological aspects. | Law — Philosophy.
    | Cognitive neuroscience. | LCGFT: Coursebooks (Law)
Classification: LCC K346 .J66 2021 (print) | LCC K346 (ebook) | DDC
    340/.19 — dc23
LC record available at https://lccn.loc.gov/2020030500
LC ebook record available at https://lccn.loc.gov/2020030501

About Wolters Kluwer Legal & Regulatory U.S.

Wolters Kluwer Legal & Regulatory U.S. delivers expert content and solutions in the areas of law, corporate compliance, health compliance, reimbursement, and legal education. Its practical solutions help customers successfully navigate the demands of a changing environment to drive their daily activities, enhance decision quality and inspire confident outcomes.

Serving customers worldwide, its legal and regulatory portfolio includes products under the Aspen Publishers, CCH Incorporated, Kluwer Law International, ftwilliam.com and MediRegs names. They are regarded as exceptional and trusted resources for general legal and practice-specific knowledge, compliance and risk management, dynamic workflow solutions, and expert commentary.

To Kelty   To Michelle   To Gabriel and Simone

O.D.J.   J.D.S.   F.X.S.

SUMMARY OF CONTENTS

CONTENTS

PREFACE

This book provides an introduction to the field of *Law and Neuroscience*.

Why neuroscience? Law regulates behavior. Behavior comes from brains. And through powerful new tools of cognitive neuroscience we are learning more than ever, faster than ever, about the complex relationships between brains, environments, mental states, and behavior. As we develop a deeper understanding of why and how we behave as we do, some rendezvous of law and neuroscience was inevitable. Cognitive neuroscience challenges law to examine many of its long-held assumptions and encourages each of us to reflect upon our own decision making, emotion regulation, and cognitive biases.

There have been a great many developments since the first edition of this book, seven years ago. There have been many new technological achievements in exploring, studying, and understanding the brain. Neuroscientific evidence is now mentioned so frequently in federal and state judicial opinions that it is no longer feasible to survey all instances. And, we reviewed over 600 of the many new publications—domestically and internationally—at the law/neuroscience intersection.

Consequently, this second edition has many major updates. We have substantially revised most chapters, in light of new scientific knowledge and legal developments. The revisions reflect current knowledge, and include new excerpts, new notes, new questions, and new advice about cutting-edge sources for further reading.

Although the superstructure of the book and the key topics remain largely the same as in the first edition, we have reordered several of the chapters based on our experiences teaching this course for optimal learning. Also, we have added a new chapter on Aging Brains.

As before, the materials—which span subjects such as lie-detection, judging, brain injury, emotions, memory, and the adolescent brain—are accessible, informative, and provocative. No prior knowledge of neuroscience is assumed or necessary. And, as before, the animating inquiry is not simply theoretical.

A rapidly increasing number of attorneys are attempting to use and defuse neuroscientific evidence in larger and larger swaths of criminal and civil law. For example, criminal defense attorneys increasingly proffer brain images, at the sentencing stage, to support arguments for mitigation. Both federal and state courts have been forced to rule on the admissibility of so-called brain-based lie detection. And the Supreme Court has considered neuroscience research in its rulings on the constitutionality of practices for sentencing juveniles. Some defendants have even successfully argued that their counsel was ineffective for failing to procure brain images as a part of their defense. On the civil side, brain images are increasingly proffered not only in tort cases, as one would expect, but also in constitutional, disability benefit, and contract cases, among others.

Judges are therefore increasingly confronted with whether to admit neuroscientific evidence. Jurors are increasingly tasked with trying to understand and evaluate it. And both legislatures and agencies are deciding what, if anything, to do in response to our expanding neuroscience knowledge base.

It is not possible to include, in these pages, everything that deserves attention. We have focused on providing the basics of brain science that lawyers, judges, and law students can use. And we have focused our coverage on a core set of fundamental questions and topics that presently animate the field.

There is no denying that neuroscience continues to present and continuously improve powerful new tools, such as in functional brain imaging. But it is also clear that, as with any tools, neuroscientific tools—and the evidence or policy shaped by and around them—can be used for good or for ill, skillfully or sloppily, and in ways that are legally and socially useful, on one hand, or irrelevant and potentially harmful, on the other. For these reasons, our book not only introduces some of the basics of how the brain works, but also highlights the delicate balance between the promise of neuroscience and the perils. Readers will be challenged to evaluate claims, evidence, and implications—both in science and in law—with care and rigor.

O.D.J., J.D.S., and F.X.S.

ACKNOWLEDGMENTS FOR THE SECOND EDITION

As before, we thank our schools, deans, and faculty colleagues for support and inspiration. For financial and institutional support we again thank the *MacArthur Foundation Research Network on Law and Neuroscience*, headquartered at Vanderbilt Law School and generously funded by grants from the John D. and Catherine T. MacArthur Foundation. We also thank the Vanderbilt University Center for Integrative & Cognitive Neuroscience.

In addition: ODJ acknowledges the support of the Glenn M. Weaver Foundation, through the Glenn M. Weaver, M.D. and Mary Ellen Weaver Chair in Law, Brain, and Behavior; JDS acknowledges the support of Robin and Richard Patton through the E. Bronson Ingram Chair of Neuroscience; and FXS acknowledges the support of the University of Minnesota Law School and the Massachusetts General Hospital Center for Law, Brain, and Behavior.

Special thanks to Quenna Stewart and Sarah Grove of Vanderbilt Law School for steadfast assistance in all aspects of this enterprise, to librarian Clanitra Nejdl of Vanderbilt Law School for research assistance, and to numerous librarians at the University of Minnesota Law School. Ms. Joni West—daughter of Herbert Weinstein (featured in Chapter 2)—provided generous and substantial insight into the life and later tribulations of her father. Journalist and author Kevin Davis generously shared his in-depth research for and manuscript of his book *The Brain Defense*, which brought many intriguing new facts and perspectives to light.

We would like to single out the following colleagues for numerous helpful insights, citations, and—often—permission to cite from their good works: Eyal Aharoni, Peter Alces, Matthew Baum, Marc Blitz, Ted Blumoff, Richard Bonnie, BJ Casey, Jennifer Chandler, Ed Cheng, Federica Coppola, Ryan Darby, Kevin Davis, Deborah Denno, Jennifer Drobac, Judy Edersheim, Ira Ellman, David Faigman, Martha Farah, Nita Farahany, Mark Fondacaro, Dov Fox, Mathew Ginther, James Giordano, Hank Greely, Betsy Grey, Valerie Hardcastle, Morris Hoffman, Judy Illes, Kent Kiehl, Adam Kolber, John Meixner, Michael Moore, Jane Moriarty, Stephen Morse, Roland Nadler, Michael Pardo, Dennis Patterson, Russell Poldrack, Adrian Raine, Valerie Reyna, Jesper Ryberg, Michael Saks, Elizabeth Scott, Adam Shniderman, Katrina Sifferd, Paige Skiba, Chris Slobogin, Larry Steinberg, Christopher Sundby, Anthony Wagner, Rick Wilson, and Gideon Yaffe.

We also thank the following students for crucial help in updating our various chapters and topics: Amber Banks, Andrea Bilbija, Julianne Campbell, Rebecca Childress, Gabriela Barriuso Clark, Warren Cormack, Michael Dunbar, Lea Gulotta, Jessica Lauren Haushalter, Brendan Johnson, Emily Lamm, Greg Maczko, Erin

Malapit, Monica Miecznikowski, Madeleine Muller, Corrine Nabors, Aubrianne Norton, Jennifer Novo, Breanna Philips, Christopher Sundby, Tevyn Waddell, Kennon Wales, Matthew Wilkinson, and Michaelene Wright. And this book as benefitted more broadly, as have we, from the eager engagement of our students, over the years, in our *Law and Neuroscience* courses.

The following sources are reprinted with permission:

American Law Institute, *Restatement of the Law Third, Torts: Liability for Physical and Emotional Harm* (2005).

Darby Aono, Gideon Yaffe & Hedy Kober, *Neuroscientific Evidence in the Courtroom: A Review*, 4 Cognitive Res. 40 (2019).

Daniel M. Bernstein & Elizabeth F. Loftus, *How to Tell If a Particular Memory Is True or False*, 4 Persp. Psychol. Sci. 370 (2009). Copyright © 2009 by Association for Psychological Science.

Marc J. Blitz, *Searching Minds by Scanning Brains: Neuroscience Technology and Constitutional Privacy Protection* (Marc J. Blitz, Jan C. Bublitz & Jane C. Moriarty eds., 2017).

Richard J. Bonnie, *Responsibility for Addiction*, 30 J. Am. Acad. Psychiatry L. 405 (2002). Copyright © 2002.

Nick Bostrom & Anders Sandberg, *Cognitive Enhancement: Methods, Ethics, Regulatory Challenges*, 15 Sci. & Engineering Ethics 311 (2009). Copyright © 2009, Springer Science & Business Media B.V.

Joshua W. Buckholtz, Valerie Reyna & Christopher Slobogin, *A Neuro-Legal Lingua Franca: Bridging Law and Neuroscience on the Issue of Self-Control*, 5 Mental Health L. & Pol'y J. 1 (2016).

Glenn R. Butterton, *How Neuroscience Technology Is Changing Our Understanding of Brain Injury, Vegetative States and the Law*, 20 N.C. J. L. & Tech. 331 (2019).

Ryan Calo, *Robotics and the Lessons of Cyberlaw*, 103 Calif. L. Rev. 513 (2015).

Samir Chopra & Laurence White, *Artificial Agents—Personhood in Law and Philosophy*, in *Proceedings of the 16th European Conference on Artificial Intelligence* 635 (2004). Copyright © 2004 by IOS Press.

Patricia Churchland, *The Big Questions: Do We Have Free Will?*, New Scientist, Nov. 18-24, 2006, at 42. Copyright © 2006 by New Scientist.

Federica Coppola, *The Brain in Solitude: An(other) Eighth Amendment Challenge to Solitary Confinement*, 6 J. Law & Biosciences 184 (2019).

Shana De Caro & Michael V. Kaplen, *Current Issues in Neurolaw*, 33 Psychiatric Clinics N. Am. 915 (2010). Copyright © 2010 by Elsevier, Inc.

Deborah W. Denno, *The Myth of the Double-Edged Sword: An Empirical Study of Neuroscience Evidence in Criminal Cases*, 56 B.C. L. Rev. 493 (2015).

David M. Eagleman, Mark A. Correro & Jyotpal Singh, *Why Neuroscience Matters for Rational Drug Policy*, 11 Minn. J. L. Sci. & Tech. 7 (2010). Copyright © 2010 by David M. Eagleman, Mark A. Correro, & Jyotpal Singh.

Joseph J. Fins, *Brain Injury: The Vegetative and Minimally Conscious States*, in *From Birth to Death and Bench to Clinic: The Hastings Center Bioethics Briefing Book for Journalists, Policymakers, and Campaigns* 15 (Mary Crowley ed., 2008). Copyright © 2008 by The Hastings Center.

Lyn M. Gaudet & Gary E. Marchant, *Under the Radar: Neuroimaging Evidence in the Criminal Courtroom*, 64 Drake L. Rev. 577 (2016).

Nancy Gertner, *Neuroscience and Sentencing*, 85 Fordham L. Rev. 533 (2016).

Paul Gewirtz, *On "I Know It When I See It"*, 105 Yale L.J. 1023 (1996).

Sara Gordon, *The Use and Abuse of Mutual-Support Programs in Drug Courts*, 2017 U. Ill. L. Rev. 1503 (2017).

Henry T. Greely, *Premarket Approval Regulation for Lie Detections: An Idea Whose Time May Be Coming*, 5 Am. J. Bioethics 50 (2005). Copyright © 2005 by Routledge.

Joshua Greene & Jonathan Cohen, *For the Law, Neuroscience Changes Nothing and Everything*, 359 Phil. Transactions Royal Soc'y B 1775 (2004). Copyright © 2004 by The Royal Society.

Joshua D. Greene & Joseph M. Paxton, *Patterns of Neural Activity Associated with Honest and Dishonest Moral Decisions*, 106 Proc. Nat'l Acad. Sci. U.S. 12506 (2009). Copyright © 2009 by National Academy of Sciences.

Betsy J. Grey, *Neuroscience and Emotional Harm in Tort Law: Rethinking the American Approach to Free-Standing Emotional Distress Claims in Law and Neuroscience*, in *Law and Neuroscience: Current Legal Issues* 203 (Michael Freeman ed., Oxford Univ. Press 2011). Copyright © 2011 by Oxford University Press. Reproduced with permission of the Licensor through PLSClear.

Jaap Hage, *Theoretical Foundations for the Responsibility of Autonomous Agents*, 25 Artificial Intelligence & L. 255 (2017).

Valerie Gray Hardcastle, M. K. Kitzmiller & Shelby Lahey, *The Impact of Neuroscience Data in Criminal Cases: Female Defendants and the Double-Edged Sword*, 21 New Crim. L. Rev. 291 (2018).

Morris B. Hoffman, *Nine Neurolaw Predictions*, 21 New Crim. L. Rev. 212 (2018).

Morris B. Hoffman, *Problem-Solving Courts and the Psycholegal Error*, 160 U. Pa. L. Rev. PENNumbra 129 (2011). Copyright © 2011 University of Pennsylvania Law Review.

Morris B. Hoffman & Frank Krueger, *The Neuroscience of Blame and Punishment*, in *Self, Culture and Consciousness* 207 (Sangeetha Menon, V.V. Binoy & Nithin Nagaraj eds., 2020).

Dietmar Hübner & Lucie White, *Neurosurgery for Psychopaths? An Ethical Analysis*, 7 Am. J. Bioethics Neurosci. 140 (2016).

Virginia Hughes, *Science in Court: Head Case*, 464 Nature 340 (2010). Copyright © 2010, Rights managed by Nature Publishing Group.

Steven E. Hyman, *The Neurobiology of Addiction: Implications for Voluntary Control of Behavior*, 7 Am. J. Bioethics 8 (2007). Copyright © 2007 by Routledge.

Irena P. Ilieva, Cayce J. Hook & Martha J. Farah, *Prescription Stimulants' Effects on Healthy Inhibitory Control, Working Memory, and Episodic Memory: A Meta-Analysis*, 27 J. Cognitive Neurosci. 1069 (2015).

Owen D. Jones & Timothy H. Goldsmith, *Law and Behavioral Biology*, 105 Colum. L. Rev. 405 (2005). Copyright © 2005 Columbia Law Review.

Kent A. Kiehl et al., *Age of Gray Matters: Neuroprediction of Recidivism*, 19 Neuroimage 813 (2018).

Adam Kolber, *Free Will as a Matter of Law*, in *Philosophical Foundations of Law and Neuroscience* 9 (Michael Pardo & Dennis Patterson eds., 2016).

Adam J. Kolber, *Therapeutic Forgetting: The Legal and Ethical Implications of Memory Dampening*, 59 Vand. L. Rev. 1561 (2006). Copyright © 2006 Vanderbilt Law Review, Adam Kolber.

Harrison A. Korn, Micah A. Johnson & Marvin M. Chun, *Neurolaw: Differential Brain Activity for Black and White Faces Predicts Damage Awards in Hypothetical Employment Discrimination Cases*, 7 Soc. Neurosci. 398 (2012). Copyright © 2012 Routledge.

Ivan S. Kotchetkov et al., *Brain-Computer Interfaces: Military, Neurosurgical, and Ethical Perspective*, 28 Neurological Focus E25 (2010). Copyright © 2010 Neurological Focus.

Adam Lamparello, *Using Cognitive Neuroscience to Predict Future Dangerousness*, 4 Colum. Hum. Rts. L. Rev. 481 (2011).

Daniel Langleben & Jane Moriarty, *Using Brain Imaging for Lie Detection: Where Science, Law, and Policy Collide*, 19 Psychol. Pub. Pol'y & L. 222 (2013).

The MacArthur Foundation Research Network on Law and Neuroscience, *G2i Knowledge Brief* (2017).

Terry A. Maroney, *The False Promise of Adolescent Brain Science in Juvenile Justice*, 85 Notre Dame L. Rev. 89 (2009). Copyright © 2009 Notre Dame Law Review.

Daniel A. Martell, *Causal Relation Between Brain Damage and Homicide: The Prosecution*, 1 Seminars Clinical Neuropsychiatry 184 (1996). Copyright © 1996 Elsevier B.V.

Helen S. Mayberg, *Medical-Legal Inferences from Functional Neuroimaging Evidence*, 1 Seminars Clinical Neuropsychiatry 195 (1996).

Michael S. Moore, *Addiction, Responsibility, and Neuroscience*, 2020 U. Ill. L. Rev. 375 (2020).

Stephen J. Morse, *Neuroscience and the Future of Personhood and Responsibility*, in *Constitution 3.0: Freedom and Technological Change* 113 (Jeffrey Rosen & Benjamin Wittes eds., 2011). Copyright © 2011 Brookings Institution.

Stephen J. Morse, *Voluntary Control of Behavior and Responsibility*, 7 Am. J. Bioethics 12 (2007). Copyright © 2007 Routledge.

Bryan Myers et al., *Psychology Weighs in on the Debate Surrounding Victim Impact Statements and Capital Sentencing: Are Emotional Jurors Really Irrational?*, 19 Fed. Sent'g Rep. 13 (2006). Copyright © 2006, published by University of California Press for Vera Institute of Justice.

Nat'l Research Council, *Identifying the Culprit: Assessing Eyewitness Identification* (2014).

Nat'l Research Council, *Adolescent Development*, in *Reforming Juvenile Justice: A Developmental Approach* 89 (2013).

Eric A. Posner, *Law and the Emotions*, 89 Geo. L. J. 1977 (2001). Copyright © 2001 Georgetown Law Review.

Norman Relkin et al., *Impulsive Homicide Associated with an Arachnoid Cyst and Unilateral Frontotemporal Cerebral Dysfunction*, 1 Seminars Clinical Neuropsychiatry 172 (1996). Copyright © Elsevier B.V.

Neil M. Richards & William D. Smart, *How Should the Law Think About Robots?*, in *Robot Law* 5 (Ryan Calo, A. Michael Froomkin & Ian Kerr eds., 2016).

Edwina L. Rissland, *Artificial Intelligence and Law: Stepping Stones to A Model of Legal Reasoning*, 99 Yale L.J. 1957 (1990).

Adina L. Roskies, Nicholas J. Shweitzer & Michael J. Saks, *Neuroimages in Court: Less Biasing Than Feared*, 17 Trends Cognitive Sci. 99 (2013). Copyright © 2013, Elsevier.

Michael J. Saks & David L. Faigman, *Expert Evidence After Daubert*, 1 Ann. Rev. L. Soc. Sci. 105 (2005).

Robert M. Sapolsky, *The Frontal Cortex and the Criminal Justice System*, 359 Phil. Transactions Royal Soc'y B 1787 (2004). Copyright © 2004, The Royal Society.

Sally Satel & Scott O. Lilienfeld, *Addiction and the Brain-Disease Fallacy*, in *Brainwashed: The Seductive Appeal of Mindless Neuroscience* 49 (2013). Copyright © 2013, Perseus Books Group.

Daniel L. Schacter, *The Seven Sins of Memory: Insights from Psychology and Cognitive Neuroscience*, 54 Am. Psychologist 182 (1999). Copyright © 1999. Reprinted with permission by the author.

Frederick Schauer, *Neuroscience, Lie-Detection, and the Law*, 14 Trends Cognitive Sci. 101 (2010). Copyright © 2010, Elsevier.

Elizabeth Scott, Natasha Duell & Laurence Steinberg, *Brain Development, Social Context, and Justice Policy*, 57 Wash. U. J. L. & Pol'y 13 (2018).

Elizabeth Scott & Thomas Grisso, *Developmental Competence and Juvenile Justice Reform*, 83 N.C. L. Rev. 793 (2005). Copyright © 2005 by the North Carolina Law Review.

Francis X. Shen, *Legislating Neuroscience: The Case of Juvenile Justice*, 46 Loy. L.A. L. Rev. 985 (2013).

ACKNOWLEDGMENTS FOR THE FIRST EDITION

This book would not have been possible without considerable and generous support, feedback, and assistance.

We first gratefully acknowledge the many scholars, both in science and in law, whose research has launched construction of the key interdisciplinary bridges that have enabled this field and this book. Many of their works are excerpted or mentioned in these pages.

For financial and institutional support we thank the *MacArthur Foundation Research Network on Law and Neuroscience*, and the *MacArthur Foundation Law and Neuroscience Project*, each generously funded by the John D. and Catherine T. MacArthur Foundation. We especially thank Laurie Garduque and Julia Stasch, of the Foundation, for a decade of enthusiasm for exploring the ways in which neuroscience might help the legal system to be more just, fair, and effective. Relatedly, we thank all the members of the *MacArthur Foundation Research Network on Law and Neuroscience* and the *MacArthur Foundation Law and Neuroscience Project* for their feedback at all stages.

We also thank *Vanderbilt Law School*, the *Vanderbilt University Center for Integrative & Cognitive Neuroscience*, and the *University of Minnesota Law School*. We extend special thanks to our respective Deans and Chairs—Christopher Guthrie, Carolyn Dever, Andrew Tomarken, and David Wippman—for their support and encouragement in this endeavor. JDS acknowledges the support of the College of Arts & Science for a semester leave of absence, and the support of Robin and Richard Patton through the *E. Bronson Ingram Chair of Neuroscience*. FXS acknowledges the support of the University of Minnesota Robina Institute of Criminal Law and Criminal Justice, as well as Tulane University Law School and the Tulane University Murphy Institute.

The *Dana Foundation* supported this book through the very thoughtful review and feedback provided on each chapter by Jane Nevins. We are also grateful for the opportunity to participate in numerous education and outreach programs enabled and facilitated by Monika Gruter Cheney, Oliver Goodenough, and *The Gruter Institute for Law and Behavioral Research*. These programs taught us much about how to communicate across disciplinary boundaries.

We are extremely grateful to the many colleagues who have reviewed, taught from, or thoughtfully critiqued earlier chapters or full drafts of this book: Peter Alces, Marc Blitz, Theodore Blumoff, Teneille Brown, Glenn Butterton, Limin Chen, Patricia Churchland, Deborah Denno, Jason Dominguez, Jennifer Drobac, David Faigman, Martha Farah, Neal Feigenson, Oliver Goodenough, Hank Greely, Joshua Greene, Betsy Grey, Tracy Gunter, Morris Hoffman, Peter Huang, Kent Kiehl, Adam Kolber, Gary Marchant, René Marois, Jane Campbell Moriarty, Stephen Morse, Emily Murphy, Ken Murray, Thomas Nadelhoffer, Amanda Pustilnik, Anna

Roe, Oliver Rollins, Susan Rushing, Michael Saks, Elizabeth Scott, Gideon Yaffe, and the anonymous reviewers. For their help in developing the chapter on Herbert Weinstein, we thank Abass Alavi, Jonathan Brodie, Antonio Damasio, Daniel Martell, Norman Relkin, and Diarmuid White.

In addition, we thank those colleagues and friends not already mentioned who have helped us to make this a better book though friendship, feedback, critique, and conversation. These include, among others too numerous to list: Kathryn Abrams, Eyal Aharoni, Jay Aronson, Susan Bandes, Mimi Belcher, James Blumstein, Richard Bonnie, Joshua Buckholtz, Silvia Bunge, BJ Casey, Kate Darling, Andre Davis, Robert Desimone, David Eagleman, Martha Farah, Nita Farahany, William Fletcher, Michael Flomenhaft, Dov Fox, Michael Gazzaniga, Apostolos Georgopoulos, Matthew Ginther, Scott Grafton, Dena Gromet, Pim Haselager, Robert Heilbronner, Yasmin Hurd, Doug Husak, Steve Hyman, William Iacono, Judy Illes, Peter Imrey, Elizabeth Janss, Ronald Kalil, Michael Kaplen, Rob Kar, David Kaye, Rob Kurzban, Adam Lamparello, Terence Lenamon, Tyler Lorig, Philip Low, Monica Luciana, Beatriz Luna, Gerard Lynch, Angus MacDonald, Robin Mackenzie, John Maloney, Andrew Mansfield, Terry Maroney, Helen Mayberg, John Meixner, Gilbert Merritt, John Mikhail, John Monahan, Read Montague, Michael Moore, Milica Mormann, Michael Neff, William Newsome, Charles O'Brien, Sandra Day O'Connor, Erin O'Hara, Cheryl Olman, Dennis Patterson, Elizabeth Phelps, The Pontifical Academy of Sciences Working Group on Neuroscience and the Human Person, Martha Presley, Fred Pritzker, Jeffrey Rachlinski, Marc Raichle, Adrian Raine, Jed Rakoff, David Redish, Jennifer Richeson, Jeffrey Rosen, Adina Roskies, Amedeo Santosuosso, Robert Sapolsky, Joseph Savirimuthu, Fred Schauer, Darren Schreiber, Nick Schweitzer, Julie Seaman, Benjamin Shannon, Dan Simon, Ken Simons, Walter Sinnott-Armstrong, Pate Skene, Chris Slobogin, Carter Snead, Tade Spranger, Laurence Steinberg, Adam Steiner, Christopher Sundby, Sherrod Taylor, Kim Taylor-Thompson, Brooke Terpening, Frank Tong, Tim Totolo, Stacey Tovino, Michael Treadway, University of Pennsylvania's Neuroscience Boot Camp participants and speakers, Mike Vandenbergh, Nicole Vincent, Anthony Wagner, Gary Watson, Amy Wax, Susan Wolf, William Woodruff, Wu Xiyu, and David Zald. And for graciously allowing us to adapt portions of their excellent glossary materials, we thank Adina Roskies, Mimi Belcher, and Stephen Morse.

More generally, we would like to acknowledge other colleagues and friends we have had the pleasure of interacting with at various neurolaw events sponsored by, among others, the *American Association for the Advancement of Science, American Bar Association, Cognitive Neuroscience Society, European Association for Neuroscience and Law, Federal Judicial Center, MGH Center for Law, Brain & Behavior, Society for Evolutionary Analysis in Law, Society for Neuroscience*, and the *University of Pennsylvania Center for Neuroscience and Society*.

We owe a special debt of gratitude to the numerous research assistants who have provided us with tremendous support. We thank: Mariam Abdel-Malek, John Arceci, Sarah Becker, Andrea Bilbija, Thomas Booms, Sam Brandao, Monisha Chakravarthy, Spencer Compton, Neal Curtis, Sean Deitrick, Jonathan Dial, Shawn Donovan, Kathryn Easterling, Jenna Farleigh, John Frost, Christopher Gilmore, Anne Gooch, Felicity Grisham, Vihra Groueva, Courtney Holliday, Eric Jackson, Lauren Bair Jacques, Annie Jwa, Michelle Kallen, Ellen Kleeman, Cameron Kruger, Kathleen Kubis, Kathryn Kuhn, Emily Larish, Ryan Lee, Amy Mandel, Jillian Mastroianni,

Lindsey Gilling McIntosh, Tim Mitchell, Andrew Nielsen, Jonathan Ord, Sonal Patel, Sadev Parikh, Sarah Pazar, Alex Payne, Sarah Prentice-Mott, Lauren Ramos, Jennifer Sauer, Alexandria Scarbrough, Michael Sherby, Bailey Spaulding, Drew Staniewski, Raquel Stringer, Jamie Lynn Thalgott, Katherine Van Deusen, Kurt Vincent, Charles Wei, Richard Weinmeyer, Jacob Westerberg, Bethany Whelan, Eun Sun Yoo, and Emily Zenger.

We are also grateful to the many students in our law and neuroscience courses at Vanderbilt, Tulane, and Minnesota. They have provided helpful critiques, suggestions, and feedback on teaching and text alike.

We thank the many people at Aspen Publishers—including Carol McGeehan, Peter Skagestad, Christine Hannan, and Patrick Cline of The Froebe Group—who provided crucial support from the inception to the completion of this project.

For support in many facets of the research for this book, we thank the Vanderbilt Law School Library staff, as well as the University of Minnesota Law School Library staff. For technology support, we thank Sean Jewett, Sergey Motorny, and the entire Vanderbilt University IT staff. For administrative work at Vanderbilt, we are grateful for consistently outstanding and helpful support from Mollie Bodin Claar, Jennifer Kilgore, and Sue Ann Scott.

We owe a special debt of gratitude to Sarah Grove and Christie Bishop, who from the first stages of this project have provided countless hours of invaluable organization and assistance.

Finally, and always, we thank our families for their love and support throughout this project. Our brains (and we hope our chapters) are better for it.

CONVENTIONS

As an interdisciplinary text, aimed at students not only in law but also in neuroscience, psychology, philosophy, and related disciplines, this coursebook presents material in a way that may be foreign to some readers.

For those unfamiliar with legal texts, and law coursebooks in particular, it is important to note that law school coursebooks are wholly unlike scientific textbooks. Indeed, they may appear more like bound class packs—collections of reprints used to introduce a range of topics. Specifically, law school coursebooks are primarily composed of provocative selections and excerpts, reflecting a variety of different source materials and viewpoints, in order to prompt probing classroom discussion and analysis.

We have adopted that customary approach. But we have supplemented it with more background information—particularly in the early chapters—than ordinarily appears. That reflects the balance we have chosen to strike between establishing basic knowledge and prompting consideration of potential legal and policy implications.

We have also generally put references into legal citation format. This differs from MLA and APA styles. For instance, in legal citation the volume in which an article appears is located ahead of the title of the journal in which it appears (rather than after it) and only the first page (rather than the full range) is cited.

For law students, most of our formatting conventions should seem familiar. We have adopted the customary coursebook approach of including ellipses to signify missing text in excerpts, but not including them to signify only missing citations. Thus, inside judicial opinions we have liberally omitted, without distracting ellipses, the frequent citations to other cases. In law review articles, we have generally not included footnotes. In the science excerpts, we have similarly omitted references without ellipses. Where footnotes remain, numbered footnotes within excerpts are from the original source and footnotes denoted with an asterisk have been inserted by us to provide additional clarification. We have also generally converted British spelling to American, and we have at times converted color graphics to black-and-white.

Many resources are available to readers interested in additional information on law and neuroscience.

To keep you up to date on recent happenings in neurolaw, the complimentary *Neurolaw News* listserv periodically circulates new developments in publications, conferences, cases, and the like. Sign up to receive it at http://www.lawneuro.org/listserv.php (Past editions available at: http://www.lawneuro.org/news.php).

A comprehensive, searchable, sortable bibliography of publications in Law & Neuroscience is also available online here: http://www.lawneuro.org/bibliography .php.

Follow the research of the *MacArthur Foundation Research Network on Law and Neuroscience* here: www.lawneuro.org.

Readers who seek further knowledge about the brain—whether at very basic or very advanced levels – have many resources available. We list many popular books, at both levels, at the end of Chapter 3 (which introduces brain structure and function).

In addition, many websites offer valuable and sometimes more visual information about the brain. The Society for Neuroscience, for instance, provides a very useful and authoritative online resource. The Society for Neuroscience was founded in 1969 and now has more than 40,000 members. It not only serves to advance understanding of the brain and the nervous system, but also promotes educational programs about the brain and informs legislators and other policy makers about the implications of neuroscience research for public policy, societal benefit, and continued scientific progress. Its website, www.sfn.org, hosts several excellent resources on basic information about the brain including Brain Facts (www.brainfacts.org).

A number of other professional organizations also provide useful information and perspective:

- Association for Psychological Science: http://www.psychologicalscience.org
- Cognitive Neuroscience Society (CNS): http://www.cogneurosociety.org/
- Society for Evolutionary Analysis in Law (SEAL): http://www.sealsite.org
- Society for Neuroeconomics: http://neuroeconomics.org
- Society for Social Neuroscience: http://s4sn.org/

You can also learn more about neuroscience and brain disorders at the National Institutes of Health (www.nih.gov), and of special interest may be the NIH Brain Research through Advancing Innovative Neurotechnologies ® (BRAIN) Initiative: https://braininitiative.nih.gov/. In addition, the websites of the various NIH Institutes may be of interest:

- National Institute on Aging: http://www.nia.nih.gov/
- National Institute on Alcohol Abuse & Alcoholism: http://www.niaaa.nih .gov/

- Eunice Kennedy Shriver National Institute of Child Health & Human Development: http://www.nichd.nih.gov
- National Institute on Drug Abuse: http://www.drugabuse.gov/
- National Institute of Mental Health: http://www.nimh.nih.gov/
- National Institute of Neurological Disorders & Stroke: http://www.ninds.nih .gov

Finally, a growing number of law and science student groups—such as those at Vanderbilt, Stanford, University of Pennsylvania, and the University of Wisconsin, to name a few, are organizing on college campuses. And if your campus doesn't have a student group yet, you can start one. . . .

LAW AND NEUROSCIENCE

INTRODUCTION

This book has five Parts. The first Part orients you to the intersections of law and neuroscience. It provides a broad and distinctly introductory view of some of the most interesting issues in neurolaw, while saving the deeper details for later Parts. Part 1 assumes no prior familiarity either with neuroscience, or with the major advantages, challenges, and limitations of using neuroscientific evidence in the legal system. In addition, this Part introduces the legal issues so that readers without extensive legal backgrounds will still find the material accessible.

In Part 1, you'll read about criminals with various brain deficiencies and debate what the legal implications should be. You'll hear from proponents, critics, and those with intermediate positions regarding the existing and future roles of neuroscience in law. And you'll begin developing your own sense of how, when, and where neuroscience can (and cannot) aid the goals of law.

Part 2 introduces the basic facts and tools of cognitive neuroscience. It provides a user-friendly overview of brain structure and brain function. It explains in an accessible way how the various brain-monitoring techniques work. And it discusses the important limits and cautions that should serve as a necessary restraint on the interpretation and use of brain data in legal proceedings.

Part 3 introduces some of the main conceptual issues in the field of Law and Neuroscience. These include: the ways law, science, and behavior interact; legal and neuroscientific perspectives on the relationship between behavior and responsibility; and the evidentiary issues that underlie decisions to proffer, admit, or reject neuroscientific evidence in a range of legal contexts.

Part 4 then turns to core themes in Law and Neuroscience. These include legal issues surrounding brain states such as death, injury, pain and distress, and addiction. These also include legal issues affected by how people think and feel, in the realms of memory, emotions, lie detection, and decision-making. The Part ends with consideration of legal issues arising from the still-maturing adolescent brain and the wiser but slower and more forgetful aging brain.

Part 5 looks to the future, which seemed so far away when we wrote the first edition. It explores the complicated legal and policy issues surrounding "cognitive enhancement"—the improvement of brain function through drugs and machines. It also provides a window into the challenges for law that flow from advances in brain-machine interfaces, neuroprosthetics, and artificial intelligence.

But first, the beginning.

PART SUMMARY

This Part:
- Introduces, in Chapter 1, a wide variety of contexts in which law and neuroscience already meet, and many ways in which they may intersect in the future.
- Illustrates, in Chapter 2, how evidence about the brain of an individual who is party to a case can raise challenging evidentiary and scientific issues.

CHAPTER 1

Law and Neuroscience: An Overview of the Issues

"You," your joys and your sorrows, your memories and your ambitions, your sense of personal identity and free will, are in fact no more than the behavior of a vast assembly of nerve cells and their associated molecules. Who you are is nothing but a pack of neurons . . . although we appear to have free will, in fact, our choices have already been predetermined for us and we cannot change that.

—Francis Crick[†]

Neuroscience has the potential to make internal contributions to legal doctrine and practice if the relation is properly understood. For now, however, such contributions are modest at best and neuroscience poses no genuine, radical challenges to concepts of personhood, responsibility, and competence.

—Stephen Morse[††]

CHAPTER SUMMARY

This chapter:
- Introduces fundamental themes to be explored in the book, and illustrates the potentially wide-ranging applications of neuroscience to law.
- Foreshadows some of the important limits to using neuroscience in legal contexts.
- Raises practical and ethical questions about the implications of neuroscience research for the courtroom, legal practice, and public policy.

INTRODUCTION

From 2009 through 2013, more than 1,700,000 publications appeared on brain and neuroscience research. According to the authors reporting this, that figure constituted 16% of the world's scientific publication output for that period.[*]

[†] Francis Crick, *The Astonishing Hypothesis* 3 (1994).

[††] Stephen Morse, *Lost in Translation? An Essay on Law and Neuroscience*, in *Neuroscience: Current Legal Issues* 562 (Michael Freeman ed., 2011).

[*] Elsevier Research Intelligence Analytical Services, *Brain Science: Mapping the Landscape of Brain and Neuroscience Research* 3 (2014).

Although not all neuroscientific studies are conducted with human participants, scientists have learned a tremendous amount about how the human brain works, how it malfunctions, and how it can be repaired and altered. This growing neuroscience knowledge base has already revolutionized medical practice. But when, why, and how can neuroscience aid *law*?

This is the central question you will encounter in this coursebook, and we will encourage you to consider a wide number of potential legal applications. We will also encourage you to maintain a critical eye. Careful scientific analysis and careful legal analysis are requisites to successfully navigating the field of neurolaw.

This introductory chapter highlights the wide variety of possible, potential, and actual intersections of neuroscience and law. Many of these, as you might guess, arise in the criminal justice context. For instance, between 2005 and 2015 alone, over 2,800 judicial opinions were published regarding neuroscientific evidence proffered by defendants.* That is a surprisingly large number, given that more than 90% of criminal cases in the United States are resolved through plea bargaining and that the vast majority of the remainder that do proceed to trial result in no published opinion whatsoever.

Yet while the basic criminal defense "my brain made me do it" has drawn disproportionate attention (presumably reflecting greater readership interest), you should see from the material in this chapter that neuroscience is commonly—probably more commonly—used in civil contexts as well. Personal injury litigators frequently rely on neurologists, for instance, and there appears to be a rapidly-growing use of neuroscientific evidence by those litigating for disability benefits. Indeed, it was lawyers on the civil side who first coined the term "neurolaw" in 1995.**

In addition to recognizing the variety of potential uses, you should also see that current and future uses of neuroscience in law are not unlimited. Although evidence suggests that the number of cases involving neuroscientific evidence is rapidly rising,*** modern brain science is still new to the legal scene. This is perhaps obvious, but it is a point worth emphasizing because the youth of the field has implications for how you read the materials in this book. Unlike some courses, in which the law is relatively fixed and has been for some time, neurolaw is comparatively new and changing. Consider that over 92% of the publications and cases included in this book were published only since 2000, with nearly 70% published since 2010 and 45% published just since the first edition of this book in 2014. As compared to the first edition, this edition contains 600 new references and citations to recent developments, with 260 new readings, including 27 new case selections.

As with other new technologies that law has confronted, the rise of modern neuroscience raises deep, recurring questions that you will ask yourself as you read this book: Is the neuroscience ready? Do we know enough to draw legally relevant conclusions? Does neuroscience tell us anything we don't already know from common

---

* Henry T. Greely & Nita A. Farahany, *Neuroscience and the Criminal Justice System,* 2 Ann. Rev. Criminology 451, 453 (2019).

** The earliest published uses of the term "neurolawyer" and "neurolaw" were in 1991 and 1995 by Attorney J. Sherrod Taylor. J. Sherrod Taylor et al., *Neuropsychologists and Neurolawyers,* 5 Neuropsychology 293, 293-305 (1991); J. Sherrod Taylor, *Neurolaw: Towards a New Medical Jurisprudence,* 9 Brain Inj. 745, 745-51 (1995).

*** *See, e.g.,* Henry T. Greely & Nita A. Farahany, *Neuroscience and the Criminal Justice System,* Ann. Rev. Criminology 2:451, 2:451-471 (2019); Nita A. Farahany, *Neuroscience and Behavioral Genetics in US Criminal Law: An Empirical Analysis,* 2 J.L. & Biosci. 485, 485-509 (2016).

sense or previous behavioral research? Are there some areas of law to which neuro-science may never be relevant? How shall we assess when law should and should not defer to neuroscientific conclusions? Are the legal actors—judges, lawyers, and leg-islators—ready and able to integrate sound neuroscience evidence into their prac-tice and deliberations? How can legal actors distinguish between neuroscientific wheat and chaff? Are the scientific researchers and medical professionals capable of communicating their ideas in ways accessible to a legal audience?

How these questions will be answered is of course unknown today. But what is known is that the future of neurolaw will likely be determined as much by legal decision-makers like yourself as it will be by scientists. Legislators, judges, lawyers, and legal scholars will decide first how to frame these policy questions and then how to answer them, based on the best information that science can provide.

This introductory chapter proceeds in two sections. In Section A you will learn about two cases, one in criminal law and one in contracts, in which attorneys offered neuroscientific evidence. As you read, consider the arguments of proponents and critics of using neuroscience in these ways—as those arguments will reoccur throughout the book. Section B discusses the rise of neurolaw as an area of legal practice, scientific research, and interdisciplinary dialogue. It also surveys the views of several scholars about some of the key legal topics on which law and neuroscience have already intersected, or might soon intersect. As you read, you should think critically and creatively about which areas of law and policy will be most, and least, affected by advances in neuroscience.

A. INTRODUCING NEUROSCIENTIFIC EVIDENCE

Virginia Hughes
Science in Court: Head Case
464 Nature 340, 340-42 (2010)

Brian Dugan, dressed in an orange jumpsuit and shackles, shuffled to the door of Northwestern Memorial Hospital in downtown Chicago, accompanied by four sher-iff deputies. It was the first time that Dugan, 52, had been anywhere near a city in 20 years. Serving two life sentences for a pair of murders he committed in the 1980s, he was now facing the prospect of the death penalty for an earlier killing.

Dugan was here on a Saturday this past September to meet one of the few people who might help him to avoid that fate: Kent Kiehl, a neuroscientist at the University of New Mexico in Albuquerque. Dugan, Kiehl, and the rest of the entourage walked the length of the hospital, crossed a walkway to another building, and took the lift down to a basement-level facility where researchers would scan Dugan's brain using functional magnetic resonance imaging (fMRI).* Todd Parrish, the imaging cen-ter's director, offered plastic zip ties to replace the shackles—no metal is allowed in the same room as the scanner's powerful magnet—but the guards said they weren't necessary. Dugan entered the machine without restraints, and Parrish locked the door—as much to keep the guards and their weapons out as to keep Dugan in.

---

* [Chapters 4 and 5 describe the fMRI method, and the Appendix carefully explains how to criti-cally evaluate publications using this method.—EDS.]

Dugan lay still inside the scanner for about 90 minutes, performing a series of cognitive control, attention, and moral decision-making tests. Afterwards, he ate a hamburger, sat through an extensive psychiatric interview, and rode back to DuPage county jail, about 50 kilometers west of Chicago.

Kiehl has been amassing data on men such as Dugan for 16 years. Their crimes are often impulsive, violent, committed in cold blood, and recalled without the slightest twinge of remorse. They are psychopaths, and they are estimated to make up as much as 1% of the adult male population and 25% of male prisoners. To date, Kiehl has used fMRI to scan more than 1,000 inmates, many from a mobile scanner set up in the courtyard of a New Mexico prison. He says that the brains of psychopaths tend to show distinct defects in the paralimbic system, a network of brain regions important for memory and regulating emotion.

Mitigating Circumstances

The purpose of the work, Kiehl says, is to eliminate the stigma against psychopaths and find them treatments so they can stop committing crimes. But Dugan's lawyers saw another purpose. During sentencing for capital crimes, the defense may present just about anything as a mitigating factor, from accounts of the defendant being abused as a child to evidence of extreme emotional disturbance. Kiehl's research could offer a persuasive argument that Dugan is a psychopath and could not control his killer impulses. After reading about Kiehl's work in the *New Yorker*, Dugan's lawyers asked Kiehl to testify and offered him the chance to scan the brain of a notorious criminal. Kiehl agreed. . . . Kiehl's decision has put him at odds with many in his profession and stirred debate among neuroscientists and lawyers.

"It is a dangerous distortion of science that sets dangerous precedents for the field," says Helen Mayberg, a neurologist at Emory University School of Medicine in Atlanta, Georgia. Mayberg, who uses brain imaging to study depression, has testified against the use of several kinds of brain scans in dozens of cases since 1992. Although other brain-imaging techniques have been used in court, it is especially hard to argue that fMRI should be, argue critics. The technique reveals changes in blood flow within the brain, thought to correlate with brain activity, and it has become popular in research. But most fMRI studies are small, unreplicated, and compare differences in the average brain activity of groups, rather than individuals, making it difficult to interpret for single cases. It is rarely used in diagnosis. Moreover, a recent scan, say some critics, wouldn't necessarily indicate Dugan's mental state when he committed his crimes.

In 1983, Dugan kidnapped 10-year-old Jeanine Nicarico, of Naperville, Illinois. He raped her in the back seat of his car and beat her to death. In 1984, he saw a 27-year-old nurse waiting at a stop light on a deserted road. He rammed into her car, raped her, and drowned her in a quarry. A year later, he plucked a 7-year-old girl from her bicycle, raped her, killed her, and left her body in a drainage ditch, weighed down with rocks.

Plea Bargaining

. . . Brain imaging has a long history in legal cases. Lawyers have often used scans as a way to tip the scale in the perpetual battle between opposing expert psychiatric witnesses. You can't control your brain waves, the theory goes, and scans are an objective measure of mental state. "The psychiatric diagnosis is still soft data—it's behavior," notes Ruben Gur, director of the Brain Behavior Center at the University of Pennsylvania in Philadelphia. "The brain scan doesn't lie. If there is tissue miss-ing from your brain, there is no way you could have manufactured it for the purpose of the trial."

Brain imaging played into the 1982 trial of John Hinckley Jr., who had attempted to assassinate U.S. President Ronald Reagan. Lawyers presented a computed tomog-raphy X-ray scan of his head, arguing that it showed slight brain shrinkage and abnormally large ventricles,* indicating a mental defect. The prosecution's expert witnesses said the scans looked normal. Whether imaging influenced the verdict is not known, but Hinckley was found not guilty by reason of insanity.

Over the next decade, lawyers gradually switched to positron emission tomogra-phy (PET), which can be used to give a measure of metabolic activity in the brain. Gur's research team has scanned dozens of patients with mental illness and hun-dreds of healthy volunteers using PET and structural MRI—a technique that looks at the static structure of the brain and is more established for diagnosis than fMRI. Through his research, he has developed algorithms that can predict whether a per-son has schizophrenia, for example, from structural MRI alone with about 80% accuracy. Gur has testified in roughly 30 criminal cases on behalf of defendants alleged to have schizophrenia or brain damage.

"We determine whether the values are normal or abnormal," Gur says. "It's a challenge to explain that to a jury, but when they understand, basically all I'm telling them is that this is not someone who's operating with a full deck. And so, they may not be eligible for the harshest punishment possible." Gur gets so many requests to testify that he has a team of psychology residents and interns to vet them. Still, he doesn't think that fMRI is reliable enough for legal settings. "If somebody asked me to debunk an fMRI testimony, it wouldn't be too hard," Gur says.

That's mainly because fMRI studies deal in average differences between groups. For example, Kiehl's work has shown that, when processing abstract words, psycho-pathic prisoners have lower activity in some brain regions than non-psychopathic prisoners and non-prisoners. But there's bound to be overlap. He has not shown, for example, that any one person showing a specific brain signature is guaranteed, with some percent certainty, to be a psychopath or behave like one. . . .

Taking the Stand

On October 29, Kiehl participated in a "Frye hearing" for Dugan's case. Based on a 1923 ruling, the hearing determines whether scientific evidence is robust enough to be admitted.** Joseph Birkett, the lead prosecutor in the Dugan case, argued that allowing the scans—the bright colors and statistical parameters of which are chosen by the researchers—might bias the jury. Some studies, prosecutors argued, have shown that neuroscientific explanations can be particularly seductive to the layperson.

---

* [Ventricles are cavities in the brain filled with fluid. This and all of the other brain structures you should know are explained in Chapter 3.—EDS.]

** [See Chapter 8 for a discussion of the evidentiary rules that govern the admissibility of expert evidence. Under *Frye* the court decides whether the proffered evidence has "gained general acceptance in the particular field in which it belongs." *Frye* is no longer the standard in many states nor in the federal courts, which apply a different rule called the *Daubert* standard. — EDS.]

The judge ultimately "cut the baby in half," says Birkett. He ruled that the jury would not be allowed to see Dugan's actual brain scans, but that Kiehl could describe them and how he interpreted them based on his research.

On November 5, Kiehl took the stand for about six hours. He described the findings of two three-hour psychiatric interviews with Dugan. Dugan had scored 38 out of a possible 40 on the Hare Psychopathy Checklist, which evaluates 20 aspects of personality and behavior through a semi-structured interview. (It was developed by Kiehl's graduate-school mentor, Robert Hare.) That puts him in the 99.5th percentile of all inmates, Kiehl says.

Using PowerPoint slides of bar graphs and cartoon brains—but not the scans—Kiehl testified that Dugan's brain, like those of psychopaths in his other studies, showed decreased levels of activity in specific areas. Prosecutors, Kiehl says, went to great lengths to sow confusion about the data. . . .

The next day, the prosecution brought a rebuttal witness: Jonathan Brodie, a psychiatrist at New York University. He refuted the imaging evidence on several grounds.

First, there was timing: Kiehl scanned Dugan 26 years after he killed Nicarico. It was impossible to know what was going on in Dugan's brain while he was committing the act, and it was perhaps not surprising that his brain would look like a murderer's after committing murder. Second, Brodie said, there was the issue with average versus individual differences. If you look at professional basketball players, most of them are tall, he told the jury, but not everyone over six foot six is a basketball player.

From a technical perspective, Kiehl's work is expertly done, says Brodie. "I have no issue with his science. I have an issue with what he did with it. I think it was just a terrible leap."

Even if fMRI could reliably diagnose psychopathy, it wouldn't necessarily reduce a defendant's culpability in the eyes of a judge or jury. Ultimately, the law is based on an individual's rational, intentional action, not brain anatomy or blood flow, says Stephen Morse, professor of law and psychiatry at the University of Pennsylvania. "Brains don't kill people. People kill people," says Morse, who also co-directs the MacArthur Foundation's Law and Neuroscience Project, which brings together scientists, lawyers, and judges to debate how brain technology should be used in legal settings.

Change of Heart

Dugan's sentencing proceedings ended four days after Brodie's testimony. The jury deliberated for less than an hour before coming back with a verdict: ten for the death penalty and two for life in prison—a death sentence requires a unanimous vote.

But while waiting for the Nicarico family to return to the courtroom, one of the jurors asked for more time and the judge agreed. The jury asked for copies of several transcripts of testimony, including Kiehl's, and went back into deliberation. The next day, all 12 jurors voted to send Dugan to his death.

Even with the unfavorable final verdict, Kiehl's testimony "turned it from a slam dunk for the prosecution into a much tougher case," says Steve Greenberg, Dugan's lawyer. . . .

Navigating Neuroscience: Who Does What?

If a lawyer needs to consult someone with expert knowledge about the brain, who should she call? The answer to this question is somewhat complex because of the variety of specialized educational degrees, areas of expertise, and titles that surround medical and scientific work on the brain. Furthermore, the prefix "neuro-" fits so well in front of so many words (like neurolaw) that it may lead to confusion about who actually works directly with the brain.

To start, it's useful to know that we have not had a meaningful sense of what the brain actually does until very recently in human history. For example, Aristotle thought the brain distilled food vapors. When the modern scientific study of the brain began in the seventeenth century, it was called "neurology." Today neurology is understood to apply particularly to an area of medicine concerned with the diagnosis and treatment of disorders of the nervous system. Thus, a "neurologist" is an MD who has specialized training to deal with disorders, such as epilepsy or Parkinson's disease, as well as traumatic brain injury. A "psychiatrist" is also an MD but with a specialization in diagnosing and treating disorders, such as schizophrenia or depression. The boundary between neurology and psychiatry blurs as we appreciate the brain basis of cognitive and emotional disorders. Thus, you will be able to find individuals who specialize in "neuropsychiatry." Other MDs are known as "radiologists"; they know how to use various technologies such as X-ray, ultrasound, computed tomography (CT), positron emission tomography (PET), and magnetic resonance imaging (MRI) to diagnose or treat diseases.

The MD degree entails the authority to deliver treatments such as prescribing drugs. The PhD degree does not entail this authority, rather it is awarded for scientific research.

The term "neuroscience" was not used before the 1970s. Before then, researchers who studied the brain and behavior earned PhDs in anatomy, physiology, or psychology. Today, many universities also grant a PhD in neuroscience. It is important to appreciate, though, that researchers investigating the brain have a generally common educational background regardless of the discipline in which their PhD is granted. Broadly speaking, neuroscientific research is conducted by individuals with a variety of labels, such as neuroscientist, neurobiologist, and even psychologist.

You will also probably encounter a "forensic psychologist" or "forensic psychiatrist." Such individuals work particularly at the intersection of law and psychology, and some subset of these professionals engage in neuroscience-related cases.

One type of PhD a lawyer might interact with in particular is referred to as a "neuropsychologist." This is a rather vague term, but in the American medical domain, it identifies individuals who perform various psychological tests to evaluate the effects or location of brain damage. Neuropsychologists, neurologists, and psychiatrists often work together on cases.

Van Middlesworth v. Century Bank & Trust Co.

No. 215512, 2000 WL 33421451 (Mich. Ct. App. May 5, 2000)

PER CURIAM. Plaintiffs commenced this action seeking specific performance of a written agreement between them and the late Harold N. Piper to purchase approximately five hundred acres of farmland and a wheat crop from Piper, and seeking damages for breach of contract. After a bench trial, the trial court found that Piper was mentally incompetent to enter the agreement, and that the circumstances were such that reasonable persons in plaintiffs' position would have been put on notice that they should inquire further regarding Piper's mental competence before proceeding with the agreement. Plaintiffs now appeal as of right, challenging the trial court's order dismissing their complaint with prejudice. We affirm.

Plaintiffs first argue that the evidence of Piper's mental incompetence in March 1995 was insufficient to provide them with notice and require them to investigate his mental ability before proceeding with the transaction. We disagree. This Court reviews the trial court's findings of fact for clear error, and defers to the trial court's resolution of factual issues, especially where it involves the credibility of witnesses. A trial court's finding of fact is clearly erroneous when, although there is evidence to support it, this Court is left with the definite and firm conviction that a mistake has been made.

. . . "The test of mental capacity to contract is whether the person in question possesses sufficient mind to understand in a reasonable manner the nature and effect of the act in which the person is engaged. To avoid a contract it must appear not only that the person was of unsound mind or insane when it was made, but that the un-soundness or insanity was of such a character that the person had no reasonable perception of the nature or terms of the contract."

Timothy Piper testified that, in the fall of 1992, Rodney Van Middlesworth dried and sold some corn for Piper pursuant to the latter's request, and after Rodney gave Piper the figures involved in the transaction and settled with him, Piper later questioned the calculations and wondered whether he had been paid enough. Rodney then came back and went over the calculations with Piper a second time. Timothy also testified that, in 1993, Rodney agreed to haul and sell part of Piper's corn crop, and Piper believed that Rodney had hauled more bushels than Piper had requested to be hauled. As a result, Piper quit hauling or selling corn for a period of time, and Rodney told Timothy that, in the future, Timothy would have to verify what Piper wanted in order to avoid any more discrepancies. Also, on one occasion Piper asked Rodney to haul a couple of loads of corn for him, and Timothy did not confirm Piper's order because the corn was not ready to haul. In January 1995, Rodney hauled two almost identically sized loads of beans to the market for Piper, receiving a separate check for each load. Piper thought he had been paid twice for the same load of beans, and it took Rodney half a day "to sort it out and make sure that he hadn't been." Rodney was also questioned about his deposition statement referring to an April 11, 1995, meeting with Piper, regarding which Rodney stated, "He acted like he didn't know what I was talking about. He acted like he had no idea what he was talking about."

Another indication that Rodney Van Middlesworth had notice that Piper was mentally incompetent occurred in relation to a police report that Piper apparently filed on April 28, 1995, accusing Rodney of assaulting him. From all that appears in the record, Piper's charge was false. When questioned about this incident at trial,

Rodney denied having told the investigating police officer on May 1, 1995, that Piper's "mind was starting to go," but he was impeached with an excerpt of his deposition testimony in which he acknowledged having made such a statement.

Although these latter incidents occurred some weeks after Piper signed the sales agreement, we believe it reasonable to assume that Rodney's expressed belief on several dates so soon after the transaction that Piper's "mind is starting to go" can be extrapolated backward in time to Piper's condition on March 13, 1995, thus constituting further indication that plaintiffs were on notice regarding Piper's possible mental incompetence.

Additionally, the trial court placed reliance on the fact that three of the four expert witnesses testified to Piper's deteriorated mental state. The first witness, a clinical psychologist, concluded from his examination that Piper's reasoning would have been significantly impaired on and around March 13, 1995 to the extent that he would not have been able to understand the offer to purchase his real estate. The second witness, a neurologist, examined the results of Piper's magnetic resonance imaging (MRI), found evidence of brain shrinkage and hardening of the arteries, and opined that the MRI was consistent with dementia both at the time of the MRI and in March 1995. The third expert witness, a physician specializing in geriatric neurology, concluded that Piper suffered from a combination of Alzheimer's disease and multi-infarct dementia, and that Piper was mentally incompetent at the time of examination as well as in March 1995. Although plaintiffs presented a psychiatric expert witness of their own who came to a contrary conclusion, we give much weight to the opinion of the trial judge who was in the best position to consider and evaluate the testimony of these witnesses. . . .

Plaintiffs argue that defense counsel's closing argument reflects defense counsel's own belief that plaintiffs had no knowledge of Piper's incompetence at the time the sales agreement was executed. During his remarks, counsel stated that he did not believe that plaintiffs "entered into those negotiations saying to themselves, 'Harold is incompetent and we are going to take advantage of him.'" Whatever counsel may have meant by these remarks, they do not negate the evidence of Piper's mental incompetence in March 1995, nor do they relieve plaintiffs of their obligation to inquire regarding Piper's competence before proceeding with the transaction. . . . Having examined counsel's statement in context, we conclude that it was not meant as a formal admission, but was rather merely part of counsel's rhetoric during argument, charitably suggesting that plaintiffs did not intend to take advantage of an incompetent old man.

Plaintiffs also contend that, even if Piper were mentally incompetent at the time of the agreement, the resulting contract is voidable, not void, and should be set aside only if its terms are unjust or unfair to Piper. However, the trial court determined that the fairness of the contract was affected due to a $75,000 discrepancy between the sale price and the price the property could have brought at auction, a below-market interest rate, and "the fact that it's the family homestead and . . . we'd have to look into the competency of anybody deeding out the family homestead."

. . . Moreover, there is no inequity in the trial court's decision to declare the agreement void because the agreement involved only an acceptance of an offer to purchase Piper's farm, and plaintiffs neither paid Piper for the farm, nor received title from him. As this Court stated in *Star Realty, Inc v. Bower*, "The integrity of written contracts must be preserved, but so must an incompetent be protected against

his own folly. . . . The evidence presented does not preponderate for specific performance as equitable relief." There was no error. . . . Affirmed.

The relationship between brain tumors and violent behavior was the subject of intense scrutiny after the 1966 mass killing perpetrated by Charles Whitman. Law professor Adam Lamparello describes the case below.

Adam Lamparello
Using Cognitive Neuroscience to Predict Future Dangerousness

42 Colum. Hum. Rts. L. Rev. 481, 496-499 (2011)

Before he killed fourteen people and wounded thirty-one at the University of Texas, Charles Whitman was described as "handsome," "fun," "high spirited" and in many respects the "all American boy." When he was twelve years old, he became one of the youngest Eagle Scouts on record and in high school, pitched for the baseball team and managed the football team. After high school he joined the Marines, where he was described as "the kind of guy you would want around if you went into combat." . . . [H]e obtained a scholarship to the University of Texas, performed volunteer work while having a part-time job as a bank teller, and was described by his supervisor as "an outstanding person, very likeable, neat, and nice looking."

Suddenly, however, Whitman began to suffer severe headaches and frequently grew angry or acted aggressively. He repeatedly wrote notes reminding himself to control his anger and to "smile." As he continued to experience increased feelings of anger, Whitman sought professional help at the University of Texas, where he admitted to have attacked his wife on two occasions. In addition, his doctor stated that "[h]is real concern is with himself at the present time. He readily admits having overwhelming periods of hostility with a very minimum of provocation. [He makes] vivid reference to thinking about going up on the tower [at the University of Texas] with a deer rifle and start shooting people [sic]." . . .

Whitman never again met with a doctor about his condition. Before climbing the tower, he composed another letter to himself. In that letter, he wrote,

> I don't quite understand what it is that compels me to type this letter. . . . I don't really understand myself these days. . . . However, lately (I can't recall when it started) I have been a victim of many unusual and irrational thoughts. These thoughts constantly recur, and it requires tremendous mental effort to concentrate. . . . I talked with a doctor once for about two hours and tried to convey to him my fears that I felt come [sic] overwhelming violent impulses. After one session I never saw the Doctor again, and since then I have been fighting my mental turmoil alone, and seemingly to no avail. *After my death I wish that an autopsy would be performed on me to see if there is any visible physical disorder.* I have had some tremendous headaches in the past and have consumed two large bottles of Excedrin in the past three months.

One day before Whitman climbed the tower at the University of Texas, he visited his mother just after midnight and followed her into her bedroom where he strangled her, stabbed her in the chest with a hunting knife, and brutally smashed the bones in her left hand. After murdering his mother, Whitman left a note saying, "I have just taken my mother's life. I am very upset over having done it . . . I am truly sorry. . . . Let there be no doubt in your mind that I loved this woman with all of my heart."

After murdering his mother, Whitman then made the decision to kill his wife, stating, "[i]t was after much thought that I decided to kill my wife, Kathy, tonight. . . . I love her dearly. . . . I cannot rationaly [sic] pinpoint any specific reason for doing this." Whitman stabbed his wife to death just several hours after he killed his mother. He then wrote another note saying,

> I imagine it appears that I bruttaly [sic] kill [sic] both of my loved ones. . . . If my life insurance policy is valid . . . [p]lease pay off all my debts. . . . Donate the rest anonymously to a mental health foundation. Maybe research can prevent further tragedies of this type.

The next day, Whitman climbed the tower at the University of Texas and started shooting, killing fourteen people and injuring thirty-one.

In the post-mortem autopsy, a "pecan-sized" Glioblastoma multiforme tumor was removed from "the right temporo-occipital" region of Whitman's brain. While acknowledging at the time that they could not definitively link Whitman's behavior to his brain tumor, the team of doctors who had worked on the report observed that "the highly malignant brain tumor conceivably could have contributed to [Whitman's] inability to control his emotions and actions."

NOTES AND QUESTIONS

1. What did the commentator mean when he said that the judge in *Dugan* "cut the baby in half" with regards to the scientific evidence? What do you think led the judge to rule that way? And, on the information here, how would you likely have approached the admissibility question? Chapter 8 on Neuroscience in the Courtroom will introduce the rules of scientific evidence in more detail. But note in the meantime that in the federal system, and in many states, the rules for admissibility are different in the guilt and sentencing phases (and are more lenient in the latter).

2. In 2014, Brian Dugan spoke with two newspaper reporters about his past acts. Over the course of multiple interviews in a three-month span, Dugan spent 12 hours with the reporters. Christy Gutowski & Steve Mills, *Serial Killer Brian Dugan Gives 1st Prison Interview: 'I Could Not Stop,'* Chi. Trib. (Dec. 13, 2014). Amongst other things, Dugan said: "I've changed to a point, but I'm still dangerous. . . . He still lives in me. . . . Nothing's changed except what I've tried to do for myself. I'm a threat to other people to a certain extent, I realize that . . . I know I'm a psychopath. I don't see anything that would have stopped me. . . ."
Describing the interview experience, the reporters observed: "When he tried to recall a detail from a crime or closed his eyes in concentration, his expression was almost menacing. On learning for the first time that a younger brother had died more than a year earlier, he appeared unmoved. But there are moments when one can almost forget that the sky-blue shirt and dark blue pants he wears are an inmate's uniform."

Many of the family members of Dugan's victims expressed no interest in hearing from him. For example, the sister of one of Dugan's victims said: "He is evil through and through."

3. Admissibility concerns often involve juror reaction to the proffered evidence. But what about judges? In 2012, Lisa G. Aspinwall, Teneille R. Brown, and James Tabery published a study with 181 U.S. state trial judges as subjects in an online experiment. The results suggest that judges' sentencing decisions may be affected by the introduction of biomechanical evidence. The researchers found that "despite the significant variability among states when it came to sentencing, the addition of a biomechanism for psychopathy significantly reduced the sentence and significantly reduced the degree to which psychopathy was rated as aggravating." Lisa G. Aspinwall et al., *The Double-Edged Sword: Does Biomechanism Increase or Decrease Judges' Sentencing of Psychopaths?*, 337 Science 846, 847 (2012). Are you surprised at this result? If the same effect were seen in actual cases, what, if anything, should the legal system do to respond? For a critique of this study, see Deborah W. Denno, *What Real-World Criminal Cases Tell Us About Genetics Evidence*, 64 Hastings L.J. 1591, 1606 (2013) ("My survey results suggest that behavioral genetics evidence either has no decipherable impact on a defendant's case or it becomes at most an effective factor alongside other variables in rendering a defendant ineligible for the death penalty. At the same time, it can be challenging to isolate the effect of any one piece of mitigating evidence when it comes to interpreting the influences on death penalty sentences.").

4. Law professor Stephen Morse has written that "[b]rains do not commit crimes; people commit crimes. This conclusion should be self-evident, but, infected and inflamed by stunning advances in our understanding of the brain, advocates all too often make moral and legal claims that the new neuroscience does not entail and cannot sustain." Stephen Morse, *Brain Overclaim Syndrome and Criminal Responsibility: A Diagnostic Note*, 3 Ohio St. J. Crim. L. 397, 397 (2006). What do you think are the likely limits of neuroscience-based defenses, either to a criminal charge or contractual dispute? If people (not brains) commit crimes and people (not brains) sign contracts, were the courts mistaken to admit brain science in their adjudication of the cases above?

5. In 2012, an Italian pediatrician, Domenico Mattiello, was accused of pedophilia. Colleagues could not understand why he acted this way: "He was a pediatrician for 30 something years and he saw tens of thousands of children and never had any problem. The question is why, at some point, did someone who has always behaved properly suddenly change so drastically?" An MRI revealed a brain tumor, and, at his defense, Dr. Mattiello argued that this brain tumor made him act in the way he did. Kate Kelland, *Neuroscience in Court: My Brain Made Me Do It*, Health News (Aug. 29, 2012). This and other international developments raise questions about comparative neurolaw. To what extent do different legal regimes and different cultural attitudes affect the role of neuroscience in law?

6. What role do you think neuroscientific evidence played in *Van Middlesworth*? What factors do you think led the defense attorneys to pursue and include such evidence? What issues would have arisen if, holding all other facts equal, the brain scans had shown nothing unusual?

7. Neuroscientist Michael Gazzaniga cautions that "exciting as the advances that neuroscience is making every day are, all of us should look with caution at how they may gradually come to be incorporated into our culture. The legal relevance of neuroscientific discoveries is only part of the picture. Might we someday want brain scans of our fiancées, business partners, or politicians, even if the results could not stand up in court?" Michael S. Gazzaniga, *Neuroscience in the Courtroom*, 304 Sci. Am. 54, 59 (2011). How might and should the legal system respond to these possible implications of neuroscience in society?

8. In *Dugan*, neuroscientist Kent Kiehl suggested that we now know much about the psychopathic brain. Should that knowledge be relevant at sentencing? Neuroscientist David Eagleman argues that "[t]he punishment has to fit the brain." *Talk of the Nation: David Eagleman Gets Inside Our Heads*, Nat'l Pub. Radio (Aug. 24, 2012). Do you agree, and what would this mean in practice? How would you define the threshold level of brain dysfunction necessary for a defendant to be considered as suffering from a brain dysfunction, and thus, as eligible for a reduced or alternative sentence? Should a defendant asserting such a claim be required to prove that he or she not only suffers from such a disorder, but also acted *because of* the disorder at the time of the crime?

9. In Chapter 10 you will read about brain injuries, including brain injuries experienced through participation in contact sports such as football. In some instances, former athletes who have suffered a brain injury find themselves as criminal defendants and argue that their brain trauma is relevant in explaining, and perhaps excusing, their violent actions. One prosecutor, in a case in which a former football player killed his girlfriend, argued that "[t]here is no psychosis fairy who magically sprinkles a dose of psychosis on this defendant. . . . The time for blaming football, the time for blaming marijuana, the time for blaming the victim is over." Melinda Henneberger, *Blaming Football in Lauren Astley's Killing*, Wash. Post (Mar. 6, 2013). Is the prosecutor's characterization of this brain-based defense a useful one? Why or why not?

10. During the confirmation hearing of now Chief Justice John Roberts, then Senator Joe Biden observed: "Can brain scans be used to determine whether a person is inclined toward criminality or violent behavior? You will rule on that." Although the issue of neuroprediction has not yet reached the courts (or the criminal justice system), perhaps one day it will. While law often looks backward to assess a mental state at a previous time, society and the criminal justice system also frequently look forward to make a prediction about an individual's likelihood of doing something bad. In 2013 a group of researchers published a study finding that anterior cingulate cortex activation, associated with a laboratory impulse control task, could aid in the prediction of future re-arrest. The researchers noted, however, that "Should the neuroimaging effects be robust to replication, they remain silent on the question of suitability in making individual-level predictions. Whether neurobiological markers should ever be used to make predictions about individual offenders' risk is a thorny question that, at the least, depends on *(i)* whether these estimates can survive particular sensitivity and specificity thresholds with the use of large random samples, *(ii)* whether they can survive a required legal standard of proof, and *(iii)* whether their use would violate offender rights." Eyal Aharoni et al., *Neuroprediction of*

Future Rearrest, 110 Proc. Nat'l Acad. Sci. 6223, 6224 (2013). How would you address these thorny issues?

11. The evidence of Charles Whitman's tumor suggests that the tumor may have "caused," or at least contributed to, his violent behavior. But experts disagree about the relationship between brain and behavior. Eva Frederick, *Experts Still Disagree on Role of Tower Shooter's Brain Tumor*, Daily Texan (July 30, 2016). One expert commented that, "[y]es, he had an aggressive, malignant tumor in his temporal lobe that could have impacted his bizarre and violent behavior. . . . However, what is often overlooked is that he came from a very abusive home, and admitted to domestic violence with his own wife prior to stabbing her. I suspect his tumor was little more than 'circumstantial.' " Gary Lavergne, whose book *A Sniper in the Tower*, describes the incident in detail, is also skeptical that Whitman's brain made him do it. Lavergne observed: "For 48 hours, [Whitman] made serial decisions in a correct order leading to the accomplishment of a goal. . . . To me his actions speak for themselves. If indeed a tumor or anything else took control of him and made him do something he didn't want to do, when did this 'seizure' of sorts start?" For further debate on brain injury and responsibility, see Micah Johnson, *How Responsible Are Killers with Brain Damage?*, Sci. Am. (Jan 30, 2018) (asking "Can murder really be a symptom of brain disease?").

B. INTERSECTIONS WITH LAW

Owen D. Jones & Anthony D. Wagner
Law and Neuroscience: Progress, Promise, and Pitfalls

in *The Cognitive Neurosciences* 1015, 1015-21 (David Poeppel, George R. Mangun & Michael S. Gazzaniga eds., 6th ed. 2020).

Introduction

Cognitive neuroscientific discoveries about mind and brain not only advance scientific theory, but also hold promise to inform, and often directly bear on, real-world problems of the human condition. This is increasingly evident at the intersection of law and neuroscience. The law often concerns itself with making judgments about human behavior, and the cognitive neurosciences aim to explain the psychological and neurobiological mechanisms that give rise to thought and action. The legal system—including legal decision makers (such as judges and juries) and legal policy makers (such as legislators)—is frequently charged with making decisions based on limited or noisy evidence. Given the challenges of doing so, the hope has naturally arisen that cognitive neuroscientific advances may yield informative evidence that facilitates fact-based legal decisions and policy.

While neuroscientific evidence, such as the presence of a neural injury or disorder, has long been a staple of tort law (the law of injuries), the remarkable neuroscientific advances made in recent decades have not gone unnoticed by the legal community. Increasingly, legal actors are offering neuroscientific evidence during litigation and citing neuroscientific studies during policy discussions. It appears that such evidence often has some influence on outcomes. In a complementary manner, cognitive neuroscientists are coming to appreciate how their approach can be leveraged to address important problems the law regularly confronts, as well as how their methods and results may be used, for better or worse, by legal actors.

In this review, we provide a high-level summary of recent activities at the inter-face of law and neuroscience, including overviews of what is happening, of the potential influences of neuroscientific evidence, and of contexts in which neurosci-ence can be useful to law. Along the way, we consider some of the legal problems on which neuroscientific data are thought, at least by some, to provide potential answers, and we highlight some illustrative cases. Throughout, the chapter reflects our view that there is a zone of suitable sense that lies somewhere between being too zealous about the long-term effects of neuroscience on law and being too skeptical that neuroscience has anything useful to offer.

Cross-field Interactions — The Emergence of "Neurolaw"

We begin by considering some of the key developments that have propelled interactions between neuroscience and law over the last ten to fifteen years.

First, as already noted, lawyers are increasingly offering neuroscientific evidence in the courtroom. In the civil (non-criminal) domain, for example, one core issue of the multi-district NFL concussion litigation concerns the neurological effects of repetitive impacts to the head. Neuroscience also appears in contexts as varied as medical malpractice litigation, on one hand, and suits seeking disability benefits, on the other. In the criminal domain, many defendants now offer evidence of brain abnormalities — such as tumors, cysts, or unusual features — to argue during the sentencing phase of a trial that they should receive a lesser punishment than would someone who acted identically, but with a "normal" brain. Former mayor of San Diego Maureen O'Connor, for instance, claimed that a tumor contributed to her gambling addiction, which in turn led to the embezzlements of which she was con-victed. The past decade has even seen attempts to enter functional brain imaging evidence purported to reveal the veracity of a defendant's testimony, a development to which we return below.

In 2007, the John D. and Catherine T. MacArthur Foundation funded the inter-disciplinary Law and Neuroscience Project (under Michael Gazzaniga, and later Owen D. Jones, Directors) to help build direct links between neuroscience, psy-chological science, academic law, and legal actors such as judges and attorneys. In 2011, the foundation funded the new Research Network on Law and Neuroscience (Owen D. Jones, Director). Over 12 years, these efforts propelled exploration of the promise and the limitations of using neuroscientific research to further the goals of criminal justice, building bridges between neuroscientists and legal scholars. Together with leading federal and state judges, teams co-designed and published dozens of legally relevant experiments, as well as many analyses and proposals for ways the legal system could use neuroscience usefully, while simultaneously mini-mizing misuses. (See www.lawneuro.org for details, including members, publica-tions, resources, and more.)

Given rapid expansion in the types and technical complexity of neuroscientific evidence available, along with the growth in their submission as evidence, cross-field education is critical. Some of this, of course, will come in the form of expert wit-nesses, when neuroscientists share knowledge with the legal system, in the context of specific litigation. But more broadly, this education often takes the form of train-ing sessions and seminars. For example, a number of organizations have offered, and judges are increasingly requesting, some basic exposure for judges in the tech-nologies, vocabularies, capabilities, and limitations of neuroscientific techniques. Over the past decade, more than 1,000 judges — along with many legal scholars, prosecutors, and defense attorneys—have participated in training sessions offered by the American Association for the Advancement of Science, the Federal Judicial Center, the MacArthur Foundation Research Network on Law and Neuroscience, and the MacArthur Law and Neuroscience Project.

Finally, burgeoning activity in law and neuroscience (sometimes called "neurolaw") is evident along other critical dimensions. To give but a few examples, for context, consider that neurolaw publications numbered barely 100 in 2005, but swelled sixteen-fold over the next decade, to over 1600 today. Across the same time span, over 150 law and neuroscience conferences and symposia were hosted, a variety of law and neuro-science societies formed around the globe, and a number of law schools and other departments started offering neurolaw courses, some using a dedicated textbook on the subject. Broader knowledge sharing has taken the forms, for instance, of cover-page articles in The New York Times Sunday Magazine (2007) and the American Bar Association Journal (2012), a multi-part television program, various radio documenta-ries and interviews, a complimentary electronic newsletter (Neurolaw News) and more than 50 neurolaw video lectures (at https://www.youtube.com/user/lawneuroorg).

Driving the Interest

There are doubtless many drivers of the increased interest in neurolaw. But at the most basic level, it arises from the intersection of: a) perennial questions that the legal system has been grappling with for generations; and b) the proliferation of new neuro-technological capabilities. Where these overlap springs the hope—or, at the very least, active curiosity—that neuroscientific tools that can be applied to humans may yield better answers to some legally relevant questions that have his-torically yielded unsatisfying or uncertain solutions.

For instance: Is this person responsible for his or her behavior? What was this person's likely mental state at the time of the act? How competent is this person? Is this person lying? What does this person remember? How accurate is this per-son's memory? Is this person really in pain, and—if so—how much? How can we improve juror and judge decisions?

And what developments have laid foundation for the hope that cognitive neuro-science can help answer these questions? For one thing, many people—including legal thinkers—increasingly recognizes that the brain is not a product of either nature or nurture, but rather necessarily exists at the intersection of genes and envi-ronments. They increasingly understand that the brain is the product of evolution-ary processes, including natural selection, that have shaped it to readily associate various environmental inputs with behavioral outputs that tended (on average, in past environments) to increase the chances of survival and reproduction. And they increasingly understand that human cognition and behavior—including both rela-tively "automatic", non-conscious phenomena (e.g., implicit racial biases) and more "controlled", conscious phenomena (e.g., planning future acts)—are products of the brain, with some emerging from functionally specialized neural processes and others from large-scale network computations.

Against this background, there also has been increasing awareness of the remark-able rate of technological progress in the neurosciences. This includes awareness of key new tools of cognitive neuroscience that provide unprecedented insights into how human minds and brains work, as well as unique opportunities to try to 'read out' from neural signals what a person is perceiving, thinking, or remembering.

These cutting-edge tools—including brain imaging methods such as positron emission tomography (PET) and functional magnetic resonance imaging (fMRI), and data analytic methods such as machine learning, as well as the combination of both kinds of methods—have yielded both striking new discoveries as well as overhyped illusory advances. In turn, cognitive neuroscience's many discoveries and advances have, for better or for worse, tantalized the legal system with the prospects of answering some of its most challenging questions, and commensurate concerns for associate risks.

Illustrative Research

In this section we provide a sampling, for general flavor, of some of legal problems on which neurolaw experiments have been published in the last decade or so. We focus on the works with which we are most familiar, given that we each served on the MacArthur Foundation Research Network on Law and Neuroscience (the "Network"). Readers interested in the broader neurolaw literature can access a sortable and searchable bibliography here: http://www.lawneuro.org/bibliography.php.

Brain-based Memory Detection

Behavioral expressions of memory serve as critical evidence for the law, including eyewitness identifications and memory-based statements about an individual's intent or frame-of-mind during a past act. Mnemonic evidence is often challenged by the opposing side, leaving the jury to decide whether to believe, and how heavily to weigh, the evidence. Given this long-standing challenge for the law, there is interest in whether neural measures can detect the presence or absence of a memory, or distinguish true from false memories. Being able to detect reliable neural signals of memory could be useful in a variety of investigative contexts, including probing the probability of deception (see next subsection).

To examine whether functional brain imaging can be used to detect real-world memories, one Network working group, led by one of us (Wagner), put cameras around the necks of undergraduate students that automatically took photos as they navigated their lives for a few weeks. Subsequently, selected photos from a subject's camera were interleaved with photos from other subjects' cameras and displayed while the subject made memory decisions during fMRI. Machine-learning techniques applied to the fMRI data—here, multivoxel pattern analyses—revealed that activity patterns in numerous cortical regions along with the medial temporal lobe can be used to classify whether the subject is viewing and recognizing photos of their past (i.e., hits) versus viewing and perceiving as new photos from someone else's camera (i.e., correct rejections). Classifier accuracy was well above chance (approaching ceiling performance in some cases) and, intriguingly, this was the case even when the classifier was applied to brain data from subjects other than the ones on which it was trained up. In addition to detecting memories for real-world autobiographical events, a lab-based study revealed high accuracy when classifying brain patterns associated with recognizing studied faces versus correctly rejecting novel faces, as well as discriminating higher confidence versus lower confidence memories.

While the above findings suggest that, under controlled experimental conditions, memory states can be detected from fMRI-measured brain patterns, initial studies also point to important boundary conditions. First, while high classification accuracy is possible (under some conditions) when discriminating recognized stimuli from stimuli perceived as novel, classification accuracy was only slightly above chance when attempting to discriminate true versus false recognition of faces. This finding converges with a wealth of other data highlighting the similarity of brain responses during true and false memory, and suggests that brain-based measures may not solve the law's frequent quandary of knowing when a witness's memory is accurate or mistaken. Second, classification accuracy was essentially at chance when applied to implicit memory—i.e., discriminating between old stimuli that a subject failed to recognize (i.e., misses) from new stimuli perceived as novel (i.e., correct rejections). Finally, the high level of fMRI-based classification of hits versus correct rejections fell to chance when subjects used cognitive countermeasures (shifting how they attended to memory) in an effort to mask their neural patterns of memory. As with the polygraph and fMRI-based lie detection (see below), potential real-world application of brain-based memory detection can be 'beat' by motivated non-compliant individuals. Thus, while extant data highlight that brain-based memory detection is possible, significant hurdles to real-world application remain.

Brain-based Lie Detection

As noted at the outset, lawyers are increasingly proffering (i.e., "offering into evidence") neuroscientific evidence, both structural and functional. In many cases, such evidence is the subject of admissibility hearings, in which a judge determines (according to state or federal law standards) whether the jury will be allowed to hear and see the evidence. For instance, in the case of *United States v. Semrau* (2010), the defendant Lorne Semrau, who ran a psychiatric group, was prosecuted for Medicare and Medicaid fraud. Although not all criminal statutes require knowledge of wrongdoing to be guilty, it is in fact one element of proving fraud that Dr. Semrau have known that what he was doing was illegal. In his defense, Dr. Semrau sought to introduce a report from the company Cephos purporting to show that an fMRI lie-detection protocol "indicated he is telling the truth in regards to not cheating or defrauding the government." Following 16 hours of hearings before a magistrate judge, the magistrate convincingly recommended to the trial judge that the evidence be excluded from the jury, due to specific flaws in the particular protocol, as well as doubt that the urged inferences could properly be drawn from the results.

With the advent of fMRI, cognitive neuroscientists are examining whether brain-based lie detection is possible. Despite some very promising studies, the prospects for legal use remain almost entirely speculative. Take-home points from the literature include: (a) laboratory-based studies predominantly use instructed or permitted lie paradigms, and have negligible stakes for failure to successfully deceive (in contrast to the stakes in real-world settings); (b) a set of frontal and parietal lobe regions are often more active during the putative "lie" versus "truth" conditions, and most evidence comes from group-based analyses that average over trials and subjects (c.f., the law requires an assessment of truthfulness about individual facts in individual brains); (c) experimental design limitations raise uncertainty as to whether these neural effects reflect responses associated with deception or whether they reflect attention and memory confounds that are unrelated to deception; and (d) countermeasures appear to alter these neural responses, suggesting that, even if associated with deception, it may be possible to mask such responses. These limitations will frequently prevent brain-based techniques from satisfying the legal standards for admissibility of scientific findings. Indeed, some of these limitations and boundary conditions, along with others, were considered in the *Semrau* case, as well as the handful of other cases in which judges decided not to admit fMRI-based "lie detection" testimony into evidence.

Detection and Classification of Mental States

Generally speaking, the government must prove, in order to get a criminal conviction, both that a defendant performed a prohibited act ("actus reus") and that he did so in one of several defined states of mind ("mens rea"). Because most crimes are matters of state law rather than federal law, the mental state definitions can vary. However, the "Model Penal Code"—which itself has no legal force—has been widely influential on the mental state definitions in most states. By its taxonomy, culpable mental states include: purposeful, knowing, reckless, and negligent—in descending sequence of severity, each with importantly different sentencing results. In Colorado, for instance, the difference between being convicted of a knowing homicide on one hand or a reckless homicide on the other could mean the difference between 14 years in prison and incarceration-free probation.

Scholars have long debated whether the knowing-versus-reckless distinction drawn by law actually exists in the brains of defendants, a concern heightened by recent behavioral work strongly suggesting that juror-like subjects have a difficult time distinguishing between the two. Consequently, another line of research seeks to explore the extent to which coupling fMRI with machine-learning algorithms could shed light on whether there is a real psychological distinction between a "knowing" frame of mind and a "reckless" frame of mind. And one Network working group, led by Gideon Yaffe, found that the combination of fMRI and machine-learning algorithms could (under laboratory conditions) predict with high accuracy whether a subject was in knowing versus in reckless frames of mind. This arguably suggests that the distinction the law had posited academically actually exists neurologically. And this is the first proof of concept that it is possible to read out a law-relevant mental state of a subject, in a scanner, in real time.

Intent and Punishment

Humans are notoriously prone to various kinds of psychological biases. At the same time, few things are more crucial to the fair administration of criminal justice than trying to ensure that jurors and judges are minimally biased in their decisions about whether or not a defendant is criminally liable (typically a decision for the jury) and, if he is, how much to punish him (typically a decision for the judge). Until recently, nothing was known about how human brains make these important decisions.

Consequently, one line of research explores the extent to which fMRI might illuminate the neural processes underlying these determinations, which could potentially be an important first step in learning how to debias them (through, for instance, more effective training interventions). A first fMRI study found correlations between guilt and punishment decisions and activity in regions commonly associated with analytic, emotional, and theory-of-mind processes. A subsequent study suggested that theory-of-mind circuitry may either gate or suppress affective neural responses, tempering the effect of emotion on punishment levels when, for instance, a perpetrator's culpability was very low, at the same time the harm he caused was very high. A third study, using repetitive transcranial magnetic stimulation (rTMS) to test the causal role of right dorsolateral prefrontal cortex, found, as predicted, that compared to sham stimulation rTMS changed the *amount* that subjects punished protagonists in scenarios, without altering how much they *blamed* those protagonists. Breaking liability and punishment decisions down into constituent steps, a Network working group led by Owen Jones recently identified distinct neural responses that separately correlate with four key components of liability/punishment decisions: 1) assessing harms; 2) discerning mental states in others; 3) integrating those two pieces of information; and 4) choosing punishment amounts.

Adolescent and Young Adult Brains

A constant challenge for legal systems is figuring how best to handle young offenders. While it has always been obvious that the very young are not as culpable for bad behavior as are the mature, legal systems have often struggled to develop juvenile justice regimes that are stable and fair. Several U.S. Supreme Court cases reflect this struggle. In *Roper v. Simmons* (2005) the Court held unconstitutional any sentence to death for a crime committed by an adolescent of 16 or 17 years old. In *Graham v. Florida* (2010), the Court similarly held it unconstitutional to sentence any juvenile offender, in a non-homicide crime, to a sentence of life imprisonment without possibility of parole. In *Miller v. Alabama* (2012) the Court went further. It held that *mandatory* life imprisonment without possibility of parole, for those under the age of 18 at the time of their crimes, was unconstitutional—even in cases of homicide. (However, the Court left open the possibility of such a sentence, if the judge were to make an individualized assessment of the particular juvenile, crime, and surrounding circumstances.) Although the role neuroscientific arguments actually played in the disposition of these cases is debatable, it is notable in itself that neuroscientific arguments about adolescent brain development were provided to the Court in each case, and cited in some of them.

Complementing structural data that suggest that full maturation of the human brain may occur as late as into one's 20s, a wealth of behavioral and functional neural data highlight the context-dependence of developmental trajectories. Importantly, these studies of adolescents and young adults might illuminate issues potentially relevant to juvenile and young adult justice. For example, potentially bearing on the legal system's challenge of deciding when and how to hold juveniles criminally responsible for their behavior, a Network working group led by B.J. Casey is exploring whether it is possible to draw meaningful lines between juveniles and young adults using fMRI and behavioral assays. In one study, fMRI data and behavioral measures from 250 juveniles and young adults examined cognitive control under affectively arousing versus neutral conditions. Among the findings was this one: the brains and behaviors of 18-to-21 year olds operate more like older adults under some environmental circumstances—specifically, when arousal and affective states are neutral—and more like juveniles in others—when arousal and affect are elevated (such as when emotion is triggered by stimuli or when performance is under peer observation). These data may have broad implications for the law, as they suggest that the age at which mature behavior may be fully realized is context dependent.

Categories of Relevance

There are at least seven contexts in which neuroscience can be relevant to law [per Jones, 2013].*

---

* [Owen D. Jones, *Seven Ways Neuroscience Aids Law*, in *Neurosciences and the Human Person: New Perspectives on Human Activities* 181 (Antonio M. Battro, Stanislas Dehaene & Wolf Singer eds., 2013).—Eds.]

Buttressing

Neuroscientific evidence, most commonly perhaps, can be used to buttress other—typically behavioral—evidence. For example, suppose a criminal defendant has raised an insanity defense. If there is behavioral evidence consistent with insanity, those data will be the most salient evidence. If it turns out that there is also evidence of an acute abnormality in brain form or function, then the latter will buttress the former. But note that the neuroscientific evidence, no matter how strong, would be insufficient on its own to build a credible insanity defense, if there were no behavioral evidence consistent with insanity to accompany it. In such a case, the buttressing effect of neuroscientific evidence would add to the weight of the behavioral evidence, not independently supplant it; that is, the brain data could support a conclusion, but not drive it.

Detecting

One of the most potent uses of neuroscience, perhaps, is its ability to detect facts that may be legally relevant. For example, in the 1992 New York case of *People v. Weinstein*, Mr. Weinstein, an executive in Manhattan, came home one day, strangled his wife, and threw her out of the couple's 12th story apartment building. After arrest Mr. Weinstein complained of headaches, which led to a discovery, through positron emission tomography, of a very large subarachnoid cyst, compressing his prefrontal cortex, known to be important for impulse control and executive function. Although it is unknown—perhaps unknowable—how much the cyst contributed to the murder, the possession by the defense of a visually powerful brain image contributed to Mr. Weinstein's plea agreement with the state. And it illustrates the extent to which neuroscientific methods for detecting brain structures and functions may uncover new legally relevant avenues to pursue. The same is true, for instance, of the extent to which brain imaging might more clearly detect injuries—or even the existence and amount of pain—in torts cases. Of course, as noted earlier, some maintain the hope that functional neuroimaging may one day enable the reliable detection of lies or legally relevant memories.

Sorting

Neuroscience might also aid the legal system in sorting individuals into different categories, for different purposes. A paradigmatic example, perhaps, would be if neuroscientific measures could reliably identify criminal addicts who were most susceptible to rehabilitative interventions. In theory, the legal system could then send some such individuals into drug rehabilitation, instead of into the general prison populations.

Predicting

Over time, neuroscience may make important contributions to law's efforts to predict various kinds of behaviors. For instance, two papers provided initial evidence that certain brain-based variations in incarcerated individuals predict some of the variance in the probability of their rearrests after release. It was a small part of the variance, and the magnitude of the effect is debated due to questions about analytic approach. Nevertheless, as parole boards, for instance, sometimes expand and revise their actuarial approaches to predicting recidivism (including age, sex, type of crime, etc.), such observations raise the possibility that at some point in the future neuroscientific measures may become relevant. Determination of if and when such application emerges will be informed by meaningful debates about how best to interpret and apply neuroprediction.

Intervening

In theory, neuroscience could aid law through the development and validation of intervention approaches. For example, if certain drug treatments prove to substantially decrease the probability of recidivism, psychopharmacological interventions may be recommended for inclusion as a condition of parole.

Of course this, like many aspects of neurolaw, can raise important ethical considerations about what trade-offs we as a society are willing to make, between perceived benefits, attendant risks and costs, and individual rights.

Explaining

Neuroscientific methods are beginning to uncover regions of the brain, neural responses, and interactions within and between regions that subserve the processes by which decisions—key to the functioning of law—are made. As discussed above when considering adolescent brain development, these could provide new insights into why and how individuals transgress the law, in criminal or civil domains. Such discoveries also could provide new insights into the experiences of individuals who have been wronged. And, as noted above, they could provide insights into the processes by which jurors and judges make their decisions. All of these might increase the knowledge base on which new behavioral interventions and legal policy are deployed in furtherance of improving decisions, and the legal consequences they create.

Challenging Assumptions in the Legal System

Neuroscience may sometimes challenge assumptions in the legal system. For example, the legal system currently assumes that solitary confinement is insufficiently damaging to the brain to constitute "cruel and unusual punishment," and thus it is not prohibited as unconstitutional. Perhaps that's right. Perhaps it isn't. The tools of neuroscience may eventually help us to know which. If the assumption is wrong, that may provide impetus for law reform.

Similarly, note that the rules of evidence can be thought of as designed to keep certain information from entering the brains of jurors, because of assumptions about how that information might affect the decisions of jurors. The evidentiary rules also reflect underlying neuroscientific assumptions about witness brains. For instance, a general rule of evidence, known as the prohibition against "hearsay," typically operates to prevent person A from testifying as to what person B said they observed, at the time of an act relevant to the trial (such as the name of a perpetrator). The logic is that (so long as person B is available), person B's testimony is deemed to be more reliable than person A's. But there are some exceptions. Among them is the exception for "excited utterances." That exception allows person A to testify as to what person B said—so long as person B was excited, and believed to be more or less blurting things out at the time. The explicit assumption underlying this rule is that person B, being in an excited state, would not have time to lie about what she was witnessing. Perhaps that's true. Perhaps it isn't. The tools of cognitive neuroscience might help us to know which. And if the assumption is wrong—with respect to this evidentiary rule or others—neuroscience may again provide potential foundation for reform.

Two Key Caveats

There are, of course, many cautions and caveats about whether neuroscientific information should directly impact legal decisions and policy and, if so, how to carefully, sensibly, and responsibly incorporate such information. For example, above we described some of the open questions and potential boundary conditions surrounding brain-based memory and lie detection. In each of the areas of research we briefly considered, as well as others being explored in by the field, additional cautions and caveats are warranted.

Here we consider two especially salient, cross-cutting caveats.

The Long Chain of Inference

First, it is not a simple thing to reason from the presence of a brain feature (a large subarachnoid cyst, for example) to the conclusion that that feature contributed meaningfully to generating or enabling a specific behavior (such as murder). Such a conclusion requires a long chain of inferences, with many potential weak links. What exactly is the brain feature at issue? How long was it there? What is known to correlate with the presence of the brain feature? What are the known causal pathways of influence? In many instances, answers to one or more of these critical questions are unknown, which greatly tempers confidence in any inferences drawn.

Unknown Frequencies of Predictors and Outcomes

Second, and relatedly, one key limitation to drawing logical and informed inferences is that the relative frequency of a feature in the population — Mr. Weinstein's cyst, for instance — is often not known. Without that information, we have no idea how many people are walking around in the population with the same feature, but without engaging in the same behavior as did the accused. Knowing the relative frequency of a predictor, as well as of the frequency of a particular outcome (i.e., the base rate), are necessary to determine the increased likelihood, if any, of engagement in an undesirable behavior given the feature in question. Without this information, proper inferences are difficult to draw. With what confidence could one say that Mr. Weinstein's cyst meaningfully, and legally, caused him to commit murder?

The issue of unknown predictor frequencies is particularly relevant given the remarkable pace of progress in neuroscientific methods in recent years. Whereas structural imaging of the human brain has been available for a few decades, and detection of a structural abnormality is often relatively straightforward for neuroradiologists, functional imaging is a more recent development and machine-learning characterization of functional patterns and their relation to cognition is at an even earlier stage. Thus, whereas some limited information is available on the relative frequencies of structural abnormalities and their relationships to altered behavior, cognitive neuroscience is only just beginning to conduct large-scale individual difference studies of the relationships between functional brain patterns (which themselves vary depending on the particulars of the analytic approach) and cognitive states and behaviors. Early work is focused on characterizing the heterogeneity evident in healthy young adults — we seem far from the point at which we can say anything about the relative frequencies of particular functional patterns in healthy individuals and their associated outcomes, let alone those of atypical patterns and states.

Legal Impact of Neuroscience Evidence

In instances where neuroscientific evidence is admitted, what are its impacts? We know that jurors are, at least sometimes, significantly affected by neuroscience evidence. For example, in the case of *State of Florida v. Grady Nelson* (2010), the defendant was quickly convicted of a murder, leaving the question to the jury by simple majority vote (under Florida death penalty law, as it was at the time) whether Mr. Nelson should be executed or given life in prison without parole. With Mr. Nelson's life hanging in the balance, the defense introduced qEEG evidence (quantified electroencephalography) in support of the inference that Mr. Nelson's brain was too abnormal to warrant his execution. By the narrowest of possible votes, the jury gave Mr. Nelson life in prison. Afterward, two jurors granted interviews indicating that the brain data had turned their prior inclinations, to vote in favor of execution, completely around.

Some members of the judiciary are increasingly invoking neuroscience in judicial opinions, sometimes drawing colleagues into public debates over its relevance. High profile examples include the U.S. Supreme Court cases of *Graham v. Florida* and *Miller v. Alabama* (mentioned earlier). And Supreme Court Justice Sotomayor recently referred to "a major neurocognitive disorder that compromises [the defendant's] decision-making abilities" in her dissent from the Court's refusal to hear the appeal in *Wessinger v. Vannoy* (2018).

Of course, given the complexity of neuroscience, one natural concern is that both judges and jurors may have a hard time understanding where it is — and equally importantly is not — relevant. Relatedly, some have expressed worry that jurors may be over-awed by the pictorial nature of some brain data, and give it more weight than it is due. Two laboratory studies investigating this phenomenon found that the images themselves appear to have no particular biasing effect on subjects — above and beyond non-pictorial neuroscientific testimony — except in the case of death penalty decisions, wherein images decreased the probability of a vote for execution.

Given the complex interactions between law and neuroscience, there is a need for reasoned consideration of the ethical and legal impacts of neuroscientific evidence.

Conclusions

The domains of science and law have very different goals. Painted with broad brush, these are the attempt to uncover truths, on one hand, and the attempt to fairly and effectively govern the behaviors of large populations, on the other. While truths may inform governance, they don't dictate it. Indeed most scholars (including ourselves) believe it impossible to argue directly from a description to a prescription without reference to other values. Put another way, explanation isn't justification. And therefore we do not expect the law will or should automatically change, or refuse to change, in light of a neuroscientific finding alone.

At the same time, advances in the cognitive neurosciences effectively guarantee a future in which the law increasingly interacts with neuroscientific evidence. Even at this relatively early stage, there is a gradual but discernible shift from nearly exclusive reliance on structural brain evidence (in cases involving any brain evidence) to increasing reliance on functional neural assays. As this shift continues to develop and accelerate, there will be divergent views on whether and when particular types of neural data should be drawn upon to inform legal decisions.

In this review, we have highlighted a few illustrative legal problems on which neuroscience research is beginning to yield potentially informative data, as well as others in which the science suggests it is premature to move from the lab to the courtroom. Concurrently, we have considered the categories of potential relevance for neuroscience evidence, along with cross-cutting caveats. The growth of neuro-law—which crucially depends on interdisciplinary interactions—has produced significant progress and suggests promise. At the same time, there is ample cause for caution, lest over-exuberance pave a path to pitfall.

NOTES AND QUESTIONS

1. As demonstrated by the quote at the beginning of the chapter by Francis Crick, many neuroscientists suggest, either explicitly or implicitly, that we are nothing more than our brains. Others see things differently. Consider, for instance, philosopher Tyler Burge's argument: "Individuals see, know, and want to make love. Brains don't. Those things are psychological—not, in any evident way, neural." Tyler Burge, Opinion, *A Real Science of Mind*, N.Y. Times (Dec. 19, 2010). Do you agree or disagree?

2. *The New York Times* published a Letter to the Editor, on April 1, 2007, in which the author, reacting to an article on Law and Neuroscience, states that "[A] form of phrenology is alive and well in the 21st century. . . . Let's get away from looking for easy answers and bumps on (or inside) the head to explain why we act as we do. The world, and we, are much more complex than that." Robert Barsky, *The Brain on the Stand*, N.Y. Times (Apr. 1, 2007). In what ways do you agree or disagree? Why?

3. In 2009, Dr. Martha Farah, a cognitive neuroscientist at the University of Pennsylvania, observed that "neuroscience is giving us increasingly powerful methods for understanding, predicting, and manipulating behavior. Every sphere of life in which the human mind plays a central role will be touched by these advances." Press Release, Univ. of Pennsylvania Center for Neuroscience & Society, *Neuroethics: Ethical, Legal, and Social Implications of Neuroscience* (Aug. 14, 2009). Neuroscientist Joshua Greene and psychologist Jonathan Cohen have similarly argued that "cognitive neuroscience, by identifying the specific mechanisms responsible for behavior, will vividly illustrate what until now could only be appreciated through esoteric theorizing: that there is something fishy about our ordinary conceptions of human action and responsibility, and that, as a result, the legal principles we have devised to reflect these conceptions may be flawed." Joshua Greene & Jonathan Cohen, *For the Law, Neuroscience Changes Nothing and Everything*, 359 Phil. Trans. R. Soc. Lond. B. 1775, 1775 (2004). What pronouncements, if any, would you make about the implications of neuroscience?

4. United States District Court Judge Jed Rakoff has observed that "as neuroscience enters the courtroom . . . [there is a] growing perception among judges that [it] has the potential to be of great service, and challenge, to a great many aspects of the law." In what ways do you think might neuroscience be of service? And when and how might it pose significant challenges to judges? Judge Rakoff has also observed that the law "has struggled both to define relevant states of mind and to devise ways of perceiving them." Can neuroscience help law in defining and

perceiving mental states? Why or why not? The SAGE Center for the Study of the Mind, *A Judge's Guide to Neuroscience: A Concise Introduction* 1, 1 (2010).

5. In addition to neuroscience researchers and treating clinicians, criminologists are also making use of neuroscience and behavioral genetics. The field of "biosocial criminology," which like neurolaw is only now emerging, seeks to integrate knowledge from the biological sciences (including genetics, evolutionary psychology, and the neurosciences) into criminology. The goal is a greater understanding of criminal behavior. *See Biosocial Criminology: New Directions in Theory and Research* (Anthony Walsh & Kevin M. Beaver eds., 2009); Michael Rocque et al., *Biosocial Criminology and Modern Crime Prevention*, 40 J. Crim. Just. 306 (2012). How might findings from biosocial criminology be relevant to the criminal justice system?

6. In his book *The Anatomy of Violence: The Biological Roots of Crime*, neurocriminologist Adrian Raine suggests that neuroscience may one day allow society to preemptively intervene into the lives (and brains) of would-be criminals. Raine asks his readers to imagine that in 2034 the government launches the program, Legal Offensive on Murder: Brain Research Operation for the Screening of Offenders, or LOMBROSO. Under this program, every adult male must have a brain scan and submit a DNA sample to the government. Using this data and algorithms that are improved over time, some of these males are labeled "Lombroso Positive" (LP). The LPs are held in a detention center (though they do have an opportunity to legally challenge the findings). LPs are retested each year and can become eligible for release back into the community. Raine further imagines, in 2040, the creation of a National Child Screening Program (NCSP), which would apply to all children aged ten years and above. Adrian Raine, *The Anatomy of Violence: The Biological Roots of Crime* (2013). The picture Raine paints is, of course, purely speculative at this point. But Raine argues that this is a realistic, and indeed likely a desirable, future. Do you agree?

7. In criminal and civil contexts, should the law permit "psychosurgery"? As legal scholars Roland Nadler and Jennifer Chandler point out, the answer is complicated because "[l]ike many other countries, the United States has a troubled history with prefrontal lobotomy." Roland Nadler & Jennifer A. Chandler, *Legal Regulation of Psychosurgery: A Fifty-State Survey*, 39 J. Legal Med. 335, 336 (2019). Nadler and Chandler conducted a 50-state survey review of current laws on psychosurgery (which in their view may be better described as "invasive neuromodulation"), and found that states vary considerably in their willingness to allow different types of psychosurgery. The authors suggest that "greater harmonization would improve the consistency of the law's efforts to protect people from the abuses of psychosurgery that legislators have rightly sought to eradicate."

8. Lie detection, the subject of a later chapter in this book, has been a focus of much neurolaw research. A 2001 editorial in *Nature Neuroscience* suggests that questions about the efficacy of neuroscience-based lie detection can "only be resolved by extensive field-testing. This seems desirable; although EEG testing may raise the specter of 'Big Brother' in the public imagination, it is in reality just another tool for determining the facts, no different in principle from handwriting, fiber, or DNA evidence. Moreover, its use by prosecutors, at least in the U.S., would be governed by the constitutional protection against self-incrimination, and its main application in the courts would probably be to argue for innocence

rather than guilt." *Forensic Neuroscience on Trial*, 4 Nature Neurosci. 1, 1 (2001). Do you agree that neuroscientific evidence is no different than handwriting, fiber, or DNA evidence? Or is neuroscience categorically different?

9. Is neuroscientific evidence special? Consider law professor Deborah Denno's commentary.

> Why wouldn't neuroscience evidence be treated like any other type of scientific evidence? This inquiry is not to suggest that neuroscience evidence should always be admitted into the courtroom, but rather to ask why the decision-making process would be any different when neuroscience is involved? My perception is that misconceptions and unfounded fears are dominating the dialogue. This pattern needs to change. We should consider neuroscience evidence to be like any other type of evidence, and let the chips fall where they may. We must take neuroscience evidence off of its pedestal (or out of its pillory, depending on one's point of view) so that we can move on from misguided debates regarding the admissibility of this evidence and instead turn our attention to the myriad other ways in which neuroscience can inform the legal system. . . .
>
> Some of the misconceptions and fears that plague neuroscience add to the complexity of using such evidence in legal settings. A main source of this complexity is the exaggerated focus that some legal commentators have on the neuroscience evidence that may be involved in a particular case even when that case includes a wide range of other types of evidence. This focus on the so-called 'deficiencies' of neuroscience diverts away attention from the flaws in other types of evidence as well as diminishes consideration of how neuroscience could improve the criminal law. . . .
>
> The recent surge of neuroscientific evidence in the criminal justice system has been accompanied by criticisms and concerns over its potential dangers and effectiveness. Yet my research shows that, while we should always be careful about the kind of evidence attorneys introduce into the courtroom, there is little basis for the unease surrounding neuroscience in particular. Indeed, neuroscience discoveries can help us reconceptualize how the criminal justice system defines and assesses defendants' mental states, for example, or assist in clarifying state jury instructions on the meaning of *mens rea*. To benefit from neuroscience in these ways, however, we must first penetrate the mystique. We must move on from misconceptions, fears, and misguided debates. We must also realize that although neuroscience brings unique insight *to* the law, there is nothing about neuroscience that merits unique treatment *by* the law.

Deborah W. Denno, *The Place for Neuroscience in Criminal Law*, in *Philosophical Foundations of Law and Neuroscience* 69, 72-81 (Dennis Patterson & Michael Pardo eds., 2016).

Morris B. Hoffman
Nine Neurolaw Predictions
21 New Crim. L. Rev. 212, 212-14 (2018)

Predictions about the impact neuroscience will have on law seem to be grouped around two extremes: it will have no impact or it will have broad and paradigm-shifting impacts. In my experience, neuroscientists tend toward the latter view, I think in part because they underestimate the difficulty of moving the battleship that is the law. Some also fail to appreciate that the law represents thousands of years of pretty good accumulated folk psychology about the human condition. Some legal scholars, by contrast, tend toward the opposite, overly pessimistic, extreme. I think many of them overestimate both the law's inertia and its pedigree. Some no doubt under-appreciate the extraordinary advances made by neuroscience in the last few decades.

. . . I try to stake out some middle ground. In the end, I think neuroscience's legal impacts in the next 50 years will likely be rather lumpy, with some significant, but not paradigm-shifting, impacts in a few discrete areas and not much impact anywhere else. I divide my nine predictions into three temporal segments: near term (next 10 years), long term (10 to 50 years in the future), and never happening:

1. In the next 10 years, neuroscience will be able to detect chronic pain accurately and reliably, and may even be able to distinguish chronic pain from malingering. This will have significant impacts on tort and disability law.

2. In the next 10 years, neuroscience will be able to diagnose many legally relevant psychiatric conditions, including several that often bear on criminal competence and insanity (such as severe schizoaffective disorder), as well as mental conditions claimed to have been caused by torts or justifying disability payments (such as PTSD). This development will not have much legal impact because most legally relevant mental conditions will continue to be diagnosed by traditional clinical methods, but it could help when experts disagree on their diagnoses.

3. Ten to 50 years from now, neuroscience will develop accurate and reliable lie detection methods, which could in theory have significant and widespread impacts for both the criminal and civil systems. Most likely, however, this development will not have significant impacts in the courtroom because the law will continue to be resistant to the admissibility of lie detection results. But it will have significant impacts pre-trial.

4. Ten to 50 years from now, neuroscience will show that some drugs seriously affect our ability to assess risk but not our ability to form intentions, and for those drugs the law may reverse its age-old rule that voluntary intoxication is a defense to purposeful crimes but not to knowing or reckless ones.

5. Ten to 50 years from now, neuroscience will demonstrate that there is no distinction between the mental states of "knowing" and "reckless" when it comes to results elements, and the criminal law may abandon the distinction.

6. Ten to 50 years from now, neuroscience will develop accurate and reliable ways of detecting autobiographical memories for faces and places. This development could theoretically have significant and widespread impacts on both civil and criminal law, but likely won't have much courtroom impact because it is a form of lie detection to which the law of evidence will continue to be resistant.

7. Ten to 50 years from now, neuroscience will be able to determine, on an individual basis, how mature a brain is, dispensing with the law's need to draw some age-based lines for things like criminal responsibility or the age of consent.

8. Neuroscience will never completely solve the mystery of addiction. Even though it may solve the puzzle of tolerance, it will not solve the riddle of dependence.

9. Neuroscience will never convince the law to abandon notions of free will or responsibility.

I make these predictions with great trepidation, fully aware not only of the special kind of schadenfreude in which we all seem to delight when our fellow humans get predictions wrong, but also of the sad fact that so many predictions, even by (maybe especially by) well-informed people, end up being spectacularly wrong. I nevertheless make the effort because . . . neuroscience is already having impacts on the law. Anything we can do to prepare broadly for future impacts seems to me to be an effort worth making.

Francis X. Shen

Law and Neuroscience 2.0

48 Ariz. St. L. J. 1043, 1045-76 (2016)

[Professor Shen considers additional possible intersections of law and neuroscience, not counting the many concerning criminal justice, brain injury, and pain. — EDS.]

Scholarship and case law have intersected with brain death, brain injury, criminal responsibility, criminal treatment, decision-making, bias, pain, evidence law, addiction, mental health law, disability law, insurance law, genetics, evolution, memory, emotions, and much more. Scholarship has been theoretical, empirical, international, and intensely interdisciplinary. New ideas have sprung forth from a variety of fields, including law and neuroeconomics, law and behavioral biology, and law and behavioral genetics. At the same time, the parallel field of neuroethics has developed a research profile that included legal issues. Cases have been heard in local counties all the way up to the Supreme Court. . . .

[In addition to the implications of neuroscience for criminal law already explored in this chapter, additional possibilities present themselves across a variety of legal domains.]

Regulation of Mobile Consumer Neurotechnology

[Beyond the fMRI technique alone,] . . . [t]he advent of smart phones, combined with advances in both brain reading and brain manipulation, has led to a great number of new products. . . .

Mobile neurotechnology such as this offers both promise and peril. On one hand, the technology may lead to improved mental health and enjoyment of life. On the other hand, the technology (and the data it collects) raises important questions concerning regulation, safety, efficacy, and privacy. While academic dialogue about some of these questions has begun, the questions above have not been sufficiently explored. . . . [Questions to address include:]

- *Efficacy:* Does the technology provide the benefits it promises, and what is known about variation in efficacy across individuals?
- *Safety:* What are the known side effects, and how do they compare to other technologies?
- *Regulation:* How, if at all, should the FDA regulate this technology? In what ways is this distinguishable from, or analogous to, existing technologies (some of which are under FDA oversight and some of which are not)?
- *Privacy:* How is brain data being stored and used by the companies processing the data for consumers? What levels of access do users have to their own data?

- *Legal:* The law regulates many types of brain modulation, for instance making it illegal to drive in certain brain states. In what ways should law account for brain changes brought on by neurofeedback and neurostimulation?
- *Ethical:* Does neurostimulation deserve special ethical attention as compared to other, more indirect, ways of modulating mental activity? . . .

Concussions in Youth and Professional Sports

In just the past ten years, all fifty states have enacted statutes related to youth sports concussions. Following this "first wave" of concussion legislation, states are beginning to revisit the issue to determine what works, what does not, and what additional reforms are needed. . . .

Legal and policy scholars have important roles to play in shaping this next wave of concussion policy. In particular, we know little about the quality of information and effectiveness of treatment provided to student-athletes, including potential disparities of treatment across ages, sports, or regions. Nor do we know if students are receiving the care they need to succeed in the classroom (i.e., "Return to Learn") after concussion incidents. Unknowns like this make it difficult to assess legal exposure for school districts and optimal regulatory structures for states to employ.

Moreover, the role of neuroscience in the assessment and treatment of TBI, both in and beyond the sports context, is developing rapidly. This raises questions about the reasonable standard of care, efficacy of reforms, and more. Legal scholars, working with a variety of other disciplines, are well positioned to lead in this area. Statutes are being re-evaluated, policies being implemented, and law suits being filed. . . . [See Chapter 10 for further discussion of sports concussions and the law. — EDS.]

Legal Implications of Early-Onset Dementia Detection

[Although much attention has focused on the implications of neuroscience for matters of juvenile justice,] . . . [i]n 2010, an estimated 4.7 million Americans aged 65 and older suffered from Alzheimer's disease ("AD"), and by 2050 this number is projected to reach 13.8 million. With no cure for Alzheimer's, there is a push toward using neuroimaging ...to identify changes in the brain that might indicate a higher-than-normal risk for developing dementia (and thus allow for behavioral and pharmacological interventions earlier.) At present, the medical consensus is that this is not ready for clinical use, but it's being used in research contexts and it seems reasonable to expect that—given consumer demands—we will see some version of early detection methodology arriving in clinics in the not too distant future.

Law, especially regulatory, insurance, and related bodies of health law, are already (and will continue to) play important roles here. For instance, the Food and Drug Administration governs the approval of methods—such as the use of PET brain scans—to detect Alzheimer's. In 2012 and again in 2013, the FDA approved drugs, in conjunction with PET imaging, for evaluation of Alzheimer's. Yet, in 2015 the FDA also intervened to stop . . . [a] company . . . from promoting an unapproved drug for dementia detection.

The attendant legal and ethical questions to these developments are numerous and challenging. . . . [See Chapter 18 for further discussion. — EDS.]

The crux of the challenge is that most law (and to date, most medicine) doesn't respond until there is a change in observed behavior. That is, we don't typically know that someone has dementia until they repeatedly show behavioral manifestations.

Early diagnosis—based on changes in brain tissue and not just static factors such as age—complicates things. An individual appears normal to her friends, and feels normal herself. But if her brain has changed (and is changing), is she still "normal" in the eyes of the law? . . .

Revisiting Brain Death and Disorders of Consciousness

In the history of law and neuroscience, debates over brain death and the law play a prominent role. The "Harvard Report" of 1968 put into motion what would eventually become the Universal Declaration of Death Act. Today, all fifty states have recognized neurological criteria for determining death. The 1980s saw a flurry of literature in both medicine and law debating the topic, and the Terri Schiavo case in the 2000s made national headlines.

Delineating the line between life and death has been a challenging medical and legal question for centuries, and it will continue to be a ripe area for neurolaw exploration. This is especially so because of new technologies that—for the first time—might allow some patients with certain disorders of consciousness (such as locked-in syndrome) to communicate via brain imaging. . . . [See Chapter 9 for further discussion.—EDS.]

Cognitive Enhancement Through Direct Brain Intervention

In the past fifteen years, much has been written by scholars on human cognitive enhancement. The possibilities are tantalizing. As neuroscientist David Eagleman says at the conclusion of his PBS series *The Brain*, "Our brains don't have to remain as we've inherited them. . . . Our species is just at the beginning of something. . . . Who we become is up to us." Who we become is up to us—but within the confines of legally permissible behavior.

Given the growing marketplace of new (if not necessarily effective) enhancement technologies, drawing legal boundaries will become increasingly important. . . . [See Chapter 19 for further discussion.—EDS.]

Privacy and Brain Hacking

Legal scholars Nita Farahany and Marc Blitz, amongst others, have begun to explore mental privacy. While at present I believe the "mind reading" capabilities of brain technologies do not raise constitutional concerns, privacy discussions will become more salient as the technology progresses. Continued discussion with privacy scholars is surely warranted.

Brain-Computer Interface invites the possibility that—just as computers can be hacked to get into your checking account—computers could be hacked to access the technology modulating your brain activity. This is an excellent place for legal thinkers to contribute, as often the BCI device manufacturers themselves "are developing devices and applications without taking much the security and privacy issues into account." . . . [See further discussion in Chapter 20.—EDS.]

Global Neurolaw

. . . To date, the bulk of scholarship (like the bulk of scholarship in many other fields) is heavily U.S. and European centric. This reflects neuroscience research more generally, which remains challenging to do in the developing world. [The following website compiles all the international neurolaw publications, from 14 countries to date, of which we are aware: https://www.lawneuro.org/internationalneurolaw.php—EDS.]

Law has become increasingly international over the past five decades, as have fields such as political science, economics, sociology, and public health. Can neurolaw do the same? It would take some paradigm-shifting work, but an energetic, creative, culturally sensitive, and interdisciplinary team could make real headway in this area.

. . . [W]ith more space, we might consider further intersections with mental health law, forensic psychiatry, pharmacology, neuroengineering and brain-machine interface, biases and decision-making, transhumanism, informed consent, property in neuronal cell lines, criminal treatment, and much more. . . .

In her article "Functional Neuroimaging and the Law"* Professor Stacey Tovino provides an overview of many potential intersections of law and neuroscience, a number of which we summarize here:

- Property
  - Might neuroscience provide insight on "property instincts" that predate legal systems, the rules of which might tend to reflect evolved and neurologically coded predispositions?
- Intellectual Property
  - To what extent are methods that combine brain scanning, machine learning, and medical diagnosis patentable?
- Torts
  - Can neuroimaging help us to identify and quantify a victim's physical and emotional pain more objectively?
- Lie Detection
  - Can neuroimaging help us to identify lies more accurately?
- Privacy
  - Should you be entitled to heightened privacy protections of your brain scans?
- Employment Law
  - Given the potential for inappropriate discrimination, should employers be prohibited from requiring a brain scan as a condition of employment, for purposes of screening? For purposes of lie detection?
- First Amendment
  - Does the First Amendment protect a person's "privacy of thought" against government intrusions, in the context of cognitive privacy, liberty, or freedom?
- Fourth Amendment
  - Under what circumstances would a government-ordered brain scan be considered unlawful search and seizure?
- Fifth Amendment
  - Does the right to remain silent, so as not to self-incriminate, extend to the right not to have one's brain scanned? Put another way: Is brain scanning evidence more like protected testimonial and communicative evidence (such as spoken words) or more like unprotected physical evidence (such as a blood test, a fingerprint, or a DNA test)?

---

* Stacey Tovino, *Functional Neuroimaging and the Law: Trends and Directions for Future Scholarship*, 7 Am. J. Bioethics 44, 44-56 (2007).

NOTES AND QUESTIONS

1. The importance and promise of neuroscientific research were prominently high-lighted when President Obama, in April 2013, announced the Brain Research through Advancing Innovative Neurotechnologies (BRAIN) initiative. For more on this initiative, see https://braininitiative.nih.gov.

2. Neurotheorist David Marr once wrote that "trying to understand perception by studying only neurons is like trying to understand bird flight by studying only feathers: it just cannot be done. In order to understand bird flight, we have to understand aerodynamics; only then do the structure of feathers and the different shapes of birds' wings make sense." David Marr, *Vision: A Computational Investigation into the Human Representation and Processing of Visual Information* 27 (1982). What else, other than the brain, might one need to study in order to understand human cognition?

3. The readings in this chapter have mentioned many new technologies and many legal issues they do or may raise. Which issues strike you as the most important for society and law to grapple with? Why? As an attorney, which would you find most useful to you, or most threatening to encounter from the other side, and why?

4. Professor Deborah Denno has argued that "a criminal justice system that is more personalized would likely be more effective, efficient, and fair and that incorporating neuroscience into the factfinding process is a particularly apt vehicle for enhancing personalization." Deborah W. Denno, *Neuroscience and the Personalization of Criminal Law*, 86 U. Chi. L. Rev. 359, 394-95 (2019). How could neuroscience improve the personalization of administering justice?

5. To ask whether "neuroscience" will affect "law" is of course actually to ask whether *specific types* of neuroscientific findings will affect *specific types* of law in *specific kinds* of legal contexts. The excerpts in this chapter identify a number of possible intersections for law and neuroscience. Before delving deeper into the neuroscience later in this coursebook, take a moment to assess your first impressions. What specific areas of law do you think are most likely to be affected by neuroscience? How and why did you identify those areas?

6. Law professor Christopher Slobogin identifies five types of neuroscience evidence that "relate to the law defining criminal liability and criminal punishment" :

> The five types, in roughly ascending order of usefulness, are as follows: (1) *Evidence of abnormality*: Evidence showing that the defendant has neurological impairment (eg brain imaging showing that the defendant has frontal lobe disorder, or [frontal lobe disorder] FLD); (2) *Cause-of-an-effect evidence*: Evidence showing that the defendant's neurological impairment is common in criminals or others who behave in an antisocial manner (eg research showing that many criminals have FLD); (3) *Effect-of-a-cause evidence*: Evidence tending to show that the defendant's neurological impairment predisposed him or her to commit the crime (eg research showing that people with FLD are more likely to commit crime than those without FLD); (4) *Individualized neuropsychological findings compared against known performance baselines*: Psychoneurological testing results showing that the defendant has behavioral impairments that are legally relevant (eg testing showing that the defendant, say one with FLD, is highly impulsive or unable to conceptualize); and (5) *Individualized neuropsychological findings compared against known performance baselines*:

Evidence showing that the defendant's impairments are similar to impairments the law has recognized as exculpatory or mitigating (eg evidence that the defendant's FLD is similar in legally relevant respects to the brain of a 14 year old).

The admissibility of neuroscience evidence should depend on which of these five categories is at issue. All five types of evidence may have what has been called 'rhetorical relevance', that is, the potential for swaying a judge or jury in the defendant's (or prosecution's) favor. But a close analysis of each type of evidence makes clear that *genuine* relevance establishes a narrower threshold. More specifically, the first two types of neuroscience evidence should often be considered immaterial at trial; whether they should be admissible at sentencing depends on the law of the jurisdiction. The other three types of neuroscience evidence are more likely to be relevant at both trial and sentencing, with the final category of evidence probably being the most persuasive. But these latter types of evidence are also much more difficult to produce than the first two. . . .

Christopher Slobogin, *Neuroscience Nuance: Dissecting the Relevance of Neuroscience in Adjudicating Criminal Culpability*, 4 J.L. & Biosci. 577, 579 (2017).

7. As brain science matures, claims about brain health are increasing as well. For instance, one brand of milk has included the following statement in their marketing materials: "Kids' brains grow incredibly fast. In fact, the brain nearly quadruples in the first five years of life. Up to 20 percent of the human brain is made of DHA, yet most kids don't get their recommended DHA from common dietary sources like fish. By making Horizon Organic Milk Plus DHA your family choice, you're bringing home all the goodness of organic plus an extra nutritional boost for growing minds and bodies." How would you evaluate such a claim? In *In re Horizon Organic Milk Plus DHA Omega-3 Mktg. & Sales Practice Litig.*, 955 F. Supp. 2d 1311 (S.D. Fla. 2013), a plaintiff class sued Dean Foods for false, misleading, and deceitful representations. The plaintiffs in the case argued that clinical cause and effect studies have found no causative link between DHA algal oil supplementation and brain health. A settlement in the case was approved in 2016.

8. Headlines such as "Brain Scanning May Be Used in Security Checks" have not been uncommon, and a 2012 review found that "the US national security establishment has come to see neuroscience as a promising and integral component of its 21st century needs." Michael N. Tennison & Jonathan D. Moreno, *Neuroscience, Ethics, and National Security: The State of the Art*, 10 PLoS Biology e1001289, e1001289 (2012). How can neuroscience contribute to governments' national security efforts?

9. Several of the selections in the section reflect concern that the government may use brain imaging to "read minds." What does it mean, in this context, to read someone's mind? And if brain-based mind reading were possible, would you see such uses as more akin to the government administering a blood test, forcing a confession, or something else?

10. Brain science could conceivably also play a role in understanding, administering, and critiquing interrogation techniques. The release of Department of Justice memorandums in 2009 detailing coercive interrogation techniques used on terrorist suspects has raised questions about the underlying science of such techniques. The premise is simple: Continuously inflicting shock, stress, anxiety, disorientation, and lack of control will induce suspects to reveal reliable information from long-term memory. But, as you will read in the chapter

on memory, this is not necessarily the case. While studies have shown that extreme stress impairs the ability to recall previously learned information and prior events, mildly stressful events in fact enhance recall. One neuroscientist suggests that "[t]he experience of capture, transport and subsequent challenging questioning would seem to be more than enough to make suspects reveal information." Shane O'Mara, *Torturing the Brain: On the Folk Psychology and Folk Neurobiology Motivating "Enhanced and Coercive Interrogation Techniques,"* 13 Trends Cognitive Sci. 497, 498 (2009). Can neuroscience help to draw the line between permissible and impermissible interrogation techniques? *See* Jonathan H. Marks, *Interrogational Neuroimaging in Counterterrorism: A "No-Brainer" or a Human Rights Hazard?*, 33 Am J.L. Med. 483 (2007).

11. The use of neuroscience in one domain of law may affect other domains as well. How might the law's definition of "disability" be affected by shifting notions of control over one's behavior? *See* Jennifer A. Chandler, *The Impact of Neuroscience in the Law: How Perceptions of Control and Responsibility Affect the Definition of Disability*, in *Neuroethics: Anticipating the Future* 570 (Judy Illes ed., 2017); Jennifer A. Chandler, *The Impact of Biological Psychiatry on the Law: Evidence, Blame and Social Solidarity*, 54 Alberta L. Rev. 831 (2017).

12. Consider that in 2002 *The Economist* wrote, "Genetics may yet threaten privacy, kill autonomy, make society homogeneous and gut the concept of human nature. But neuroscience could do all of these things first." *The Ethics of Brain Science: Open Your Mind*, The Economist (May 23, 2002). Do you agree? Do you still agree after reading Stephen J. Morse, *Avoiding Irrational Neurolaw Exuberance: A Plea for Neuromodesty*, 62 Mercer L. Rev. 837 (2011)?

13. Given rapid advances in brain scanning technology, it would be easy to believe that the intersection of law and neuroscience is a relatively recent phenomenon. In fact, it long predates the origin of the words "neuroscience" (attributed to Francis Schmitt in 1962) and "neurolaw" (attributed to Sherrod Taylor in 1991). As Professor Shen detailed, there were foundational medico-legal dialogues in the 19th and 20th centuries including the following: use of the polygraph for lie detection beginning in the 1920s, electro-encephalography evidence introduced in the 1950s; a controversy over psychosurgery for violence prevention in the 1960s and 1970s; and the use of neuroscience in personal injury litigation at least as early as the 1980s. Francis X. Shen, *The Overlooked History of Neurolaw*, 85 Fordham L. Rev. 667 (2016). Today, the admissibility of neuroscientific testimony regarding brain injury (for instance) is believed to be "generally accepted in most jurisdictions." Bruce H. Stern & Jeffrey A. Brown, *Litigating Brain Injuries* §6:1 (2015).

FURTHER READING

Owen D. Jones & Francis X. Shen, *Law & Neuroscience: What, Why, and Where to Begin – A Knowledge Brief of the MacArthur Foundation Research Network on Law and Neuroscience* (2017).

Francis X. Shen, *The Overlooked History of Neurolaw*, 85 Fordham L. Rev. 667 (2016).

Jeffrey Rosen, *The Brain on the Stand*, N.Y. Times Mag. (Mar. 11, 2007).

Henry T. Greely, *Law and the Revolution in Neuroscience: An Early Look at the Field*, 42 Akron L. Rev. 687 (2009).

Henry T. Greely & Nita A. Farahany, *Neuroscience and the Criminal Justice System*, 2 Ann. Rev. Criminology 451 (2019).

Nita A. Farahany, *Neuroscience and Behavioral Genetics in US Criminal Law: An Empirical Analysis*, 2 J.L. & Biosci. 485 (2016).

Law and Neuroscience: Current Legal Issues (Michael Freeman ed., 2011).

International Neurolaw: A Comparative Analysis (Tade M. Spranger ed., 2012).

A Primer on Criminal Law and Neuroscience: A Contribution of the Law and Neuroscience Project, Supported by the MacArthur Foundation (Stephen J. Morse & Adina L. Roskies eds., 2013).

Henry T. Greely & Anthony Wagner, *Reference Guide on Neuroscience*, in Fed. Judicial Center, *Reference Manual on Scientific Evidence* 747 (3d ed. 2012).

Owen D. Jones & Francis X. Shen, *Law and Neuroscience in the United States*, in *International Neurolaw: A Comparative Analysis* 349 (Tade M. Spranger ed., 2012).

Oliver R. Goodenough & Micaela Tucker, *Law and Cognitive Neuroscience*, 6 Ann. Rev. L. Soc. Sci. 61 (2010).

Owen D. Jones et al., *Law and Neuroscience*, 33 J. Neurosci. 17624 (2013).

Owen D. Jones, Read Montague & Gideon Yaffe, *Detecting Mens Rea in the Brain*, 169 U. Pa. L. Rev. (forthcoming 2020).

Philosophical Foundations of Law and Neuroscience (Dennis Patterson & Michael S. Pardo eds., 2016).

The SAGE Center for the Study of the Mind, *A Judge's Guide to Neuroscience: A Concise Introduction* (2010).

Michael S. Pardo & Dennis Patterson, *Minds, Brains, and Law: The Conceptual Foundations of Law and Neuroscience* (2013).

Handbook on Psychopathy and Law (Kent Kiehl & Walter Sinnott-Armstrong eds., 2013).

Law, Mind and Brain (Michael Freeman & Oliver R. Goodenough eds., 2009).

Francis X. Shen, *The Law and Neuroscience Bibliography: Navigating the Emerging Field of Neurolaw*, 38 Int'l J. Legal Info. 352 (2010).

Laura Stephens Khoshbin & Shahram Khoshbin, *Imaging the Mind, Minding the Image: An Historical Introduction to Brain Imaging and the Law*, 33 Am. J.L. & Med. 171 (2007).

Neuroimaging in Forensic Psychiatry: From the Clinic to the Courtroom (Joseph R. Simpson ed., 2012).

Owen D. Jones, *Seven Ways Neuroscience Aids Law*, in *Neurosciences and the Human Person: New Perspectives on Human Activities* 181 (Antonio M. Battro, Stanislas Dehaene & Wolf Singer eds., 2013).

Peter A. Alces, *The Moral Conflict of Law & Neuroscience* (2018).

Law & The Brain (Semir Zeki & Oliver Goodenough eds., 2006).

Susan M. Wolf, *Neurolaw: The Big Question*, 8 Am. J. Bioethics 21 (2008).

David Eagleman, *The Brain on Trial*, The Atlantic (June 7, 2011).

Stacey Tovino, *Functional Neuroimaging and the Law: Trends and Directions for Future Scholarship*, 7 Am. J. Bioethics 44 (2007).

Neuroscience and the Law: Brain, Mind, and the Scales of Justice (Brent Garland ed., 2004).

William R. Uttal, *Neuroscience in the Courtroom: What Every Lawyer Should Know About the Mind and the Brain* (2008).

William R. Uttal, *The New Phrenology: The Limits of Localizing Cognitive Processes in the Brain* (2001).

Erica Beecher-Monas & Edgar Garcia-Rill, *Fundamentals of Neuroscience and Law: Square Peg, Round Hole* (2020).

Michael Moore, *Mechanical Choices: The Responsibility of the Human Machine* (2020).

CHAPTER 2

The Case of the Murdering Brain

I think the age of scanning has dawned in our courtrooms. This is not a technological genie we are going to be able to put back in the bottle.
— Zachary Weiss, prosecutor in the *Weinstein* case[†]

I think it's a misuse of the technology and a grandiose claim that a resting PET scan is a predictor of behavior.
— Dr. Jonathan Brodie, expert witness for the prosecution in the *Weinstein* case[††]

CHAPTER SUMMARY

This chapter:
- Introduces *People v. Weinstein*, a landmark criminal case that raised threshold questions about the use of brain imaging evidence in trials.
- Presents multiple and competing perspectives on the *Weinstein* case through the writings and recollections of the presiding judge, defense counsel, prosecutor, and testifying experts.
- Invites comparisons to more recent cases in which an accused murderer proffers neuroscientific evidence as a part of his defense.

INTRODUCTION

In the previous chapter, you were briefly introduced to "Mr. Weinstein's Cyst" and the brain-based legal defense Mr. Weinstein used. In this chapter, we explore that case in depth. The case is important historically because it arose in 1991, well before the term "neurolaw" was widely circulating, and well before the majority of law and

---

[†] Zachary Weiss, *The Legal Admissibility of Positron Emission Tomography Scans in Criminal Cases:* People v. Spyder Cystkopf, 1 Seminars Clinical Neuropsychiatry 202, 209 (1996). [To protect his anonymity, commentators originally used the pseudonym Spyder Cystkopf to refer to Weinstein. To improve clarity in this chapter, we have replaced all Cystkopf references to Weinstein. Professor Stephen Morse recalls the origin of the term: "The term 'arachnoid' is derived from the spiderweb-like [blood vessels] that anatomically mark this lining. Thus, Spyder Cystkopf (cyst head)." (Personal communication with authors.) —EDS.]

[††] Quoted in J. Rojas-Burke, *PET Scans Advance as Tools in Insanity Defense*, 34 J. Nuclear Med. 13N, 13N (1993).

neuroscience scholarship was written. In that year New York ad salesman Herbert Weinstein was accused of strangling his wife and then throwing her out of their high-rise apartment window in order to make it look like a suicide. Her body was found on the ground outside the building. Although Weinstein ultimately admitted to the bad acts, he argued in court that—because of a mental defect—he did not appreciate the wrongfulness of his actions when he strangled his wife. The *M'Naghten* test for insanity (the standard by which Weinstein was held in New York) requires a finding of this inability to appreciate right from wrong in order to be found not guilty by reason of insanity.

Weinstein was certainly not the first defendant accused of murder to make an insanity defense. But Weinstein's defense team was the first in New York to proffer brain imaging evidence to support such a claim. Weinstein underwent MRI and positron emission tomography (PET) brain imaging and, as you'll read below, the judge in the case had to decide whether to allow these scans into evidence. The debates over admissibility raise a number of questions that will recur throughout the book: Is the evidence relevant? Is it unduly prejudicial? Is the scientific technology well enough developed for a particular legal application, e.g., as evidence of insanity? How is explanation of behavior related to legal excuse?

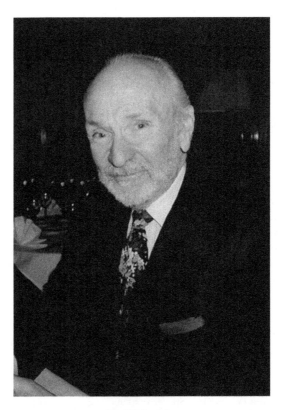

Mr. Weinstein
Courtesy of Joni West

As you consider questions such as these, try to understand exactly why the defense team wanted to use the evidence, precisely what information the evidence conveyed, and the details of the judge's evidentiary ruling. While doing so, notice that the defense proffered individualized neuroscientific evidence as relevant to the defendant's brain specifically. This is in contrast to the use in litigation of *group-based* evidence (i.e., not from the litigants themselves), such as the adolescent brain development evidence that will be discussed in Chapter 17. How courts should treat individualized versus group-based evidence is another recurring theme in the coursebook.

This chapter proceeds in three sections. In Section A you will read the New York court's ruling on the admissibility of the PET scan evidence. The case illustrates the challenges that lawyers, both for prosecution and defense, are likely to face in brain-based criminal defenses. The case raises the question: What, exactly, was going on inside Mr. Weinstein's brain, and what caused him to murder his wife? In Section B you'll read two different answers to these questions, first an analysis by Weinstein's treating physician (who testified for the defense) and then a report from an expert retained by the prosecution. In Section C you will read about the legal implications of this case.

A. PEOPLE v. WEINSTEIN

People v. Weinstein
156 Misc. 2d 34 (N.Y. Sup. Ct. 1992)

CARRUTHERS, J. Herbert Weinstein stands indicted for the crime of murder in the second degree. The indictment alleges that Weinstein murdered his wife, Barbara, on January 7, 1991. Weinstein allegedly strangled his wife in their 12th floor apartment in Manhattan, and then threw her body from a window to make her death appear to be a suicide.

Weinstein's attorney has filed notice that the defense at trial will be that Weinstein lacked criminal responsibility for killing his wife due to mental disease or defect. Evidence to support this defense includes scans of Weinstein's brain obtained through positron emission tomography (PET) and the results of skin conductance response (SCR) tests of his autonomic nervous system. The PET scans were obtained after Weinstein's indictment. The purpose of the scans was to enable neurologists and psychiatrists to study images that depict how Weinstein's brain functions metabolically in its various regions. In accordance with the applicable protocol, a radioactive substance called flourine-18 deoxyglucose was injected into Weinstein's body several minutes before each scan was made. In each instance, when this substance reached Weinstein's brain, it was metabolized, to a point, in the same way that glucose is metabolized. The human brain uses glucose as its energy source. The radioactivity that then was emitted from Weinstein's brain during the metabolic process was captured by a highly sophisticated monitoring device. The device, in each scan, converted this radioactivity into images that showed how well or ill each region of Weinstein's brain was performing metabolically. Weinstein's PET scans confirmed that a cyst exists within the arachnoid membrane, one of the brain's protective coverings. This arachnoid cyst is an abnormality that was first detected by

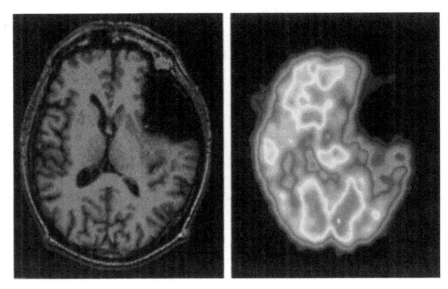

Figure 1.   MRI (left) and PET (right) scans of Herbert Weinstein's brain. The MRI image shows the internal structure of the brain. The PET image shows the amount of glucose metabolism, with higher metabolism in the whiter areas and lower metabolism in the darker areas. The large, dark region in the upper right of each image is the large cyst that displaced and damaged brain tissue. The cyst was actually in the left frontal lobe of the brain. The arrangement of right-left in this figure follows medical imaging convention, as if you are viewing the patient from beneath, with face at the top. Thus, the actual left side of the brain is on the right in the figure. Chapter 4 explains these methods and conventions. Scans performed by Abass Alavi of the University of Pennsylvania and originally published in J. Rojas-Burke, *PET Scans Advance as Tools in Insanity Defense*, 34 J. Nuclear Med. 13N, 13N (1993).

images of brain structure obtained by an MRI machine. The PET scans also showed metabolic imbalances exist in areas of the brain near the cyst and opposite it.*

The SCR tests of Weinstein's autonomic system were performed, also after indictment, at the neurological laboratory of the University of Iowa. The physicians at this laboratory are the first to use SCR tests of the autonomic nervous system as a means of indicating the existence of lesions in the frontal lobes of the brain. During the tests, a machine similar to a polygraph is used to measure a person's galvanic skin responses while that person is shown a series of photographs depicting scenes ranging in emotional content from the serene to the shocking. Unlike more familiar polygraph tests, SCR tests are not used as a purported means of determining whether a person is telling the truth. Weinstein's SCR results were consistent with those of tested individuals who were confirmed as having lesions in the frontal lobes of their brains.

---

* [Although subarachnoid cysts like this are within the skull (and might, therefore, be referred to as being in the brain), technically the cyst impinged on the brain by compressing those areas of the brain underneath it. Such compression causes neurons to stop functioning normally, or to stop functioning altogether.—Eds.]

PET scans and SCR test results, according to Weinstein's attorney, are factors that a psychiatrist will rely upon at trial to explain his diagnosis that, due to mental disease or defect, Weinstein was not criminally responsible for the death of his wife. The psychiatrist will explain that his diagnosis is also based upon physical and neuropsychological tests, his interviews of Weinstein, as well as other information available to him. The District Attorney has moved for an order precluding Weinstein's attorney from offering at trial any testimony or other evidence concerning the PET scans and SCR test results, arguing that PET and SCR technology have not been shown to be sufficiently reliable as diagnostic devices for brain abnormalities so as to warrant the admission of such evidence at the trial of a criminal case. Pursuant to this court's order, a pretrial hearing was held upon this motion. Many physicians, including neurologists, psychiatrists, and experts in nuclear medicine, testified at this hearing. The court resolves below the issues raised by the District Attorney's motion.

I.

Almost 70 years ago James Alphonso Frye was tried for murder in Washington, D.C. During the trial his attorney offered as corroboration for Frye's exculpatory statements the results of a "systolic blood pressure deception test" performed on Frye prior to trial. The trial court refused to admit the test results. Frye was convicted. On appeal, Frye's principal argument was that the trial court erroneously excluded relevant evidence of a scientific nature. The Circuit Court of Appeals affirmed Frye's conviction. It held that the trial court's exclusion of the test results was correct, finding that the systolic blood pressure deception test had not gained "general acceptance" among authorities in the fields of physiology and psychology. (*Frye v. United States*, 293 F 1013, 1014 [D.C. Cir. 1923].) The court stated its full holding as follows: "Just when a scientific principle or discovery crosses the line between the experimental and demonstrable stages is difficult to define. Somewhere in this twilight zone the evidential force of the principle must be recognized, and while courts will go a long way in admitting expert testimony deduced from a well-recognized scientific principle or discovery, the thing from which the deduction is made must be sufficiently established to have gained general acceptance in the particular field in which it belongs." (*Supra*, at 1014.)

The "general acceptance" test of *Frye* for the admission of scientific evidence at trial is the standard most often used by courts throughout the United States.* Those who support continued reliance upon the *Frye* test argue: it guarantees that in any particular case independent experts will exist who can be called upon to carefully examine a scientific opinion; that it promotes uniformity of judicial decisions with respect to the admission of scientific evidence; and that it protects juries from being misled by expert opinions that may be couched in formidable scientific terminology but that are based on fanciful theories.

The *Frye* test is not without detractors. Its critics most frequently argue: that the identification of the appropriate discipline or professional field can be problematical, because many scientific techniques cut across several disciplines; that the

---

* [Some states still employ the *Frye* standard, but federal courts and many states have since adopted the *Daubert* test, discussed in detail in Chapter 8, Neuroscience in the Courtroom: Assessing Scientific Evidence. — EDS.]

percentage of experts in a field who must accept the technique before it can be accorded the status of "general acceptance" is unclear; and that the delay between the introduction of a scientific technique and its recognition as generally accepted prevents reliable evidence from being heard in court. Perhaps the potential for undue restrictiveness under the *Frye* test occasions the sharpest criticism. . . .

The courts of New York, including the Court of Appeals, regularly apply the *Frye* test in cases involving novel scientific evidence. They have done so where such evidence concerned physical phenomena and measurements. They have also employed the *Frye* test where psychological or physiological theories were offered as a novel means of explaining human behavior. The case law thus demonstrates the existence of a judicial policy in this State to favor the *Frye* test due to its strengths and despite its potential for undue restrictiveness.

The judicial policy in New York favoring the *Frye* test might seem to require its application to all issues regarding the admissibility of the novel scientific evidence that Weinstein wishes to offer at his trial, PET and SCR. However, application of the *Frye* test is complicated by the fact that Weinstein's defense at trial will be the affirmative defense that he was not responsible for his conduct due to mental disease or defect. The PET and SCR evidence is to be offered in partial support of Weinstein's psychiatrist's opinion that his cognitive ability was so impaired that when he allegedly killed his wife he lacked substantial capacity to know or appreciate either the nature and consequences of his conduct or that his conduct was wrong.

When a defendant in a criminal case interposes the insanity defense, he may offer at trial the testimony of psychiatric experts to support it. Should Weinstein present such evidence, as his counsel says he shall, the People must be accorded an opportunity to present their own psychiatric experts in rebuttal. The permissible scope of the testimony of psychiatric experts on the subject of diagnostic opinion in an insanity defense case is set out in [New York Criminal Procedure Law] CPL 60.55(1). . . .

The wording of the second paragraph of section 60.55 (1) is virtually identical to a provision of the Model Penal Code, one of the sources from which the Penal Law is derived. Section 4.07(4) of the Model Penal Code states, in pertinent part, that a psychiatrist or other expert who testifies in an insanity defense case "shall be permitted to make any explanation reasonably serving to clarify his diagnosis and opinion and may be cross-examined as to any matter bearing on his competency or credibility or the validity of his diagnosis or opinion." It is instructive that the intent of the drafters of this model statute was to foster a full airing of reasonable psychiatric opinions in insanity defense cases. As the Explanatory Note to this provision states, section 4.07(4) was designed to free psychiatric experts from those evidentiary restrictions that would otherwise inhibit or prevent them from thoroughly explaining to a jury what they know of a defendant's mental condition: "Subsection (4), which indicates the sort of testimony experts may give, is meant to eliminate artificial constraints on psychiatric testimony by allowing the experts to testify fully in terms comprehensible to the jury about their conclusions and the basis for those conclusions." . . .

It is thus clear that both section 4.07(4) of the Model Penal Code and New York's CPL 60.55(1) are aimed at permitting psychiatric experts to testify concerning information that reasonably serves to clarify and support the diagnosis. Indeed, the touchstone of both provisions is reasonableness.

To arrive at a valid diagnostic opinion, a psychiatric expert is entitled under the norms of the profession to consider such sources of background information as the statements of the defendant and witnesses, police reports, hospital records, and results of all relevant neuropsychological and medical tests performed upon the defendant. It is hardly surprising, then, that in forming a diagnosis psychiatrists and psychologists do consider technical and scientific material that, while relevant and reasonable, has not been accorded general acceptance in their disciplines. In fact, during the hearing in the case at bar, Doctor Norman Relkin, one of the defendant's experts, observed that "there are hundreds and thousands of tests that we use which wouldn't meet that criteria [of general acceptance], that a physician uses in making his diagnosis." Doctor Daniel Martell, the forensic psychologist called by the People, alluded to this very point when he testified that the clinical judgment of a diagnostician is, in part, "based on the clinician's accumulated experience over the years that he or she has been in practice, and every clinician learns from that process." Thus, a requirement that each diagnostic test administered to a defendant in an insanity defense case pass muster under the *Frye* test might well impair, in contravention of section 60.55(1), the ability of a psychiatric expert "to make any explanation reasonably serving to clarify his diagnosis and opinion."

Having stated that the *Frye* test is inapplicable under section 60.55(1) to evidence relating to the diagnostic tests employed by psychiatric experts in insanity cases, this court must now state that it would be a mistake to conclude that the statute's test of reasonableness completely supersedes the *Frye* test in these cases. It does not. Section 60.55(1) loosens only the restrictions that might otherwise be placed upon a psychiatric expert's ability at trial to provide a reasonable explanation for the diagnosis and opinion about the defendant's mental state. The statute does not by its terms affect such matters as the standard that must be met to justify a psychiatric expert's testimony that a mental disease or syndrome does in fact exist or that a psychological or physiological theory serves to explain human behavior.

Unlike the diagnosis of a patient, which, in large measure, is based upon the clinical judgment of a psychiatrist or psychologist that is formed by information particular to that patient, such issues as whether a mental disease or syndrome exists or whether a theory validly explains conduct are matters susceptible to controlled research studies, to debate by a cross-section of experts in the field, and, if warranted, to general acceptance. Thus, courts in New York readily have applied the *Frye* test in determining the latter, overarching issues. . . .

To recapitulate: in an insanity defense case, the existence of a mental disease or syndrome or the validity of a theory of human behavior must be generally accepted in the field of psychiatry or psychology before experts may discuss such matters in their testimony at trial. If general acceptance has been attained, a psychiatric expert then "must be permitted" to state a diagnosis and to give a reasonable explanation for a finding that the defendant does or does not suffer from the mental disease, or that that person is or is not affected by the syndrome, or that a theory of human behavior does or does not explain the defendant's conduct.

II.

The evidence adduced at the hearing showed that Weinstein's brain is abnormal due to the presence of the arachnoid cyst, the attendant displacement of the left frontal lobe, and firm indications of metabolic imbalance near the cyst and the regions of the brain opposite it. The defendant's experts testified at length about these matters. Doctor Jonathan Brodie, the People's expert, also acknowledged in his testimony that Weinstein's brain is abnormal, "[b]ecause there is evidence of a cyst in the brain from the MRI results. Once you have a sack in the skull, it's going to compress the brain and make it look abnormal." Doctor Brodie testified, too, that Weinstein's brain exhibited "an abnormality in his regional glucose metabolism."

The frontal lobes of the human brain—the general region where Weinstein's abnormalities are most apparent—control the so-called executive functions. The ability to reason and to plan constitute the most important of these functions. The frontal lobes, in other words, are the seat of man's cognitive powers. According to the evidence at the hearing, damage to the frontal lobes can adversely affect a person's reasoning capabilities. Putting it another way, as did Doctor Daniel Martell, . . . damage to the frontal lobes may be signaled by an erosion of a person's powers of judgment, insight, and foresight. These are matters that are generally accepted as valid in the fields of psychiatry, psychology, and neurology.

Defense counsel intends to call at trial a psychiatrist to testify that the moment Weinstein allegedly killed his wife, he lacked the cognitive ability to understand the nature and consequences of his conduct or that his conduct was wrong. The psychiatrist is prepared to testify that Weinstein's cognitive power was impaired at that instant, in part, by organic brain damage. Defense counsel states that this opinion is to be based upon many sources of information, including PET and SCR test results. As noted above, the admissibility of the results of these tests depends upon whether it would be reasonable for the psychiatrist to consider these results with other available information in forming a diagnosis that Weinstein's cognitive ability was so impaired at the time he allegedly killed his wife that he was not responsible for his conduct.

PET is a highly advanced form of medical technology. Doctor Abass Alavi, a pioneer in the development and uses of PET, testified that PET has been employed as both a research tool and a diagnostic device for several years. PET's use for purposes of obtaining images depicting the metabolic functioning of various organs, including the brain, has been the subject of review articles in major medical publications. . . . As discussed earlier in this opinion, general acceptance of a diagnostic device or technique—the *Frye* test's requirement for admissibility—is a more stringent standard than the test or reasonableness that is applicable, by virtue of CPL 60.55(1), to insanity defense cases in New York. Thus, a diagnostician's consideration of Weinstein's PET test results, insofar as they depict the existence of both the cyst and the metabolic imbalances in Weinstein's brain, is, a fortiori, reasonable. The District Attorney argues that the complex mathematical formulae used to quantify the results of PET tests have not gained general acceptance in relevant technological and medical fields. Doctor Alavi's testimony supports this argument. However, the evidence shows that the formulae are used with regularity by PET experts and that the results are relied upon by them. Consequently, in forming a diagnosis, a psychiatrist in an insanity defense case could reasonably consider the quantitative results derived by application of the formulae to raw data.

According to Doctor Norman Relkin, SCR tests are routinely used to diagnose dysfunction of the autonomic nervous system. They have not been widely used as a means of diagnosing damage to the frontal lobes of the brain. The latter point does not mean, however, that a psychiatrist would be acting unreasonably in including the results of such tests in the data base used to make such a diagnosis. Although SCR tests do not directly evince frontal lobe dysfunction, experiments performed on 50 subjects at the neurological laboratory at the University of Iowa indicate that SCR tests can be used successfully to distinguish patients with abnormalities in the frontal lobes from normals and from patients with damage in other areas of the brain. The results of these experiments were reported in a medical journal by the chief of the Iowa laboratory, Doctor Antonio Damasio, a neurologist who, according to Doctor Relkin, is highly regarded in the profession.

It would seem unreasonable for a psychiatrist to rely exclusively on SCR tests as a basis for concluding that a particular patient suffered from frontal lobe damage. The Damasio report does not merit such complete reliance, given the fact that the number of persons tested was relatively small. However, because Doctor Damasio's reputation as a scientist is good, because the experiments were performed according to a carefully devised protocol, and because the results were peer reviewed prior to their publication, a psychiatrist would be reasonable in considering the results of the SCR tests as a form of corroboration of other, more definitive tests, namely PET and MRI, that clearly show abnormalities in Weinstein's left frontal lobe. . . .

IV.

Having discussed what is admissible evidence, brief reference should be made to certain theories relating to human behavior that may not be mentioned in testimony at the trial. Evidence concerning these theories is not admissible because they have not been generally accepted as valid in the fields of psychiatry, psychology, and neurology. The first of these theories is that arachnoid cysts directly cause violence. Doctor Martell testified categorically that this theory was not generally accepted, noting that he had seen no scientific research to support it. Doctor Relkin, the defendant's witness, appeared to agree. Another theory that has not been generally accepted is that reduced levels of glucose metabolism in the frontal lobes of the brain directly cause violence. In his brief, the defendant disavows any intention to rely on this theory at trial. As he states, "[w]ith respect to hypometabolism causing violence, it is critical for the Court to recognize that it is a completely false issue." This position is fully justified by the record. The only evidence offered in support of the theory was a preliminary research report: . . . The report concerned four patients, each of whom had a history of purposeless violent behavior. PET scans showed hypometabolism in the frontal lobes. However, each of the four patients also had long-standing personality disorders apparently resulting from such problems as alcoholism and drug abuse. It cannot be definitively stated that the behavioral problems of these four patients was due to hypometabolism and not to their personality disorders, a fact that the authors of the report fully recognized. Doctor Brodie, the People's witness, trained the report's principal author, Doctor Nora Volkow, in PET scanning. He testified that her report was published because the four cases were "potentially of interest," and that the findings were "potentially to be further investigated." Thus, a conclusion based upon Volkow and Tancredi's report that hypometabolism in the frontal lobes causes violence would be entirely premature and not at the level of general acceptance in the relevant scientific disciplines. . . .

While cognitive problems might render a person unable to choose a proper behavioral response in a moment of stress, it has not been shown that experts in the relevant disciplines generally accept the theory that aberrant behavior can be the product of a person's history of reward and punishment responses as encoded in the autonomic nervous system. Rather, Doctor Damasio appears to have first proposed this theory in his research report as a "possible" explanation of the phenomena that his team observed during reported SCR studies.

The foregoing constitutes the court's decision on the evidentiary issues raised by the District Attorney's motion. The parties are ordered to comply with the rulings expressed within this decision should PET and SCR test results be offered in evidence at trial.

NOTES AND QUESTIONS

1. Would it affect your analysis of this case if Mr. Weinstein had been a gambling addict and was relying on his wife's funds to feed the addiction and pay off his debts? What if Mr. Weinstein had visited the Hemlock Society (a group that promoted the right to commit suicide) sometime prior to making the crime scene look like his wife had taken her own life? Because the case did not go to trial, the full picture of facts remains incomplete. We do know that Mr. Weinstein and his wife did gamble (though whether it was problematic is contested), and we do know he visited the Hemlock Society (though whether for a nefarious reason or because of the chronic illness of a family member remains contested).

2. If you were the prosecutor in this case, how would Judge Carruthers' evidentiary ruling affect your strategy and tactics? If you were defense counsel?

3. After the admissibility ruling, Weinstein agreed to a plea deal of manslaughter, with a prison sentence of 7 to 21 years. "The district attorney had sought a murder conviction, which would have landed [Weinstein] in prison for 25 years to life. Given the grim details of the crime," Weinstein's lawyer "doubted that jurors would have much sympathy for an insanity defense and might go ahead and convict Mr. Weinstein of murder or at best seek the lesser charge of manslaughter—in spite of the PET evidence...." Weinstein's lawyer suggested that "the prosecutor would never have agreed to a plea if the judge had excluded the PET evidence." J. Rojas-Burke, *PET Scans Advance as Tools in Insanity Defense*, 34 J. Nuclear Med. 13N, 26N (1993). Was this a better deal for prosecution or defense, in your view?

4. Why did Weinstein accept a plea deal? Dr. Norman Relkin offers an intriguing suggestion: "[Weinstein] stated that this was because of the anticipated cost of continuing his legal defense. When I asked him what he saw himself doing when his sentence ended 7-21 years from now, HW said (then age 68), 'Sales. There will always be a need for people who can do billboard advertising.' I have always wondered whether the brain dysfunction that led HW to commit an impulsive act of homicide also caused him to accept a less than favorable plea bargain for a 68-year-old. If so, that provides an O'Henryesque twist to his story." (Personal communication with authors). Under what circumstances do you think that defendants who are alleging their insanity should be allowed to accept a plea bargain that is, as here, against the advice of counsel?

5. *Postscript.* Herbert Weinstein entered the New York prison system in 1993, and despite good behavior and advancing age, he was repeatedly denied parole. He filed suit to challenge the parole board's decision and found favor with the court.

In 2005 Judge Shirley Kornreich found that Weinstein "is now 79 years old and ill. He is blessed with family and friends willing to provide him with support and a home upon release and enough funds to make him self-sufficient. The Board's unfounded conclusory statement that 'there is a reasonable probability that [petitioner] would not live and remain at liberty without violating the law' and that his 'release is thus not presently compatible with the public safety and welfare,' is but an empty recitation of the statutory exception. Without any reasons, much less the required detailed reasons, and with a record which suggests otherwise, the finding is irrational bordering on impropriety." *Weinstein v. Dennison*, 801 N.Y.S.2d 244, 251 (N.Y. Sup. Ct. 2005). After remand, Weinstein was finally given conditional release to parole in December 2006. On parole, Weinstein lived in Tuxedo Park, New York, where he passed away on June 22, 2009.

6. When and how do you think evidence of brain anatomy and/or brain function should inform the question of whether a defendant is insane, and therefore not criminally responsible (or not criminally responsible for reasons other than insanity)? To what extent is your opinion informed by, or should it be informed by, data on the percentage of the population that has similar cysts, or worse ones, and don't strangle and defenestrate their spouses? What if the data isn't yet known? To learn more about arachnoid cysts, visit the resources of the National Institute of Neurological Disorders and Stroke.

7. How would evidence of either a violent or pacifistic past for Weinstein affect your thinking about this case?

8. Is there any kind of brain abnormality that, in your view, should as a matter of sound policy entitle a defendant to a rebuttable presumption that he is not criminally responsible? If you were to think so, how would you approach categorizing it? By region? By importance? By percentage of brain tissue (e.g., 10%, 30%, 80%) affected? By relationship between the region affected and the prohibited act?

9. How should evidence of structural or functional brain abnormalities be weighed in comparison to observational evidence (e.g., testimony from fact witnesses) and clinical evidence (e.g., conclusions of an examining psychiatrist)? For example, do you think brain images that reveal structural lesions are likely to be more persuasive to a jury than evidence of behavioral disorders (which may be a consequence of a lesion)? What about functional abnormalities in the absence of structural defects? What if brain scanning evidence and clinical evidence conflict?

10. Diarmuid White, attorney for defendant Herbert Weinstein, reflected back on the case in this way: "This was the most demanding case I ever worked on because I had to be able to examine these scientific witnesses at a hearing—these people were geniuses in fields I knew nothing about." (Personal communication with authors). How, as a lawyer, would you prepare for these types of challenges?

11. Dr. Gary Tucker, who edited a special volume on the *Weinstein* case, observed that: "The most difficult questions in neuropsychiatry pertain to the determination of causality: (1) Is the lesion which is seen in the MRI the cause of the observed symptoms or behavior? (2) Is the focal temporal slowing noted in the EEG indicative of a seizure disorder? (3) Could this mild head injury have caused such a marked behavior change? . . . Certainly, all of the new imaging techniques and functional evaluations of the central nervous system are providing us with 'abnormalities' for which we have, as yet, no clear brain-behavior

correlation or even a neuropathological referent. Consequently, we are frequently confronted with a 'pathologic' finding that may or may not be related to the 'pathology' we are attempting to investigate. While we are used to tolerating such ambiguity, the legal system is not." Gary J. Tucker, *Introduction*, 1 Seminars Clinical Neuropsychiatry 169, 169 (1996). What would it mean for the legal system to tolerate such ambiguity? Should it?

12. Consider Dr. Helen Mayberg's reflections on *Weinstein*:

> [The *Weinstein* case] exemplifies the premature use and potentially prejudicial nature of a PET scan abnormality when presented as a key piece of evidence linking regional brain dysfunction to a specific behavior. In this case, the behavior was impulsive violence resulting in murder, and the PET scan was believed to provide important corroborative evidence of orbital frontal dysfunction critical to the defendant's defense. The MRI scan clearly demonstrated a large, chronic, left-sided subarachnoid cyst with thinning of the underlying bone, compression of the adjacent temporal lobe, and extension into the frontal fossa. Unambiguous left-sided hypometabolism of the cyst was seen on two resting FDG PET studies. In addition, significant, but more subtle, metabolic changes were demonstrated in adjacent areas of frontal and temporal cortex. These regional metabolic abnormalities, in combination with results from skin conductance and social fluency testing, were used to argue that the crime was caused by an organic impulsive-control disorder, despite no previous history of aggression or impulsivity. Furthermore, no data are available as to the sensitivity or specificity of these or any PET scan or neuropsychological test findings for these particular behaviors.
>
> Because of the perceived experimental nature of PET scanning, an evidentiary hearing was held to determine their admissibility. The issue in this case was not whether FDG PET scans provide a reliable measure of brain glucose metabolism. They do, and this was emphasized in the judge's ruling. The more substantive issue was the causative relationship between the structure lesion, the PET scan changes, and the criminal behavior in question. The sensitivity and specificity of frontotemporal hypometabolism for impulsivity or violence is unknown. There are no published controlled PET studies of either episodic violence or subarachnoid cysts. More specifically, there are no imaging studies of cyst patients with and without violence. The judge acknowledged the lack of any generally accepted studies regarding the neurological localization of violent behavior (especially the absence of replicated, controlled imaging studies) and ruled that, although the PET scans could be used to show regional hypometabolism, no cause-and-effect relationships between frontal abnormalities and specific behavioral disturbances, including violence, could be offered at trial. Although this decision appeared to severely restrict the use of the PET scan evidence in this case, the mere introduction of the scans would still be predicted to strongly influence a jury.
>
> In retrospect, the push to introduce the PET scans, which required a lengthy evidentiary hearing, now seems particularly ironic, because the defendant is currently serving a 25-year term after an unexpected plea bargain made before the start of trial. It has been suggested that the time and considerable expense required to pursue the admissibility of the PET scans influenced this abrupt decision, which was made against the recommendations of his defense counsel. With this turn of events, none of the neurological, neuropsychological, or imaging evidence was ever argued in court, and one can only speculate as to the likely impact the PET scan evidence and the overall mental defect strategy originally planned by the defense might have had on a jury, had they been given the opportunity to hear the evidence.

Helen S. Mayberg, *Medical-Legal Inferences from Functional Neuroimaging Evidence*, 1 Seminars Clinical Neuropsychiatry 195, 199-200 (1996). How do these perspectives change your initial reactions to the case, if at all?

B. INSIDE THE MURDERING BRAIN

What, exactly, was going on inside Herbert Weinstein's head when he killed his wife? Although no one knows for sure, at the evidentiary hearing experts for the prosecution and for the defense offered their opinions. In this section we present those opinions, which include discussion of Weinstein's brain and its relationship to his behavior.

Norman Relkin et al.
Impulsive Homicide Associated with an Arachnoid Cyst and Unilateral Frontotemporal Cerebral Dysfunction
1 Seminars Clinical Neuropsychiatry 172, 178-82 (1996)

Several aspects of [Herbert Weinstein's] presentation alerted us to the possible presence of underlying brain dysfunction. His act of homicide constituted a clear departure from past behaviors, which in an elderly individual is not infrequently a symptom of incipient systemic, neurologic or psychiatric illness. He had suffered unexplained neurological deficits of several months duration earlier in life, increasing the likelihood that he possessed an abnormal brain substrate. He also showed a striking inability to express emotions such as remorse in a heartfelt manner and showed limited insight into the motivations for his isolated act of violence. While various psychodynamic or psychosocial explanations could be forwarded to explain these deficiencies, the incongruity of an impulsive act of homicide committed by a previously nonviolent, elderly individual led us to carry out further testing. . . .

In our opinion, [Weinstein's] isolated episode of violent behavior and his constricted emotionality are most consistent with damage to the prefrontal cortex. It was for this reason that we asked him to undergo further testing using a psychophysiological paradigm sensitive to symptomatic ventral frontal dysfunction. It was by no means a foregone conclusion that his autonomic responses would be abnormal, or that they would in any way resemble those observed after bilateral parenchymal orbital frontal injury. The fact that his autonomic responses on this paradigm precisely replicated those observed in individuals with disorders of social conduct secondary to orbital frontal injury provided a strong indication that the corticolimbic systems in this region of his brain were abnormal.

Armed with these observations, we considered the possibility of a relationship between [Weinstein's] violent behavior and his focal cerebral dysfunction. His own account suggests that he reacted in what might be construed as a reflexively aggressive manner when confronted by the novel, threatening circumstances of his wife's scratching attack on his face. This is consonant with one of the known effects of prefrontal dysfunction, namely, a predisposition to stimulus-bound aggression. The dissociation between [Weinstein's] actions and his emotional experience, as well as his subsequent lack of expression of heartfelt remorse is also consistent with expected effects of injury to the prefrontal limbic system. . . .

CONCLUSIONS

In the present case, a violent and impulsive act of homicide was committed by an elderly individual who had previously avoided all forms of aggression. Although no overt psychiatric pathology was evident, his constricted emotionality, his lack of insight into his motivations for strangling his wife, his past history of an unexplained neuro-event and subtly decreased dexterity in his dominant right hand provided the impetus for further neuropsychiatric evaluation. He was found to have a large, albeit common intracerebral cyst in the left sylvian fissure and structural deformation of neighboring left frontal, temporal and insular regions. Comparison of earlier angiography results and current MRI findings suggested that the cyst had enlarged during his adult life. EEG and PET studies further indicated the presence of left frontotemporal dysfunction, and he was found to have abnormal autonomic responses to affectively charged visual stimuli in a pattern previously observed in patients with focal orbital frontal pathology. The presence of structural, cerebral metabolic, psychologic and functional abnormalities in cortico-limbic structures essential to the regulation of aggressivity suggests the possibility that his homicidal actions may constitute stimulus-bound aggression. The novel, threatening nature of his wife's scratching attack and the necessity it created for an immediate response, may have reduced or eliminated [Weinstein's] opportunity to develop the alternative responses strategies that he appears quite capable of bringing to bear in other circumstances. By this formulation, his actions provide an extreme and unfortunate example of how an innate behavioral response (stimulus-bound aggression) can be triggered by environmental contingencies (a scratching attack) and lead to disastrous consequences (homicide) when the normal mechanisms for restraining such behaviors fail in the context of ventral prefrontal dysfunction.

[Herbert Weinstein's] case leads us to recommend that greater attention be paid to neurobehavioral symptoms in patients with large or expanding intracranial cysts, particularly those in the Sylvian fissure. We share Wortis' sentiment that "interest in the biological determinants of violent behavior should not serve as a means of getting away with murder." It is important to acknowledge that some brain lesions can heighten the inherent predisposition for aggressive behavior whereas others are less likely to do so. In a small percentage of cases, appropriate neurosurgical, pharmacological and/or psychotherapeutic interventions may reduce or even eliminate the adverse behavioral consequences of such lesions. The legal system can play an important role in determining whether or not such treatment is made available. It is therefore essential for counselors, judges, juries, and the public to keep an open mind when confronted by neuropsychiatric findings in the courtroom, and for experts to provide balanced and responsible testimony, permitting the relevance of such findings (or the lack thereof) to be considered on a case-by-case basis.

Daniel A. Martell

Causal Relation Between Brain Damage and Homicide: The Prosecution
1 Seminars Clinical Neuropsychiatry 184, 187-92 (1996)

Analysis of the Case.   My involvement in [*Weinstein*] began with a series of conversations with the prosecutor. Most of the data described above had already been obtained through discovery when I began to work on the case. I was the first expert he had retained, and one of the first things he wanted was an analysis of the chain of inference being used by the defense, identification of the possible weaknesses in that chain, and input as to other appropriate experts to help address those weaknesses. As I saw it at that point, the chain of inference was as follows:

1. Some undetermined but documented neurological event, quite possibly related to his congenital cyst, occurred in 1948 at age 22.

2. There was current evidence of the arachnoid cyst on MRI.

3. There was a hypothesis that the cyst had grown, based on negative findings of arterial displacement in 1948, versus positive MRI findings in 1991.

4. There was a claim that the cyst was causing impairment in the functioning of the frontal lobes.

5. There was a claim that the instant offense reflects the growth of that cyst and its effects on the defendant's behavior, that is, with resulting impairment in social functioning, judgment, and behavior, otherwise known as a frontal lobe syndrome.

6. The claim was supported by the following functional evidence:
   a. Neuropsychological test findings
   b. Frontal hypometabolism on PET
   c. SCR experiments
   d. Forensic psychiatric opinion

I evaluated the weaknesses in the chain of inference as follows: First, there was no doubt that the defendant had a neurological abnormality. The key question was what the behavioral impact of that abnormality might be. My most fundamental concern with the defense theory was what I perceived to be a misrepresentation of evidence of possible volitional impairment to support an opinion on the purely cognitive right/wrong standard of New York's *M'Naghten*-based insanity test. Dr Damasio's somatic marker theory, it seemed to me, went rather directly to the issue of volitional impairment rather than to the right/wrong test at issue in this case.

The Damasio opinion suggested that the defendant knew cognitively the right thing to do, but could not properly make choices to control his behavior (volition), because of the putative effects of the cyst on his frontal lobe functioning. In a jurisdiction with a volitional prong to its insanity defense, this would certainly have been a viable way to go, but not under the New York standard. Dr Schwartz's opinion then seemed a matter of semantic sleight-of-hand, twisting what was essentially a volitional defense arbitrarily to fit the appreciation of wrongfulness standard of the New York insanity test.

This suggested to me that the defense might attempt to wow the jury with lots of impressive high-tech pictures of the defendant's brain and then tap-dance over the real insanity issue. Simultaneously, I was concerned that the potentially prejudicial impact of some of the neuroscientific data would outweigh its probative value in the case. For example, I was concerned about the SCR experiments, because (1) SCR is not generally accepted as a method of testing for frontal lobe dysfunction; and (2) criminals, psychopaths, prisoners, and delinquents without acquired brain damage and subsequent behavioral changes are also known to be hyporeactive in autonomic arousal. I was also concerned about the PET findings because of the lack of data on PET and violence. There is only one published study in this area that examined only four violent subjects using PET and other brain scanning methods. Although the study is very interesting, even its authors acknowledge that there are too many confounding factors in the design to permit any conclusions about PET and violent behavior. Yet in this case, PET findings were being used as evidence to suggest that brain dysfunction played a causative role in this violent crime.

Strategy.   On the basis of this analysis, it seemed to me that there were three primary questions to be pursued. The first involved putting all the neurological issues aside for a moment, and taking a long hard look at what was going on in the life of this couple around the time of the crime, and specifically what the defendant was thinking, feeling, and experiencing at the time of the crime itself. In this way it would be possible to address what he "knew" or "appreciated" pursuant to the New York State insanity test. Call this the "right from wrong" question. The second strategy, returning to the neurological issues, would be to look for evidence of brain impairment not only in the test data and within the crime itself, but also in the larger context of the defendant's life. If he had sustained brain damage sufficient to produce murder as a symptom, then surely there would be other, less dramatic evidence of impairment. Homicide alone would be insufficient evidence of behavioral impairment in the presence of real brain damage of the magnitude alluded to by the defense. Call this the "ecological validity" question. The final strategy was to explore the scientific status of key elements of the neuroscientific evidence, in particular the PET scans and the SCR experiments, with an eye toward challenging their admissibility at trial. Call this the "admissibility" question. I discuss each of these questions and how they were pursued in the course of my consultation. . . .

Addressing the Strategic Questions.   First, I went to the library. I obtained all the literature I could find on arachnoid cysts, galvanic skin response, and PET, particularly as they had to do with violence, aggression, or crime. This I shared with the District Attorney, as well as giving him some of my own relevant publications. I also recommended that the DA find a top expert in PET and neuroimaging, a forensic neurologist, and a forensic psychiatrist. He retained two of the three.

He retained the services of Jonathan Brodie, MD, a professor of psychiatry and the director of the NYU/Brookhaven National Laboratory PET program. Dr. Brodie testified at the Frye hearing about the current state of the art in PET research. The DA also retained Alan Tuckman, MD, a forensic psychiatrist in private practice, who evaluated the defendant and prepared a report on the insanity issue. Dr. Tuckman concluded that at the time of the crime, the defendant:

> . . . certainly was fully aware of his actions and knew and appreciated the nature and consequences of his behavior. . . . There is no evidence at all that [Weinstein] acted without conscious and purposeful intent. All of the neurologic tests and psychological testing lend no basis at all to conclude that there existed an organic cause for this behavior.

The "Right from Wrong" Question: Evaluation of the Defendant.   In the course of my evaluation, I had two opportunities to interview the defendant, Mr. [Herbert Weinstein], for a total of seven hours. His attorney, Mr. Diarmuid White, was present throughout both interviews. I met with them on January 24, 1992[,] for three hours, and again on March 9, 1992[,] for four hours. My request to videotape the examinations was declined by the defendant. During the course of these examinations, I administered the clinical interview for Hare's Psychopathy Checklist Revised, and a small number of neuropsychological tests that he had not been given previously.

I also developed two separate case-specific structured interview protocols that I used to organize my questions and notes.

Interviewing of the defendant showed what I believed to be clear evidence that he knew what he was doing at the time he killed his wife, and that he was aware that it was wrong. In my report, I detailed his verbatim responses to questions about his actions, thoughts, and feelings during each stage of the crime: the fight and strangulation; while staging the crime scene and destroying evidence; while throwing her body out of the window; while staging what he described as a "charade" by going to the neighbors on the pretense of "looking for" his wife; while attempting to fool the police; and even during his ultimate confession. At each of these points, I could find no evidence that he did not know or appreciate what he was doing or that it was wrong. His statements all pointed in quite the opposite direction.

The "Ecological Validity" Question: Analysis of Data Sources.   I explained to the DA that I would need a number of things to address this issue. Before examining the defendant, I asked for access to all of the evidence discovered in the case, from the crime scene photographs to the SCR tracings, including all the raw data from each of the doctors who had examined the defendant. It is my practice to request access to all of the available evidence in each of my cases, because I have found that a careful review of as much data as possible always bears fruit in terms of supporting or refuting the claims being made.

Often, data from these "secondary" sources of information are more reliable than those obtained from "primary" sources, such as the defendant, who may or may not be a truthful or reliable informant, for various reasons. Also, the secondary data sources help me to gain a clearer idea of the reality of the crime itself, what was happening in the lives of the principles during and around the time of the crime, and how the defendant was behaving before, during, and after the offense.

. . . I thought I needed to find an objective way to probe his everyday behavior over time in the real world, to look for any evidence of behavioral impairment, evidence that would not be colored by his report or that of his friends and family. Therefore, I asked the DA to petition the court for access to the defendant's personal writings, journals, datebooks, calendars, checkbook records, and financial records for the past several years.

This request was granted by the court, with the proviso that the raw material not be shared directly with the District Attorney. The requested materials were provided directly by the defendant's attorney, including: (1) date books, schedules, and personal itineraries for the period from January 1, 1989 through December 31, 1991 and (2) personal financial records for the period from November 1, 1988 through July 15, 1991.

Mr. [Weinstein's] insanity defense was based on an arachnoid cyst that he claimed was affecting the normal functioning of the left side of his brain. His defense team claimed that his cyst had been growing, thus suggesting a progressive disease process. If this were true, then there should have been evidence of either behavioral impairment or changes in his behavior over time. Specifically, given the location of his cyst, the expected impairments or changes would be reflected in (1) the organization, planning, and control of his behavior, and in (2) memory and language functioning.

To assess potential changes in his behavior in these areas, I reviewed materials that he had kept regularly for a three-year period before and surrounding the time of the offense. These records provided some of the best documentation possible with which to (1) evaluate his level of everyday functioning in these areas and (2) document any significant change or deviation in his behavior patterns over time that might have occurred because of any progressive deterioration or change in his brain status.

This analysis showed no evidence of impairment or change in his management of his everyday affairs, as described in detail on pages 51 and 52 of my report. However, these records did show substantial gambling losses at Atlantic City casinos—which supported a possible diagnosis of pathological gambling. They also showed appointments with the Hemlock Society, a group devoted to suicide, in the weeks before his wife's murder. I thought this was significant in light of the fact that he had staged the crime scene to look like his wife had committed suicide. These findings began to suggest a possible motive for the crime other than an uncontrollable organic rage attack, as well as providing evidence that some degree of forethought or planning may have been involved.

NOTES AND QUESTIONS

1. Brain scanning at the time of the *Weinstein* case was not an inexpensive proposition, and today it remains relatively costly. The scan itself costs between $1,000 and $3,000. But significant additional costs are typically incurred for professional interpretation of the results and expert presentation at trial. For a more detailed discussion of current legal uses of PET and SPECT, see Susan E. Rushing, Daniel E. Pryma & Daniel D. Langleben, *PET and SPECT*, in *Neuroimaging in Forensic Psychiatry: From the Clinic to the Courtroom* 3-26 (Joseph R. Simpson ed., 2012). At what price would the cost of neuroimaging cease to be prohibitive in criminal cases? If it came to be widely used by wealthy defendants, how would you respond to arguments about disadvantages to poor defendants?

2. How should the legal system assess the merits of different neuroimaging techniques? Dr. Abass Alavi, whose brain scans of Herbert Weinstein appeared earlier in the chapter and who testified in the case, offers this perspective on the value of functional imaging:

> While structural imaging with either CT or MRI has been of great value for specialties in medicine such as surgery and radiation therapy, the impact of molecular imaging with either SPECT or PET has been much wider in scope. By now, it has become evident that most diseases and disorders are initiated at the molecular level and may or may not eventually translate to structural abnormalities. Thus, relying on structural imaging alone may prevent accurate detection, and therefore, allow for early interventions for many serious disorders such as cancer and cardiovascular diseases. But structural imaging techniques are quite insensitive for demonstrating the efficacy of most drugs soon after they are initiated, and as such, are inadequate for guiding the clinicians about their decision about adopting alternate therapies. In contrast, molecular imaging techniques allow detecting failure early on, and therefore, allow shifting to other drugs. Finally, structural imaging techniques are non-specific and cannot differentiate between active and inactive processes.
>
> Molecular imaging, particularly with PET, has overcome many of these deficiencies and truly has had a major impact in patient care over the past three decades.

There is a great deal of debate among physicians about the role of PET in the court. Some colleagues believe that there is no role for this type of imaging in the legal system and heavily defended their position in the past. In the other extreme, there are colleagues who have heavily emphasized the importance of PET for various purposes in the court system. Unfortunately, both groups that have taken extreme positions have hampered optimal use of this technology over the past two decades. I strongly believe that there is a compromise between the two groups and future court decisions will be substantially influenced by optimal utilization of this technique. I believe that any modality that has clinical applications should be of value in the legal system. In other words, those who are suffering from serious consequences of either inherited or acquired brain disorders and are unable to function in a normal manner in society should benefit from use of these technologies for civilized treatment in the modern societies. Therefore someone who commits a crime due to his/her uncontrolled behavior as validated by imaging techniques would not be subjected to the same type of punishments set aside for individuals who intentionally and viciously hurt and affect other people's lives.

Personal communication with authors.

3. Did Weinstein have a "hidden drive" because of his cyst? Neuroscientist David Eagleman has written that "[w]hen your biology changes, so can your decision-making and your desires. . . . Although acting on such drives is popularly thought to be a free choice, the most cursory examination of the evidence demonstrates the limits of that assumption. . . . Hidden drives and desires can lurk undetected behind the neural machinery of socialization." David Eagleman, *The Brain on Trial*, Atlantic, July-Aug. 2011, at 112, 114.

4. Dr. Jonathan Brodie, who testified for the prosecution, commented that in the *Weinstein* case: "The guy has a cyst, the PET was abnormal, [but] that has nothing to do with the fact he threw his wife out the window." Is this conclusion, as stated, fair? What evidence would be necessary to support it? And to what extent does this highlight important reflection on who bears the burden of proof?

5. On the subject of satisfying burdens of proof, consider this reflection of Dr. Richard Restak, a neurologist and a guest editor of a special volume on the *Weinstein* case:

[N]europsychiatric determinations in the courtroom are fraught with social, moral, and even political considerations. Some would argue that the presence of a neurological lesion in relevant areas, principally the frontal lobes and its immediate connections, is sufficient to establish mitigation. To do so, however, three questions would need to be answered in the affirmative. If brain damage exists, does it produce a deficit in the individual's ability to conform his or her behavior to the demands of the law? Secondly, is the resulting deficit a contributing cause of the defendant's actions? Finally, and most importantly, can a persuasive argument be made that absent the defect produced by the brain lesion, the criminal action would never have taken place? This final criteria is especially difficult to meet because the more complex and symbolically meaningful behaviors and emotions, especially love, hate, and aggression, among others, are mediated by many brain areas and a plethora of neurotransmitter interactions. And, of course, disturbances in these aspects of the personality are always multidetermined because of social, political, and other environmental factors. Most importantly, no necessary correlation has ever been established between a brain abnormality, however reliably demonstrated, and the carrying out of murder or other violent actions.

Another source of difficulty stems from the differences between what lawyers and judges accept as proof as compared with the more empirical approaches of the neuropsychiatrist. The former have little tolerance for speculation, whereas neuropsychiatrists perform their best service by setting up hypotheses and testing them out. Certainly the neuropsychiatric literature is filled with terms such as "could represent," "possible mechanisms," "it is conceivable," "the possibility is strong," "it raises intriguing possibilities," and "these findings may reflect." (All of these phrases were excerpted from a single paper selected at random from a peer-reviewed journal of neuropsychiatry). The courtroom, however, demands as a threshold determination that the proposed explanation be at least "more likely than not." In most instances, a neuropsychiatrist will be asked to conform his or her opinion to an even more stringent criteria: Do you hold your opinion within a reasonable degree of medical certainty, i.e., do you think it more likely than not that absent the alleged brain disease this criminal act would not have occurred?

Richard M. Restak, *Brain Damage and Legal Responsibility*, 1 Seminars Clinical Neuropsychiatry 170, 171 (1996).

6. The differences that Dr. Restak notes above between legal standards of proof and scientific and medical standards of proof are important to note. One reason for the differing standards is that law must typically render an opinion, and thus if the scientific evidence is excluded from consideration it will rely on the other evidence on the record. Admissibility in the law's eye, then, is in part about a comparison between the value of the proffered evidence vis-à-vis the next-best alternative. Law professor Frederick Schauer makes the following point in the context of brain-based lie detection:

Compared to What? In law, as in science, a crucial question is, "compared to what?" And this question can usefully be applied to determining witness veracity in courts of law. Traditionally, the legal system has left the assessment of witness credibility and veracity to the scientifically-unaided determination of the trier of fact, but just what mechanisms do judges and juries use to make these determinations? We know that jurors often use characteristics other than the content of what a witness says to evaluate the truth of a witness's claim, including factors such as whether a witness looks up or down, fidgets, speaks slowly or quickly, and speaks with apparent confidence; and we know that such factors are at best highly unreliable and at worst random. . . .

We can now reframe our question. The question is not, or at least not only, whether fMRI-based lie detection is reliable enough in the abstract to be used in court. Rather, it is whether there are sound reasons to prohibit the use of evidence of witness veracity that is likely better, and is at least no worse, than the evidence of witness veracity that now dominates the litigation process. The choice is not between very good evidence of veracity and inferior fMRI evidence; it is between less good—bad, if you will—fMRI evidence and the even worse evidence that is not only permitted, but also forms the core of the common law trial process. And although it is sometimes a weak argument for a conclusion that something else is worse, if the something else is unlikely to change and the improvement is plausible, then the argument is not so weak after all.

Frederick Schauer, *Can Bad Science Be Good Evidence? Neuroscience, Lie Detection, and Beyond*, 95 Cornell L. Rev. 1191, 1213-14 (2010).

7. *Weinstein, redux.* On February 20, 2010, the American Association for the Advancement of Science (AAAS) presented *The Brain on Trial: Neuroscience Evidence in the Courtroom* during a half-day session within a four-day AAAS annual

meeting in San Diego, California. The demonstration involved a real judge, Judge Luis A. Rodriguez, from the Orange County Superior Court, hearing arguments regarding MRI evidence. The cast of characters—actual neurologists and lawyers—provided testimony regarding the admissibility of an MRI scan. In a fact pattern similar to the *Weinstein* case, the defendant in the mock trial, a fictitious Mr. Johnson, was accused of killing his ex-girlfriend with a frying pan following an argument. The evidence presented to the jury (composed of all the audience members, attendees of the annual meeting) was that witnesses saw the defendant enter the victim's apartment and heard their arguing, that the defendant's DNA was found on the victim's fingertips, and that the defendant's fingerprints were found on the frying pan. At issue was an MRI scan of the defendant that showed a large lesion in his frontal lobe area. The judge heard admissibility arguments outside the presence of the jurors. The defense submitted the MRI scan to support their argument that the defendant was not capable of the premeditation and intent necessary for first-degree murder. The defense attorney argued the evidence of frontal lobe damage presented in the MRI scan, in conjunction with past studies of people exhibiting criminal behavior after frontal lobe damage, could cast reasonable doubt on the defendant's ability to form the requisite intent and premeditation required for first-degree murder. The prosecution argued that while the defendant had an abnormality in the frontal lobe area, many non-criminals could have the equivalent abnormality. Behavioral evidence of the defendant, such as defendant's difficulty forming intent in other aspects of his life—like getting dressed, taking care of himself, and so forth—was not offered in conjunction with the scan. Therefore, the prosecution concluded, the MRI did not provide statistically relevant evidence and would only confuse the jury. The judge decided to admit the evidence and allow the jury to decide on its weight and applicability. After hearing neurologists give testimony from both sides regarding the MRI scan, the jury found the defendant guilty of second-degree murder, but not first-degree murder.

8. At the crux of Judge Carruthers' challenge in *Weinstein* was the question of how to appropriately recognize that, even if most experts evaluating Weinstein would not integrate brain imaging into their assessment, this particular expert did. In the decades since *Weinstein*, how frequently do forensic psychiatrists rely on brain imaging in formulating their opinions on legal issues such as insanity? Forensic psychiatrist Manish A. Fozdar observes:

> How far have we come since *People v. Weinstein* with the use of brain imaging (structural and functional) evidence to palpate the heartbeat of the trial: namely, whether the defendant knew right from wrong or was capable of conforming his actions according to the requirements of the law? The answer, unfortunately, is not very far. Whereas neuroimaging research has been central in revealing the deep-seated mysteries of the brain, these revelations have not shed much light on the areas of free will, morality, and behavioral responses to environmental stimuli. The activation of a brain region on functional imaging such as the PET scan does not mean that the activated brain region correlates with a specific behavior. A single area of the brain may be two or three different areas working simultaneously. In fact, one of the fascinating findings of modern neuroscience research has been the discovery that the brain is an organ that is operational through parallel circuitry in different regions and that these circuits are interconnected. . . .

Neuroscience can contribute greatly to the forensic practice. Neuroscientists and clinicians should take a visible role in informing the legal community and the public of newly gained insights into brain functioning. They must speak out loudly against the misuse of neuroscience in the courtroom. Neuroscientific evidence alone should not be offered to assert the inability to form the requisite intent to commit the crime.

Manish A. Fozdar, *The Relevance of Modern Neuroscience to Forensic Psychiatry Practice*, 44 J. Am. Acad. Psychiatry & L. 145, 147, 150 (2016).

9. *Weinstein* was decided in 1992. Decades later, what is the state of neuroscience research on the murdering brain? In short, the underlying neurobiology of violence generally, and murder in particular, remains unclear. *See* Brigitte Vallabhajosula, *Murder in the Courtroom: The Cognitive Neuroscience of Violence* (2015). Neuroscientist Adrian Raine, who has scanned brains of murderers and compared them to brains of matched normal controls, has argued that "the most important neurobiological process that underlies so many different forms of antisocial, aggressive, violent, conduct-disordered, and psychopathic criminal behaviors . . . is functional impairment to the neural circuit underlying morality." Adrian Raine, *The Neuromoral Theory of Antisocial, Violent, and Psychopathic Behavior*, 277 Psychiatry Research 64, 64 (2019). At the same time, Raine recognizes that "grand theories of criminal behavior which claim for one predominating cause must be humbled by the empirical reality that offending is a complex jigsaw puzzle made up of many different causal pieces that do not fit neatly together. The neuromoral theory is but one piece, consisting at best of a limited number of inter-related neural elements in a much larger cortical and subcortical space." *Id.* at 68.

C. NEUROSCIENCE AND LEGAL EXCUSE

Weinstein is notable because of the novel scientific information allowed into evidence. But whether it marks the dawn of the age of scanning evidence in courtrooms remains to be seen. As you will see throughout this coursebook, just because a particular type of evidence is advanced, accepted, and clinically useful, it does not necessarily follow that it is legally relevant. In this section the authors consider the question of relevance in the criminal context.

Zachary Weiss
The Legal Admissibility of Positron Emission Tomography Scans in Criminal Cases: People v. Spyder Cystkopf
1 Seminars Clinical Neuropsychiatry 202, 202-10 (1996)

I can truthfully say that until five years ago I had no special interest in the subject of the admissibility of positron emission tomographic (PET) scans in criminal cases. The sole reason I can claim any acquaintance with the subject (and my knowledge, like that of most lawyers who find themselves thrust into areas beyond their technical competence, is not very wide and less than an inch deep) is that one day I had the misfortune to "pick up" a murder case called *People v.* [*Weinstein*]. . . .

In September of 1992, I was given a series of medical and psychiatric reports. In toto, they concluded that [Weinstein] had an arachnoid cyst on his left temporal lobe that was exerting a mass effect on his left frontal lobe. This mass effect was leading to "hypometabolism" in [Weinstein's] left frontal lobe. This in turn made him unable to determine the difference between right and wrong at the time he strangled his wife.

The "hypometabolism" in his frontal lobe was supposedly shown by a functional brain imaging device known as a positron emission tomograph or PET scan. With the report describing the results of this PET scan were a series of images. These pictures were cross-sectional views of the [Weinstein] brain. I was quite struck by the beauty of these pictures—seas of blue and gray punctuated by islands of red, yellow, and white.

As I looked at these pictures, I had a premonition about the future of criminal insanity cases. No longer would experts wrangle over whether a defendant satisfied the diagnostic criteria for a mental illness. Social models of mental illness would be replaced by biological ones. In place of learned swearing contests, there would be pretty pictures. These pictures would be tangible and presumptive proof of a mental disease or defect. Indeed, if mental illness can be reduced to biology, I mused, traditional legal tests of insanity, using philosophical notions of free will and moral knowledge to assess blameworthiness, would fall by the wayside as well.

These musings quickly gave way to paranoia. The last thing I wanted was to have a defense attorney flashing pictures of [Weinstein's] brain in front of an impressionable injury. Some people, of course, did not share my fear. My immediate supervisor at the time, a very canny trial lawyer, had a dartboard in his office. On hearing about [Weinstein's] defense, he picked up a dart and flicked it at the dartboard— announcing as he did so that this was a rich man's defense. He opined that a New York jury would find it ridiculous, and threw me out of his office. Ultimately, my supervisor was proved a prophet when [Weinstein] pled guilty to manslaughter in large measure, his attorney informed me, because he no longer had the money to mount a psychiatric defense.

Nonetheless, I filed a motion for a *Frye* hearing. My argument was that it was not yet "generally accepted" in the neuroscientific community that these pretty pictures were accurate and reliable depictions of cerebral metabolism or that the "hypometabolism" in the frontal lobes caused or was associated with frontal lobe dysfunction. The judge granted the motion, and a hearing was held. . . .

I discovered during the hearing that PET scanners are not of uniform design, and that the rate constants plugged into the Sokoloff equation are not the same from laboratory to laboratory. Remarkably, all of the experts seemed to think this did not matter. However, in a number of other areas, I was given pause.

. . . [E]ven if you can take an "accurate picture" of brain metabolism, one is left with the question of the relationship between the "picture" and the human behavior the "picture" purports to explain.

If one thing was established in the hearing, it was that at the time there was not a single existing experimental study showing a convincing relationship between low metabolic values in the frontal lobe and frontal lobe dysfunction, which would lead to an inability to control one's impulses or appreciate the difference between "right and wrong." Every expert who testified admitted as much. From a PET standpoint, nothing is really known about the metabolic substrates of violence in the human brain.

Nonetheless, after the hearing, Justice Carruthers wrote an opinion permitting the defendant's psychiatric expert to testify about his reliance on this evidence. . . . Justice Carruthers's opinion is, I believe, not well reasoned. The evidentiary rule he construed in [Weinstein] is found in many states. Its purpose, I submit, was not to permit an expert to base his opinion on unreliable and invalid scientific evidence but to allow experts to outline their reasoning to juries. It is a procedural rule, not a substantive one.

The upshot of the opinion in *People v.* [*Weinstein*] is to give PET scan evidence a safe harbor as long as it is part of the evidence a psychiatric expert relies on in reaching his or her opinion. I find it difficult to believe that the New York legislature or the drafters of the Model Penal Code intended to displace evidentiary doctrines designed to assure the reception of valid and reliable scientific evidence in insanity cases, while leaving them intact in all other cases. Certainly, the concerns that are reflected in these rules are just as pressing in insanity cases. There seems no principled reason to accord them special treatment. . . .

In my opinion, there is no question that this use of a PET scan — to prove criminal insanity or some sort of diminished capacity by associating blobs with brain regions — is one that will at this point not even come close to satisfying either the *Frye* rule or the flexible *Daubert* inquiry.*

The fact that the courtroom door should be barred to this sort of crude associationism, of course, does not mean that courts will do so. If I were forced to hazard a prediction, I think the age of scanning has dawned in our courtrooms. This is not a technological genie we are going to be able to put back in the bottle. It will be the rare judge in a murder case who will limit a defendant's use of this kind of evidence, no matter how unreliable. It will be the rare prosecutor, for reasons I outlined earlier, who will want to move to limit this evidence. Defense lawyers with visions of acquittal swimming in their head are unlikely to exercise any principled restraint.

Stephen J. Morse
Brain and Blame
84 Geo. L.J. 527, 531-47 (1996)

The "fundamental psycholegal error" is the mistaken belief that if science or common sense identifies a cause for human action, including mental or physical disorders, then the conduct is necessarily excused. But causation is neither an excuse per se nor the equivalent of compulsion, which is an excusing condition. . . .

All phenomena of the universe are presumably caused by the necessary and sufficient conditions that produce them. If causation were an excuse, no one would be responsible for any conduct, and society would not be concerned with moral and legal responsibility and excuse. . . .

[Weinstein] was not raising a "standard" insanity defense, because he lacked a diagnosis of major mental disorder and grossly psychotic symptoms. Both are usually

---

* [These two rules are discussed in Chapter 8. — EDS.]

practically required to support an insanity defense, and the law sometimes requires the presence of severe mental disorder to raise the defense. Nevertheless, I believe that [Weinstein] raised a colorable insanity claim. No diagnosis or symptoms necessarily entail that the agent is not legally responsible, as the American Psychiatric Association's official diagnostic manual admits. The genuine basis for the excuse is nonculpable irrationality. [Weinstein] should be excused if he can demonstrate that the tumor (or anything else) rendered him nonculpably irrational when he killed his wife, even if his mental state does not fit traditional definitions of major mental disorder. . . .

The impressive theorizing and extensive medical and psychological findings about [Weinstein] are unlikely to provide precise data concerning the level of his impairment in the capacity for rational conduct. There is no quantitative scale with which to compare him to normal or abnormal populations. All we know is that there is some defect of indeterminate real-world effect. Although the uncharacteristic homicidal behavior was not inconsistent with the defect, we cannot even be sure that the defect played a causal role in the conduct. Opinions that it did or that it did not are both speculations, not confirmed scientific or clinical fact. Opinions based on the theory and findings that [Weinstein] did or did not appreciate the wrongfulness of his conduct, or that it was or was not impossible for him to do so, are similarly speculative, not fact. Indeed, these are moral and legal conclusions, rather than clinical or scientific opinions.

. . . [Herbert Weinstein's] capacity for rational conduct on the day he killed his wife is the crucial issue. It is relevant but not dispositive that he had an abnormality that may have affected this capacity. Medical and psychological evidence may help us decide if his capacity was affected, but it is not very precise evidence about incapacity, and it is surely not dispositive of the legal issue. . . .

NOTES AND QUESTIONS

1. For a book-length investigation of the *Weinstein* case, with many new details and insights, see Kevin Davis, *The Brain Defense: Murder in Manhattan and the Dawn of Neuroscience in America's Courtrooms* (2017). Davis observes:

   Neuroscience alone cannot absolve someone of committing murder—or any crime—or pinpoint the cause of a single act or demonstrate that someone is legally insane. But accepting that our behavior can be influenced by brain injuries, disease, genetics, and other abnormalities does have a place in our legal system, and neuroscience is an important adjunct that can be used responsibly to support it. The ancient Greek ideal of a justice systems that holds people accountable for their actions, yet also strives to understand the mind of the offender, is a worthy model from which to build. Modern science empowers us to evaluate criminal defendants more fully and compassionately, which is not incompatible with holding them responsible or protecting society from those who can do harm.

   On what points do you agree or disagree, and why?
2. Ms. Joni West, daughter of Mr. Weinstein, is currently writing a book about her father's case. The book will provide personal observations of her father, and provide potentially relevant details that have been overlooked, such as a prior history of amnesia and other neurological problems that required several

weeks of hospitalization when he was in his twenties. The book will also contest some of the bases for expert opinions about him, including whether he had a gambling problem, whether he stood to gain financially from his wife's death, and the reasons for contacting the Hemlock Society. In the meantime, Ms. West has observed: "To the neuroscientists, you ARE your brain while to lawyers and psychiatrists, you are your mental states." (E-mail to Owen Jones, February 22, 2017.) How would you describe the implications — as well as similarities and dissimilarities — between these two perspectives? To what extent might this explain or predict miscommunication between the fields, and with what prospects for reconciliation?

3. Weiss suggests that perhaps images should be inadmissible because they can be unfairly prejudicial. Assess that line of reasoning both generally and in light of Federal Rule of Evidence 403, which states that "[t]he court may exclude relevant evidence if its probative value is substantially outweighed by a danger of one or more of the following: unfair prejudice, confusing the issues, misleading the jury, undue delay, wasting time, or needlessly presenting cumulative evidence."

4. The *Weinstein* case is exceptional because it was one of the first to make such central use of neuroimaging in a criminal defense. But might the exceptional become the routine in future cases of this nature? Psychiatrist Joseph Simpson wrote in 2012 that "the field of forensic psychiatry is approaching a crossroads. As neuroimaging becomes more reliable, standardized and informative, attempts to use its results in civil and criminal proceedings of all types will increase dramatically." *Neuroimaging in Forensic Psychiatry: From the Clinic to the Courtroom* xv-xvi (Joseph R. Simpson ed., 2012). On the basis of what you know so far, what do you see as the most likely future for neuroimaging as a tool in the criminal justice system?

5. Scientists and lawyers may have differing perspectives on cases such as *Weinstein*. Dr. Richard Restak concludes: "It seems appropriate to give the legal experts the final words . . . because, whatever the merits of neuropsychiatry in the clinic, its relevance in the courtroom remains a legal and not a medical determination." Do you agree with this characterization, and if so, are you comfortable with it — why or why not?

6. If one stipulates that particular damage to the frontal lobes impairs moral reasoning in the way the defense in *Weinstein* suggests, should it matter how the individual came to have the damage? For instance, consider the case of the brain at high altitudes. Research has shown that mountain climbers can experience permanent brain injury when ascending peaks as low as 15,780 feet. *See* Nicolás Fayed et al., *Evidence of Brain Damage After High-Altitude Climbing by Means of Magnetic Resonance Imaging*, 119 Am. J. Med. 168.e1 (2006). These injuries are thought to be a result of hypoxia (low blood-oxygen level), although a vascular component of high-altitude sickness may also be responsible. Climbers in the Fayed et al. study experienced transient memory loss and other cognitive deficits. Suppose a mountain climber throws his climbing buddy off the mountain. Could he successfully claim that, due to his altitude-induced brain damage, he lacked the requisite *mens rea*? What if he had an MRI that displayed frontal lobe lesions? What if he was a professional mountain climber with no visible lesions? In addition, pilots have historically experienced altitude

sickness in unpressurized cabin situations or while riding hot-air balloons at high altitudes. Pilot behavior at unpressurized altitudes of 16,000 feet has been compared to intoxication, with people experiencing euphoria and disorientation. If a pilot was found guilty of sexually harassing his co-pilot, but could show the plane had improper pressurization, would a defense of temporary insanity strike you as colorable?

7. What if Mr. Weinstein had learned of his tumor three years earlier, was told that this could very well impair his impulse control, had been offered treatment to remove the cyst, but refused the procedure? Should this affect how the law treats him? Should the law impose an affirmative duty on those who know of such brain abnormalities to take precautions that prevent their brain disorders from leading to violence? For instance, if they're available and proven to be effective and safe, should an individual be required to take drugs? What if they are effective but safety risks are not minimal?

8. Law professor Jane Campbell Moriarty observes that: "Neuroscience may help improve opinions about blameworthiness by providing more science-based support for diagnoses, as happened with the nurses discussed at the beginning of this Article. And neuroscience may also encourage the judicial system to reject the stereotypes and myths that have shaped our current insanity defense doctrines and embrace a more humane way of dealing with the mentally ill and brain-injured criminal defendants." Jane Campbell Moriarty, *Seeing Voices: Potential Neuroscience Contributions to a Reconstruction of Legal Insanity*, 85 Fordham L. Rev. 599, 618 (2016). What might neuroscience offer to a reconsideration of the insanity defense such as the one Weinstein offered, and what further neuroscience research would be required?

9. Should brain surgery ever be a consideration, or a requirement, for parole? Dr. Shelley Batts speculates that:

> [N]euroimaging evidence might provide insight for parole hearings, especially if a tumor or lesion that had been argued to be affecting behavior had been surgically removed. If the behavior had been judged to be improved, the chance of reoffending might be low. This observation is reflected in the case of a 40 year old man who experienced sudden and uncontrollable pedophilia which was later thought to be caused by an egg-sized tumor in the orbitofrontal cortex. After the tumor was successfully removed, the urges disappeared and he successfully completed a therapy program. When the tumor began to re-grow, the behavior once again returned, and when the tumor was again removed, so did the urges. Consistent with other reports of prefrontal damage, the man knew that the urges and behavior was morally wrong, yet he was still unable to stop himself. This leads to another question: Should people who are biologically unable to control their behavior, or predisposed to anti-social behavior, be released from custody if the behavior can return as a result of the disorder? . . . Neurological follow-up visits could become mandatory for offenders who suffered from a lesion that could recur.

Shelley Batts, *Brain Lesions and Their Implications in Criminal Responsibility*, 27 Behav. Sci. L. 261, 270 (2009).

10. Is there a compromise to be struck between prosecution and defense arguments in cases like *Weinstein*? Should the law have a "semi-voluntary" category? What would the effects of such a category be? Consider this argument:

[T]he voluntary act requirement should be simplified and consist of three parts: (1) voluntary acts, (2) involuntary acts, and (3) semi-voluntary acts. Semi-voluntary acts would incorporate cases that have previously been shoehorned into the first two categories. The result of integrating increasing knowledge about the unconscious into the criminal law will mean that individuals will be held both more and less responsible than the conventional understanding. . . .

A key issue [is] whether Weinstein's behavior could constitute a threat to the safety or welfare of the community. While most arachnoid cysts are congenital—suggesting that Weinstein had the cyst since birth—they "are not usually considered to be lesions that promote abnormal aggression." Rather, large cysts, like Weinstein's, are associated with a range of relatively benign complaints, such as headaches, dizziness, or mental impairments; some people have no symptoms whatsoever. Until Weinstein killed his wife, he showed no overt symptoms linked to the cyst, apart from a period at age 22 when he had two months of headaches with an unexplained cause. He also has not committed additional acts of violence while serving his prison sentence. Alternatively, some evidence indicates that Weinstein could be a danger. Weinstein's cyst expanded during his adult life, suggesting it may be a factor in later life problems. While in prison, he may not confront the kinds of "novel and threatening" environments that apparently contributed to his violence toward his wife. How would Weinstein act upon release when he is in a less controlled environment? . . .

Weinstein's background of neurological disorders and compulsive gambling indicates that he could be dangerous in the future, despite his age and history of nonviolence. . . . For example, Norman Relkin, a behavioral neurologist who conducted a range of tests on Weinstein, contended that Weinstein's "volitional freedom was compromised by the cyst," in ways that affected his conscious awareness and ability to "know" what he was doing. As Relkin explained, "an important step in the process of 'knowing' is disturbed in such patients, relating to the perception of 'gut feelings' and their integration with other components of conscious experience." This assertion does not suggest complete involuntariness on Weinstein's part; nor does it necessarily indicate insanity. [Denno thus suggests a "semi-voluntary category" as "a compromise between the two, relying on the new consciousness research."]

Deborah W. Denno, *Crime and Consciousness: Science and Involuntary Acts*, 87 Minn. L. Rev. 269, 274, 380-81 (2002).

FURTHER READING

Further Proceedings in the *Weinstein* Case:

Weinstein v. Dennison, 801 N.Y.S.2d 244 (N.Y. Sup. Ct. 2005).

Additional Commentary on the *Weinstein* Case:

Kevin Davis, *The Brain Defense: Murder in Manhattan and the Dawn of Neuroscience in America's Courtrooms* (2017).

J. Rojas-Burke, *PET Scans Advance as Tools in Insanity Defense*, 34 J. Nuclear Med. 13N (1993).

Helen S. Mayberg, *Medical-Legal Inferences from Functional Neuroimaging Evidence*, 1 Seminars Clinical Neuropsychiatry 195 (1996).

Robert E. Dauer, *Evidentiary Admissibility of Evidence of Neurodiagnostic Testing Showing Frontal Brain Lesion as a Defense in a Criminal Homicide Trial*, 1 Seminars Clinical Neuropsychiatry 211 (1996).

Richard M. Restak, *Brain Damage and Legal Responsibility*, 1 Seminars Clinical Neuropsychiatry 170 (1996).

Deborah W. Denno, *Crime and Consciousness: Science and Involuntary Acts*, 87 Minn. L. Rev. 269 (2002).

Jennifer Kulynych, *Psychiatric Neuroimaging Evidence: A High-Tech Crystal Ball?*, 49 Stan. L. Rev. 1249 (1997).

PART 2

FUNDAMENTALS OF COGNITIVE NEUROSCIENCE

At this point, you should be developing a sense of the kinds of issues that can arise at the law and neuroscience intersection, the contexts in which they arise, why those issues arise, and how they can play out.

Before exploring those issues further, Part 2 provides the basic background and essential tools you need to understand the fundamental biology and technology of brain sciences. This will not be as intimidating as you might think. Our goal as authors is not for readers to become entry-level neuroscientists, which would be entirely unrealistic (and also entirely unnecessary). Our goal is to help readers to develop informed ways of understanding and thinking about the intersections of law and neuroscience. For aspiring attorneys, for example, this should provide the same basic, starting familiarity as one gets in other law school courses, upon which further experience in practice later builds.

For these reasons, Part 2 provides a tour, from the ground floor up, of how the brain is built and how it operates, as well as the techniques we use to study and treat it. Moreover, in one of this book's most important chapters, we detail the limitations of neuroscience and cognitive neuroscience methods that should temper overzealous interpretations of evidence — by oneself or opposing counsel.

PART SUMMARY

This Part:
- Surveys, in Chapter 3, basic information about the structure and function of the brain.
- Introduces, in Chapter 4, the technologies for monitoring and manipulating the human brain.
- Identifies, in Chapter 5, particular limits and cautions in interpreting brain imaging evidence. Those seeking further information on how to read and understand a brain imaging study will find a user-friendly example, with explanatory annotations, in the Appendix.

CHAPTER 3

Brain Structure and Brain Function

We saw that an exact knowledge of the structure of the brain was of supreme interest. . . . To know the brain, we said, is equivalent to ascertaining the material course of thought and will. . . .

—Santiago Ramon y Cajal[†]

Your brain is a network of neurons, bursting with electrical activity flowing through your synapses. Makes you think, doesn't it?

—Anonymous

CHAPTER SUMMARY

This chapter:

- Introduces the basic vocabulary needed to describe and explain the parts of the brain that are most salient in legal contexts.
- Introduces basic concepts of brain function.
- Introduces the types of cells in the nervous system and summarizes how neurons signal to each other.

INTRODUCTION

How do we maintain such exquisite control of the body in walking, talking, and riding bicycles? How do we feel disgust or dread, joy or pain? How do we think of theorems, compose music, or learn laws? Understanding brain structure and function can help us answer questions like these. Neuroscience research has accumulated many layers of detail and complexity. Don't panic. This chapter will survey only the basic fundamentals necessary to deal with the legal topics explored in this coursebook. These fundamentals will provide the foundation on which a lawyer can build a more specialized knowledge base to succeed in neurolaw. Even without a background in neuroscience, biology, or psychology, reading this chapter provides the foundation on which to understand and discuss the cases and reading material that

---

† Santiago Ramón y Cajal, *Recollections of My Life* 305 (E. Horne Craigie & Juan Cano trans., MIT Press 1989) (1937). Ramón y Cajal won the Nobel Prize in Physiology or Medicine in 1906 for his pioneering descriptions of the fine structure of the nervous system.

comprise the remainder of the coursebook. We will focus on basic terminology and concepts and avoid overwhelming detail. Those wishing to read more about particular brain structures should consult the resources listed at the end of this chapter.

Most students without a science background enter this course with some trepidation, worrying that they will be out of their depth. If you feel this way, you are in good company. You will be introduced to new terminology and basic facts about the brain. We assure you that you *can* learn what you need to know to be successful in navigating the intersection of law and neuroscience, to appreciate both the promise and the limitations of neuroscience in the legal arena, and to debate the ethical implications of scientific advances. You will finish knowing vastly more than the average lawyer about the relationship between the brain and behavior. You will also learn what questions to ask and what sources to consult when issues arise in your future practice.

To begin, you should recognize that you already know more about brain structure than you think you do. You already know that your brain is in your head, and, like your head, it has a top and bottom, a left and right, an inside and an outside. You already know that your brain has different parts. And you likely already appreciate that different parts of the brain have different functions.

You also probably know that your brain has two sides (called "hemispheres"), and that the two sides have different specialized functions. You probably already know (perhaps from TV commercials hawking mood-altering drugs) that your brain function depends on specific chemical processes. You may also know that your brain function also depends on electrical processes. And you probably know that brains are built from a very large number of cells called *neurons*.

Given all of this knowledge, we only need to fill in some details. This chapter will begin with a description of the *structure* of the human brain, starting with its large-scale structure followed by smaller scales of organization. This will be followed by a description of brain *function*. But as you begin examining the rather impersonal diagrams and photographs of a human brain,* keep in mind that the disembodied brain in the photograph once belonged to a living, breathing person who, like Hamlet's poor Yorick, was likely "a fellow of infinite jest, of most excellent fancy," who was distressed or amazed at the end. The organic dynamics of your brain enable your learning and locution as a student as well as the excitement or anxiousness you may be experiencing right now.

Just as when you began learning law, some things will seem familiar, and some will be foreign. And, again, as with law, some of what's foreign is written in Latin or Greek. The good news is that the meanings underlying the foreign-sounding terms are generally far less intimidating than they seem. Early anatomists named things according to how they looked — their location and shape, their color and texture — using descriptions just like you would use, such as "front," "big," "dark," and "dense." Later, other anatomists used arbitrary numbers or abbreviations to identify different areas of the brain, much like ZIP codes. With these naming schemes scientists began to sort out the many parts of the brain.

---

* Images of humans' and other species' brains are readily found on the Internet. To introduce the variety of brains in different species including human, we invite you to visit www.brainmuseum.org. An atlas of the human brain with many clearly diagrammed figures can be found at www.thehumanbrain.info.

You should also understand that the terminology of the nervous system has a history that makes some terms peculiar but resistant to change. Just as it can take a while to become acquainted with street names in a new city, brain terminology takes a little getting used to. But just as you can learn to navigate a new city quickly, with some exposure, instruction, and effort, the basic layout of the brain will rapidly become familiar. To aid in this process, new terms-of-art will be announced in *italics*, and every italicized word or term will be found in the glossary at the end of the book.

The chapter has several sections. Section A will introduce the terms used to describe location in the brain. Section B will describe the functional and anatomical subsystems of the brain. Section C will introduce the cells that comprise the brain, *neurons* and *glia*. Section D frames brain function in its evolutionary context. Section E will survey the organization of the human *cerebral cortex* (cerebral refers to brain and cortex refers to outer-covering like the bark of a tree) with basic explanations for the function of each lobe. The diverse functions of the brain structures buried beneath the cerebral cortex will then be summarized in Section F. Section G briefly overviews the function of blood supply to the brain. It is important to understand how critical the blood supply is for normal brain function and to understand what functional brain imaging measures. Lastly Section H explains in more detail how neurons signal to one another.

A. ORIENTATION AND LOCATION IN THE BRAIN

To be proficient in speaking about the human brain, one must be able to describe the region to which one is referring. Anatomists use special terms for describing spatial relations in the human brain. The necessity for these terms arises from the fact that our brains are three-dimensional objects that are often viewed from many different angles. To a neurosurgeon operating on an upright subject, down and to the left will mean something substantially different than it would to anyone viewing brain images taken from a body lying face up. Specialized terms exist to remove ambiguity in brain anatomy, just as "north" or "south" have a more permanent meaning than "left" or "right."

Geographers use two perpendicular axes — longitude (the north-south axis) and latitude (the east-west axis) — to describe locations on the surface of Earth. Anatomists use particular coordinate systems when referring to the human body and the brain. But unlike geography, these systems have three elements because we need to locate interior as well as surface features.

Specifically, we use three perpendicular axes to describe positions in the three dimensions of the brain. As shown in Figure 3.1, the three axes are (a) the *anterior-posterior*, (b) the *dorsal-ventral*, and (c) the *medial-lateral*.

The anterior-posterior axis runs from front to back. Two other terms are also used: *rostral* and *caudal*. Rostral refers to the nose, so it is synonymous with anterior. Caudal refers to the tail, so it is synonymous with posterior. Thus, the front of the head (the forehead) is the anterior (rostral) pole, and the rear of the head is the posterior (caudal) pole. The forehead is anterior (or rostral) to the ears, and the back of the head is posterior (or caudal) to the ears.

The dorsal-ventral axis runs from top to bottom. Two other terms are also used: *superior* and *inferior*. Thus, the top of the head is dorsal (superior) to the chin.

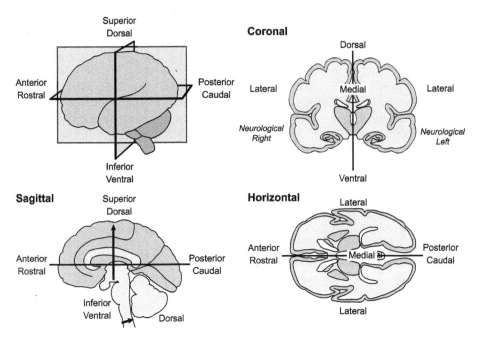

Figure 3.1   Orientation and position in the human brain.   The top-left panel illustrates the orientations of the major planes of each section and labels the terms for describing position in the front-to-back and the top-to-bottom axes. The bottom-left panel illustrates a simplified sagittal section through the center midline of the brain. The vertical line in the coronal section below indicates the location of this section. Location in the front-to-back and top-to-bottom axes is labeled. The orientation of the dorsal-ventral axis changes from approximately horizontal in the spinal cord to vertical in the brain. The top-right panel illustrates a simplified coronal section through the brain at the level indicated by the vertical arrow in the sagittal section above. Location in the top-to-bottom and left-right axes is labeled. Note that neurologists label left-right as if the brain section is in the patient facing you. The bottom-right panel illustrates a simplified horizontal section through the brain at the level indicated by the horizontal line in the sagittal section above. Location in the front-to-back and left-right axes is labeled.

The nose is ventral (inferior) to the eyes. The dorsal-ventral axis is also used to describe the bodies of other animals. For example, we refer to the dorsal fins of fish. Similarly, the top of a fish's head is dorsal to the bottom. As you know, the human head is rotated 90 degrees from the axis of the body because we stand up, so the top of the head points toward the sky while our back points toward the horizon. Nevertheless, the dorsal-ventral axis is applied to both the brain and the spinal cord.

The medial-lateral axis runs left to right, but it is referenced also to the natural symmetry of the human body. Medial refers to the middle, and lateral refers to the side. The ears are lateral to the nose. The nose is medial to the eyes.

The three axes define three perpendicular planes (Figure 3.1). The *coronal* plane is a slice through the brain, perpendicular to the anterior-posterior axis. Locations in the coronal plane are identified as dorsal-ventral (toward the top or bottom) and medial-lateral (toward the middle or side), as well as left-right.

Before going further, you need to know something important about "left" and "right." When you look at the coronal section in Figure 3.1, you would likely describe the left side of the brain as being on the left side of the image. But you must be aware that radiologists reverse this. For a radiologist the right side of the brain is on the left side of the image and vice versa. The reason for this is simple—radiologists prefer to see the image as it would appear in a patient who is facing them, or as if they are looking at them from the bottom. Knowing this convention is significant because when you look at coronal or horizontal sections in publications, you need to know whether the authors are using the radiological convention. In many current scientific brain-imaging studies the radiological convention is no longer used. And it can make all the difference in consequences for the brain whether some malformation or damage is on the left or right side.

The *sagittal* plane is a slice through the brain perpendicular to a medial-lateral line. Locations in the sagittal plane are identified as dorsal-ventral and anterior-posterior. The midsagittal plane is directly down the center, the most medial part of the brain.

The *horizontal* plane is a slice through the brain, perpendicular to the dorsal-ventral axis. Locations in the horizontal plane are identified as anterior-posterior (or rostral-caudal) and medial-lateral. As with the coronal plane, when you look at horizontal sections in publications, you need to know whether the authors are using the radiological convention.

We suggest that you mark these pages for reference when you encounter these terms in the chapters to come. If you really want to master this brain terminology, we advise you to practice drawing Figure 3.1 from memory with all of the labels. After a few attempts, they will become as familiar as *mens rea* or *pro se*.

B. SUBSYSTEMS OF THE NERVOUS SYSTEM

Although the brain is considered a single "organ" of the body, it consists of a stunningly complex and beautiful collection of structures and circuits that ultimately guide and control behavior through connections with the senses in ears and eyes, the muscles in limbs and heart, and the glands in brain and body. The brain has been compared to a computer because it has inputs and outputs, and it transforms and stores "information."* As you know, computers are built from diverse electrical components connected in complex circuits. An electrical circuit consists of the paths of wires connecting different components to one another to perform the designed function; if the wires become disconnected or happen to be connected in the wrong way, then the device will not work as designed or at all. Brain circuits consist of cells called *neurons* and *glia*. Unlike electrical devices in which wires are separate from the device components, neurons are both the processing units and the connections, while glia support the function of the neurons. The brain consists

---

* Metaphors are useful but should be recognized for what they are. The brain is not actually a computer. Scientists in each era of history analogize the brain to the most advanced technology of the time. Before the computer, the brain was analogized a hard-wired telephone exchange, and before that, to a hydraulic system. Today, researchers think about the brain as a Bayesian network.

of numerous complex circuits that work in concert to accomplish the various functions that keep you alive and make you who you are.

We now provide an overview of the major subsystems of the human brain. We will describe both functional (Figure 3.2) and anatomical (Figure 3.3) subdivisions. However, keep in mind that while subdividing is useful for exposition, the subsystems function in highly integrated ways. The brain enables us to perceive the world outside and within our body, to plan actions and to control our behavior. These functions require coordinated processes in the cerebral cortex, the thalamus, basal ganglia, cerebellum, brainstem (consisting of midbrain, pons, and medulla), and spinal cord.

The brain responds to sensory input from outside in the world and from inside the body. From the outside, the brain is sensitive to distant stimuli conveyed through light and sound. The brain is also sensitive to local stimuli that contact the body through taste and touch. From the inside, the brain is sensitive to inputs from sensors in the muscles, joints, and gut so that it responds to stimuli within the body such as stomach or bladder distension.

The brain has two major streams of output. The brain controls the heart, the gut, and various glands in the body; it is necessary for the basic functions of sustaining life. The brain also controls the various muscles that move the face, the limbs, and the rest of the body. It should be clear that our brains are embedded in the stream of events that we experience. Thus, the actions produced by the brain through the body will result in changes in our senses of the external and internal environments. For example, if you shift gaze from this page to another location in your environment, you will see something else. Similarly, if you run as fast as you can for a few minutes, the rates of your respiration and heartbeat will increase, and your sweat glands will help cool your body. Your brain senses if you are hungry or thirsty and motivates actions to satisfy those drives. Your brain senses if you are anxious, excited, or fearful. Your brain also senses if you are bored or tired and can control itself to sustain attention for at least another page or two. Your brain not only controls your body—it also controls itself.

Circuits in the *cerebral cortex* and associated structures analyze the signals conveyed by the sensory system. The brain generates body movements to respond to sensory stimulation, internal states, and goals through two major systems that neuroscientists refer to as the *motor system*. The first controls the muscles that move the limbs, the face, and the eyes. This system is typically under voluntary control and produces the range of activities we do like walking and talking, reading and writing.

The second controls internal organs like the glands, gut, and heart. This motor system is also referred to as the *autonomic* or visceral system and is further divided into *sympathetic* and *parasympathetic* subsystems. It is an oversimplification, but we can say that the sympathetic subsystem organizes fight-flight responses, and the parasympathetic subsystem organizes rest-and-digest maintenance. The sympathetic nervous system diverts blood flow from the gastrointestinal system to the skeletal muscles and lungs, increases heart rate, and dilates the pupils. In contrast, the parasympathetic nervous system diverts blood flow to the gastrointestinal tract and slows the heart rate.

How do all of these systems communicate with one another so effectively? The answer, in a word, is neurons. The centrality of the neuron—also known as a "nerve cell"—is why the field of brain science is called *neuro*science, and it's why we label the human communication network the "nervous system." The nervous system

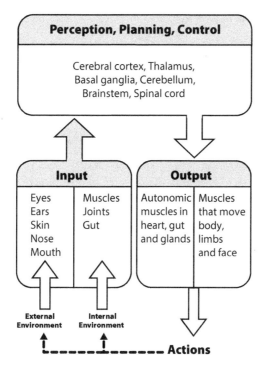

Figure 3.2   Functional subdivisions of human brain.   Details in Text.

refers to a system of nerve cells, communicating with one another to produce perception, emotion, thought, and action.

Neuroscientists divide the nervous system into two subsystems: the *central nervous system* (CNS), consisting of the brain and the spinal cord, and the *peripheral nervous system* (PNS), consisting of everything else—that is, the nerves that communicate with sensory receptors, muscles, internal body organs, and glands. The autonomic nervous system can be classified as part of the PNS. Not being protected by the skull or spinal column, the nerves in the PNS are more exposed to potential for injury, so they can regrow if crushed or cut. In contrast, nerves in the CNS will not regrow. This is why significant damage to the spinal cord or brain commonly results in permanent disabilities.

The CNS is so important to life that evolution has endowed it with extensive protection. That protection begins with the skull in which the brain rests. You already know that the skulls of different animals have different shapes; in all cases, form serves function. The spinal cord, likewise, is surrounded by the flexible column of spinal bones and muscle. Within the encasing bones of the skull and spine, the CNS is protected by another collection of structures called the *meninges*. The meninges are composed of three layers. The outer layer is the *dura mater*, a leather-like tissue inside the bone. The inner layer is the *pia mater*, a delicate film that seals the surface of the brain. The middle layer is the *arachnoid mater*, a web-like substance connecting pia mater to dura mater. While the meninges are essential for protecting the brain, they can also lead to brain damage; the cyst that developed in Weinstein's brain arose from excessive growth of the arachnoid mater.

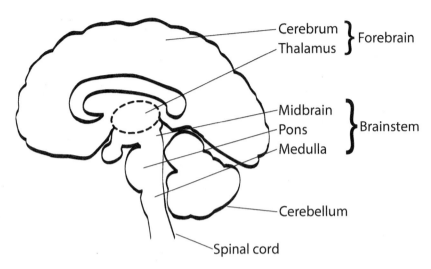

Figure 3.3   Structural subdivisions of the central nervous system.   Details in text.

The brain and spinal cord are bathed by and suspended in cerebrospinal fluid contained within the meninges. This fluid provides additional mechanical and metabolic support for the brain. However, because the human brain is floating in the skull, when the head moves violently, the brain can slosh against the bone like a plate of Jell-O dropping to the floor. Other animals that naturally bang their heads, like a woodpecker or a ram, have smoother interior skull surfaces and less space between brain and skull to allow less sloshing. The medical and legal implications of human brain sloshing are considered in Chapter 10.

Neuroscientists recognize three broad subdivisions of the CNS: the *forebrain*, *brainstem*, and *spinal cord*. The forebrain consists of the *cerebral cortex* and the *thalamus*. The brainstem consists of the *midbrain, pons, cerebellum*, and *medulla oblongata*. The spinal cord exits the skull and extends nearly to the end of the spinal column. Take a moment to review Figures 3.2 and 3.3. As you will see, this is not as complicated as its description in prose might suggest.

C. CELLS OF THE NERVOUS SYSTEM

The CNS is comprised of two major types of cells: *neurons* and *glia*. Brain function arises from neurons communicating with each other, as well as with glands and muscles throughout the body. What neurons communicate (their outputs, so to speak) depends on the pattern of influences (inputs) they receive from other neurons. These processes and interactions are facilitated and supported in various ways by glia (which is derived from the Greek word for "glue").

1. Neurons

Neurons come in many shapes and sizes, but, as illustrated in Figure 3.4 they all have three main parts: (1) the *cell body*, (2) the *axon*, and (3) the *dendrites*. The cell

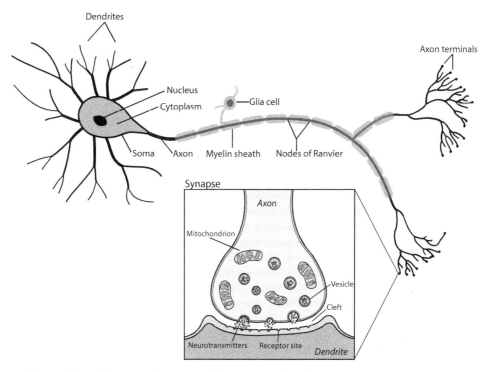

Figure 3.4   The general structure of a neuron.   Details in text.

body (also called the *soma*) encloses the nucleus in which genes regulate protein production and other organelles that organize and sustain the chemical reactions that keep the cell alive and performing its functions.

A single *axon* exiting the cell body is the output end of the neuron, enabling it to communicate with other neurons, glands, or muscles. This communication can happen because neurons have the special property of *excitability*. That is, they respond to a stimulus (like a pinch or an electric shock) by generating a *nerve impulse*. Another term for nerve impulse is *action potential*. Nerve impulses are rapid on-off signals that are sparked at the cell body and are transmitted to the multiple ends of the axon. This means that nerve impulses from a single neuron are amplified as the axon branches and excites hundreds or even thousands of other neurons or muscle fibers or gland cells.

The speed at which nerve impulses travel along axons is not immeasurably fast; it is about 20 to 50 meters per second, depending on the size of the axon. In fact, nerve impulse transmission is slow enough that the difference in communication time between the hand and brain versus the foot and brain can be measured reliably. Nerve impulses are transmitted more rapidly if axons are wrapped in a *myelin sheath* interrupted by periodic nodes.

Axons come in many sizes and shapes. Some axons are microscopically short, reaching only to the dendrites of nearby neurons (a distance of less than 100 micrometers or 0.004 inches). Other axons are very long, extending from the top of the brain to the spinal cord or all the way from the spinal cord to far-distant muscles in the feet or fingers. When they reach their targets, they produce branches to contact with specific neurons, muscle fibers, or gland cells.

Neurons receive inputs from axons on their *dendrites*—resembling the branches of trees. Dendrites are the input end of the neuron, receiving signals from other neurons and translating these into electrical signals that are transmitted through a main trunk into the cell body. The signals from multiple input neurons are integrated by the dendrites, and a neuron signals the completion of that integration by producing a nerve impulse that is transmitted along the axon to its terminals, making contact with other neurons (or muscles or glands). Different kinds of neurons have diverse shapes and sizes of dendrites through which they accomplish their specialized functions. Neuroscientists continue to discover surprising, new features of dendrite form and function that enable intelligence.

Axons contact neurons, muscles, and glands at specialized sites called *synapses*. At each synapse there is a tiny gap (known as the *synaptic cleft*) that separates the axon of a transmitting neuron from the dendrite of the receiving neuron. The axon of the first neuron influences the dendrite of the second neuron by releasing a *neurotransmitter* that floats like springtime pollen in this gap. Neurotransmitters are small molecules that are stored in the terminal of the transmitting neuron in small spheres called *vesicles*. *Neurotransmission* occurs when the contents of these vesicles are released into the synaptic cleft; this is caused by the arrival of a nerve impulse at the axon terminal. The neurotransmitter molecules diffuse across the cleft until they encounter *receptors* that are embedded in the receiving neuron's dendrites. The binding of the neurotransmitter to the receptor (like a key in a lock) triggers other events within the receiving neuron that constitute the communication. The neurotransmitter molecules do not remain in the synaptic cleft for very long. Several processes remove them; these include being taken back into the axon terminal to use again and being decomposed by other chemical processes in the synapse.

The human brain has roughly 86 billion neurons, which connect to one another in complex and intricate ways. A typical neuron has a "social circle" of direct connections with 1,000-10,000 other neurons. By responding *selectively* to the inputs that they receive, neurons can be said to interpret the pattern of inputs—similar to the way that a computer processes information through a nested series of "if-then" rules.

Different neurons with different neurotransmitters convey different kinds of influence. The specific nature of these influences will be described further below. Before proceeding, though, let's make an important point. Many authors and scientists write about neurons "processing information" or "signaling." These terms are natural consequences of adopting the metaphor that the brain is like a computer. In fact, scientists have a very specialized, quantitative definition of "information" that is used for devices like cell phones and computers, and this quantity can be used to describe neuron processes. However, it is crucial to remember that describing the brain as a computer is only a metaphor; it is not the final scientific theory of brain function. The reason this is important is that the metaphor can encourage an insidious form of dualism in which statements about information processing by neurons presume some kind of homunculus (or ghost in the machine) that "reads" that information. There is no homunculus; it's only neurons through and through.

With billions of neurons, each connected to thousands of other neurons, your brain has hundreds of trillions of synapses. And while you are born with (by and large) all of the neurons you will ever have, your synapses do not remain static over time. From the moment you were born, your brain was engaged in *synaptic plasticity*—a process whereby the synapses that are strengthened through use survive and those that are weakened through disuse are pruned. Which synapses survive depends crucially on the interaction of genes and the environment in which a child is raised. Insights about this early synaptic plasticity have played a role in policy proposals to provide educational and social services in the birth to three-year age period.

The final structure of the brain is a record of its evolutionary and developmental history. The cell bodies of neurons are not randomly spread throughout the CNS. Instead, they are organized into dense collections that bring their dendrites into close proximity with one another to receive inputs from axons of particular neurons. Where neuron cell bodies are densely packed with their surrounding dendrites and associated glia cells appears like *gray matter* to anatomists, and where myelinated axons are densely packed appears as *white matter*. The cerebral cortex is one example of a dense collection of neurons, or gray matter, surrounding the white matter formed by the axons running to and from the cerebral cortex. In the interior of the brain are other collections of neuron cell bodies or gray matter that we will describe below.

2. Glia

Glial cells (from the Greek word for "glue") support and enhance the function of neurons. Neuroscientists distinguish different kinds of glial cells. But for this course it is enough to appreciate that one kind of glia forms the myelin sheath around axons to enhance the speed of nerve impulse transmission, while another kind of glia facilitates synaptic transmission by absorbing neurotransmitters and connecting neurons to blood vessels.

While glial cells provide essential functions in the brain, they are also susceptible to uncontrolled division resulting in cancerous growths, called *gliomas*. Gliomas are the most common type of brain tumor and are incredibly lethal. One side effect of a growth resulting from a glioma can be behavioral effects due to impingement on certain brain structures.

D. WHERE BRAINS COME FROM

Much could be said about how brains came to be on this planet. But we will emphasize just two particular ideas. First, brains exist because certain kinds of organisms (mammals, say, as distinct from flowers) have a body plan that—absent a nervous system that coordinates bodily functions and associates perceptions with actions—would lie immobile and quickly die. At the most fundamental level, brains enable sensitivity to and mobility in the complex and challenging environments in which they must navigate to find food and mates and avoid predators. In short, brains enable behavior.

Second, inquiries about the brain, like inquiries about all other features of organisms, including their behaviors, are divisible into separate "why" and "how" questions. These are often conflated by the unwary. Biologists often refer to the "why" questions as being about the evolutionary history of features (how they came over generations to exist as they do) while referring to "how" questions as being about detailed mechanisms (what are the physical and chemical pathways by which such a thing exists?). Biologists typically label the "why" questions as inquiries into the "ultimate causes" of a feature, in contrast to the "how" inquiries into the so-called "proximate causes."*

To illustrate, suppose you were interested in the phenomenon of a male robin singing in the spring. From the perspective of ultimate or evolutionary causation, birds sing in the spring because it was more effective in translating energy into successful mating opportunities (by advertising health, strength, interest, and location) than many of the alternatives, such as singing exclusively in the low-food depths of winter, or responding to the coming of spring only with stubborn silence, one-legged hopping, or the like. That is, the ultimate cause of singing behavior is derived from the fact that the remote ancestors of today's singing males—through their singing—claimed territory, attracted mates, and left more offspring than did contemporaries not predisposed to sing. To the extent that the ability to sing and the urge to respond to certain environmental cues with singing were influenced by genetically heritable predispositions, the proportion of male robins in successive generations that sang inevitably increased over time until we now observe the trait to be typical of males of the species. In contrast, from the perspective of proximate or mechanistic causation, birds sing because the lengthening of the day triggers hormonal changes that in turn prompt the bird's body to contract muscles in ways that pass air over vocal cords shaped in ways that result in air vibrations perceived as a song. Both kinds of causes operate simultaneously—whether you are talking about bird brains or human brains.

So, why and how do our brains function the way they do? To begin to answer this question, we must frame it within an evolutionary history extending over millions of years, as well as a more recent social history over tens or hundreds of thousands of years. We must also appreciate the fact that our brain shares much in common with the brains of other primates. Diverse primate species separated from common ancestors by tens of millions of years have very different sizes of brains that nonetheless share common principles of structure and function.

While bearing certain similarities with the brains of other species, the primate brain is nonetheless structurally distinct in numerous fundamental ways from other mammal brains such as those of carnivores (cats and dogs) and rodents (rats and mice). As a result of the similarity among primate brains, nonhuman primates exhibit many "human" traits, such as cooperation, deception, aversion to inequity, and even some psychological quirks often thought to be uniquely human, such as the endowment effect (a propensity to value something just received at more than one would have "paid" to acquire it an instant ago). Because of these commonalities, scientists gain important insights into the human brain from studies of nonhuman primates (among other species). And, this, coupled with the rise of modern technologies for investigating both non-human and human brains, has afforded remarkable advances in our understanding of the why's and how's of brain structures and functions.

---

* The law's term of art "proximate cause"—though similar in its content—has a quite distinct origin and implication.

E. ORGANIZATION OF THE HUMAN CEREBRAL CORTEX

We now jump up from the microscopic realm to a scale that you may find more comfortable: the larger features of the brain landscape. After a brief overview for general orientation, we will consider each of the four main *lobes* of the cerebral cortex.

First, though, a word about brain size. Across the animal kingdom, brains come in many shapes and a wide range of sizes. It makes no sense to ask which brain is smartest, for the brain of every species does just what it must for the survival of the individuals in that species. Among humans, total brain volume varies from as small as 1,100 to over 2,300 cubic centimeters. A recent, very careful, and unbiased study of a sample of more than 13,000 human brains found a weak but positive association between total brain volume and fluid intelligence and also educational attainment.* The results account for sex, age, height, socioeconomic status, and population structure.

1. Overview

The cerebral cortex is necessary for memory, attention, awareness, language, thought, and consciousness. The importance of the cerebral cortex for the law should be clear when you appreciate that it is necessary for reasoning, problem solving, planning, and impulse control, not to mention basic sensory processing (like reading this text). Thus, as you can imagine, many of the legal cases involving neuroscience are concerned with activity somewhere in the cerebral cortex. The cerebral cortex is a thin layer of neurons on the surface of the brain, typically around 3 millimeters thick (roughly the height of the letters on this page).

In humans, like other large-brained animals, the cerebral cortex is densely folded such that nearly two-thirds of the cortex is submerged into the grooves that give the brain its characteristically wrinkled appearance. The grooves are called *sulci* (singular is *sulcus*), while the exposed surface parts of the rippling folds of cortex are referred to as *gyri* (singular is *gyrus*). This folding and crumpling is necessary to fit the approximately 325 square inches (that's a large pizza) of cerebral cortex into the confines of the skull.

The cerebral cortex has two apparently symmetrical hemispheres: left and right. Each hemisphere is divided into four lobes that are defined by the most prominent sulci and are also associated with different functional properties that will be reviewed later in the chapter.

The four lobes of the cerebral cortex are the *frontal, parietal, temporal,* and *occipital* (Figure 3.5). The names of the four lobes derive from the names of the different bones of the skull that overlay them. They can all be understood, and easily distinguished, by learning the location of three key features: (a) the *central sulcus;* (b) the *lateral sulcus* (also known as the Sylvian fissure); and (c) the *preoccipital notch.*

The frontal and parietal lobes are located on opposite sides of the *central sulcus,* which is a major sulcus (indeed one of the longest, straightest, and most visible grooves) that runs across the medial-lateral axis in the center of the cortex. If you remember some of the orientation terminology from earlier in the chapter, you will

---

* Gideon Nave et al., *Are Bigger Brains Smarter? Evidence from a Large-Scale Preregistered Study,* 30 Psychol. Sci. 43 (2019).

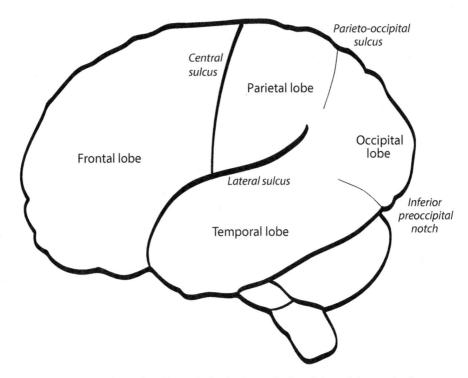

Figure 3.5   Locations of and boundaries between the four lobes of the cerebral cortex. Other structures are not labeled.

see that the frontal lobe is anterior of the sulcus and the parietal lobe is posterior to the sulcus. The temporal lobe is separated from the frontal lobe by the *lateral sulcus,* one of the most prominent structures in the human brain. The lateral sulcus also partially separates the temporal lobe from the parietal lobe. Finally, the occipital lobe, which is located at the posterior extreme of the cerebral cortex, is separated from the parietal lobe by the *parieto-occipital sulcus* and from the temporal lobe by the *preoccipital notch* (which, unlike the central and lateral sulci, is more visible from the rear of the brain than it is from the side).

As mentioned earlier, the cerebral cortex is composed of two nearly identical hemispheres. The *longitudinal fissure* separates the two hemispheres. And the two hemispheres are connected by bundles of axons called *commissures,* the largest being the *corpus callosum,* consisting of 250 million axons that interconnect the two hemispheres. With certain exceptions, the processing of sensory stimuli and the control of movement take place in the opposite side of the brain. For example, movements of the left hand are initiated in the right hemisphere (and vice versa), and the processing of visual information from the right visual field occurs in the left hemisphere (and vice versa). In humans the two hemispheres are specialized for particular functions. In general, the left hemisphere is responsible for language, for example, and the right hemisphere is responsible for navigating in space.

We will now describe in a little more detail the organization and function of different parts of the cerebral cortex. We appreciate the complexity of this information

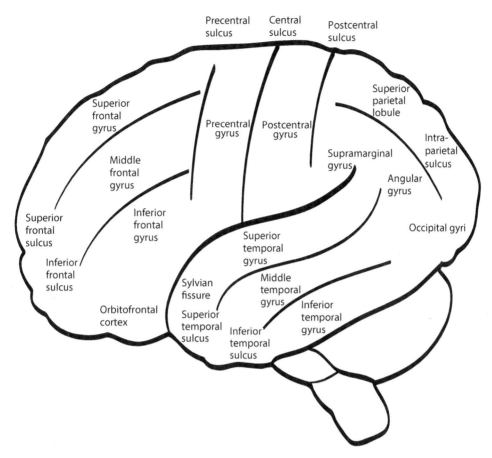

Figure 3.6   Major *gyri* and *sulci* of the human cerebral cortex.

for the novice, but we remind you that if your brain weren't this complex, you couldn't be in law school.

2. Frontal Lobe

In humans, the frontal lobe is the largest of all, supporting our unique ability to behave so flexibly, to navigate complex social relationships, to communicate with symbols through speech, art and music, to contemplate mindboggling options, and to plan further into the future than any other species on the planet. The frontal lobe is organized into four major gyri: precentral, superior frontal, middle frontal, and inferior frontal (see Figure 3.6). Based on function, the frontal lobe can be divided into three broad areas: the primary motor cortex, the secondary motor cortex, and the prefrontal cortex.

The *primary motor area* occupies the caudal end (remember that means: toward the rear) of the frontal lobes, nestled in the central sulcus. The primary motor area is necessary for producing organized, coordinated movements of the body such as speech, as well as reaching, grasping, and manipulating. The axons of certain neurons in primary motor cortex extend to the brainstem and spinal cord to communicate with (*innervate*) the neurons that in turn communicate with the muscles of the face and limbs. The pattern of this communication is organized such that there is a "map" of the body in the primary motor cortex, with places there corresponding to places in and around the body.

Two secondary motor areas are anterior to the primary motor cortex. One is called the *supplementary motor area*, and the other is known as the *premotor area*. These areas are responsible for higher level planning of movements in coordination with events in the world and ongoing movements that may be occurring in an extended sequence (as, for example, when you type a paper).

Anterior to these secondary motor areas lies the expansive *prefrontal cortex (PFC)*, comprising the cortical regions that will be encountered most frequently in this coursebook. Those regions of PFC are known by their locations: dorsolateral, ventrolateral, ventromedial, and orbitofrontal.

The PFC is regarded as the "CEO" of the brain in that it connects with many other areas of the cerebral cortex and every structure beneath the cerebral cortex that will be described below. The PFC is responsible for the highest-level control of behavior.

The first indication that the PFC played this role was the result of a freak accident in 1848 involving a man named Phineas Gage. An unintended explosion propelled an iron rod through Gage's head, entering below his left eye and exiting the top of his skull. The entire left frontal lobe was destroyed, though the right hemisphere remained intact. Descriptions of Gage's behavior following the accident indicated that he suffered from an inability to exercise any form of behavioral restraint. He was described this way:

Navigating the Prefrontal Cortex You will encounter the PFC many times in this coursebook. You will see discussion of the following four subregions of the PFC: the dorsolateral, ventrolateral, ventromedial, and orbitofrontal. Thus, it's worth taking a few minutes now to study these different parts of the PFC. Imagine you have to explain in a brief where your client's PFC injury was in detail. Armed with what you learned earlier in this chapter, you should be able to translate the four PFC subregions into rough locations in the brain. For example, dorsolateral is a combination of "dorsal" (top) and "lateral" (side) — in the same way that the compass direction "northwest" is a combination of "north" and "west" — such that the dorsolateral region of the PFC is roughly the upper side area of the PFC. Using the same approach, take a moment to describe where each of the other regions are. Which is just above the eyes?

> The equilibrium or balance, so to speak, between his intellectual faculties and animal propensities, seems to have been destroyed. He is fitful, irreverent, indulging at times in the grossest profanity (which was not previously his custom), manifesting but little deference for his fellows, impatient of restraint or advice when it conflicts with his desires, at times pertinaciously obstinate, yet capricious and vacillating, devising many plans of future operations, which are no sooner arranged than they are abandoned in turn for others appearing more feasible. . . . In this regard his mind was radically changed, so decidedly that his friends and acquaintances said he was "no longer Gage."

John Martyn Harlow, *Recovery from the Passage of an Iron Bar Through the Head*, 2 Pub. Mass. Med. Soc. 327, 339-40 (1868).

Extensive research has confirmed the impression, illustrated by this case, that the PFC is critical for the ability to predict outcomes, delay gratification, compare multiple options, assess risk, adapt to changing rules and goals, and redirect attention based on new information. However, each of these functions is accomplished by different parts of the prefrontal cortex, so let us consider them in turn.

Dorsolateral prefrontal cortex (commonly abbreviated DLPFC) has been associated with attentional control, decision-making, the integration of information, high-level control of behavior, working memory of items during planning and deliberation, and inductive reasoning. The DLPFC is critical for our ability to think abstractly so as to anticipate and simulate events that either might not necessarily be true or might not be occurring in the present. An example of this would be predicting the outcome of future events based on hypothetical situations. Research has demonstrated a contribution of this region (and related regions) to fluid intelligence.

Ventrolateral PFC (VLPFC) occupies the most lateral and ventral portion of the PFC. This region of cortex in the left hemisphere includes an area known as *Broca's area* that is responsible for generating speech.* Research has also described a region that contributes to responding to surprising stimuli, often through inhibiting ongoing actions. This region contributes to regulating movements in response to arbitrary cues.

Ventromedial PFC (VMPFC) and *orbitofrontal PFC* (OFPFC) have been linked to motivation, decision-making, and judgment. VMPFC and OFPFC have distinct connections and functions.

VMPFC contributes importantly to cognitive, emotional, and social functions that are commonly disrupted in mental illness. More specifically, VMPFC is important for reward- and value-based decision-making. It is also crucial for generation and regulation of negative emotion, i.e., "counting to ten." In addition, VMPFC contributes to social cognition including recognizing facial expressions of emotion and supporting theory-of-mind. Impairments of VMPFC have been associated with many psychiatric disorders including depression, posttraumatic stress disorder, addiction, social anxiety disorder, bipolar disorder, schizophrenia, and attention-deficit/hyperactivity disorder. Disorders of this region have also been implicated in the impairments of moral reasoning, empathy, and social cognition of individuals rating high on scales of psychopathy.

OFPFC receives basic olfactory information and more refined information from the other senses, plus signals about hunger and thirst. It is also sensitive to emotional and social information. OFPFC integrates this information about outer and inner states to influence behavior. Individuals with disconnected or damaged OFPFC tend to exhibit increased extroversion, restlessness, and euphoria, and aggressive or impulsive tendencies worsen. A popular early theory about OFPFC suggested that this region interprets changes in bodily state during emotional experiences, such as elevated heart rate or churning stomach, as cues to avoid excessively risky or unwanted actions. Further research has expanded and clarified our understanding. OFPFC signals the value, ranging from aversive to rewarding in the context of uncertainty and risk, of items in the environment associated with the cost or effort

---

* Broca's area and Wernicke's area (see below) are almost always in the left hemisphere of right-handed individuals, especially males. If you are left-handed, then it is possible that language production and comprehension depends more on the right hemisphere.

of actions necessary to acquire or avoid them. It contributes to comparing different kinds of consequences on a common scale (do you prefer to finish reading this
chapter or eat that apple?). Given the arbitrary nature of payoffs, OFPFC is also
important for learning the relationships between actions and consequences, especially under risk and uncertainty. OFPFC helps encode rules and strategies as well
as regret upon recognition that an alternative action would have been more beneficial. Crucial for law and neuroscience, these functions are expressed in organizing social interactions and regulating emotional responses. For example, disrupted
interactions between OFPFC and VMPFC and amygdala, which can disrupt the ability to learn about social rewards, have been associated with psychopathic traits like
reduced emotional reactivity and empathy.

3. Insula

Buried in the lateral sulcus of the brain is a cortical region known as the insula.
Being less accessible than other brain regions, rather less is known about the
insula. Interest in and information about the insula increased when neuroimaging
studies (explained in Chapter 4) found activation during an unexpectedly diverse
variety of conditions and tasks. Because the insula is so relevant in Chapter 11 on
Pain and Distress, Chapter 12 on Addicted Brains, and Chapter 16 on Judging,
we will survey its functions in more detail. In short, when you "follow your gut"
in deciding an uncertain course of action, or ruminate with stomach-churning,
heart-racing, dry-throat anxiety, or agonize about how much the visit to the dentist
will hurt, or feel someone else's pain, or contemplate moral dilemmas, you can
thank your insula for linking internal body states to external situations and resulting actions.

We will describe four broad functions supported by different subregions in the
insula. These diverse functions are enabled through connections organized across
the insula with cortical areas in the frontal (in particular the anterior cingulate cortex, described below in the section on the Limbic System), orbital frontal (in particular, olfactory), parietal (in particular, somatosensory areas), and temporal lobes.

First, the insula contributes to perception of internal body states and autonomic responses to those states. This sensitivity to visceral state is known as *interoception*. Electrical stimulation of the insula causes changes in respiration, heart rate,
blood pressure, and saliva production, as well as stomach churning and vomiting. Neuroimaging indicates that the insula becomes activated when participants
become aware of thirst, heartbeat, and distention of the esophagus, stomach, bladder, and rectum. The insula is also essentially involved in pain perception, known as
nociception. Electrical stimulation of the insula causes uncomfortable or even painful
tingling, burning, or numbness of the face, arm, or hand. Neuroimaging studies
associate activation of the insula with perception of heat/cold and the severity of
painful stimulation. Damage to or removal of the insula can result in reduced or
altered pain perception. The insula is involved as well in higher-level auditory perception, including sensitivity to loud sounds. More directly, the insula is critically
involved in processing the intensity, quality, and affective value of taste stimuli plus
anticipation of and attention to tastes and smells. To summarize, the insula receives
diverse information about the internal state of the body and influences physiological processes to maintain the healthiest state possible.

Second, being a central node in responding to visceral signals about the body, the insula is thought to play a crucial role in arousal and subjective feelings associated with emotions. Neuroimaging studies have found activation of the insula upon viewing disgusting, frightening, happy, sad, or sexual images. Damage to the insula can result in abnormal experience of the emotion, apathy, or anxiety. Through its role in self-awareness of internal body states, the insula is also crucial for recognition of emotion in others and empathy supporting social interactions. Neuroimaging studies describe activation of the insula upon viewing others in pain and also to expressions of disgust, fear, anxiety, and happiness in others. Indeed, the insula supports feelings of disgust at unfairness in economic or similar exchanges. This capacity is altered or eliminated following damage to the insula. With its representations of internal body states and connections with orbitofrontal cortex, the insula is thought to contribute to decision-making under risk and uncertainty. When reason cannot resolve alternatives, emotions, hunches, and the gut must lead the way. Neuroimaging studies report activation of the insula during tasks requiring responses under risk, uncertainty, and conflicting impulses, often in parallel with anterior cingulate cortex. Damage to the insula can impair decision-making in these conditions.

Third, the insula contributes to responding appropriately to multiple, even conflicting internal and external stimuli. In neuroimaging studies, the insula is one of the most commonly observed activations, usually in association with anterior cingulate cortex. It is commonly activated when novel stimuli are presented, regardless of sensory modality, presumably to identify the most relevant among multiple competing internal and external stimuli, especially when performing a task that calls on greater cognitive control.

4. Temporal Lobe

Another important source of inputs to the frontal lobe is the temporal lobe. In general, the temporal lobe provides information about the identity of objects, supporting memory and recognition.

The primary auditory processing cortex is located in the temporal lobe near the posterior extreme of the lateral fissure. As is the case in the primary somatosensory processing area, the processing of auditory input does not end with the primary auditory cortex. As previously mentioned, certain vision processing for guiding movements in space occurs in the parietal lobes of the brain. Complementary vision processing for recognizing objects like faces occurs in the temporal lobes. The recognition of all of the complex objects in our lives requires learning, and the temporal lobes also contain structures that are essential for forming and retrieving memories. Damage to the temporal lobes commonly results in impaired recognition of objects such as faces, even of family members.

5. Parietal Lobe

Generally speaking, the parietal lobe's main function is to synthesize the senses of vision, hearing, touch, and balance to guide body movements in space. Circuits in the parietal lobe support your ability to reach for that cup of coffee while holding this book, or to aim the gun accurately before pulling that trigger.

From where does the frontal lobe receive the information that it evaluates? One rich source of information is the parietal lobe. The parietal lobe provides sensory guidance for the actions, like reaching and grasping, produced by the frontal lobe. That guidance integrates information across the senses into a unified framework to guide action in space and time.

Primary somatosensory cortex occupies the rostral end of the parietal lobe, nestled in the central sulcus, adjacent to primary motor cortex. This cortical area is responsible for our sense of touch, pain, temperature, and limb position. Different nerve pathways beginning at different receptors convey these different sensory modalities with different speeds. This is why when a person hits her thumb with a hammer, she feels the sensation of the pressure of the object against her thumb before she feels the pain.

Beyond the sense of touch, the parietal lobe, traditionally part of the *association cortex*, is involved in cognitive processes. Areas in the association cortex are neither specifically motor nor exclusively sensory in function. Neuroscientists surmise that the association cortex is where converging inputs catalyze everything from coordinated complex body movements to creativity to social cognition. The organizing of convergent information for different tasks and abilities is accomplished in a variety of subregions. Some of these regions are involved in visual orienting and attention to guide actions through our spatial environment. Accordingly, damage to these regions renders the patient unable to notice objects in the environment even though they can see them just fine. Other regions are involved in speech comprehension. Accordingly, damage to a region located in the *supramarginal gyrus*, also known as *Wernicke's area*, impairs speech comprehension. Yet another region, known as the *temporoparietal junction* (TPJ), is involved in what psychologists call "theory of mind." Accordingly, damage to the TPJ renders patients challenged to interpret the thoughts, intentions, and desires of others.

The medial surface of the parietal lobe is known as the *precuneus*. This cortical region contributes to self-awareness, episodic memory including contextual associations, the allocation of visual attention in space, and mental imagery. It is identified as a central node in the default network, a collection of cortical areas that are coordinated during wakeful resting.

6. Occipital Lobe

The occipital lobe is the smallest of the lobes in the human cerebral cortex. It is the visual processing center of the mammalian brain. The primary visual cortex is located at the posterior pole of the occipital lobe and is surrounded by a variety of other areas that perform more complex analyses of the visual image. Thus, damage to the posterior pole results in profound loss of vision, while damage to more rostral regions results in more subtle problems with visual perception. For example, damage restricted to a small region that is specialized for perception of visual motion renders patients incapable of seeing the continuity of motion even though they can see the color, shape, and location of objects.

The scientific study of perception investigates basic questions about how sensitive we are to the presence of stimuli in the different sensory modalities (vision, hearing, touch, smell, taste) and about how well we can discriminate different stimuli. In considering the function of the parts of the brain that accomplish sensation, it is important to appreciate that they can be fooled. Psychologists have discovered many illusions that illustrate just how much of our perception of the world is constructed by the brain.*

It is easy to see why perception is legally relevant. What a witness hears, or what you hear when a client is explaining her case to you, are central to legal practice. The *limits* of perception are also highly relevant in many legal contexts. For example, at what distance can one reliably discriminate the faces of different individuals? Perception varies with experience. For example, the ability to discriminate among objects (like cars) varies with the amount of experience one has viewing and considering such objects.

Another essential fact about perception is that we are bombarded by many more stimuli than we can respond to. Therefore, perception is selective. In short, we perceive those few objects to which we pay attention.

F. ORGANIZATION OF SUBCORTICAL SYSTEMS

We noted earlier that the cerebral cortex is a relatively thin layer of neurons folded over the surface of the brain. When the early anatomists peeled away the cerebral cortex and underlying white matter, they discovered many other collections of neuron cell bodies arranged in various ways from the forebrain to the brainstem. They are known as "subcortical" structures, because, if you were to drill into someone's head from the skull, you would find these other structures "beneath" the cortex.

This section surveys the major subcortical structures. Subcortical structures can be organized into functional subdivisions or into anatomical subdivisions. We will do both by describing two functional systems (the *limbic system* and the *basal ganglia*) and these anatomical subdivisions (*thalamus, hypothalamus* plus *pituitary gland, brainstem* including *cerebellum, pons, medulla oblongata,* and the spinal cord). This section of the chapter probes a deeper level of detail than the previous sections, but the detail is provided so that when you encounter these structures later in the book, you can refer back to this section to be reminded of their location and function.

1. Limbic System

Researchers formulated the term *limbic system* in the early 1950s to organize their understanding of the function of a diverse group of structures. The word "limbic" was derived from the Latin word for "border" and was originally used to label structures at the border between the cerebral hemispheres and subcortical structures. Some scientists believe that the term is obsolete, and newer, more accurate classifications have been developed. Nevertheless, you should be familiar with the term limbic system because it remains in common usage outside neuroscience and will be used in studies that will be described in later chapters. We will focus on just three of the many structures that compose the limbic system—the *amygdala, hippocampus,* and *cingulate cortex.*

---

* Many websites display visual illusions. We like this one: www.michaelbach.de/ot.

Two functions mediated by the limbic system are memory and emotion. The hippocampus (named by the Greek word for sea horse, with which it shares a stunning resemblance) is a prominent structure in the medial temporal lobe. The hippocampus with nearby regions is responsible for episodic memory. Episodic memory can be thought of as memory of past "episodes" of personal experiences, such as what you had for breakfast and where you parked your car. You will learn in Chapter 13 that human memory is not a perfect digital recorder on which you simply press the rewind button to replay previous episodes in your life. Humans with damage to the hippocampus and surrounding tissue are unable to form new biographical memories and also may have trouble recalling memories of past events before they experienced the unfortunate damage. Impaired formation of memories is called *anterograde amnesia*, and impaired recall of memories is called *retrograde amnesia*. We have all experienced how emotional arousal during an event seems to enhance recollection of that event. Our memories are formed and retrieved wrapped in an emotional package that helps organize the content with the context of the memory. This association between emotion and memory is mediated by the amygdala (named by the Greek word for almond, which it resembles). It is a dense collection of neurons nestled in the rostral tip of the temporal lobes. The amygdala and hippocampus work together to add emotional tone to episodic memories, such as your first kiss or a traumatic experience. For example, if the experience of a stimulus is associated with a fear response, then the amygdala recreates the fear response at a much later point in time upon the reappearance of the original stimulus or even something only resembling the initial stimulus. For instance, if a fast-moving object is headed your way, you want to immediately move out of its way. Your fear response (i.e., the fear you attach to memories of previous objects coming quickly at you) allows you react quickly.

The balance of emotion and memory is complex. On the one hand, the association can become so strong that a fear response, for example, results in inappropriately excessive responses. Often this association will continue despite substantial experience indicating that the association is invalid, and without the subject's awareness that the association has been formed. The neurological inability to extinguish the association has been interpreted as insufficient "top-down" control exerted on the amygdala by regions in the PFC. The phrase "top-down" is used here as it is in a business context—the PFC (as "CEO" of the brain) has the responsibility to determine when certain fear associations are useful (e.g., take cover when you hear a bomb explode on the battlefield) and when they are not (e.g., you don't need to hide under your desk every time you hear the trash truck rumbling outside). The result of this deficient extinction ability is thought to lead to the anxiety disorder known as post-traumatic stress disorder (PTSD). As you will read in subsequent chapters, personal injury litigation and criminal defense now sometimes invoke a client's PTSD diagnosis.

On the other hand, in some cases too much emotional arousal during a traumatic event can reduce the ability to recall the memories of the event. Such disagreement has found its way into the courtroom. For instance, in the trial of a Bosnian-Croatian soldier accused of abuse of a female prisoner, the defense called expert witnesses who testified that the woman's memories were inaccurate due her traumatic experiences. The experts brought in by the prosecution, however, suggested precisely the opposite, that she remembered more vividly and accurately her traumatic ordeals. You will read more about cases like these in the chapter on memory (Chapter 13).

The final part to introduce is the cingulate cortex. While it could have been reviewed in the section on regions of the cerebral cortex, this cortical region is included in this section because it has been historically and conceptually identified with the limbic system. The cingulate cortex encircles the corpus callosum on the midline of the brain, spanning beneath the frontal and parietal lobes. Two major subdivisions are recognized: the anterior cingulate cortex (ACC) and posterior cingulate cortex. We will focus on the ACC.

The ACC has become an area of significant research interest in the last 30 years with the introduction of brain imaging. As neuroscientists investigated other cortical structures using neuroimaging methods, they found that the ACC, usually coupled with the insula, was activated during a broad variety of cognitive tasks and emotional conditions. The caudal-dorsal and rostral-ventral segments of the ACC have distinguishable functions. The caudal-dorsal region is more involved in cognitive and executive processes. The rostral-ventral region is involved in emotional processes.

Overall, the ACC has been associated with monitoring behavior by judging the consequences of actions, evaluating choices based on expected value, evaluating choices in social interactions, including making moral judgments or producing lies, and in planning body movements in complex situations. The ACC is also responsive to physical pain, social pain, and empathic pain as well as emotional distress.

The role of ACC in regulating emotion has led to experimental therapy of electrical stimulation to treat depression. While debate continues about the function of the ACC, one plausible hypothesis states that the ACC is generally sensitive to the difficulty of a task when errors are likely and mobilizes through connections with the prefrontal cortex the resources necessary to withhold undesirable actions and perform the task correctly.

2. Basal Ganglia

The *basal ganglia* area is a collection of about a half-dozen separate but connected groups of neurons in the center of the brain that form a circuit to regulate movement, emotion, and thought. The term "basal" refers to its location deep in the brain, and the term "ganglia" refers to a dense collection of neuron cell bodies beneath the cerebral cortex. The basal ganglia were originally identified entirely with the motor system of the brain because of its essential role in producing movements of the body. This function is highlighted by the fact that the symptoms of Parkinson's disease and Huntington's disease arise from the death of specific neurons in the basal ganglia.

The basal ganglia circuitry is now recognized to play an equally important role in the control of cognition, emotion, and motivation as evidenced, for example, by its contribution to the establishment of habits that can become extreme in, for example, addiction or obsessive-compulsive disorder. A key component of the basal ganglia for responding to rewards is the *nucleus accumbens.*

3. Thalamus

The thalamus is located in the center of the brain, beneath the cortex, surrounded by (and part of) the limbic system and basal ganglia. Neuroscientists describe the thalamus, perched atop the brainstem, as the gateway to the cerebral cortex. The thalamus consists of neurons that receive inputs from many other parts of the brain and send axons to the cerebral cortex. Different parts of the thalamus are connected with different parts of the cerebral cortex in a very organized manner. The different parts of the thalamus receive inputs from either different sensory pathways or from other parts of the brain, such as the limbic system, the basal ganglia, the cerebellum, and the brainstem. Thus, cortical areas in occipital, temporal, and parietal lobes that perform visual processing receive input from parts of the thalamus that themselves receive input from neurons in the eye. Accordingly, a stroke of this part of the thalamus results in problems with visual perception. Likewise, cortical areas in the frontal lobe that produce body movements receive input from parts of the thalamus that themselves receive input from neurons in the basal ganglia and cerebellum. A stroke damaging this part of the thalamus results in problems of movement and planning.

4. Hypothalamus & Pituitary Gland

Beneath the thalamus is the hypothalamus ("hypo" means below). The hypothalamus consists of different subdivisions that maintain the internal state of the body. This includes body temperature, hunger, thirst, and sexual drive. It also is involved in maintaining synchronization of sleep and the day-night (circadian) rhythms. Neuroscientists say that the hypothalamus maintains the body's state of *homeostasis*. This is accomplished through neural connections with the autonomic nervous system and hormone signals through the pituitary gland. The latter has been called the "master gland of the body," because it releases hormones that modulate a wide variety of body functions by controlling, in turn, the functions of other glands throughout the body.

5. Brainstem — Cerebellum, Pons, & Medulla

The brainstem is located between the forebrain and the spinal cord. We can divide the brainstem into parts: the *cerebellum*, the *pons*, and the *medulla oblongata* (often referred to simply as the medulla).

The cerebellum ("small brain") is the conspicuous structure hanging beneath the occipital lobe (Figure 3.3). The cerebellum is connected to the rest of the brain through neurons in the pons. The pons is a bulbous part appearing to wrap around the brainstem. The cerebellum is necessary to produce precisely timed and coordinated movements. It is also involved in coordinating thoughts.

The pons and medulla consist of axons traveling down to and up from the spinal cord as well as collections of neurons that are necessary for the most basic control of heartbeat, breathing, and consciousness, as well as reflexive actions like vomiting, coughing, sneezing, and swallowing. When we consider the topic of brain death in a subsequent chapter, we will learn how important the status of the brainstem is when evaluating brain death.

6. Spinal Cord

As we mentioned at the beginning of this chapter, the central nervous system (CNS) is composed of the brain and the spinal cord. Like the brain, the spinal cord is sheathed in meninges, which provide protection along with the spine. The *spinal cord* travels from the end of the medulla oblongata through the spinal column, ending near the bottom of the spine.

The spinal cord consists of the axons mediating the two-way transmission of motor signals from the brain to the body and sensory signals from the body to the brain. These two paths are separate in the spinal column, with the motor outputs running down the ventral side and the sensory neurons rising up the dorsal side. These axons surround a central core of sensory neurons that receive inputs from the body, motor neurons that make muscles contract to produce body movements, and intermediate inhibitory and excitatory neurons that regulate the function of these neurons. These spinal cord circuits can operate independently of the cerebral cortex, and this provides for rapid reflexes that occur substantially faster than they would if the signal had to be conducted to the brain and back. The skin and muscles of the body are connected in an orderly map with the spinal cord; the arms are connected to the part of the spinal cord closer to the brain, and the legs are connected to the part of the spinal cord further from the brain. This is why damage to the spinal cord typically only affects the parts of the body connected to the spinal cord caudal to the damaged point.

G. BLOOD SUPPLY TO THE BRAIN

It should be evident by now that the brain does *a lot* of work. From keeping your heart beating, to helping you answer questions on an exam, your brain is working around the clock. You might be wondering at this point what types of fuel the brain needs to accomplish all of this work. The brain relies on oxygen and glucose supplied by blood flow. Comprising just 1/40th of body mass, the brain consumes 1/5th of all the body's oxygen. The human brain contains 60,000 miles of blood vessels, large and small. Neuron function and blood flow are very closely related; neurons influence blood vessel size through certain glial cells.

Arteries deliver oxygenated blood, glucose, and other nutrients to brain tissue. Veins take deoxygenated blood and the by-products of metabolism, such as carbon dioxide and lactic acid, back to the heart and respiratory system. The seemingly miraculous images of brain function that are so important for neurolaw are derived from tiny differences in the magnetic properties of oxygenated and deoxygenated blood, or by an indirect measure of metabolic activity in which radioactive tracers are injected to visually see relative levels of glucose uptake.

The blood supply to the brain is divided into anterior and posterior arteries. The two main pairs of arteries are the internal carotid arteries and vertebral arteries. Pairs of arteries communicating across the midline interconnect the anterior and posterior blood supplies of each hemisphere. This connection of arteries forms a circuit that balances blood pressure and provides a path for blood flow to both hemispheres even if one of the major supply arteries becomes occluded. The arteries split into anterior, middle, and posterior branches that further split into smaller and smaller branches to supply cortical and subcortical tissue.

The blood that has released oxygen and absorbed waste products collects in the venous drainage system. This consists of a superficial system and a deep system. The superficial system is composed of gaps called sinuses beneath the dura. One very prominent example is the superior sagittal sinus located between the cerebral hemispheres. The deep venous drainage is composed of veins inside the deep structures of the brain. Smaller veins combine to flow into larger veins that join the confluence of the sinuses that send blood to the heart through the two jugular veins.

The brain is exceedingly susceptible to compromises of its blood supply, so the cerebral circulatory system has many safeguards. Failure of these safeguards results in *cerebrovascular accidents*, commonly known as strokes. The particular pattern of brain damage following a stroke will depend on which blood vessels are damaged. Blood vessel branching patterns vary across individuals, so even strokes in individuals affecting arteries of the same name can produce somewhat different patterns of symptoms.

H. HOW NEURONS COMMUNICATE

This section will describe more of the basics about how circuits of neurons function. No survey of brain function would be complete without this information. As noted above, nervous systems work through the interactions of neurons with other neurons, sensory receptors, muscles, and glands. Neuroscientists differentiate between major types of neurons on the basis of what type of signal the neuron sends and what distance the signal travels. Some neurons have axons that project to structures other than where their cell body resides. For example, neurons located in the frontal lobe of the cerebral cortex send axons to the spinal cord to produce body movements. Also, neurons in one area of the cerebral cortex send axons to many other cortical areas. These are just two of the numerous connections that neuroscientists have described. Another pattern of connection is the feedback loop; most brain structures that send an axon somewhere get an axon back from that place.

Neuroscientists have also found neurons that communicate only locally within structures. These tend to be smaller neurons with axons that connect only to neurons in the local vicinity of the cell body. These local circuit neurons are important for tuning the state of activation of the larger neurons that project to other structures.

Scientists sort neurons into three major categories, based on the nature of the output messages sent to other neurons. Neurons in the first category are called *excitatory*, those in the second category are called *inhibitory*, and those in the third category are called *modulatory*. Every neuron receives a diverse collection of excitatory, inhibitory, and modulatory inputs. Whether that neuron produces an impulse depends on the pattern of these three inputs over time and over the space of the dendritic tree in complicated ways that are progressively well understood but well beyond the scope of this introduction.

Excitatory neurons commonly use a neurotransmitter called *glutamate*. When glutamate binds to receptors in the dendrites of receiving neurons, processes occur that increase the probability that the post-synaptic neuron becomes active immediately. Most neurons that communicate across structures are excitatory. (This is the same glutamate that is in monosodium glutamate, more commonly known as MSG.)

Inhibitory neurons commonly use a neurotransmitter called *GABA* (gamma-amino butyric acid). When GABA binds to receptors in the dendrites of receiving neurons, processes occur that decrease the probability that the post-synaptic neuron becomes active immediately. Most neurons that communicate within a local region are inhibitory.

Modulatory neurons have longer term and more subtle effects that can either increase or decrease the likelihood of a post-synaptic neuron becoming active in response to excitatory and inhibitory inputs. Modulatory neurons can be understood to tune the balance of activation in many neurons comprising a circuit or system or even the whole brain. These neurons use a variety of neurotransmitters, some of which you may have heard of. The major modulatory neurotransmitters are *dopamine, norepinephrine,* and *serotonin.* The cell bodies of these neurons are concentrated in the brainstem, and their axons travel and branch very broadly throughout subcortical structures and the cerebral cortex. Thus, they have very broad influence. These neurotransmitters are the targets of drugs that affect thought, movement, and mood.

We will now describe the mechanics of synaptic transmission. Once again, this will be a superficial survey of basic principles. With only a few exceptions that need not concern us, every neuron signals with only one neurotransmitter. We will treat the process of synaptic transmission as equivalent for all types of neurons.

When a nerve impulse reaches an axon terminal, it causes the vesicles storing the neurotransmitter to release their contents into the synaptic cleft. The neurotransmitters diffuse and eventually may bind to a receptor located in the membrane of the post-synaptic neuron. What happens next dictates whether the neurotransmitter effect is excitatory, inhibitory, or modulatory. It is excitatory if it changes the state of the neuron such that it becomes more likely to produce a nerve impulse. It is inhibitory if it changes the state of the neuron such that it becomes less likely to produce a nerve impulse. Both of these effects occur through the receptor changing the state of the membrane in the dendrite to make it either *depolarize* (if excitatory) or *hyperpolarize* (if inhibitory).

In contrast to this direct effect, modulatory neurotransmitters exert their influence through *second messenger* systems within the post-synaptic neuron. These systems are called second messenger because the binding of the neurotransmitter to the receptor causes a cascade of chemical reactions within the neuron that amplifies in magnitude and duration the influence of the neurotransmitter. Researchers have studied a variety of second messenger systems, and they remain the focus of intense research because they are likely sites of drug influence. Ultimately, these second messenger systems influence the inner workings of the neuron in ways that can either increase or decrease the responsiveness to other influences. Through second messenger systems, a given neurotransmitter can have a range of effects. For example, dopamine is heavily concentrated in the basal ganglia where it has both excitatory and inhibitory effects on different neurons depending on the type of receptor in the respective neurons. Because they have such spatially and temporally distributed effects, modulatory neurotransmitter systems have been identified with general aspects of behavior such as reward, sleep-wake cycle, and mood.

Once the neurotransmitter has been released into the synaptic cleft, it cannot be left to act forever or the signaling would not be a signal anymore. Three major mechanisms exist to remove neurotransmitters from the synapse to limit their duration of action. First, specific enzymes may convert the neurotransmitter to a chemical that will no longer bind to the receptor. Second, the neurotransmitter molecule may be taken up into the presynaptic membrane; this reuptake process allows the neurotransmitter molecule to be recycled and released again. Third, certain neurotransmitters can be removed by glia.

The complex interaction of neurotransmitters and their receptors change the likelihood that a neural signal will pass between one or another neuron. Through processes like these, brains can reconfigure their neural networks at astonishing speed and in unimaginable combinations to support activities like thinking, feeling, and learning.

FURTHER READING

Neuroscience is such a popular topic that many introductory books have been authored such as:

> Rita Carter, *The Human Brain Book: An Illustrated Guide to its Structure, Function, and Disorders* (2014).

Neuroscience is taught in undergraduate and graduate courses from textbooks like these:

> Dale Purves et al., *Neuroscience* (6th ed. 2017).
> Eric Kandel, James Schwartz & Thomas Jessell, *Principles of Neural Science* (5th ed. 2012).
> Larry R. Squire et al., *Fundamental Neuroscience* (4th ed. 2012).
> Marie T. Banich & Rebecca J. Compton, *Cognitive Neuroscience* (4th ed. 2018).
> Mark F. Bear, Barry W. Connors & Michael A. Paradiso, *Neuroscience: Exploring the Brain* (4th ed. 2015).
> Michael Gazzaniga, Richard B. Ivry & George R. Mangun, *Cognitive Neuroscience: The Biology of the Mind* (5th ed. 2018).

The history of neuroscience is full of fascinating people, events, and insights covered in books like these:

> Andrew P. Wickens, *A History of the Brain: From Stone Age Surgery to Modern Neuroscience* (2014).
> Mitchell Glickstein, *Neuroscience: A Historical Introduction* (2014).
> Matthew Cobb, *The Idea of the Brain: The Past and Future of Neuroscience* (2020).

Neuroanatomy is complex, but these books make it simpler:

> Marion C. Diamond & Arnold B. Scheibel, *The Human Brain Coloring Book* (1985).
> Adam Fish, *Neuroanatomy: Draw It to Know It* (2d ed. 2012).
> Suzana Herculano-Houzel, *The Human Advantage: How Our Brains Became Remarkable* (2017).

Online Resources:

We recommend www.brainfacts.org because it is supported by the Society for Neuroscience. The Society for Neuroscience was founded in 1969 and now has more than 40,000 members. It not only serves to advance understanding of the brain and the nervous system, but also promotes educational programs about the brain and informs legislators and other policymakers about the implications of neuroscience research for public policy, societal benefit, and continued scientific progress. BrainFacts.org includes an interactive 3D brain.

You can learn about the activities and accomplishments of the Allen Institute for Brain Science at https://alleninstitute.org.

You can also learn more about neuroscience and brain disorders at the websites of the National Science Foundation and various National Institutes of Health such as:

Nat'l Sci. Found., Understanding the Brain, https://www.nsf.gov/news/special_reports/brain.

Nat'l Inst. on Aging, http://www.nia.nih.gov.

Nat'l Inst. on Alcohol Abuse & Alcoholism, http://www.niaaa.nih.gov.

Eunice Kennedy Shriver Nat'l Inst. of Child Health & Human Dev., http://www.nichd.nih.gov.

Nat'l Inst. on Drug Abuse, http://www.drugabuse.gov.

Nat'l Inst. of Mental Health, http://www.nimh.nih.gov.

Nat'l Inst. of Neurological Disorders & Stroke, http://www.ninds.nih.gov.

Finally, the Dana Foundation's website includes a number of accessible publications about brain science, at www.dana.org.

CHAPTER 4

Brain Monitoring and Manipulation

Today, . . . the Neurocentric Age is more deeply entrenched than ever. At the beginning of the twenty-first century, thousands of neuroscientists . . . continue to dismantle the brain, but they don't have to pull it from a corpse to do so. Instead, they can scan the positronic glow of neurons recalling the faces of friends, searching for a word, generating anger or bliss, or reading the minds of others.
 —Carl Zimmer[†]

Few scientific developments have been more striking than the ability to image the functioning human brain. . . . Like the maps used by early explorers, our current understanding of brain function is riddled with errors, inconsistencies, and puzzles deserving of solution. Yet the difficulty in understanding the brain has only added to the excitement of the quest.
 —Scott A. Huettel, Allen W. Song, & Gregory McCarthy[††]

CHAPTER SUMMARY

This chapter:
- Introduces techniques used to look at the structure and function of the brain.
- Introduces manipulations of the brain including surgery, specialized activation and disruption techniques, and psychoactive drugs.
- Introduces basic experimental designs used to assess behavior and mental states during brain imaging or manipulation.

INTRODUCTION

Much of what we know about how the human brain works was discovered in experiments with non-human animals because these permit invasive techniques to probe brain function. Historically, the main way to understand human brain function was to investigate the particular impairments that followed from damage to a part of the

---

[†] Carl Zimmer, *Soul Made Flesh* 7 (2004).
[††] Scott A. Huettel, Allen W. Song & Gregory McCarthy, *Functional Magnetic Resonance Imaging* 1 (1st ed. 2004).

brain by a stroke or some other accident. Traditionally, the only way to know with certainty where the damage happened was to look at the brain after the patient died.

In the last 30 years, imaging techniques have revolutionized medicine and neuroscience by giving physicians and researchers the ability to create images of the structure of the brain. These images allow for localization of abnormalities in the brain caused by cancer, stroke, degeneration, traumatic brain injury, and the like. As you will see in subsequent chapters, courts have been encountering this type of imaging evidence.

In the 1980s and 1990s new technologies for probing brain function were invented that revealed patterns of the energy utilization in the brain. Experimental psychologists employed these methods with their array of tests used to study behavior and mental representations. Through this research our understanding of human brain function increased tremendously—beyond the scope of a simple summary that can be offered here. These advances have created powerful and dramatic opportunities (for better or for worse) for the introduction of this information about brain function into legal proceedings. Many believe that neuroscience may in some contexts usefully contribute to assessments of truth-telling, memories, pain and disability, competency, and criminal responsibility, to name just a few. Future possibilities may be even more extensive, as access to neuroimaging becomes more widespread and as neuroimaging datasets grow significantly in size and participant diversity.

Another dynamic area of neuroscience discovery has described methods to change the brain. Historically, the most powerful ways to change the brain have been through nutrition and education—as well as through drugs like stimulants (caffeine) and hallucinogens (mushrooms). Modern neuroscience offers specific drugs and devices to manipulate the brain through targeted stimulation or inhibition of particular neurotransmitter systems and brain centers.

Neuroscientists, physicists, and engineers are also exploring new ways to manipulate the brain through the use of light. The breakthrough method known as "optogenetics" is a method for very specific manipulation of the activation state of very particular groups of neurons. This is accomplished using sophisticated genetic methods to place specific kinds of ion channels in the membrane of particular neurons. The ion channels have the special property of being controlled by light. Thus, when a researcher shines the appropriate light on the tissue, only the neurons with the genetically modified channel are affected. The effect can be inhibition or excitation. It has been used successfully in experiments with rodents, but it is less useful in experiments with monkeys at the present time.

The purpose of this chapter is to explain the basics of the most widely utilized brain monitoring and manipulation techniques so that you can recognize the results provided by the methods and understand how they are produced. This will prepare you to ask the right questions when such information arises in a legal setting. The next chapter will consider in more detail the limitations and cautions that should be kept in mind when considering such findings. Also, the Appendix provides a detailed guide on how to read an fMRI brain imaging study.

The chapter proceeds in four sections. In Section A we review techniques for visualizing the structure of a living human's brain. In Section B we introduce techniques for visualizing how those structures are functioning. In Section C we discuss the research strategies that are employed to harness imaging technology for better understanding human cognition. In Section D we conclude with a discussion of direct interventions to modify human brain function.

A. BRAIN STRUCTURE

This section reviews four techniques available for visualizing the structure of a living human's brain.

1. X-Ray

In 1895, German physicist Wilhelm Röntgen was investigating the nature of cathode tube emissions. He noticed that when he shone the emitted rays onto a distant wall, a glow was seen even though solid objects blocked the path of the rays. He proposed that the glow was the result of a novel type of penetrating radiation, what was later termed the *X-ray*. To illustrate his findings, he published an image of the bones in his wife's hand with her wedding ring.

X-rays are familiar, especially if you have ever had a broken bone. X-rays have very high spatial resolution (about 0.1 mm), but they lack contrast. The electromagnetic waves that result in the X-ray image are absorbed to varying degrees by bone, brain, and other tissues. Being less dense than other structures in the body, the brain does not show up clearly on an X-ray image. This variable absorption results in dark images when reflected against objects with little density, and lighter grey or even white when reflected against objects with greater density. Bones appear white in an X-ray image because they are the densest material in the body.

While physicians have used X-rays to locate bone injuries for many years, new technology was developed to use X-rays to visualize soft tissues to some degree. Thus, X-ray technology can be helpful to detect cysts or tumors in the brain. Moreover, by introducing dyes with higher densities to increase the visual contrast, blood vessels can be observed.

2. Computed Axial Tomography

X-ray images are two-dimensional slices. *Computed Axial Tomography* (CAT or CT) computes the three-dimensional shape of the interior structure of the head from X-ray slices from all angles around the head. The math is complicated, but the concept is simple. If you wanted to determine the position of each person in a glass room, you would need to walk all the way around to view each perspective. From the collection of two-dimensional X-ray patterns, it is possible to reconstruct the three-dimensional composition of the interior of the head. Like X-ray images, high-density regions like bone are light, and low-density regions are dark. The typical spatial resolution for CT scanners is ~1 cm. After the technology's advent in the early 1970s, CT scans became the standard of care for detection and diagnosis of neurological damage. Although complications from CT scans are rare, some patients can have severe reactions to dyes injected to visualize blood vessels.

3. Magnetic Resonance Imaging

Magnetic Resonance Imaging (MRI), first used on humans in 1977, provides images of the brain with great anatomical detail. Unlike other imaging technology, MRI uses no damaging radiation or injected tracers, making the procedure non-invasive and safe. MRI reveals the inner structure of the brain with much more resolution than CT.

MRI takes advantage of the magnetic characteristics of the atoms that make up our bodies (and everything else). Atoms consist of a nucleus made of protons and neutrons surrounded by electrons. The protons spin on an axis; this makes them very tiny, weak magnets. The MRI scanner consists of a very large, powerful magnet shaped into a tube with a very thick wall. Magnet strength is measured in units of *Tesla* (T). While some advanced research centers have 7.5T magnets, and one university even has a 10.5T magnet, MRI scanners used today are typically either 1.5T or 3T. To appreciate the magnitude, a 3T magnet is roughly 80,000 times stronger than the Earth's magnetic field. So, if you were to walk into the room containing the magnet, you could feel the keys in your pocket pulled toward the magnet. This is why the procedure for MRI requires you to leave all metal outside the room. Similarly, when placed into the scanner, the axis of rotation of the trillions and trillions of subatomic particles of the brain becomes aligned with the axis of the magnetic field just as compass needles align to Earth's magnetic field.

This alignment sets the stage for the MRI measurement. Patterns of periodic radio wave energy pulses are applied to the tissue. These pulses are just large enough to knock the protons in water molecules out of alignment with the magnet. However, like a spinning top that returns to its upright axis when it is wobbled, the axis of the spinning protons realigns with the magnetic field. As they realign, they release energy that is detected by sensors positioned around the head.

Now, here's the amazing part that makes MRI work. The amount of time to realign and the amount of radio wave energy released by each proton is proportional to the environment in which the proton spins. Recall from Chapter 3 that the CNS is organized into gray matter, consisting of the cell bodies and dendrites of neurons and glia, and white matter, consisting of the myelinated axons of the neurons running from one part of the brain to another. It happens to be the case that the spinning proton realignment takes different amounts of time in gray and white matter. By mapping the pattern of radio wave energy throughout the head, the scanner calculates a three-dimensional representation of the brain's internal structure that distinguishes gray matter from white matter and any other structures that may be present.

To analyze MRI signals, the scanner divides the brain into a three-dimensional grid, something like the pixels of computer display monitors. In fact, these three-dimensional boxes are called *voxels*, short for volumetric pixels. Each voxel is 2 or 3 mm on each side, the size of a small pea, although newer methods resolve less than 1 mm. To appreciate this scale, recall that the cerebral cortex is just 2-3 mm thick.

MRI images provide a much clearer image of the brain than is possible with CT scans. Therefore, MRI scans make it possible to see the individual sulci and gyri of the cerebral cortex, the impressive size of the corpus callosum, and the fine detail of small, subcortical structures, such as the basal ganglia. The spatial resolution of MRI images depends on the strength of the magnetic field and other components of the system. A 1.5T system produces images with a resolution of 1 mm. In addition, by adjusting various parameters of the process, it is possible to create images emphasizing different aspects of brain structure.

In clinical care, MRI is used primarily to visualize brain structure and pathologies such as tumors, cysts, and brain injury. More recently, anatomical MRI images have been introduced in the courtroom as evidence for claims of brain damage. It is important, therefore, to appreciate the factors that affect the quality of MRI images. On the one hand, the quality of the MRI system such as magnet strength and numerous other technical features can produce higher or lower quality images that emphasize different aspects of brain structure. So, when you evaluate an MRI image critically, you need to ask questions about the settings of the equipment.

On the other hand, recall that the MRI process works by detecting the location of protons aligning faster or slower after being wobbled. If the head of the subject lying in the scanner moves, then this determination of location will be inaccurate, and the image will be blurrier. This is why researchers are always pleading with their subjects to lie still. Scientists have developed methods to correct for head movement in the scanner, but the corrections are never as good as a perfectly still head. Head movements are especially an issue when higher resolution images are produced, because they require longer scan times. So, when you evaluate an MRI image critically, you need to ask if the person was very still when the scan was done. Of course, if the person being scanned wishes to be uncooperative for some reason, then by simply moving her head slightly, the individual will corrupt the image.

Finally, as a practical matter, the MRI scanning process can be stressful and expensive. First, to get an MRI scan, you must lay within the rather narrow tube in the center of the magnet. Many people feel anxious or claustrophobic. Second, as noted above, high-resolution scans can take as long as 30 minutes throughout which you must lay perfectly still. Third, the machine is very loud when the energy pulses are produced. Subjects are usually given earplugs. Fourth, MRI images cannot be obtained from people with magnetic metal in their body; this includes pacemakers, joint replacements, and cochlear implants. Machinists who have small metal shavings embedded in their skin after years in the shop are also disqualified for MRI scans. Finally, MRI equipment is expensive to obtain and maintain, so the scans are costly.

4. Diffusion Tensor Imaging

Diffusion Tensor Imaging (DTI) is a method that relies on the same MRI equipment but extracts even more information. DTI is used to make inferences about the axon pathways passing through the white matter. DTI has been used in conjunction with MRI to study the developing and adolescent brain, where the formation of connections between neurons is of tremendous importance.

As with MRI, the mathematics of DTI is complicated, but the concept is simple. By way of analogy, recall the way water flows through a hose. The velocity of the water is higher along the axis of the tube than perpendicular to the axis. DTI is based on a similar observation. Axons are actually tubes through which the fluids of the neuron flow. So, by measuring the direction of diffusion of the water molecules with the spinning protons, it is possible to find parts of the brain where the diffusion or flow of the water is higher or lower. The diffusion is lower in the gray matter because the axons are not very well aligned. The diffusion is higher in the white matter where bundles of axons are aligned. When regions of high diffusion are found, the orientation of that diffusion can be determined. The DTI measure is found in each voxel. By tracing the direction of diffusion through neighboring voxels, in some cases it is possible to connect the dots and trace an axon bundle from one end to the other. For example, in the corpus callosum, the diffusion direction is all in the medial-lateral axis because that is how all the axon bundles are oriented.

Scientists are developing evermore complex and effective algorithms to trace the axon bundles more accurately because this provides the opportunity to examine the pattern of connections within living human brains. For example, recent work has used deep neural networks to resolve the structure found in DTI scans. The connectivity analysis has limits, though. One of the most severe is sorting out voxels where fiber pathways cross over each other. So this information is very useful and exciting, but it must be interpreted with caution. Given the current state of the art, for assessing traumatic brain injury, DTI is sensitive at the group level but is not yet reliable at the individual level. As discussed in Chapter 10, courts are now considering whether DTI evidence should be admissible as evidence of mild Traumatic Brain Injury.

Even if its ability to trace connections in the brain remains limited, DTI provides other information in the simple magnitude of directional diffusion. Thus, one can map the brain according to where directional diffusion is high or low. One can also compare brains on this measure. For example, researchers have found that the magnitude of directional diffusion in white matter changes as the brain develops through early life.

B. BRAIN FUNCTION

1. Introduction

CT and MRI provide information about the structure of the brain, but they do not provide information about activation within the brain. An array of other technologies is used to investigate brain function. These noninvasive methods measure either electrical signals from the surface of the head or local changes of blood oxygen levels. The relationship is complex and uncertain between either of these indirect measures and the nerve impulses and synaptic signals produced in the circuits introduced in Chapter 3. Collectively these methods have been referred to as *functional neuroimaging.*

The information collected with functional neuroimaging must be interpreted in the context of the processes occurring in the brain while the measurements are obtained. As you learned in Chapter 3, the occurrence of brain processes creates perceptions, emotions, and plans—indeed all of human psychology. Therefore, to obtain interpretable functional imaging data, the psychological testing conditions must be designed very carefully.

One of the earliest and still common approaches to reporting functional imaging data involves creating a map of how different parts of the brain appear active in different tasks or states such as moving a finger, looking at pictures of faces, reading lists of nouns, thinking of verbs that go with those nouns, imagining playing tennis, weighing purchasing options, considering moral dilemmas, and determining whether a defendant is guilty. This can lead to conclusions that claim to pinpoint particular mental processes to distinct regions of the brain. This has been criticized as a modern form of phrenology, an idea popular over a century ago that claimed to map unique function to discrete areas of the cerebral cortex. As you learned in Chapter 3, the brain works because it is organized into many complex circuits spanning cortical and subcortical centers. Thus, although different parts of the brain contribute to different functions, do not be seduced by the fallacy of *exclusive* localization of complex function—as if single parts of the brain do just one thing.

Each technique used for neuroimaging has pros and cons. Each opens a window of a particular range of space and time. Recording the nerve impulses in single neurons provides the highest resolution in space and time, but this requires invasive methods that can be employed only in serious clinical conditions in humans. The noninvasive methods sacrifice resolution in time and space but expose function of the living human brain. If interpretations remain limited within the bounds of the techniques, then the evidence obtained from each should converge on a unified and more nearly correct understanding of brain function as it produces behavior.

2. Measuring Brain Electrical Signals

You learned in Chapter 3 that neurons signal to each other through nerve impulses. By inserting small electrical probes into the brain, the impulses from individual neurons can be recorded (referred to as *single-unit recordings*), as can the impulses from populations of tens or hundreds of neurons in a small region (referred to as *multi-unit recordings*). These electrical probes can also measure the fluctuations of electrical potentials associated with synaptic transmission in the local region (*local field potentials*). Although commonly obtained in animal research studies, these measurements are also obtained from human patients during certain types of brain surgery to treat disorders such as Parkinson's disease or epilepsy. The patients are usually awake and interacting with physicians during surgery to help the surgeons locate the particular regions of the brain necessary for the treatment. Most patients give prior consent for research use of the recordings, so information like that summarized in Chapter 3 can be obtained. The patterns of activity measured in the human brain are not different from what is observed in animal studies. This engenders confidence that measurements of human brain signals can be compared usefully to what is found in more rigorously controlled experiments with animals.

As you will learn in Chapter 20, these electrical probes are used for brain-machine interfaces that enable the deaf to hear, the paralyzed to move, and other applications. One of the limits of the current generation of electrical probes is the damage that they cause when they are inserted into the brain and the response of the immune system to the foreign body. Consequently, many researchers are testing other materials and smaller probes that can detect neuron impulses but cause less or no damage. Probes have been developed with diameters comparable to the cell bodies of the cells in the brain (25 micrometers). When such thin probes are inserted, they slide between rather than tear through the blood vessels and other brain tissue.

Now, while it is typically not possible to insert probes into the brains of humans, a weak electrical signal can be recorded from the surface of the head. This recording method is known as the *electroencephalograph*. You can decipher the term into "electro," meaning electrical, "encephalo," meaning brain, and "graph," meaning plot for display and measurement. You can abbreviate it as EEG, but many refer to this signal as a brainwave. Closely related to the EEG is the *magnetoencephalograph* (MEG). To understand EEG and MEG, we need to review the basic physics of electromagnetism. Electrical current happens when charged particles move in a circuit. The amount of current that can flow depends on the electrical potential, also known as voltage, that is present. If there is no voltage, it's like a dead battery; no charge can flow, so no work can be done to run a flashlight, a computer or a brain. When current flows, an electrical field can be measured, and with every electric field, an associated magnetic field is also created. You can learn how this is so in physics textbooks, but for our purposes this should be enough background information.

You learned in Chapter 3 that most of the neurons in the cerebral cortex are called pyramidal neurons because they have a pyramid-shaped cell body with an elongated dendrite stretching up toward the pia surface. When the elongated pyramidal neurons are depolarized by their synaptic inputs, they become tiny batteries with a positive and a negative end. When millions of these neurons become polarized, they create an electrical field of sufficient strength to be measured on the surface of the head. This randomly oscillating electrical potential, the EEG, can be measured with relatively inexpensive equipment. Much more expensive equipment can measure the magnetic field associated with the electric field, the MEG. The EEG and the MEG are two ways of recording the same brain processes, and, being less expensive, EEG is used much more commonly in the legal arena.

The EEG is obtained by placing small metal disks on the scalp of a participant. A recording device measures the millionth of a volt electrical potential between each disk and a reference probe, usually on the earlobes. The recording disks are typically placed on the head according to an international convention known as the 10-20 (or 10-10) system. The numbers refer to the distances between recording disks, being either 20% or 10% of the total front-back or right-left distance of the skull. Each recording disk location is labeled according to the cortical lobe beneath the site, e.g., pre-frontal (Fp), frontal (F), temporal (T), parietal (P), occipital (O). Sites over the right hemisphere are indexed by even numbers, and those over the left, by odd. Sites on the midline are indexed as "z." An attorney dealing with a case involving EEG and fMRI measurements will benefit from knowing how the "10-20" convention maps onto brain structures observed with MRI across individuals. These publications provide this information: Masako Okamoto et al., *Three-Dimensional Probabilistic Anatomical Cranio-Cerebral Correlation via the International 10-20 System Oriented for Transcranial Functional Brain Mapping*, 21 Neuroimage 99 (2004); L. Koessler et al., *Automated Cortical Projection of EEG Sensors: Anatomical Correlation via the International 10-10 System*, 46 Neuroimage 64 (2009).

The EEG detects randomly rhythmic fluctuations of electrical signals produced by the brain that oscillate between peaks and troughs. Researchers measure the interval between or frequency of successive peaks and troughs. The frequency is measured in units of cycles-per-second (also known as Hertz or Hz).* They also measure the amplitude from the peaks to the troughs in units of microvolts (millionths of a volt). The frequency and amplitude of the EEG oscillation varies with behavioral state. When subjects are alert, the EEG shows higher frequency and lower amplitude. As the subject/brain relaxes, the EEG shows lower frequency and higher amplitude. As the subject/brain goes to sleep, the EEG shows even

---

* To facilitate communication between researchers, the frequency ranges of EEG have been given an arbitrary nomenclature, which is shown here for your reference. The unit of measurement of frequency is named for the German scientist, Hertz, and is abbreviated Hz. One Hz is one cycle per second.

Frequency range	Up to 4 Hz	4 to 8 Hz	8 to 13 Hz	13 to 30 Hz	30 to 100 Hz
Name	Delta	Theta	Alpha	Beta	Gamma

lower frequency and higher amplitude; however, the waves are interrupted with intermittent high frequency and high amplitude signals called spindles. When the subject/brain suffers an epileptic seizure, the EEG exhibits pronounced series of high amplitude spikes. The information obtained from the EEG is invaluable for diagnosing and monitoring the treatment of epilepsy, sleep disorders, and other neurological diseases. The EEG is also used to assess brain death in some states because a brain that cannot produce EEG cannot produce behavior or consciousness. As you will learn in Chapter 9, this has important implications for the status of a person as living or dead, which touches on areas of the law such as wills, trusts, and estates, as well as insurance.

A recent and particularly exciting development is the use of EEG in prosthetic devices. In Chapter 20 you will learn how sophisticated computer algorithms can read the brainwaves from a person who is totally paralyzed to guide a cursor on a computer monitor and to write emails, for example.

Before the development of inexpensive, powerful computers, EEG data were recorded on very long strips of paper, and investigators did measurements by hand. As digital EEG recording and analysis became possible, a form of computer analysis has been developed known as quantitative EEG (QEEG). As described above, the EEG consists of rhythmic fluctuations. QEEG simply employs well-established algorithms to decompose the fluctuations into different frequency components.* The EEG is usually recorded from an array of dozens of electrical contacts arranged around the head. Based on what you learned in Chapter 3, it should not be a surprise that the brainwaves recorded over different regions of the brain differ in various ways.

The QEEG approach plots the magnitude of the different frequency components on an image of the head, usually in vivid colors. Some call this a "brain map," but you should appreciate that it is an image constructed from mathematical calculations performed on the brainwaves. These mathematical calculations are only loosely related to the operations that the brain actually performs. Nevertheless, researchers have found that the frequency content of the brainwaves varies with the location of the recording contacts and mental state. They have also found that the QEEG pattern varies across individuals but seems to be replicable when measured at different times from the same individual. Researchers are seeking to develop a database of the natural variability of QEEG patterns against which to judge deviations that may be informative clinically for diagnosis or measuring effects of medications. Many investigators employ the QEEG approach for research studies, and some businesses provide access to this measurement for commercial purposes. In the neurolaw arena, as you will see in Chapter 8, courts are weighing the admissibility of QEEG in novel legal contexts.

Sophisticated computer analysis permits another approach using EEG that has been much more informative scientifically. Consider a participant responding to stimuli to perform a task such as pressing the right button when the stimulus

---

* If you remember sine waves from mathematics, then you can appreciate that the EEG can be decomposed into a collection of sine waves with different frequencies and amplitudes. The quantitative characterization of that collection of sine waves is just what QEEG does. If you don't remember sine waves, then you can think of QEEG as decomposing a musical chord into which keys on a piano were struck and how hard.

displayed is an "O" and the left button when it is an "X" (or pressing the right button if judging an act as purposive and the left if reckless). Embedded in the rhythmic fluctuations of the EEG recording from the participant are small signals related to presentation of stimuli, production of responses and other cognitive processes. By using a computer to remove the random noise in the EEG recorded over dozens of testing trials, investigators can measure the smaller electrical signals related to the events of the task. The noise is removed by measuring the EEG synchronized on one of the events in the testing trial (like presentation of the stimulus or pressing the button), so the signal that is known as an *event-related potential* (ERP). The more trials that can be sampled, the more reliable the ERP signal because they arise from the summed polarization of large groups of neurons responding collectively to the events. Scientists have described ERPs related to sensory processes, attention, memory, intention, body movements, and monitoring of consequences. In other words, all of the cognitive processes described in Chapter 3 have associated ERPs through which the brain correlates can be studied.

The scientific foundation of ERPs is much stronger than that of QEEG. ERPs are commonly used in clinical settings. ERPs measured with visual stimuli, for example, are of particular importance in detecting multiple sclerosis, a disease arising from loss of axonal myelination. When demyelination occurs in the optic nerve, the early peaks of a visual ERP are delayed. In neurolaw, as we will see in Chapter 15, some have proposed using ERP measures for lie detection.

EEG provides good information about the timing of brain processes because it can measure neural events with millisecond (1/1,000th of a second) resolution. On the other hand, it lacks resolution in space, so it is difficult to determine where in the brain particular EEG signals arise. It is a very common tool, though, because EEG data can be obtained using equipment that is much less expensive than that necessary for the two neuroimaging tools discussed next.

3. Positron Emission Tomography and Single Photon Emission Computed Tomography

The techniques discussed in the next two sections assess neural events indirectly through their metabolic consequences. These metabolic consequences are measured through local changes in blood flow and oxygen utilization. Blood flow delivers oxygen and glucose, the basic sustenance of neurons and glia, so when certain regions are more active and thus more demanding of energy, blood flow will redirect oxygen and glucose toward these regions. Techniques based on these indirect measures are popular because they result in vivid two-dimensional or three-dimensional images of brain activity.

Positron Emission Tomography (PET) requires injecting a radioactive tracer into a subject's blood stream. Different tracers offer different pictures of brain function. Some tracers reveal the locations of specific neurotransmitter receptors. Such a tracer will flow to all parts of the body but will collect where the receptors are located in the brain. For example, a PET tracer targeting dopamine receptors will collect in the striatum of the basal ganglia. Being radioactive, the tracer emits subatomic particles as they degrade. These particles are detected by an array of sensors that provide information used to reconstruct the three-dimensional location from which the particle was emitted in the brain.

Other tracers reveal locations where neuron activation is higher than elsewhere. A PET tracer with radioactive glucose or oxygen is injected into the subject's blood stream, and the scan is done while she is engaged in a sensory, motor, or cognitive task. In this situation, more blood will flow to parts of the brain with more neural activity and more oxygen or glucose will be consumed. Hence, the regions with the most active neurons will have preferential accumulation of the tracer. Regions of more or less blood flow are identified by the detection of more or fewer particle emissions.

To obtain more information about the role of brain areas in performing experimental tasks, the tracer is administered twice: once during a control condition and once during an experimental condition. The difference in blood flow between the testing conditions measures the degree of involvement of different parts of the brain in a given experimental task. Thus, for example, if the experimental condition involves presentation of visual stimuli and the control condition is darkness, then the brain image will show elevated blood flow in visual processing areas in occipital cortex. On the other hand, if the experimental condition involves generating verbs in response to nouns and the control condition is just repeating nouns, then the brain image will show elevated blood flow in language processing and production areas in temporal and frontal cortex. Finally, if the experimental condition involves imagining producing a sequence of finger movements and the control condition is actually producing the sequence of finger movements, then the brain image will show elevated blood flow in an area of frontal cortex responsible for planning movements. In Chapter 9 we will learn that these patterns of activation can be used to infer whether an individual who is unresponsive is actually alert and aware.

The major advantage of PET is obtaining information about local processes in the human brain. This information is more elaborate than just blood flow because PET allows researchers to use different kinds of radioactive tracers. As noted above, the tracers can be incorporated into compounds used naturally by the brain (such as glucose or water to look at metabolic use) or into molecules that bind to receptors or other sites of drug action. For example, the location and density of dopamine receptors can be measured with PET. Thus, PET can be used to trace the pathway of any compound in the human brain as long as it can be labeled with a radioactive tracer. New tracers are being synthesized to explore various molecules and processes with dozens in clinical use and hundreds in research use. The most common tracer used for clinical PET scanning is *fluorodeoxyglucose* (also called FDG) because it reveals the utilization of glucose. Researchers have also used PET to obtain images of the location where particular neurotransmitters such as dopamine are more concentrated.

PET has many disadvantages. First, radioactive tracers must be injected into the blood stream. Beyond the potential health risks posed by the radiation, a facility must have the equipment and expertise necessary to produce the radioactive tracers because they degrade at a rapid rate. Second, the resolution of PET in time is very low because ~40 seconds is needed to count enough particles to derive the map of brain activity. Rapid changes in brain state that could be observed through EEG or MEG will be invisible to PET. Third, the spatial resolution of the activity maps is very coarse, on the order of centimeters. Consequently, variation across individual neurons or local circuits that could be observed with single-unit recordings will be blurred by PET.

With the development of functional MRI (described below), the use of PET in research has decreased to some extent. Still, PET offers particular advantages for diagnosis of brain disease. In neurolaw, PET scans have been allowed in criminal trials as evidence, as we saw in Chapter 2 to locate a cyst in the skull of Herbert Weinstein.

We close this section by introducing a method that approximates PET. *Single Photon Emission Computed Tomography* (SPECT) traces the emission of a radioactive tracer injected into the bloodstream. Unlike PET, though, SPECT uses tracers that do not decay rapidly. Using SPECT, researchers effectively take a snapshot of brain activity at the moment the tracers are injected. Thus, relative to PET, SPECT has less spatial resolution and no timing resolution. However, SPECT is more affordable and thus more widely available, so it may appear more often in neurolaw cases.

4. Functional MRI

Functional Magnetic Resonance Imaging (fMRI) is a specialized application of MR technology to measure levels of brain activity indirectly through changes in oxygen carried by regional blood flow. You learned above that MRI is based on the magnetic spin properties of atoms in the brain. Recall now that blood transports oxygen from the lungs to the body using a protein called *hemoglobin*. Oxygen binds to hemoglobin (becoming *oxyhemoglobin*) in the lungs and transports it to the organs of the body where it is released from hemoglobin (becoming *deoxyhemoglobin*). fMRI is based on the fortunate fact that oxyhemoglobin is not magnetic and deoxyhemoglobin *is* magnetic and perturbs the local magnetic field. This difference is the basis of fMRI, because the scanner can detect regions with more oxyhemoglobin relative to deoxyhemoglobin as a consequence of demands from neural activity. This signal is called the *blood-oxygenation level-dependent* (BOLD) signal.

The typical fMRI study uses roughly 200,000 voxels, 100,000 of which enclose the cerebral cortex and underlying white matter. The BOLD signal measured in each voxel is compared between a baseline period and an active period. This is just like the comparison described for PET above. To create the fMRI image, a color is assigned to each voxel according to the magnitude of the BOLD signal during a test period compared to the magnitude of the BOLD signal during a control baseline period. While the color assignments are completely arbitrary, it has become standard to use warm hues (red and yellow) to represent increased BOLD and cool hues (blue and green) to represent decreased BOLD. Because the data are so complex, researchers continue to develop different ways to visualize brain circuits and patterns of activation, appreciating that different conclusions can be derived from different ways of analyzing and showing the data.

The description of the method here will be as simplified as the procedure is not. Because this method is becoming so important for law, though, you should know what is actually done. Particular limitations of this technique are considered in more depth in the next chapter and in the Appendix.

One of the most important things to know is this: fMRI images, with "hot" and "cold" spots, are not just photographs of the brain. fMRI brain images are constructed through a complex sequence of computerized analytical steps. One of the first is called *slice-timing correction*. The entire brain is scanned in a series of successively measured two-dimensional slices. Accordingly, the last slice is obtained after the first in the sequence. Slice-timing correction accounts for this time difference across the brain scan slices. This is particularly important for event-related designs in which the BOLD signal changes are measured relative to particular testing events. Another processing step is *motion correction*, which adjusts for incidental head movements produced during the scan. Next, if the scans from multiple individuals will be compared directly, then differences in brain size and shape must be accounted for. This is accomplished through *coregistration*, which involves adjusting the size and shape of different parts of individual brains to bring them into registration with each other. Commonly, this is done by transforming each subject's brain to match the size and shape of a standard brain, like distorting each person's face to map it onto one standard face. A French physician named Talairach established a popular standard based on postmortem sections of a 60-year-old female. She happened to have a smaller-than-average brain, though, so most subjects' brains must be adjusted considerably, and that introduces some error. Such standards of measurement are necessary for science, and the error introduced from these standardization procedures is well known and accounted for. However, an fMRI scan used in a neurolaw context is usually of a single individual. Finally, the raw BOLD signals have incidental, noisy variation across the voxels, so another processing step involves smoothing across voxels to remove the random noise.

Once all of that pre-processing is done, the real analysis can begin. Many approaches have been developed for discovering voxels or sets of voxels that exhibit more or less BOLD signal in relation to testing events and inferred mental states. You should appreciate that increased BOLD happens when both excitatory and inhibitory neurons are more active. In other words, higher BOLD should not be confused with higher neural excitation even though the BOLD signal is so often referred to simply as "activation."

One popular approach is known as a *general-linear model* (GLM). A GLM identifies voxels with BOLD signal changes that relate to specific events in a task. Typically, this analysis results in patterns of voxels located in particular parts of the brain that have BOLD signal changes that are statistically related to a testing variable such as a task condition or an experimental or diagnostic group. A second approach is known as *independent component analysis*. Independent component analysis describes how different regions interact with each other instead of which region has more or less BOLD signal. A third powerful approach is known as *multi-voxel pattern analysis* (MVPA). MVPA searches for patterns of BOLD signal across all or many voxels throughout the brain. This approach is sometimes referred to as "brain reading" because different voxel patterns can be used to distinguish specific mental states. The computer tools for this analysis originate from a specialty in artificial intelligence known as machine learning.

Brain images differ from photographs in other ways too. The brain images one sees are nearly always comparisons (often referred to as contrasts) between two different behavioral states. In "activation paradigms," for instance, subject responses are typically measured and compared between two or more task conditions during a series of scans conducted in a single experimental session. Regional differences in the measured signal between various tasks are considered to reflect differences in the amount of local neuronal activity associated with performance of those tasks. However, the fMRI signal is very weak and can be corrupted by numerous problems with the machine (such as gradual changes of the strength of the magnetic field) and with the subject (for example, moving the head). Hence, a relatively standard set of "pre-processing" steps is performed to prepare the data for the actual analysis. These steps include accounting for incidental movements of the subject's head, for incidental distortions in the strength of the magnetic field through the brain and smoothing the signal through time and across adjacent voxels to remove incidental noise.

A multitude of approaches to analyzing fMRI data have been developed, and more are invented every year as this method develops further. One approach employs basic statistical methods to identify voxels in which the BOLD signal varies significantly with specific events or experimental manipulations. Such a finding is then interpreted as an indication of a regionally-specific "activation" associated with an experimental condition or group. The locations where BOLD signal changes are of most interest are referred to as *regions of interest* (ROI). Other approaches seek to identify networks of brain regions that collectively co-vary with condition or group. Yet another approach takes advantage of differences between individual subjects to identify differences in patterns of brain activation.

fMRI has significant advantages relative to PET. First, fMRI uses signals intrinsic to the brain rather than signals originating from exogenous, radioactive probes. This means that subjects can be tested repeatedly with fMRI, providing the opportunity to obtain more data from each individual. Second, fMRI offers greater spatial resolution than PET (a few millimeters compared to almost a centimeter), allowing more clarity about the location of brain damage or other events. Third, fMRI offers better temporal resolution than PET (a few seconds compared to many seconds or minutes), affording more informative studies of cognitive processes as described in the next section.

To be clear, the temporal resolution of fMRI lags far behind the ERP measurements described above. To address this, researchers are combining EEG and fMRI in the same subjects. Based on these advantages MRI devices have become ubiquitous in clinical settings. Recall that in Chapter 1 you learned of a vivid neurolaw application of fMRI research with convicted criminals using a device carried to prisons in a tractor trailer.

Scientists continue to gain better understanding of the signals measured by fMRI and are seeking to improve the spatial and functional resolution of fMRI. On the one hand, recent research has drawn attention to the BOLD signal that can be measured in the white matter of the brain. A weaker signal that has actually been ignored until the late 2010s, the BOLD signal in white matter might improve the accuracy of tracing connections in the human brain. On the other hand, researchers are developing substances, either particular chemicals or genetically modified proteins, that can be delivered into the brain safely and then visualized through MR imaging. Referred to as molecular fMRI, the resulting signals will measure particular aspects of neuron signaling instead of the complex coupling between neural activity and blood flow.

5. Functional Near-Infrared Spectroscopy

Like fMRI, *functional near-infrared spectroscopy* (fNIRS) measures brain activity noninvasively through the hemodynamic signal associated with neuron behavior. The method is based on the fact that skin, bone, and brain tissue are mostly transparent to near-infrared light, but hemoglobin absorbs the light strongly. Hence, the amount of light absorbed will vary with the volume, flow and oxygenation of the blood through which the light passes. The signal is the same as that used for a pulse oximeter that may be put on your finger when you visit the hospital or clinic. fNIRS is accomplished by placing a band or cap on the head to position light emitters and detectors. Unlike fMRI, it detects signals only near the surface of the skull because it measures the absorption of near infrared light that is shined into the head. Nevertheless, the signal is good enough to control brain-machine interfaces. Further unlike fMRI, the equipment necessary to obtain this measure are inexpensive and portable.

6. Field-Based and Point-of-Care Neuroimaging

To date, if you wanted a brain scan you had to go to a hospital or scientific research facility. But the advent of cheaper, portable neuroimaging means that neuroimaging will soon be utilized as a field-based research tool and at the point of care. Already researchers are taking mobile EEG and fNIRS into the field, allowing for real-time measurement of brain activity as children learn, athletes play sports, and bikers pedal around the city. One study even put EEG recording devices on an entire classroom of students to measure how the brain processes dynamic group interactions. In addition, researchers are now developing methods for mobile PET, mobile MEG, and even mobile MRI.

As described above, MRI traditionally requires a large, heavy scanner, powerful magnet, liquid helium for cooling, and a dedicated room with radiofrequency (RF) shielding, sound proofing, and a large power supply. To date, "mobile MRI" has meant placing a traditional MRI machine on a flat-bed trailer and driving it to a new location, then imaging under many of the same constraints as in conventional MRI. New advances in engineering, physics, and AI offer new possibilities for brain data acquisition. It is expected that clinical-grade magnetic resonance images (with high spatial and contrast resolution, equivalent to those generated by MRI with 1.5T magnetic field strength) can be produced from machines that are much smaller; that sit in a room without RF shielding; run on batteries, power generator, or a standard 120-V outlet; and that do not require an elaborate helium cooling system.

High-quality MR images are produced using one of two strategies. The first, called "ultra-low field" MRI, uses a smaller, less powerful magnet to acquire imaging data, and then relies upon advanced techniques to extract signals from noisy data. In 2020, the company Hyperfine received FDA 510(k) clearance for its bedside MRI system. The founder of the company remarked that they had realized their "dream to create a portable, affordable MRI system. . . . [We've] built something astonishing, something disruptive."* Other disruptive neuroimaging technologies are also being pursued. For instance, the NIH BRAIN Initiative has funded research on portable "high field" MRI, which retains the high signal-to-noise ratio of 1.5T, even while reducing the size of the magnet. Although the resulting magnetic field is very nonuniform, new RF pulse and image reconstruction strategies are being developed.

Mobile neuroimaging raises tantalizing possibilities. As a direct to consumer (DTC) technology, some business plans envision a brain scanner in every pharmacy. For researchers, mobile neuroimaging will allow for new research designs and for access to underserved and geographically remote populations. What about the law?

---

* Press Release, Hyperfine, *World's First Bedside MRI System Receives FDA 510(k) Clearance* (Feb. 12, 2020).

Could brain scanners also be located in police stations, prisons, and courtrooms? Mobile neuroimaging technologies raise unique ethical and legal questions because existing recommendations have assumed that this equipment would be located within a medical or research facility and have not yet considered their use in a highly mobile context and as a potential DTC service.

C. TASK DESIGN IN FUNCTIONAL IMAGING

1. Introduction

The brain is constantly active, blood is always flowing, and most of the brain's regulation of blood flow is not related to particular tasks or cognitive states. Accordingly, a BOLD signal in a brain area in and of itself tells us that the cells in that area are functioning—but what does that function actually mean? How do we know whether someone is in pain, is remembering a vivid memory, or is exercising self-control? Answering questions like these are not easy, and as the next chapter explores, one should use great caution in evaluating research that claims to do mind reading. But cognitive neuroscientists are making important advances, and to understand how they are doing this we need to review experimental design.

Researchers use many experimental designs. But one described below is the *block design* study, using *subtraction* techniques. In block designs, subjects lie flat in the scanner while they see alternating blocks (groups) of images or text on the screen in front of them. The blocks are designed so that the only difference between them identifies the cognitive process of interest. For example, an experimenter might alternate between showing the subject a set of images of places and a set of images of faces. The researcher compares the brain activity of the subject when she is looking at places versus when she is looking at faces. This comparison is carried out by "subtracting" the brain activity while looking at places from the activity while looking at faces. The differences found after the subtraction are thought to be the additional brain activity for processing faces or places.

Similar designs have been used for investigating complex cognitive states like intentions, even states as mysterious as "love." But whether such designs are truly informative and appropriate for a given mental state remains an open question. Experimental design should be scrutinized just as carefully as the technology used to carry out the experiment. This section provides a general introduction to the details of those designs.

2. Functional Decomposition and Experimental Design

Complex cognitive tasks are composed of numerous sub-operations. For instance, most commonly a subject receives instructions (e.g., press this key after one stimulus and another key after a different stimulus), perceives stimuli (perhaps the different stimuli are difficult to distinguish), performs certain cognitive operations (such as remembering the instructions), and responds overtly in some prescribed way (pressing this and not that key). *Functional decomposition* refers to the conceptual breakdown of a task into its component operations, carving the task at its functional joints.

Carefully planned functional decomposition lies at the heart of successful neuroimaging experiments. The ideal experiment creates conditions that hold most functional components as fixed as possible and manipulate just one variable at a time. In this way, differences in activation between scan conditions can be clearly attributed to the manipulated variable. The experimental design must be informed by knowledge derived from previous psychological studies of the component operations and their relationships.

3. Task Types

Three types of tasks are used in neuroimaging activation studies. (1) The target task requires the participant to perform the sequence of operations of interest (e.g., decide whether a scenario explained in a short paragraph is a crime). (2) The comparison task requires participants to perform a sequence of operations that differs from the target task in a critical and informative manner (e.g., decide whether the same scenario involves a male or a female actor); more than one comparison task may be necessary. (3) The baseline task requires the participant to perform a very basic sequence of operations (or even nothing at all) (e.g., read a paragraph of the same length as the experimental scenarios to control for the eye movements and basic comprehension that occur during reading).

Investigators then contrast the activation in different parts of the brain between the different types of task. The contrast of brain activation between the target or comparison tasks and the baseline tasks reveals the brain regions that are involved in accomplishing the additional operations (like interpreting a scenario as opposed to just moving eyes and reading). If the baseline task is not designed correctly, then the activation observed in the target and comparison tasks can be misleading. For example, if the baseline task required simply fixing gaze on a single letter in the middle of the screen, then the brain activation in the target and comparison tasks would be derived not only from the operations of reading and interpreting the scenario but also simply moving the eyes.

The contrast of brain activation between the target and comparison tasks is intended to reveal the brain regions that are involved in accomplishing the specific operation of interest (in this case, judging guilt versus innocence), while accounting for all of the other operations necessary to perform the overall task (moving eyes, sitting upright, breathing, etc.). If the comparison task is not designed correctly, then the activation observed in the target task can be misleading. For example, if the comparison task required simply reading a paragraph silently, then the brain activation in the target task could be derived not only from the operation of judging guilt versus innocence but also from just interpreting the text.

Selection of the tasks involved in a study is critically important, strongly affecting its interpretability and outcome. Baseline tasks are typically chosen to be simple operations that lack the demands of the target and comparison tasks. Many researchers use baseline tasks in all their studies, regardless of the study's goal. This makes it easier to begin to find common patterns of activation across numerous studies and allows the possibility of future meta-analyses. Regardless of the choice of baseline task, it is of primary importance to be aware of the cognitive operations required by that task, as well as others in which the subject might engage.

Comparison tasks are more complex, requiring most high-level operations chosen because either they differ in some specific way from the target task or because they share important features with the target task, or both. The choice of comparison tasks is a major determinant of the ultimate perspicuity and value of a study: Careful choice of tasks can go far in disclosing the functional roles of one or a few brain regions, while inappropriate choice of tasks can result in a study that fails to answer any specific cognitive question.

4. Blocked Designs

The ability of fMRI to acquire data in brief time slices confers important advantages over other imaging methods, such as PET. Blocked designs are necessary in PET and used to be common in fMRI but are becoming less so. In blocked designs, subjects perform one type of task for a period or "block" of time (in fMRI usually between 10 and 30 seconds, and in PET for several minutes), e.g., decide whether a scenario explained in a short paragraph is a crime. Then they switch to another type of task, e.g., decide whether the same scenario involves a male or a female actor. Blocked designs are relatively easy to analyze, for the data are averaged across blocks of the same task type and subtracted from data averaged across blocks of a different task type. The resulting activation pattern can be compared with a control condition when the subject is either not doing the task or doing some other sort of task. The information one gains from such studies reflects aggregate differences in brain activity in different regions between the two task periods.

Blocked designs have some serious limitations, however. Some tasks are performed differently when one knows exactly what sort of task one has to perform, and the ability to distinguish between different trials is lost. Thus, certain kinds of information regarding differences in task or performance cannot be investigated by this method, such as differences between correct and error trials. In other words, blocked designs limit the specificity with which brain activation can be associated with particular cognitive processes.

5. Event-Related Designs

A marked improvement over the blocked design, called *event-related design*, takes advantage of the temporal resolution available with fMRI. Event-related designs are more powerful than blocked designs for exploring cognitive function and describing more subtle differences in task performance. Hence, it is now widely used. An event-related experimental design measures the BOLD signal synchronized on various events during a task such as presentation of the short paragraph to read and production of the response reporting whether it describes a crime or whether the actor is male or female. The signal is then averaged across many experimental trials so that the random fluctuations of the BOLD signal that are unrelated to the brain processes performing the task cancel out, leaving the systematic variation of the BOLD signal that is related to performance of the task. The fMRI response to an event starts after 1-2 seconds, peaks at 5-6 seconds, and returns to the starting level after 12-20 seconds. Although this is much slower than event-related EEG and MEG, it is still fast enough to provide useful information if the task events are designed properly.

Different types of trials (target, comparison, and baseline) can be randomly inter-leaved. After the data are collected, computers sort, align and average the BOLD signal for each type of trial. The location and timing of the BOLD signal occurring immediately before or after task events is contrasted across trial types to draw con-clusions about the brain processes occurring during the tasks. This approach can reveal differences in brain activation related to, for example, the types of stimuli, whether or not the subject performed correctly, and the time taken to respond. Event-related designs are typically analyzed by correlating activation patterns with mathematical models of task performance that incorporate various task-related aspects of the experiment, such as stimulus onset, response timing, response type, etc. The models are based on functional decompositions; the validity of the results will depend on the accuracy of the models.

6. Multi-Voxel Pattern Analysis

The procedures described above emphasize the magnitude and timing of BOLD activation in particular parts of the brain, referred to as *regions of interest* (ROI). More recently, an entirely different analysis approach has been devised that exam-ines the pattern of activation across the voxels throughout a brain region or even the entire brain. This is known as *multi-voxel pattern analysis* (MVPA). This analysis includes the BOLD signal in all the voxels during the various conditions in the experimental trials. Particular statistical methods then use the information in all the voxels to discriminate between the task conditions. This approach provides greater sensitivity to detect BOLD pattern differences between testing conditions than the conventional ROI analyses. MVPA results are often offered in terms of "brain read-ing," whereby particular mental states or representational content is decoded from fMRI activity patterns.

D. HUMAN BRAIN MANIPULATION

This section explores different ways—temporary and permanent, planned and unplanned—by which the human brain is manipulated. Subsection 1 examines how brain lesions have been used to study mechanisms of disease, as well as more generally how the brain works together as a whole. In particular, it focuses on surgi-cally created lesions, some techniques that are obsolete and others that are still used today in the treatment of certain diseases. The next subsections describe techniques that researchers use to temporarily improve or disrupt brain function. Finally, we survey briefly the use of drugs to manipulate brain function.

1. Brain Damage

The brain can be damaged in many ways. A localized area of damage is referred to as a *lesion*. Brain lesions occur due to "insults" like stroke (blockage or bursting of blood vessels), tumors (cancerous growth of neurons, of glia, or of meninges), cysts (cavities between the skull and brain formed by the meninges that fill with cerebrospinal fluid or air), and traumatic injuries (like the tamping iron blown through Phineas Gage's head). Traumatic injuries can be very localized (such as penetrating gun shots) or diffuse (concussions). Common causes of traumatic brain injury include falls and automobile accidents. In addition, the wars in Iraq and Afghanistan have resulted in a large increase in patients with *closed head injuries* as a result of concussions suffered during explosions. Brain damage may also result from participation in contact sports. Degenerative diseases such as Alzheimer's, Huntington's, and Parkinson's result from loss of neurons in particular parts of the brain.

Historically, some of the first insights into brain function were obtained by correlating the site of the lesion with the type of changes of behavior. Often the location of the brain damage could not be determined until after death because the non-invasive imaging methods described above were not available. Nevertheless, particular patterns of symptoms were described. Neurologists and psychiatrists distinguish *positive symptoms* from *negative symptoms*. Positive symptoms are abnormal behaviors resulting from the brain damage. Examples include abnormal movements such as the tremor and rigidity of Parkinson's disease or the hallucinations of psychosis. Negative symptoms are absent or deficient behaviors resulting from the brain damage. Examples include blindness or paralysis consequent to a stroke damaging visual or motor cortex. Brain damage symptoms can be categorized as perceptual, motor, cognitive, and mood. Damage to the primary sensory areas of the cerebral cortex and associated structures results in outright loss of sensation such as loss of hearing or vision. Damage to higher-order sensory areas in the parietal and temporal lobes results in more complex perceptual disorders such as disorientation in space and lack of recognition of complex objects including faces and speech.

Damage to the movement systems of the brain result in another pattern of symptoms. Neurologists distinguish *lower motor neuron* symptoms from *upper motor neuron* symptoms. Lower motor neuron signs include the weakness, atrophy, and reduced or absent reflexes consequent to damage to the spinal cord or neurons innervating the muscles (as in muscular dystrophy or Lou Gehrig's disease). Upper motor neuron signs occur in groups of muscles (like the side of the face or a whole arm) without atrophy and increased reflexes consequent to damage in the brain that removes control over the spinal cord.

Damage to primary motor cortex and associated structures results in a pattern of symptoms, referred to as *hemiplegia*, that include loss of voluntary movement with changes in postural tone and reflexes on one side of the body. The problems are found on the side of the body opposite the hemisphere with the lesion because of the pattern of nerve pathways between brain and body.

Damage to higher order motor structures result in syndromes collectively referred to as *apraxia* that is the inability to produce a movement that is not due to paralysis but instead seems to be a loss of a specific skill. The various forms of apraxia occur depending on the particular site of the lesion. Examples include misuse of objects due to lack of recognition, difficulty with complex patterns or sequences of movements, inability to use objects for their intended purpose.

Damage to the basal ganglia results in particular patterns of symptoms including tremors (involuntary oscillatory movements), athetosis (slow, writhing movements of fingers and hand), chorea (abrupt movements of limb and facial muscles), ballism (violent, flailing movements), and dystonia (persistent abnormal posture).

Damage to structures associated with the limbic system results in more complex patterns of symptoms, including memory loss, mood changes including depression and anxiety, and poor judgment in decision-making. Post-traumatic stress disorder may arise from disordered functioning of parts of the limbic system. Also, research is suggesting that disordered functioning of parts of the limbic system and associated structures is a basis of criminal psychopathy.

You might imagine that a lesion restricted to a particular part of the brain disrupts only one mental operation. You would be wrong, though, because the brain is so massively interconnected that a particular symptom could arise following damage to different parts of the brain. Consider an automobile engine. Either allowing the spark plugs to decay or cutting the gas line will cause the car to stop running, but it doesn't mean that these two disrupted parts do the same thing—rather, their removal has similar consequences. On the other hand, damage at one location can have widespread consequences. In an automobile engine a dead battery will prevent the engine from starting, the radio from playing, and the doors from unlocking.

Obvious ethical considerations do not allow researchers to produce controlled lesions within the human brain; therefore, researchers study large groups of patients with similar patterns of brain damage and map the particular patient-to-patient variations onto a common brain to discover any correlation between damaged regions and the loss of a particular function.

The diagnosis of brain damage is often uncertain due to variability in the location, extent, and duration of the lesion. To use stroke patients as an example, factors that can vary between patients include how long ago the stroke occurred, which artery within the brain was blocked, what areas were cut off from blood supply because of the blockage, whether other arteries compensated to provide an alternative supply of blood to that particular region, and how much brain circuits adapted to the insult.

Particular kinds of brain damage can also have therapeutic effects. Neurosurgeons intentionally produce lesions to treat a variety of disorders. One obvious example is the treatment of epilepsy by removing the tissue sparking the seizure.

Such treatments are not without negative side effects. For example, many years ago neurosurgeons removed parts of the medial temporal lobe, including the hippocampus, to eliminate seizures, but they stopped this treatment when it was discovered that it leaves the patient with profound *amnesia*, an inability to form new memories. More notorious and ineffective is the "psycho-surgery," known as the *frontal lobotomy*. This involved severing the connections between prefrontal cortex and the rest of the brain. It peaked in popularity in the mid-20th century as a treatment for disorders ranging from depression to schizophrenia because it seemed to reduce the negative symptoms of anxiety, severe depression, and manic-depressive psychosis. However, other normal functions were also often affected, such as empathy, performance of normal household and work duties, and sexual propriety. Consequently, this procedure is no longer performed except in very rare circumstances when all other treatment options have failed.

We cannot leave the topic of brain damage without calling attention to *brain plasticity*. The brain can repair itself, sometimes to an amazing extent. Through various mechanisms the brain adapts to certain kinds of insult. The discovery of brain plasticity has had many important therapeutic consequences.

For example, amputees who have lost, say, an arm experience "phantom limb" pain—pain in the limb that is no longer there. Researchers have discovered that this can happen because the brain's map of the body changes after a limb is lost; neurons once devoted to the lost limb begin to respond to stimulation of neighboring parts of the body. As a result, some patients who have lost an arm experience sensation on the arm when the face is touched. This discovery has led to a potential therapy for phantom limb pain, offering patients a mirror in which they visually perceive their missing limb as normal.

Also, if stroke patients who lose function of one limb are forced to use that limb, then they recover more function than they would otherwise. The recovery may not be complete, but it is more than it would have been without the challenging exercises.

Finally, a neuroprosthetic treatment for profoundly deaf individuals uses a cochlear implant to pick up sounds and transmit electrical signals directly to the auditory nerve in the cochlea. Plasticity in the brain is believed to be crucial for patients to learn to make sense of the unusual sensory inputs.

2. Transcranial Magnetic Stimulation

Transcranial magnetic stimulation (TMS) is a noninvasive method for either activating or inactivating parts of the cerebral cortex. Those undergoing TMS have a figure-eight-shaped device placed near their head, and when the device is pulsed, brain stimulation occurs. To understand how it works, recall that every electrical field has an associated magnetic field and vice versa. TMS happens when a very powerful magnetic field is generated by the figure-eight device located somewhere on the head. The electric field associated with this induced magnetic field passes through the scalp, skull, and dura mater to influence neural activity beneath the coil. The area of cerebral cortex affected is estimated at 1.0-1.5 cm³, and the influence does not extend beneath the cerebral cortex.

Whether TMS activates or inhibits neurons varies for reasons that remain uncertain, but the influences of TMS can be vivid and reliable. For example, TMS over visual cortex elicits perception of light flashes. TMS over the hand representation in motor cortex elicits discrete twitches of the fingers. TMS targeted to other cortical areas can impair function, inducing temporary blindness or paralysis, loss of recognition of different letters, or an inability to read words. Thus, in some cases, TMS is described as producing a temporary lesion. The variability of the effects of TMS is believed to be a result of the geometry of the cortex beneath the skull and the nature of the networks involved.

Originally, TMS was limited to single brief pulses of stimulation. Subsequently, *repetitive TMS* (rTMS) was found to be safe when properly executed. Single-pulse TMS has short-lasting effects, but rTMS can have much longer duration effects, lasting even beyond the end of the stimulation. In the clinic, TMS has been used to assess the strength of connection between the primary motor cortex and the muscles to evaluate damage from insults such as stroke, multiple sclerosis, amyotrophic lateral sclerosis, and spinal cord injuries. Also, some investigators have reported therapeutic effects of rTMS in cases of major depression.

TMS has many limitations. First and most notable, perhaps, is that the electric field that activates neurons also activates the overlying muscles causing possibly uncomfortable contractions of scalp and facial muscles. Second, when TMS is done with longer trains of pulses, it can cause seizures. Third, although TMS is delivered to a particular location, its influence occurs through changes in brain circuitry of an unknown scale. To explore this, neuroscientists have worked to obtain fMRI data (with an incredibly strong magnet), following TMS (with an incredibly strong magnetic field) to investigate how stimulation of one part of the cortex influences

BOLD activation in other parts of the cortex. Ultimately, though, TMS cannot influence brain processes with the precision of localization that can be accomplished with invasive techniques.

3. Transcranial Direct Current Stimulation

Transcranial direct current stimulation (tDCS) is another noninvasive method for influencing larger regions of the cerebral cortex. Whereas TMS involves pulses of very intense stimulation, tDCS involves sustained weak stimulation at levels corresponding to an automobile battery. A person undergoing tDCS has two small, wet sponges placed on the head, one over the brain region of interest and the other over a remote location like the shoulder, neck, or cheek to complete the electrical circuit. Wires connect the sponges to the device that delivers the desired magnitude, duration, and polarity of stimulation. The effects of the stimulation can vary according to whether the positive or negative pole of the device is connected to the sponge over the brain. It is thought that when the negative electrode (cathode) is located over the brain region, it hyperpolarizes neurons, making them less responsive. In contrast, when the positive electrode (anode) is located over the brain region, it depolarizes neurons, making them more responsive. However, research is continuing to understand the actual complexity of effects.

tDCS seems to be less risky than TMS with few relatively minor side effects. Indeed, for just a few hundred dollars you can purchase an apparatus to apply tDCS to your own brain. tDCS has been shown to influence perception, attention, movement, and decision-making. Importantly, tDCS often has prolonged effects after the stimulation period is finished. The general approach has been explored for over a century, but in the last several years interest has renewed for research and potential therapies.

4. Direct Brain Stimulation

Electrical stimulation to elicit responses has been used since the 1800s to investigate brain function. For example, the function of different parts of the human cerebral cortex has been described in fascinating detail through discoveries that stimulating different parts elicits markedly different effects. Electrically stimulating the occipital lobe elicits discrete sensory experiences such as flashes of light. Stimulating parts of the temporal lobe elicits more complex perceptions like autobiographical memories. Meanwhile, stimulating the primary motor cortex in the frontal lobe elicits movements like twitches of a finger, while stimulating the supplementary motor area elicits the feeling of willing a movement. Findings like these highlight the profound connection between brain function and our mental experiences. For surgical treatment of epilepsy, electrical stimulation of the brain is essential to locate centers responsible for language (that should not be removed) and centers sparking the seizure (that should be removed).

Electrical stimulation of subcortical structures can also be very powerful. For example, stimulating around the amygdala elicits a phenomenon called *sham rage* in animals characterized by biting, clawing, hissing, arching the back, and violently attacking vulnerable items in the environments. Meanwhile, stimulation in the base of the brain around a bundle of dopamine fibers passing to the limbic system is experienced as an incredibly potent reward that animals will work to earn to the exclusion of food and water. Both of these phenomena have been described in humans as well as animals.

Electrical stimulation of subcortical structures has also proven amazingly effective therapeutically. *Deep brain stimulation* (DBS) refers to electrical stimulation of structures deep in the brain to treat particular symptoms. This requires surgical insertion of electrodes attached by a thin wire to a battery implanted near the collarbone. Extensive anatomical and physiological testing in animal models guided the therapeutic effect of DBS of a particular part of the basal ganglia for treating Parkinson's disease. DBS is now employed commonly in patients for whom the effectiveness of L-DOPA therapy (see below) has diminished, and clinical research is investigating the use of DBS before drugs. Subsequent research has reported beneficial effects of DBS of anterior cingulate cortex to treat major depression. Remarkably, the symptoms of the disease remit immediately upon turning on the stimulation — the tremor and rigidity of Parkinson's patients subsides, and the black cloud lifts from chronically depressed patients. As discussed in Chapter 20, a host of ethical and legal issues are raised by the advent of implantable neurotechnology.

The previous examples have emphasized the specificity of effects of electrical stimulation of particular parts of the brain. The final example we will consider is referred to as *electroconvulsive therapy*, which involves stimulation of the whole brain. Complete seizures are induced in anesthetized patients to treat profound psychiatric disorders. Even though the mechanism of the therapeutic effect is not understood, electroconvulsive therapy can be effective for treating clinical depression in some individuals who have not responded to other treatments.

5. Pharmacological Manipulation

You learned in Chapter 3 how signaling between neurons involves the release of and response to neurotransmitter molecules at synapses. Synaptic transmission occurs through several steps, each of which can be manipulated pharmacologically. In this section we review some of the ways in which brain, and thus behavior, can be affected by drug use. We must emphasize, however, that at present the complex web of relationships between drugs, brain, and behavior remains incompletely understood. While many of these mysteries may one day be solved, it may take considerable time. This is why, for instance, some large pharmaceutical companies have reduced their present investments in mind-altering drugs. In spite of current limitations about how, it is clear that certain drugs do modify brain function.

Drugs that facilitate or impede neurotransmission can improve or impair perception, movement, memory, and mood. Drugs that influence mental processes are called *psychoactive drugs*. Humans have used such drugs for centuries, e.g., caffeine, cocaine, and cannabis. Modern neuroscience has provided many other psychoactive drugs motivated by the prevailing view that psychiatric disorders arise from improper functioning of specific brain neurotransmitter systems. You should also appreciate that other drugs can influence the brain by promoting birth of neurons and influencing the expression of genes.

Drugs that affect the brain have been categorized as follows:

- *Anesthetics* or *hypnotics* are given to create a reversible loss of sensation, commonly for the purpose of a surgical procedure. Whereas local anesthetics, like lidocaine, prevent sensation from a limited part of the body, general anesthetics eliminate consciousness. One kind of general anesthetic is a gas that has its effects as long as it is inhaled. Other general anesthetics, exemplified by Propofol, are given intravenously to induce anesthesia quickly.

- *Antidepressants* and *anxiolytics* (anti-anxiety) are prescribed to treat depression and anxiety. Exemplified by Prozac, this group includes drugs that reduce the reuptake of serotonin into the synapse and are thus called *selective serotonin reuptake inhibitors* (SSRIs).

- *Antipsychotics* are prescribed to treat psychotic disorders, such as schizophrenia. Exemplified by Haldol, one type of antipsychotic blocks the effect of dopamine at the synapse. A common side effect of Haldol is impaired production of movements due to the blockage of dopamine in the basal ganglia. Exemplified by Clozapine, atypical antipsychotics influence serotonin as well as dopamine neurotransmission.

- Drugs to treat cognitive disorders are diverse. *Methylphenidate* and *Adderall* are prescribed to treat ADHD. *Modafinil* is prescribed to treat narcolepsy and has been suggested to be helpful for ADHD. Antidementia drugs such as acetylcholinesterase inhibitors are prescribed to treat the symptoms of Alzheimer's disease. Some of these and related drugs have been suggested as cognition enhancing agents.

- The major drug to treat movement disorders such as Parkinson's disease is L-DOPA, a substance that crosses the blood-brain barrier and is converted into dopamine.

- *Analgesics* are prescribed to treat pain. Exemplified by morphine, these drugs bind to particular neurotransmitter receptors called endorphins.

- *Antiepileptic* drugs are given to prevent various forms of seizures. Exemplified by phenytoin, some of these drugs impede the propagation of nerve impulses. Others, such as benzodiazepines, enhance the GABA inhibition in the brain.

- Recreational psychoactive drugs are used to change perception and mood for entertainment or, perhaps, enlightenment. *Psychostimulants*, exemplified by cocaine, amphetamine, and Ecstasy inhibit the reuptake and enhance the release of norepinephrine, dopamine, and serotonin. *Narcotics*, exemplified by heroin, produce a sense of euphoria by activating the natural opiate receptors in the brain. *Psychedelics*, exemplified by LSD and mescaline, seem to affect serotonin neurotransmission. The effective compound in cannabis, referred to as THC, is an agonist for a specific second-messenger synaptic system that ultimately inhibits release of certain neurotransmitters. Alcohol affects brain processes in a variety of complex ways. Nicotine in the brain seems to regulate the release of numerous other neurotransmitters.

An important aspect of psychoactive drugs is their addictive properties. Addiction will be considered in detail in Chapter 12, but let's preview what is understood about some of the basic mechanisms. Cocaine, for example, activates dopamine receptors, leading to a sense of satisfaction. However, later the dopamine system rebounds leading to a sense of dissatisfaction worse than before the cocaine was taken. Consuming more cocaine leads to a weaker sense of satisfaction because the dopamine system develops a tolerance for the drug. Consequently, progressively more must be consumed each time to achieve equivalent senses of satisfaction. However, each consumption produces the rebound, leading to ever deeper dissatisfaction, so the downward spiral into addiction proceeds.

FURTHER READING

General:

Olaf Sporns, *Networks of the Brain* (2011).

EEG and QEEG:

Steven J. Luck, *An Introduction to Event-Related Potential Technique* (2d ed. 2014).

The Oxford Handbook of Event-Related Potential Components (Steven J. Luck & Emily S. Kappenman eds., 2011).

Introduction to Quantitative EEG and Neurofeedback: Advanced Theory and Applications (Thomas H. Budzynski et al. eds., 2d ed. 2009).

PET and SPECT:

Michael J. Posner & Marcus E. Raichle, *Images of Mind* (1997).

MRI and fMRI:

Geoffrey K. Aguirre, *Functional Neuroimaging: Technical, Logical, and Social Perspectives*, 44 Hastings Ctr. Rep. S8 (2014).

Scott A. Huettel et al., *Functional Magnetic Resonance Imaging* (3d ed. 2014).

The Oxford Handbook of Functional Brain Imaging in Neuropsychology and Cognitive Neurosciences (Andrew C. Papanicolaou ed., 2017).

Richard E. Passingham & James B. Rowe, *A Short Guide to Brain Imaging: The Neuroscience of Human Cognition* (2015).

Russell A. Poldrack & Martha J. Farah, *Progress and Challenges in Probing the Human Brain*, 526 Nature 371 (2015).

Neurosynth (neurosynth.org) is a platform where you can explore patterns of brain activation observed with many kinds of stimuli, conditions, or tasks. As of February 2020, the site includes nearly 51,000 activations reported in over 14,000 separately published studies to describe functional connectivity and coactivation maps for over 150,000 brain locations. You can examine meta-analyses with 1,335 terms and view whole-brain maps of expression levels of numerous human genes. You can also navigate with your cursor to locations in the brain and learn the name of a given structure, the conditions in which that region is activated, and the other brain regions with which it is associated.

Mobile Neuroimaging:

Francis X. Shen et al., *Ethical Issues Posed by Field Research Using Highly Portable and Cloud-Enabled Neuroimaging*, 105 Neuron 771 (2020).

Mathieu Sarracanie et al., *Low-Cost High-Performance MRI*, 5 Sci. Rep. 1 (2015).

TMS and tDCS:

Practical Guide to Transcranial Direct Current Stimulation: Principles, Procedures and Applications (Helena Knotkova et al. eds., 2019).

Brain Damage:

Oliver Sacks, *The Man Who Mistook His Wife for a Hat: And Other Clinical Tales* (1998).

Pharmacology:

Leslie Iversen et al., *Introduction to Neuropsychopharmacology* (2008).

CHAPTER 5

Limits and Cautions

fMRI is not and will never be a mind reader, as some of the proponents of decoding-based methods suggest, nor is it a worthless and non-informative "neophrenology" that is condemned to fail, as has been occasionally argued.

—Nikos Logothetis[†]

Understanding the brain by looking at images of it strikes me as akin to deciphering a computer by where the casing feels hot. You may locate the hard drive, but you'll never know what the 1s and 0s are.

—Anonymous comment[††]

CHAPTER SUMMARY

This chapter:
- Introduces basic limitations of noninvasive measures of brain function.
- Highlights several principles that can help effectively evaluate and critique functional brain imaging evidence.
- Presents critical perspectives on exaggerated claims about neuroscience.

INTRODUCTION

You have learned about the major noninvasive techniques available to measure human brain function—fMRI and EEG (with QEEG). These methods yield dazzling visual images that are informative to trained scientists and seem persuasive if not conclusive to laypeople. But having read the previous chapter, you now also know that neuro-images are the product of a process involving many steps of statistical and graphical choices.

Because the end result is an image that researchers can use to illustrate patterns of brain activation associated with complex and, crucially, uniquely human abilities, it is no wonder that we are amazed. When we see a colorful brain image purporting to be "our brain in love," we take a second look. When we see headlines suggesting that the government can use neuroscientific technologies to read our minds, we shudder. But are such hopes and fears about neuroscience justified?

[†] Nikos Logothetis, *What We Can and Cannot Do with fMRI*, 453 Nature 869, 869 (2008).
[††] *Reader Rants and Raves*, Wired (July 21, 2008) (excerpting a comment by user docbmac).

This chapter goes beyond the colorful images, and beneath the sensational head-lines, to scrutinize what brain-imaging neuroscience can—and *cannot*—do for law. The Appendix provides specific details beyond those summarized in this chapter.

A vivid reminder of the need for caution comes from an Atlantic salmon. In 2010 a group of neuroscientists published a paper in which they reported fMRI brain activation in a dead Atlantic salmon.* The researchers treated the salmon in the scanner just as they treated their human participants—they asked the salmon, like other participants, to adopt the point of view of a person shown on the screen.

Standard analysis of the data found several regions displaying increased activa-tion when the expired salmon was exposed to pictures of humans in different social-emotional situations, compared to control periods without pictures. How can this be? In fact, the observed activation was due entirely to "noise" in the fMRI signal, which achieved statistical significance only by happenstance.

When modest statistical corrections were applied to correct this noise and limit the false positives (a statistical false alarm to be discussed later in this chapter), the differential activation was no longer significant. In other words, when the thresh-old for statistical significance was appropriately elevated, the dead salmon's brain showed, as expected, no regions of increased activation.

For the practitioner and consumer of neurolaw, the tongue-in-cheek salmon experiment illustrates an important point: Brain-imaging data is meaningful only if carefully acquired, analyzed, and interpreted. Of course, the dead salmon's brain activation is easy to refute. But in typical research experiments or clinical evalua-tions, we do not have such strong prior expectations. Indeed, the very reason the testing is being undertaken is typically to ascertain whether there is a real difference between two conditions or whether a certain part of the brain is active in a particu-lar way. How, then, can one have confidence in reported findings and proffered brain evidence?

The goal of this chapter is not to demean the validity of noninvasive brain measurements. Indeed, to do so would render a coursebook about law and neu-roscience curiously irrelevant. Instead, the goal of this chapter is to inoculate you from being overwhelmed or overawed by evidence provided by these techniques. Although glaring cautionary tales like that of the dead salmon might suggest that noninvasive measurements of brain function are fatally unreliable, the outlook for neuroscientific evidence is more positive than negative, especially in light of new developments since the first edition of this book. While this chapter aims to throw a bucket of cold water on the *uncritical* acceptance of information from noninva-sive measures of brain function, such measures—carefully analyzed and properly understood—can be incredibly informative and useful. Consequently, their accu-racy and applications are growing. Hence, we do not advocate that the law entirely discard fMRI and EEG measures of brain function. Rather, we desire to shape their effective and judicious incorporation into the legal community with knowledge of the limitations of such methods.

---

* Craig Bennett et al., *Neural Correlates of Interspecies Perspective Taking in the Post-Mortem Atlantic Salmon: An Argument for Proper Multiple Comparisons Correction*, 1 J. Serendipitous & Unexpected Results 1 (2010).

The chapter proceeds in three sections. Section A surveys the general and unavoidable limitations and appropriate cautions in the interpretation of fMRI and EEG findings. Section B surveys in more detail particular measurement limitations of fMRI and EEG with QEEG. Section C explores concerns about overreaching claims about what neuroscience can do for law and for society more broadly.

A. GENERAL LIMITS AND CAUTIONS

1. Functional Magnetic Resonance Imaging

Owen D. Jones et al.
Brain Imaging for Legal Thinkers: A Guide for the Perplexed
2009 Stan. Tech. L. Rev. 5, 11-14

We can now turn to discuss key concepts about brain imaging that legal thinkers should know:

1. Anatomical imaging and functional imaging are importantly different.

Two anatomical images, taken one minute apart, will ordinarily look indistinguishable. Yet two functional images, from data collected one minute apart, could look completely different. One reason this is so is simply that, in the latter case, brain activity changes rapidly. Another reason is because fMRI brain images are built statistically, not recorded photographically. In the typical fMRI case, hundreds of recordings are made of each voxel in the brain, at slightly different times (e.g., every two seconds). Each recording of each voxel within a given trial is analogous to a single frame in a movie. Learning what happens within each voxel, over time, is akin to watching motion seem to emerge from the observation of successive snapshots that comprise a moving picture. But that metaphor only captures part of the fMRI technique, because there are subsequently many repeat recordings of that voxel, under similar conditions, on many consecutive trials — the results of which are typically then averaged across trials. Complicating matters further is that there are about one hundred thousand voxels within the brain, and what typically matters is how neural activity within those voxels is varying over time, in relation to some task the subject(s) undertake while being scanned. Furthermore, within each voxel are millions of neurons of different types, interacting in ways that could be mechanistically different but indistinguishable from the measure of fMRI. In the end, fMRI brain images lay the result of any one of many possible statistical tests overtop of an anatomical image of a selected slice of the brain. That is, an fMRI image is a composite of an anatomical image, of the researcher's choosing, and a statistical representation of the brain activity in that image, also of the researcher's choosing.

2. Functional brain imaging is not mind reading.

There is more to a thought than blood flow and oxygen. fMRI is very good at discovering where brain tissue is active (commonly by highlighting differences between brain activations during different cognitive tasks). But these differences are not thoughts. fMRI can show differences in brain activation across locations, across time, and across tasks. But that often does not enable any reliable conclusion about precisely what a person is thinking.

3. Scanners don't create fMRI brain images; people create fMRI brain images.

Images are only as good as the manner in which the researcher designed the specific task or experiment, deployed the machine, collected the data, analyzed the results, and generated the images. It is important to remember that fMRI images are the result of a process about a process. Multiple choices and multiple steps go into determining exactly what data will be collected, how, and when—as well as into how the data will be analyzed and how it will be presented.

4. Group-averaged and individual brain images are importantly different.

Most brain imaging research is directed toward understanding how *the average brain*, within a subject population, is activated during different tasks. This is not the same as saying either that all brains performing the same task activate in the average way, or saying that the activation of a single brain can tell us anything meaningful about the appearance of the average brain. Consequently:

- Do not assume that the scan of any individual is necessarily representative of any group.
- Do not assume that the averaged scan of any group will necessarily be representative of any individual.

5. There is no inherent meaning to the color on an fMRI brain image.

fMRI does not detect colors in the brain. fMRI images use colors of whatever segment of the rainbow the researcher prefers—to signify *the result of a statistical test.* By convention, the brighter the color (say, yellow compared to) the greater the statistical significance of the differences in brain activity between two conditions. Put another way, the brighter the color, the less likely it is that the differences in brain activity in that voxel or region, between two different cognitive tasks, was due to chance alone. As with any color-coded representation, accurate interpretation requires knowing exactly what each color represents in absolute terms. The researcher specifies what each color will represent, and this matters. Yellow might mean that there is only one chance in one thousand that the difference between brain activations in this voxel, between condition, is due to random chance. Or yellow might mean that there is one chance in twenty that the difference is due to random chance.

6. fMRI brain images do not speak for themselves.

No fMRI brain image has automatic, self-evident significance. Even well-designed, well-executed, properly analyzed, properly generated images must have their import, in context, interpreted.

7. Classification of an anatomical or behavioral feature of the brain as normal or abnormal is not a simple thing.

Because we have learned a great deal about the brain, from dissection, imaging, and the like, we have some confidence about what a typical brain looks like, and how a typical brain functions. But even without full anatomical scans of everyone on the planet, we know there is considerable variation—both anatomically and functionally—within some general parameters. That means that it can be (with some exceptions, such as a bullet lodged in the brain) difficult to say with precision *how uncommon* a given feature or functional pattern may be, even if it appears to be atypical. Base rates for anatomical or functional conditions are often unknown. For example: suppose brain images show that a defendant has an abnormal brain feature. We often do not have any idea how many people with nearly identical abnormalities do not behave as the defendant did. . . .

8. Even when an atypical feature of function is identified, understanding the meaning of that is considerably complex.

Brain images can show unique features and functions of a person's brain. But their meaning is rarely self-evident. Determining which of those are important, and how, depends not only on the legal context for which the images are offered, but also on expert analysis of what the images do and do not mean. For example, suppose that measurement of the fMRI-detected signal during a given cognitive task indicates that a person has less neural activity in a given region than does the average person. Does that mean that the person is somehow cognitively impaired in that region? Or might it alternatively indicate that the person has more expertise or experience than average, requiring less cognitive effort?

9. Correlation is (still) not causation.

The fact that two things vary in parallel tells us little about whether the two are necessarily causally related and, if so, which causes which. For example, suppose brain imaging reveals that seventy percent of inmates on death row for homicide have atypical brain activation in a given region, compared with normal, unincarcerated subjects. That statistic does not mean that the brain activation pattern causes homicidal behavior. It might mean that having murdered affects brain activations, or that being incarcerated for long periods of time affects brain activations, or something else entirely.

10. Today's brain is not yesterday's brain.

In all but the most fanciful of contexts, a brain scan likely takes place long after the behavior (such as criminal activity) that gives rise to the scan. Drawing causal inferences is therefore further complicated. People's brains change with age and experience. And some proportion of the population will develop atypical anatomical or functional conditions over time. If a defendant is scanned six months or six years after the act in question, and the scan detects an abnormality, it is not a simple matter to conclude with confidence that the same abnormality was present at the time in question or—even if one assumes so, arguendo—that it would have meaningfully affected behavior.

11. Scanners (in theory) detect what they are built, programmed, and instructed to detect, in the way they are built, programmed, and instructed to detect it.

Scanners are highly complex and individualized pieces of machinery. So (as in other areas of science) are the people who calibrate, program, operate, and interpret collected data. It is important to recognize that the product of these intersecting complexities may or may not be reliable, generalizable, and replicable.

12. fMRI brain imaging enables inferences about the mind, built on the detection of physiological functions believed to be reliably associated with brain activity.

It is important to remember that fMRI does not provide a direct measure of neuronal activity—as do, for example, invasive techniques that measure single neuron recording. fMRI detects fluctuations in oxygen concentrations thought to be reliably associated with neuronal activity. But the precise relationship between metabolic demands and neuronal function remains poorly understood.

Even if regional activations in brain images reflect true neural activity, it should also be kept in mind that our ability to confidently infer the cognitive process that must have led to such regional activation is highly constrained. This is because neuroscientists still understand so little about what the various regions of the human brain contribute to a particular cognitive function.

2. Electroencephalography

Many of the challenges inherent in fMRI data acquisition and analysis exist for EEG and QEEG, as well. As you recall, EEG measures cumulative electrical potential on the surface of the head instead of blood oxygenation within the brain. Thus, it is a more direct measure of brain function that does not suffer from the seconds-long time lag of the fMRI blood oxygen signal. The magnitude of the EEG signal, referred to as *polarization*, varies with mental state, such as being asleep or alert, and in association with responses to stimuli in experimental testing. To facilitate comprehension, we will parallel the previous excerpt as we review key concepts to know about EEG.

1. The anatomical sources of EEG signals are difficult to specify.

EEG does not provide information about brain structure, but the structure of the brain is crucially important for the nature of the EEG signal. The EEG measured on the surface of the head originates in the electrical potentials associated with synaptic processes changing the state of pyramidal neurons in the cerebral cortex. The magnitude of the electrical potential measured on the surface varies with the angle of the neurons in the sulci and gyri of the cortex. The EEG measured on the surface of the head originates from the electrical currents flowing in large areas of the cerebral cortex. However, it is impossible to calculate exactly where in the brain these currents are located. In spite of this, various mathematical approaches and physical and biological intuitions permit some estimates of the source location of EEG signals.

2. EEG measurements are not mind reading, but they do relate to mental states.

Scientists have identified reliable associations between particular mental operations and the magnitude and timecourse of EEG. The frequency content and magnitude of the EEG varies systematically with level of consciousness, with higher frequency and lower magnitude during alert states and lower frequency and higher magnitude during sleep. The form of the EEG is violently dramatic during epileptic seizures. An EEG with no variation of electrical potential is a useful sign of brain death.

In psychological testing conditions, the EEG can be averaged over many testing trials and synchronized on different testing events, such as presentation of a stimulus or initiation of a body movement. These averaged EEG are called *event-related potentials*. For example, the magnitude of the average EEG around 200 milliseconds (ms) after a visual stimulus is presented differs if participants are paying attention to that stimulus as compared to them simply viewing it. Around 300 ms after a stimulus is presented the magnitude of the EEG is modulated by how unexpected a stimulus is and how much you notice and remember about it. Preceding actions, the EEG slowly increases in polarization until the body movement is made whereupon the EEG changes back to a neutral state. Finally, the magnitude of the average EEG after an action varies according to the consequences of the action. Besides modulating at different times in association with different mental operations, the various event-related potential components vary in magnitude over the surface of the head. Some ERP components have larger magnitudes over the occipital lobe, for instance, and others have larger magnitudes over the frontal lobes. None of these event-related potentials can be detected without averaging over dozens, if not hundreds, of testing trials. In legally relevant settings it is difficult to obtain such extensive data.

QEEG decomposes EEG into different frequency bands, and maps of the various frequency bands are constructed over the surface of the head. Think of the EEG as a musical chord played on a piano and the QEEG as a measure of which keys (frequencies) were struck with what strength. Some researchers have identified associations between patterns of EEG frequency bands across the head and particular mental states. However, a particular pattern of EEG frequency bands cannot be taken as a certain sign that a particular mental state is occurring.

3. Amplifiers don't create EEG brain images; people create EEG brain images. Consequently, there is no inherent meaning to the color of an EEG map.

One of the alluring aspects of QEEG is that it allows one to produce a color map of the EEG frequency bands across the head. When presented in graphic color, these maps seem to bear some relation to the patterns of activation displayed after fMRI measurements. As noted above, though, the colors used and how they are made to gradually change in these plots is up to the investigator to specify. Accordingly, small absolute differences in the magnitude of EEG frequency bands can be made to appear much larger through the use of colors that we resolve as distinctly different.

4. Group-averaged and individual data are different.

The general timing and spatial pattern of EEG signals associated with different mental states is fairly consistent among individuals. This regularity is the basis of the scientific studies that are performed. However, because the EEG originates primarily from the pyramidal neurons aligned in the cerebral cortex, and because the precise folding pattern of each person's cerebral cortex is different, the timing and magnitude of the EEG measured on each person will have variation. The magnitude of this natural variation has not been quantified systematically.

Further variation in EEG signals can occur when measurements are obtained across days. Some of this variation arises from idiosyncrasies in how the electrodes are placed on the scalp. Some of the variation can also arise from differences in alertness and engagement of the participant across testing sessions.

5. EEG and QEEG maps do not speak for themselves.

As noted above for images derived from fMRI measurements, the maps of EEG magnitude or frequency content cannot be interpreted without the context of the state of the participant (e.g., awake, asleep, dreaming) and what the participant was doing (e.g., simply resting or performing a particular task).

6. Classification of EEG signals as normal or abnormal is not simple.

As noted above for fMRI measurements, the magnitude of variation of EEG and QEEG signal patterns varies across individuals. Some studies have quantified EEG and QEEG measures across healthy normal individuals over time and found less variation across repeated measurements from one individual than across individuals. However, these studies have not thoroughly quantified the nature and magnitude of variation in EEG and QEEG measures across gender, race, and age. Numerous studies have characterized EEG and QEEG differences between individuals with various neurological and psychiatric disorders and healthy counterparts. In most cases, a measure may be significantly different on average between the groups, but the range of variation of that measure overlaps between the groups. Therefore, unless an individual's particular measure is extremely high or low, it can be impossible to specify reliably in which group the individual belongs. In some conditions, like certain types of epilepsy, the EEG signatures are very distinct, but in most conditions, like schizophrenia and depression, the EEG differences are very subtle. Therefore, a conclusion that a particular individual's EEG pattern is meaningfully abnormal must be considered with caution and skepticism.

7. Even when an atypical EEG signal is identified, its relationship to mental states and behavior is uncertain.

As described in Chapter 4 and above, particular measures of EEG have been associated with particular mental states or processes such as attention, working memory, volition, and sensitivity to consequences. However, scientific findings do not support strong inverse conclusions about disordered mental states from abnormal EEG signals. Furthermore, inferences about relationships between EEG measures and mental states cannot be considered reliable unless suitably controlled behavioral testing procedures are used to independently manipulate or probe the given mental state or process. Scientific studies collect data with a controlled set of testing conditions, e.g., different kinds of stimuli or responses, measured in numerous testing trials to obtain reliable average measurements. As you will see in Chapter 15 on lie detection, the use of an event-related potential measure for lie detection is questionable when the data are collected with too few testing trials with too few and uncontrolled stimuli. In short, without concomitant psychological testing, EEG measurements can support no strong conclusions about mental states and processes. This is especially problematic for QEEG measurements obtained when individuals are doing nothing in particular.

8. Correlation is (still) not causation.

As noted above for fMRI, the association between abnormal EEG and abnormal behavior may not be one-directional. The abnormal EEG could be a consequence of a long period of abnormal behavior.

9. Today's brain is not yesterday's brain.

As noted above for fMRI, brain scans almost never happen during commission of a crime. Even if scientists identify EEG signatures of *mens rea*, it is very unlikely that the brain state can be measured during the planning and commission of the crime.

10. EEG systems measure what they are built to measure.

As noted, the EEG signal bears a more direct relationship to brain function than the blood oxygen signal of fMRI. However, because the measurement is obtained noninvasively, it remains indirect. EEG systems vary in certain ways that may or may not be relevant for a particular case. Some systems sample EEG signals from just a dozen or so locations on the head, while other systems sample EEG signals from 64, 128, or even 256 locations covering the head. More electrodes generally provide better information about potential sources within the brain responsible for a given EEG signal. However, to assess the presence, timing and magnitude of certain mental states and processes, fewer than a dozen electrodes, and perhaps even just a couple, are needed.

NOTES AND QUESTIONS

1. Statistical analyses of noisy and variable measurements (like measurements of brain and behavior) have demonstrated two fundamental types of errors that occur. The first, called a *false positive* (also called Type I error), occurs if a statistically significant experimental effect is identified when in fact none actually exists. The second, called a *false negative* (Type II error), occurs when a true effect is not identified. To understand these errors, consider a household smoke detector. Smoke detectors are designed to be quite sensitive, so they can be set off by very small amounts of smoke, such as from burnt toast. Assuming that the goal of a smoke detector is to sound alarms for serious house fires, and not minor annoyances like burnt toast, then an alarm triggered by the toast is a false alarm because in fact the house was not on fire. Now imagine a careless homeowner who has unknowingly allowed the batteries in their smoke detector to expire. In this case the alarm would fail to sound even if a significant house fire is burning near the detector. This failure to signal a fire would be a false negative. What legal implications do you see for these two types of errors?

2. Statisticians distinguish *sensitivity* and *specificity.* Sensitivity measures the proportion of actual positives that are correctly identified as such (e.g., the percentage of sick people who are correctly identified as having some illness). The fewer false negatives, the higher the sensitivity. Specificity measures the proportion of negatives that are correctly identified (e.g., the percentage of healthy people who are correctly identified as not having the condition). The fewer false positives, the higher the specificity. In real world settings, like medical diagnosis or airport security, 100% sensitivity (i.e., predict all people from the sick group as sick) with 100% specificity (i.e., predict no one from the healthy group as sick) is impossible. Consequently, a risk-benefit analysis is undertaken, and a trade-off is made by enacting policies that set categorization thresholds higher or lower. For example, if one wishes to avoid any threat to safety, airport screening scanners can be adjusted to trigger on low-risk items like belt buckles and keys (low specificity) so as to reduce the probability of missing high-risk items like knives and guns (high sensitivity). What risk-benefit policy do you think should govern

application of fMRI and EEG measures in criminal law? What about personal injury claims? Social security disability? National security?

B. METHODOLOGICAL AND ANALYTICAL LIMITATIONS OF fMRI

1. Limitations in Measurement

Functional brain imaging utilizing fMRI has proven to be a very informative tool for research and many applications. However, you must appreciate the limitations of the technology.*

The main advantages of fMRI include noninvasiveness, reasonably good spatial resolution, acceptable temporal resolution, and the opportunity to obtain a view of the entire brain. Still, as neuroscientist Nikos Logothetis explains, fMRI has profound limitations beyond the basic physics or sophisticated engineering. A limitation will not be resolved just by increasing the power of the scanners. These more basic limitations arise from the indirect and coarse nature of the fMRI signal relative to the very dense and precise functional organization of the brain and also due to inappropriate experimental protocols that ignore this organization.

The main disadvantage is that fMRI measures a signal derived from the metabolism associated with the activity of thousands or tens of thousands of neurons. Consequently, the spatial and temporal specificity of this signal is limited by physical and biological constraints. The typical voxel size has been 3 mm × 3 mm × 3 mm, although improved technology allows for voxels that are fractions of a millimeter ($<0.5 \times 0.5 \times 0.5$ mm). Even so, fMRI voxels are packed with neurons, glia, blood vessels, and blood cells. One cubic millimeter in the human cerebral cortex contains ~25,000 neurons with around 10,000,000,000 synapses, as well as 4 km of axons and 0.4 km of dendrites. Less than 3% of this volume is occupied by blood vessels. Thus, a 3 x 3 x 3 mm^3 fMRI voxel in the cerebral cortex will contain ~675,000 neurons, more than 2.7×10^{11} synapses, over 100 km of axons, and over 10 km of dendrites. Some authors have compared fMRI to measurements of the heat coming from different locations on a computer—perhaps you could deduce something about the operation of the computer, but without monitoring the individual circuit elements, you could not learn just how the computer works.

As detailed in Chapter 4, fMRI studies commonly use two basic experimental designs. Logothetis emphasizes a basic limitation of the logic of the *block design* in which the pattern and magnitude of the BOLD signal during a task condition (e.g., generating verbs associated with a list of nouns) are compared to those during a control condition (e.g., just reading the nouns). The BOLD activation in each voxel during the test condition is subtracted from that in the control condition, revealing voxels with enhanced or reduced BOLD signal. Logothetis notes that a necessary assumption underlying this approach is that a single cognitive process can be inserted into a task without affecting the remainder. Psychologists concluded many years ago that this assumption is generally unjustified because the mind does not

---

* These few paragraphs summarize key points from the following article: Nikos K. Logothetis, *What We Can and What We Cannot Do with fMRI*, 453 Nature 869 (2008).

have such discrete modules or operations. He also explains that the brain consists of networks of neurons subserving different functions but overlapping within voxels, but the fMRI signal cannot resolve such subtle differences at the cellular level.

Logothetis also notes the complexity to be considered before drawing the conclusion that activation of a given brain region means that it is truly involved in the task at hand. Much of the complexity involves biological and physical details that need not concern us here. You should understand this, though. Observing an increase in the BOLD signal in a voxel does not guarantee that the neurons with axons exiting that voxel are necessarily generating more nerve impulses. The BOLD signal is a signature of the metabolic consumption in a part of the brain, and that consumption increases when excitatory neurons produce more impulses, but it also increases when inhibitory neurons prevent the excitatory neurons from producing more impulses. Thus, when you read about "fMRI activation" in some brain region, remember this does not necessarily mean that more nerve impulses are being sent from that brain region to other parts of the brain.

NOTES AND QUESTIONS

1. Imagine you are given a laptop and a variety of devices that can measure things like heat, sound, and vibration. What noninvasive measurements could you make that would provide information about the operation of a computer? What would you be unable to learn about the operation of the computer with such measurements?

2. Imagine you have a device that remotely measures local temperature in a room full of people who are engaged in various conversations. The device is sensitive enough to detect the elevated temperature emitted from speakers as they exhale. What could you infer from the measurements using this device? What limitations of those inferences do you recognize?

2. Limitations of fMRI Analysis Procedures

The previous excerpt surveyed some of the technical and conceptual problems with fMRI. This section summarizes the problems inherent in the various fMRI analysis procedures. One of the most salient points to take away is that what is found in an fMRI study depends very much on how the data are analyzed.

a. The dangers of multiple analysis alternatives

Joshua Carp

On the Plurality of (Methodological) Worlds: Estimating the Analytic Flexibility of fMRI Experiments

6 Frontiers Neurosci. 149, 1, 12 (2012)

How likely are published findings in the functional neuroimaging literature to be false? According to a recent mathematical model, the potential for false positives increases with the flexibility of analysis methods. Functional MRI (fMRI) experiments can be analyzed using a large number of commonly used tools, with little consensus on how, when, or whether to apply each one. This situation may lead to

substantial variability in analysis outcomes. Thus, the present study sought to estimate the flexibility of neuroimaging analysis by submitting a single event-related
fMRI experiment to a large number of unique analysis procedures. Ten analysis
steps for which multiple strategies appear in the literature were identified, and two
to four strategies were enumerated for each step. Considering all possible combinations of these strategies yielded 6,912 unique analysis pipelines. Activation maps
from each pipeline were corrected for multiple comparisons using five thresholding
approaches, yielding 34,560 significance maps. While some outcomes were relatively
consistent across pipelines, others showed substantial methods-related variability in
activation strength, location, and extent. Some analysis decisions contributed to this
variability more than others, and different decisions were associated with distinct
patterns of variability across the brain. Qualitative outcomes also varied with analysis
parameters: many contrasts yielded significant activation under some pipelines but
not others. Altogether, these results reveal considerable flexibility in the analysis of
fMRI experiments. This observation, when combined with mathematical simulations linking analytic flexibility with elevated false positive rates, suggests that false
positive results may be more prevalent than expected in the literature. This risk of
inflated false positive rates may be mitigated by constraining the flexibility of analytic choices or by abstaining from selective analysis reporting.

How common are false positive results in the functional neuroimaging literature? Among functional MRI (fMRI) studies that apply statistical correction for
multiple comparisons, most use a nominal false positive rate of 5%. However, [one
research team estimates] that between 10 and 40% of fMRI activation results are
false positives. Furthermore, recent empirical and mathematical modeling studies
argue that the true incidence of false positives may far exceed the nominal rate in
the broader scientific literature. Indeed, under certain conditions, research findings are more likely to be false than true.

. . . While some research outcomes were relatively stable across analysis pipelines,
others varied widely from one pipeline to another. Given the extent of this variability, a motivated researcher determined to find significant activation in practically
any brain region will very likely succeed—as will another researcher determined to
find null results in the same region. To mitigate the effects of this flexibility on the
prevalence of false positive results, investigators should either determine analysis
pipelines *a priori* or identify optimal pipelines using data-driven metrics. If researchers use multiple pipelines to analyze a single experiment, the results of all pipelines
should be reported—including those that yielded unfavorable results. If implemented, these steps could significantly improve the reproducibility of research in
the fMRI literature.

NOTES AND QUESTIONS

1. To better understand how conclusions from neuroimaging studies crucially
depend on specific analyses used, consider a study published in 2007. The
authors collected MRI data (static, not functional) from schizophrenic patients
and non-schizophrenic controls using a 1.5T scanner. After some standard
post-processing of the data, the authors transmitted the unanalyzed data sets to
nine different labs for analysis. The labs were only told that the data came from
two different groups and that they should use their typical MRI data analysis

approach to distinguish the individuals in each group. Would you be surprised to learn that the findings from the different labs overlapped only minimally? This led the authors of the study to conclude that "just because one method finds a particular difference, it does NOT mean that there were NO other differences—a fact that can be easily overlooked. This study therefore also highlights the extreme difficulty in interpreting differences in reported results obtained by different labs where there may be differences in the subjects recruited, or in the methods chosen to analyze the data, or indeed both." Derek K. Jones, *What Happens When Nine Different Groups Analyze the Same DT-MRI Data Set Using Voxel-Based Methods?*, 15 Proc. Int'l Soc. Mag. Reson. Med. 74 (2007). A study published in 2020 by members of the Neuroimaging Analysis Replication and Prediction Study similarly found that "analysis of a single fMRI dataset by 70 independent analysis teams, all of whom using different analysis pipelines, revealed substantial variability in reported binary results, with high levels of disagreement across teams for most of the tested hypotheses." The study went on to observe that this "substantial amount of analytical variability, and the subsequent variability of reported hypothesis results with the same data, demonstrates that steps need to be taken to improve the reproducibility of data analysis outcomes." Rotem Botvinik-Nezer et al., *Variability in the Analysis of a Single Neuroimaging Dataset by Many Teams*, 582 Nature 84 (2020).

2. Some measurements of the human adult are roughly the same over time. Measuring the size of our hands and feet will produce roughly the same measurement week-to-week and month-to-month. But researchers have found much more variation in an individual's brain activity pattern across different fMRI scanning sessions. That is, if you scan John doing a particular behavioral task in January, March, and May—or even simply on Monday, Tuesday, and Wednesday—you might not get the same activation patterns. It is not hard to see why this might be a problem for the types of legal uses of fMRI suggested in this book. What if the defendant's brain scan in January wasn't the same as his brain scan in July, or again in December? Is relying on results from a single scan—as almost all of the cases you will read in this book do—the equivalent of building a case on a lucky (or unlucky) draw from a deck of cards? In light of such possibilities, what should courts do? Keep in mind the high cost of conducting and analyzing data from an fMRI scan. For more on this issue, consider these publications that have compared the replicability of fMRI findings across time and laboratories:

a. AmanPreet Badhwar et al., *Multivariate Consistency of Resting-State fMRI Connectivity Maps Acquired on a Single Individual Over 2.5 Years, 13 sites and 3 vendors*, 205 NeuroImage 116210 (2020). This study quantified the consistency of resting state fMRI connectivity maps obtained from one adult cognitively healthy volunteer scanned repeatedly at 13 sites on scanners from three vendors (General Electric, Philips, and Siemens) over 2.5 years. On a scale of 0.0 (worst) to 1.0 (best) the consistency of the connectivity maps ranged from 0.3 to 0.8. Consistency was higher among scans at different times. Consistency was lower across scans at different locations and using scanners from different vendors.

b. BJ Casey et al., *Reproducibility of fMRI Results Across Four Institutions Using a Spatial Working Memory Task*, 8 Neuroimage 249 (1998). These investigators compared fMRI (of that era) obtained at four institutions from healthy adults

performing a standard task testing people's ability to remember briefly a location in space. They found common general regions of interest in dorsolateral
prefrontal and posterior parietal cortex.

c. David J. McGonigle et al., *Variability in fMRI: An Examination of Intersession
Differences*, 11 Neuroimage 708 (2000). These investigators compared fMRI (of
that era) obtained from one healthy adult in 99 sessions over two months consisting of 33 repetitions of simple motor, visual, and cognitive paradigms. They
accounted statistically for the variability across sessions and testing conditions
and found that the activation of many voxels was particular to sessions. The
authors showed meaningful variability of activation across voxels both within
sessions and between sessions and concluded that erroneous conclusions can
be drawn from data obtained from a single session from a single subject.

d. Stephen M. Smith et al., *Variability in fMRI: A Re-Examination of Inter-Session
Differences*, 24 Human Brain Mapping 248 (2005). These investigators performed new analyses of the data reported by McGonigle et al. in the 2000 paper
just considered. They reported that fMRI variability across sessions was of similar
magnitude to that within sessions. They also showed that the amount of variability observed across scanning sessions is affected by the methods of analysis. They
advocated caution in the interpretation of data obtained in a single session.

e. Bram B. Zandbelt et al., *Within-Subject Variation in BOLD-fMRI Signal Changes
Across Repeated Measurements: Quantification and Implications for Sample Size*, 42
NeuroImage 196 (2008). These investigators compared fMRI data collected
from ten healthy subjects performing a simple motor task in three sessions,
separated by one week. They found large variation in individual activation
levels, in individual voxels and in regions of interest. Based on the magnitude
of variation, the authors provide sample size estimations needed for repeated
measurement studies.

f. Maxwell L. Elliott et al., *What Is the Test-Retest Reliability of Common Task-Functional
MRI Measures? New Empirical Evidence and a Meta-Analysis*, 31 Psychological
Sci. 792 (2020). These investigators demonstrated poor reliability of task-
fMRI measures through a meta-analysis of 90 experiments and test-retest reliabilities of activation in specific regions of interest across 11 common fMRI
tasks collected by the Human Connectome Project and the Dunedin Study.
The authors concluded that current task-fMRI measures are not suitable
for individual-differences research and suggest ways to improve task-fMRI
reliability.

b. The risk of false positives in fMRI data

The dead salmon study highlights the risks of multiple statistical comparisons within
a set of data. Even if appropriate corrections for multiple comparisons are applied,
the massive quantities of data generated by a typical fMRI study can still create analytical pitfalls. One such problem, which was labeled "voodoo correlations," generated a flurry of discussion among researchers using fMRI technology to study the
neural substrates of human emotion and personality.

Edward Vul and colleagues observed that several high-profile articles in the field
of social neuroscience had reported very strong correlations between personality measures (based on self-report questionnaires) and brain activity as measured
by fMRI. Edward Vul et al., *Puzzlingly High Correlations in fMRI Studies of Emotion,
Personality, and Social Cognition*, 4 Persp. on Psychol. Sci. 274 (2009).

Vul et al., intrigued by the suspiciously high correlations, calculated the theoretical upper limit for correlations between personality measure and fMRI data. According to their calculations, many of the correlations reported in social neuroscience articles exceeded this upper limit.* So how did these exceedingly high correlations arise? Vul and colleagues argued that it was the result of what they termed the *nonindependence error*, which occurred during the data analysis portion of the fMRI studies.

The nonindependence error is subtle even to scientists in the field and even more elusive to those without a strong statistics background. To illustrate the problem more vividly, Vul and colleagues used an example from another domain. They identified a weather station whose temperature readings predict daily changes in the value of a specific set of stocks with a correlation of r = -0.87. They arrived at -0.87 by separately computing the correlation between the readings of the weather station in Adak Island, AK, with each of the 3,315 financial instruments available for the New York Stock Exchange between November 18 and December 3, 2008. They then averaged the correlation values of the stocks whose correlation exceeded a particular threshold, thus yielding the correlation value of -0.87. Should you pay for this investment strategy? Probably not. Of the 3,315 stocks assessed, some correlated with the Adak Island temperature measurements simply by chance—and if we select just those (as our selection process would do), there is no doubt we would find a high average correlation. Thus, the final measure (the average correlation of a subset of stocks) was not independent of the selection criteria (how stocks were chosen). This, in essence, is the nonindependence error.

After identifying this potential error, Vul and colleagues evaluated the results of more than 50 peer-reviewed articles in social neuroscience to determine how often this alleged error was committed. They reported that more than half of the articles contained some form of the nonindependence error and argued that the presence of this error cast serious doubts on the validity of those studies. Vul and colleagues' claims sparked a barrage of commentary on the nonindependence error, both in the scientific community and in the popular press. In fact, so much discussion and correspondence were generated that the journal *Perspectives on Psychological Science* published several commentaries by other social neuroscientists alongside the original article followed by Vul and colleagues' response to those commentaries.

Unsurprisingly, the social neuroscience community responded primarily with strong critiques of Vul et al.'s arguments and conclusions. The following excerpt highlights several of the most prominent criticisms.

Matthew D. Lieberman et al.

Correlations in Social Neuroscience Aren't Voodoo: Commentary on Vul et al.

4 Persp. on Psychol. Sci. 299, 305-06 (2009)

Because social neuroscience has garnered a lot of attention in a short period of time, singling it out for criticism may make for better headlines. As this article makes clear, however, Vul et al.'s criticisms rest on shaky ground at best.

---

* Vul et al.'s proposed upper limit has been disputed. *See, e.g.,* Craig M. Bennett & Michael M. Miller, *How Reliable Are the Results from Functional Magnetic Resonance Imaging?*, 1191 Annals N.Y. Acad. Sci. 133 (2010). However, it is undisputed that (1) an upper limit for the correlation of personality measures and fMRI does exist and (2) this limit can be calculated.

Vul et al. describe a two-step inferential procedure that would be bad science if anyone did it, but as far as we know, nobody does. They used a survey to assess which authors use this method, but they did not include any questions that would actually assess whether the nonindependence error had occurred. As long as standard procedures for addressing the issue of multiple comparisons are applied in a reasonable sample size, large correlations will occur by chance only rarely, and most observed effects will reflect true underlying relationships. Vul et al.'s own meta-analysis suggests that the nonindependent correlations are only modestly inflated, calling into question the use of labels such as "spurious" and "untrustworthy." Finally, Vul et al. make incorrect assumptions when attempting to use average expected reliabilities to inform on the theoretically possible observed correlations.

Ultimately, we should all be mindful that the effect sizes from whole-brain analyses are likely to be inflated, but confident in the knowledge that such correlations reflect meaningful relationships between psychological and neural variables to the extent that valid multiple comparisons procedures are used. There are various ways to balance the concerns of false positive results and sensitivity to true effects, and social neuroscience correlations use widely accepted practices from cognitive neuroscience. These practices will no doubt continue to evolve. In the meantime, we'll keep doing the science of exploring how the brain interacts with the social and emotional worlds we live in.

Statistical challenges with the analysis of data acquired from functional brain imaging are being further identified and addressed by the research community. For example, a 2015 study performed nearly 3 million analyses on resting-state fMRI data from 499 healthy individuals. While they should have found 5% false positives, they found that the most common software packages for fMRI analysis gave false positive results in as many as 70% of tests. Anders Eklund et al., *Cluster Failure: Why fMRI Inferences for Spatial Extent Have Inflated False-Positive Rates*, 113 Proc. Nat'l Acad. Sci. U.S. 7900, 7900 (2016). Perhaps unsurprisingly, news media highlighted the finding with headlines referring to a bug in fMRI software that might invalidate years of brain research. But the research community is addressing these problems with improved approaches and greater appreciation of publication bias and the utility of improved transparency through measures like preregistering studies. *See* Balazs Aczel et al., *A Consensus-Based Transparency Checklist*, 4 Nature Hum. Behav. 4 (2020).

NOTES AND QUESTIONS

1. "A long-standing problem in fMRI research concerns the potential pitfalls of reverse inference. As an example, it is well established that the human amygdala responds more strongly to fear related stimuli than to neutral stimuli, but it does not logically follow that if the amygdala is more active in a given situation that the person is necessarily experiencing fear. If the amygdala's response varies along other dimensions as well, such as the emotional intensity, ambiguity, or predictive value of a stimulus, then it will be difficult to make strong inferences from the level of amygdala activity alone." Frank Tong & Michael S. Pratte, *Decoding Patterns of Human Brain Activity*, 63 Ann. Rev. Psychol. 483, 497 (2012). As you

read subsequent chapters that explain how fMRI measures have been used to support inferences about, for example, whether a person is not telling the truth, ask yourself whether reverse inference is being applied.

2. How do the technical issues summarized in the last two sections affect your sense of how brain imaging might best be used, if at all, in legal contexts?

3. A brain imaging study reported greater fMRI activation of the amygdala in response to images of African-American faces as compared to Caucasian faces that was correlated with the participants' racial evaluation, as measured by a psychological test. Elizabeth A. Phelps et al., *Performance on Indirect Measures of Race Evaluation Predicts Amygdala Activity*, 12 J. Cogn. Neurosci. 729 (2000). *See also* Adam M. Chekroud et al., *A Review of Neuroimaging Studies of Race-Related Prejudice: Does Amygdala Response Reflect Threat?* 8 Frontiers Hum. Neurosci. 179 (2014). Would you advocate using such information in the *voir dire* process? What problems can you anticipate in such an application?

4. What are corrected and uncorrected statistics? This example, offered by Daniel Bor (www.danielbor.com/dilemma-weak-neuroimaging), should help to clarify.

> Imagine that you are running an experiment to see if corporate bankers have lower empathy than the normal population, by giving them and a control group an empathy questionnaire. Low and behold, the bankers do have a lower average empathy score, but it's only a little bit lower. How can you tell whether this is just some random result, or that bankers really do have lower empathy? This is the point where statistical testing enters the frame.
>
> Classically, a statistical test will churn out a probability that you would have gotten the same result, just by chance. If it is lower than some threshold, commonly probability (or p) = 0.05, or a 1 in 20 chance, then because this is really very unlikely, we'd conclude that the test has passed, the result is significant, and that bankers really do have a lower empathy score than normal people. All well and good, but what if you also tested your control group against politicians, estate agents, CEOs and so on? In fact, let's say you tested your control group against 20 different professions, and the banker group was the only one that was "significant." Now we have a problem, because if we rerun a test 20 times, it is likely to be positive (under this p = 0.05 threshold at least) one of those times, *just by chance*.
>
> As an analogy, say Joe Superstitious flips a coin four times in a row, willing it with all his might to fall on heads four times in a row (with 1 in 16 odds, so pretty close to p = 0.05). But the first time it's just a mix of heads and tails. He tells himself that he was just getting warmed up, so let's ignore this round. So he tries again, and this time it's three heads and a tail—or so nearly there. His mojo must be building! The third time it's almost all tails, well that was because he was a bit distracted by a car horn outside. So he tries again, and again and again. Then, as if by magic, on the 20th attempt, he gets all four heads. Joe Superstitious proudly concludes that he is in fact very skilled at telekinesis, puts the coin in his pocket and saunters off.
>
> Joe Superstitious was obviously flawed in his thinking, but the reason is actually because he was using uncorrected statistics, just as the empathy study would have been if it concluded that bankers are less empathic than normal people. If you do multiple tests, you normally have to apply some mathematical correction to take account of how many tests you ran. One simple yet popular method of correction (known as a Bonferroni correction) involves dividing the probability your statistical test outputs by the number of tests you've done in total. So for the bankers to be significantly lower than the control at a p = 0.05 criterion, the statistical test would

have had to output a probability of p = 0.0025 (p = 0.05/20), which only occurs 1 in 400 times by chance.

Daniel Bor, *The Dilemma of Weak Neuroimaging Papers*, Daniel Bor: Neuroimaging Blog (Mar. 8, 2012).

5. If scientists can be challenged with reasoning about statistics, what about lawyers and the lay public? Some scholars have called attention to the problem of statistical illiteracy in health care, journalism, politics, and education. *See* Gerd Gigerenzer et al., *Helping Doctors and Patients Make Sense of Health Statistics*, 8 Psychol. Sci. Pub. Int. 53 (2008); John Monahan, Editorial, *Statistical Literacy: A Prerequisite for Evidence-Based Medicine*, 8 Psychol. Sci. Pub. Int. i (2008). Fortunately, particular training and exercises can improve anyone's statistical reasoning. Peter Sedlmeier & Gerd Gigerenzer, *Teaching Bayesian Reasoning in Less Than Two Hours*, 130 J. Experimental Psychol. 380 (2001).

6. There is an emerging body of literature suggesting that poverty is related to brain function. *See, e.g.,* Martha J. Farah, *Socioeconomic Status and the Brain: Prospects for Neuroscience-Informed Policy*, 19 Nature Reviews Neuro. 428 (2018); Martha J. Farah, *The Neuroscience of Socioeconomic Status: Correlates, Causes, and Consequences*, 96 Neuron 56 (2017). Given this new body of research, is it problematic that most neuroimaging studies to date have relied upon participants who are not representative of the population along socioeconomic indicators? *See* Francis X. Shen, *Is There an Ethical Duty to Report the Socioeconomic Status of Research Participants in Human Neuroscience Research?*, Presentation at the Annual Meeting of the Society for Neuroscience (Oct. 19, 2019) (finding that "99% of published human neuroimaging studies supported by NIH BRAIN do not report the socioeconomic status of the study participants.").

7. A 2020 headline read, "Google Publishes Largest Ever High-Resolution Map of Brain Connectivity." The sub-headline, however, grounded the headline in reality: "It's a fruit fly brain, but it's still impressive." Headlines like this catch our attention, and they accurately communicate that impressive strides are being made in understand the brain. Advances in understanding the non-human brain are enabled through a variety of the *invasive* methods reviewed in Chapter 4. But however impressive these studies may be, mapping connectivity in the fruit fly brain makes little immediate contribution to the legally relevant questions explored in this book. As neuroscience research on non-human animals improves—facilitated by methods that are not ethically permissible on humans—courts may be confronted with the challenge of how, if at all, to infer legally relevant conclusions about humans from non-human animal research findings. James Vincent, *Google Publishes Largest Ever High-Resolution Map of Brain Connectivity*, The Verge (Jan. 22, 2020).

C. CRITICAL PERSPECTIVES

As the amount of neuroscience in law, society, and mainstream media quickly grows, separating wheat from chaff will become increasingly important. Neuroscience is a powerful science, but maintaining realistic expectations is important. In this section we present several critiques, each aimed at a different facet of brain overclaim.

Joseph H. Baskin, Judith G. Edersheim & Bruce H. Price

Is a Picture Worth a Thousand Words? Neuroimaging in the Courtroom

33 Am. J.L. & Med. 239, 240, 268-69 (2007)

While "scientific" brain imaging appears to offer greater objectivity, current brain imaging techniques, by themselves, may be no more objective than the modalities that came before them. . . .

Data from fMRI, SPECT, and PET scans can be referenced and presented in dazzling multimedia displays that may inflate the scientific credibility of the information presented. Imaging, available in brilliant colors, with its apparent simplicity and vividness, accompanied by exotic names for brain regions, can prove irresistible to many defense attorneys, judges, and jurors. Sophisticated clinicians may present oversimplified, contradictory testimony that may be met with naïve acceptance or considerable skepticism by judges, juries, and society in general. The psychiatric or neurological expert who uses brain imaging in the courtroom must be careful to acknowledge the limitations of the technology, to resist inflating the meaning of the images, and to be more circumspect and less definitive than retaining counsel might prefer.

. . . No image to date can identify thoughts or ascribe motive. Images cannot distinguish thought from deed and have little, if any, predictive power.

What then can we conclude regarding the use of structural and functional imaging technology in the courtroom? Science is so uncharted at present that it is best to limit the legal use of neuroimaging to the elucidation of known structural correlates of neurological insult and the resulting inability to control behavior. These include instances in which the correlation between brain injury and behavior is specifically identified, well researched, and supported by other diagnostic modalities. The technical information derived from a brain image should be given added weight in assisting the fact finder in reaching a decision when it is complementary to other specific and neurologic data presented. Neuroimaging should not stand alone.

. . . [I]n the final analysis, criminal responsibility may be more of a moral question than scientific one. Even with further advances, neuroscience will supplement but not entirely supplant existing criteria of responsibility within moral and legal domains.

Teneille Brown & Emily Murphy

Through a Scanner Darkly: Functional Neuroimaging as Evidence of a Criminal Defendant's Past Mental States

62 Stan. L. Rev. 1119, 1204-08 (2010)

The familiar story is one of weak circumstantial evidence and impressive scientific findings. The combination of these elements may be a powerful prescription for injustice: scientific evidence seems so compelling that it could sway even the most skeptical juror and convince him that the elements of a weak case are proved beyond a reasonable doubt. If, on the other hand, the defendant catches the court's sympathies, then the junk science may swing in the opposite direction and make a weak defense appear stronger. This story has played out before with phrenology, the polygraph, and countless other forensic technologies that have since been discredited.

Improper reliance on each of these untested and unreliable technologies has led to unjust outcomes.

These older forensic technologies all have the window dressings of science. Each supplies the court with lab coat-wearing experts who will speak to analyses of "matching" criteria with confidence that their methods are sound. But despite popular appeal, phrenology, polygraphy, and fingerprint and handwriting analysis have never had the ringing endorsement of mainstream physical or biological sciences. In addition, empirical studies have confirmed that there is little reliability or validity in many of these methodologies. However, unlike these sensationalized forensic sciences, functional neuroimaging has the imprimatur of the scientific research community. Indeed, it is difficult to open a copy of Nature or Science without eyeing several colorful functional brain images.

Perhaps, then, the once fledgling field of genetics can provide a more appropriate analogy. So long as genetic samples are not contaminated, the ability to exclude someone from a suspect list based on modern DNA testing is fairly robust. Even so, recall that it took many years for DNA evidence to arrive at the presently-understood state of fallible yet scientifically-valid evidence. However, before the lab standards and analytical models were fully vetted, suspects were unfortunately charged based on DNA samples that were later found to have been carelessly analyzed.

Science can appear to be beyond the reach of human distortion. As a result, the more the scientific evidence relies on complex technologies like computers or imaging devices, the greater the risk that it may be endowed with powers to solve difficult legal questions. Litigants have long used this fact to their advantage, stretching scientific findings in order to retrofit them to legal conclusions. This may be what is happening with fMRI. The device is not yet capable of capturing past mental states, but because the criminal law is sometimes desperate to prove the unprovable, there will almost surely be an increase in proffered evidence and testimony based on this new technology. However, until fMRI is able to reliably capture past mental states, this evidence should not be admissible for such purposes either under FRE 403 or under local standards for admissibility of scientific evidence.

APPENDIX: CHECKLIST FOR JUDGES CONFRONTED WITH FUNCTIONAL NEUROIMAGING EVIDENCE

It is possible that the validity and probative value of fMRI in assessing mental states will improve in the future. It is also possible that the public understanding of the inferential leaps required by functional imaging techniques will progress such that the technology carries less risk of unfair prejudice. In the event that these twin events occur, judges and opposing counsel may appreciate having access to a simple checklist of questions that they can pose when deciding whether to admit fMRI evidence. Although our thesis is addressed to functional brain images used to prove mens rea, this checklist could also be applied to fMRI used as evidence of lie detection and other mental states.

General questions to ask counsel seeking to introduce functional neuroimaging evidence:

(a) Behavioral task. What is the particular behavior assessed during the scan? Why was the particular behavioral task chosen? Is it well supported in the psychological literature as best capturing this type of mental state? Did the subject perform the behavioral task adequately? Is the task vulnerable to manipulation, countermeasures, or malingering? Are the subject's behavioral data within or significantly outside the normal distribution of performance on the task?

(b) Controls. How were the controls selected to be in the control group? Are they the correct reference class? What sort of testing was done on the controls to make sure that they were in fact, "normal"? Is the sample size large enough to capture normal variance between subjects?

(c) Variance. Can you show us the brain scans of the control group, and are there significant differences among the individuals in this group? How much difference between individuals do we see?

(d) Image construction. Please walk us through the process for developing the image. How did you go from the raw data in the scanner to the color picture of the brain? Can you provide the raw data and exact methodology to an independent party for verification of the image creation process?

(e) Alternative explanations. What are possible alternate explanations for this behavior and corresponding neural activation correlates (i.e., expertise in the task, medication status, drug abuse history, hormonal fluctuations, language or motor limitation, etc.)?

(f) Purpose of fMRI evidence. What justifies the introduction of this brain image over evidence of the accused's behavior at the time of the crime?

(g) Statistical threshold. What statistical threshold was used to create the image? Why was it used?

(h) Causal connection. Is there a known or hypothesized mechanism causally connecting any perceived brain abnormality to a functional deficit? Do we have any data on the incidence of reduced metabolic or hemodynamic activity of this kind resulting in this type of cognitive deficit?

NOTES AND QUESTIONS

1. Although this chapter has focused on neuroscience specifically, it is important to remember that all empirical research necessarily involves various limitations. One interesting observation is that the effect sizes of some published results seem to decline over time. This is known as the "decline effect," and it could be the result of regression to the mean, i.e., the first result was particularly large (and hence most subsequent effect sizes are smaller). But as psychologist Jonathan Schooler has pointed out, we remain in the dark on the decline effect because we don't typically have access to unpublished results. Jonathan Schooler, *Unpublished Results Hide the Decline Effect*, 470 Nature 437 (2011). This is not a new problem, nor is it limited to the natural sciences. See, for instance, this particularly jabbing view of the extent to which data can be mined until gems appear: Edward E. Leamer, *Let's Take the Con Out of Econometrics*, 73 Am. Econ. Rev. 31 (1983).

2. Neuroscientific evidence is often presented along with behavioral genetics, leading to a similar claim: My genes made me do it. The use of genetic evidence as part of a criminal defense raises similar concerns about what (if any) legal inferences can be drawn. *See* Judith G. Edersheim, Bruce H. Price & Jordan

W. Smoller, *Your Honor, My Genes Made Me Do It*, Wall St. J., Oct. 22, 2012, at A21, arguing that

> You can't isolate a single gene from an individual and claim that it causes a complex human behavior such as violence. Genes don't operate in isolation but interact with social environments and other genes, and we often don't understand how gene variants operate in the working brain. Yet if we have learned anything over the past 100 years of violence research, it is that human violence is a complicated and multifactorial behavior and is not now—and may never be—reduced to a series of genetic variations or mutations. . . . [U]ntil we can make well-founded, scientifically sound and legally relevant links between genes, brains and behaviors, judges, juries and the public should be wary of neuroscience in the courtroom.

3. Consider the view of one critic:

> It's not hard to understand why neuroscience is so appealing. We all seek shortcuts to enlightenment. It's reassuring to believe that brain images and machine analysis will reveal the fundamental truth about our minds and their contents. But as the neuro doubters make plain, we may be asking too much of neuroscience, expecting that its explanations will be definitive.

Alissa Quart, *Neuroscience: Under Attack*, N.Y. Times (Nov. 23, 2012). Another critic has similarly written:

> [T]he "neural" explanation has become a gold standard of non-fiction exegesis, adding its own brand of computer-assisted lab-coat bling to a whole new industry of intellectual quackery that affects to elucidate even complex sociocultural phenomena. . . ."
>
> Happily, a new branch of the neuroscience explains everything genre may be created at any time by the simple expedient of adding the prefix "neuro" to whatever you are talking about. Thus, "neuroeconomics" is the latest in a long line of rhetorical attempts to sell the dismal science as a hard one; "molecular gastronomy" has now been trumped in the scientised gluttony stakes by "neurogastronomy"; students of Republican and Democratic brains are doing "neuropolitics"; literature academics practise "neurocriticism." There is "neurotheology," "neuromagic" (according to Sleights of Mind, an amusing book about how conjurors exploit perceptual bias) and even "neuromarketing." Hoping it's not too late to jump on the bandwagon, I have decided to announce that I, too, am skilled in the newly minted fields of neuroprocrastination and neuroflâneurship.

Steven Poole, *Your Brain on Pseudoscience: The Rise of Popular Neurobollocks*, New Statesman (Sept. 6, 2012). Are such criticisms on point? Overstated? Understated? What do and should we expect of neuroscience? Is neuroscience useless to law if it is not definitive?

It would be easy to take away from this chapter the notion that results from brain imaging are so variable, so complicated, and so uncertain that such results cannot be employed usefully by law. But that would be a mistake. The key idea to take away is that neuroscience research is most useful to law when it is carefully done and accurately interpreted. The debates over how best to conduct experiments and how best to interpret their findings and their limitations will continue in neuroscience, just as they do in other fields. By exposing you to some of the major issues in those debates, this chapter should equip you to be an informed consumer of neuroscientific information—neither overskeptical nor overzealous.

4. Structural neuroimaging evidence is sometimes used forensically to buttress other evidence of insanity. For a review of the literature, and suggestions for how to avoid misinterpreting such evidence, see Cristina Scarpazza et al., *The Charm of Structural Neuroimaging in Insanity Evaluations: Guidelines to Avoid Misinterpretation of the Findings*, 8 Translational Psychiatry 1 (2018).

5. In practice, forensic psychiatrists strike a balance when determining whether neuroimaging is appropriate in the courtroom. For commentary, see Gerben Meynen, *Forensic Psychiatry and Neurolaw: Description, Developments, and Debates*, 65 Int. J.L. & Psychiatry 101345, 5 (2019) (arguing that "Naïve use of neuro-tools for legal and forensic purposes will do more harm than good. At the same time, neglect of potentially helpful neuroscientific insights and techniques — under the motto of 'being very cautious' — may also have negative consequences for the justice system, and for forensic psychiatric evaluations in particular.")

With the next chapter, we start the transition from this trio of introductory brain science chapters to a trio of chapters detailing some of the crucial conceptual issues in neurolaw. As part of that transition, the next chapter encourages you to think about the intersection of law, science, and behavior generally, before we delve, in the subsequent chapters, into issues specific to the intersection of law and neuroscience.

Before beginning the next chapter, this is a good point at which to pause and do the following: (1) Without doing any research, prepare one paragraph offering your opinion on the similarities and differences between what law does and what science does. That is: compare the disciplines of law and science. (2) Without doing any research, prepare one paragraph offering your opinion on the nature of the relationship between law and human behavior. (Put another way: what is your view on how the concepts of "law" and "behavior" relate to each other?). (3) Without doing any research, prepare one paragraph giving your considered opinion/description of where behavior comes from. Taking a few moments to gather your thoughts on these questions will significantly aid your engagement with the coming chapters.

FURTHER READING

General Concerns, Limitations, and Procedures:

Russell A. Poldrack, *The New Mind Readers: What Neuroimaging Can and Cannot Reveal about Our Thoughts* (2018).

Ralph Adolphs, *The Unsolved Problems of Neuroscience*, 19 Trends Cognitive. Sci. 173 (2015).

John T. Cacioppo et al., *Just Because You're Imaging the Brain Doesn't Mean You Can Stop Using Your Head: A Primer and Set of First Principles*, 85 J. Personality & Soc. Psychol. 650 (2003).

Julien Dubois & Ralph Adolphs, *Building a Science of Individual Differences from fMRI*, 20 Trends Cognitive Sci. 425 (2016).

Gregory A. Miller, *Mistreating Psychology in the Decades of the Brain*, 5 Perspectives Psychol. Sci. 716 (2010).

Russell A. Poldrack, Jeanette A. Mumford & Thomas E. Nichols, *Handbook of Functional MRI Data Analysis* (2011).

Issues Concerning Risk of False Positives:

Nikolaus Kriegeskorte et al., *Circular Analysis in Systems Neuroscience: The Dangers of Double Dipping*, 12 Nature Neurosci. 535 (2009).

Craig M. Bennett & Michael M. Miller, *How Reliable are the Results from Functional Magnetic Resonance Imaging?*, 1191 Annals N.Y. Acad. Sci. 133 (2010).

Improved Procedures:

Russell A. Poldrack et al., *Guidelines for Reporting an fMRI Study*, 40 NeuroImage 409 (2007).

Russell A. Poldrack et al., *Scanning the Horizon: Towards Transparent and Reproducible Neuroimaging Research*, 18 Nature Reviews Neurosci. 115 (2017).

Andreas Keil et al., *Committee Report: Publication Guidelines and Recommendations for Studies Using Electroencephalography and Magnetoencephalography*, 51 Psychophysiology 1 (2014).

PART 3

BRAIN, BEHAVIOR, AND RESPONSIBILITY

To this point, we have taken a broad look at many intersections—both existing and potential—of law and neuroscience. We've considered a classic criminal case in which an individual defendant claimed that his murderous act could be traced, with important legal consequences, to interference with his normal brain function by a large cyst. And you've had an introduction to brain structures and functions, brain-monitoring and manipulations, and important limitations you should know about current technologies and how to interpret their findings.

You should, at this point, see the tension between sweeping possibilities and constraining realities. On one hand, the ability of new technologies to reveal information about brain structure and brain function, through noninvasive means, is an important step forward in understanding the relationships between brain and behavior, and between human cognition and the human condition. On the other hand, not even the longest technological stride can take us very far down the branching roads of legal complexity, where social constructs like "responsibility" reside and where tradeoffs between the ideals of individualized justice and the realities of imperfect information force hard choices that science alone cannot resolve.

Deciding how lawyers can or should use neuroscience, or how they might best defend against its use, requires a sound foundation in the legal contexts that make neuroscience arguably relevant to law, as well as in the rapidly advancing neuroscientific contexts that highlight both the promise and the limitations of neuroscience. To provide you with a deeper appreciation of how neuroscience is being invoked in legal arenas today (for better and for worse), and to develop more sophisticated critical thinking about possible uses in the future, this Part proceeds in three contextualizing steps.

PART SUMMARY

This Part:
- Explores, in Chapter 6, the interrelationships of law, science, and behavior.
- Compares and contrasts, in Chapter 7, legal and neuroscientific views on the mechanisms of human decision-making and behavior, as well as potential legal implications.
- Illustrates, in Chapter 8, various evidentiary issues relating to the use of neuroscientific evidence in the courtroom.

CHAPTER 6

Relationships of Law, Science, and Behavior

[P]eople have argued for years—does science make progress, and then the law has to conform, or does the law set the system, and then science has to follow it? It's probably a mixture of both. In the end, science . . . seeks for truth. In the end law seeks for truth. And in the end, both of us use our disciplines to shape our destiny and to ensure human progress, and we must do this together.
—Justice Anthony Kennedy[†]

Building more robust behavioral models to serve as solid fulcra for the lever of law requires, among other things, integrating existing social science and humanities models of human behavior with life science models.
—Owen D. Jones & Timothy H. Goldsmith[††]

CHAPTER SUMMARY

This chapter:
- Compares and contrasts the domains of law and science.
- Considers the development of "behavioral models" relevant to law, examining the ways in which science can illuminate law's behavioral models.
- Explores the questions law asks about behaviors, at both group and individual levels.

A. LAW AND SCIENCE

To understand the current uses of neuroscience in law, as well as potential future uses, we must evaluate how law and science relate to one another and what science has revealed about human behavior. This chapter addresses those issues.

First, let's consider similarities and differences between law and science as fields of human endeavor. As you did the exercise at the end of the prior chapter, you likely

---

[†] Allan Sobel, *The Intersection of Law and Science: Foreword*, 54 Drake L. Rev. 591, 596 (2006) (quoting Justice Anthony Kennedy, AJS Launch of Institute of Forensic Science and Public Policy and National Commission on Forensic Science and Public Policy 25-26 (Nov. 10, 2005) (transcript available at The Opperman Center at Drake University)).

[††] *Law and Behavioral Biology*, 105 Colum. L. Rev. 405, 421 (2005).

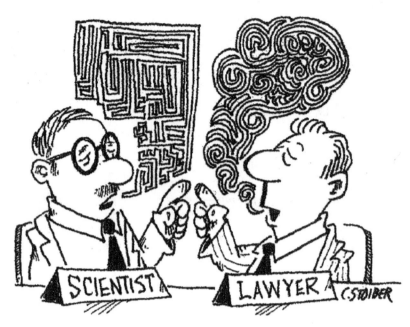

Figure 6.1   The language of science meets the language of law.   Copyright Carlton Stoiber, Washington, D.C.

concluded (with accompanying clusters of caveats) that—generally speaking—law and science are both tools that society uses to order the world, to answer important (albeit different) questions, and to resolve various kinds of disputes. Both require logical reasoning and both depend, in large measure, on acquired or demonstrated facts. Both include processes for seeking truths.

You likely also concluded that there are many differences between law and science. Whereas law is principally prescriptive, reflecting and supplying normative positions, science is principally descriptive, eschewing normative goals in furtherance of truth-seeking. (As before, there are, of course, many caveats.) Whereas law focuses on advancing the social order, science focuses on advancing knowledge. Whereas law regulates human behavior, science seeks (among other things) to understand and explain it. Legal methods and scientific methods are distinct. Whereas law is often deductive, applying general principles to specific cases, science is generally inductive, trying to derive general principles from individual bits of data. And the goals of law are as varied as the goals of humankind, while the goals of science are to illuminate the causes, machineries, and "laws" of nature—without necessarily giving humanity primacy of place.

The list of differences goes on. And there is a rich literature about how law and science relate to one another; how their practitioners understand (and often do not understand) one another; and how they work together when, as is often the case, they must.

For present purposes, it is enough to appreciate that what law does is often informed by many disciplines, including scientific knowledge. The extent to which science is useful in a particular context is often hotly debated. And when there is agreement on its usefulness, there can still be and often are sharp disagreements—even among science experts—on what the current state of scientific knowledge is and how it can or cannot bear on matters of legal import.

What we explore, in this book, is how a particular kind of science—neuroscience—may and may not usefully aid legal purposes. As evident in the chapters to follow, we take a broad view of what constitutes law, including discussion of common law, statutory law, administrative regulation, and legal decision-making, to name just a few. In these and other legal contexts, determining the relevance of neuroscience requires some reflection on law's relationship to behavior, on one hand, and science's impressive but necessarily imperfect abilities to illuminate the causes and complexities of that behavior, on the other.

B. CONNECTING LAW, SCIENCE, AND BEHAVIOR

On first encounter, combining the neurological complexity of brains with the technological complexity of brain imaging machines and the systemic complexity of law might seem bewildering and intimidating. What connects these things, exactly? And how is a lawyer (who, perhaps like most lawyers, has no deep scientific background) to make sense of it all?

To see the connections, let's simply start at the beginning. It should be clear that neuroscience is relevant to law only when it provides information that helps the legal system—or in some cases a litigant—make better, fairer, more accurate, more informed, more effective, or more efficient decisions. Can neuroscience do this? The answer depends, in part, on the context. Let's consider two.

The first context operates in the domain of *individualized* resolution of legal issues or conflicts, such as through civil and criminal litigation. Here, lawyers face the narrow and pragmatic questions (as did Weinstein's lawyers in Chapter 2): How can I best serve my client's interests? And is there something in neuroscience that can help me help my client?

The second context operates in the broader domain of *groups*. Here, policymakers of various sorts face the broad questions about how law should treat entire categories of people, such as juveniles, addicts, the LGBTQ community, those earning more (or less) than certain incomes, the sick but poor, those with mental illness, the married, or young males and females during wartime. Is there something in neuroscience that can help us decide how law can and should identify such groups, draw boundaries around or within such groups, and decide how best to treat, punish, or incentivize such groups?

1. The Level of the Group

Let's take these two contexts in reverse order, so that we may survey the forest before the trees. Thinking first at the broader level of groups, legal decision-makers must contemplate large communities of people, defined within the jurisdictional boundaries of states and nations. At this level, the challenge to law is one of providing fair, efficient, prosperous, stable, and peaceful governance. And that challenge is at base, necessarily, about how humans do or should behave.

Why is human behavior so central to legal governance? Because one primary purpose of the legal system is to engage with the fact that people are not *already* behaving in precisely the manner that existing or desired norms suggest. If people weren't occasionally inappropriately violent, for example, we would need no legal machinery for investigating, prosecuting, and incarcerating those who batter or kill. If everyone naturally drove on the right, there'd be no need to require that they do. If parties never breached contracts (or at least never failed, when they did so, to quickly satisfy aggrieved parties) and never behaved in ways reflecting inconsistent interpretations of contract terms, the Contracts course wouldn't be taught in every law school. And so on, through the rules for behavioral modification that we call Property, Torts, Civil Procedure, and all the rest.

There are many ways to think about this relationship between law and behavior. One common way is to view the legal system as machinery for deploying carrots and sticks in socially useful ways. Carrots (such as tax incentives to leave your old clothes at a local charity for distribution to the poor) essentially entice those who are not already doing so to behave in a way that, by fulfilling a self-interest, also serves a societal interest. Sticks (such as the use of police powers to constrain liberty and movement through incarceration) can remove and punish those who behave badly and deter them—and others who might behave similarly—from similar behavior in the future.

But there are limitations to characterizing law this way. For example, this approach neglects the process by which the legal system must make choices that connect legal responses to behavior. The legal system must not only decide which behaviors to encourage and which to discourage, but must also decide how to effect those preferences. Should law meet undesirable behavior with a slap on the wrist, changes to tax laws, shaming sanctions, fines, imprisonment, or something else entirely? What informs law's choices among options?

A better way to think of the legal system, perhaps, is as a lever for moving human behavior in directions it would not ordinarily go on its own. This image has limitations too. For example, law not only influences human behavior, it's also, itself, a form of human behavior. And there are schools of thought that see some legal activity, such as punishment, as its own categorical good quite apart from its utility in changing future behavior. Nonetheless, this lever metaphor has one significant advantage: It focuses attention on the importance to law of having a solid fulcrum. A fulcrum, you will recall, is the crucial support on which a lever rests.

In the sense we're using it here, the fulcrum is a "behavioral model"—the sum total of all our best thinking, experience, and knowledge about how and why people behave as they do. In the same way that a real lever is ineffective without a strong fulcrum against which to lean, the legal system can rarely be more effective than its model of human behavior is accurate. An inaccurate model bends and breaks under the pressure a legal regime subjects it to—because the assumptions law makes about how people will respond to particular legal interventions will be incorrect. The behavioral model is the thing that suggests to us: If law moves this way, behavior will move that way, and not some other entirely unintended third way.

In other words, every legal intervention reflects assumptions about human behavior that inevitably vary in accuracy. And, all else equal, the more accurate the model of human behavior, the more behavioral modification bang we get for each interventionist legal buck.

We're not to neuroscience yet, but you can probably see that we're on our way there. Because where do our models of human behavior come from, and what populates them? They come from a variety of sources, including observation, experience, trial and error, self-reflection, projection, logic, and intuitions.

Everyone has some basic and operational beliefs about how and why people behave as they do and what sorts of things are likely to increase the chances that they will behave differently. It would be hard to succeed on this planet without them. Some of these beliefs are informed by the Humanities. (Try reading *The Odyssey* without learning a little something about human behavior.) Some of these beliefs derive from religious and spiritual traditions. And some of these beliefs are informed by advances in one or more of the Social Sciences, such as Sociology or Economics.

The legal system, by and large, follows this social trend in supplementing human experience, traditions, and intuitions with the teachings of the Humanities and the Social Sciences. There is only one problem. And it is a big one. It is that human behaviors don't come pre-sorted into those that can, for instance, be illuminated through Sociology (rather than other disciplines) and those that, instead, are in the rightful domain of Economics, etc. As in the parable of the first time an elephant was encountered by blind men—each of whom thought the elephant to be either like a tree-trunk, a rope, or a spear, depending on whether he felt a leg, tail, or tusk—behavior as a whole, like reality as a whole, is not reasonably susceptible of parsing into exclusive disciplinary domains.

The next reading explores some implications of this, including the need, in many contexts, to add behavioral biology (a supercategory that includes neuroscience) into the model.

Owen D. Jones & Timothy H. Goldsmith
Law and Behavioral Biology
105 Colum. L. Rev. 405, 405-09 (2005)

INTRODUCTION

In all but a few universities, human behavior is studied by social scientists in one set of buildings, while the behavior of every species except humans is studied by life scientists in other buildings. There are reasons for this—but few good ones.

The division reflects a long history of scholarly traditions moving on separate tracks. To be sure, there are gains from specialization. But there are also losses from impeded exchange of knowledge, insufficient synergy, and a scholarly isolation that allows cross disciplinary inconsistencies to lurk unnoticed. These in turn enable longstanding but disciplinarily constricted conceptions of human behavior to harden into the received truths of the next academic generation.

This poses increasingly significant problems for legal thinkers, for human behavior is the very currency in which law deals. Helping to govern how humans behave and interact with one another, in their myriad individual and collective ventures and misadventures, is a—perhaps the—principal reason law exists. Law consequently has an unending need for improved understandings of how and why humans behave as they do.

Yet there is no widespread consensus in law that a deeper understanding of the causes of human behavior is really necessary for the day-to-day work. And among those who consider a deeper understanding desirable, there is no standard method for seeking, extracting, and developing that information from among the ranging disciplines. Viewed as a whole, the process by which law informs itself about the *causes* of human behavior (as distinct from the effects and patterns of human behavior) is haphazard, idiosyncratic, and unsystematic. When legal thinkers do look to other disciplines for updated theories and findings about causes, most tend to focus principally on social sciences such as economics, psychology, or political science, sometimes supplemented by a sprinkling of philosophy, sociology, or passing references to "human nature." This focus has, of course, often been productive. But not everyone holds the same truths to be self-evident.

We see four problems. First, law still struggles to induce people to behave more constructively. This, coupled with explicit calls from some legal quarters for a more comprehensive behavioral science, strongly suggests that existing perspectives on behavior are incomplete and insufficiently satisfying. Second, when it does look to other disciplines for insights concerning a given behavior, law commonly incorporates the perspective of one discipline at a time, rather than pursuing a synthesis of perspectives that may be more accurate and more useful. Third, the favored perspective on the causes of human behavior often reflects ephemeral enthusiasms wafted on the politics of the moment. Fourth, by focusing almost exclusively on the social sciences (sometimes supplemented by the humanities), legal thinkers have generally ignored an array of interdisciplinary approaches that are rapidly changing the way we understand how the mind works and what it means to be human.

Failure to attend to this new knowledge can lead to importantly incorrect assumptions about the causes of human behaviors, as well as to missed opportunities for improvements in law's ability to regulate behavior. For example, it is common to assume that virtually all behavior relevant to law arises exclusively through environmental, cultural pathways. This assumption overlooks essential components of causation that underlie the behaviors law seeks to address and also obscures important patterns of behavior that offer both knowledge and utility. That, in turn, risks law's anachronism, and it is limited, limiting, and costly—as well as avoidable.

It is avoidable, in part, because there is gathering momentum within universities for interdisciplinary work, including that which explores the human mind. And it is avoidable, in particular, because the important melding of perspectives and techniques now occurring in the behavioral sciences is increasingly accessible to legal scholars. Just as exploring the moon or Mars requires the integrated efforts of physicists, astronomers, geologists, engineers, chemists, and physiologists, it is increasingly clear that exploring and understanding the human mind requires the integrated, interdisciplinary efforts of cognitive scientists, neuroscientists, and evolutionary biologists as well as social scientists in psychology, anthropology, economics, and related disciplines. Empirical findings from different disciplines increasingly point toward similar conclusions that reflect a converging understanding of behavior. In principle, this synergy is valuable because it enables us to synthesize a coherent whole greater than the sum of its parts. It can help us to understand realities underlying behavior in a more subtle, comprehensive, and sophisticated way.

Some legal scholars have begun to deploy insights from behavioral biology to address existing problems in law.[3] . . .

---

3 This work goes by a variety of names, such as evolutionary analysis in law, law and biology, law and behavioral research, and the like. One of us (Jones) maintains a bibliography of works in this area that can be accessed through the webpage of the Society for Evolutionary Analysis in Law (SEAL), https://www.vanderbilt.edu/seal.

I. LAW, BEHAVIOR, AND BEHAVIORAL MODELS

Until about forty years ago, legal thinkers were firm in the conviction that law was an autonomous discipline.[5] Law was a subject "properly entrusted to persons trained in law and in nothing else,"[6] who could draw to sufficient effect upon general intelligence, general education, legal texts, and the experiential wisdom developed early in law practice. The decline of that parochial view has coincided with the rise of the many "law and" subjects familiar today. Law is increasingly seen, at least in large measure, as a consumer and applier of knowledge that other disciplines offer. . . .

Some efforts have proved more enduring than others. . . . [O]ur claim is not that law and behavioral biology should compete with other disciplines for dominant influence. The study of biology is, after all, the study of how multiple causal influences interact in organisms and their behavior. Our claim is therefore necessarily more modest: Behavioral biology provides one important component of many necessary to any firm foundation for understanding human behavior. . . .

A. The Relationship Between Law and Behavior

One view — perhaps the most common one — is that law attempts many things, only one subset of which concerns behavior. Law allocates property, it reduces injuries, it provides justice, and it also both prohibits some behaviors and mandates others. From a broader perspective, however, one can make a strong case that all law exists to effect changes in human behavior.

Allocating property rights, for example, is meaningless except to the extent it defines how people may and may not behave with respect to owned things. Reducing injuries involves inducing those who have unjustifiably caused harm to behave differently in the future — for example, by taking more care or designing safer products. Procedural rules govern how people will coordinate their behavior during formal contests over conflicts. Constitutional law prescribes how people in branches of government may and may not behave toward each other, and may and may not behave toward the governed. Contract law ensures that people who behaved a certain way in the past (creating obligation) will behave a particular way in the future (performing or paying compensation) — all so that still other people will have requisite confidence to engage in future transactional behavior with yet other people. Providing justice almost inevitably results in important changes in behavior, as the essence of injustice is unfair or improper treatment of one party at the hands of another. And criminal and civil fines are among the ways we induce people to behave as society wants. Examples could of course be multiplied.

B. The Relationship Between Law and Behavioral Models

We can consider law effective when it gets its job done, and efficient when it does so with minimum waste. If the enterprise of law is, in the main, to change human behavior according to socially percolated preferences, then its ability to deploy legal tools to effect these changes at the least cost to society often (though importantly not always) depends on the accuracy of the behavioral models on which law relies.

---

5 *See generally* Richard A. Posner, *The Decline of Law as an Autonomous Discipline: 1962-1987*, 100 Harv. L. Rev. 761 (1987).

6 *Id.* at 762.

By "behavioral models" we refer to the combination of knowledge, intuition, and experience that enables us collectively to expect that, when law takes a given action, people will likely respond in patterns consistent with law's intent.

In the context of a given behavior of interest, a sound behavioral model should include, at a minimum, two features. It should include the impressions we have, arising from empirical observations, about how people actually behave in response to various changes in the legal environment, and it should also include, whenever possible, prevailing theoretical and empirical understandings of *why* people will behave the way the behavioral model anticipates. . . .

The key point at the outset is that a good behavioral model makes predictions about the ways environmental inputs will affect behavioral outputs not only on the basis of raw observational data, but also by connecting the data with explanatory, causal theories that enable not only a greater understanding of phenomena already observed, but also useful extrapolations into new contexts. Although it is possible to learn a fair amount about how people behave solely through multiple iterations of trial and error, that approach is not very practical. Not only is it inefficient, but it also has no theoretical foundation from which to generate promising hypotheses to be tested. Even if it worked reasonably well, this approach would not be particularly satisfying, for it affords no sense of the distance between what has been achieved and what is achievable. In short, it neither provides nor leads to any deep and generative understanding of human behavior, either generally or specifically.

In current legal education, it is not only possible but also common to study torts, criminal law, contracts, and all the rest without ever pausing to specifically consider the behavioral models on which different legal approaches within these subjects rely. Moreover, we suspect it is only the exceedingly rare judge, legislator, professor, or member of law enforcement who considers this question explicitly. One might therefore wonder whether law really uses any behavioral models at all.

The answer, we believe, must clearly be yes. We all live in contexts thick with human behavior. The better we understand people—what they are like, how they behave, when they will respond to circumstances with one set of reactions instead of others, and within what general ranges of behavior they will act—the better we can navigate the insistent challenges of social living. Our understanding may grow as a product of cultural experience, but even that experience is processed by and reflected in brains that evolved in highly social environments. We therefore carry with us—partly for evolutionary reasons, and whether we are aware of them or not—assumptions about human nature that serve to make sense of social actions.

What is true in life is no less true in law. The legal system is immersed in behavioral models, some open, most hidden. Every time a judge pronounces sentence, every time Congress passes a law, every time an agency establishes penalties for transgressions, every time parties maneuver through threats of litigation, people are acting with a theory about what will happen in the minds of other people. As surely as all legal activities reflect assumptions about how people's behavior will respond to particular environmental circumstances, these aggregated assumptions constitute behavioral models, however hidden from conscious view.

To put the relationship metaphorically, law is a lever for moving behavior that has a model of human behavior as its fulcrum. That fulcrum consists of what we think we know about how and why people behave as they do, and it therefore incorporates the aggregated insights that underlie our prediction that if law moves this way behavior will move that way, and not some other way. Consequently, law can generally obtain no more leverage on human behaviors it seeks to change than the accuracy of its behavioral model allows. Since a soft fulcrum provides poor support, the success of every legal system necessarily depends, in part, on the solidity—the accuracy, robustness, and predictive power—of the behavioral model on which it relies.

C. Contemporary Behavioral Models

It remains to be considered, then, how well law's behavioral models serve as fulcra for the levers of law. Although it is possible to make some generalizations, it is not a simple matter to assess the quality and relative solidity of existing behavioral models. There are at least four reasons.

First, as alluded to earlier, the behavioral models on which law relies are rarely explicit. . . .

Second, behavioral models almost certainly vary somewhat by jurisdiction. The collective legal systems of the United States obviously do not reflect a coordinated effort to deploy a common and consistent national model of behavior. Nor does it appear likely that any single constituent jurisdiction, state or local, actually deploys a consistent approach to behavioral models across all or even many areas of law.

Third, behavioral models vary considerably across behaviors. Looking across the many facets of law's endeavors, it is unavoidably obvious that law rarely attempts to connect—let alone crosscheck for consistency—assumptions that underlie its approaches to different behaviors. Law's pattern—though often reasonably effective—is generally ad hoc and narrowly reactive. It addresses accidental pool drownings of infants here, driving while intoxicated there, underreporting income somewhere else, and sexual aggression, overfishing, jaywalking, market coordination, and discovery rules still elsewhere, with isolated focus.

Fourth, there has been to date no concerted effort to systematically develop a science for fairly, reliably, and correctly inferring, deducing, and otherwise extracting from legislative, judicial, and executive actions the specific set of assumptions on which each legal action lies. Nor, since that would be an obvious prerequisite, has there been a subsequent metastudy of how the behavioral models aggregating these assumptions compare with one another on various relevant dimensions, such as content of assumptions, accuracy of assumptions, and effectiveness of programs based on the assumptions. . . .

Existing behavioral models are multiple in number, diffuse in kind, indistinct in form, and inconsistent in content. The general impression one gets from reading and observing legal activity is that there is no consistent set of assumptions about human behavior that has been drawn from relevant scholarly disciplines. There is little to suggest that behavioral models do anything more regularized than shift according to varying emphases on such things as emotions, perceptions, rational choice, heuristics and biases, and political movements.

Even in the absence of a conclusive study, most legal thinkers likely agree that to the extent law relies on behavioral models, these reflect varying amalgamations of trial and error, intuition, observation, experience, self-reflection, path dependence, imitation, the influence of various disciplines that appeal at any given moment, and hope. . . .

Despite these several challenges, it is still possible to generalize that law's behavioral models are imperfect and to offer at least some partial diagnosis for why this may be true. First, and least surprisingly, we know law is imperfect because there are so many ways in which efforts to channel human behavior fail daily. Without minimizing law's many successes, which are in part responsible (alongside nonlegal norms, technological advances, cultural practices, religions, and other cultural practices) for the internal stability of many human societies, no one could seriously entertain the argument that legal systems are not in need of improvement.

Second, and more to the point, at least some large measure of law's failings can be attributed to weaknesses in the behavioral models law deploys to regulate behavior. . . .

There are doubtless many areas in which these and other perspectives on behavioral models could be improved. But in this Article we focus on one, which happens to be an elephant in the room. However else they may be aligned, law's behavioral models are aligned in this: their nearly wholesale omission of life science perspectives on where behavior comes from, how it emerges, what processes give rise to its patterns, and how multiple causal influences will intersect to affect it.

We do not, of course, mean to suggest that biology has played no role in law. In the broad sense, biology has become central to myriad legal questions, such as those addressing reproductive technology, environmental resources, forensic identification, genetically modified foods, and property rights in biotechnology industries. . . .

We are referring, instead, to the near-total absence of recognition in legal thinking that all behavior, and all the brain activity that perceives and directs it, are fundamentally biological phenomena, rendering the study of behavioral biology manifestly relevant to any deep and current understanding of how and why humans behave in ways important to law. Phrased this way, some might object that everyone knows that the brain is involved in behavior and that actions occur as a function of muscle contractions, themselves biological in origin. But that is a very superficial nod to the biology of human behavior. . . .

There is already a large body of nearly untapped literature in behavioral biology that is rich in theory and increasingly robust in empirical work. Over the last few years, it has been growing at an extraordinary rate. Given law's focus on behavior, it is regrettable that law's behavioral models have for so long omitted life science perspectives. Neglect may be attributable to path dependence, the overspecialization of scholars, and the attendant balkanization of subjects within most universities. It may be a product of demonstrably false dichotomies—such as "nature versus nurture"—taking misleading hold in the public's mind, suggesting that the set of biological influences excludes the set of cultural influences. It probably is a function of the fact that so few trained in law have also been trained in science generally, or biology specifically. It is almost certainly also a product of a variety of misunderstandings, as well as both reasonable and unreasonable fears about what biological knowledge does and can legitimately say about human behavior, and about what the political implications—for racism, sexism, genetic determinism, and other evils—might be, whether based on use or misuse of biological information.

At the broadest level, however, law's relationship to science and technology is complex and often problematic.[30] Science is routinely ignored, misunderstood, or improperly invoked by judges, legislators, agency personnel, and other

---

30 *See generally* David L. Faigman, *Laboratory of Justice: The Supreme Court's 200-Year Struggle to Integrate Science and the Law* (2004).

policymakers.[31] Well-known examples include litigation contexts in which the underlying scientific claims are largely undemonstrated or in which error rates are far higher than courts acknowledge, such as those involving lie detectors, handwriting, bitemarks, toolmarks, arson, visual identification of individuals, and even fingerprints.[32] Courts frequently misunderstand or misapply statistical research and are confronted with the efforts of parties to introduce as science what some refer to as "junk science." Experts have called law reform efforts reflecting a large gap between legislative assumptions and empirical data "breathtakingly negligent."[35] And Congress has been known to empanel commissions charged with recommending legal approaches to a technology without bothering to include any experts on the technology itself.

In the context of law and biology generally, science often is similarly ignored, misunderstood, or improperly invoked. The breast implant litigation famously ignored medical findings, including negative results. The notorious Delaney Amendment established a scientifically ridiculous policy of zero tolerance for carcinogens. Tort reform, particularly medical malpractice reform, regularly proceeds on the basis of assumptions contrary to data. And in the environmental context, legislators routinely legislate as if difficult matters of science were simple.

In the context of law and behavioral biology, more specifically, the situation is often equally grim. The discordant clash of law and science has been especially obvious in cases involving mental illness. Clinical predictions of future dangerousness are often untrustworthy, despite their often unskeptical use in law. Courts typically assume that individualized evaluations and predictions by clinical psychologists and psychiatrists, parole officials, and others are more accurate than statistical profiles, even though those assumptions are predominantly wrong.

More disturbingly, the operation of the legal system often reflects outdated and incorrect assumptions about behavior that—even when they do not yield clear errors—often forgo opportunities for improvement. To mention just a few examples to be explored in Part III, outdated assumptions about the processes that shape human behavior generally can obscure patterns relevant to law, such as those evident in instances of child abuse. Outdated assumptions about the causal influences on human behavior can lead to false dichotomies, such as those evident in the law's treatment of sexual aggression. Outdated assumptions can cause us to overlook factors relevant to cost-benefit calculations. And outdated assumptions about how the brain operates can yield analytic missteps, such as are present in the law and behavioral economics approach to irrational behavior.

D. The Relationship Between Behavioral Models and Behavioral Biology

So if law is about changing behavior, changing behavior requires sound behavioral models, and our behavioral models are evidently incomplete, then by what process might they be improved so as to serve as a more solid fulcrum for the lever of law? We do not have a full answer. But we have a partial one. . . . Building more robust behavioral models to serve as solid fulcra for the lever of law requires, among

---

31 *See generally* David L. Faigman, *Legal Alchemy: The Use and Misuse of Science in the Law* 53-54 (1999).
32 *See generally Science in the Law: Forensic Science Issues* (David L. Faigman et al. eds., 2002).
35 *See, e.g.,* Teresa A. Sullivan et al., *As We Forgive Our Debtors: Bankruptcy and Consumer Credit in America* 336 (1989).

other things, integrating existing social science and humanities models of human behavior with life science models.

Such an integrative approach should offer some gains in both the effectiveness and efficiency of law for the simple reason that biology addresses some unrecognized or underrecognized influences on behavior that in fact exist. It is important to distinguish biology, in this respect, from disciplines such as those constituting the humanities that—however useful they may be—are generally more interpretive or normative than scientific. Biology is not a discipline that simply offers one way of looking at human behavior—though it does offer that, too. Biology provides a process for uncovering scientific facts about what influences human behavior, why, and how. . . .

While existing social science and humanities approaches focus exclusively on the influences of environmental features (such as cultural norms) on human behavior, modern science makes unequivocally clear that the complexity of the causal influences underlying that behavior cannot be captured by simplistic models that focus on environmental features alone. Gaining an improved understanding of that complexity requires attention to biology because (1) all theories of human behavior are ultimately theories about the brain; (2) the brain is a computational organ that works on physical principles; and (3) modern biology makes forcefully clear that the brain's design, function, and behavioral outputs are all products of gene-environment interactions that have been shaped through time by various evolutionary and developmental processes. . . .

What does it mean to integrate life science and behavioral biology perspectives into models of human behavior? It means considering the ways in which the fields of evolutionary biology, behavioral genetics, cognitive psychology, and neuroscience (the last two of which are often referred to in intersection as "cognitive neuroscience") provide useful contributions toward understanding the complexities of human behavior.

Although it is beyond the scope of this book to provide detailed introductions to each of these, it is worth your being aware, at a minimum, that:

- Evolutionary biology explores the ways in which various evolutionary processes, including natural selection, can and have shaped human bodies (including brains) and behavioral predispositions across time. Although you are probably already aware of the term generally, you should at this point also be aware that "natural selection" describes the inevitable result of any system that combines: (1) heritable traits; (2) variations in those traits; and (3) differential reproduction as a function of bearing those traits. In a nutshell, those traits that contribute more effectively toward survival and reproduction than do contemporaneous traits exhibited by other organisms will tend to appear in increasingly large proportions of subsequent generations (all else equal). Significant changes to the environments that members of a species encounter can lead to mismatches between features that humans evolved to have and features it would now, in the current environment, be better to have.
- Behavioral genetics is a subset of genetics that studies the influence of genes on behaviors. It is essential to note that, in all but a few cases, the presence of a gene does not alone determine whether a particular behavior will or will

not manifest in someone. The overwhelming majority of behaviors are the product of gene/environment interactions (just as the area of a rectangle is the product of both its length and its width*) such that genetic potentiality may manifest only in the presence of certain environmental conditions.

- Cognitive psychology scientifically investigates mental states such as perception, memory, decision-making, and intention. Subsequent chapters on memory and decision-making will introduce this in more detail.
- Neuroscience is a subfield of biology and medicine (and, increasingly, other fields such as physics, chemistry) that explores what the brain is made of, how it works, and how it can be treated through surgical or drug interventions. The scope of neuroscience is vast, ranging from molecules in invertebrates to whole brain systems in humans.

In this book we are concerned principally with the existing and potential implications of cognitive neuroscience—the study of the structure and function of the nervous system underlying mental processes—for law. And, in this subsection, we have thus far explored the conceptual framework in which it may be relevant when law addresses behavior at the broad community or group levels. In the next section, we highlight the significance of applying neuroscience to questions about specific individuals. As should be obvious, however, the distinctions between group- and individual-level applications are not perfectly divisible. There are many overlaps between them, and the legal system must often grapple with the vexing problem of using group-based data in individual-level adjudication.

2. The Level of the Individual

We stated earlier that the usefulness of science to law is not automatic, but rather depends on the ability of a science to usefully inform a specific legal decision. What are some of the legal questions law encounters as to which—at least on first blush—science might have some individually relevant contributions to make?

Here, it helps to imagine litigation over issues that instead of being relevant to entire populations (e.g. how should we use the tools of law to reduce the incidence of violence in America?) address very fact- and person-specific problems. This is the domain of, for example, contests over a will provision, prosecution for the killing of a spouse found in bed with another, a claim for compensatory monies following injuries sustained in a car accident, and the like.

In these kinds of contexts the legal system is called upon to resolve highly individualized issues such as:

- Was this decedent legally competent at the time she executed her most recent will?
- Should this defendant be held criminally responsible for his prohibited behavior?
- What was this person's mental state, at the time of the act?
- Did the defendant really intend to defraud the government, or was he just careless?

---

* [The rectangle metaphor for nature/nurture interactions originated with psychologist O.E. Hebb. — EDS.]

- What capacity did this person have to act differently than she did?
- How injured is this person's brain?
- How much pain and distress is the litigant feeling?
- Is this person mentally ill?
- Was this person competent to contract?
- What does this person remember?
- How accurate is this person's memory?
- Is this person telling the truth?
- Should an inmate receive treatment, and if so what kind? For a particular addiction?
- If released from custody, will this person commit another violent crime?
- Was this plaintiff's mental distress caused by the defendant or by something else?

To answer each of these and similar questions, the legal system makes official, legally-operative pronouncements about what the facts are (or will be considered to have been). Because these questions are both deeply complicated and vitally important, parties draw on wide varieties of scientific literature and expert testimony in efforts to inform and influence judge and juror thinking. The machinery of the legal and regulatory systems also relies heavily, and sometimes without transparency, on individualized assessment. Pre-sentence reports in the criminal justice system are but one example.

How can the legal system best connect research on groups to legally relevant questions about individuals? Consider the suggestion offered in the next reading.

The MacArthur Foundation Research Network on Law and Neuroscience
G2i: A Knowledge Brief
(2017)

There's a good chance that if you take an aspirin, your headache will disappear. Then again, it might not.

Decades of clinical trials conducted with hundreds of thousands of ordinary headache sufferers confirm that the humble aspirin really works. So, why isn't your headache budging? The answer, or a version of it, is usually somewhere on the package insert: individual results may vary. The longer version of the marketing shorthand is this: Even the best science—science characterized by rich data collected from multiple experimental subjects or events and over multiple trials or experiments—frequently can tell us little, if anything at all, about the individual case.

Science seeks to understand general phenomena, not particular instances. Scientists typically don't attempt to infer from group or population-based data (or "G") to a particular individual (or "i"). Answering the individual question simply isn't part of the everyday scientific enterprise. That's why the applied science that is part of our everyday lives—whether in the form of drugs, diagnostic tests, or weather forecasts—doesn't come with a promise. It comes with a probability.

G2i IN THE COURTS: MUDDLING THROUGH

The challenge of reasoning from group data to make decisions about individuals—a process we call "G2i"—is endemic in the modern courtroom. As in everyday life, that challenge is also frequently ignored, underestimated, or misunderstood.

Neuroscientists offer evidence that, on average, adolescents are less developmentally mature than adults. Cognitive psychologists testify to factors that contribute to eyewitness misidentification. Psychiatrists identify factors associated with "future dangerousness." In each case, experts offer general statements about the empirical world based on aggregate data across groups of individuals. The courts, however, are typically looking for answers specific to the case at hand: Is or was *this* defendant developmentally mature? Was *this* eyewitness's identification accurate? Will this defendant be violent in the future?

Courts are generally guided by one of two cases when it comes to admitting—or excluding—scientific evidence. Established in 1923, the *Frye* test asks whether the scientific methods supporting the expert opinions are generally accepted in the particular fields from which they come. Seventy years later, the Supreme Court ruled that the applicable federal rules of evidence replaced *Frye* test with a validity test. Under that approach, first established in the case of *Daubert v. Merrell Dow Pharmaceuticals, Inc.,* courts must determine whether the methods and principles underlying the expert opinion are reliable and valid.* Today, *Daubert* is the rule in all federal cases. Most states have adopted it, as well, and many others have been influenced by its reasoning. Neither *Frye* nor *Daubert,* however, speak directly to G2i.

Courts are daily confronted with admissibility issues, some of which involve the existence of the general phenomenon (i.e., "G") and others the question of whether a particular case is an instance of that general phenomenon (i.e., "i"). For instance, research might indicate that a particular abnormality in a part of the brain called the amygdala is associated with psychopathy. But many psychopaths have normal amygdalae and many non-psychopaths have abnormal amygdalae. So although, on average, psychopaths might have more abnormal amygdalae than nonpsychopaths, a particular person's amygdala is not diagnostic of psychopathy.

Unfortunately, courts have yet to carefully consider the implications of G2i for their admissibility decisions. In some areas, courts limit an expert's testimony to the general phenomenon. They insist that whether the case at hand is an instance of that phenomenon is exclusively a jury question, and thus not an appropriate subject of expert opinion. In other cases, in contrast, courts hold that expert evidence must be provided on *both* the group-data issue, i.e., that the phenomenon exists, and what is called the "diagnostic" issue, i.e., that this case is an instance of that phenomenon.

Courts' treatment of expert testimony on factors that might lower the accuracy of eyewitness identifications illustrates the "phenomenon only" approach. Courts generally permit eyewitness experts to testify about factors, such as cross-race identifications or stress, that might negatively affect accuracy. They do not permit testimony, however, on whether a particular identification was accurate or not. In *United States v. Smith,*** for instance, the court explained that the value of this general testimony was educative: "Educating the jury about this research . . . is an important step along the road to using improved scientific knowledge to create more accurate and fair legal proceedings." The testimony was not, the *Smith* court emphasized, diagnostic: "Applying this research to the facts of the case is within the sole province of the jury."

---

* [We will return to the *Frye* and *Daubert* tests in Chapter 8: Neuroscience in the Courtroom.—EDS.]
** [*United States v. Smith,* 621 F. Supp. 2d 1207 (M.D. Ala. 2009)—EDS.]

Yet in a host of other cases, the courts either demand or permit experts to offer diagnostic opinions on whether the case at hand is an instance of some legally relevant phenomenon. In medical causation cases, for example, a plaintiff must introduce expert testimony on both "G" and "i". A plaintiff claiming that benzene exposure caused his or her leukemia, for instance, would have to introduce both general scientific evidence that benzene causes leukemia and scientific diagnostic evidence that exposure to benzene specifically caused his or her leukemia. In cases involving forensic identification—ranging from fingerprints to firearms—the courts generally allow experts to testify to both "G" and "i". Thus, a firearms expert typically testifies that certain marks on cartridge cases are associated with a group of firearms and, additionally, that the marks on the cartridge case found at the crime scene were made by a specific gun.

Unfortunately, the cases in which the courts insist on, or permit, diagnostic testimony do not necessarily align with scientists' ability to offer valid diagnostic opinions. It is exceedingly difficult to determine whether a particular case of leukemia is attributable to benzene exposure, and it's impossible to say that the marks on a cartridge case came from a particular gun. A key insight of G2i, then, is that courts should assess an expert's ability to provide empirical framework evidence separately from his or her ability to provide diagnostic evidence.

KNOWLEDGE AND ITS LIMITS: THE ADOLESCENT BRAIN

Three decisions of the United States Supreme Court illustrate both how far we have come and how far we still have to go in understanding the limitations of scientific inference. All three cases involved grouplevel behavioral and neuroscience research that demonstrates that the brain, with its concomitant developmental capacities, does not fully mature until the early 20s.

In *Roper v. Simmons* (2005), the Court held that the Eighth Amendment did not permit imposing the death penalty on a defendant who had killed prior to his eighteenth birthday.* Writing for the majority, Justice Kennedy implicitly acknowledged that justice must take into account both the validity of the "G"—the empirical evidence that on average the adolescent is not developmentally mature—and the difficulty of the "i," that is, of knowing whether a particular adolescent is mature or not.

"[T]he differences between juvenile and adult offenders," Kennedy wrote, "are too marked and well understood to risk allowing a youthful person to receive the death penalty despite insufficient culpability." Drawing a line at 18 years of age, the Court allowed, was arbitrary but necessary under the circumstances. "It is difficult even for expert psychologists to differentiate between the juvenile offender whose crime reflects unfortunate yet transient immaturity, and the rare juvenile offender whose crime reflects irreparable corruption," he wrote.

In *Graham v Florida* (2009), the Court extended this reasoning to another set of juvenile offenders, those facing life without parole for crimes other than homicide. The decision, like the one in *Roper*, was categorical, applying to all individuals below the age of 18 at the time the crime was committed. Again, the Court explained, "even if we were to assume that some juvenile nonhomicide offenders . . . merit

---

* [We will return to the three U.S. Supreme Court cases, mentioned in these paragraphs, in Chapter 17: Adolescent Brains. — EDS.]

a life without parole sentence, it does not follow that courts taking a case-by-case proportionality approach could with sufficient accuracy distinguish the few incorrigible juvenile offenders from the many that have the capacity for change."

Finally, in *Miller v. Alabama* (2013), the Court concluded that the Eighth Amendment also prohibits mandatory life without parole for juveniles convicted of homicide. Citing both *Roper* and *Graham*, once again the Court's decision referenced scientific findings that "both lessened a child's 'moral culpability' and enhanced the prospect that, as the years go by and neurological development occurs, his 'deficiencies will be reformed.'" It also reiterated the previously noted difficulty of distinguishing between "transient immaturity" and "irreparable corruption."

Yet in *Miller*, the Court declined to "foreclose a sentencer's ability" to make that distinction. That is, unlike *Roper* and *Graham*, *Miller* gave courts the option of sentencing youthful offenders to life without parole on a case-by-case basis, despite the fact that there is no available neuroscience research to aid such a determination. There is no neural signature for maturity, no single psychological test that directly reveals how well developed an individual person is. Justice Kagan, writing for the *Miller* Court, did note the incongruity between the earlier cases of *Roper* and *Graham* and the one before her. She believed that the scientific studies regarding the average maturity of adolescents might create something of a presumption against Life Without Parole sentences for youthful offenders. As she put it, "appropriate occasions for sentencing juveniles to this harshest possible penalty will be uncommon."

Do the inherent challenges of G2i, then, constitute an unbridgeable gulf between science and the law? We think not. Although G2i decsribes a fundamental divide between the two disciplines, and perhaps no single structure is available to bridge it—at least, not yet—it's a division that might be managed effectively.

Effective management will depend both on paying attention to the specific legal context and on the science that might be available at the time in each of those contexts. Consider, for example, the issue raised by the *Miller* case. The Court found that the state of the science indicated legally relevant differences in maturity between adolescents and adults, which supported its ruling that it was unconstitutional to sentence adolescent homicide offenders to mandatory life in prison. The science on adolescents as a group thus helped establish the constitutional rule. But, as a practical matter, courts must now sentence individual adolescents. Almost certainly, at sentencing the parties will seek to introduce "scientific" expert testimony that supports their side—for the defendant, that he was developmentally immature at the time of the crime and, for the prosecution, that the defendant was as developmentally mature as an average adult when he committed the crime.

Should courts admit this form of diagnostic expert evidence? The answer rests on a G2i evaluation and, specifically, whether the scientific foundation is sound enough to permit a valid opinion about the individual case. If the answer is no, other evidence, evidence from non-experts (i.e., family, friends, police, victims, etc.) can still be introduced to demonstrate the defendant's level of developmental maturity at the time of the crime. Just as in the case of eyewitness identification research, the general framework research on adolescent behavioral and brain development is valuable and admissible. Whether a particular individual is or is not mature continues to be a pivotal legal issue, but may not be one that science can answer with any certainty.

MANAGING THE G2i DIVIDE

Managing G2i requires, foremost, the active involvement of both legal scholars and scientists.

For the courts, adopting just two key best practices will help reduce the complexity that contemporary science has added to the already complex adjudicative task. First, courts must begin their consideration of scientific evidence by focusing on both whether it is "good"—that is, meets certain evidentiary standards—and on what it's good *for*. Every case involving expert evidence involves a choice: admit testimony about the general phenomenon, or admit such general testimony *and* diagnostic testimony. The first decision is separate from the second. Furthermore, diagnostic testimony cannot be admissible unless the testimony on the general phenomenon is also admissible; evidence that something is an instance of a larger phenomenon presumes that the larger phenomenon itself exists.

Second, only after the court has decided whether the expert testimony concerns a general phenomenon, or concerns whether a particular case is an instance of that phenomenon, should it determine whether that testimony is admissible. While few courts realize it, the primary criteria derived from Daubert— i.e., relevance, qualifications, scientific validity, added value or helpfulness, and unfair prejudice—operate differently depending on how the evidence is to be used.

For scientists, and the experts who testify to the science, a host of issues should be paramount. The process of reasoning from group data to individual cases, of course, is principally a scientific one and, more particularly, a matter of statistical inference. The scientific community might begin by asking which methods or tools might be available or could be developed to facilitate the process. The issue of G2i reasoning is not unique to the courtroom. Meteorologists study storms, but we want to know whether a storm will hit during our commute tomorrow morning. Medical researchers study the effectiveness of drugs, but we want to know whether a particular drug will relieve our headache or, possibly, cause some side effects. Ordinarily, the G2i issue is translated into group statistical terms: "there's a 60 percent chance it will be raining at 8:30 a.m. tomorrow." In court, decision makers often need to translate those probabilities into more categorical terms, such as guilty/not guilty, liable/not liable, mature/not mature, and causation/no causation. Scientists could assist the process considerably by helping courts understand and translate the probabilities derived from group data to help legal decision makers decide individual cases.

Scientific advances in understanding the challenges of G2i, however, might not be far off. For instance, we may be on the cusp of an explosion of high-quality "precision" science in realms from neuroscience to genetics to nanotechnology. One tantalizing promise of science in the 21st century is knowledge at the level of the individual, and the challenge for courts in the 21st century is to distinguish between that promise and reality. Developing and refining a more sophisticated understanding of science, along with evidentiary guidelines that reflect that understanding, will enable the courts to meet that challenge now and in the decades to come.

C. TALKING ACROSS DISCIPLINES

Given deepening knowledge and increasing specialization, it is not easy for people to talk across disciplines. And the domains of law and science are particularly far apart, when considering the very different educational backgrounds, knowledge bases, and procedures. But the specific meanings of words and phrases can cause particular problems. Not only because law and science have obvious terms of art—such as *res ipsa loquitur* or *right dorsolateral prefrontal cortex*. But also because there are many terms of art that both fields use in entirely different ways. For example, the word "trial" makes a lawyer think of a courtroom procedure, while the same word makes a scientist think of an experiment (or a piece of it). Hearing the word "normative," a lawyer will typically think of an "ought" proposition (on the order of "norms"), while a scientist often thinks of a statistical distribution (relating to a "normal distribution").

Keeping this in mind, consider the following proposal (illustrated with a neuro-law application) for aiding lawyer-neuroscientist communications.

Joshua W. Buckholtz, Valerie Reyna & Christopher Slobogin
A Neuro-Legal Lingua Franca:
Bridging Law and Neuroscience on the Issue of Self-Control
5 Mental Health L. & Pol'y J. 1, 1-29 (2016)

ABSTRACT

This article argues that if the law wants the full benefits of neuro-scientific knowledge, it should attempt to develop a lingua franca—a method of communication understandable to both scientists and lawyers—based on neuro-scientific concepts. As a demonstration of such an attempt, we describe . . . how the criminal law's concept of self-control might be operationalized using constructs, domains, processes and tasks familiar to neuroscientists.

I. NEUROSCIENCE AND SELF-CONTROL

Many of us have an intuitive sense that, though we may not be able to define self-control precisely, we know it (or really, its absence) when we see it. . . . The underlying assumption is that some individuals, by quirk of brain or biology, lack this capacity, either generally or under certain circumstances. To a cognitive neuroscientist, this conceptualization poses three fundamental problems.

First, it treats self-control as if it were a unitary capacity, when in fact there are many distinct (i.e., dissociable) cognitive and socio-emotional capacities that comprise what we understand as "self-control." Our folk understanding of self-control fails to account for the fact that we can observe preserved function in one capacity and poor function in another seemingly related function. . . .

Second, while legal standards recognize some degree of variability among people, they assume that a valid, objective distinction between "able" and "deficient" or "normal" and "abnormal" individuals exists. In truth, individuals vary continuously with respect to many (if not most) cognitive capacities. . . . Complicating matters further, for most capacities relevant to self-control, we lack the large-scale normative datasets that would be required to make a reasonable comparison of an individual's capacity to that of the rest of the population (as we can do, for example, with I.Q.). . . .

Third, even assuming we can identify legally relevant capacities and identify where in the population distribution a given individual falls with respect to those capacities, that information would not answer the normative question of whether a person crosses the threshold into "deficient" or "abnormal." [I]f this decision is made in the absence of compelling scientific data, the law must recognize the arbitrary nature of any such cut- point.

With these caveats in mind, we outline below a basic neuroscientific framework for thinking about self-control. . . . Cognitive neuroscientists often consider relationships among brain, mind, and behavior in terms of "constructs," "domains," "processes," and "tasks." Here, we offer some working definitions. *Constructs* refer to concepts that cannot be directly observed, but that plausibly describe a phenomenon of interest—here self-control. *Domains* reflect distinct branches or subdivisions of a construct; the self-control domains considered in this article are impulsive action, impulsive choice, and behavioral flexibility. Within a domain, there may be several *processes*, which can be thought of as specific types of mental operations or computations. Within the domain of impulsive action, for instance, neuroscientists might conceive of several processes, including motor response cancellation and motor response suppression. Finally, such processes can be measured through performance on *tasks*—experimental paradigms that are designed to index specific cognitive processes (or domains of processes)—although, as made clear below, process-task mappings are often fuzzy.

A. Self-Control Domains: Action, Choice, and Flexibility

Behavioral and neurobiological data suggest that self-control is not a unitary construct. [A]vailable data highlight three legally relevant self-control domains: action, choice, and behavioral flexibility. Here, we refer to self-control deficits in these three domains as "impulsive action," "impulsive choice," and "behavioral inflexibility," respectively.

1. Impulsive Action

The self-control domain of action involves processes that enable people to use external cues to inhibit "pre-potent" (habitual or dominant) motor responses. For example, "action suppression" is thought to support the ability to prevent the generation of a motor response when an external cue indicates that it is no longer appropriate. . . .

A second process within this domain, often called "action cancellation," is thought to be crucial to the ability to use new information from the environment to inhibit the execution of a motor response once it has been initiated. . . .

2. Impulsive Choice

From decisions about life insurance plans and 401k investments to choosing what (or what not) to eat for dinner, humans are constantly faced with choices that require weighing the benefits of a decision against its costs. Impulsive choice refers to a deficit in the ability to appropriately weigh the costs, benefits, and consequences of one's actions when making a decision. Processes within this domain may be complicated by the nature of the costs and benefits that need to be integrated in order to make a decision. . . .

Depending on the particular kind of cost, impulsive choice failures lead to problems with delaying gratification (i.e. greater sensitivity to immediate rewards or to the cost of delaying a reward) or to increased risk-taking (i.e. greater sensitivity to the prospect of greater rewards or lower sensitivity to the prospect of bad outcomes) . . . .

3. Behavioral Inflexibility

A third domain of self-control—flexibility—includes processes that enable an individual to marshal their attentional resources to achieve a goal, particularly in the face of interference, and to adapt their decisions to changing rules and dynamic feedback. The interference suppression process refers to the capacity to suppress the influence of distracting information while focusing attention to perform a task. . . .

Set shifting and task switching tasks index another flexibility process—adaptability to rule changes. . . .

Finally, reversal learning tasks require an individual to use dynamic feedback to override learned stimulus-response associations. . . .

4. Related Constructs

Two additional constructs with conceptual links to self-control warrant mention because of their likely relevance to the law. The first, *sensation-seeking*, describes a desire for excitement or biological arousal that makes it more difficult to suppress risky or dangerous behaviors. . . . High levels of both impulsivity (low self- control) and sensation-seeking are found in substance abusers. . . .

Another relevant construct pertains to *mental representations* at the time of a decision. According to Fuzzy Trace Theory (FTT) people form two types of mental representations about an event: verbatim and gist traces. Gist traces are "fuzzy" representations of an event because they focus on its bottom-line meaning, whereas verbatim traces are detailed representations of an event. . . . This focus on gist highlights core values and reduces susceptibility to interference from distractions, thereby decreasing maladaptive decision-making. More generally, changes in mental representations enhance self-control without requiring greater willpower.

B. Caveats

While cognitive psychology and neuroscience research have made great strides in identifying self-control related cognitive processes and the neural circuits that serve them, several significant caveats are worth noting. First, our understanding of the . . . cognitive architecture of self-control is still impoverished. Neuroscientists and cognitive scientists use experimental tasks that they think map on to the processes described above, but they are still unclear about the selectivity of those mappings, or indeed, whether the cognitive processes we suspect the tasks measure truly "carve nature at the joints." . . .

Furthermore, even discrete processes . . . likely interact, both with each other and with affective and motivational context. . . .

Two final methodological problems are particularly salient in the legal setting. The first is that lab-based measures of self-control of the type we have described may not predict self-control in the real world. . . .

Also of concern is that neuroscience data, like most scientific data, is group-based. . . .

However, the translation of general scientific findings into information that is useful in an individual case is far from straightforward, a complicated inferential process that has been called the "G2i" problem. . . .

This means that, as of now, even the best experimental *tasks* are not useful as *tests* for determining capacity in any individual defendant. . . .

II. SELF-CONTROL IN THE COURTROOM:
EVIDENTIARY CONSIDERATIONS

With this brief background on the law and science of self-control in mind, imagine a man named John is charged with murder and wants to argue that he has "a substantial inability to conform [his] behavior to the requirements of the law," language found in both insanity doctrine and sentencing law. Assume that the methodological and conceptual problems just described are resolved (a big assumption, but one that is necessary to get to the issues we want to discuss). Assume further that John performs "poorly" on tests measuring response inhibition, action cancellation, delay discounting, and response reversal and that we can be sure John was not malingering during the testing process (another big assumption). Are the results of those tests relevant to the legal claim? The answer to that question requires answers to three sub-questions: the *type* of impairment the law considers salient, the *degree* of impairment the law considers salient, and the extent to which the law is willing to adopt a true lingua franca.

A. Type of Impairment

As of now, the first sub-question—the type of neurocognitive impairment that the law considers relevant—is impossible to answer, because the law's language is incompatible with cognitive and neuro-scientific measurement. Legal language referring to "substantial incapacity to conform behavior," "irresistible impulses," or "extreme mental or emotional stress" does not map well onto any of the self-control processes we have described. If legal policymakers want to take advantage of cognitive and neuro-scientific knowledge they will need to engage in hard thinking about whether difficulty in inhibiting one's responses, choosing long-range goals over short ones or any of the other self-control processes detailed above should affect legal liability.

Unfortunately, formal legal doctrine defining criminal liability does not track even the rough distinctions that moral philosophers and social psychologists have developed. The relevant case law on the volitional prong of the insanity defense—the basis of the claim John is making—usually focuses on the spontaneity of the conduct, with an emphasis on the degree of planning evidenced by the defendant or the rationality of the conduct, sometimes captured through the conceit of asking whether the act would have occurred had a police officer been standing nearby. . . . Similarly, case law defining premeditation speaks both of the need to show deliberation and "cool reflection" at the same time it insists that an act can be premeditated even if the decision to engage in it is instantaneous. Self-control in the provocation context, if defined at all, is usually simply described as "extreme mental or emotional stress" or an act of "sudden passion."

Formal legal pronouncements about the relevance of self-control in the sentencing context are somewhat more useful. For instance, in *Graham v. Florida* the Supreme Court supported its decision that mandatory life-without-parole sentences for juvenile offenders are unconstitutional by noting that juveniles have "[d]ifficulty in weighing long-term consequences" and thus have a "corresponding impulsiveness." In concluding that people with intellectual disability should not be eligible for the death penalty in *Atkins v. Virginia*, the Court spoke of these individuals' "diminished capacities to understand and process information, to . . . abstract from mistakes and learn from experience, . . . to control impulses." . . . Even when citing scientific findings related to self-control, the law's governing doctrine remains vague.

B. Degree of Impairment

Even if some or all of neuroscientists' findings on self-control are considered legally pertinent, however, a second determination will have to be made about *how much* impairment in the relevant self-control domains is required to affect the legal determination. The assumption above was that John performed poorly on his self-control tasks, but the word "poorly" was not defined. If John's case were tried today, neurologists or psychiatrists testifying on his behalf would likely make statements to the effect that, based on their experience and their evaluation of John, his capacity to appreciate the wrongfulness of his conduct was "significantly impaired" or, alternatively, his capacity to control his behavior was, "within a reasonable degree of psychological certainty," significantly compromised. Unfortunately, this type of testimony is close to meaningless.

If such data were available then a lingua franca in the self-control setting might identify "cut points," or the number of standard deviations below which a person is considered seriously impaired for legal purposes. There is precedent for this approach. In *Castaneda v. Partida* the Supreme Court had to decide whether, in a jurisdiction that was 79.1% Latino/a, the fact that only 339 out of 870 jury pool members were Latino/a constituted a prima facie violation of the equal protection clause. To answer that question, the Court resorted to statistical analysis, stating that "[a]s a general rule for such large samples, if the difference between the expected value and the observed number is greater than two or three standard deviations, then the hypothesis that the jury drawing was random would be suspect to a social scientist." The Court noted that the standard deviation on the facts of *Castaneda* was 12, and went on to hold that a prima facie case of discrimination had been made out.

A second Supreme Court case that adopted scientific concepts, in a context more closely related to the self-control inquiry, is *Hall v. Florida*, decided in 2014. Twelve years earlier, in *Atkins v. Virginia*, the Court had held that executing people with intellectual disability is unconstitutional even when they have intentionally killed another [because] it concluded that such people are less likely to be able to "process the information of the possibility of execution as a penalty and, as a result, control their conduct based upon that information." In *Hall*, the Court reaffirmed that holding and held that, in defining intellectual disability for purposes of *Atkins'* exemption, the states must adhere to the American Psychiatric Association's formulation of that condition, which, inter alia, provides that a person is intellectually disabled if he or she has an IQ score that is "approximately two standard deviations or more below the population mean, including a margin for measurement error (general 5% points)". In other words, the Court was willing to incorporate a scientific definition into a legal culpability principle.

After *Castaneda* and *Hall*, the lingua franca in jury selection and death penalty cases speaks in terms of standard deviations. In the self-control context, the law could take a similar approach. . . .

C. Potential Objections

Would the law be willing to adopt such a lingua franca? Although *Casteneda* and *Hall* demonstrate that courts are sometimes willing to move in that direction, lawyers have often resisted "trial by mathematics," especially in connection with legal issues that go to substantive liability, for at least three reasons. First, there is a justifiable distrust of numbers. In the self-control context, until cognitive science and neuroscience can demonstrate they possess the empirical foundation needed for compelling individual inference, the law should be hesitant to invite them into the courtroom.

Second, there is a valid concern that, even if the science is solid, attempting to fashion a lingua franca with it might tempt the law to compromise its normative premises. After *Atkins*, for instance, legal scholars worried that the diagnosis of intellectual disability, developed primarily for treatment purposes, did not mesh with the law's focus on blameworthiness. . . .

Less justifiably, the legal system is also squeamish about reducing culpability determinations to probabilities and other quantified concepts. . . . The most likely explanation for this adamant position is the concern that giving significant weight to scientific data—and to scientists— has the effect of reducing the law's power to control the scope of the inquiry. . . .

III. THE PATH FORWARD

The relationship between neuroscience and criminal law is still in its infancy. If neuroscience is to be maximally useful to law, it is imperative that both disciplines work *proactively* to develop a coherent framework for dealing with neuro-scientific evidence, rather than reactively responding in an ad hoc manner each time such evidence is considered in the courts. Here, we focus on self-control [and] propose that . . . the law adopt a lingua franca that relies on cognitive and neuro-scientific definitions in articulating the relevant concepts.

What might this lingua franca look like? While we believe that the details must reflect the outcome of an iterative, multilateral process that is open to all relevant stakeholders (e.g. legal scholars, judges, litigators, cognitive scientists, neuroscientists, and forensic clinicians), a few concrete goals can be outlined. . . . First, a lingua franca of self-control should facilitate objective classification of legal standards according to scientifically meaningful criteria. In practice, this process would begin with an exhaustive survey of case law, legal opinions, state penal codes, and law review articles, with the goal of generating a definitive list of self-control standards applied in courtrooms.

The next step would involve identifying sets of experimental paradigms that putatively operationalize and quantify the capacities described by each selected legal standard. . . . The outcome of this stage would be a hypothetical task-standard map.

The validity of such maps could be assessed by surveying state and federal judges (perhaps through the National Center for State Courts, the Administrative Office of U.S. Courts, and the Federal Judges Association) to measure the degree of agreement among jurists about the relationship between standards and measures. Behavioral scientists would translate methodological details into comprehensible text for jurists, who would in turn indicate the degree to which they believe each paradigm measures the mapped legal standard. . . .

Crucially, such a lingua franca must demarcate specific legal standards for which there is consistent agreement that no viable scientific operationalization exists, or for which the law indicates it neither desires nor requires scientific evidence to adjudicate. The legitimacy of the lingua franca enterprise rests largely on this third step. . . .

[I]f the law wishes, or intends to permit, the use of cognitive and neuro-scientific evidence to make inferences about legally germane aspects of mind and brain, legal policymakers must work with scientists to ensure that their constructs map on to scientific valid data.

IV. CONCLUSION

The underlying premise of this article is that if the law wants the full benefits of neuro-scientific knowledge, it needs to develop a lingua franca based on neuro-scientific concepts. In doing so, the law should be mindful of the limits of scientific inference (particularly as it pertains to legally relevant individual-level assessment) and alert to the fact that, despite semantic similarities, scientific constructs often do not track with its normative precepts. But the law should not resist a neuro-scientific lingua franca simply because it conflicts with legal sensitivities or surrenders too much power to scientists.

The effort in this article to reconcile legal standards for self-control with current neuro-scientific insights is unavoidably preliminary in nature. Such efforts must begin now because of the accelerating pace with which neuroscience evidence is being introduced in the courts. Until such efforts bear fruit, law and neuroscience will continue its high-stakes game of charades, each making stabbing guesses at what the other means, while citizens' lives and freedom hang in the balance.

The literature on when and how science is relevant to determining facts in litigation is vast. The important thing to recognize at this stage is that law *must* make hard decisions, and it is the necessity of resolving these questions that drives the search for better ways of answering them. Some of these better ways involve science. And some of those science contexts involve neuroscience. There are many in law who hope that the combination of legal need and dramatic scientific advancement will generate, at long last, some clear answers to hard questions.

But as we will see later in the book, that hope can be only partly vindicated and must be coupled with caution, given the extent to which neuroscience, like any science, pairs new information with necessarily remaining uncertainties. In the meantime, the next chapter will compare and contrast law's existing assumptions about human behavior and responsibility with the emerging knowledge from neuroscientific perspectives.

NOTES AND QUESTIONS

1. How would you compare and describe the processes that drive change in law and in science?
2. Which would you say is more "black and white," and which more "shades of gray," law or science? Why? How, if at all, does your answer vary by context?
3. Do you agree that legal systems actually depend on and need behavioral models? What are the best arguments to the contrary?
4. How would you describe the costs to society when legal policymakers have (frequently) no backgrounds in the sciences of behavior—such as biology, psychology, or neuroscience?
5. Choose a problem in law (e.g., insider trading, rape, breach of contract). Where, in your view, does law get the content to populate its behavioral models? To what extent does it matter whether that content is accurate or not?

6. Law, both in the United States and elsewhere, has at many points explicitly or implicitly used religious sources to inform its views about human motivations. To what extent are such sources valid ways of understanding the human condition? If religious sources are different from scientific sources, are they better, worse, or just different?

7. What would a more scientific approach to legislation look like?

8. You are daily surrounded by people, and could not navigate your world without some internal models of how you expect others to behave. How would you describe the origins and bases of your own models of human behavior?

9. What kind of training have you had previously in science? What kind of scientific knowledge, if any, do you think all lawyers should possess? If you had to learn quickly about a field of science for a new case, where and how would you start your research?

10. Critique the statement: "The love of complexity without reductionism makes art; the love of complexity with reductionism makes science." Edward O. Wilson, *Consilience: The Unity of Knowledge* (1999). What does it mean to appropriately reduce, on one hand, and to over-reduce, on the other? How should the legal system distinguish between the two?

11. An important concept known as "the naturalistic fallacy" states the claim that one cannot legitimately derive a normative conclusion from descriptive propositions alone. That is, one cannot directly (without reference to separate values) derive an "ought" from an "is"—as in the hypothetical statement, "What is natural is good." To what extent do you agree or disagree? And how neatly, or not, does this distinction map on to the differences between law and science? For discussion of subtleties of the naturalistic fallacy, see Patricia Churchland, *Braintrust: What Neuroscience Tells Us About Morality* (2012). For more, as applied to neuroscience, see Selim Berker, *The Normative Insignificance of Neuroscience*, 37 Phil. & Pub. Aff. 293 (2009).

12. Risk assessment is used pervasively in the legal system. One landmark study, led by Professor John Monahan at the University of Virginia, was *Rethinking Risk Assessment: The MacArthur Study of Mental Disorder and Violence* (2001). Studies such as this have led one scholar to conclude that "risk assessment has established a new scientific paradigm that is in a position to reshape much of practice." Jonathan Simon, *Reversal of Fortune: The Resurgence of Individual Risk Assessment in Criminal Justice*, 1 Ann. Rev. L. & Soc. Sci. 397, 417 (2005). Should neuroscience play a role in future risk-assessment tools? How should authorities balance group-based predictions versus individualized clinical assessment? For a review of how neuroscience might contribute to the prediction of violent behavior, see Russell A. Poldrack et al., *Predicting Violent Behavior: What Can Neuroscience Add?*, 22 Trends Cogn. Sci. 111 (2018).

13. Carl Sagan wrote that "we live in a society exquisitely dependent on science and technology, in which hardly anyone knows anything about science and technology." How close is society, in your view, to the optimal respect for science generally, and neuroscience specifically? Carl Sagan, *Why We Need to Understand Science*, Parade Magazine (Sept. 10, 1989), at 6.

14. One important way in which law may foster or inhibit scientific practice is through regulation and funding of scientific research. At first blush it may appear that law has the upper hand in that lawmakers can decide when, how,

and how much to fund scientific enterprises. But does the government really shape the course of science so dramatically? Even without government funding, will scientific pursuits persist (and perhaps even thrive)? Can a government or its citizenry stop scientific progress?

15. What does it mean for a lawyer to use science "correctly" or "morally" or "responsibly"? If using "bad" science improves client outcomes, is it necessarily "bad" for them to use the science? And should lawyers necessarily try to check all of their confirmation biases? How does a lawyer's zealous advocacy for a client differ from a scientist's dispassionate investigation of scientific truth? What can be said about policymakers? Former Congressman (and PhD scientist) Vernon Ehlers once observed: "I've learned over the years that if another member of Congress comes to me and asks me a question about science and I give them an answer which as far as I know is scientifically correct, and if the answer I give that person agrees with the previous assumptions the person has made about it, I am the world's greatest scientist, and they will go around quoting me to other members. . . . However, if my statement disagrees with their intrinsic, intuitive belief, I'm a lousy scientist and they will never quote me." Edward W. Lempinen, *Vernon Ehlers, Congressman and Physicist, Urges Scientists and Engineers to Join the Political Process*, Am. Ass'n Advancement Sci. (June 2, 2010). Do we turn to science to challenge our existing beliefs or to confirm them?

16. In an influential article, Kenneth Culp Davis distinguished "legislative facts," which are facts bearing on broad matters of policy, from "adjudicative facts," which bear only on a particular litigation. Kenneth Culp Davis, *An Approach to Problems of Evidence in the Administrative Process*, 55 Harv. L. Rev. 364 (1942). How useful do you find that distinction when thinking about the intersections of law and science? For critique of this distinction, and the proposal of an also influential alternative "social frameworks" approach that would incorporate into adjudication "general conclusions from social science research" (such as that evaluating the reliability of eyewitness testimony generally), see Laurens Walker & John Monahan, *Social Frameworks: A New Use of Social Science in Law*, 73 Va. L. Rev. 559 (1987).

17. With respect to the so-called "G2i" (group to individual) problem, how would you most succinctly describe it to a friend? How would you best summarize, then, the approach described in the G2i Knowledge Brief?

18. What are your reactions to the proposal for a "Neuro-Legal" lingua franca? One challenge in developing a universally applicable language to bridge the law/science divide is that law, unlike science, varies greatly across nations and cultures. The properties of neuronal signaling are the same in every country. The same cannot be said for the properties of the law. Can these differences be overcome?

FURTHER READING

Science Generally:

David Goodstein, *How Science Works*, in *Reference Manual on Scientific Evidence* 37 (3d ed. 2011).

Law and Science:

David L. Faigman, John Monahan & Christopher Slobogin, *Group to Individual (G2i) Inference in Scientific Expert Testimony*, 81 U. Chi. L. Rev. 417 (2014).

David Faigman et al., *Science in the Law* (2002).

David Faigman, *Legal Alchemy: The Use and Misuse of Science in the Law* (2000).

Tal Golan, *Laws of Men and Laws of Nature: The History of Scientific Expert Testimony in England and America* (2007).

Nat'l Res. Council of the Nat'l Acad. of Sci., *Strengthening Forensic Science in the United States: A Path Forward* 7 (2009).

Sheila Jasanoff, *Science at the Bar: Law, Science, and Technology in America* (1997).

Steven Goldberg, *Culture Clash: Law and Science in America* (1996).

Evolutionary Biology:

Dustin R. Rubenstein & John Alcock, *Animal Behavior* (11th ed. 2019).

John Cartwright, *Evolution and Human Behavior* (3d ed. 2016).

Mark Kirkpatrick & Douglas Futuyma, *Evolutionary Biology* (4th ed. 2017).

Timothy Goldsmith & William Zimmerman, *Biology, Evolution, and Human Nature* (2000).

Evolutionary Psychology:

The Handbook of Evolutionary Psychology (David M. Buss ed., 2d ed. 2015).

Behavioral Genetics:

Robert Plomin et al., *Behavioral Genetics* (6th ed. 2017).

Catherine Baker, *Behavioral Genetics: An Introduction to How Genes and Environments Interact Through Development to Shape Differences in Mood, Personality, and Intelligence* (2004).

Cognitive Psychology:

Psychological Science and the Law (Neil Brewer & Amy Bradfield Douglass eds., 2019).

E. Bruce Goldstein, *Cognitive Psychology: Connecting Mind, Research and Everyday Experience with Coglab Manual* (5th ed. 2019).

John R. Anderson, *Cognitive Psychology and Its Implications* (9th ed. 2020).

Daniel Reisberg, *Cognition: Exploring the Science of the Mind* (7th ed. 2018).

Behavioral Economics:

Handbook of Behavioral Economics: Foundations and Applications 2 (B. Douglas Bernheim, Stefano DellaVigna & David Laibson eds., 2018).

Daniel Kahneman, *Thinking, Fast and Slow* (2011).

Advances in Behavioral Economics (Colin F. Camerer, George Loewenstein & Matthew Rabin eds., 2004)

Unifying Disciplines:

Edward O. Wilson, *Consilience: The Unity of Knowledge* (1999).

Steven Pinker, *The Blank Slate: The Modern Denial of Human Nature* (2002).

CHAPTER 7

Behavior, Responsibility, and Punishment: Views from Law and Neuroscience

Genetics may yet threaten privacy, kill autonomy, make society homogeneous and gut the concept of human nature. But neuroscience could do all of these things first.

—The Economist[†]

I'm not a fatalist. But even if I were, what could I do about it?

—Emo Phillips[††]

CHAPTER SUMMARY

This chapter:
- Surveys invocations of cognitive neuroscience in philosophical and legal debates about determinism, free will, and the relationship between mind and brain.
- Highlights the extent to which doctrines of legal responsibility rely on "folk psychology" notions about the causes of human action.
- Explores views—from neuroscientists and from legal thinkers—on whether the implications of cognitive neuroscience on notions of human agency should prompt reconsideration and reform of current approaches to legal responsibility and criminal punishment.

INTRODUCTION

Chapter 6 discussed the relationships between law, science, and behavior. In this chapter, we begin to focus on how and where law and neuroscience overlap—and, equally important, where they don't. To begin opening up this complex interaction, consider the man described in this next reading.

[†] *The Ethics of Brain Science: Open Your Mind,* Economist, May 25, 2002, at 93.
[††] Quoted in Daniel C. Dennett, *Freedom Evolves* 12 (2004).

Patricia Churchland
The Big Questions: Do We Have Free Will?
New Scientist, Nov. 18-24, 2006, at 42, 42

In 2003, the *Archives of Neurology* carried a startling clinical report.* A middle-aged Virginian man with no history of any misdemeanor began to stash child pornography and sexually molest his 8-year-old stepdaughter. Placed in the court system, his sexual behavior became increasingly compulsive. Eventually, after repeatedly complaining of headaches and vertigo, he was sent for a brain scan. It showed a large but benign tumor in the frontal area of his brain, invading the septum and hypothalamus-regions known to regulate sexual behavior.

After removal of the tumor, his sexual interests returned to normal. Months later, his sexual focus on young girls rekindled, and a new scan revealed that bits of tissue missed in the surgery had grown into a sizeable tumor. Surgery once again restored his behavioral profile to "normal."

This case renders concrete the issue of free will. Did the man have free will? Was he responsible for his behavior? Can a tumor usurp one's free will?

———————

Dr. Churchland's passage raises many important questions. For example:

1. How did you (and should you) interpret such evidence?

2. What do you think is the probability that the tumor caused the behavior? Why, specifically?

3. What do you mean by "caused," precisely, in this context?

4. If you think the tumor probably did play some causal role in the behavior, how do you think the legal system should respond?

5. Is this man different in kind, or just in degree, from every other offender?

6. Do you see the potential causal role for the tumor as relevant during guilt determination? Sentencing? Both? Neither? Why?

7. What about potential civil liability? Should a victim's recovery be affected by the presence of the perpetrator's tumor?

These questions are not easily answered. And, for a start, all require some consideration of law's present starting point. So in Section A we consider law's view of the person. In Section B we examine the implications of neuroscientific "determinism" for free will and legal responsibility. In Section C we explore whether reconceptualizing humans as bundles of neurons should prompt reevaluation of various legal notions, such as retributivism. In Section D we turn attention to punishment, examining whether neuroscience challenges the use of particular punishments such as solitary confinement and whether new neurointerventions can be ethically justified. Throughout this chapter, we use the criminal law to illustrate legal responsibility. But as later chapters in this book will show, debates about brains, behavior, and responsibility are important to many non-criminal legal contexts as well.

———————

* [Jeffrey M. Burns & Russell H. Swerdlow, *Right Orbitofrontal Tumor with Pedophilia Symptom and Constructional Apraxia Sign*, 60 Archives Neurology 437, 437-40 (2003).—EDS.]

A. LAW'S VIEW OF THE PERSON

Stephen J. Morse
Neuroscience and the Future of Personhood and Responsibility
in *Constitution 3.0: Freedom and Technological Change* 113, 115-22
(Jeffrey Rosen & Benjamin Wittes eds., 2011)

The law's concern with justifying and protecting liberty and autonomy is deeply rooted in the conception of rational personhood. Human beings are part of the physical universe and subject to the laws of that universe, but, as far as we know, we are the only creatures on earth capable of acting fully for reasons and self-consciously. Only human beings are genuinely reason-responsive and live in societies that are in part governed by behavior-guiding norms. Only human beings have projects that are essential to living a good life. Only human beings have expectations of each other and require justification for interference in each other's lives that will prevent the pursuit of projects and seeking the good. We are the only creatures to whom the questions Why did you do that? and How should we behave are properly addressed, and only human beings hurt and kill each other in response to the answers to such questions. As a consequence of this view of ourselves, human beings typically have developed rich sets of interpersonal, social attitudes, practices, and institutions, including those that deal with the risk we present to each other. Among these are the practice of holding others morally and legally responsible, which depends on our attitudes and expectations about deserved praise and blame, and our practices and institutions that express those attitudes, such as reward and punishment.

There is little evidence at present that neuroscience, especially functional imaging, and genetic evidence are being introduced routinely in criminal cases outside of capital sentencing proceedings. It may well happen in the near future, however, especially as the technology becomes more broadly available and less expensive. So it's worth considering in detail neuroscience's radical challenge to responsibility, which treats people as "victims of neuronal circumstances" or the like. If this view of personhood is correct, it would indeed undermine all ordinary conceptions of responsibility and even the coherence of law itself.

CURRENT CRIMINAL JUSTICE: PERSONS, REASONS AND RESPONSIBILITY

Criminal law presupposes a "folk psychological" view of the person and behavior. This psychological theory explains behavior in part by mental states such as desires, beliefs, intentions, willings, and plans. Biological, other psychological and sociological variables also play a causal role, but folk psychology considers mental states fundamental to a full causal explanation and understanding of human action. Lawyers, philosophers and scientists argue about the definitions of mental states and theories of action, but that does not undermine the general claim that mental states are fundamental. Indeed, the arguments and evidence disputants use to convince others presuppose the folk psychological view of the person. Brains don't convince each other; people do. Folk psychology presupposes only that human action will at least be rationalizable by mental-state explanations or that it will be responsive to reasons, including incentives, under the right conditions. For example, the folk psychological explanation for why you are reading this chapter is, roughly, that you desire to understand the relation of neuroscience to criminal responsibility, you believe that reading the chapter will help fulfill that desire, and thus you formed the intention to read it.

Brief reflection should indicate that the law's psychology must be a folk psychological theory, a view of the person as a conscious (and potentially self-conscious) creature who forms and acts on intentions that are the product of the person's other mental states. We are the sort of creatures that can act for and respond to reasons. The law treats persons generally as intentional creatures and not simply as mechanistic forces of nature.

Law is primarily action-guiding and could not guide people directly and indirectly unless people could use rules as premises in their reasoning about how they should behave. Otherwise, law as an action-guiding system of rules would be useless, and perhaps incoherent. Legal rules are action-guiding primarily because they provide an agent with good moral or prudential reasons for forbearance or action. Human behavior can be modified by means other than influencing deliberation and human beings do not always deliberate before they act. Nonetheless, the law presupposes folk psychology, even when we most habitually follow the legal rules.

The legal view of the person does not hold that people must always reason or consistently behave rationally according to some pre-ordained, normative notion of rationality. Rather the law's view is that people are capable of acting for reasons and are capable of minimal rationality according to predominantly conventional, socially constructed standards. The type of rationality the law requires is the ordinary person's commonsense view of rationality, not the technical notion that might be acceptable within the disciplines of economics, philosophy, psychology, computer science, and the like.

Virtually everything for which agents deserve to be praised, blamed, rewarded, or punished is the product of mental causation and, in principle, responsive to reason, including incentives. Machines may cause harm, but they cannot do wrong and they cannot violate expectations about how people ought to live together. Machines do not deserve praise, blame, reward, punishment, concern or respect because they exist or because of the results they cause. Only people, intentional agents with the potential to act, can violate expectations of what they owe each other and only people can do wrong.

Many scientists and some philosophers of mind and action consider folk psychology to be a primitive or pre-scientific view of human behavior. For the foreseeable future, however, the law will be based on the folk psychological model of the person and behavior described. Until and unless scientific discoveries convince us that our view of ourselves is radically wrong, the basic explanatory apparatus of folk-psychology will remain central. It is vital that we not lose sight of this model lest we fall into confusion when various claims based on neuroscience or genetics are made. If any science is to have appropriate influence on current law and legal decision-making, it must be relevant to and translated into the law's folk psychological framework.

All of the law's doctrinal criteria for criminal responsibility are folk psychological. Begin with the definitional criteria, the "elements" of crime. The "voluntary" act requirement is defined, roughly, as an intentional bodily movement (or omission in cases in which the person has a duty to act) done in a reasonably integrated state of consciousness. Other than crimes of strict liability, all crimes also require a culpable further mental state, such as purpose, knowledge or recklessness. All affirmative defenses of justification and excuse involve an inquiry into the person's mental state, such as the belief that self-defensive force was necessary or the lack of knowledge of right from wrong.

Our concepts of criminal responsibility follow logically from the nature of law itself and its folk psychological concept of the person and action. The general capacity for rationality is the primary condition for responsibility and the lack of that capacity is the primary condition for excusing a person. If human beings were not rational creatures who could understand the good reasons for action and were not capable of conforming to legal requirements through intentional action or forbearance, the law could not adequately guide action. Legally responsible agents are therefore people who have the general capacity to grasp and be guided by good reason in particular legal contexts.

In cases of excuse, the agent who has done something wrong acts for a reason, but is either not capable of rationality generally or is incapable on the specific occasion in question. This explains, for example, why young children and some people with mental disorders are not held responsible. How much lack of capacity is necessary to find the agent not responsible is a moral, social, political, and ultimately legal issue. It is not a scientific, medical, psychological, or psychiatric issue.

Compulsion or coercion is also an excusing condition. Literal compulsion exists when the person's bodily movement is a pure mechanism that is not rationalizable by the agent's desires, beliefs and intentions. These cases defeat the requirement of a "voluntary" act. For example, a tremor or spasm produced by a neurological disorder that causes harm is not an action because it is not intentional and it therefore defeats the ascription of a voluntary act. Metaphorical compulsion exists when the agent acts intentionally, but in response to some hard choice imposed on the agent through no fault of his or her own. For example, if a miscreant holds a gun to an agent's head and threatens to kill her unless she kills another innocent person, it would be wrong to kill under these circumstances, . . . [but] the law may decide as a normative matter to excuse the act because the agent was motivated by a threat so great that it would be supremely difficult for most citizens to resist. Cases involving internal compulsive states are more difficult to conceptualize because it is difficult to define "loss of control." The cases that most fit this category are "disorders of desire," such as addictions and sexual disorders. The question is why these acting agents lack control but other people with strong desires do not? In any case, if the person frequently yields to his or her apparently very strong desires at great social, occupational, or legal cost to herself, the agent will often say that she could not help herself, that she was not in control, and that an excuse or mitigation was therefore warranted.

The criminal law's criteria for responsibility and excuse rest on acts and mental states. In contrast, the criteria of neuroscience are mechanistic: neural structure and function. Conceptually, the apparent chasm between those two types of discourse should be bridgeable, albeit with difficulty. The brain enables the mind. If your brain is dead, you are dead, you have no mind, and you do not behave at all. Therefore, facts we learn about brains in general or about a specific brain in principle could provide useful information about mental states and human capacities, both in general and in specific cases. While some people doubt this premise, for present purposes, let us assume that what we learn about the brain and nervous system can be potentially helpful in resolving questions of criminal responsibility.

The question is when the new neuroscience is legally relevant because it makes some given proposition about criminal responsibility more or less likely to be true. Any legal criterion must be established independently, and biological evidence must be translated into the criminal law's folk psychological criteria. That is, the expert must be able to explain precisely how the neuroevidence bears on whether the agent acted, formed a required mens rea, or met the criteria for an excusing condition. If the evidence is not directly relevant, the expert should be able to explain the chain of inference from the indirect evidence to the law's criteria.

At present, we lack the neuroscientific sophistication necessary to be genuinely legally relevant. The neuroscience of cognition and interpersonal behavior is largely in its infancy and what we know now is quite coarse grained and correlational, rather than causal. We lack the ability neurally to identify the content of a person's legally relevant mental states, such as whether the defendant acted intentionally or knowingly, but we are increasingly learning about the relationship between brain structure and function and behavioral capacities, such as executive functioning. And these are relevant to broader judgments about responsibility. Over time, these problems may ease, as imaging and other techniques become less expensive and more accurate, and as the sophistication of the science increases.

DANGEROUS DISTRACTIONS

It is important quickly to dispose of two dangerous distractions that neuroscience is thought to pose to ascriptions of criminal responsibility. The first is the threat of determinism. Many people think that neuroscience will prove once and for all that determinism (or something like it) is true and that we therefore lack free will and cannot be responsible. In this respect, however, neuroscience provides no new challenge to criminal responsibility. It cannot prove that determinism is true and it is simply the determinism du jour, grabbing the attention previously given to psychological or genetic determinism. This challenge is not a problem for criminal law because free will plays no doctrinal role in criminal law and it is not genuinely foundational for criminal responsibility. Nor is determinism inconsistent with the folk psychological view of the person. Moreover, there is a traditional, respectable philosophical reconciliation of responsibility and the truth of determinism called "compatibilism."

Related confusions are the view that causes are per se excusing, whether they are biological, psychological or sociological, or that causation is the equivalent of compulsion. If causation were per se an excusing condition or the equivalent of compulsion, then no one or everyone would be responsible because we live in a causal universe, which includes human action. Various causes can produce genuine excusing condition, such as lack of rational or control capacity, but then it is the excusing condition, not causation, that is doing the legal work.

In contrast, the new neuroscientific challenge to personhood, exemplified by treating [a person] as a victim of neuronal circumstances, is not saved by compatibilism or by the recognition that causation as an excuse cannot explain our practices, which hold most people responsible but excuse some. The radical challenge brain science poses threatens to undermine the very notions of agency that are presupposed by compatibilism and that are genuinely foundational for responsibility and for the coherence of law itself.

THE DISAPPEARING PERSON

At present, the law's official position — that conscious, intentional, rational, and uncompelled agents may properly be held responsible — is justified. But what if neuroscience or some other discipline demonstrates convincingly that humans are not the type of creatures we think we are? Asking a creature or a mechanistic force that does not act to answer to charges does not make sense. If humans are not intentional creatures who act for reasons and whose mental states play a causal role in our behavior, then the foundational facts for responsibility ascriptions are mistaken. If it is true that we are all automatons, then no one is an agent and no one can be responsible. If the concept of mental causation that underlies folk psychology and current conceptions of responsibility is false, our responsibility practices, and many others, would appear unjustifiable.

This claim is not a strawperson, as neuroscientists Joshua Greene and Jonathan Cohen illustrate . . . [in an excerpt below — EDS.].

Greene and Cohen are not alone among thoughtful people in making such claims. The seriousness of science's potential challenge to the traditional foundations of law and morality is best summed up in the title of an eminent psychologist's recent book, *The Illusion of Conscious Will*. If Greene and Cohen are right, cases that involve alleged abnormalities are really indistinguishable from any other case and thus represent just the tip of the iceberg that will sink our current criminal justice system. In this view, we are all "merely victims of neuronal circumstances."

But are we? Is the rich explanatory apparatus of intentionality simply a post hoc rationalization the brains of hapless homo sapiens construct to explain what their brains have already done? Will the criminal justice system as we know it wither away as an outmoded relic of a prescientific and cruel age? If so, not only criminal law is in peril. What will be the fate of contracts, for example, when a biological machine that was formerly called a person claims that it should not be bound because it did not make a contract? The contract is also simply the outcome of various neuronal circumstances.

This picture of human activity exerts a strong pull on the popular, educated imagination too. In an ingenious recent study, investigators were able to predict accurately based on which part of the brain was physiologically active whether a shopper-subject would or would not make a purchase. This study was reported in the Science Times section of the *New York Times*. The story's spin began with its title: "Findings: The Voices in My Head Say 'Buy It!' Why Argue?" It reflects once again the mechanistic view of human activity. What people do is simply a product of brain regions and neurotransmitters. The person disappears. There is no shopper. There is only a brain in a mall.

The law's fundamental presuppositions about personhood and action are indeed open to profound objection. Action and consciousness are scientific and conceptual mysteries. We do not know how the brain enables the mind, and we do not know how action is possible. At most we have hypotheses or a priori arguments. Moreover, causation by mental states seems to depend on now largely discredited mind-brain dualism that treats minds and brains as separate entities that are somehow in communication with one another. How can such tenuously understood concepts be justifiable premises for legal practices such as blaming and punishing? And if our picture of ourselves is wrong, as many neuroscientists claim, then our responsibility practices are morally unjustified according to any moral theory we currently embrace.

Given how little we know about the brain-mind and brain-action connections, to claim based on neuroscience that we should radically change our picture of ourselves and our practices is a form of neuroarrogance. Although I predict that we will see far more numerous attempts to introduce neuroevidence in the future, the dystopia that Greene and Cohen predict is not likely to come to pass. There is little reason at present to believe that we are not agents.

Most scientists and philosophers of science are physicalists and monists; they believe, as I do, that all material and non-material elements begin with matter subject to the universe's physical laws and that we do not have minds or souls independent of our bodies. But theorists such as Greene and Cohen go a step further. They appear to assume the validity of a complete reduction of mental states to brain states at the level of (apparently) neural networks. Indeed, the complete post-Enlightenment project of reducing all phenomena to the most basic physical building blocks is controversial even among physicalist monists and most probably is a chimera. Almost certainly, a complete explanation of human behavior will have to use multiple fields and multiple levels within each field. The complete reductionists have to explain how molecules, which have no intentionality or temporal sense, produce intentional creatures with a sense of past, present and future that guides our lives.

It is also possible that if we do ever discover how the brain enables the mind, this discovery will so profoundly alter our understanding of ourselves as biological creatures that all moral and political notions will change. Nevertheless, this argument is different from claiming that we are not agents, that our mental states do no explanatory work. . . .

Uri Maoz & Gideon Yaffe
What Does Recent Neuroscience Tell Us About Criminal Responsibility?
3 J.L. & Biosci. 120, 123-24 (2016)

Potentially, a neuroscientific result could show that a class of people, or perhaps, even, an individual person, fails to meet, or succeeds in meeting, one of the necessary conditions of criminal responsibility. If it could be shown, for instance, that people with orbitofrontal tumors like [the Virginia Man's] typically meet the law's criteria for insanity, then such research would provide some support for the claim that [the man with the orbitofrontal tumor] was not criminally responsible for his behavior by supporting the claim that he had an insanity defense. We would not know that for sure; [he] would need to be examined. But still, such a result would provide some support for the claim that [he] is not criminally responsible. Notice that such a result would not extend to everyone who engages in criminal behavior. Some states of the brain—[e.g.,] low ACC activity—that (when in the right environment) give rise to criminal behavior might do so without it being the case that the agent meets the law's criterion for insanity. Sanity, like insanity, depends on capacities that brains have. And criminal behavior by the sane, like such behavior on the part of the insane, has its source in the brain. But, still, if the neural sources of insanity can be identified, that would be of potential use to the legal system. For example, a better understanding of the neural basis of capacities underlying criminal responsibility might shed new light on the standards that we apply for individuals having or lacking criminal responsibility.

In addition, neuroscientific studies might illuminate the neural mechanisms that underlie those features of people in virtue of which they are criminally responsible for their behavior. And so they would help us to understand criminal responsibility better, without thereby supporting an argument for or against holding any person or class of people criminally responsible. While knowing more about a problem can be a first step to solving it, knowing more might be valuable simply because it involves knowing more. In the same way that the knowledge that the neuroscience of memory provides is of value even before we make use of it to treat memory disorders, or to improve our memories, if neuroscience can help us to understand the neural nature of criminally responsible behavior, that would be of value, even if we cannot use such knowledge to reduce crime or increase justice. Such results would add to human knowledge not just of the brain but of one of the most socially important phenomena to which the brain gives rise: crimes for which people are responsible and deserving of punishment.

[After reviewing relevant neuroscience research, the authors conclude that] . . . the work that has been done to date is just the smallest drop in the bucket. So far, very little is known about the brain that is of significance for understanding criminal responsibility.

NOTES AND QUESTIONS

1. Do you find Morse's description and analysis of the criminal law implications of neuroscience accurate and persuasive? Why or why not?
2. Would you extend these arguments beyond criminal responsibility, to apply to responsibility in tort as well?
3. What predictions does this view make about the way law evolves over time?
4. What do you see as the likely result when neuroscience meets folk psychology?
5. Although Morse critiques neuroarrogance, common ground is found in the belief that "we do not have minds or souls independent of our bodies." This belief is a departure from traditional religious views, still shared by a majority of Americans. Does embrace of neurolaw, even in a more modest form as Morse advocates for, necessarily require rejection of the soul?

B. DETERMINISM

Morse considers determinism to be the first of two "dangerous distractions." Consider the following view:

> Free will has long been a fraught concept among philosophers and theologians. Now neuroscience is entering the fray. For centuries, the idea that we are the authors of our own actions, beliefs, and desires has remained central to our sense of self. We choose whom to love, what thoughts to think, which impulses to resist. Or do we?
>
> Neuroscience suggests something else. . . . What's at stake? Just about everything: morality, law, religion, our understanding of accountability and personal accomplishment, even what it means to be human.

Editorial, *Is Free Will an Illusion?*, Chron. Rev., Mar. 18, 2012, at B6. As you will see in the excerpts below, some believe that neuroscientific findings put traditional concepts of free will, moral responsibility, and legal responsibility in jeopardy. As you read the views excerpted below, it will be useful to keep in mind three distinct reactions to this challenge.

One reaction, known as *incompatibilism*, holds that that because the universe is deterministic, it allows no room at all for free will. Adherents to its opposite reaction, known as *compatibilism*, reject the determinism/free-will dichotomy as false, believing that meaningful quanta of free will exist, even within a universe that operates according to materialistic and deterministic principles. A third reaction, known as *metaphysical libertarianism*, rejects that the universe is determined, thereby affording expansive room for free will.

Owen D. Jones
The End of (Discussing) Free Will
Chron. Rev., Mar. 18, 2012, at B9

The problem with free will is that we keep dwelling on it. Really, this has to stop. Free will is to human behavior what a perfect vacuum is to terrestrial physics—a largely abstract endpoint from which to begin thinking, before immediately moving on to consider and confront the practical frictions of daily existence.

I do get it. People don't *like* to be caused. It conflicts with their preference to be fully self-actualized. So it is understandable that, at base, free-will discussions tend to center on whether people have the ability to make choices uncaused by anything other than themselves. But there's a clear answer: They don't. Will is as free as lunch. (If you doubt, just try willing yourself out of love, lust, anger, or jealousy.)

All animals are choice machines for two simple reasons. First, no organism can behave in all physically possible ways simultaneously. Second, alternative courses are not all equal. At any given moment, there are far more ways to behave disastrously than successfully (just as there are more ways to break a machine than to fix it). So persistence of existence consistently depends on one's ability to choose nondisastrous courses of action.

Yet (indeed, fortunately) that choosing is channeled. Choices are initially constrained by the obvious—the time one has to decide, and the volume of brain tissue one can deploy to the task. Choices are also constrained by things we have long suspected but which science now increasingly clarifies.

For example, human brains are not general-purpose processors, idly awaiting culture's activating infusion of consciousness. Evolutionary processes pre-equip brains in all species with some information-processing predispositions. Generally speaking, these increase the probabilities that some combinations of environmental circumstances—immediate physical and social factors, contexts, and the like—will yield one subset of possible (and generally nondisastrous) behaviors rather than others.

Also, we now know that brains, though remarkable and often malleable, are functionally specialized. That is, different brain regions have evolved to do different things—even though they generally do more than one thing. As a consequence, impairments to specific areas of the brain—through injury or disease, for example—an impede normal human decision-making. And those impediments can, in turn, relax inhibitions, increase impulsive and addictive behaviors, alter the ability to make moral judgments, or otherwise leave a person situated dissimilarly from the rest of the population.

Which brings us to law. How will insights from the brain sciences affect the ways we assess a person's responsibility for bad behavior? Answer: only somewhat, but sometimes significantly. Many people assume that legal responsibility requires free will, such that an absence of free will necessarily implies an absence of responsibility. Not true, as many scholars have amply demonstrated. Full, complete, utterly unconstrained freedom to choose among available actions might be nice to have, but it is not in fact necessary for a fair and functioning legal system.

This is not to say that *degrees* of freedom are irrelevant to law. Science hasn't killed free will. But it has clarified various factors—social, economic, cultural, and biological in nature—that constrain it.

The existence of constraints very rarely excuses behavior, as when a person in an epileptic fit hits someone. But evidence of brain-based constraints—which can vary from small to large—can be, and indeed have been, relevant in determining the severity of punishment. For example, some jurors in a recent Florida case reported that evidence of abnormal brain functioning warranted a murderer spending his life in prison, instead of being executed.

All behaviors have causes, and all choices are constrained. We need to accept this and adapt. Brain sciences are revealing complex and interconnected pathways by which the information-processing activities of multiple brain regions coalesce to influence human decision-making. But this poses an advantage—neither a threat nor a revolutionary transition—to the legal system. In the near term, these complexities are more likely to inform than to utterly transform law's justice-driven efforts to treat people fairly and effectively.

Michael S. Gazzaniga
Free Will Is an Illusion, but You're Still Responsible for Your Actions
Chron. Rev., Mar. 18, 2012, at B7

Neuroscience reveals that the concept of free will is without meaning. . . . [N]euroscience, with its ever-increasing mechanistic understanding of how the brain enables mind, suggests that there is no one thing in us pulling the levers and in charge. . . . But brain determinism has no relevance to the concept of personal responsibility.

The exquisite machine that generates our mental life also lives in a social world and develops rules for living within a social network. For the social network to function, each person assigns each other person responsibility for his or her actions. There are rules for traffic that exist and are only understood and adopted when cars interact. It is the same for human interactions. Just as we would not try to understand traffic by studying the mechanics of cars, we should not try to understand brains to understand the idea of responsibility. Responsibility exists at a different level of organization: the social level, not in our determined brains.

Paul Bloom
Free Will Does Not Exist. So What?
Chron. Rev., Mar. 18, 2012, at B10

Most of all, the deterministic nature of the universe is fully compatible with the existence of conscious deliberation and rational thought. These (physical and determined) processes can influence our actions and our thoughts, in the same way that the (physical and determined) workings of a computer can influence its output. It is wrong, then, to think that one can escape from the world of physical causation—but it is not wrong to think that one can think, that we can mull over arguments, weigh the options, and sometimes come to a conclusion. After all, what are you doing now?

Patricia Churchland
The Big Questions: Do We Have Free Will?
New Scientist, Nov. 18-24, 2006, at 42, 42-45

I suggest that free will, as traditionally understood, needs modification. Because of its importance in society, any description of free will updated to fit what we know about the nervous system must also reflect our social need for a working concept of responsibility.

Think about what we mean by "free will." As with all concepts, we learn the meaning of this from examples. We learn what to count as fair, or mean-spirited, or voluntary by being given sterling examples of people doing things that are fair, or mean-spirited or voluntary. . . . Our understanding is balanced by contrasting cases-actions that are obviously not freely chosen: a dreaming man who strangles his wife, the toddler who wets his pants, a startle response to a thunderclap, or a coerced confession. From such prototypes, brains manage to extract a common enough meaning so that we can talk about free will tolerably well.

As well as prototypical cases, there are outlying cases beset with ambiguity, daunting complexity and background cultural differences. Here, the status of an action—freely chosen or not—has no clear answer, and such cases often come before the courts. Andrea Yates, the Texas mother who drowned her five children in a bathtub, was unquestionably psychotic, though her actions were methodical and purposeful, unlike the erratic movements of someone suffering an epileptic seizure. She understood that her actions were against the law, and telephoned the police to say so. Outside of our usual ken, this sort of case divides opinion. The way we currently think about free will, there may be no right answer as to whether she exercised it.

A rigid philosophical tradition claims that no choice is free unless it is uncaused: that is, unless the "will" is exercised independently of all causal influences—in a causal vacuum. In some unexplained fashion, the will—a thing that allegedly stands aloof from brain-based causality—makes an unconstrained choice. The problem is that choices are made by brains, and brains operate causally; that is, they go from one state to the next as a function of antecedent conditions. Moreover, though brains make decisions, there is no discrete brain structure or neural network which qualifies as "the will" let alone a neural structure operating in a causal vacuum. The unavoidable conclusion is that a philosophy dedicated to uncaused choice is as unrealistic as a philosophy dedicated to a flat Earth.

To begin to update our ideas of free will, I suggest we first shift the debate away from the puzzling metaphysics of causal vacuums to the neurobiology of self-control. The nature of self-control and the ways it can be compromised may be a more fruitful avenue to understand cases such as the Virginian man* and Andrea Yates than trying to force the issue of "freely chosen or not."

Self-control can come in many degrees, shades, and styles. We have little direct control over autonomic functions such as blood pressure, heart rate and digestion, but vastly more control over behavior that is organized by the cortex of the brain. Self-control is mediated by pathways in the prefrontal cortex, shaped by structures regulating emotions and drives. . . .

Ulysses famously bound himself to the mast of his ship to avoid seduction by the sirens, and monkeys will deviate from a direct route to avoid a temptation known to be troublesome. This is the prefrontal cortex using cognition for impulse control.

Self-control also allows us to make sense of difficult cases where free will is unhelpful. Self-control may be diminished in persons with brain lesions or tumors. Self-control is also diminished during an epileptic seizure, while intoxicated or under anaesthesia. . . .

How do neural networks achieve these effects that we call self-control, and what is different in the brain when self-control functions are impaired? Although little is known so far about the exact nature of the mechanisms, relevant experimental details have begun to pour in from many directions: on the properties of neurons sensitive to reward and punishment, on the generation of fear responses by neurons in the amygdala, and on the response profiles of "decision" neurons in parietal regions of cortex when the animal makes a choice. . . .

These sorts of discoveries promise that eventually we will understand, at least in general terms, the neurobiological profile of a brain that has normal levels of control, and how it differs from a brain that has compromised control.

So is anyone ever responsible for anything? Civil life requires it be so. . . .

NOTES AND QUESTIONS

1. Where and how do the views above overlap? Differ?
2. With which of the perspectives do you most closely identify, and with what implications for whether you are an incompatibilist, compatibilist, or metaphysical libertarian?
3. Consider this passage: "I found myself . . . looking down on the face of the dead man. I hadn't consciously thought about doing that—but when it became apparent what my body was up to, I didn't veto the action either." Robert J. Sawyer, *Mindscan* 138 (2005). To what extent does this suggest an important distinction between "free will" and "free won't"? For more on this subject, see Michael S. Gazzaniga, *Who's in Charge?: Free Will and the Science of the Brain* (2011).
4. Consider the two examples mentioned thus far of individuals who committed serious crimes against children: the Virginia man who molested his stepdaughter,

---

* [The reference is to the Virginian pedophile in the chapter-opening excerpt.—EDS.]

and Andrea Yates, the woman who methodically drowned her five children. If you were forced to absolve one, whom would you absolve? Why? Can you reconcile that choice, in a principled way, with neuroscientific perspectives? Does that matter?

5. Stephen J. Morse has argued: "There is no bright line between free and unfree choices. Harder and easier choices are arranged along a continuum of choice: there is no scientifically dictated cutting point where legal and moral responsibility begins or ends." *The Twilight of Welfare Criminology*, 49 S. Cal. L. Rev. 1247, 1253 (1976). Do you agree or disagree? Why or why not? Must the law define cut points?

6. Does society need to maintain a belief in free will? Philosopher Paul Nestor argues that the answer is yes:

> Criminal responsibility with its presumption of free will serves both social and truth-seeking demands of justice. From a social perspective, it is indeed difficult to conceive of the emergence of partnerships and groups without members sharing in the belief, experience, or intuition that their actions are caused by free will. . . . [S]ystems of criminal justice help human societies to maintain important forms of cooperation. The doctrine of criminal responsibility fits with a brain-culture co-evolution model that posits free will as a core element of human cooperation and justice. . . . [F]or the moral questions of fairness and justice, and for the ultimate legal question of criminal responsibility, these matters are best left to the collective wisdom of the court.

Paul G. Nestor, *In Defense of Free Will: Neuroscience and Criminal Responsibility*, 65 Int'l J.L. & Psychiatry 101344 (2019).

7. Will neuroscience uncover the neural circuitry of free will? In 2018, a group of neuroscientists took a step in this direction. R. Ryan Darby et al., *Lesion Network Localization of Free Will*, 115 Proc. Nat'l Acad. Sci. U.S. 10792, 10792-96 (2018). Here is a brief description of their study and tentative conclusions:

> Recent investigations [of free will by neuroscientists have] . . . focused on understanding this perception, dividing it into two processes: the intention or motivation to act, referred to as volition, and the sense of responsibility for one's action, referred to as agency. . . .
>
> . . . [P]atients with brain lesions in specific locations can experience profound disruptions in volition and agency. For example, patients with akinetic mutism lack the motivation to move or speak, while patients with alien limb syndrome feel that their movement is generated by someone else. These lesion induced syndromes are often used as paradigmatic examples of disrupted volition and agency, respectively. . . .
>
> . . . First, we test whether lesions in different brain locations causing akinetic mutism and alien limb are part of the same functionally connected brain network. Second, we test for specificity by comparing our results to those for lesions causing similar physical symptoms, but with intact perception of volition and agency. Finally, we test whether our localizations of volition and agency based on focal brain lesions align with brain stimulation sites altering free will perception and neuroimaging abnormalities in psychiatric patients with disordered free will perception. . . .
>
> Our results show that lesions that disrupt free will perception occur in different brain locations but localize to common brain networks. Specifically, we show

that lesions that disrupt volition, causing akinetic mutism or abulia, are part of a common brain network defined by connectivity to the ACC. Lesions that disrupt agency, causing alien limb, are part of a common brain network defined by connectivity to the precuneus. Finally, we show that our lesion-based localization of volition and agency aligns well with brain stimulation sites that disrupt free will perception and neuroimaging abnormalities in psychiatric patients with disordered free will perception. . . .

 . . . It remains unknown whether the network of brain regions we identify as related to free will for movements is the same as that important for moral decision making, as prior studies have suggested important differences.

Whether this study, and others like it, are real challenges to folk psychological conceptions of free will, however, is not clear. Consider this commentary on the study:

> How much this [study . . .] begins to explain criminality . . . seems still very much open to question because . . . the vast majority of patients with impairments in theory of mind or value-based decision-making are not criminals. In a way this is good news for folk psychology and jurisprudence: our concepts of moral responsibility and free will are not challenged by these data, since neither the brain lesions nor the lesion network maps explain criminality.
>
> Presumably this is so because the many other ingredients that need to come into play refer to factors outside the brain. Genes, upbringing, provocation, alcohol and drugs, and other factors that cause momentary emotions and lapses in control, are all going to act through the brain but may not be easily mapped onto the brain. Only by gaining a firm handle on these other factors can we understand the substrate on which a focal brain lesion could cause criminal behavior. . . .

Ralph Adolphs, Jan Gläscher & Daniel Tranel, *Searching for the Neural Causes of Criminal Behavior*, 115 Proc. Nat'l Acad. Sci. U.S. 451, 452 (2018).

C. THE DISAPPEARING PERSON

A second "dangerous distraction"—in Morse's view—is the case of the "disappearing person," wherein the very notion of personhood is winnowed by the view, incorrect in Morse's opinion, that to identify a cause is to identify an excuse. Consider this passage (to which the Morse excerpt above refers). As you read, consider: Do you find Greene/Cohen, Sapolsky, or Morse more persuasive on these issues? Or do you disagree with all of them?

Joshua Greene & Jonathan Cohen
For the Law, Neuroscience Changes Nothing and Everything
359 Phil. Transactions Royal Soc'y B 1775, 1775-84 (2004)

1. INTRODUCTION

The law takes a long-standing interest in the mind. In most criminal cases, a successful conviction requires the prosecution to establish not only that the defendant engaged in proscribed behavior, but also that the misdeed in question was the product of *mens rea*, a "guilty mind." Narrowly interpreted, *mens rea* refers to the intention to commit a criminal act, but the term has a looser interpretation by which it refers to all mental states consistent with moral and/or legal blame. . . . Thus, for centuries, many legal issues have turned on the question: "what was he thinking?" . . .

Given the law's . . . concern for mental states, along with its preference for "hard" evidence, it is no surprise that interest in the potential legal implications of cognitive neuroscience abounds. But does our emerging understanding of the mind as brain really have any deep implications for the law? . . . Some have argued . . . that new neuroscience contributes nothing more than new details and that existing legal principles can handle anything that neuroscience will throw our way in the foreseeable future.

. . . Existing legal principles make virtually no assumptions about the neural bases of criminal behavior, and as a result they can comfortably assimilate new neuroscience without much in the way of conceptual upheaval. . . . We maintain, however, that our operative legal principles exist because they more or less adequately capture an intuitive sense of justice. In our view, neuroscience will challenge and ultimately reshape our intuitive sense(s) of justice. New neuroscience will affect the way we view the law, not by furnishing us with new ideas or arguments about the nature of human action, but by breathing new life into old ones. Cognitive neuroscience, by identifying the specific mechanisms responsible for behavior, will vividly illustrate what until now could only be appreciated through esoteric theorizing: that there is something fishy about our ordinary conceptions of human action and responsibility, and that, as a result, the legal principles we have devised to reflect these conceptions may be flawed.

Our argument runs as follows: first, we draw a familiar distinction between the consequentialist justification for state punishment, according to which punishment is merely an instrument for promoting future social welfare, and the retributivist justification for punishment, according to which the principal aim of punishment is to give people what they deserve based on their past actions. We observe that the common-sense approach to moral and legal responsibility has consequentialist elements, but is largely retributivist. Unlike the consequentialist justification for punishment, the retributivist justification relies, either explicitly or implicitly, on a demanding . . . conception of free will. We therefore consider the standard responses to the philosophical problem of free will. "Libertarians" (no relation to the political philosophy) and "hard determinists" agree on "incompatibilism," the thesis that free will and determinism are incompatible, but they disagree about whether determinism is true, or near enough true to preclude free will. Libertarians believe that we have free will because determinism is false, and hard determinists believe that we lack free will because determinism is (approximately) true. "Compatibilists," in contrast to libertarians and hard determinists, argue that free will and determinism are perfectly compatible.

We argue that current legal doctrine, although officially compatibilist, is ultimately grounded in intuitions that are incompatibilist and, more specifically, libertarian. In other words, the law *says* that it presupposes nothing more than a metaphysically modest notion of free will that is perfectly compatible with determinism. However, we argue that the law's intuitive support is ultimately grounded in a metaphysically overambitious, libertarian notion of free will that is threatened by determinism and, more pointedly, by forthcoming cognitive neuroscience. At present, the gap between what the law officially cares about and what people really care about is only revealed occasionally when vivid scientific information about the causes of criminal behavior leads people to doubt certain individuals' capacity for moral and legal responsibility, despite the fact that this information is irrelevant according to the law's stated principles. We argue that new neuroscience will continue to highlight and widen this gap. That is, new neuroscience will undermine people's common sense, libertarian conception of free will and the retributivist thinking that depends on it, both of which have heretofore been shielded by the inaccessibility of sophisticated thinking about the mind and its neural basis.

The net effect of this influx of scientific information will be a rejection of free will as it is ordinarily conceived, with important ramifications for the law. As noted above, our criminal justice system is largely retributivist. We argue that retributivism, despite its unstable marriage to compatibilist philosophy in the letter of the law, ultimately depends on an intuitive, libertarian notion of free will that is undermined by science. Therefore, with the rejection of common-sense conceptions of free will comes the rejection of retributivism and an ensuing shift towards a consequentialist approach to punishment, i.e. one aimed at promoting future welfare rather than meting out just deserts. Because consequentialist approaches to punishment remain viable in the absence of common-sense free will, we need not give up on moral and legal responsibility. . . . We can, however, recognize that free will, as conceptualized by the folk psychology system, is an illusion and structure our society accordingly by rejecting retributivist legal principles that derive their intuitive force from this illusion.

2. TWO THEORIES OF PUNISHMENT: CONSEQUENTIALISM AND RETRIBUTIVISIM

There are two standard justifications for legal punishment. According to the forward-looking, consequentialist theory, . . . punishment is justified by its future beneficial effects. Chief among them are the prevention of future crime through the deterrent effect of the law and the containment of dangerous individuals. Few would deny that the deterrence of future crime and the protection of the public are legitimate justifications for punishment. The controversy surrounding consequentialist theories concerns their serviceability as *complete* normative theories of punishment. Most theorists find them inadequate in this regard, and many argue that consequentialism fundamentally mischaracterizes the primary justification for punishment, which, these critics argue, is retribution. As a result, they claim, consequentialist theories justify intuitively unfair forms of punishment, if not in practice then in principle. One problem is that of Draconian penalties. It is possible, for example, that imposing the death penalty for parking violations would maximize aggregate welfare by reducing parking violations to near zero. But, retributivists claim, whether or not this is a good idea does not depend on the balance of costs and benefits. It is simply wrong to kill someone for double parking. A related problem is that of punishing the innocent. It is possible that, under certain circumstances, falsely convicting an innocent person would have a salutary deterrent effect, enough to justify that person's suffering, etc. Critics also note that, so far as deterrence is concerned, it is the *threat* of punishment that is justified and not the punishment itself. Thus, consequentialism might justify letting murderers and rapists off the hook so long as their punishment could be convincingly faked. . . .

The backward-looking, retributivist account does a better job of capturing these intuitions. Its fundamental principle is simple: in the absence of mitigating circumstances, people who engage in criminal behavior *deserve* to be punished, and that is why we punish them. Some would explicate this theory in terms of criminals' forfeiting rights, others in terms of the rights of the victimized, whereas others would appeal to the violation of a hypothetical social contract, and so on. Retributivist theories come in many flavors, but these distinctions need not concern us here. What is important for our purposes is that retributivism captures the intuitive idea that we legitimately punish to give people what they deserve based on their past actions — in proportion to their "internal wickedness," to use Kant's phrase — and not, primarily, to promote social welfare in the future.

The retributivist perspective is widespread, both in the explicit views of legal theorists and implicitly in common sense. There are two primary motivations for questioning retributivist theory. The first, which will not concern us here, comes from a prior commitment to a broader consequentialist moral theory. The second comes from skepticism regarding the notion of desert, grounded in a broader skepticism about the possibility of free will in a deterministic or mechanistic world.

3. FREE WILL AND RETRIBUTIVISM

The problem of free will is old and has many formulations. Here is one, drawing on a more detailed and exacting formulation by Peter Van Inwagen: determinism is true if the world is such that its current state is completely determined by (i) the laws of physics and (ii) past states of the world. Intuitively, the idea is that a deterministic universe starts however it starts and then ticks along like clockwork from there. Given a set of prior conditions in the universe and a set of physical laws that completely govern the way the universe evolves, there is only one way that things can actually proceed. . . .

There are three standard responses to the problem of free will. The first, known as "hard determinism," accepts the incompatibility of free will and determinism ("incompatibilism"), and asserts determinism, thus rejecting free will. The second response is libertarianism (again, no relation to the political philosophy), which accepts incompatibilism, but denies that determinism is true. This may seem like a promising approach. After all, has not modern physics shown us that the universe is *in*deterministic? The problem here is that the sort of indeterminism afforded by modern physics is not the sort the libertarian needs or desires. If it turns out that your ordering soup is completely determined by the laws of physics, the state of the universe 10,000 years ago, *and* the outcomes of myriad subatomic coin flips, your appetizer is no more freely chosen than before. Indeed, it is *randomly* chosen, which is no help to the libertarian. What about some other kind of indeterminism? What if, somewhere deep in the brain, there are mysterious events that operate independently of the ordinary laws of physics and that are somehow tied to the will of the brain's owner? In light of the available evidence, this is highly unlikely. Say what you will about the "hard problem" of consciousness, there is not a shred of scientific evidence to support the existence of *causally effective* processes in the mind or brain that violate the laws of physics. In our opinion, any scientifically respectable discussion of free will requires the rejection of what Strawson famously called the "panicky metaphysics" of libertarianism.

Finally, we come to the dominant view among philosophers and legal theorists: compatibilism. Compatibilists concede that some notions of free will may require indefensible, panicky metaphysics, but maintain that the kinds of free will "worth wanting," to use Dennett's phrase, are perfectly compatible with determinism. Compatibilist theories vary, but all compatibilists agree that free will is a perfectly natural, scientifically respectable phenomenon and part of the ordinary human condition. They also agree that free will can be undermined by various kinds of psychological deficit, e.g. mental illness or "infancy." Thus, according to this view, a freely willed action is one that is made using the right sort of psychology—rational, free of delusion, etc.

Compatibilists make some compelling arguments. After all, is it not obvious that we have free will? Could science plausibly deny the obvious fact that I am free to raise my hand *at will?* For many people, such simple observations make the reality of free will non-negotiable. But at the same time, many such people concede that determinism, or something like it, is a live possibility. And if free will is obviously real, but determinism is debatable, then the reality of free will must not hinge on the rejection of determinism. That is, free will and determinism must be compatible. Many compatibilists skeptically ask what would it mean to give up on free will. Were we to give it up, wouldn't we have to immediately reinvent it? Does not every decision involve an implicit commitment to the idea of free will? And how else would we distinguish between ordinary rational adults and other individuals, such as young children and the mentally ill, whose will—or whatever you want to call it—is clearly compromised? Free will, compatibilists argue, is here to stay, and the challenge for science is to figure out how exactly it works and not to peddle silly arguments that deny the undeniable.

The forward-looking-consequentialist approach to punishment works with all three responses to the problem of free will, including hard determinism. This is because consequentialists are not concerned with whether anyone is really innocent or guilty in some ultimate sense that might depend on people's having free will, but only with the likely effects of punishment. (Of course, one might wonder what it means for a hard determinist to justify any sort of choice. We will return to this issue in §8.) The retributivist approach, by contrast, is plausibly regarded as requiring free will and the rejection of hard determinism. Retributivists want to know whether the defendant truly *deserves* to be punished. Assuming one can deserve to be punished only for actions that are freely willed, hard determinism implies that no one really deserves to be punished. Thus, hard determinism combined with retributivism requires the elimination of all punishment, which does not seem reasonable. This leaves retributivists with two options: compatibilism and libertarianism. Libertarianism, for reasons given above, and despite its intuitive appeal, is scientifically suspect. At the very least, the law should not depend on it. It seems, then, that retributivism requires compatibilism. Accordingly, the standard legal account of punishment is compatibilist.

[The authors discuss, among other things, the views of those who claim that neuroscience will change nothing of significance in the law.—EDS.]

6. NEUROSCIENCE AND THE TRANSPARENT BOTTLENECK

We have argued that, contrary to legal and philosophical orthodoxy, determinism really does threaten free will and responsibility as we intuitively understand them. It is just that most of us, including most philosophers and legal theorists, have yet to appreciate it. This controversial opinion amounts to an empirical prediction that may or may not hold: as more and more scientific facts come in, providing increasingly vivid illustrations of what the human mind is really like, more and more people will develop moral intuitions that are at odds with our current social practices.

Neuroscience has a special role to play in this process for the following reason. As long as the mind remains a black box, there will always be a donkey on which to pin dualist and libertarian intuitions. For a long time, philosophical arguments have persuaded some people that human action has purely mechanical causes, but not everyone cares for philosophical arguments. Arguments are nice, but physical demonstrations are far more compelling. What neuroscience does, and will continue to do at an accelerated pace, is elucidate the 'when', 'where' and 'how' of the mechanical processes that cause behavior. It is one thing to deny that human decision-making is purely mechanical when your opponent offers only a general, philosophical argument. It is quite another to hold your ground when your opponent can make detailed predictions about how these mechanical processes work, complete with images of the brain structures involved and equations that describe their function.

Thus, neuroscience holds the promise of turning the black box of the mind into a *transparent bottleneck*. There are many causes that impinge on behavior, but all of them—from the genes you inherited, to the pain in your lower back, to the advice your grandmother gave you when you were six—must exert their influence through the brain. Thus, your brain serves as a bottleneck for all the forces spread throughout the universe of your past that affect who you are and what you do. Moreover, this bottleneck contains the events that are, intuitively, most critical for moral and legal responsibility, and we may soon be able to observe them closely.

At some time in the future we may have extremely high-resolution scanners that can simultaneously track the neural activity and connectivity of every neuron in a human brain, along with computers and software that can analyze and organize these data. Imagine, for example, watching a film of your brain choosing between soup and salad. The analysis software highlights the neurons pushing for soup in red and the neurons pushing for salad in blue. You zoom in and slow down the film, allowing yourself to trace the cause-and-effect relationships between individual neurons—the mind's clockwork revealed in arbitrary detail. You find the tipping-point moment at which the blue neurons in your prefrontal cortex out-fire the red neurons, seizing control of your pre-motor cortex and causing you to say, 'I will have the salad, please'.

At some further point this sort of brainware may be very widespread, with a high-resolution brain scanner in every classroom. People may grow up completely used to the idea that every decision is a thoroughly mechanical process, the outcome of which is completely determined by the results of prior mechanical processes. What will such people think as they sit in their jury boxes? Suppose a man has killed his wife in a jealous rage. Will jurors of the future wonder whether the defendant acted in that moment *of his own free will*? Will they wonder if it was *really him* who killed his wife rather than his *uncontrollable anger*? Will they ask whether he *could have done otherwise*? Whether he really *deserves* to be punished, or if he is just a victim of unfortunate circumstances? We submit that these questions, which seem so important today, will lose their grip in an age when the mechanical nature of human decision-making is fully appreciated. The law will continue to punish misdeeds, as it must for practical reasons, but the idea of distinguishing the truly, deeply guilty from those who are merely victims of neuronal circumstances will, we submit, seem pointless.

At least in our more reflective moments. Our intuitive sense of free will runs quite deep, and it is possible that we will never be able to fully talk ourselves out of it. . . .

8. FREE WILL, RESPONSIBILITY AND CONSEQUENTIALISM

Even if there is no intuitively satisfying solution to the problem of free will, it does not follow that there is no correct view of the matter. Ours is as follows: when it comes to the issue of free will itself, hard determinism is mostly correct. Free will, as we ordinarily understand it, is an illusion. However, it does not follow from the fact that free will is an illusion that there is no legitimate place for responsibility. Recall from §2 that there are two general justifications for holding people legally responsible for their actions. The retributive justification, by which the goal of punishment is to give people what they really deserve, does depend on this dubious notion of free will. However, the consequentialist approach does not require a belief in free will at all. As consequentialists, we can hold people responsible for crimes simply because doing so has, on balance, beneficial effects through deterrence, containment, etc. It is sometimes said that if we do not believe in free will then we cannot legitimately punish anyone and that society must dissolve into anarchy. In a less hysterical vein, Daniel Wegner argues that free will, while illusory, is a necessary fiction for the maintenance of our social structure. We disagree. There are perfectly good, forward-looking justifications for punishing criminals that do not depend on metaphysical fictions. (Wegner's observations may apply best to the personal sphere: see below.)

The vindication of responsibility in the absence of free will means that there is more than a grain of truth in compatibilism. The consequentialist approach to responsibility generates a derivative notion of free will that we can embrace. In the name of producing better consequences, we will want to make several distinctions among various actions and agents. To begin, we will want to distinguish the various classes of people who cannot be deterred by the law from those who can. That is, we will recognize many of the 'diminished capacity' excuses that the law currently recognizes such as infancy and insanity. We will also recognize familiar justifications such those associated with crimes committed under duress (e.g. threat of death). If we like, then, we can say that the actions of rational people operating free from duress, etc. are free actions, and that such people are exercising their free will.

At this point, compatibilists such as Daniel Dennett may claim victory: "what more could one want from free will?" In a word: retributivism. We have argued that commonsense retributivism really does depend on a notion of free will that is scientifically suspect. Intuitively, we want to punish those people who truly deserve it, but whenever the causes of someone's bad behavior are made sufficiently vivid, we no longer see that person as truly deserving of punishment. This insight is expressed by the old French proverb: "to know all is to forgive all." It is also expressed in the teachings of religious figures, such as Jesus and Buddha, who preach a message of universal compassion. Neuroscience can make this message more compelling by vividly illustrating the mechanical nature of human action.

Our penal system is highly counter-productive from a consequentialist perspective, especially in the USA, and yet it remains in place because retributivist principles have a powerful moral and political appeal. It is possible, however, that neuroscience will change these moral intuitions by undermining the intuitive, libertarian conceptions of free will on which retributivism depends.

As advocates of consequentialist legal reform, it behooves us to briefly respond to the three standard criticisms levied against consequentialist theories of punishment. First, it is claimed that consequentialism would justify extreme overpunishing. As noted above, it is possible in principle that the goal of deterrence would justify punishing parking violations with the death penalty or framing innocent people to make examples of them. Here, the standard response is adequate. The idea that such practices could, in the real world, make society happier on balance is absurd. Second, it is claimed that consequentialism justifies extreme underpunishment. In response to some versions of this objection, our response is the same as above. Deceptive practices such as a policy of faking punishment cannot survive in a free society, and a free society is required for the pursuit of most consequentialist ends. In other cases consequentialism may advocate more lenient punishments for people who, intuitively, deserve worse. Here, we maintain that a deeper understanding of human action and human nature will lead people—more of them, at any rate—to abandon these retributivist intuitions. Our response is much the same to the third and most general criticism of consequentialist punishment, which is that even when consequentialism gets the punishment policy right, it does so for the wrong reasons. These supposedly right reasons are reasons that we reject, however intuitive and natural they may feel. They are, we maintain, grounded in a metaphysical view of human action that is scientifically dubious and therefore an unfit basis for public policy in a pluralistic society.

Finally, as defenders of hard determinism and a consequentialist approach to responsibility, we should briefly address some standard concerns about the rejection of free will and conceptions of responsibility that depend on it. First, does not the fact that you can raise your hand "at will" prove that free will is real? Not in the sense that matters. As Daniel Wegner has argued, our first-person sense of ourselves as having free will may be a systematic illusion. And from a third-person perspective, we simply do not assume that anyone who exhibits voluntary control over his body is free in the relevant sense, as in the case of Mr. Puppet.

A more serious challenge is the claim that our commitments to free will and retributivism are simply inescapable for all practical purposes. Regarding free will, one might wonder whether one can so much as make a decision without implicitly assuming that one is free to choose among one's apparent options. Regarding responsibility and punishment, one might wonder if it is humanly possible to deny our retributive impulses. This challenge is bolstered by recent work in the behavioral sciences suggesting that an intuitive sense of fairness runs deep in our primate lineage and that an adaptive tendency towards retributive punishment may have been a crucial development in the biological and cultural evolution of human sociality. Recent neuroscientific findings have added further support to this view, suggesting that the impulse to exact punishment may be driven by phylogentically old mechanisms in the brain. These mechanisms may be an efficient and perhaps essential, device for maintaining social stability. If retributivism runs that deep and is that useful, one might wonder whether we have any serious hope of, or reason for, getting rid of it. Have we any real choice but to see one another as free agents who deserve to be rewarded and punished for our past behaviors?

We offer the following analogy: modern physics tells us that space is curved. Nevertheless, it may be impossible for us to see the world as anything other than flatly Euclidean in our day-to-day lives. And there are, no doubt, deep evolutionary explanations for our Euclidean tendencies. Does it then follow that we are forever bound by our innate Euclidean psychology? The answer depends on the domain of life in question. In navigating the aisles of the grocery store, an intuitive, Euclidean representation of space is not only adequate, but probably inevitable. However, when we are, for example, planning the launch of a spacecraft, we can and should make use of relativistic physical principles that are less intuitive but more accurate. In other words, a Euclidean perspective is not necessary for *all* practical purposes, and the same may be true for our implicit commitment to free will and retributivism. For most day-to-day purposes it may be pointless or impossible to view ourselves or others in this detached sort of way. But—and this is the crucial point—it may not be pointless or impossible to adopt this perspective when one is deciding what the criminal law should be or whether a given defendant should be put to death for his crimes. These may be special situations, analogous to those routinely encountered by "rocket scientists," in which the counter-intuitive truth that we legitimately ignore most of the time can and should be acknowledged.

Finally, there is the worry that to reject free will is to render all of life pointless: why would you bother with anything if it has all long since been determined? The answer is that you will bother because you are a human, and that is what humans do. Even if you decide, as part of a little intellectual exercise, that you are going to sit around and do nothing because you have concluded that you have no free will, you are eventually going to get up and make yourself a sandwich. And if you do not, you have got bigger problems than philosophy can fix.

Robert M. Sapolsky
The Frontal Cortex and the Criminal Justice System
359 Phil. Transactions Royal Soc'y B 1787, 1787-94 (2004)

1. INTRODUCTION

[S]ome findings in neuroscience should seem nothing short of flabbergasting to any intelligent person. In some instances, these findings must challenge our sense of self. . . . [N]eurobiology is beginning to provide the first hints of mechanistic explanations for our personalities, propensities and passions.

These insights can be of extraordinary relevance, in that neurobiology often must inform some of our decision-making. Is a loved one, sunk in a depression so severe that she cannot function, a case of a disease whose biochemical basis is as "real" as is the biochemistry of, say, diabetes, or is she merely indulging herself? Is a child doing poorly at school because he is unmotivated and slow, or because there is a neurobiologically based learning disability? Is a friend, edging towards a serious problem with substance abuse, displaying a simple lack of discipline, or suffering from problems with the neurochemistry of reward? . . .

Arguably, the most important arena in which a greater knowledge of neuroscience is needed is the criminal justice system. In some cases, the criminal justice system has accommodated well the lessons of neurobiology. If someone with epilepsy, in the course of a seizure, flails and strikes another person, that epileptic would never be considered to have criminally assaulted the person who they struck. But in earlier times, that is exactly what would have been concluded, and epilepsy was often assumed to be a case of retributive demonic possession. Instead, we are now a century or two into readily dealing with the alternative view of, "it is not him, it is his disease." . . .

. . . [T]he criminal justice system in the USA has been dominated increasingly by a view that an inability to tell right from wrong is the sole basis of an acceptable insanity defense. I will now examine how contemporary neuroscience strongly argues against this trend. Instead, we have come to understand increasingly the organic basis of impaired impulse control.

[The author surveys literature concerning the relationship between impulse control problems and damage to a region of the brain—the prefrontal cortex (or "PFC")—that is known to be importantly involved in (among other things) choosing the harder but analytically "more correct" course of action.—EDS.]

. . . We have come to recognize numerous realms in which a biological abnormality gives rise to aberrant behavior. And such recognition has often then given rise to an expectation that people now exert higher-order control over that abnormality. For example, as noted, we would never consider an epileptic violent who strikes someone in the process of a seizure: "it is not him; it is his disease." However, we expect that epileptic to not drive a car if their seizures are uncontrolled. Or we are coming to understand the neurochemistry of context-dependence relapse into drug dependency in organisms. Thus, we have come to expect ex-addicts to avoid the settings in which they previously abused drugs.

There is a false dichotomy in this manner of thinking. It is as if we artificially demarcate an area in which biology dominates: yes, there is something organic that gives rise to this person having uncontrolled and synchronous neuronal discharges (i.e. a seizure), or who has certain pathways potentiated that project onto dopamine-releasing 'pleasure' pathways (one theory about the neurochemistry of substance abuse relapse). But it is as if, with that area of organic impairment identified and given credence, we expect it to be bounded, and for the rest of our "us-ness," replete with free will, to now shoulder the responsibility of keeping that organic impairment within the confines of its boundaries. It cannot possibly work this way. What the literature about the PFC shows is that there is a reductive, materialistic neurobiology to the containment, resulting in the potential for volitional control to be impaired just as unambiguously as any other aspect of brain function. It is possible to know the difference between right and wrong but, for reasons of organic impairment, to not be able to do the right thing.

The most obvious implication of this concerns how individuals with demonstrable PFC damage are treated in the criminal justice system. As the simplest conclusion, everything about this realm of contemporary neurobiology argues against the retrenchment back towards a sole reliance on *M'Naghten* that has gone on in recent decades.*

Amid the seeming obviousness of this conclusion, there is always a valid counterpoint that can be raised: there are individuals with substantial amounts of PFC damage who, nonetheless, do not commit crimes. At present, knowing that someone has sustained PFC damage does not give much power in predicting whether that person's disinhibition will take the form of serial murder or merely being unable to praise a nearly inedible meal prepared by a host. This seems to weaken the "volition can be organically impaired, just like any other aspect of brain function" argument; in these interstices of unpredictability seem to dwell free will.

However, we can begin to imagine tree diagrams of variables that, with each new layer, add more predictive power. We can already see two layers in the realm of PFC function. The first layer might query, "PFC: normal or damaged?" (while recognizing that this is a false dichotomy). The second might then query, "if damaged: damaged in childhood or later?" This same structure of increasing predictive power was shown in a recent, landmark study concerning clinical depression . . . [that] generates an impressive predictive power as to which adults succumb to clinical depression. If free will lurks in those interstices, those crawl spaces are certainly shrinking.

A second way in which findings about the PFC are relevant to the criminal justice system concerns individuals who have committed grotesquely violent, sociopathic crimes, but who have no demonstrable PFC damage. Initially, it seems a fatuous tautology to say that there must be an organic abnormality in such cases — "it is only an organically abnormal brain that produces abnormal behavior" — and that we simply lack sufficiently sensitive techniques for demonstrating it. However, it must be emphasized that most of the neurobiological techniques used to demonstrate PFC abnormalities in humans (predominantly structural and functional brain imaging)

---

* The *M'Naghten* standard refers to a test for legal insanity that requires the defense to show that at the time of the offense the defendant could not appreciate right from wrong. This test is sometimes referred to as the "cognitive" insanity test, as contrasted with a "volitional" test in which defendants have to show only that they could not control their impulses (even if they knew what they were doing was wrong). The *M'Naghten* test originated from an 1843 English case in which Daniel M'Naghten was charged with attempting to kill the English Prime Minister. *M'Naghten's Case,* 10 Cl. & Fin. 200, 8 Eng. Rep. 718 (1843). M'Naghten was acquitted by reason of insanity, and the *M'Naghten* test became widely adopted by courts in both England and the United States. *See* Richard Moran, *Knowing Right from Wrong: The Insanity Defense of Daniel McNaughtan* (1981).

did not exist a decade or two ago. It would be the height of hubris to think that we have already learned how to detect the most subtle ways in which PFC damage impairs volitional control. Instead, we probably cannot even imagine yet the ways in which biology can go awry and impair the sorts of volitional control that helps define who we are.

At the most disturbing level, findings about the PFC are relevant to the criminal justice system with respect to those of us with a normal PFC and who have never behaved criminally. It is here that the tendency of science to function in continua comes up against the legal culture of jury decisions. Among sociopaths without overt PFC damage, the smaller the volume of the PFC, the greater the tendency towards aggressive and antisocial behavior. Similarly, as noted, among humans with no neurological impairments or histories of antisocial behavior, the greater the level of metabolic activity in parts of the PFC, the lower the activity of the amygdala. There is little support for the idea that over the range of PFC function, there is a discontinuity, a transition that allows one to dichotomize between a healthy PFC in an individual expected to have a complete capacity to regulate behavior, and a damaged PFC in someone who cannot regulate their behavior. The dichotomy does not exist.

A conclusion like this makes sense to neurobiologists, but may seem alien to legal scholars. The emphasis on continua seems to hold the danger of a world of criminal justice in which there is no blame and only prior causes. Whereas it is true that, at a logical extreme, a neurobiological framework may indeed eliminate blame, it does not eliminate the need for forceful intervention in the face of violence or antisocial behavior. To understand is not to forgive or to do nothing; whereas you do not ponder whether to forgive a car that, because of problems with its brakes, has injured someone, you nevertheless protect society from it.

Legal scholars have objected to this type of thinking for a related reason, as well. In this view, it is desirable for a criminal justice system to operate with a presumption of responsibility because, "to treat persons otherwise is to treat them as less than human." There is a certain appealing purity to this. But although it may seem dehumanizing to medicalize people into being broken cars, it can still be vastly more humane than moralizing them into being sinners.

NOTES AND QUESTIONS

1. Are the views of Greene/Cohen and Sapolsky radical, reasonable, or both? Would it be fair to characterize Greene/Cohen and Sapolsky, or either of those excerpts, as a plea for greater recognition that humans are victims of neuronal circumstances? How would you describe the main implications they draw for law from neuroscientific perspectives? Given that, do you find the views of Greene/Cohen, Sapolsky, or Morse more appealing? For what reasons?

2. How persuasive do you find Sapolsky's argument for medicalizing criminal justice?

3. What are your reactions to Sapolsky's and Greene/Cohen's arguments for abandoning retributivist approaches to criminal justice in favor of consequentialist ones? Why?

4. What evidence would be required for you to reach the conclusion that a defendant did not have the requisite prefrontal resources to be responsible for her

crime? How would you determine that a defendant's moral engine was broken beyond repair? Would it affect your decisions about culpability, mitigation, or both?

5. Is hard determinism completely incompatible with retributivism? To what extent is free will necessary to justify retributive justice?

6. Greene and Cohen argue (in another passage) that "syndromes and other causes do not have excusing force unless they sufficiently diminish rationality in the context in question." Would prefrontal cortex damage and its resulting impaired volitional control that Sapolsky describes meet that requirement of sufficiently diminished rationality?

7. In a critique of Greene and Cohen's argument, law professor Michael Pardo and philosopher Dennis Patterson have pointed out that if criminal defendants are victims of their neuronal circumstances, then so too are legal policy makers and academics critiquing the criminal justice system. They pose the following hypothetical:

> Imagine a group of open-minded policy makers faced with the task of constructing a justified system of legal punishment. They listen to and take seriously the arguments of Greene and Cohen regarding retributivism, hard determinism, and neuroscience. At the end of the day, they could evaluate the various claims and reasons for them, deliberate about the various avenues open to them and the benefits and costs of each, and then choose a course of action that they think is justified or more justified than the alternatives. Or they could simply sit back and wait for their neurons to make the decision for them. Or they could flip a coin. For the normative project of justifying criminal punishment, these distinctions matter a great deal to the issue of whether the criminal punishment that followed would be justified and legitimate. From the perspective of Greene and Cohen, however, these differences ultimately do not matter (just as they do not matter at the level of criminal responsibility.) If no one is *really* blameworthy or praiseworthy, justified or unjustified, then the same goes for the lawmakers who decide how and when to distribute punishment. If it is just causally determined neuronal activity all the way down, and if the folk psychological explanations of punishment behavior are founded on an illusion, then for purposes of moral evaluation *it does not matter why anyone choose to engage in criminal punishment or how they do so.* The same goes for theorists engaged in the normative project of critiquing and defending possible policies regarding the distribution of criminal punishment. If so, then one wonders why they bothered to make the argument.

Michael S. Pardo & Dennis Patterson, *Minds, Brains, and Law: The Conceptual Foundations of Law and Neuroscience* 206-07 (2013).

8. Is it possible to find a middle ground between the viewpoint of Stephen Morse, on one hand, and the viewpoints of Greene/Cohen and Sapolsky, on the other? Philosophers Tyler Fagan, Katrina Sifferd, and William Hirstein believe the answer is yes. *See* William Hirstein et al., *Responsible Brains: Neuroscience, Law, and Human Culpability* (2018). Is the argument below persuasive as a solution to the neuroscience and legal responsibility debate:

> We occupy a middle ground. . . . We believe folk conceptions of agency and responsibility can be reconciled with the notion that human beings are physical objects, and that any mistaken assumptions about human decision making can be revised without much disruption to the structure of responsibility assessments. The

folk-psychological concepts that underpin assessment of responsibility—by which mental capacities and states are attributed as part of determining the level of blame or punishment that constitutes an appropriate response to a particular action—do not seem undermined by the brute fact that these capacities and states are realized in the brain. Nor, however, does neuroscience hold merely "limited and indirect" relevance to responsibility; it is rather a powerful tool integrating scientific and folk perspectives into a fuller, more accurate picture of human agency. . . .

Although a full articulation of [our] . . . theory would be outside this chapter's scope, our central claim is that the folk and legal concepts underpinning the structure of criminal offenses and verdicts implicitly refer to a particular set of cognitive functions that reside primarily in the prefrontal lobes of the brain. These cognitive functions have become known as the executive functions.

In general, executive functions activate when we go out of our routine mode and plan more complicated actions, but they may also activate when the stakes are high, or when special care is needed in performing an action. While executive functions are accomplished by large brain networks, typically spanning several cortical areas and supported by additional subcortical areas, they reside primarily in the brain's prefrontal cortex. These functions, we contend, allow for the cognitive and volitional capacities necessary to the "normative competence" the law must impute to any person it judges to be fit for criminal punishment. Only a person with (at least) a minimal level of executive functioning can qualify as normatively competent, we argue—and only the normatively competent can be properly held responsible for their actions, because only such persons have the fair opportunity to adhere to legal and moral rules. . . .

. . . [T]he basic schema of our theory of criminal responsibility . . . [is that] . . . a person is responsible for criminal illegal act, omission, or consequence only if:

1. They have a minimal working set of executive functions, and
2. They performed the act, and/or caused the consequence, or failed to act to prevent it, and
3. Their executive processes either played an appropriate role in bringing about the action, omission, or consequence or should have played an appropriate role in preventing it.

These criteria are not jointly sufficient for criminal responsibility, but each is necessary. . . . Our chosen term for this basic capacity—minimal working set (MWS)—denotes the idea that a person needs a certain level of executive function to be the subject of responsibility attributions, and that level of total function must be achieved by the executive functions working together in an effective way. . . .

Tyler K. Fagan, Katrina Sifferd & William Hirstein, *Juvenile Self-Control and Legal Responsibility: Building a Scalar Standard*, in *Surrounding Self-Control* 334 (Alfred R. Mele ed., 2020).

9. What is your reaction to the following reasoning?

Imagine this futuristic courtroom scene. The defence barrister stands up, and pointing to his client in the dock, makes this plea: "The case against Mr X must be dismissed. He cannot be held responsible for smashing Mr Y's face into a pulp. He is not guilty, it was his brain that did it. Blame not Mr X, but his overactive amygdala." . . . [Yet t]hose who blame the brain should be challenged as to why they stop at the brain when they seek the causes of bad behaviour. Since the brain is a physical object, it is wired into nature at large. "My brain made me do it" must mean (ultimately) that "The Big Bang" made me do it. . . . And there is a contradiction built into the plea of neuromitigation. The claim "my brain made me do it" suggests that I am not my brain; even that my brain is some kind of alien force. one of the founding notions of neurolaw, however, is that the person is the brain. If I were my brain, then "My brain made me do it" would boil down to "I made me do it" and that would hardly get me off the hook.

Raymond Tallis, *Why Blame Me? It Was All My Brain's Fault*, Times (London), Oct. 24, 2007, at 17.

10. "[Sam] Harris [author of a book titled *Free Will*] predicts that a declaration by the scientific community that free will is an illusion would set off 'a culture war far more belligerent than the one that has been waged on the subject of evolution.'" Editorial, *Is Free Will an Illusion?*, Chron. Rev., Mar. 18, 2012, at B6. What do you think of that prediction?

11. Philosopher Nicole Vincent argues that there is good reason to use neuroimaging to aid in individualized assessment of responsibility. She recognizes ten challenges to this proposal but argues that all of these challenges can be addressed. As you consider this list, do you agree?

> [T]en worries and problems with the suggestion that neuroimaging can help us to individually assess people's responsibility: (1) that not all people with abnormal brains commit crimes; (2) that our understanding of how the human brain works is still very rudimentary; (3) that brain plasticity might make it difficult to diagnose who has which capacities; (4) that methodological and technological problems with current neuroimaging techniques cast doubt over the usefulness of neuroimaging data; (5) that we can't go back in time and check what capacities a person had at the time when they committed their crime; (6) that neuroimaging evidence for a person's incapacity may actually damn them even harder rather than exculpating them; (7) that social factors, and not just neurological impairments, also play some role in determining our behaviour; (8) that responsibility assessments also depend in part on normative assumptions which are at least partially independent of what cognitive neuroscience tells us about the human mind; (9) that people might be responsible for their own incapacity and thus that they might be responsible for what they do on account of that; and (10) that people who know about their own incapacities may be responsible for what they do if they fail to avoid situations in which those incapacities may become a problem.

Nicole A. Vincent, *Neuroimaging and Responsibility Assessments*, 4 Neuroethics 35, 42 (2011).

12. How should the advent of probabilistic biomarkers—for instance, identified genetic profiles or brain differences related to violent behavior—be incorporated into a legal system that relies upon binary outcomes, such as guilty or not guilty? Psychiatrist Matthew Baum argues that the law should revisit its reliance on strict categorical structures, and even if categorical thinking is not eliminated, "then we can still reconceptualize many of these categorical distinctions as probabilistic in a Bayesian sense. . . . Within this probabilistic framework, the degree to which biomarkers are relevant to legal responsibility is governed by the strength of their claims on the likelihood of one of the legally relevant excusing or mitigating conditions, or the degree of doubt they introduce in the interpretation of other

evidence." Matthew L. Baum, *The Neuroethics of Biomarkers* 137 (2016). Does neuroscience challenge the law to abandon its categorical distinctions and adopt a more probabilistic, sliding scale approach to adjudication of criminal responsibility?

13. Consider this statement: "There is something more to being a person than biology can tell us." Steven K. Erickson, *Blaming the Brain*, 11 Minn. J.L. Sci. & Tech. 27, 77 (2010). To what extent do you agree or disagree, and why? To what extent could neuroscience be thought to ever shift crime policy "from a legal framework to one engineered by science"? What would be the hallmarks of such a shift? What would be the appropriate legal response?

14. Neuroscientist Benjamin Libet performed a landmark study showing that when a subject has been instructed to flick his wrist at will and to note the time at which he decides to do so, neural signals leading to the movement actually precede the subject's conscious awareness that he is about to do so. Benjamin Libet, *Do We Have Free Will?*, 6 J. Consciousness Stud. 47 (1999) (summarizing this study). A great deal of commentary has debated whether or not these findings are meaningful, both scientifically and normatively. If neuroscience shows conclusively that brain processes precede (and cause) the experience of "will," in what sense are human agents free? For further exploration of the controversies over the implications of Libet's work, see *Conscious Will and Responsibility: A Tribute to Benjamin Libet* (Walter Sinnott-Armstrong & Lynn Nadel eds., 2010).

15. Neuroscientist David Eagleman and attorney Sarah Isgur Flores suggest that systems of law should be consistent with contemporary brain science. To measure this congruence, they propose a "neurocompatibility index," which states:

> Criminal jurisprudence is often driven more by intuition and political needs than by evidence-based science. . . . [The] neurocompatibility index sets up a series of guidelines by which governments and policy-makers can consider the inclusion of modern science into their criminal justice system [and includes these criteria]:
>
> > understanding of mental illness
> > meaningful methods for rehabilitation
> > individualized sentencing based on risk assessment
> > eyewitness identification standards
> > specialized court systems (mental health, drug, juvenile)
> > incentive structuring based on behavioral economics
> > a minimum standard of science education for policy-makers. . . .

David M. Eagleman & Sarah Isgur Flores, *Defining a Neurocompatibility Index for Criminal Justice Systems: A Framework to Align Social Policy with Modern Brain Science*, in *The Law of the Future and the Future of Law: Volume II* 161, 161-72 (Sam Muller et al. eds., 2012). Is an index such as this a useful lens through which to view the justice system?

As you will see in the excerpts that follow, 15 years after Greene/Cohen and Sapolsky published their seminal papers, there remains much disagreement amongst legal scholars, philosophers, psychologists, and neuroscientists about whether, and how, neuroscience should change the law.

Adam J. Kolber
Free Will as a Matter of Law
in *Philosophical Foundations of Law and Neuroscience* 9, 10-24
(Dennis Patterson & Michael S. Pardo eds., 2016)

Stephen Morse and Paul Litton offer an alternative, compatibilist interpretation of criminal law. On their view, defendants can be punished because they can be responsible for their actions even if they are not responsible for all of the causes that make them act. Such an interpretation is consistent with the criminal law in the sense that no significant body of cases or statutes clearly contradicts it. But given that the intent underlying the criminal law is quite possibly at odds with their compatibilist interpretation, its mere consistency with cases and statutes provides a relatively weak *legal* reason to adopt it. If there is any weighty argument in favor of the compatibilist interpretation, it derives from highly contested policy or philosophical grounds about the nature of free will that have been debated for centuries.

To the extent that the philosophical debate is likely to remain unsettled, arguments about the current state of the law take on increased importance. And the view that the criminal law was never intended to apply to mechanistic humans is at least as plausible as, if not more plausible than, the view that the law was intended to punish in a compatibilist fashion. . . .

B. THE LAW'S DUALISTIC VIEW OF MIND AND BRAIN

Under the modern scientific worldview, we live in a physical universe. The universe is composed of atoms and other matter that follow physical laws. In principle, human choices and actions can be explained in terms of the interaction of matter in the universe, including the matter in our brains. Free will sceptics believe that the mechanistic nature of the universe leaves no room for free will, while compatibilists believe it does.

The law does not obviously adopt either approach. Indeed, the law says little if anything explicitly about the nature of free will in the sense that concerns us here. At least on its surface, the law treats people as morally responsible, invoking notions of retribution in criminal codes and at sentencing. But, it seems, the law has never explicitly tried to square responsibility with the mechanistic nature of the universe. . . .

C. THE PLAUSIBILITY OF SOUL-BASED LIBERTARIAN INFUSION

By claiming that criminal law can plausibly be interpreted in soul-based libertarian terms, I am in no way defending the truth of soul-based libertarianism. Legal interpretations are sometimes touted for their fidelity to law: how closely they fit with traditional sources of law like statutes, cases, the intentions of legislators and judges, and so on. Call this the legal component of an interpretation. Interpretations may also be touted for their superiority on policy, ethical or metaphysical grounds independent of specific legal authority. Call this thepolicy component of an interpretation. Since I make no claims here about the underlying moral or social issues related to the free will debate, my focus is on the legal component of the interpretation, unencumbered by the policy component.

Even as a legal matter, I merely claim that soul-based libertarianism is a plausible interpretation and not necessarily the best or only valid interpretation of criminal law. . . . [Kolber reviews a series of reasons to be cautious about advancing this interpretation.—EDS.]

Let me suggest an analogy for the unconvinced. Stephen Morse, as I shall soon discuss, defends a compatibilist interpretation of criminal law. He believes that mental state terms can be satisfied even if a person is caused to have a particular mental state by factors beyond his control. But Morse recognizes a possibility, albeit small, that neuroscience could someday show that our intentions are not what we think they are. Maybe our intentions really have no causal effect on our conduct and are merely epiphenomenal. Perhaps I only experience what I think of as the intention to go to a store after my brain has already put in place the steps by which I will in fact proceed to the store. If so, Morse concedes, we are not the creatures we currently take ourselves to be and ought not to be held morally responsible.

Now suppose that the neuroscientific community definitively proves that all intentions are epiphenomenal, and Morse is the judge in a case against a person charged with an intentional crime. Clearly, Morse would not consider such a person morally responsible. But would he use his view of morality to dictate the legal result? Judges are supposed to go beyond their own policy preferences, so Morse might plausibly ask whether the crafters of the law would consider a mental state 'intentional' were it found to be entirely epiphenomenal. In other words, regardless of our individual policy preferences, the legal doctrine of mens rea may contain background assumptions, including perhaps the denial of epiphenomenalism. And if the denial of epiphenomenalism is a plausible background assumption, then the acceptance of contra-causal free will might be as well. . . .

ii. Reply to Morse

In recent writing, however, Morse clarifies that he is not arguing that the law overtly embraces compatibilism but simply that, on its face, it is *consistent* with compatibilism. Sharing my speculation about the views of lawmakers, he states that he 'does not claim that judges and legislators throughout the centuries of development of modern criminal law explicitly adopted the compatibilist position in the metaphysical debate about determinism, free will, and responsibility. Far from it'. Indeed, he recognizes that '[c]riminal law doctrine is fully consistent with metaphysical libertarianism', even noting that '[m]ost criminal justice actors are probably implicitly libertarian and believe that we somehow have contra-causal free will'. So, Morse could accept my soul-based libertarian interpretation of current law and offer compatibilism as a reinterpretation of criminal law to save it from its outdated metaphysics.

Importantly, however, if Morse merely claims that compatibilism is consistent with the law, there is no strong *legal* reason to favor it. Lots of theories are consistent with the law. The strength of the compatibilist interpretation would derive not from any traditional legal source per se but only from its debatable strength on policy grounds. In other words, to convince us to adopt a compatibilist interpretation of criminal law, you have to convince us to believe in compatibilism. That is no easy task, considering that debate over free will has been going on for centuries. . . .

Natalie S. Gordon & Mark R. Fondacaro
Rethinking the Voluntary Act Requirement: Implications from Neuroscience and Behavioral Science Research
36 Behav. Sci. & L. 426, 426-27 (2018)

A judgment of criminal responsibility in the American legal system generally requires that both a voluntary act and a culpable mental state at the time of the offense be proven beyond a reasonable doubt. Yet the voluntariness of the prohibited act, or actus reus, is typically not proven at all. . . .

This presumption that illegal acts are committed voluntarily and typically with an ill will is at the core of the retributive, evil-doer theory of crime that forms the primary foundation and justification for criminal punishment in the United States. Retributive punishment is grounded in a moral judgment model of criminal responsibility. Inherent in this moral judgment model is the assumption that the lion's share of human behavior is guided by conscious awareness and the rational capacity to choose whether to voluntarily conform one's behavior to the requirements of the law. . . .

However, recent research in neuroscience and the behavioral sciences suggests that this core assumption underlying retributive justifications for punishment is seriously flawed. . . .

We argue that the legal system can indeed maintain its ability to hold people responsible for their criminal behavior once the justification for punishment is shifted toward more forward-looking consequentialist responses to crime. Our argument is threefold.

First, we argue, consistent with the views of many in the scientific community, that scientific progress in understanding the interrelated biological, psychological, and social influences on human behavior will increasingly shrink the homunculus at the core of the autonomous individual that the legal system now relies on to explain, judge, and punish criminal behavior.

Second, we argue that empirically suspect presumptions of voluntariness and individual autonomy are not necessary requirements for holding individuals responsible for their legally prohibited conduct once responsibility is untethered from retributive justifications for punishment. All societies establish rules and norms to guide individual and social behavior. Violations of these rules and norms can be identified and judged without resort to unverified legal presumptions about voluntariness and human autonomy.

Third, we propose reconstructing notions of responsibility and punishment within an empirically based, consequentialist framework that does not rely on empirically suspect presumptions about human behavior. Instead, our framework eliminates the "voluntariness" prong of the actus reus requirement, redefines it as a "legally prohibited act," and restores its centrality to judgments of legal responsibility. By replacing moral judgments of criminal responsibility with social judgments of "legally prohibited acts," we seek to reconceptualize responsibility as a social construct (rather than a personal attribute). In turn, this reconceptualization paves the way for more constructive evidence-based responses to crime aimed at rehabilitation, recidivism reduction, and risk management rather than retributive punishment grounded in principles of just desert. . . .

Peter A. Alces
The Moral Conflict of Law and Neuroscience
3-4, 33-37, 252-53 (2018)

The thesis here is simple: If emerging brain science reshapes what we understand to be the meaning of being human, then that same brain science must reshape our law, from the moral foundations up. . . .

. . . Law, perhaps uniquely in human affairs, depends on morality: We would not brook immoral law; from at least one perspective immoral law might even be an oxymoron. So the moral conflict of law and neuroscience is a worthwhile, and, indeed, particularly important juncture at which to measure the impact of neuroscience on what it means to be human. . . .

Though the science is, by some measures, young, it is not naïve. We do not need to know what every single neuron is doing and precisely how networks of neurons cooperate in order to appreciate challenges to conceptions we have taken for granted, but which may warrant reconsideration in light of enhanced empirical understanding. . . .

. . . [T]he premise of the arguments developed here are resolutely deterministic. . . . [W]e are the product of forces that act on us—and only the product, not the producer of such causes. So it would not matter if something like choice intervened when the human agent acts: If that choice is determined by nature and nurture, there is no basis for morality independent of those forces. And since we are not morally responsible for the formative forces that determine us, there is no "we" responsible for the consequences of those choices. The law assumes that moral responsibility, and so it is no surprise that legal doctrine often fails. It is built on a false premise. . . . [O]nce we come to understand that human agents are determined, not possessing free will, normative philosophies positing stuff like moral realism are revealed as vacuous, and human institutions such as legal doctrine, founded on and justified by those normative philosophies, are undermined. [Here, I explore that undermining, and try] to answer the "what if" question: What if neuroscientific insights, broadly construed, confirm that human agents are determined creatures, without free will in any meaningful moral sense? What happens to our legal doctrine when the normative premise of our legal doctrine, noninstrumentalism, fails? . . .

There is . . . nothing mysterious, nothing holy, about justice. . . . Neuroscience explains justice as it explains everything else about human agency, in mechanical terms, and that is true even if we have not yet figured out all the mechanics. That may be, for some, even for most, the cause of an awakening. And the coming age, an Age of Realization, may be the rudest awakening yet.

Dennis Patterson
Review of **The Moral Conflict of Law and Neuroscience**
by Peter A. Alces
5 J.L. & Biosci. 440, 441-56 (2018)

Alces' book is the strongest statement yet from those who argue for the view that the mind is the brain and we are just our brain. Advocates of the materialist and reductionist persuasion sometimes suffer from what Stephen Morse has described as 'Brain Overclaim Syndrome.' . . . Professor Alces seems to suffer more than most. In his eagerness to convince the reader of his mechanistic view of humanity, Alces fails to marshall the facts and arguments needed to sustain even his milder claims. The reason for this is quite simple: neuroscience simply has not progressed to the point where it can even tell us how the brain enables the mind. . . .

. . . Alces thinks that all human action can be reduced to what goes on in the brain. . . . Reducing human action to what goes on in the brain runs afoul of the Act/Object fallacy. The fallacy is a failure to recognize that there is a difference between what one thinks about and the activity of thinking about it. . . . Alces writes as if virtually all human practices can be reduced to neuronal activity, as if somehow the practice of, say, mathematics is just a matter of what goes on in the brain of mathematicians. This is a very strong and controversial claim for which he provides no arguments. . . .

Can we derive ought from is? Do the conclusions of neuroscience, by themselves, dictate normative conclusions? Alces thinks so but there is a considerable literature to the contrary. . . .

. . . Alces overclaims to a surprising degree. Neuroscience is a rapidly growing but young science. Its primary investigative tool, the fMRI, has substantial technical challenges that, in time, will be overcome. But many of the problems in the field of law and neuroscience are conceptual: we simply don't know how to relate scientific developments to conceptual and legal questions. Much work needs to be done. Alces' book will contribute to the discussion, if only for the force with which his case is made. But enthusiasm is no substitute for clear thinking. The book is a prime example of neuromania.

Peter A. Alces
'Neurophobia', a Reply to Patterson
5 J.L. & Biosci. 457, 458-59 (2018)

No one, and certainly not I, has ever concluded that we can now determine from a brain scan *without more* whether someone is, in fact, a psychopath. *Empirically* we cannot know, yet; there is no conceptual barrier to our eventually overcoming that empirical limitation. 'Moral Conflict' is considerate throughout of the current empirical limitations. . . .

I am not sure Patterson appreciates what it means to understand human agency in mechanical terms: 'Alces likens blaming humans for their actions to blaming a car for not starting. . . . Humans, like the cars they drive, are purely mechanical devices that occasionally require repair but benefit not at all from praise or blame.' I never suggest that human agents cannot benefit from praise or blame. In fact, the opposite is true. Patterson's confusion is a product of his conclusion that because humans respond to reasons they are not mechanistic. Reasons are just another 'cause', empirically but not conceptually different from other more obviously mechanical causes. . . .

Ultimately it becomes clear that Patterson's problem is neither with my particular argument nor with the authorities I have collected nor even with how I have presented them. He simply refuses to believe that neuroscience can tell us anything about human agency so far as law is concerned. That is 'neurophobia'. . . . The persistent problem for philosopher-neurophobes is that they cannot explain how their philosophy 'helps'. . . .

The law can steer through the straits of neuromania and neurophobia. We must appreciate the limitations of the science as well as problematic doctrine and misplaced enthusiasm for non-instrumental normative theory that is inconsiderate of the nature of human agency neuroscientific insights can reveal.

NOTES AND QUESTIONS

1. Alces and Patterson disagree about the implications of neuroscience for law. But both agree that neuroscience research will continue to expand. Is there any set of future neuroscience research findings that could resolve this dispute one way or the other?

2. As many authors recognize, retribution is at the core of many criminal justice systems. Where does the retributive impulse come from? Stephen Koppel and Mark Fondacaro suggest that neuroscience provides an answer: "The picture that begins to emerge [from review of relevant neuroscience on moral decision-making] is of a highly complex, biologically hard-wired network of regions in the brain, shaped by evolution so as to produce automatic moral assessments; and when a moral wrong has occurred, to engender retributive emotions that promote a punishment response." The authors further argue that "[i]n order to move criminal justice policy forward, it will therefore be necessary to de-legitimate retribution as a justification of punishment." Do you agree? Stephen Koppel & Mark R. Fondacaro, *The Retribution Heuristic*, in *The Routledge Handbook of Criminal Justice Ethics* 244, 247, 254 (2016). *See also* Mark R. Fondacaro & Megan J. O'Toole, *American Punitiveness and Mass Incarceration: Psychological Perspectives on Retributive and Consequentialist Responses to Crime*, 18 New Crim. L. Rev. 477 (2015).

3. Kolber discusses the work of law professor Paul Litton, who argues that "[o]n the best interpretation of criminal law, its responsibility requirements are compatibilist. . . . Reason does not exist to interpret the law's responsibility criteria as reflecting either incompatibilist view, hard determinism, or libertarianism." Paul Litton, *Is Psychological Research on Self-Control Relevant to Criminal Law*, 11 Ohio St. J. Crim. L. 725, 742 (2014).

D. PUNISHMENT AND NEUROINTERVENTION

Beyond determination of guilt and innocence, neuroscience also raises questions about how, if found guilty, an offender should be punished. In this section we explore first whether neuroscience has legal import in debates over the constitutionality of prolonged solitary confinement. We then turn to the use of neuroscience-informed rehabilitative techniques, examining contemporary proposals in light of historical considerations. We conclude with an examination of the potential of neuroscience to aid in prediction of recidivism, thus affecting sentencing, parole, and probation decisions.

1. Solitary Confinement

Francis X. Shen

Neuroscience, Artificial Intelligence, and the Case Against Solitary Confinement

21 Vand. J. Ent. & Tech. L. 937, 967-69 (2019)

B. NEUROSCIENCE AND SOLITARY CONFINEMENT LITIGATION

[S]cholars and scientists alike have . . . recognized that neuroscience may be a valuable tool to support constitutional challenges to the practice of solitary confinement. For instance, reflecting on how neuroscience might affect the law, psychologists Arielle Baskin-Sommers and Karelle Fonteneau have suggested that "[t]he first area in which findings from neuroscience may be applied to affect correctional change is with regard to the excessive and unrestricted use of segregation or solitary confinement." . . . Neuroscientist Huda Akil has made a similar argument [see below]. . . .

Given this enthusiasm for neuroscience in solitary confinement litigation, advocates in several recent cases have added it to their litigation strategy. A prominent example is *Ashker v. Brown*, a federal class action lawsuit in California brought by a class of prisoners held in the Security Housing Unit (SHU) at California's Pelican Bay State Prison. In *Ashker*, each prisoner spent ten years or more in solitary confinement. After many years of litigation, the case reached a settlement in 2015. Recognized as a "landmark settlement," the agreement ended indefinite solitary confinement for gang validation and minor rule infractions.

Ashker was notable for its utilization of brain experts. Matthew Lieberman, a neuroscientist at the University of California, Los Angeles, filed an expert report on behalf of the plaintiffs in 2015 [see below]. Lieberman argued that humans have a basic need for "social connection," and that the social pain of isolation is "registered by the brain as a type of genuine pain, just as any other forms of physical pain are." Dacher Keltner, a psychologist at University of California, Berkeley, also filed an expert report that relied heavily on the brain science of touch. Keltner argued that a lack of touch has detrimental physiological effects on inmates' brains and bodies.

It is not possible to isolate the specific added value from neuroscience's role in the *Ashker* settlement. Other factors, such as multiple hunger strikes and much additional (nonbrain) evidence on the conditions and effects of solitary confinement surely played a significant role as well. Yet it seems plausible that the neuroscience contributed, at least marginally and perhaps more substantially, in shaping the settlement's dialogue. . . .

Expert Report of Matthew D. Lieberman at 3-10

Ashker v. Governor of California

N.D. Cal. (2015), Case No.: 4:09-cv-05796-CW

I am a Professor of Psychology, Psychiatry and Biobehavioral Sciences at University of California, Los Angeles (UCLA). I am also Director of the Social Cognitive Neuroscience Laboratory at UCLA. . . .

My work broadly focuses on the intersection of social psychology and neuroscience and my early research is often associated with the founding of the field of social cognitive neuroscience. Most of the research in my laboratory uses functional magnetic resonance imaging (fMRI) to examine individuals' brain responses while thinking about or interacting with other people. . . .

C. WHAT IS THE RELATIONSHIP BETWEEN HOW THE BRAIN PROCESSES "SOCIAL PAIN" AND "PHYSICAL PAIN"?

There is considerable evidence that has accumulated in mammalian and human research to suggest that the mammalian brain evolved to process social pain (i.e. the painful feelings associated with potential or actual social rejection, loss, or isolation) repurposing some of the same neural and neurochemical processes invoked during physical pain. . . .

The lionshare of the data bearing on the hypothesis of overlap between social and physical pain comes from fMRI studies focusing on dACC and AI activity—the regions associated with physical pain distress. In collaboration with Naomi Eisenberger, I conducted the first fMRI study of social pain (Eisenberger, Lieberman, & Williams, 2003) published in the journal Science. We observed that when people played a video game that involves tossing a ball with two other people and then were excluded from the game there was selectively increased neural activity in the dACC and AI. Additionally, both of these regions showed increased activity proportionate to the subjective feelings of social pain felt by each participant. If an individual reported feeling high levels of social pain then they showed more activity in dACC and AI than another individual who felt low levels of social pain. This work has been cited more than 2000 times and has been replicated dozens of times in labs around the world. . . .

In summary, just as humans have basic needs for food, water, shelter, and sleep, they also have need for social connection. . . . Failure to provide for this need for social connection is likely to have various undesirable consequences. . . . [T]he social pain associated with social deprivation is registered by the brain as a type of genuine pain, just as other forms of physical pain are. . . . To the extent that such needs are not being met at the Pelican Bay SHU, this would serve as a major thread, both short-term and long-term, to the physical and mental well-being of those incarcerated there.

Jules Lobel & Huda Akil
Law & Neuroscience: The Case of Solitary Confinement
147 Daedalus 61, 64-68 (2018)

The neuroscientific insight that mental pain and harm are sometimes the result of or correlated with brain damage or abnormalities may also play an important role in constitutional jurisprudence addressing American prison systems' practices of prolonged solitary confinement.

The . . . use of neuroscience [to challenge the constitutionality of solitary confinement is] . . . similar to the role neuroscience played in the Eighth Amendment challenge to the execution of juveniles, wherein the Court viewed scientific evidence not as an independent basis for decision, but as evidence that would tend to confirm the conclusion that prolonged solitary confinement caused serious mental and physical harm to the brain to a degree prohibited by the Constitution. . . .

Using neuroscience in the prisoner context, however, . . . [faces] substantial obstacles. The most important was that neuroscientists had never studied the brains of prisoners and, therefore, no studies directly on point existed. Moreover, the possibility that neuroscientists could do significant scientific studies of the Pelican Bay prisoners was remote. To demonstrate conclusively that solitary confinement alters the brain, a study would have to use one of two types of design. The optimal design would be longitudinal and would require gathering baseline brain imaging data on prisoners before they were placed in solitary confinement followed by periodic testing to ascertain changes in brain structure and function. To be certain that such changes were associated with isolation and not with prison life in general, similar observations of well-matched control subjects (of similar age, sex, mental ability, and ideally criminal offense history) would have to be taken over the same period of time. An additional control group of subjects equally well-matched on crucial variables but not incarcerated would also be useful since this would enable the parsing of the effects of the general stress of prison life from the additional impact of social isolation, physical inactivity, and other distresses of solitary housing. . . .

Not only would the cost of doing such a study be massive and untenable for a public interest lawsuit, but even if the necessary funds could be raised, prison officials do not allow scientists into the prison to do studies, and, absent an unlikely court order, the plan would not be workable. Thus, using neuroscience to aid the Court in understanding how prolonged solitary confinement affected the brain . . . [requires] drawing on extant knowledge and theory and extrapolating from what scientists know generally about the brain to the situation in which these prisoners found themselves. . . .

Federica Coppola

***The Brain in Solitude: An (Other) Eighth Amendment Challenge to
Solitary Confinement***

6 J.L. & Biosci. 184, 214-18 (2019)

SOLITARY CONFINEMENT IS PER SE CRUEL AND UNUSUAL PUNISHMENT

The body of neuroscientific research on the vital importance of social interaction for brain morphology and function in combination with the insights into the damaging effects of social isolation and environmental deprivation for the brain, mind, and behavior could reinvigorate challenges to solitary confinement.

While more precise empirical answers are needed to fully comprehend the variety and extent of the implications of solitary confinement for the brain and behavior, yet existing evidence can provide additional empirical support to challenge the crux of solitary confinement: extreme isolation. . . .

. . . First, the core feature of solitary confinement—extreme isolation or social and environmental deprivation—fails to meet the current conditions standard. Second, there is a manifest imbalance between the generalized traumatic and potentially permanent implications of social and environmental deprivation and the penological purposes of prison that solitary confinement is intended to serve.

Furthermore, and more broadly, solitary confinement is antithetical to all justifications for punishment. Acknowledging that solitary confinement fails to meet any relevant Eighth Amendment requirement implies that solitary confinement is innately unconstitutional. . . .

FAILURE TO MEET CURRENT CONDITIONS STANDARD

The body of neuroscientific research on the effects of socio-environmental deprivation on the brain presents a strong empirical premise for the normative argument that socioenvironmental deprivation (or extreme isolation)—the crux of solitary confinement—qualifies as an Eighth Amendment violation under all prongs of the current conditions standard.

Social Interaction and Environmental Stimulation as Basic Human Needs

Consistent with evolutionary perspectives, neuroscientific research has provided a compelling argument for qualifying social interaction as a basic human survival need on par with other identifiable physical needs, such as water, or food, or shelter . . . that social interaction and environmental stimulation are "but for" conditions for physiological brain function. As such, depriving human beings of social contact and environmental stimulation is equivalent to depriving them of their very own nature.

Acknowledging the vital importance of social interaction in enriched environments implies that forcing individuals into isolation in tiny, environmentally poor cells is sufficient per se to deprive them of basic human needs. Accordingly, single material conditions of solitary confinement (e.g. the lack of heating, proper bedding, or winter clothing) should be viewed as circumstances that aggravate and are therefore parasitic to an underlying condition—extreme isolation—that is alone sufficient to constitute a serious deprivation of basic human needs.

Importantly, including social interaction and environmental stimulation in the range of basic human needs also impugns the substantial equivalence by the Courts between normal confinement and solitary confinement. . . .

. . . [S]uch equivalence fails to consider that extreme isolation is the condition that renders the two types of confinement materially different. This difference emerges precisely from the fact that solitary confinement deprives individuals of a survival need that normal confinement guarantees. Considering this fundamental distinguishing aspect and the consequences that it entails, normal and solitary confinement cannot at all be placed on the same level. Rather, the evaluation of solitary confinement should be based upon its own criteria, which should systematically recognize social interaction as a fundamental need rather than a mere privilege.

Socio-Environmental Deprivation (Extreme Isolation) Entails an
Objectively Serious Risk of Physical Harm

If the vital role of social interaction and environmental stimulation for human brain and behavior is not sufficient to establish them as basic physical needs, evidence of risks that socio-environmental deprivation imposes on the brain add ample weight and encourage a reconsideration of the "objectively serious risk of substantial harm" requirement in relation to solitary confinement. . . .

. . . First, socio-environmental deprivation does entail an objectively serious risk of physical harm that is on par of food or sleep deprivation. Even if the harm that solitary confinement imposes on the brain translates into mental deterioration, and is therefore mental, it is also undeniable that "the type of severe psychological deterioration observed in solitary confinement is due to physical harms imposed on the brain." As such, it is ultimately physical.

Second, the harm that solitary confinement imposes on the brain underpins a number of long-lasting or potentially permanent mental, physical, and physiological conditions. Therefore, the possible harms of solitary confinement are not only disfiguring but also potentially permanent. Last, and perhaps most importantly, the risk of such physical harms may manifest even after a short period of extreme isolation. As mentioned, (neuro)science has not yet determined with sufficient precision how long an individual can spend in isolation without undergoing irreversible brain damage. However, there is a consensus across scientific disciplines (including neuroscience) that the amount of time that an individual spends in socio-environmentally deprived conditions positively correlates to the degree of risk that he or she will deteriorate neurologically, physiologically, psychologically, and physically. . . .

. . . When acknowledging that the core condition of solitary confinement, namely extreme isolation, amounts per se to a wanton and unnecessary infliction of pain and constitutes cruel and unusual punishment, the subjective prong of the test loses its raison d'etre and becomes superfluous. Given the growing general awareness of the objective damages linked with solitary confinement, proof of socio-environmental deprivation is sufficient to infer that prison officials acted with deliberate indifference, as extremely isolating a prisoner is essentially depriving him or her of a basic human need and entails an objectively serious and well-known risk of harm. Therefore, a fact finder could conclude that by keeping a prisoner is solitary confinement in spite of the obvious health risks, both physical and psychological, the prison staff acted with deliberate indifference to the substantial risk of consequent harm. . . .

2. Neurointerventions for Criminal Rehabilitation

Oliva Choy, Adrian Raine & Roy H. Hamilton

Stimulation of the Prefrontal Cortex Reduces Intentions to Commit Aggression: A Randomized, Double-Blind, Placebo-Controlled, Stratified, Parallel-Group Trial

38 J. Neurosci. 6505, 6505-11 (2018)

Prefrontal brain impairment is one of the best-replicated risk factors for aggressive behavior. . . . [But] little is known about the causal role of the prefrontal cortex on aggressive behavior. Conclusions from extant research on the neural foundations of aggression have largely been correlational. . . . Given the association between prefrontal impairments and aggression, this study tests the hypothesis that upregulating the prefrontal cortex using tDCS will reduce intent to commit an aggressive act. . . .

[The study design involved 86 participants in a double-blind, placebo-controlled, stratified, randomized trial. The researchers gave the treatment group a tDCS intervention, and for the control group put them through the same procedure only with no electricity flowing (what the research community calls a "sham intervention"). A day after the tDCS and sham sessions, the researchers followed up with each participant to have them read and respond to two hypothetical vignettes. One vignette described a physical assault, and the other a sexual assault, and participants were asked their anticipated likelihood (on a scale of 0-100%) of committing the aggressive act. — EDS.]

. . . Individuals who underwent bilateral anodal stimulation of the DLPFC using tDCS reported a lower likelihood of committing an aggressive physical and sexual assault 1 d after stimulation compared with a sham control group. The treatment–aggressive intent relationship was partly accounted for by enhanced perception that the aggressive acts were more morally wrong, resulting from prefrontal upregulation. Findings help to strengthen conclusions from neurological, neuroimaging, and neuropsychological research by documenting experimentally the role of the prefrontal cortex on the likelihood of engaging in aggression and the perception of such acts as morally wrong. . . .

There has been increasing discussion of biological interventions on antisocial and aggressive behavior in both children and adults. Our initial findings, which are limited to intentions to commit aggression and moral judgment, require extensive replication. Nevertheless, among other etiological mechanisms, the role of biological factors on the development of antisocial behavior, including aggression, has been increasingly acknowledged. It has been suggested that treatment programs will be improved by considering biological mechanisms that potentially regulate aggression. Thus, it can be argued that further investigation of basic science trials on tDCS may potentially offer a promising new biological approach for reducing aggression, which is a major public health problem and a feature of a variety of mental disorders, including antisocial personality disorder, intermittent explosive disorder, conduct disorder, and borderline personality disorder. . . .

Dietmar Hübner & Lucie White
Neurosurgery for Psychopaths? An Ethical Analysis
7 Am. J. Bioethics Neurosci. 140, 142-43 (2016)

Recent advances in modern neuroscience have encouraged considerations concerning . . . neurosurgical interventions in delinquents classified as "psychopathic." . . . [T]he prospect of such techniques emerging is plausible enough to warrant discussion and evaluation . . . and their basic normative implications can be carved out notwithstanding their still visionary nature. . . .

The current state of [deep brain stimulation] DBS research and practice suggests that testing or applying this technique in psychopaths with the aim of modifying their behavior would, at least at present, constitute a highly burdensome and risky procedure. Its performance would amount to a major intervention, entailing intense physical strain and possible psychological traumatization, while its inadvertent consequences might be severe, including physiological complications as well as undesired changes in personality. Whether and when this procedure is ethically justified will crucially depend on the questions of whether there is an individual medical benefit to be expected for the subject of the intervention and of whether she gives her voluntary informed consent to that procedure. This holds both for research settings and for prospective "therapies." . . .

For DBS in psychopathic inmates to be justified, whether it is regarded as research or therapy, it must be accompanied by a realistic chance of a considerable individual medical benefit to the persons involved. . . .

. . . [A] closer investigation reveals that an individual medical benefit cannot obtain in the case at issue: A psychopath may have a "disease" or a "disorder" by some commonsensical or medical-psychiatric standard. But DBS cannot be thought to constitute an individual medical benefit for the psychopath, even if it "alleviates" or "cures" her condition. . . .

As stated in the preceding, some scholars doubt that psychopathy should be classified as a "disease" or "disorder" in the first place, rather than as a set of traits and behaviors that may be undesirable from a social point of view, but that do not imply any kind of health impairment on the side of the subject. Others are skeptical that this condition might be altered, contending that psychopathy is too deeply embedded in a subject's personality to allow for any successful intervention (see second section).

In both cases, the criterion of individual medical benefit could not be met: When there is no disease or disorder an intervention cannot be medical, and when there is no success to be expected, there will be no benefit. For the sake of argument, however, we shall assume that both conditions are met, that is, that psychopaths display some sort of "pathology," in a tenable sense, and that DBS experiments or treatments promise some sort of "remedy," at least in terms of reducing or eradicating psychopathy's most pressing symptoms of deviant behavior.

Even this being granted, however, it does not imply that a psychopath who is subject to DBS in either experiment or therapy could expect an individual medical benefit from the procedure. This seemingly strange constellation is due to the fact that individual medical benefit requires release from, or prevention of, subjective suffering on the side of the person concerned. It does not obtain from the mere elimination, or avoidance, of some objective condition that society declares undesirable (even for good reasons). . . .

This lack of subjective suffering and, consequently, of individual medical benefit implies that DBS on imprisoned psychopaths fails to meet an essential ethical standard for both research and therapy. . . .

Jesper Ryberg

Deep Brain Stimulation, Psychopaths, and Punishment

7 Am. J. Bioethics Neurosci. 168, 168-69 (2016)

What Hübner and White (2016) suggest is that there are strong reasons to believe that the use of deep brain stimulation (DBS) as a method of treating imprisoned psychopaths cannot be ethically justified. More precisely, the authors argue, first, that, once the psychopathic personality structure is adequately understood, there are reasons to doubt that DBS involves an "individual medical benefit" for the psychopath and, second, that the idea that an imprisoned psychopath can provide "voluntary informed consent" to such a treatment should be rejected. . . .

. . . What the authors fail to consider is the possibility that DBS could be used as a punishment (or as part of a punishment scheme). If this is the case, then it seems that the two arguments against the use of DBS lose their force. Surely it is not plausible to contend that a punishment must involve an "individual benefit" for the person who is being punished. In fact, what characterizes a punishment is usually quite the opposite. And it is most certainly not the case that a punishment requires "voluntary informed consent." But does this idea of using DBS as part of a punishment scheme constitute a genuine option? At first glance, several objections might come to mind.

First, it might be held that DBS constitutes a treatment (or perhaps a kind of enhancement), while a punishment involves suffering or deprivation. This is no doubt correct. . . . However, it is not clear that DBS cannot satisfy this suffering clause. . . . [T]here is no reason to believe that the possibility of using DBS as part of a punishment can be rejected by reference to the suffering clause of the punishment definition.

Second, it might be objected that, even if it is correct that DBS in one way or another may satisfy the suffering clause, this is still not sufficient to establish that DBS treatment can properly serve the function as a punishment. [But] . . . [i]t is very hard indeed to believe that a semantic theory can be provided to the effect that a punishment in the form of DBS treatment—if appropriately imposed—can never serve a communicative function while this function is well served by all standard types of punishment. . . .

In sum, none of the preceding objections succeeds in blocking the possibility that DBS could serve the function of a punishment that could be inflicted upon the psychopath in response to the crime he or she has committed. . . . [T]his is clearly not tantamount to holding that DBS should be used as punishment. Whether this is the case would require much more comprehensive considerations. . . . [T]he aim here has been much more modest, namely, to direct attention to the possibility that DBS could be used as a punishment, and to underline that the fact that Hübner and White ignore this possibility implies that the step—from the premises concerning "an individual medical benefit" and "voluntary informed consent" to the conclusion that the use of DBS techniques on psychopaths cannot be justified—becomes premature.

Adam B. Shniderman & Lauren B. Solberg

Cosmetic Psychopharmacology for Prisoners: Reducing Crime and Recidivism Through Cognitive Intervention

8 Neuroethics 315, 318-21 (2015)

Significant legal questions arise from any proposal to mandate [cognitive intervention] CI therapy for a convicted criminal. The standards that must be satisfied and the legality of CI may be contingent upon whether CI is punishment or treatment. Ultimately, CI may be neither punishment nor treatment, and instead enhancement, in which case the criminal justice system will find itself in uncharted waters as we have found no legal precedent or statutes to provide guidance on the legality of enhancement. . . .

LEGAL CHALLENGES

Legal Challenges to CI as Punishment

If CI were considered part of an offender's punishment the Eighth Amendment of the U.S. Constitution's proscription against cruel and unusual punishment may prove a difficult barrier to overcome. Chemical castration of convicted sex offenders provides an analogue to examine the implications of CI as an element of punishment and the subsequent Eighth Amendment implications. Chemical castration works by drastically reducing the level of testosterone, subsequently reducing sex drive. Chemical castration may be mandated as a part of sentencing or offered as a condition of release. Legal scholars have argued that chemical castration is a pharmaceutical intervention designed to incapacitate the offender, eliminating not only the deviant sexual behavior for which the offender was convicted but all sexual behavior. This incapacitation of the offender is a sort of biological imprisonment. For nearly five decades, chemical castration has been administered to convicted sex offenders, with relatively little judicial scrutiny. This lack of judicial scrutiny may be attributable to widespread fear and disdain for these offenders. . . .

While castration laws have largely escaped litigation, scholars and civil rights advocates have expressed significant concerns over the constitutionality of chemical castration. . . . Perhaps most useful for understanding the legality of CI, Stinneford contends that a punishment must meet two criteria for constitutionality: it must not be designed to control capacities fundamental to human dignity (e.g., reason and free will); and it must not treat the offender's suffering with indifference According to his analysis, the very purpose of chemical castration is to control an offender's mind and body, and is therefore unconstitutional. . . .

. . . [T]he exact nature of the CI used could be the largest determinant in whether CI is constitutional under Stinneford's proposed analysis. Interventions that truly increase cognitive abilities (e.g., reducing impulsivity), rather than simply eliminating a targeted behavior (e.g., chemical castration) may be said to have less of an incapacitative aim and more of a restorative aim, making the intervention less legally problematic and potentially more ethically sound.

Legal Challenges to CI as Treatment

If CI therapy is deemed treatment or medical care, the analysis and framework for considering its legality is significantly different than if it is simply to be used for enhancement purposes. Prisoners must be offered the right to seek medical care and at the same time, like non-incarcerated individuals, inmates are usually free to decline treatment. . . . However, because prisoners are not entirely autonomous, there are some instances in which it has been deemed legal, and by some ethical as well, to mandate that they receive treatment. . . .

ETHICAL CHALLENGES

In addition to the legal challenges of mandating cognitive intervention, there are myriad ethical issues that must be considered before implementing programs that offer cognitive intervention to prisoners. The foundation of these ethical issues are Beauchamp and Childress' four fundamental principles of bioethics: respect for autonomy, or respecting the ability of individuals to make their own informed decisions; beneficence, or providing benefits; non-maleficence, or avoiding harm; and justice, or distributing benefits, risks, and costs equitably. . . .

3. Prediction of Future Criminal Behavior

Kent A. Kiehl et al.
Age of Gray Matters: Neuroprediction of Recidivism
19 NeuroImage 813, 813-22 (2018)

A practical approach for differentiating risk levels among offenders is to develop algorithms that identify variables that predict how likely inmates are to commit another crime after their release from prison. . . .

Developments in bio-psycho-social models have identified risk variables with strong relevance to antisocial behavior. . . . Chronological age, however, may be an imprecise measure in these risk equations. That is, within the spectrum of all 25-year olds, some of the cohort may be lower than average risk and some may be higher than average risk to re-offend. In other words, chronological age does not account for individual differences in the physiological and neurocognitive aging processes. Recent developments have shown that biological aging of the brain can be quantified using MRI techniques. . . .

. . . Here, we extend this work by developing a brain-based model of age using multivariate analyses of structural MRI data and apply this method to improve prediction of antisocial outcomes. Specifically, we test whether our brain-age measures improve the accuracy of prediction models for rearrest over and above chronological age and other variables used in our prior analyses (Aharoni et al., 2013). To our knowledge, this is the first attempt to develop a brain maturation model to distinguish individuals who are more or less likely to re-offend following release from prison. . . .

[The study involved 1,332 male offenders, ages 12-65, as well as a second sample of 93 male offenders, ages 20-52. Recidivism data was derived from official arrest records. MRI brain data was obtained for each of these individuals, and the research team examined the relationship between gray matter volume and chronological age of participants. The predictive model derived from analysis of the first sample allowed the researchers to test the efficacy of their model out-of-sample with the second set of participants (none of whom were in the first sample.) — EDS.]

We confirmed hypotheses that structural brain components related to age would distinguish offenders who are likely to re-offend from those who do not re-offend. Brain-age measures accounted for almost four times the variance in the risk equation for rearrest than did chronological age. Brain-age incrementally added to risk outcomes that included other psychological and behavioral variables and, when neural age was included in the model with chronological age, chronological age was not necessary in predicting rearrest. Reduced gray matter volume and density were identified as significant predictors of both neural age and rearrest. Specifically, reduced gray matter in bilateral anterior/lateral temporal lobes, amygdala, and inferior/orbital frontal cortex was helpful in predicting rearrest. This is the first prospective study to report brain-age measures predict re-offending.

The temporal pole was identified in both volume and density measures as useful in predicting age and rearrest. The temporal pole is considered to be a paralimbic region, lying between the amygdala and orbitofrontal cortex. Anterior and medial temporal lobe damage is classically involved in Klüver–Bucy syndrome, and atrophy of this region is typically implicated in frontotemporal dementia. Both of these conditions involve symptoms that include changes in personality and socially inappropriate behavior. . . .

In the present sample, those who recidivated had lower volume in the temporal pole than did those who did not re-offend. It is reasonable to suspect that individuals who have lower volume of the temporal pole may be relatively limited in their ability to couple emotional responses to cues from their environment, leading to deficits in mentalizing the actions of others, or theory of mind. These inferred limitations might contribute to poor decision-making and poor outcomes (i.e., crime). . . .

Importantly, a combination of variables was most useful in predicting rearrest in the present sample. Psychopathy scores and anterior cingulate activity elicited from a Go/No Go task had previously demonstrated utility in predicting rearrest. By combining structural MRI data to these measures, several additional neural regions were identified which uniquely contribute to improving prediction models. Further, structural variation in these regions was a better indicator of future reoffending than was chronological age. . . .

. . . [T]his study represents an incremental step in demonstrating the utility of brain measures for their practical predictive value; however, these findings should not be considered apart from a number of important limitations and ethical considerations. . . . Ethical considerations abound in using brain-derived information to make decisions about individuals' freedom, based on improved, but still-imperfect prediction models. . . .

NOTES AND QUESTIONS

1. Many rehabilitative programs in prisons are aimed at improving decision -making in the incarcerated population. How can such programs be justified if one adopts the reductionist view that the neurons of these offenders produced their actions, as opposed to freely chosen decision-making?

2. Research on inmates is both ethically and practically difficult. Research on inmates in solitary confinement even more so. Given the barriers of conducting neuroscience research on inmates in prolonged solitary confinement, can neuroscience ever make a meaningful contribution to legal challenges to solitary confinement? Should courts consider evidence from studies of non-human animals in similar, though not identical, conditions of confinement? For a review of the psychological effects of prolonged solitary confinement, see Craig Haney, *The Psychological Effects of Solitary Confinement: A Systematic Critique*, 47 Crime & Just. 365 (2018).

3. Hübner/White and Ryberg disagree about whether the use of deep brain stimulation for offenders can be justified. Which argument is more persuasive? How should we conceptualize the use of neurointerventions on criminals—as treatment, punishment, or something else?

4. What is your gut reaction to the proposed use of biomedical approaches to criminal rehabilitation? What would the public think? For data on this question, see Robin Whitehead & Jennifer A. Chandler, *Biocriminal Justice: Exploring Public Attitudes to Criminal Rehabilitation Using Biomedical Treatments*, 13 Neuroethics 55 (2020).

5. Commenting on the tDCS research described above, senior author Adrian Raine observed: "This is not the magic bullet that's going to wipe away aggression and crime. . . . But could transcranial direct-current stimulation be offered as an intervention technique for first-time offenders to reduce their likelihood of recommitting a violent act?" Shubham Sharma, *Intent to Commit Violence, Sexual Assault Reduces by Zapping Brain with Current*, Int'l Bus. Times (July 4, 2018).

6. In 1949, the Nobel Prize in physiology or medicine was awarded to Portuguese neurologist António Egas Moniz for his discovery of the prefrontal lobotomy. This invention prompted one law student to write: "[P]sychosurgery has startling

implications for rehabilitation . . . and it is proving successful in an increasing number of cases. Perfection of so relatively simple and inexpensive a rehabilitative technique as the prefrontal lobotomy promises to be a major contribution to the cure of criminals." *Toward Rehabilitation of Criminals: Appraisal of Statutory Treatment of Mentally Disordered Recidivists*, 57 Yale L.J. 1085, 1097-98 (1948). As new direct brain interventions are developed, by what standards should they be evaluated before being implemented for rehabilitative purposes in the criminal justice system?

7. The Kiehl et al. (2018) study excerpted above presents research on brain-based prediction of recidivism, and it builds on previous work from the same group. *See* Eyal Aharoni et al., *Neuroprediction of Future Rearrest*, 110 Proc. Nat'l Acad. Sci. U.S. 6223 (2013); Eyal Aharoni et al., *Predictive Accuracy in the Neuroprediction of Rearrest*, 9 Soc. Neurosci. 332 (2014); Vaughn R. Steele et al., *Multimodal Imaging Measures Predict Re-Arrest*, 9 Frontiers Hum. Neurosci. 425 (2015); Lyn M. Gaudet et al., *Can Neuroscience Help Predict Future Antisocial Behavior?*, 85 Fordham L. Rev. 503 (2016). *See also* Vaughn R. Steele et al., *Machine Learning of Structural Magnetic Resonance Imaging Predicts Psychopathic Traits in Adolescent Offenders*, 145 Neuroimage 265 (2017).

8. The prospect of brain-based interventions for criminal offenders is not new. In the 1960s and 1970s, for instance, several groups proposed the use of psychosurgery as a cure for criminals. For discussion and critique of psychosurgery, see Amanda C. Pustilnik, *Violence on the Brain: A Critique of Neuroscience in Criminal Law*, 44 Wake Forest L. Rev. 183 (2009); Francis X. Shen, *The Overlooked History of Neurolaw*, 85 Fordham L. Rev. 667, 682 (2016); Carlin Meyer, *Brain, Gender, Law: A Cautionary Tale*, 53 N.Y.L. Sch. L. Rev. 995, 997 (2009) ("The U.S. legal system has a long history of romance with brain science—often junk science."); Nicole Hahn Rafter, *Seeing and Believing: Images of Heredity in Biological Theories of Crime*, 67 Brook. L. Rev. 71, 76 (2001).

Law professor Emily Murphy, recognizing this history, argues that new attempts at neurointervention should be viewed through a critical lens:

> California has a not-so-distant history of therapeutic interference in the brains of criminal offenders. UCLA hosted the "Violence Project" in the early 1970's, and there are reports of experimental psychosurgery in the Vacaville state correctional facility in the same time period.[1] These programs were designed to take advantage of cutting-edge understanding in psychology and neuroscience to fix a politically problematic crisis in rising crime rates. Such efforts were reportedly abandoned after political backlash against abusive research and treatment practices.[2] This historical context, coupled with present-day procedures that may give an undue sense of sophistication, should make the criminal justice system particularly cautious about adopting new and potentially invasive neuroscience technologies even if guided by the legitimate and compassionate goals of treating public health problems and promoting public safety. . . .
>
> Advances in neuroscience (leading to long-lasting or permanent effects after acute administration or that have collateral consequences of memory or personality modification) shift the burdens on informed consent in two crucial ways. First, they require a person to be able to rationally consider long-term and uncertain outcomes with respect to fundamental issues of identity and agency. Second, they heighten the risk of therapeutic misconception by offering scientifically sophisticated treatments with potentially variable outcomes. Hypothetically, a defendant may be too quick

to waive important constitutional rights because he thinks that a new neurotechnology might cure his addiction, when in fact, outcomes may be different or less than hoped for and relapse results in criminal punishment anyway such that he may have been better off in the adversarial system. It seems doubtful that defense counsel would be well-equipped to advise a client, as the "best interests" calculus would become significantly more complex and uncertain. This is but one of many potentially risky scenarios that advances in neuroscience technologies to treat addiction and antisocial behavior may present. Rather than simplifying addiction treatment with advanced technology and greasing the wheels of drug court functioning, such novel therapies complicate the analysis about appropriate balances between relinquishing rights and accepting increasingly invasive interventions in exchange. . . .

Emily R. Murphy, *Paved with Good Intentions: Sentencing Alternatives from Neuroscience and the Policy of Problem-Solving Courts*, 37 L. & Psychol. Rev. 83, 84, 115-16 (2013).

FURTHER READING

On Free Will and Responsibility:

Daniel M. Wegner, *The Illusion of Conscious Will* (2002).

Hilary Bok, *Freedom and Responsibility* (1998).

Alfred R. Mele, *Effective Intentions: The Power of Conscious Will* (2009).

Michael S. Moore, *Responsible Choices, Desert-Based Legal Institutions, and the Challenges of Contemporary Neuroscience*, 29 Soc. Phil. & Pol'y 233 (2012).

Michael S. Moore, *Mechanical Choices: The Responsibility of the Human Machine* (2020).

Joshua Greene, *Moral Tribes: Emotion, Reason, and the Gap Between Us and Them* (2013).

Kadri Vihvelin, *Causes, Laws, and Free Will: Why Determinism Doesn't Matter* (2013).

Selim Berker, *The Normative Insignificance of Neuroscience*, 37 Phil. & Pub. Aff. 293 (2009).

Michael S. Pardo & Dennis Patterson, *Minds, Brains, and Law: The Conceptual Foundations of Law and Neuroscience* (2013).

Michael S. Pardo & Dennis Patterson, *Philosophical Foundations of Law and Neuroscience*, 2010 U. Ill. L. Rev. 1211 (2010).

Neuroscience and Legal Responsibility (Nicole A. Vincent ed., 2013).

Neurolaw and Responsibility for Action Concepts, Crimes, and Courts (Bebhinn Donnelly-Lazarov ed., 2018).

Michael S. Gazzaniga, *Who's in Charge? Free Will and the Science of the Brain* (2011).

Bruce A. Arrigo, *Punishment, Freedom, and the Culture of Control: The Case of Brain Imaging and the Law*, 33 Am. J.L. & Med. 457 (2007).

Stephen J. Morse, *The Non-Problem of Free Will in Forensic Psychiatry and Psychology*, 25 Behav. Sci. & L. 203 (2007).

Stephen J. Morse, *Determinism and the Death of Folk Psychology: Two Challenges to Responsibility from Neuroscience*, 9 Minn. J.L. Sci. & Tech. 1 (2008).

Stephen J. Morse, *Neuroscience, Free Will, and Criminal Responsibility*, in *Free Will and the Brain: Neuroscientific, Philosophical, and Legal Perspectives* 251 (Walter Glannon ed., 2015).

Stephen J. Morse, *The Neuroscientific Non-Challenge to Meaning, Morals, and Purpose*, in *Neuroexistentialism: Meaning, Morals, and Purpose in the Age of Neuroscience* 333 (Gregg D. Caruso & Owen Flanagan eds., 2018).

Stephen J. Morse, *The Inevitable Mind in the Age of Neuroscience*, in *Philosophical Foundations of Law and Neuroscience* 29 (Dennis Patterson & Michael S. Pardo eds., 2016).

William Hirstein, Katrina L. Sifferd & Tyler K. Fagan, *Responsible Brains: Neuroscience, Law, and Human Culpability* (2018).

Conscious Will and Responsibility: A Tribute to Benjamin Libet (Walter Sinnott-Armstrong & Lynn Nadel eds., 2010).

On the Folk Psychology of Intentionality:

Bertram F. Malle & Joshua Knobe, *The Folk Concept of Intentionality*, 33 J. Experimental Psychol. 101 (1997).

Joshua Knobe, *The Concept of Intentional Action: A Case Study in the Uses of Folk Psychology*, 130 Phil. Stud. 203 (2006).

In Addition:

Azim F. Shariff et al., *Free Will and Punishment: A Mechanistic View of Human Nature Reduces Retribution*, 25 Psychol. Sci. 1563 (2014).

Frank Krueger et al., *An fMRI Investigation of the Effects of Belief in Free Will on Third-Party Punishment*, 9 Soc. Cognitive & Affective Neurosci. 1143 (2014).

Steven K. Erickson, *Blaming the Brain*, 11 Minn. J.L. Sci. & Tech. 27 (2010).

O. Carter Snead, *Neuroimaging and the "Complexity" of Capital Punishment*, 82 N.Y.U. L. Rev. 1265 (2007).

Theodore Y. Blumoff, *The Neuropsychology of Justifications and Excuses: Some Problematic Cases of Self-Defense, Duress, and Provocation*, 50 Jurimetrics 391 (2010).

Dean Mobbs, Hakwan C. Lau, Owen D. Jones & Christopher D. Frith, *Law, Responsibility, and the Brain*, 5 PLoS Biology 693 (2007).

Andrea L. Glenn & Adrian Raine, *Neurocriminology: Implications for the Punishment, Prediction and Prevention of Criminal Behavior*, 15 Nature Revs. Neurosci. 54 (2014).

Carl F. Craver, *Explaining the Brain: Mechanisms and the Mosaic Unity of Neuroscience* (2007).

Neuroexistentialism: Meaning, Morals, and Purpose in the Age of Neuroscience (Gregg D. Caruso & Owen Flanagan eds., 2017).

On Neurointerventions:

Neurointerventions and the Law: Regulating Human Mental Capacity (Nicole A. Vincent, Thomas Nadelhoffer & Allan McCay eds., 2020).

Jesper Ryberg, *Neurointerventions, Crime, and Punishment: Ethical Considerations* (2019).

Treatment for Crime: Philosophical Essays on Neurointerventions in Criminal Justice (David Birks & Thomas Douglas eds., 2018).

CHAPTER 8

Neuroscience in the Courtroom: Assessing Scientific Evidence

Just when a scientific principle or discovery crosses the line between the experimental and demonstrable stages is difficult to define. Somewhere in this twilight zone the evidential force of the principle must be recognized. . . .

— Associate Justice Josiah Alexander Van Orsdel,
Frye v. United States (writing for the majority)[†]

Science can — and should — inform the legal system about facts, including facts about degrees of reliability and the extent of experimental validity, but the ultimate normative and institutional question of whether and when, if at all, a given degree of validity or reliability is sufficient for some legal or forensic purpose is a legal and not a scientific question.

— Frederick Schauer[††]

CHAPTER SUMMARY

This chapter:
- Introduces the basic rules for admitting scientific evidence in courtroom proceedings.
- Discusses how courts apply the rules of evidence to neuroscientific evidence in order to arrive at decisions about general acceptance, probative value, prejudice, relevance, and admissibility.
- Reviews research on the effect of neuroimaging evidence on jurors.

INTRODUCTION

Although neuroscience, law, and society intersect in many important ways, both in and outside the courtroom, the introduction of neuroscientific evidence in court raises a unique set of questions that can only be answered with reference to specific evidentiary rules. You have already seen such rules in action in previous chapters. In Chapter 1 you read about the capital sentencing of Brian Dugan, during which the judge allowed expert neuroscience testimony about Dugan's brain, but prevented

---

[†] *Frye v. United States*, 293 F. 1013, 1014 (D.C. Cir. 1923).
[††] Frederick Schauer, *Can Bad Science Be Good Evidence? Neuroscience, Lie Detection, and Beyond,* 95 Cornell L. Rev. 1191, 1192 (2010).

the expert from showing brain images directly to the jury. In Chapter 2 you read the evidentiary hearing on the admissibility of brain scan evidence proffered by Herbert Weinstein.

By now you should recognize that the court's evidentiary considerations will vary according to the specific science in question, the legal uses for which the evidence is proffered, and the applicable evidentiary rules. For instance, the barriers to admissibility of expert evidence during the guilt phase of a criminal trial are much greater than at the sentencing phase. Moreover, courts sometimes modify their admissibility analysis in civil versus criminal contexts. You will continue to see evidentiary rules in action in subsequent chapters. For those students who need additional background on the law of evidence more generally, we recommend several sources at the end of the chapter. For additional discussion of the limitations of certain neuroscientific techniques, refer back to Part 2 of this book on the Fundamentals of Cognitive Neuroscience, as well as the Appendix on fMRI.

In this chapter, we provide an introduction to the rules that govern the admissibility of expert evidence in U.S. courtrooms, with a focus on specific considerations most relevant to neuroscientific evidence. Section A presents data and commentary on what we know about historical and current use of neuroscience in court. Section B introduces *Frye v. United States*, a 1923 case that is the first of two landmark developments in scientific evidence. The *Frye* case established "general acceptance" as a litmus for admissibility. Section C presents subsequent and relevant rules from the Federal Rules of Evidence, originally enacted by Congress in 1975. Section C then presents the second landmark moment, the "*Daubert* trilogy," a series of three Supreme Court cases regarding the admissibility of scientific evidence: *Daubert v. Merrell Dow Pharmaceuticals* (1993), *General Electric Co. v. Joiner* (1997), and *Kumho Tire Co., Ltd. v. Carmichael* (1999); *Daubert* established the so-called "gatekeeper" approach, in which trial judges, at least in theory, should engage more actively in screening proffered scientific testimony. *Joiner* held that abuse of discretion is the appropriate standard of appellate review for district court admissibility decisions. *Kumho Tire* clarified that *Daubert* applied both to "scientific" knowledge as well as other technical and specialized knowledge.

You should be aware that the precise evidentiary rules, and of course the case law applying those rules, varies markedly by jurisdiction. For instance, the federal courts employ the *Daubert* standard, and most state courts have now adopted rules based on *Daubert*, as well. But some states still rely on the earlier *Frye* "general acceptance" test. And still other states have blended the two, in what some call a "*Fraubert*" standard. Moreover, in most jurisdictions neither *Daubert* nor *Frye* are applicable to evidence that a judge considers at sentencing. It is also worth noting that we focus here only on evidence in U.S. courtrooms, which rely on an adversarial model and a lay jury as the fact finder. In legal systems that employ an inquisitorial model, the evidentiary rules are much different.

Given this variation in evidentiary standards, our goal is not to introduce you to every type of evidentiary standard, but rather to focus on basic principles. In subsequent chapters, we discuss more specific standards and apply them to different kinds of neuroscientific evidence. For instance, the chapter on brain injury reviews cases concerning the admissibility of diffusion tensor imaging evidence in brain injury cases, and the chapter on lie detection reviews in detail a *Daubert* hearing relating to the introduction of fMRI lie-detection evidence.

With the basic principles in place, the chapter then proceeds to a series of cases that illustrate how courts have put these rules into practice in different legal contexts. We present, in Section D, material from the case of Grady Nelson, who proffered brain-based evidence in his capital sentencing proceedings. We present, in Section E, cases from non-criminal contexts.

In many of these cases, courts have expressed a concern that jurors may be unduly persuaded by brain images. Thus, in Section F we review a small but growing body of literature studying the effects of brain images on juror and judge decision-making. Along the way, you will encounter descriptions of various neuroscientific techniques. Do not get bogged down in the technical details, and as needed refer back to the introductory science text in Part 2. In this chapter, focus attention on the foundational evidentiary issues.

A. NEUROSCIENCE IN THE COURTROOM

Darby Aono, Gideon Yaffe & Hedy Kober
Neuroscientific Evidence in the Courtroom: A Review
4 Cogn. Res. Principles & Implications 40 (2019)

NEUROSCIENCE IN THE MODERN COURTROOM

Along with its development in scientific contexts, the opportunity for neuroscience to be used as evidence in criminal trials has predictably increased since the turn of the century. Theoretically, neuroscientific evidence (broadly construed as any information related to the brain) can be used like any other type of evidence to establish or dispute any claim in a criminal case. It could be used, for example, to support or cast doubt on the testimony of an expert, to support or rebut a medical diagnosis, to corroborate a defendant's testimony about his frame of mind at the time of the crime, to establish that a defendant's conduct caused severe harm, or used demonstratively to help the judge or jury understand some other kind of evidence, and so on. In practice, the standard described in the prior section regulates the admission of such evidence in various courtrooms.

Meixner (2016) reviewed the use of neuroscientific evidence in criminal trials from 2005 to 2012 in the US, Canada, the Netherlands, England, and Wales. Summarizing prior findings, he reported that the use of neuroscientific evidence has increased at similar rates across all studied jurisdictions, with a sharp upwards slope from 2005 that levels off in around 2010. The absolute number of US cases involving neuroscientific evidence, however, has been significantly higher than the other jurisdictions.

In an analysis of US cases between 2005 and 2012, Farahany (2016) reported that 1585 judicial opinions from criminal cases mentioned the defense's use of neuroscientific or genetic evidence. In 2012 alone, there were 250 judicial opinions written in which the criminal defendant argued (successfully or otherwise) that their "brain made them do it". In another analysis, Farahany determined that neuroscientific and genetic evidence was introduced in 5% of all murder trials and 25% of all death penalty trials in 2012 (Farahany, 2016). In fact, 15% of the 1585 judicial opinions reviewed discussed such evidence specifically. It should be noted, however, that only a fraction of all criminal cases go to trial and end in guilty verdicts. Of these cases, only a fraction reach appellate court and subsequently generate written opinions. Therefore, this set of judicial opinions may not be representative of all cases, or even all cases that go to trial.

Denno (2015) provided a nuanced view of how neuroscience is used in criminal trials with her review of 553 criminal cases that presented neuroscientific evidence between 1992 and 2012. Two thirds (66.18%) of the cases began as death penalty cases, while 24.23% were cases in which either life or significant prison sentences (10+ years) were possible outcomes for the defendant. In nearly all cases, neuroscientific material was presented as mitigating evidence by the defense; in only 7% of cases was it presented as aggravating evidence by the prosecution. Although Denno did not quantify the claim, she reported that, across defense cases, neuroscientific evidence was often used to bolster a diagnosis that was already confirmed by a medical professional (Denno, 2015). Such diagnoses included substance use disorders, schizophrenia, depression, and organic brain damage (among others). However, in many cases neuroscientific evidence was used to suggest the existence of a "mental or behavioral" disorder that was not otherwise diagnosed. Interestingly, 63.29% of the reviewed cases specifically involved a form of neuroimaging evidence, including MRI, PET, and CT scans.

A particularly intriguing subset of the cases reviewed by Denno (2015) were those in which a defendant was convicted and subsequently argued that they had received "ineffective assistance of counsel" thanks to their attorney's failure to introduce neuroscientific evidence. In *Strickland v. Washington* (1984), the Supreme Court ruled that in order for defendants to successfully appeal on account of ineffective assistance of counsel they must show that their attorneys performed below an "objective standard of reasonableness," and that there was "a reasonable probability that, but for counsel's unprofessional errors, the result of the proceeding would have been different."

Such *Strickland* claims appeared in 53% of the cases reviewed by Denno (2015). Importantly, 87% of these *Strickland* claims included arguments that defense counsel presented insufficient neuroscientific evidence. Furthermore, 27.65% of the reported *Strickland* claims were successful (an extraordinarily high rate), with defense counsel's inadequate use of neuroscientific evidence forming the basis of all but one successful claim. This success rate is especially striking given that *Strickland* claims are typically unsuccessful. For example, Benner (2009) reported a 4% success rate for all *Strickland* claims in California over a 10-year period. This difference in success rates likely stems from the types of cases reported by Denno (2015), namely, cases in which neuroscientific evidence was presented in the first place. Indeed, defendants who had a reason to introduce neuroscientific evidence in their original court cases (presumably due to neurological or mental abnormalities) may be more likely to successfully establish ineffective assistance of counsel compared with neurologically typical defendants. However, this high success rate may still suggest that the law is beginning to require defense lawyers to introduce neuroscientific evidence when it might prove valuable to the defendant's case. . . .

The *Journal of Law and the Biosciences* published four empirical studies, reporting on the use of neuroscientific evidence in the United States, Canada, the Netherlands, and England and Wales. The excerpts below present some of the key findings with regard to neuroimaging evidence from each of the studies, as well as related commentary that appeared in the Journal.

Nita A. Farahany
*Neuroscience and Behavioral Genetics in U.S. Criminal Law: An
Empirical Analysis*
2 J.L. & Biosci. 485, 486-95 (2015)

Over the past decade, the outcomes of hundreds of criminal cases have been influenced by neurobiological data. Over 1585 judicial opinions issued between 2005 and 2012 discuss the use of neurobiological evidence by criminal defendants to bolster their criminal defense. In 2012 alone, over 250 judicial opinions—more than double the number in 2007—cited defendants arguing in some form or another that their 'brains made them do it'. Approximately 5 per cent of all murder trials and 25 per cent of death penalty trials feature criminal defendants making a bid for lower responsibility or lighter punishment using neurobiological data. While these claims often overstate the science, used responsibly neurobiological evidence has the potential to improve the accuracy and decrease errors in the criminal justice system. . . .

[D]ecrying the use of neurobiological evidence in criminal law seems both futile and counterproductive; neuroscience is already entrenched in the US legal system. . . .

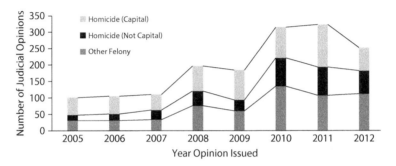

Graph 1. Judicial opinions discussing neurobiological introduced by criminal defendants 2005-12. (Homicide) (capital) are murder cases in which the prosecutor sought the death penalty. Homicide (not capital) are some degree of homicide (murder, manslaughter) cases in which the death penalty was not at issue. Other felony cases are those in which the defendant was not charged with homicide.) @ [Nita Farahany] 2016. This image/content is not covered by the terms of the Creative Commons licence of this publication. For permission to reuse, please contact the rights holder.

Notably, only about 15 per cent of the cases where neurobiological evidence was raised in the sample had any form of brain scanning discussed in the opinion. A large proportion of the cases (nearly 40 per cent) have no discussion of neurological testing in the opinion, even though the defendant staked their defense in part on a claim that 'his brain made him do it'. Of course, it's entirely possible that the judicial opinion did not discuss the specifics of testing that actually was introduced in the criminal case, so this is a conservative estimate of testing introduced.

In the 15 per cent of cases that included a discussion of brain scanning in the opinion, the type of scanning was most often MRI or CAT scans, rather than more sophisticated functional neuroimaging such as EEG, SPECT, or fMRI scanning (see Graph 5). Functional magnetic resonance imaging (fMRI) was discussed in about 2 per cent of the 15 per cent of scanning cases, but in each of the cases the fMRI evidence was not admitted into the case for further consideration because of concerns about scientific reliability, credibility, or relevance. . . .

Jennifer A. Chandler
The Use of Neuroscientific Evidence in Canadian Criminal Proceedings
2 J.L. & Biosci. 550, 551-58 (2015)

The database 'All Canadian Court Cases' within the Canadian legal service LexisNexis Quicklaw was used to search Canadian case law for reported cases involving the use of neuroscientific evidence in the five-year period between 2008 and 2012. . . .

This filtering process produced a set of 279 cases, which were read more closely for inclusion in the database. In the course of analyzing these cases, it became apparent that judges mentioned neuroscientific evidence in a range of different ways. This included discussions in which evidence of brain injury or cognitive impairment linked to some neurological cause was accepted as bearing upon an offender's responsibility, capacity, risk of recidivism, or prospects for rehabilitation ('evidence impact'). There were 133 cases in which discussions of this type occurred. . . .

Over the five years reviewed in this study, there appears to be an upward trend in the number of cases in which evidence of brain injury or cognitive impairment linked to some neurological cause was accepted as bearing upon an offender's responsibility, capacity, risk of recidivism, or prospects for rehabilitation ('evidence impact'). . . .

The three most common types of neuroscientific evidence mentioned in the set in each of the five years for which the data are being presented were evidence of prenatal alcohol exposure [fetal alcohol spectrum disorder ('FASD'), fetal alcohol effects ('FAE'), or alcohol-related neurodevelopmental disorder ('ARND')], traumatic brain injuries ('TBI'), and neuropsychological testing. . . . Brain imaging and electroencephalography were infrequently mentioned in the set of cases. A supplementary search of the same database of Canadian case law updated to August, 2014 reveals only two cases making reference to fMRI or functional magnetic resonance imaging, neither of which involve a criminal matter. . . .

Paul Catley & Lisa Claydon
The Use of Neuroscientific Evidence in the Courtroom by Those Accused of Criminal Offenses in England and Wales
2 J.L. & Biosci. 510, 517-22 (2015)

In the period covered by the research [2005-2012], we identified 204 reported cases in which neuroscientific evidence was used (or appeared from the case report to have been used) by those accused of criminal offenses [in England and Wales]. The evidence was used to appeal against conviction, to appeal against sentence and for other purposes including resisting extradition, resisting prosecution appeals that the sentence imposed was unduly lenient, seeking to have bail conditions lifted, and by prisoners seeking recategorization.

Over the period under examination, there was a marked increase in the number of reported cases in which neuroscientific evidence was presented by those accused of criminal offenses. In the period 2005-08, each year the maximum number of reported cases did not exceed 21, and the annual average was just under 17. From 2009 to 2012, the lowest number of cases any year was 25 and the annual average doubled to just over 34. . . .

The main ways in which the neuroscientific evidence is being used is to appeal against conviction (61 cases, 29.9 per cent of the cases), to appeal against sentence

(92 cases, 45.1 per cent), or to appeal against both conviction and sentence (20 cases, 9.8 per cent). The largest groupings amongst the remaining cases were where individuals were resisting extradition (11 cases, 5.4 per cent), and cases where they were resisting prosecution appeals against allegedly unduly lenient sentences (8 cases, 3.9 per cent). . . .

Almost half of appellants using neuroscientific evidence to appeal against sentence succeeded, at least partially. In most of these cases, the neuroscientific evidence formed at least part of the reasons for their success. In 10 cases, the neuro-scientific evidence appeared to be the main reason for the appellant succeeding in having the sentence reduced. . . .

C.H. de Kogel & E.J.M.C. Westgeest

Neuroscientific and Behavioral Genetic Information in Criminal Cases in the Netherlands

2 J.L. & Biosci. 580, 580-600 (2015)

Neuroscientific information and techniques have found their way into the courts of the Netherlands . . . Decisions in criminal cases published in the years 2000-12 were searched in the Dutch case law database of *'Rechtspraak.nl.'*. . . . Considered as neuro-scientific information is information from (1) assessment of the brain with imaging techniques (such as **MRI, SPECT, PET**) or **EEG**, neuro-endocrinological assessment ([e.g.] hormones, neuropeptides), (2) neuropsychological assessment, or (3) refer-ring to a certain neurobiological predisposition or damage of the brain. . . .

Neuroscientific information [was] . . . introduced in 207 of the cases. . . . In most of the cases found, serious offenses and long sentences are at issue, although a wide range of offenses and penalties occur. . . .

In the largest category of the criminal cases found, neuroscientific information is introduced in relation to the question to what extent the defendant can be held accountable for the offense. The consequences of damage to the pre-frontal brain for the behavioral choices the person had at the time of the offense are a theme in several of the cases. . . . In 15 of the criminal cases, we found, neuroscientific information is explicitly mentioned in relation to the criminal recidivism risk of the defendant. . . .

In the majority of the cases found, neuroscientific information is introduced as mitigating information in sentencing. In such cases, there is often a presump-tion that the defendant has a mental disorder or defective development that may have limited his responsibility for his criminal actions, and in which neurobiological aspects may play a role. . . .

Matthew Ginther

Neuroscience or Neurospeculation? Peer Commentary on Four Articles Examining the Prevalence of Neuroscience in Criminal Cases Around the World

3 J.L. & Biosci. 324, 325-26 (2016)

[Each of the four articles] concludes that the use of neuroscience in the courts of each respective jurisdiction is increasing at a relatively rapid pace. However, my review of their methods and results leads me to a different conclusion: there is no evidence supporting the conclusion that neuroscience is yet being introduced in trial courts, in any meaningful quantity.

The divergence in opinion rests not on semantics, but on what I think is a widespread misclassification of analyses or opinions using neuroimaging and 'neurojargon' as constituting neuroscience. I believe that in these four articles the authors have made this same common mistake by implicitly classifying evidence as neuroscience so long as the experts providing the evidence couched their opinions with a focus on specific brain systems or purported to base their opinions on brain images. . . .

KEEPING THE SCIENCE IN NEUROSCIENCE

. . . [T]here is a central tenet that underlies all of science: the requirement that knowledge be based on systemic observations of the world that result in predictions that can be tested and falsified. This focus on empiricism is the defining feature of the scientific method, and it is what allows scientists to differentiate between scientific knowledge and mere conjecture, opinion, and speculation. . . .

A common misunderstanding about science is that it results from the use of technologically advanced techniques. . . .

The contrast between the use of science and the use of technology figures prominently in the four *Journal of Law and the Biosciences* studies. The methods employed—which were largely homogenous across the studies—did not isolate cases where neuroscience was introduced insomuch as they isolated cases where brain imaging technology or neurojargon was used. Each study defined a case as 'involving neuroscience' if it contained at least one of a family of key words, such as Brain, EEG, fMRI, and CT Scan. No study examined whether the use of these technologies was consistent with the rigors of the scientific method, or in other words, actually constituted 'neuroscience.' . . .

By itself, a brain scan is no more scientific than the careful measurements of the bumps on an individual's skull—a practice called phrenology that was once considered cutting edge brain science, but now widely considered bizarre. . . .

John B. Meixner, Jr.
The Use of Neuroscience Evidence in Criminal Proceedings
3 J.L. & Biosci. 330, 333-34 (2016)

These exciting studies tee up a number of questions for follow-up work. . . .

First, . . . a critical question becomes: how is this evidence treated in court *once it is there* by judges and other legal decision makers? Do they know how to consider it properly? Do they spend time analyzing it? Do they merely defer to experts in assessing its admissibility or weight? Even beginning to answer these questions, of course, is an extremely difficult task, as they involve much more subjective decisions than the ones made by coders in these studies, and likely vary substantially be context. . . .

A second difficult, but important, avenue for follow-up work involves questions about the *value* of neuroscience evidence, both in terms of broad litigation outcomes and evidence-specific outcomes. When neuroscience evidence is offered, is it often taken seriously? What are the arguments made by the attorneys both for and against its inclusion? Which arguments do judges tend to accept? And when neuroscience evidence is introduced into evidence, is it important in shaping outcomes? In which direction? . . .

Last, similar research in the civil arena would be extremely illuminating. Neuroscience's application to the law is often discussed in the criminal context, but, as others have noted, the potential civil applications of neuroscience evidence are many, particularly in terms of measuring pain, memory or other cognitive deficits, or other brain injuries that might be alleged in a tort claim. A better understanding of how similar evidence is used in those contexts would help researchers understand potential applications for their work. . . .

Deborah W. Denno

*The Myth of the Double-Edged Sword: An Empirical Study
of Neuroscience Evidence in Criminal Cases*

56 B.C. L. Rev. 493, 498-508 (2015)

I have conducted an unprecedented empirical study ("Neuroscience Study" or "Study") of all criminal cases (totaling 800 cases) that addressed neuroscience evidence over the course of two decades (1992-2012). The Neuroscience Study provides, for the first time, extensive and systematic empirical data that show how neuroscience evidence is used in courtrooms. These data enable us to look beyond assumptions and misconceptions, particularly the myth of the double-edged sword. . . .

The Study . . . uncovers a criminal justice system that is surprisingly willing to accept and comprehend both the strengths and limitations of neuroscience evidence in ways that clearly discredit the myth of the double-edged sword. Rather than simply furthering current theoretical debates, this Study suggests that the substance of such debates should change. Indeed, the results of the Neuroscience Study spur a straightforward, yet perhaps unexpected, conclusion: the key question we should be asking is not *whether* neuroscience evidence should be used in the criminal justice system, but rather *how* and *why*. . . .

The Neuroscience Study's 800 cases . . . fall into three categories: 247 cases (30.88%) concern neuroscience evidence as it pertains to the victim, primarily to prove the extent of a victim's brain injury; 514 cases (64.25%) concern neuroscience evidence as it pertains to the defendant; and thirty-nine cases (4.88%) concern neuroscience evidence as it pertains to both the defendant and the victim because the brains of one or more individuals in both the "victim" and "defendant" categories were examined. The focus of this Article is on the cases in the latter two categories—"defendant" and "both victim and defendant"—which comprise 553 cases or 69.13% of the total data set of 800 cases. . . .

The vast majority of the . . . [cases] involve defendants convicted of murder. . . . 366 cases or 66.18% . . . began as capital cases in which the defendant was eligible for the death penalty even if that sentence was later reduced. Defendants in the remaining cases (187 cases or 33.82%) faced disproportionately severe sentences. Among these non-death penalty cases, less than half (80 cases or 42.78%) were given a sentence of life either with or without the possibility of parole. . . . In sum, . . . neuroscience evidence is typically used in cases where defendants face the death penalty, a life sentence, or a substantial prison sentence.

[N]euroscience evidence is employed at different stages of cases. . . . [N]euroscience evidence is usually offered to mitigate punishments in the way that traditional criminal law has always allowed, especially in the penalty phases of death penalty trials. This finding is noteworthy because it controverts the popular image of neuroscience evidence as a double-edged sword—one that will either get defendants off the hook altogether or unfairly brand them as posing a future danger to society. To the contrary, . . . neuroscience evidence is typically introduced for well-established legal purposes—to provide fact-finders with more complete, reliable, and precise information when determining a defendant's fate. . . .

[T]he most prevalent mental and behavioral disorders ascribed to defendants by way of neuroscience evidence include disorders of adult personality and behavior, mental and behavioral disorders due to psychoactive substance abuse, schizophrenia, schizotypal and delusional disorder, and organic mental disorders. . . .

Neuroscience evidence supporting the confirmed diagnoses include a swath of tests encompassing both imaging and non-imaging techniques. [see chart 4] . . .

[O]ver one-half . . . of the 553 defendants raised a *Strickland* [ineffective assistance of counsel] claim during litigation. . . . nearly all successful *Strickland* claims were based on an attorney's failure to appropriately investigate, gather, or understand neuroscience evidence—as opposed to any one of a number of other types of ineffective assistance of counsel claims. . . .

Chart 4
Use or Discussion of Brain Imaging Technology by Number of Cases*
553 Total Cases

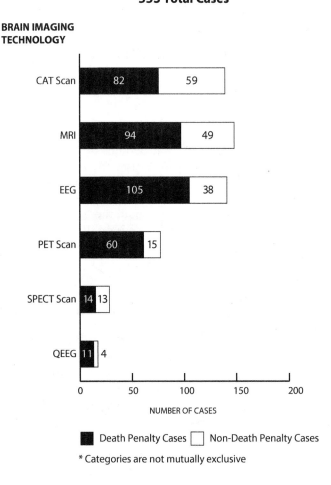

* Categories are not mutually exclusive

Lyn M. Gaudet & Gary E. Marchant
Under the Radar: Neuroimaging Evidence in the Criminal Courtroom
64 Drake L. Rev. 577, 594-654 (2016)

The present study builds on and extends the findings of Professors Denno and Faharnay in significant ways. First, this study provides an updated analysis, including cases through 2015, whereas the previous studies included cases through 2012. . . . Second, the present study more narrowly focuses only on criminal cases involving neuroimaging evidence. . . .

This study identified and analyzed reported criminal cases involving neuroimaging published through the end of 2015. Cases were identified using searches of the Westlaw database and then were analyzed to ensure they involved the use or attempted use of neuroimaging evidence of a defendant in a criminal case. . . . A total of 361 criminal cases were identified and analyzed. The cases were categorized into three groups depending on the primary use for which the neuroimaging evidence was intended in the trial: (1) guilt phase, 134 cases; (2) penalty or sentencing phase, 171 cases; or (3) competency, 56 cases. . . .

Neuroimaging evidence has been and is being admitted in the guilt phase to support a number of arguments, primarily to rebut intent or to support an insanity, mental disease, or mental defect defense. . . .

A second set of cases relating to the guilt phase involves those where the defendant sought funds from the court for neuroimaging or sought a continuance or stay of the trial in order to obtain a brain scan. The posture of the funding request cases are such that, in those cases where the trial court grants funds for a brain scan, there is unlikely to be any appeal and thus, no reported opinion. Therefore, the only cases reported are those where the defendant was originally denied funding by the trial court and has appealed that decision to an appellate court. . . .

Over the last ten years, evidence of brain damage and dysfunction has become increasingly common in the sentencing phase of capital cases. In the majority of the cases identified through Westlaw, evidence of defendants' brain abnormalities, damage, or dysfunction—established via various brain scan techniques and presented by expert testimony—was admitted during the penalty phase, but the defendant's death sentence was nonetheless upheld on appeal. . . .

Compared to the number of cases in the two previous categories, a relatively small number of appellate cases have been reported that implicate neuroimaging evidence with a defendant's competency to stand trial or change a plea. . . .

From the cases included in this Article, some generalizations can be made about the impact neuroimaging evidence has actually had at the various stages of a trial. First, there has been a steady upward trend in the number of criminal cases considering neuroimaging evidence. . . .

Second (and not surprisingly given the caveats of the methodology of using reported cases where the defendant lost at trial and then appealed), in general, neuroimaging tests have not been successfully used to establish incompetency or to rebut guilt. . . .

Third, in recent years there has been somewhat of a shift from arguments about whether neuroimaging evidence is relevant and admissible in criminal defense cases to a focus on the substantive results of the neuroimaging. This trend is demonstrated by the recent phenomenon in which courts have increasingly relied on neuroimaging results showing no evidence of organic brain damage to reject defenses or mitigation claims by defendants. . . .

Valerie Gray Hardcastle, M. K. Kitzmiller & Shelby Lahey
The Impact of Neuroscience Data in Criminal Cases: Female Defendants and the Double-Edged Sword
21 New Crim. L. Rev. 291, 292-308 (2018)

Historically, courts have been wary about using expert testimony. . . . [n]onetheless, in 1881, in one of the first insanity defenses in the country, forensic psychiatrist Dr. Edward Charles Spitzka testified at Charles J. Guiteau's trial for the assassination of President Garfield that "Guiteau is not only now insane, but that he was never anything else," and he stated that the condition was due to "a congenital malformation of the brain." The opposing side opined that Guiteau was only pretending to be insane for the purposes of the trial. Dr. John Gray, superintendent for the New York Utica Asylum, testified for the prosecution that Guiteau acted only out of "wounded vanity and disappointment." Bound up with this disagreement was the question of how and whether the brain abnormalities relate to criminal acts and behavior. This dialog continues today. . . .

Nowadays, neuroscience data are increasingly used in legal cases to support claims of decreased culpability—either supporting an NGRI defense (not guilty by reason of insanity) or as a mitigating circumstance in determining the appropriate finding or sentence. . . .

Although some articles have appeared in law journals recently regarding the use of neuroscience in the criminal justice system in general, this article represents the first to examine how these data might influence juries and judges in their assessments of the facts of a crime and in their assignments of punishment for female defendants. Though this is a preliminary analysis, it does set the questions for future research in this area. . . .

This study includes appellate criminal cases with judicial decisions released from October 1, 2015, through April 30, 2016, that reference brain data in the decision. Searches on the WestLaw database using the parameters "brain OR neuro!" resulted in well over 2,000 cataloged appellate decisions released during the study timeframe. Decisions that referenced only brain data from victims were eliminated, as were pro forma decisions that reduced or remanded sentences for minors . . . That left 692 appellate decisions citing brain data in the judicial finding. Of those, 27 had female defendants (or 4%) and 665 were male (96%). Paralleling previous studies, we find that the brain data proffered in cases of severe and premeditated violence are received and used in exactly the same manner as other sorts of evidence, which is to say that they are generally not successful in mitigating the outcome of the trial.

Women account for approximately 7 percent of the total U.S. prison population; 4 hence, women are underrepresented among those who have access to or use brain data in criminal proceedings to bolster claims of competency, mitigation, or innocence. As a result, it has been thus far impossible to run quantitative analyses testing whether neuroscience data in criminal cases are differentially successful, depending on the gender of the defendant. . . .

In 18 of the cases involving female defendants, the women were convicted of a violent crime. Thirteen were convicted of murder, attempted murder, or manslaughter; three of assault; and two of burglary or armed robbery. In the remaining cases, four lost their parental rights; three involved driving under the influence; one concerned fraud; and one was a case of animal neglect and abuse. Four of the

30 female defendants (11%) were minors when the crimes they were accused of committing occurred. . . .

[Based on case study analysis presented in the article,] [i]t is our contention that the use of neuroscience by defense counsel for women, although comparatively less common than with men, can and does backfire. We are less confident in Denno's (2015) conclusion that neuroscience data are not used as a "double-edged sword — one that will either get defendants off the hook altogether or unfairly brand them as posing a future danger to society", especially where women are concerned. Although we find no evidence that the courts *explicitly* used brain data to draw any conclusions about future dangerousness, we do find suggestions that such data can and do "[enhance] a defendant's blameworthiness" (Denno, 2015, p. 544), particularly as the data underscore the judges' or juries' underlying sentiments or biases regarding what sort of women are likely to do bad things. In other words, neuroscience data can bolster confirmation bias, which can lead to "liberation" from other legal and cognitive constraints. . . .

NOTES AND QUESTIONS

1. The studies excerpted above provide evidence on the current use of neuroscience in court. What will the future hold? Consider one prediction:

   My prediction is that neuroscientific evidence is likely to play a similar role in courtroom adjudication as instant replay does in sports. It will be used sparingly, but critically, when the stakes are high and the case is at a borderline. To carry the analogy further, the value of instant replay in sports depends on the technology available. If the camera angle did not, or could not, capture the play then video replay will be of little use. Some judgment calls in sports are, by rule, not reviewable. Similarly, if the neuroscience technology is not available, or cannot add useful information, it will be of little use in the courtroom. . . . The analogy to instant replay is not perfect, but it's useful because it reminds us that neurolaw cases need not be numerous to be noteworthy. . . .

   Francis X. Shen, *Neuroscientific Evidence as Instant Replay*, 3 J.L. & Biosci. 343, 349 (2016).

2. On the basis of empirical analysis of neuroscience in cases to date, Denno argues that "[o]nly very rarely is neuroscience evidence employed by prosecutors in rebuttal to suggest that defendants will engage in future dangerous behavior and therefore deserve more punishment." Deborah W. Denno, *How Prosecutors and Defense Attorneys Differ in Their Use of Neuroscience Evidence*, 85 Fordham L. Rev. 453, 459 (2016). Yet, Denno also finds that in shaken baby syndrome (SBS) cases, reliance on "a [child] victim's brain injury essentially enable[s] the prosecution to concoct the defendant's level of intent from a complex and convoluted science in which the victim has no (or limited) external signs of injury." Deborah W. Denno, *Concocting Criminal Intent*, 105 Geo. L.J. 323, 326 (2017). Denno's "study of SBS cases revealed that the diagnosis of SBS alone often successfully serves as the sole foundation for a prosecutor's case, with no proof of the defendant's act or intent beyond the victim's brain scan and accompanying medical expert testimony. . . . SBS cases therefore present a troubling circumstance in which prosecutors seem to be afforded free rein, by both the court

and the defense, to manufacture intent from neuroscience evidence admitted solely for medical purposes to present the victim's injury." *Id.* at 329. Denno concludes that "[e]ach time science seemingly brings criminal law forward in terms of a more sophisticated understanding of a defendant's mental state or a victim's injury, it can set the criminal law back if that science is wrongly applied." *Id.* at 331. Given these different uses of neuroscience, do you see more promise, or more peril, in the future introduction of neuroscientific evidence into the courtroom?

3. John Meixner's review of neuroscientific evidence in competency hearings finds that, at present, "the use of neuroscience is relatively infrequent and circumscribed—limited to data indicating the presence of brain injury, and often for the purpose of buttressing already-present behavioral data regarding competency." John B. Meixner, *Neuroscience and Mental Competency: Current Uses and Future Potential*, 81 Alb. L. Rev. 995, 1013 (2018). Meixner points out that, as distinct from the use of neuroscience in criminal mens rea inquiries to look *back* at past mental states, competency evaluations concern *current* brain functioning. Meixner asks: What role might neuroscience play in future competency evaluations? How would you answer this question?

4. The same type of evidence may be treated differently by courts depending on its proffered use. As law professor Jane Campbell Moriarty observes:

> To date, there have been few substantive challenges to the reliability or general acceptance of X-rays, MRI, EEG and CT scan technology—provided the technology is being used to perform the functions for which the majority of neuroscientists think it is appropriate: identification of physiological structures, trauma, and certain illnesses. . . . By comparison, courts disfavor neuroimaging evidence that provides only the starting point from which the expert can leap to a behavioral interpretation. Courts are generally unwilling to accept neuroimages as legal proof of the behavior or cognitive abilities of a person with frontal lobe damage. . . . With respect to the newer forms of neuroimaging, courts have been hesitant—and rightly so—to make sweeping statements about the evidentiary reliability of PET and SPECT scans, fMRI and the elusive P300 wave until more data is generated and the neuroscientists reach some degree of cohesiveness on the subjects. We are not yet there. These neuroimages have remarkable potential for forensic use, but they are too new, too uncertain, and too laden with troubling questions to earn easy admission to the courts. . . .

Jane Campbell Moriarty, *Flickering Admissibility: Neuroimaging Evidence in the U.S. Courts*, 26 Behav. Sci. & L. 36, 47-48 (2008).

5. What if brain scans are *normal* or inconclusive? Could that be relevant evidence? If so, of what? *See* Valerie Gray Hardcastle & Edward Lamb, *What Difference Do Brain Images Make in U.S. Criminal Trials?*, 24 J. Evaluation Clinical Prac. 909, 914 (2018) (finding that "The percentage of appellate cases in which the decision was favorable to the defendant mirrored those of decisions without proffered brain scan data. Moreover, 67% of the scans admitted showed either normal brain structures or were inconclusive.")

6. Although the popular image of a trial involves a jury, many cases involve a "bench trial," where the judge serves as the sole fact finder. In a bench trial, how might admissibility decisions about expert evidence be different? In a study of PET and

SPECT evidence in the courtroom, law professor Neal Feigenson observes the following:

> [O]n more than two-fifths (85 of 133, 63.9%) of the occasions on which this expert evidence has been at issue, its proponents have presented or sought to present it not to juries but to judges alone (e.g., proceedings before administrative law judges or relating to non-jury issues such as requests for injunctive relief or determinations of competency to stand trial). . . . PET and/or SPECT evidence has been admitted in more than four-fifths (73 of 89, 82.0%) of cases in which it has either been admitted or excluded. This perhaps surprisingly high admissibility rate may be due in part to the large proportion of bench proceedings: when a judge sits without a jury, there is no jury to protect from evidence deemed insufficiently reliable; instead, the judge typically hears the evidence and then decides how much weight to give it. Indeed, in cases in which PET and/or SPECT evidence has been admitted or excluded, it has been admitted at a significantly higher rate in proceedings before judges (44 of 46, 95.7%) than in those before juries (29 of 43, 67.5%). . . .

Neal Feigenson, *Brain Imaging and Courtroom Evidence: On the Admissibility and Persuasiveness of fMRI*, 2 Int'l J.L. Context 233, 237 (2006).

B. *FRYE* AND THE "GENERAL ACCEPTANCE" TEST

Frye v. United States

293 F. 1013 (D.C. Cir. 1923)

VAN ORSDEL, Associate Justice. Appellant, defendant below, was convicted of the crime of murder in the second degree, and from the judgment prosecutes this appeal.

A single assignment of error is presented for our consideration. In the course of the trial counsel for defendant offered an expert witness to testify to the result of a deception test made upon defendant. The test is described as the systolic blood pressure deception test. It is asserted that blood pressure is influenced by change in the emotions of the witness, and that the systolic blood pressure rises are brought about by nervous impulses sent to the sympathetic branch of the autonomic nervous system. Scientific experiments, it is claimed, have demonstrated that fear, rage, and pain always produce a rise of systolic blood pressure, and that conscious deception or falsehood, concealment of facts, or guilt of crime, accompanied by fear of detection when the person is under examination, raises the systolic blood pressure in a curve, which corresponds exactly to the struggle going on in the subject's mind, between fear and attempted control of that fear, as the examination touches the vital points in respect of which he is attempting to deceive the examiner.

In other words, the theory seems to be that truth is spontaneous, and comes without conscious effort, while the utterance of a falsehood requires a conscious effort, which is reflected in the blood pressure. The rise thus produced is easily detected and distinguished from the rise produced by mere fear of the examination itself. In the former instance, the pressure rises higher than in the latter, and is more pronounced as the examination proceeds, while in the latter case, if the subject is telling the truth, the pressure registers highest at the beginning of the examination, and gradually diminishes as the examination proceeds.

Prior to the trial defendant was subjected to this deception test, and counsel offered the scientist who conducted the test as an expert to testify to the results obtained. The offer was objected to by counsel for the government, and the court sustained the objection. Counsel for defendant then offered to have the proffered witness conduct a test in the presence of the jury. This also was denied.

Counsel for defendant, in their able presentation of the novel question involved, correctly state in their brief that no cases directly in point have been found. The broad ground, however, upon which they plant their case, is succinctly stated in their brief as follows:

The rule is that the opinions of experts or skilled witnesses are admissible in evidence in those cases in which the matter of inquiry is such that inexperienced persons are unlikely to prove capable of forming a correct judgment upon it, for the reason that the subject-matter so far partakes of a science, art, or trade as to require a previous habit or experience or study in it, in order to acquire a knowledge of it. When the question involved does not lie within the range of common experience or common knowledge, but requires special experience or special knowledge, then the opinions of witnesses skilled in that particular science, art, or trade to which the question relates are admissible in evidence.

Numerous cases are cited in support of this rule. Just when a scientific principle or discovery crosses the line between the experimental and demonstrable stages is difficult to define. Somewhere in this twilight zone the evidential force of the principle must be recognized, and while courts will go a long way in admitting expert testimony deduced from a well-recognized scientific principle or discovery, the thing from which the deduction is made must be sufficiently established to have gained general acceptance in the particular field in which it belongs.

We think the systolic blood pressure deception test has not yet gained such standing and scientific recognition among physiological and psychological authorities as would justify the courts in admitting expert testimony deduced from the discovery, development, and experiments thus far made.

The judgment is affirmed.

C. THE FEDERAL RULES OF EVIDENCE

Federal Rules of Evidence

Originally enacted by Congress in 1975, and presented here as amended to December 1, 2019

Rule 401. Test for Relevant Evidence

Evidence is relevant if:
(a) it has any tendency to make a fact more or less probable than it would be without the evidence; and
(b) the fact is of consequence in determining the action.

Rule 402. General Admissibility of Relevant Evidence

Relevant evidence is admissible unless any of the following provides otherwise:
• the United States Constitution;
• a federal statute;

- these rules; or
- other rules prescribed by the Supreme Court.

Irrelevant evidence is not admissible.

Rule 403. Excluding Relevant Evidence for Prejudice, Confusion, Waste of Time, or Other Reasons

The court may exclude relevant evidence if its probative value is substantially outweighed by a danger of one or more of the following: unfair prejudice, confusing the issues, misleading the jury, undue delay, wasting time, or needlessly presenting cumulative evidence.

Rule 702. Testimony by Expert Witnesses

A witness who is qualified as an expert by knowledge, skill, experience, training, or education may testify in the form of an opinion or otherwise if:

(a) the expert's scientific, technical, or other specialized knowledge will help the trier of fact to understand the evidence or to determine a fact in issue;

(b) the testimony is based on sufficient facts or data;

(c) the testimony is the product of reliable principles and methods; and

(d) the expert has reliably applied the principles and methods to the facts of the case.

Rule 703. Bases of an Expert's Opinion Testimony

An expert may base an opinion on facts or data in the case that the expert has been made aware of or personally observed. If experts in the particular field would reasonably rely on those kinds of facts or data in forming an opinion on the subject, they need not be admissible for the opinion to be admitted. But if the facts or data would otherwise be inadmissible, the proponent of the opinion may disclose them to the jury only if their probative value in helping the jury evaluate the opinion substantially outweighs their prejudicial effect.

Rule 704. Opinion on an Ultimate Issue

(a) In General—Not Automatically Objectionable. An opinion is not objectionable just because it embraces an ultimate issue.

(b) Exception. In a criminal case, an expert witness must not state an opinion about whether the defendant did or did not have a mental state or condition that constitutes an element of the crime charged or of a defense. Those matters are for the trier of fact alone.

Rule 706. Court-Appointed Expert Witnesses

(a) Appointment Process. On a party's motion or on its own, the court may order the parties to show cause why expert witnesses should not be appointed and may ask the parties to submit nominations. The court may appoint any expert that the parties agree on and any of its own choosing. But the court may only appoint someone who consents to act.

(b) Expert's Role. The court must inform the expert of the expert's duties. The court may do so in writing and have a copy filed with the clerk or may do so orally at a conference in which the parties have an opportunity to participate. The expert:

(1) must advise the parties of any findings the expert makes;

(2) may be deposed by any party;

(3) may be called to testify by the court or any party; and

(4) may be cross-examined by any party, including the party that called the expert.

(c) Compensation. The expert is entitled to a reasonable compensation, as set by the court. The compensation is payable as follows:

(1) in a criminal case or in a civil case involving just compensation under the Fifth Amendment, from any funds that are provided by law; and

(2) in any other civil case, by the parties in the proportion and at the time that the court directs—and the compensation is then charged like other costs.

(d) Disclosing the Appointment to the Jury. The court may authorize disclosure to the jury that the court appointed the expert.

(e) Parties' Choice of Their Own Experts. This rule does not limit a party in calling its own experts.

D. THE *DAUBERT* TRILOGY AND THE "GATEKEEPER" APPROACH

Daubert v. Merrell Dow Pharma., Inc.

509 U.S. 579 (1993)

Justice BLACKMUN delivered the opinion of the Court. In this case we are called upon to determine the standard for admitting expert scientific testimony in a federal trial.

I

Petitioners Jason Daubert and Eric Schuller are minor children born with serious birth defects. They and their parents sued respondent in California state court, alleging that the birth defects had been caused by the mothers' ingestion of Bendectin, a prescription antinausea drug marketed by respondent. Respondent removed the suits to federal court on diversity grounds.

After extensive discovery, respondent moved for summary judgment, contending that Bendectin does not cause birth defects in humans and that petitioners would be unable to come forward with any admissible evidence that it does. In support of its motion, respondent submitted an affidavit of Steven H. Lamm, physician and epidemiologist, who is a well-credentialed expert on the risks from exposure to various chemical substances. Doctor Lamm stated that he had reviewed all the literature on Bendectin and human birth defects—more than 30 published studies involving over 130,000 patients. No study had found Bendectin to be a human teratogen (*i.e.*, a substance capable of causing malformations in fetuses). On the basis of this review, Doctor Lamm concluded that maternal use of Bendectin during the first trimester of pregnancy has not been shown to be a risk factor for human birth defects.

Petitioners did not (and do not) contest this characterization of the published record regarding Bendectin. Instead, they responded to respondent's motion with the testimony of eight experts of their own, each of whom also possessed impressive credentials. These experts had concluded that Bendectin can cause birth defects. Their conclusions were based upon "in vitro" (test tube) and "in vivo" (live) animal studies that found a link between Bendectin and malformations; pharmacological studies of the chemical structure of Bendectin that purported to show similarities between the structure of the drug and that of other substances known to cause birth defects; and the "reanalysis" of previously published epidemiological (human statistical) studies.

The District Court granted respondent's motion for summary judgment. The court stated that scientific evidence is admissible only if the principle upon which it is based is "'sufficiently established to have general acceptance in the field to which it belongs.'" The court concluded that petitioners' evidence did not meet this standard. Given the vast body of epidemiological data concerning Bendectin, the court held, expert opinion which is not based on epidemiological evidence is not admissible to establish causation. Thus, the animal-cell studies, live-animal studies, and chemical-structure analyses on which petitioners had relied could not raise by themselves a reasonably disputable jury issue regarding causation. Petitioners' epidemiological analyses, based as they were on recalculations of data in previously published studies that had found no causal link between the drug and birth defects, were ruled to be inadmissible because they had not been published or subjected to peer review.

The United States Court of Appeals for the Ninth Circuit affirmed. Citing *Frye v. United States*, the court stated that expert opinion based on a scientific technique is inadmissible unless the technique is "generally accepted" as reliable in the relevant scientific community. The court declared that expert opinion based on a methodology that diverges "significantly from the procedures accepted by recognized authorities in the field . . . cannot be shown to be 'generally accepted as a reliable technique.'"

. . . Contending that reanalysis is generally accepted by the scientific community only when it is subjected to verification and scrutiny by others in the field, the Court of Appeals rejected petitioners' reanalyses as "unpublished, not subjected to the normal peer review process and generated solely for use in litigation." The court concluded that petitioners' evidence provided an insufficient foundation to allow admission of expert testimony that Bendectin caused their injuries and, accordingly, that petitioners could not satisfy their burden of proving causation at trial.

We granted certiorari, in light of sharp divisions among the courts regarding the proper standard for the admission of expert testimony.

II

A

In the 70 years since its formulation in the *Frye* case, the "general acceptance" test has been the dominant standard for determining the admissibility of novel scientific evidence at trial. Although under increasing attack of late, the rule continues to be followed by a majority of courts, including the Ninth Circuit.

The *Frye* test has its origin in a short and citation-free 1923 decision concerning the admissibility of evidence derived from a systolic blood pressure deception test, a crude precursor to the polygraph machine. In what has become a famous (perhaps infamous) passage, the then Court of Appeals for the District of Columbia described the device and its operation and declared:

> "Just when a scientific principle or discovery crosses the line between the experimental and demonstrable stages is difficult to define. Somewhere in this twilight zone the

evidential force of the principle must be recognized, and while courts will go a long way in admitting expert testimony deduced from a well-recognized scientific principle or discovery, *the thing from which the deduction is made must be sufficiently established to have gained general acceptance in the particular field in which it belongs.*" 54 App. D.C., at 47, 293 F., at 1014 (emphasis added).

Because the deception test had "not yet gained such standing and scientific recognition among physiological and psychological authorities as would justify the courts in admitting expert testimony deduced from the discovery, development, and experiments thus far made," evidence of its results was ruled inadmissible.

The merits of the *Frye* test have been much debated, and scholarship on its proper scope and application is legion. Petitioners' primary attack, however, is not on the content but on the continuing authority of the rule. They contend that the *Frye* test was superseded by the adoption of the Federal Rules of Evidence. We agree.

We interpret the legislatively enacted Federal Rules of Evidence as we would any statute. Rule 402 provides the baseline: "All relevant evidence is admissible, except as otherwise provided by the Constitution of the United States, by Act of Congress, by these rules, or by other rules prescribed by the Supreme Court pursuant to statutory authority. Evidence which is not relevant is not admissible."

"Relevant evidence" is defined as that which has "any tendency to make the existence of any fact that is of consequence to the determination of the action more probable or less probable than it would be without the evidence." Rule 401. The Rule's basic standard of relevance thus is a liberal one. . . .

Here there is a specific Rule that speaks to the contested issue. Rule 702, governing expert testimony, provides:

> "If scientific, technical, or other specialized knowledge will assist the trier of fact to understand the evidence or to determine a fact in issue, a witness qualified as an expert by knowledge, skill, experience, training, or education, may testify thereto in the form of an opinion or otherwise."

Nothing in the text of this Rule establishes "general acceptance" as an absolute prerequisite to admissibility. Nor does respondent present any clear indication that Rule 702 or the Rules as a whole were intended to incorporate a "general acceptance" standard. The drafting history makes no mention of *Frye*, and a rigid "general acceptance" requirement would be at odds with the "liberal thrust" of the Federal Rules and their "general approach of relaxing the traditional barriers to 'opinion' testimony." Given the Rules' permissive backdrop and their inclusion of a specific rule on expert testimony that does not mention " 'general acceptance,' " the assertion that the Rules somehow assimilated *Frye* is unconvincing. *Frye* made "general acceptance" the exclusive test for admitting expert scientific testimony. That austere standard, absent from, and incompatible with, the Federal Rules of Evidence, should not be applied in federal trials.

B

That the *Frye* test was displaced by the Rules of Evidence does not mean, however, that the Rules themselves place no limits on the admissibility of purportedly scientific evidence. Nor is the trial judge disabled from screening such evidence. To the contrary, under the Rules the trial judge must ensure that any and all scientific testimony or evidence admitted is not only relevant, but reliable.

The primary locus of this obligation is Rule 702, which clearly contemplates some degree of regulation of the subjects and theories about which an expert may testify. "*If scientific, technical, or other specialized knowledge will assist the trier of fact* to understand the evidence or to determine a fact in issue" an expert "may testify thereto." (emphasis added). The subject of an expert's testimony must be "scientific . . . knowledge." The adjective "scientific" implies a grounding in the methods and procedures of science. Similarly, the word "knowledge" connotes more than subjective belief or unsupported speculation. The term "applies to any body of known facts or to any body of ideas inferred from such facts or accepted as truths on good grounds." Of course, it would be unreasonable to conclude that the subject of scientific testimony must be "known" to a certainty; arguably, there are no certainties in science. See, e.g., Brief for Nicolaas Bloembergen et al. as Amici Curiae 9 ("Indeed, scientists do not assert that they know what is immutably 'true'—they are committed to searching for new, temporary, theories to explain, as best they can, phenomena"); Brief for American Association for the Advancement of Science et al. as Amici Curiae 7-8 ("Science is not an encyclopedic body of knowledge about the universe. Instead, it represents a process for proposing and refining theoretical explanations about the world that are subject to further testing and refinement" (emphasis in original)). But, in order to qualify as "scientific knowledge," an inference or assertion must be derived by the scientific method. Proposed testimony must be supported by appropriate validation—i.e., "good grounds," based on what is known. In short, the requirement that an expert's testimony pertain to "scientific knowledge" establishes a standard of evidentiary reliability.

Rule 702 further requires that the evidence or testimony "assist the trier of fact to understand the evidence or to determine a fact in issue." This condition goes primarily to relevance. "Expert testimony which does not relate to any issue in the case is not relevant and, ergo, non-helpful." The consideration has been aptly described by Judge Becker as one of "fit." "Fit" is not always obvious, and scientific validity for one purpose is not necessarily scientific validity for other, unrelated purposes. The study of the phases of the moon, for example, may provide valid scientific "knowledge" about whether a certain night was dark, and if darkness is a fact in issue, the knowledge will assist the trier of fact. However (absent creditable grounds supporting such a link), evidence that the moon was full on a certain night will not assist the trier of fact in determining whether an individual was unusually likely to have behaved irrationally on that night. Rule 702's "helpfulness" standard requires a valid scientific connection to the pertinent inquiry as a precondition to admissibility.

That these requirements are embodied in Rule 702 is not surprising. Unlike an ordinary witness, see Rule 701, an expert is permitted wide latitude to offer opinions, including those that are not based on firsthand knowledge or observation. See Rules 702 and 703. Presumably, this relaxation of the usual requirement of firsthand knowledge—a rule which represents "a 'most pervasive manifestation' of the common law insistence upon 'the most reliable sources of information,'"—is premised on an assumption that the expert's opinion will have a reliable basis in the knowledge and experience of his discipline.

Faced with a proffer of expert scientific testimony, then, the trial judge must determine at the outset, pursuant to Rule 104(a), whether the expert is proposing to testify to (1) scientific knowledge that (2) will assist the trier of fact to understand or determine a fact in issue. This entails a preliminary assessment of whether the reasoning or methodology underlying the testimony is scientifically valid and of whether that reasoning or methodology properly can be applied to the facts in issue. We are confident that federal judges possess the capacity to undertake this review. Many factors will bear on the inquiry, and we do not presume to set out a definitive checklist or test. But some general observations are appropriate.

Ordinarily, a key question to be answered in determining whether a theory or technique is scientific knowledge that will assist the trier of fact will be whether it can be (and has been) tested. "Scientific methodology today is based on generating hypotheses and testing them to see if they can be falsified; indeed, this methodology is what distinguishes science from other fields of human inquiry."

Another pertinent consideration is whether the theory or technique has been subjected to peer review and publication. Publication (which is but one element of peer review) is not a *sine qua non* of admissibility; it does not necessarily correlate with reliability, and in some instances well-grounded but innovative theories will not have been published. Some propositions, moreover, are too particular, too new, or of too limited interest to be published. But submission to the scrutiny of the scientific community is a component of "good science," in part because it increases the likelihood that substantive flaws in methodology will be detected. The fact of publication (or lack thereof) in a peer reviewed journal thus will be a relevant, though not dispositive, consideration in assessing the scientific validity of a particular technique or methodology on which an opinion is premised.

Additionally, in the case of a particular scientific technique, the court ordinarily should consider the known or potential rate of error, and the existence and maintenance of standards controlling the technique's operation.

Finally, "general acceptance" can yet have a bearing on the inquiry. A "reliability assessment does not require, although it does permit, explicit identification of a relevant scientific community and an express determination of a particular degree of acceptance within that community." Widespread acceptance can be an important factor in ruling particular evidence admissible, and "a known technique which has been able to attract only minimal support within the community," may properly be viewed with skepticism.

The inquiry envisioned by Rule 702 is, we emphasize, a flexible one. Its overarching subject is the scientific validity and thus the evidentiary relevance and reliability—of the principles that underlie a proposed submission. The focus, of course, must be solely on principles and methodology, not on the conclusions that they generate.

Throughout, a judge assessing a proffer of expert scientific testimony under Rule 702 should also be mindful of other applicable rules. Rule 703 provides that expert opinions based on otherwise inadmissible hearsay are to be admitted only if the facts or data are "of a type reasonably relied upon by experts in the particular field in forming opinions or inferences upon the subject." Rule 706 allows the court at its discretion to procure the assistance of an expert of its own choosing. Finally, Rule 403 permits the exclusion of relevant evidence "if its probative value is substantially outweighed by the danger of unfair prejudice, confusion of the issues, or misleading the jury. . . ." Judge Weinstein has explained: "Expert evidence can be both powerful and quite misleading because of the difficulty in evaluating it. Because of this risk, the judge in weighing possible prejudice against probative force under Rule 403 of the present rules exercises more control over experts than over lay witnesses."

III

We conclude by briefly addressing what appear to be two underlying concerns of the parties and *amici* in this case. Respondent expresses apprehension that abandonment of "general acceptance" as the exclusive requirement for admission will result in a "free-for-all" in which befuddled juries are confounded by absurd and irrational pseudoscientific assertions. In this regard respondent seems to us to be overly pessimistic about the capabilities of the jury and of the adversary system generally. Vigorous cross-examination, presentation of contrary evidence, and careful instruction on the burden of proof are the traditional and appropriate means of attacking shaky but admissible evidence. Additionally, in the event the trial court concludes that the scintilla of evidence presented supporting a position is insufficient to allow a reasonable juror to conclude that the position more likely than not is true, the court remains free to direct a judgment, and likewise to grant summary judgment. These conventional devices, rather than wholesale exclusion under an uncompromising "general acceptance" test, are the appropriate safeguards where the basis of scientific testimony meets the standards of Rule 702.

Petitioners and, to a greater extent, their *amici* exhibit a different concern. They suggest that recognition of a screening role for the judge that allows for the exclusion of "invalid" evidence will sanction a stifling and repressive scientific orthodoxy and will be inimical to the search for truth. It is true that open debate is an essential part of both legal and scientific analyses. Yet there are important differences between the quest for truth in the courtroom and the quest for truth in the laboratory. Scientific conclusions are subject to perpetual revision. Law, on the other hand, must resolve disputes finally and quickly. The scientific project is advanced by broad and wide-ranging consideration of a multitude of hypotheses, for those that are incorrect will eventually be shown to be so, and that in itself is an advance. Conjectures that are probably wrong are of little use, however, in the project of reaching a quick, final, and binding legal judgment—often of great consequence—about a particular set of events in the past. We recognize that, in practice, a gatekeeping role for the judge, no matter how flexible, inevitably on occasion will prevent the jury from learning of authentic insights and innovations. That, nevertheless, is the balance that is struck by Rules of Evidence designed not for the exhaustive search for cosmic understanding but for the particularized resolution of legal disputes.

IV

To summarize: "General acceptance" is not a necessary precondition to the admissibility of scientific evidence under the Federal Rules of Evidence, but the Rules of Evidence—especially Rule 702—do assign to the trial judge the task of ensuring that an expert's testimony both rests on a reliable foundation and is relevant to the task at hand. Pertinent evidence based on scientifically valid principles will satisfy those demands.

The inquiries of the District Court and the Court of Appeals focused almost exclusively on "general acceptance," as gauged by publication and the decisions of other courts. Accordingly, the judgment of the Court of Appeals is vacated, and the case is remanded for further proceedings consistent with this opinion.

Gen. Elec. Co. v. Joiner

522 U.S. 136 (1997)

Chief Justice REHNQUIST delivered the opinion of the Court.*

We granted certiorari in this case to determine what standard an appellate court should apply in reviewing a trial court's decision to admit or exclude expert testimony under *Daubert v. Merrell Dow Pharmaceuticals, Inc.* We hold that abuse of discretion is the appropriate standard. We apply this standard and conclude that the District Court in this case did not abuse its discretion when it excluded certain proffered expert testimony.

I

Respondent Robert Joiner . . . [worked a job that] required him to work with and around the City's electrical transformers, which used a mineral-oil-based dielectric fluid as a coolant. Joiner often had to stick his hands and arms into the fluid to make repairs. . . .In 1983 the City discovered that the fluid in some of the transformers was contaminated with polychlorinated biphenyls (PCB's). PCB's are widely considered to be hazardous to human health. . . .

Joiner was diagnosed with small-cell lung cancer in 1991. He sued petitioners in Georgia state court the following year. Petitioner Monsanto manufactured PCB's from 1935 to 1977; petitioners General Electric and Westinghouse Electric manufactured transformers and dielectric fluid. In his complaint Joiner linked his development of cancer to his exposure to PCB's and their derivatives, polychlorinated dibenzofurans (furans) and polychlorinated dibenzodioxins (dioxins). Joiner had been a smoker for approximately eight years, his parents had both been smokers, and there was a history of lung cancer in his family. He was thus perhaps already at a heightened risk of developing lung cancer eventually. The suit alleged that his exposure to PCB's "promoted" his cancer; had it not been for his exposure to these substances, his cancer would not have developed for many years, if at all.

Petitioners removed the case to federal court. Once there, they moved for summary judgment. They contended that (1) there was no evidence that Joiner suffered significant exposure to PCB's, furans, or dioxins, and (2) there was no admissible scientific evidence that PCB's promoted Joiner's cancer. Joiner responded that there were numerous disputed factual issues that required resolution by a jury. He relied largely on the testimony of expert witnesses. In depositions, his experts had testified that PCB's alone can promote cancer and that furans and dioxins can also promote cancer. They opined that since Joiner had been exposed to PCB's, furans, and dioxins, such exposure was likely responsible for Joiner's cancer.

The District Court ruled that there was a genuine issue of material fact as to whether Joiner had been exposed to PCB's. But it nevertheless granted summary judgment for petitioners because (1) there was no genuine issue as to whether Joiner had been exposed to furans and dioxins, and (2) the testimony of Joiner's experts

---

* [Chief Justice REHNQUIST delivered the opinion for a unanimous Court with respect to Parts I and II, and the opinion of the Court with respect to Part III. — EDS.]

had failed to show that there was a link between exposure to PCB's and small-cell lung cancer. The court believed that the testimony of respondent's experts to the contrary did not rise above "subjective belief or unsupported speculation." 864 F. Supp. 1310, 1326 (N.D. Ga. 1994). Their testimony was therefore inadmissible.

The Court of Appeals for the Eleventh Circuit reversed. 78 F.3d 524 (1996). It held that "[b]ecause the Federal Rules of Evidence governing expert testimony display a preference for admissibility, we apply a particularly stringent standard of review to the trial judge's exclusion of expert testimony." *Id.*, at 529. Applying that standard, the Court of Appeals held that the District Court had erred in excluding the testimony of Joiner's expert witnesses. The District Court had made two fundamental errors. First, it excluded the experts' testimony because it "drew different conclusions from the research than did each of the experts." The Court of Appeals opined that a district court should limit its role to determining the "legal reliability of proffered expert testimony, leaving the jury to decide the correctness of competing expert opinions." *Id.* at 533. Second, the District Court had held that there was no genuine issue of material fact as to whether Joiner had been exposed to furans and dioxins. This was also incorrect, said the Court of Appeals, because testimony in the record supported the proposition that there had been such exposure.

We granted petitioners' petition for a writ of certiorari, and we now reverse.

II

Petitioners challenge the standard applied by the Court of Appeals. . . . They argue that that court should have applied traditional "abuse-of-discretion" review. Respondent agrees that abuse of discretion is the correct standard of review. . . . He argues, however, that it is perfectly reasonable for appellate courts to give particular attention to those decisions that are outcome determinative.

We have held that abuse of discretion is the proper standard of review of a district court's evidentiary rulings. . . . The Court of Appeals suggested that *Daubert* somehow altered this general rule in the context of a district court's decision to exclude scientific evidence. But *Daubert* did not address the standard of appellate review for evidentiary rulings at all. It did hold that the "austere" *Frye* standard of "general acceptance" had not been carried over into the Federal Rules of Evidence. . . .

[W]hile the Federal Rules of Evidence allow district courts to admit a somewhat broader range of scientific testimony than would have been admissible under *Frye*, they leave in place the "gatekeeper" role of the trial judge in screening such evidence. A court of appeals applying "abuse-of-discretion" review to such rulings may not categorically distinguish between rulings allowing expert testimony and rulings disallowing it. . . .

We hold that the Court of Appeals erred in its review of the exclusion of Joiner's experts' testimony. In applying an overly "stringent" review to that ruling, it failed to give the trial court the deference that is the hallmark of abuse-of-discretion review. . . .

[The Court went on to apply this standard to the facts in *Joiner*, writing that ". . . a proper application of the correct standard of review here indicates that the District Court did not abuse its discretion." — EDS.]

Kumho Tire Co., Ltd. v. Carmichael
526 U.S. 137 (1999)

Justice BREYER delivered the opinion of the Court.

In *Daubert*, this Court focused upon the admissibility of scientific expert testimony. . . . The Court . . . discussed certain . . . factors, such as testing, peer review, error rates, and "acceptability" in the relevant scientific community, some or all of which might prove helpful in determining the reliability of a particular scientific "theory or technique." *Id.*, at 593-594, 113 S. Ct. 2786.

This case requires us to decide how *Daubert* applies to the testimony of engineers and other experts who are not scientists. We conclude that *Daubert*'s general holding—setting forth the trial judge's general "gatekeeping" obligation—applies not only to testimony based on "scientific" knowledge, but also to testimony based on "technical" and "other specialized" knowledge. See Fed. Rule Evid. 702. We also conclude that a trial court may consider one or more of the more specific factors that *Daubert* mentioned when doing so will help determine that testimony's reliability. But, as the Court stated in *Daubert*, the test of reliability is "flexible," and *Daubert*'s list of specific factors neither necessarily nor exclusively applies to all experts or in every case. Rather, the law grants a district court the same broad latitude when it decides how to determine reliability as it enjoys in respect to its ultimate reliability determination. Applying these standards, we determine that the District Court's decision in this case—not to admit certain expert testimony—was within its discretion and therefore lawful. . . .

Michael J. Saks & David L. Faigman
Expert Evidence After Daubert
1 Ann. Rev. L. Soc. Sci. 105, 105-17 (2005)

The law of expert testimony provides a lens through which many aspects of modern legal practice can be studied. Every jurisdiction that confronts devising a rule of admission for expert evidence must resolve two basic matters. First, how strict should the rule be? Should it be liberal and allow testimony from virtually all who claim expertise, stopping short perhaps of astrologers and tea-leaf readers? Or should it be conservative and demand rigorous proof of experts' claims of expertise? The second matter that a jurisdiction must resolve is where the real axis of decision-making will be. Should courts defer to the professionals in the field from which the experts come, or should they evaluate the quality of the expert opinion for themselves? Implicit in the answers that a particular jurisdiction gives to these two, largely independent, matters are numerous beliefs about legal process and beyond, including its faith in the adversarial process, its confidence in judicial competence, its trust of the jury system, and even its philosophy and sociology of science and empirical knowledge. . . .

THE MEANING OF *DAUBERT*

In essence, the *Daubert* trilogy adopts a changed perspective and relocates the axis of decision. With the old commercial marketplace test, judges piggy-backed onto what consumers seemed to think about a proffered expertise and expert. Under *Frye*'s general acceptance test, judges took a rough nose count and deferred to what the producers of knowledge thought about the knowledge they had to offer. *Daubert* finally places the obligation to evaluate the evidence where one might have expected it to be all along: on the judges themselves. For empirical or scientific proffers, *Daubert* requires judges to evaluate the research findings and methods supporting expert evidence and the principles used to extrapolate from that research to the task at hand (Risinger 2000a). And for nonscience expertise (that is, expertise on questions that are seldom the topic of systematic empirical investigation), courts might have to develop new criteria for evaluating the soundness of proffered expert evidence. . . .

Daubert, in many respects, appeared to be a revolutionary decision. . . . The core principle of *Daubert* is its changed focus from *Frye*'s deference to the experts to a more active judicial evaluation of a particular field's claims of expertise. . . .

The basic challenge for trial courts in the area of expert testimony is to define the boundary between admissible and inadmissible evidence. As the *Kumho Tire* Court understood, the definition of adequate science is only a subpart of this greater task. Expertise comes to court in myriad forms, ranging from the most traditionally rigorous fields, such as physics, to the most traditionally lax, such as clinical medicine. Some experts dress in the guise of science, such as forensic document examiners, whereas others claim expertise by virtue of experience alone, such as police officers. The one thing all these ostensible experts have in common is their claim to opinions that are relevant and sufficiently accurate to be helpful to the trier of fact. . . .

[But *Daubert*] has left much that still needs to be done. The four *Daubert* factors offer some guidance regarding a large proportion of experts, particularly those from professional fields in which quantitative empirical methods can be, and ordinarily are, employed. The Court in *Kumho Tire*, however, made no attempt to offer similar sorts of criteria for evaluating experts for whom some or all of the *Daubert* criteria might not be decisive or sufficient. Auto mechanics, historians, accountants, clinical medical doctors, and scores of others have traditionally testified but would not be able to meet one or more *Daubert* criteria. Clearly, the Court and the Rules of Evidence contemplate that many experts from these fields would still be permitted to testify, but, at the same time, trial courts must in some way determine if the bases for the opinions they intend to offer are sufficiently valid to admit. . . .

EXPERTISE AND PROCEDURAL CONSIDERATIONS

Ordinarily, rulings regarding the admissibility of evidence are firmly within the trial court's discretion. The principal reason for this is that trial courts are in a better position than appellate courts to screen evidence, an essential part of conducting a trial. In *Joiner* and *Kumho Tire*, the Supreme Court followed the conventional wisdom and held that appellate courts owe substantial deference to the trial court, both in the criteria used to assess the validity of proffered expertise (*Kumho Tire*) and the ultimate admissibility decision (*Joiner*). Under the *Daubert* trilogy, rulings on expert evidence, like other evidentiary rulings, can be overturned on appeal only for an abuse of discretion. This approach makes jurisprudential sense if expert evidence is like other kinds of evidence, but it is not.

Some questions are case specific, whereas others are relevant across a broad spectrum of cases. For example, whether or not a car in a particular case went though a red light has no implications for what color a traffic light was in other cases. But if "Which color grants a driver the right of way?" has a different answer from case to case, that would be arbitrary and lawless. Questions of fact, which typically affect only the case before the court and do not have meaning for other future cases, can be altered on appeal only when clear error is found. In contrast, matters of law, which apply across cases, are reviewed de novo. This differential treatment grants deference on some kinds of questions and consistency on other kinds, and facilitates judicial efficiency along with the rule of law: Once green is declared by a legislature or appellate court to indicate go, that question is decided for all trial courts in the jurisdiction.

Similarly, in most evidentiary contexts, admissibility decisions are case specific. Scientific evidence, however, does not conform to this traditional wisdom. Many scientific findings transcend individual cases. Questions such as whether Bendectin is a teratogen, smoking causes lung cancer, or polygraphs detect lying do not, in principle, vary from case to case. . . .

Monahan and Walker, writing before the *Daubert* decisions, were the first to explore the implications of this insight.[*] Monahan and Walker argue that although facts and law differ in that one is positive and the other normative, facts sometimes share an important similarity with law: Some factual issues are case specific and some transcend individual cases. The Monahan-Walker analysis has procedural implications. Facts that are trans-case in nature should be treated much as law is treated: Subject to de novo review on appeal, courts are not obligated to rely on the record developed by the parties but can engage in their own inquiries, and the holdings of higher courts should be binding on lower courts. . . .

Jane Campbell Moriarty & Daniel D. Langleben
Who Speaks for Neuroscience? Neuroimaging Evidence and Courtroom Expertise
68 Case W. Res. L. Rev. 783, 795-99 (2018)

Most of the academic analysis about functional neuroimaging evidence arises from the *Daubert* trilogy's focus on methods used in research, the relationship and distance between data and conclusions, and the "fit" of the proposed testimony to the issue in dispute. To date, little attention has been given to the role of expert qualifications in most scholarship, both because witness expertise historically has been a low hurdle, and because of the more acute concerns about legal reliability and the profound implications of such evidence.

Federal Rule of Evidence 702, the template for most state evidence rules, provides that a witness may be qualified as an expert by "knowledge, skill, experience, training, or education." Written in the disjunctive, the rule permits an expert to be qualified in multiple ways and envisions various types of expertise. Generally, however, there is a discernable relationship between an expert's qualifications and expertise: The more technical the specialized knowledge and the less comprehensible it is to the jury, the more likely the court is to be demanding about qualifications. The nature of the expert's opinion will determine the required qualifications,

---

[*] [*See* Laurens Walker & John Monahan, *Social Frameworks: A New Use of Social Science in Law*, 73 Va. L. Rev. 559 (1987). — EDS.]

whether academic or experiential, but it should rise to a "meaningful threshold of expertise."

Recognizing that expertise is often a question of weight of the evidence rather than admissibility, some courts have set the bar exceptionally low for qualifications, stating that experts need only "possess skill or knowledge greater than the average layman." Other courts opine that experts need to be neither "blue-ribbon practitioners" with "optimal qualification [s]," nor even "highly qualified in order to testify about a given issue." Despite the rhetoric, many courts in the post-Daubert era have employed a more rigorous standard, often in complex civil cases involving medical device and malpractice or in toxic tort cases. . . .

The wide-ranging pursuits of the neuroscience field include intersecting and often overlapping areas of expertise among psychologists, research scientists, and various categories of physicians. Yet, lawyers and judges are not always aware—nor could they be—of the general boundaries of expertise and the precise boundaries of expertise in a given matter on a specific issue.

The well-credentialed researchers producing neuroimaging data might seem to be qualified as experts in court, given their extensive knowledge of the studies, methods used, data generated, study limitations, and error rates; and to the extent that is the scope of their testimony, they are likely well-qualified. But the analysis becomes difficult when one separates the question of knowledge of neuroimaging research from the diagnostic use of such evidence in a given individual. Evaluating the proposed testimony vis-à-vis the matter at issue, i.e., the "task at hand," presents difficult questions of legal expertise in cases involving functional neuroimaging of an individual.

Three categories of professionals—physicians, psychologists, and doctoral-level research scientists—usually conduct functional neuroimaging research that relates to mental health issues. These doctoral-level scientists design the studies and oversee data collection, review the statistical analysis, and draft the findings, usually in the form of publication in peer-reviewed scientific journals. The research scientists may have degrees in one of many subspecialties of psychology, a PhD in a biomedical field such as Neuroscience, Physiology, Chemistry, Physics, or even Computer Science and Engineering. As many research scientists are far removed from the actual clinical practice of medicine or even psychology that may employ such research, their qualifications are usually insufficient to discuss the applicability of the research studies to an individual case. As a general matter, non-physician researchers are not qualified or licensed to prescribe or interpret functional neuroimages diagnostically. Thus, application of those studies to a given individual—which is often at issue in legal disputes—is generally outside of their area of competence. . . .

There are . . . overlapping areas of expertise and differing opinion about the roles of psychiatrists and psychologists both in and out of the courtroom. As many psychological and neuroscience researchers spend most of their careers using functional neuroimaging, they often have greater knowledge of the functional neuroimaging research than those practicing psychiatrists, neurologists, and radiologists who do little or no neuroimaging research. Given these complementary areas of expertise, in is not surprising that courts are not focusing on the distinctions among physicians, clinical psychologists, and research scientists. While all three specialties might be qualified to testify about aspects of functional neuroimaging, there are limits to each profession's qualifications. . . .

Nancy Gertner
Neuroscience and Sentencing
85 Fordham L. Rev. 533, 541-44 (2016)

II. THE SENTENCING CONTEXT: GOOD ENOUGH EVIDENCE

The context in which sentencing decisions are made has not materially changed from the days of rehabilitation, even as sentencing shifted from a purely discretionary system to a mandatory, structured one. It is a setting in which evidence, including expert evidence, is not tested as rigorously as it is at trials, with important implications for neuroscience and the new rehabilitation.

When rehabilitation was the dominant philosophy, there were few if any limits on the information that the judge was supposed to have. It made no more sense to limit the kind of information that a judge could receive and rely on at sentencing in exercising his "clinical" role—to cure the "moral disease"—than to limit the information available to a medical doctor in determining a diagnosis. Over time, different standards of proof and evidence evolved between the trial stage and the sentencing stage.

The trial stage is the stage of constitutional rights, formal evidentiary rules, and proof beyond a reasonable doubt. At sentencing, the rules of evidence do not apply. Hearsay and character evidence is admissible. The standard of proof is the lowest in the criminal justice system: a fair preponderance of the evidence. Additionally, the risk of error is allocated differently at trials and at sentencing. Many of the rules of evidence applicable at trial are justified by the concern that a presumptively innocent man not be convicted; the risk of error is on the prosecution. In some cases, potentially probative evidence is excluded, not simply based on the risk of a wrongful conviction, but also based on concerns about the decision maker, a lay jury. Character evidence, particularly evidence of prior crimes, is excluded because the jury may overvalue it, finding a propensity to commit crimes, which is inconsistent with the presumption of innocence. But once a defendant is convicted, the rules change: the constitutional protections are minimal, the emphasis shifts from protecting the innocent to seeking the truth, and the decision maker is a judge, presumed to be capable of separating the wheat from the chaff without the need for the usual rules. In this very different setting, the floodgates are open to all sorts of evidence, including bad character evidence, evidence of the defendant's remorse, prior crimes charged and uncharged, and even acquitted conduct.

Significantly, *Daubert* does not apply at sentencing. The standard at sentencing is that the evidence must have "sufficient indicia of reliability to support its probable accuracy," nothing like Federal Rule of Evidence 702 and its attendant decisional law. While the scholarly literature is replete with criticisms of the application of Daubert in trial settings, expert testimony at sentencing raises even more significant problems. For example, Dean David Faigman and others have described the "G2i" problem: the problem of drawing inappropriate inferences about individuals from group data. Inferences from group data, however, are frequently admitted in individual sentencing proceedings in the form of actuarial data about risk assessment, testimony about recidivism rates, or general experiential accounts about gang behavior. Indeed, because this is a setting in which folk generalizations about character, deterrence, and recidivism are too often bandied about, it is unlikely that a court would strictly limit expert testimony on "G2i" grounds even as a matter of judicial discretion.

Neuroscience testimony could well be offered by prosecutors to show aggravating factors and by defense lawyers to show mitigating factors. While Professor Deborah Denno's longitudinal studies found no instance of the prosecution using neurogenetic evidence as an aggravating factor in capital cases, the past may not predict the future, particularly in noncapital cases where the rules are more relaxed. After all, federal courts did not enhance procedural protections in non-capital sentencing, even as sentences have increased. In effect, there is capital sentencing, with some protections, and the "ordinary sentencing," largely without.

The rules of relevance also are considerably more relaxed at sentencing. At trial, to determine the relevance of a particular brain defect, a court would be concerned about the causal relationship between it and the crime at issue. But at sentencing, the issues are broader. It does not matter whether the defendant's addiction caused his illegal behavior, ostensibly a trial question. The issue is whether his addiction impairs his potential for rehabilitation, a sentencing question. A judge might sentence an addict who committed a bank robbery differently than someone who is not an addict, even if that addiction did not cause the crime, because what it takes to restore his life may be different. The brain lesion identified by a neurologist may not have diminished the defendant's capacity to commit the crime, but it could be an impediment to his ability to recover from the consequences of his conviction.

In short, neuroscience offers considerable promise . . . but considerable dangers, in a setting [criminal sentencing] that, until now, has not been geared toward a critical examination of the evidence. . . .

NOTES AND QUESTIONS

1. Commentators typically refer to the "*Daubert* factors." Review the case, and list the factors that courts should consider for admissibility. How many are there? Which factors seem more or less important in the context of neuroscientific evidence?

2. In his dissent in *Daubert,* Justice Rehnquist wrote:

> "General observations" by this Court customarily carry great weight with lower federal courts, but the ones offered here suffer from the flaw common to most such observations—they are not applied to deciding whether or not particular testimony was or was not admissible, and therefore they tend to be not only general, but vague and abstract. . . . Twenty-two amicus briefs have been filed in the case, and indeed the Court's opinion contains no less than 37 citations to amicus briefs and other secondary sources. The various briefs filed in this case are markedly different from typical briefs . . . they deal with definitions of scientific knowledge, scientific method, scientific validity, and peer review—in short, matters far afield from the expertise of judges. I defer to no one in my confidence in federal judges; but I am at a loss to know what is meant when it is said that the scientific status of a theory depends on its "falsifiability," and I suspect some of them will be, too. I do not doubt that Rule 702 confides to the judge some gatekeeping responsibility in deciding questions of the admissibility of proffered expert testimony. But I do not think it imposes on them either the obligation or the authority to become amateur scientists in order to perform that role. . . .

Given that their expertise is law and not science, what role should judges (or Supreme Court Justices) play in determining the admissibility of scientific evidence? Justice Rehnquist subsequently authored the *Joiner* decision, excerpted above. Is Justice Rehnquist's *Joiner* opinion consistent with his reasoning in *Daubert*?

3. Federal Judge Bernice Donald warns that: "as nascent neurotechnology wriggles its way into criminal and civil court . . . we must take proactive steps to confront such challenges and develop well-prepared and well-reasoned responses to address them." Hon. Bernice B. Donald, *On the Brain: Neuroscience and Its Implications for the Criminal Justice System*, 30 Crim. Just. 1 (2015). What steps should judges take to prepare themselves to perform their gatekeeping role for brain evidence?

4. What if a piece of evidence is probative, but also potentially very prejudicial? Consider this argument:

> The *Daubert* Court devoted relatively little attention to the balance of probative value and unfair prejudice encapsulated in Rule 403. In time, however, this Rule might prove to be one of the most important tools lower courts have for managing scientific evidence. Because of the typically blunt nature of the concept of scientific validity, courts are likely to use Rule 403 to sharpen their gatekeeping function. Under Rules 702 and 104(a), judges must decide whether the proponent of scientific evidence has demonstrated the validity of the scientific basis for the testimony by a preponderance of the evidence. In many cases, however, while judges might find scientific evidence to be "valid," they might believe that it is not valid enough, in light of the dangers associated with its use.
>
> Consider the example of expert testimony reporting the results of a polygraph examination. Polygraphy might be offered for a wide variety of purposes and admitted in a wide variety of ways. It is typically offered to attack or support the veracity of witnesses, ranging from criminal defendants to non-party witnesses in civil cases. Courts respond to these proffers using rules ranging from *per se* exclusion to case-by-case evaluation. But in all of these contexts, Rule 403 provides the blueprint.
>
> Although the research supporting the validity of polygraphy remains controversial, significant research has been conducted on the validity and reliability of polygraph tests. Despite the flaws associated with this research, a court could reasonably conclude that some form of polygraphy was more likely than not valid. But few courts, if any, would complete their scrutiny there.
>
> Polygraphy is a potentially awesome technique that might displace jurors' traditional task of evaluating credibility. A large percentage of courts and observers fear the overwhelming impact polygraphy might have, causing jurors to overlook the significant errors associated with even the best application of the technology. The regulation of this technology is largely accomplished through the balancing mechanism provided by Rule 403.
>
> Virtually all other forms of scientific evidence present similar difficulties and opportunities. Therefore, for instance, some courts permit hypnotically refreshed recall so long as the witness' statements are recorded before hypnosis and any testimony at trial is limited to those facts recalled prior to hypnosis; some courts view psychiatric predictions of violence as more problematic at the capital sentencing stage of trials than in ordinary civil commitment proceedings; courts overwhelmingly find that the little probative value they consider expert testimony on the unreliability of eyewitness identification to have is easily outweighed by unfair prejudice. Whether explicit or, more often, implicit, Rule 403 is an integral part of admissibility decisions surrounding scientific expert testimony. . . .

David L. Faigman et al., *Modern Scientific Evidence: The Law and Science of Expert Testimony: Expert Testimony and Rule 403* §1:36 (2019-2020 ed.).

5. In *Daubert*, the Court suggested that cross-examination is the best way to test shaky but admissible evidence. But are attorneys prepared to cross-examine medical experts effectively? For a discussion of the considerations involved, see Stewart M. Casper, *Cross-Examination of the Defense Expert in a Traumatic Brain Injury Case—No Perry Mason Moments*, 1 Ann. 2008 Am. Ass'n. Just. CLE 1103 (2008).

6. The excerpt from Jane Campbell Moriarty and Daniel Langleben serves as a reminder that *who* testifies about neuroscience evidence matters. Moriarty and Langleben consider the differences between clinical psychologists, physicians, neuroscience researchers, and other professionals involved in neuroscience research and clinical practice. For instance, for what type of expert testimony should an MD be required?

7. As Judge (Ret.) Nancy Gertner's essay reminds us, *Daubert* does not apply at sentencing. Rather, the standard for admitting expert evidence is "sufficient indicia of reliability to support its probable accuracy." How would you apply this standard to the evidence you've read about in previous chapters?

8. Although the advent of neuroimaging evidence is relatively new, courts have had to rule for many years on the admissibility of psychological "syndrome" evidence. For instance, lawyers have proffered evidence related to battered woman syndrome, combat stress syndrome, and rape trauma syndrome, amongst others. Christopher Slobogin, *Psychological Syndromes and Criminal Responsibility*, 6 Ann. Rev. L. & Soc. Sci. 109 (2010). Will brain evidence enhance syndrome evidence? Replace it?

9. Is *Daubert* an effective framework for evaluating neuroscientific evidence? Neuroscientist and neuroethics scholar James Giordano, with co-author Timothy Brindley, argues that we need new frameworks:

> We opine that the fundamental issue is the correlative nature of neuroscience. It remains debatable whether current iterations of neuroimaging—either alone or in concert with other approaches—can "fully" demonstrate valid proxies of cognition, emotion, and/or behavior. Neuroscience cannot provide the incontrovertible rigor of a "DNA test" to validate thought, intent, innocence, or culpability. Thus, *Daubert's* criteria of objectivity, and ultimately reliability, would still be questionable—at least on some level. But does that—or should that—rule out the value and utility of neurotechnologically based/derived information in legal contexts? We think not. Perhaps what is needed is a new look at what neuroscientific techniques and technologies can actually do, and what types of descriptive, inferential, and/or discriminative information these approaches can provide within the needs and scope of the law. . . .
>
> The development of such standards and metrics [to replace *Daubert*] would be a work-in-progress, given the pace and extent of neuroscientific and neurotechnological research, and would necessarily conjoin the neuroscientific, neuroethics, and legal communities in coordinated efforts to parameterize testing methods and results in ways that would allow uniform conditions, which would then meet and uphold minimum thresholds for admissibility in court. . . .

Timothy Brindley & James Giordano, *Neuroimaging: Correlation, Validity, Value, and Admissibility:* Daubert *—and Reliability—Revisited*, 5 Am. J. Bioethics Neurosc. 48, 49 (2014). *See also* Katherine Shats, Timothy Brindley & James Giordano, *Don't Ask a Neuroscientist About Phases of the Moon: Applying Appropriate Evidence Law to the Use of Neuroscience in the Courtroom*, 25 Cambridge Q. Healthcare Ethics 712 (2016).

10. Could neuroscience inform the construction and application of the Rules of
    Evidence. Consider this perspective on Rule 403 and gruesome evidence:

> Is there a methodology to reduce arbitrariness and avoid evidence that "pro-
> vokes an emotional response in the jury or otherwise tends to affect adversely
> the jury's attitude toward the defendant wholly apart from its judgment. . . ?"
> . . . Physiological studies using fMRI investigate the way in which gruesome evi-
> dence affects the perceiver's brain. In one study, participants read passages that
> described crimes. These were manipulated to evoke either weak or strong dis-
> gust. Not only did those participants who received the strong disgust materials
> dole out significantly more punishment, they also showed a decrease in activity
> in the regions of the brain that are usually active during logical reasoning and
> moral judgment. . . .

Jules Epstein & Suzanne Mannes, *"Gruesome" Evidence, Science, and Rule 403*,
Judicial Edge (March 17, 2016).

E. CRIMINAL SENTENCING: THE CASE OF GRADY NELSON

In Chapter 2 you read about the case of Herbert Weinstein, who proffered PET scan
evidence at the guilt phase to support his insanity defense. But to date neuroscientific evidence has appeared more frequently at the sentencing (or "penalty") phase
of criminal proceedings. In this section we illustrate sentencing phase evidentiary
considerations through the case of Grady Nelson, who proffered QEEG evidence
during his capital sentencing proceedings.*

In 2010 in Florida, Nelson was convicted of stabbing his wife 60 times, then slash-
ing her throat. He was also convicted of sexually assaulting his stepchildren: a stepdaughter, age 11, and a stepson, age 13. He stabbed each of the children on the day
he killed his wife, though both children survived. He had previously been convicted
of raping a seven-year-old girl.

Prosecutors in the case sought the death penalty for Nelson, and the sentencing
phase started in November 2010, with a verdict reached in December of that year. In
Florida, a 12-person jury sits for the death penalty phase, and at that time a simple
majority (7 of the 12) was enough to obtain a death sentence. Anything less than a
7-5 split for guilt resulted in life without parole.

Central to Grady Nelson's defense was the introduction of QEEG evidence. In
the materials that follow, we present in chronological sequence excerpts from: (1)
the State's motion to exclude the QEEG evidence; (2) the Defense's reply brief in
support of admitting it; (3) the trial judge's ruling on the admissibility of the evidence; and (4) direct and cross-examination of the Defense's star scientific witness.
We conclude with the disposition of the case, including quotes from actual jurors.

Although it may be tempting to jump to the end, we encourage you to work
through these materials sequentially. Doing so and pausing at each stage to think
through what strategies *you* would use and what legal conclusions *you* would draw,
will allow for considerable reflection on neuroscience in the courtroom.

---

* *State v. Nelson*, No. F05-000846 (11th Fla. Cir. Ct. Dec. 2, 2010).

State of Florida
Motion to Exclude Testimony Regarding Quantitative Electroencephalograms (QEEG)
October 5, 2010

THE STATE OF FLORIDA ("State"), by and through undersigned counsel, hereby moves this Court to exclude any testimony regarding a quantitative electroencephalogram (QEEG) performed on Defendant and any opinion based on such testing and deny the admissibility of such evidence. As grounds, therefore, the State states:

1. This matter is now before this Court for the penalty phase proceedings after the Defendant's conviction for First Degree Murder.
2. Defendant has listed Dr. Robert Thatcher, Ph.D. as a witness in this proceeding. The State has reason to believe that Dr. Thatcher plans to testify to his opinion of Defendant's mental state based on a QEEG administered by Dr. Gerald Gluck, Ph.D. Furthermore, the State believes that at the penalty phase itself the Defendant will also seek to introduce the testimony of Dr. Gerald Gluck that as a result of the QEEG, he believes the defendant has brain dysfunction. . . .
3. . . .Dr. Gluck was deposed on September 27, 2010 and Dr. Thatcher was deposed on October 4, 2010. Dr. Thatcher confirmed in his deposition that since 2001 his sole income has derived from his position as President and owner of Applied Neuroscience, Inc., the company that develops, manufactures, and distributes the software with which Dr. Gluck edited and interpreted the QEEG evaluation of the Defendant. . . .
5. The *Frye* test for admissibility of new and novel scientific evidence applies to a defendant's expert in a capital case in the penalty phases in the same manner it applies to a State expert. The QEEG testing is new and novel scientific evidence. Testimony regarding QEEG test results and opinions based on such results have been routinely excluded from court proceedings because QEEG testing is not generally accepted in the scientific community and is considered unreliable. E.g., *Nadell v. Las Vegas Metro. Police Dep't*, 268 F.3d 924, 927-28 (9th Cir. 2001) (QEEG testimony not admissible since it is not generally accepted in scientific community due to subjectivity, high rate of false positives, and lack of adequate peer review).
6. In fact, Florida Sixth Judicial Circuit Judge Robert J. Morris, Jr., granted the State's motion in limine (nearly identical to the instant motion) to preclude the introduction of the QEEG in a death penalty post conviction case, ruling that QEEG results and opinions based on them were not admissible in a post conviction evidentiary hearing specifically finding that the QEEG did not satisfy *Frye*. . . .
7. The scientific literature also does not support admission of QEEG testimony. . . .
8. The Florida Supreme Court has held that before new scientific evidence is admissible, the proponent of the evidence must prove by a preponderance of the evidence that both the underlying scientific principles and the testing procedure used to apply those principles are generally accepted in the scientific community. . . .
9. Dr. Robert Thatcher's financial interest is directly linked to the success of the QEEG admissibility. . . . As such and for the reasons to be argued in court, under *Frye*, QEEG evidence does not meet the standard for admissibility of scientific evidence. . . .

Defendant's Motion Opposing Frye Hearing
October 4, 2010

The Defendant, Grady Nelson, by and through undersigned counsel, hereby requests that this Court allow the jury to hear the opinions of defense psychological experts because their opinion testimony is not subject to *Frye* and the underlying QEEG technology is not new or novel; alternatively, if found to be new or novel, QEEG technology almost certainly would pass a *Frye* challenge because it is widely accepted in its relevant scientific community. As ground in support, the Defendant states:

1. Dr. Gerald Gluck administered a QEEG test on the Defendant. This test was administered in conjunction with an evaluation of the patient's history. The results are attached as Exhibit A.
2. Based on the opinion and experience of these experts, the results of the QEEG are highly consistent with brain wave activity found by other researchers to be associated with pre-natal alcohol exposure, loss of cognitive function consistent [with] traumatic brain injury, and early childhood abuse. These results were consistent with the Defendant's history.
3. The QEEG software used was the Neuroguide software and databases, developed by Dr. Thatcher.
4. In 2004, the FDA examined the reliability of Neuroguide software in assisting with the diagnoses of mild traumatic brain injury and registered its use for such.
5. Since 2000, QEEG testing to assist in diagnosing mild traumatic brain injury is used as part of a core clinical battery of testing as part of the Defense and Veterans Head Injury Program throughout the country as well as by the United States Department of Veteran Affairs and Department of Defense to determine which soldiers are capable of returning to the battlefield and which are not. . . .
8. The State is expected to challenge the Defense experts psychological evaluation of the Defendant with the opinions of a neurologist as to the use of QEEG in the field of neurology. . . .

[The Defendant's motion went on to argue the following points. — EDS.]

I. *Frye* is inapplicable because the opinions and conclusions of a defense expert are based on experience as well as scientific principles that are not new or novel.

The purpose of QEEG is to aide in the diagnosis of psychological or neurological condition. Like most medical tests, including CT scans and MRIs, these tests are used as an adjunct to give more information in treating a patient. . . . In Florida, expert testimony does not always need to be *Frye* tested to be admissible. Only the underlying scientific principles, not the opinions drawn from those principles, is subject to *Frye*. *Frye* testing applies to new or novel scientific techniques. . . .

Just as a bone marrow transplant should not be done based only on a blood test, or open heart surgery performed on the basis of an EKG, a QEEG is not the sole basis for a diagnosis. Here, the opinions of the expert are based on his interpretation of the results of the QEEG using his experience and training, the history of the Defendant, as well as published studies linking his opinions to certain brain wave patterns. The QEEG was used to aide in the formulations of the opinions, and should not be excluded any more than any other diagnostic aid. The jury should have the opportunity to decide the weight of those opinions.

II. A *Frye* analysis would almost certainly find the QEEG reliable because it is generally accepted in the relevant scientific community.

QEEG would almost certainly pass a *Frye* analysis because QEEG is generally accepted for statistical brain evaluation and as a diagnostic aide in the relevant scientific community of psychologists, psychiatrists, non-neurological medical doctors, neuropsychologists, clinical Ph.D. neuroscientists, and other trained individuals. . . .

The relevant scientific community for QEEG consists of psychologists, psychiatrists, non-neurological medical doctors, neuropsychologists, clinical Ph.D. neuroscientists, and other trained individuals. In the field of neurology, QEEG is not as widely accepted and is used by a small but growing number of neurologists.

In Florida, the method of determining the size of the relevant scientific community is not clearly defined. One Florida court has suggested that the relevant scientific community "should include a broader group of clinical and experimental psychologist and psychiatrists, and not merely the group of licensed professional who are making a living by relying on these tests." Another *Frye* jurisdiction suggests that the relevant community is those who espouse and use the technology.

However, it is clear that within that community, scientific unanimity is not a requirement. . . . [The brief went on to cite a number of cases in which QEEG evidence was admitted. — EDS.]

NOTES AND QUESTIONS

1. At the time of Nelson's capital sentencing, a simple majority of the 12-person jury was all that was required to recommend a sentence of death. But in 2016, the United States Supreme Court ruled that Florida's capital sentencing scheme violated the Sixth Amendment because it required the judge alone, and not the jury, to find the existence of an aggravating circumstance. *Hurst v. Fla.*, 136 S. Ct. 616 (2016). Subsequently, the Supreme Court of Florida held that "the Supreme Court's decision in *Hurst v. Florida* requires that all the critical findings necessary before the trial court may consider imposing a sentence of death must be found unanimously by the jury." *Hurst v. State*, 202 So. 3d 40, 44 (Fla. 2016). The Florida legislature updated its death penalty statute to read that, "If the jury has recommended a sentence of . . . Death, the court, after considering each aggravating factor found by the jury and all mitigating circumstances, may impose a sentence of life imprisonment without the possibility of parole or a sentence of death. The court may consider only an aggravating factor that was unanimously found to exist by the jury." Fla. Stat. Ann. § 921.141 (2020). But as of this writing in 2020, current law remains in flux because, in January 2020, the Supreme Court of Florida reversed course and ruled that:

   > The *Hurst v. State* requirement of a unanimous jury recommendation . . . finds no support in [relevant case law]. . . . As we have explained, the Supreme Court in *Spaziano* upheld the constitutionality under the Sixth Amendment of a Florida judge imposing a death sentence even in the face of a jury recommendation of life—a jury override. It necessarily follows that the Sixth Amendment, as interpreted in *Spaziano*, does not require any jury recommendation of death, much less a unanimous one. . . .

   State v. Poole, No. SC18-245, 2020 WL 3116597, at * 12 (Fla. Jan. 23, 2020).

2. Before reading the Judge's ruling in this case, evaluate the argument of each party. Would you admit the QEEG evidence? What additional information, if any, would you want to know?

3. When a brief makes claims about the use of a particular neuroscientific method or technology, how should opposing parties respond? For instance, in a portion of the Defendant's Motion Opposing *Frye* Hearing not reproduced above, a claim was made that "[o]ver 76,000 peer-reviewed QEEG articles have been published since January 1998 with multiple authors from the fields of psychology, psychiatry, and neuropsychology." However, a search in 2020 on PubMed with the keyword "QEEG" produced only 1,031 hits, dating back to 1978. Restricting this to human studies produced 812 hits since 1978. A search of "quantitative EEG" with the human filter produced only 3,758 hits. The chart below plots annual and cumulative counts from this search. Meanwhile, a PubMed search with keyword "EEG" in human studies returned 134,063 hits, going back to 1945, and 76,886 hits since 1998.

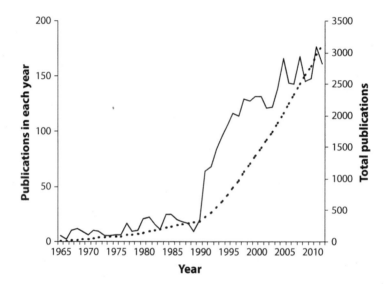

4. In this case, the defense expert, Dr. Thatcher, had previously published on the legal admissibility of QEEG evidence. Robert W. Thatcher, Carl J. Biver & Duane North, *Quantitative EEG and the* Frye *and* Daubert *Standards of Admissibility*, 34 Clin. Electroencephalography 39 (2003). What weight should be given to such publications?

5. In a 2013 ruling on DNA patenting, Supreme Court Justice Thomas, writing for a unanimous majority, began his opinion by describing some relevant background science in detail. Justice Scalia wrote separately to note that while he joined the judgment of the Court, he could not join the portions of the opinion that went "into fine details of molecular biology. I am unable to affirm those details on my own knowledge or even my own belief." *Ass'n for Molecular Pathology v. Myriad Genetics, Inc.*, 133 S. Ct. 2107, 2120 (2013). Although you will learn much about the brain in the next few chapters, at this point in the course, do you feel you have the requisite scientific knowledge to make a ruling on this evidentiary question?

What are the general limits of the judiciary in evaluating and referring in written opinions to neuroscientific evidence? When, if ever, should judges state on the record that they do not adequately understand or believe in a particular body of scientific work? And what bearing should this have on admissibility decisions?

6. The Nelson case was decided in 2010. In 1997, an expert review conducted by the American Academy of Neurology found that, "Although much scientific literature has been produced after decades of research in this field, there remains controversy about the clinical role of QEEG analysis techniques." The American Academy of Neurology specifically concluded:

> On the basis of current clinical literature, opinions of most experts, and proposed rationales for their use, QEEG remains investigational for clinical use in postconcussion syndrome, mild or moderate head injury, learning disability, attention disorders, schizophrenia, depression, alcoholism, and drug abuse. . . .
>
> On the basis of clinical and scientific evidence, opinions of most experts, and the technical and methodologic shortcomings, QEEG is not recommended for use in civil or criminal judicial proceedings.

How, if at all, does the AAN's report affect your analysis of the admissibility of the evidence in this particular legal context? See Marc Nuwer, *Assessment of Digital EEG, Quantitative EEG, and EEG Brain Mapping: Report of the American Academy of Neurology and the American Clinical Neurophysiology Society*, 49 Neurology 277, 285 (1997).

Transcript of Oral Ruling on *Frye* Hearing
Florida v. Nelson

No. F05-00846, 11th Cir. (Oct. 22, 2010)

HOGAN-SCOLA, C.J. . . . I'll have to tell you that I went back and looked at my notes again, I looked at the pleadings of both parties, and I reviewed actually a lot of the articles submitted by both sides.

And it's clear to me, though it wasn't when we started this hearing—it was my understanding at the beginning that the position of the state was that QEEG was new or novel science, and after reviewing everything, I totally disagree with that, but I don't think after the hearing that that was the State's position, but if it still is I do not think that QEEG is new or novel science.

I think at the end of the hearing that the State's position was it is only new or novel in its application to TBI or traumatic brain injury and diagnosing it. But I think it's quite clear from Dr. Thatcher's testimony as well as from the submissions, the articles I read submitted by both experts, that no one is going to come in and say that the computer spits out a diagnosis.

What happens is that raw data is taken in the form of an EEG. It is segmented by artifacting and the submission into a computer program of which there are some numerous varieties, and I don't think the computer programs are new or novel science either.

I think they are used by neuroscientists in all areas, in all fields in this modern day, and that's my take from both the testimony and the articles that I looked at.

And that what Dr. Thatcher says—and I'm assuming what Dr. Gluck will do, and we won't know until he comes in and testifies—he says that they use other adjunctive neurological tools such as a clinical evaluation as people in neuroscience do and they look at the computerized data and say this is consistent with the report of the patient or subject, or it is inconsistent or it is consistent in this regard and inconsistent and in another regard.

So, clearly this is not so much a hard science, but one of the softer sciences attempting to just use one more way of analyzing the data that they get, because the human brain is so complex, and it's going to take us centuries more to understand everything about it.

But my take on this is that the Judge's job in the being a gatekeeper is to decide — the Third or the Supreme Court, wherever this goes, may decide that I am totally wrong and I would appreciate guidance on this — but everything I have heard, the methodologies are sound, the techniques are sound, the science is sound.

Because experts disagree does not mean that tools and techniques are unreliable, and I think that there is — I am satisfied by the preponderance of the evidence that the techniques and methodologies are sound and that the acceptance is wide enough. There's not unanimous acceptance. There are clearly detractors and dissenters and Dr. Epstein is one of those.

But it was interesting because I saw so many reliances by Dr. Epstein on the QEEG and, of course, not to diagnosis or treat TBI but I saw his usage being widespread enough that I feel comfortable that the average juror can figure out what they believe and disbelieve, just like any other battle of the experts, and that's what it's going to come down to. So, I'm going to allow the defense to put on the evidence of the QEEG, and that's my findings and my ruling.

NOTES AND QUESTIONS

1. To what extent did your own anticipated ruling overlap with Judge Hogan-Scola's?
2. Why does the judge invoke the "hard science" and "soft science" labels? Are these helpful?

Having ruled that the evidence was admissible, both the Prosecution and Defense called experts related to the QEEG evidence. One of the central issues was the relevant scientific community for assessing general acceptance. The Defense called Dr. Robert Thatcher, who was mentioned above. The Prosecution called Dr. Charles Epstein, a neurologist at Emory University. The excerpts below illustrate their competing views.

Direct Examination of Dr. Thatcher by Defense Attorney Terry Lenamon

Q: Doctor, let's talk about the relevant scientific community involved with the QEEG. Who uses QEEG today and what is it used for?
A: The primary users of QEEG are psychiatrists, neuropsychiatrists, clinical psychologists, clinical and neuropsychologists and clinical neuroscientists.
Q: And what is it used for, Doctor?
A: And there's a few neurologists that use it, but very few. It's used to evaluate a patient that has, presents to a clinician a problem such as depression or attention

disorder or autism, and the clinician uses that measure of the quantitative EEG along with other assessments, it could be neuropsychological or whatever assessments they use to derive a diagnosis and to put together a treatment.

Q: So, this is a tool that's used to assist these practitioners?

A: That's correct.

Q: Including clinicians like Dr. Gluck?

A: Yes.

Q: And who—I know you've talked about this in some detail, but just to clarify, who actually conducts the research in the QEEG? The names of the organizations in the field?

A: Well, they are—almost every major university has quantitative EEG. So, graduate students in psychology, graduate students in neuroscience, medical students in psychiatry; and neuropsychologists, neuropsychiatrists and medical schools; they do most of it in medical schools and universities. And there's also research done by clinicians and they are able to put together data from a group of their own patients. It's usually done in collaboration with somebody at a research institution, and then there are clinicians who actually will do research themselves.

Q: And which journals publish articles on the QEEG?

A: Well, there's many. There's a journal called Clinical Neurophysiology, Neuro Imaging, Human Brain Mapping, Science, Nature, you know, Experimental Neurology. Many, many journals.

Q: And who is the audience that views these journals and reads these articles and relies on these articles?

A: It's primarily the users of the technology, which is psychiatrists, neuropsychologists, neuropsychiatrists, clinical psychologists, clinical neuroscientists.

Q: And are these articles peer-reviewed as you talked about before?

A: Yes, they are. . . .

Q: . . . [T]here are two schools of thought on the QEEG, two sides, they are divided. Can you talk to that issue with the Judge?

A: Well, there's just one organization that, that I know of, and that's the American Academy of Neurology. And it's really a very small group of individuals within the American Academy of Neurology. So, out of a large universe of 12,000 to 15,000 users of quantitative EEG, there's a very small handful of people actually that are opposed to the use of computers to evaluate the human electroencephalogram. . . .

Testimony of Dr. Epstein, Questions by Assistant State Attorney Mendez

Q: Would it be reliable, assuming the data was reliable, would it be proper or is it—would it be proper within the relevant scientific community to utilize the QEEG to diagnose any brain dysfunction or neurological disorder?

A: Let me clarify that for my answer. There is only one relevant community for the diagnosis of disease. There's only one group of people specifically and extensively trained in the diagnosis of disease and that is MDs. And in that community, it would not . . . be proper. . . .

Q: In the relevant scientific community do they endorse utilizing the QEEG for diagnosis of traumatic brain injury or another neurological disorders?

A: No.

Q: Does the American Academy of Neurology endorse diagnosing traumatic brain injury or neurological disorders via the QEEG?

A: No.

Q: Does the ACNS endorse utilizing the QEEG to diagnose traumatic brain injury or another neurological disorders?

A: No. It does endorse it as a [sic] adjunct in certain specific settings such as helping to pick out possible epileptic spikes for 24 hours. . . .

Q: Now, in your review of Dr. Thatcher's testimony, do you determine whether or not the peer-review articles that he talked about, who are they primarily authored by in terms of supporting his NeuroGuide software or the use of QEEG as reliable under a *Frye* or *Daubert* context?

A: Those are two different questions, actually, and I don't want to waste time but I need to clarify the difference. One can say that radiology is a reliable and valid field with hundreds of thousands of papers without arguing . . . that a specific x-ray technique is thereby automatically validated for specific use. One could not say, "I have invented an x-ray to read your in mind and it's validate because there's hundreds of thousands of papers on x-rays." The specific technique must be validated on its own. So, the gross field of QEEG can be highly valid and reliable for research without that extending from the general to the specific techniques. There's a very simple way to validate a specific technique. It's called a class one randomized double blind clinical study, and no such study has been performed with Dr. Thatcher's technique or any other relevant to closed head injury, so it would not be accepted . . . [by the] FDA or by doctors who diagnose disease.

Q: So, if the X-ray of the stomach is valid for diagnosing cancer, does it mean that an X-ray of the knee is valid in diagnosing arthritis?

A: That's exactly the point. One cannot argue from one specific to another, or from the general to the specific. Each application must stand on its [own]. . . .

NOTES AND QUESTIONS

1. If you were the prosecutor, what questions would you have asked the expert witnesses (on direct and on cross-examination)? How would you have designed your closing argument?

2. In his closing statement at the sentencing phase, attorney Lenamon told the jury that at the time of the stabbing, Grady Nelson's "brain was broken, and it was broken because of drugs and booze. . . ." How would you have responded to such a statement if you were a juror in this case? How would you have responded to the neuroscientific evidence presented? In the actual case, several jurors went on record with the *Miami Herald* to explain the effect of the scientific evidence on their decision-making:

    Delores Cannon, a hospital secretary, said she leaned toward death until the technology was presented. "But then when it came in, the facts about the QEEG, some of us changed our mind," she said.

    John Howard, an airport fleet services worker, said he, too, was ready to recommend death. "It turned my decision all the way around," Howard said the QEEG [sic]. "The technology really swayed me. . . . After seeing the brain scans, I was convinced this guy had some sort of brain problem."

But Leon Benbow, a retired mailman, said he voted for life not because of the QEEG but because he wanted Nelson to rot in prison with the stigma of being a child rapist.

"All that testimony, that was a waste of taxpayer money. That's phony," Benbow said of the QEEG, adding: "There's nothing wrong with that guy's brain."

David Ovalle, *Novel Defense Helps Spare Perpetrator of Grisly Murder*, Miami Herald (Dec. 11, 2010).

3. How would your evaluation of the evidence presented by Dr. Thatcher change if it were shown that the research publications he cites in support of his QEEG method are not recognized as influential by other researchers?

4. How would your evaluation of the QEEG evidence presented by Dr. Thatcher change if you learned that his conclusions were based on a sample of less than 15 minutes derived from a 45-minute recording session?

5. Dr. Thatcher performed an analysis of Nelson's QEEG called Low Resolution Brain Tomography (LORETA) that is supposed to infer the location within the brain from which EEG signals originate. On the basis of these results, Dr. Thatcher concluded that Nelson had abnormalities in a region of the frontal lobe called the anterior cingulate and a region of the temporal lobe called the parahippocampal gyrus. How would your evaluation of this QEEG evidence change if you understood that the LORETA results amount to a best guess based on numerous biological and physical assumptions and that many neuroscientists do not believe such results are reliable?

6. Thatcher reports "over activation of the frontal lobes and prefrontal cortex" that he relates to "social judgment and inhibition." He then refers to two research studies to explain that prenatal alcohol exposure is related to "increased aggression, decreased inhibition and judgment." Do you find this line of thought convincing?

7. Would your evaluation of the QEEG evidence change if you learned that modern neuroscience does not identify a single function with a given brain region? In fact, the various functions that are understood in psychological terms (like memory, attention, emotion, etc.) require the coordinated activation of circuits running throughout many overlapping brain regions.

8. It was estimated that the cost of Nelson's defense over five years and two trials was $1.5 million, and $200,000 was spent on experts for the penalty phase by the defense. Attorney Lenamon commented that, "The state of Florida wants to take somebody's life. If they're going to take someone's life, that person should be represented by the best lawyers and best resources possible." But Miami-Dade State Attorney Katherine Fernández Rundle expressed concern: "I'm very disappointed that the courts are not more mindful of controlling costs, especially where there seems to be so much waste on something that is so experimental." David Ovalle, *Novel Defense Helps Spare Perpetrator of Grisly Murder*, Miami Herald (Dec. 11, 2010). How will/should the cost of neuroscientific evidence contribute to its use in court? What if a technology costs $1 million to deploy? What if it costs $100? How should cost be balanced with relevance and reliability?

9. The *Frye* decision recognized that admissibility decisions would be difficult, as it's unclear "[j]ust when a scientific principle or discovery crosses the line between the experimental and demonstrable stages. . . ." Should the line be drawn differently, and if so, how, when the stakes are higher?

10. The applicable evidentiary rules in Florida at the time of the Nelson case required a *Frye* standard to be used at the penalty phase. But in 2013, the Florida legislature adopted the *Daubert* standards. Would the Nelson case have come out differently under *Daubert*? Note that in many states, and in the federal system, neither *Daubert* nor *Frye* directly apply at sentencing. In federal court sentencing, for instance, the Federal Rules of Evidence are not applicable. Rather, "Evidence does not have to be admissible at a trial in order to be considered in a sentencing hearing, which is not governed by the rules of evidence." *United States v. McIlrath*, 512 F.3d 421, 425 (7th Cir. 2008). However, the Federal Sentencing Guidelines Manual does provide judges with some direction on what factors they can consider when sentencing:

    > (a) When any factor important to the sentencing determination is reasonably in dispute, the parties shall be given an adequate opportunity to present information to the court regarding that factor. In resolving any dispute concerning a factor important to the sentencing determination, the court may consider relevant information without regard to its admissibility under the rules of evidence applicable at trial, provided that the information has sufficient indicia of reliability to support its probable accuracy. . . .

    Chapter Six—Sentencing Procedures, Plea Agreements, and Crime Victims' Rights. Part A—Sentencing Procedures §6A1.3. Resolution of Disputed Factors. How would you have applied this standard—whether the "information has sufficient indicia of reliability to support its probable accuracy"—in the Grady Nelson case?

11. How should neuroscientific evidence be used in the context of predicting future dangerousness and the determination of involuntary commitment? One scholar has proposed "that offenders with brain injuries who manifest violent tendencies be subject to involuntary confinement either during or after their sentence." Adam Lamparello, *Using Cognitive Neuroscience to Predict Future Dangerousness*, 42 Colum. Hum. Rts. L. Rev. 481, 519 (2011). But in response, it has been argued that "neuroscience does not offer us anything new that cannot be responsibly incorporated into existing substantive criminal law doctrine." Steven K. Erickson, *The Limits of Neurolaw*, 11 Hous. J. Health L. & Pol'y 303, 304 (2012). Another scholar offered this critique:

    > [T]he fact that individual assessments of criminality and violence must be made in specific cases implies that there should be no opposition to the search for better and more precise tools that may facilitate predictions of future dangerousness. But the argument in this critique has been (1) that fMRI techniques do not qualify as such tools; (2) that it is fallacious to conceptualize violence and criminality as "just so" products of brain states; and (3) that there are significant risks involved in reducing problems of violence to individual brains, risks which have been and may well in the future be distributed unequally and borne disproportionately by those already experiencing significant social disadvantages. . . .

    Daniel S. Goldberg, *Against Reductionism in Law & Neuroscience* at *Mental Health Symposium: Critical Responses to Lamparo Article*, 11 Hous. J. Health L. & Pol'y 321, 346 (2012). What role should neuroimaging play in civil commitment proceedings? Should the evidentiary bar be higher, lower, or the same as those used in other criminal contexts?

12. In *People v. Goldstein*, 14 A.D.3d 32 (N.Y. App. Div. 2004), the appellate court reviewed a case regarding a defendant that pushed a woman off a platform and into the path of an oncoming subway train, killing her. Defendant appealed his charge of second-degree murder, claiming, among other things, that the trial court erred when it precluded his PET scan. The PET scan was offered in support of defendant's expert witness's claim that defendant was insane due to his schizophrenic condition. The defendant offered the PET scan as evidence "material to one of the ultimate issues in the case since it would have supported an expert's opinion that defendant's brain physically manifested schizophrenia in the form of a 'massive reduction in metabolism in the frontal lobe and the basal ganglia.'" The court excluded the evidence because the prosecution's expert witness had already testified defendant was schizophrenic. In addition, the court, relying on a recommendation by the special master appointed by the court, held the PET scan did not conclusively prove schizophrenia, but could only show an abnormality in the brain, which, in either case, would not be probative of the key issue of the insanity defense, i.e., whether defendant comprehended either the nature and consequences of his actions or that his actions were wrong, since a diagnosis of schizophrenia does not preclude per se that defendant is capable of such comprehension. Could a PET scan be introduced for reasons other than establishing schizophrenia? Does demonstrating an abnormality in the brain inform jurors' judgment of defendant's ability to distinguish right from wrong?

F. NEUROIMAGING AND INEFFECTIVE ASSISTANCE OF COUNSEL

Attorneys must make many strategic decisions in a trial about what evidence to present to the jury. For instance, will the defendant testify or not? With the advent of neuroimaging evidence, attorneys must sometimes now weigh a new consideration: Should they try to show the jury brain images? This leads to a related question: If they decide not to invoke brain science, and their client loses, is it ineffective assistance of counsel? The cases below show how courts are beginning to answer this question in different contexts.

Pinholster v. Ayers

590 F.3d 651 (9th Cir. 2009)

SMITH, JR., C.J. Scott Lynn Pinholster (Pinholster) was sentenced to death after a jury convicted him of double murder with a knife in the course of a home robbery and burglary. After exhausting his state remedies, Pinholster sought a writ of habeas corpus in federal district court in which he alleged, among other claims, ineffective assistance of counsel at both the guilt and penalty phases of his trial. . . .

B. AVAILABLE MITIGATION EVIDENCE

Although the State's aggravating evidence was severely detrimental to Pinholster's case, the record reflects that the harmful effect of that evidence could have been significantly mitigated had Pinholster's trial counsel performed competently. Instead, the only mitigation evidence introduced by defense counsel at the penalty phase was the inaccurate, damaging testimony of Pinholster's mother, Brashear. If counsel had conducted even a minimally adequate investigation, however, they would have found a trove of additional mitigation evidence that would have humanized Pinholster to the jury and, at the same time, contradicted Brashear's misleading version of events. This omitted, but readily available, evidence also would have done much to counter the State's aggravating evidence, which Brashear's testimony failed to rebut or even address. . . .

First, counsel would have discovered evidence of the organic basis for Pinholster's mental health troubles that developed as a result of his traumatic childhood head injuries. During the penalty phase, Brashear testified that when Pinholster was two, she injured his head "quite badly" when she accidentally ran over him with her car. The accident nearly tore off one of his ears. She also testified that, when he was four or five, she had a car accident in which his head went through the windshield. Pinholster's counsel, however, failed to present any medical evidence regarding the consequences of those injuries. As a result, the State argued to an uninformed jury that these injuries were insignificant: "He was run over by a car when he was three years old. That's very unfortunate. There is no evidence of any brain damage. A lot of children get dropped, fall from their cribs or whatever. A couple of years later he went through a car window, not hospitalized, got medical care." . . .

The evidence [also] demonstrates beyond a doubt that Pinholster suffered from epilepsy from a young age. Pinholster was first diagnosed with epilepsy and treated with anti-seizure medication when he was only nine years old, and he frequently suffered complex partial and grand mal seizures thereafter. Dr. Olson concluded that the two car accidents damaged the frontal lobes of Pinholster's brain, an injury that frequently causes impulsive behaviors. This damage, Dr. Olson explained, was evidenced both by Pinholster's epilepsy and by his abnormal EEG reading as a child. Dr. Vinogradov similarly concluded that Pinholster's childhood head injuries resulted in organic, pre-frontal brain damage that changed his personality and explained his aggressive, violent, and antisocial behavior, while Dr. Stalberg characterized the injuries as possibly "devastating" and likewise connected them to Pinholster's epilepsy.

This additional medical evidence would have helped counter the State's aggravation case in three respects. First, evidence that Pinholster's brain damage may have influenced, or even caused, his behavior at the time of the crime may have led jurors to conclude that he was less morally culpable at the time of the offense, and at least one juror may have been inclined to refrain from voting in favor of a capital sentence. Evidence of organic brain injury in other cases has led juries to consider whether because a defendant's "behavior was physically compelled . . . his moral culpability would have been reduced." For this reason, evidence of serious mental health problems, including organic brain damage, is "precisely the type of evidence that we have found critical for a jury to consider when deciding whether to impose a death sentence.". . .

Second, properly presented evidence of Pinholster's brain injury, and its profound effect on his behavior, could have altered the jury's impressions of his detrimental guilt phase testimony and of his boastful, disrespectful demeanor by indicating an organic basis for his inappropriate expressions and for his tendency to exaggerate his past. In this way, "in the hands of a competent attorney," the harmful evidence provided by Pinholster's trial testimony and by his offensive manner could actually "have been used to support [his] claims of dysfunctional upbringing and continuing mental disorder."

Third, evidence of Pinholster's organic brain injury would have humanized him in the eyes of the jury, even if the jury concluded that his brain injury was not responsible for his actions during his commission of the crime. It is not necessary that there be a direct causal connection between a defendant's brain injury and the crime he commits for the existence of that injury to serve as a humanizing and therefore mitigating factor during sentencing. The very existence of organic neurological problems may serve as mitigating evidence at sentencing by eliciting sympathy or, at the very least, some degree of understanding from the sentencer. Though the dissent mocks the fact that counsel did not attempt to humanize Pinholster, the Supreme Court clearly considers humanizing an important part of penalty-phase mitigation in a death penalty case.

Bench v. State

431 P.3d 929 (Okla. Crim. App. 2018)

LUMPKIN, P.J. Appellant, Miles Sterling Bench, was tried by jury and convicted of First Degree Murder. . . . The jury found the presence of two aggravating circumstances: 1) the murder was especially heinous, atrocious, or cruel, and 2) the defendant posed a continuing threat to society, and set punishment as death. . . . Appellant now appeals his conviction and sentence. . . .

FACTS

Appellant began working at the Teepee Totem convenience store in the town of Velma, Stephens County in May of 2012. He was twenty-one years old. Appellant lived outside of town with his grandparents. . . .

After three weeks of training, Appellant began to close the store by himself. On June 6th, Jenson drove Appellant to work. They visited for 2 hours beforehand and discussed Appellant's plan to go to California so Appellant could be a mixed martial arts ("MMA") fighter. Jenson dropped Appellant off shortly before 2:00 p.m. Other than a sore throat, Appellant seemed absolutely normal to Jenson that day.

Sixteen-year-old Braylee Henry drove into Velma around 7:30 p.m. to get an item from the grocery store. After completing this task, Henry went into the Teepee Totem to get some candy and a soda fountain drink. Through Appellant's admissions to his psychological expert, we know that Appellant attacked Henry while she was filing a cup at the fountain. He struck Henry and took her to the ground. He strangled Henry with a choke hold and dragged her into the store's stockroom.

Henry played basketball for her school and was in good shape. Once inside the storeroom, she fought back. Appellant attacked Henry a second time. He repeatedly hit her. Appellant brutally beat Henry's head, face, neck, and chest. Appellant dragged Henry across the room causing her head to strike the floor. He stomped on her head, neck, arm, and upper back with his shoe. Appellant's prolonged savagery resulted in Henry's death. She asphyxiated on the blood in her lungs and died from the blunt force trauma to her head and neck.

Appellant then took steps to conceal what he had done and flee to California. He put a sack around Henry's head and placed her body inside a shopping cart. Appellant covered Henry's body with boxes, pushed the cart out to Henry's car, and placed her body inside the back seat. . . . He drove Henry's car to a semi-secluded area on his grandparent's land and removed her body from the car. . . . He dragged Henry's body to a muddy spot in the field and partially covered it with dirt and vegetation. . . .

[Bench was arrested later that day and brought in for questioning.] . . . Forensic testing revealed that Henry's DNA profile matched the DNA profile of the blood discovered in the storeroom. Similarly, Henry's profile matched the DNA profile of the blood found on Appellant's shoes. . . .

ALLEGATIONS OF INEFFECTIVE ASSISTANCE OF COUNSEL

Appellant . . . asserts in his application that counsel was ineffective for failing to investigate and present neuro-imaging evidence in both stages of the trial. He cites to two different exhibits to his application in support of this claim.

Appellant refers us to Exhibit "5" to his application for evidentiary hearing. This exhibit is the affidavit of William Werner Orrison, M.D., the Chief of Neuroradiology at Simon Med Imaging Centers in Las Vegas, New Mexico. Dr. Orrison asserts that he received the MRI data from Appellant's evaluation at the University of Oklahoma Medical Center. He alleges that Appellant has anomalies in four different areas of his brain but does not relate those anomalies to Appellant's behavior in any way. Dr. Orrison does not directly correlate these alleged anomalies with any mental defect disorder, disease, condition or illness. He has not set forth any diagnosis of Appellant. Instead, Dr. Orrison simply relates the problems which can result if a patient has an anatomical abnormality in the specified areas of the brain.

Appellant further refers us to Exhibit "6" to his application for evidentiary hearing. This exhibit is the affidavit of Jason Paulus Kerkmans, J.D., the Associate Director of MINDSET. Mr. Kerkmans asserts that MINDSET's protocol exam is sufficient to identify a wide range of structural brain abnormalities or deviations which may be of behavioral and clinical significance. He further asserts that additional imaging is necessary because Appellant's current MRI imaging data is not adequate to permit the full MINDSET protocol.

We find that Appellant has not established prejudice from counsel's omission to present neuro-imaging evidence at trial. The courts have not accepted diagnosis of psychological conditions through neuro-imaging as sufficiently reliable to be admissible under the Daubert standard. This is because neuro-imaging methods cannot readily determine whether a defendant knew right from wrong, maintained criminal intent or suffered from a psychological condition like schizophrenia at the time of the criminal act. Thus, the proffered neuro-imaging evidence would have been cumulative to the other evidence in Appellant's defense. . . .

[T]he evidence at trial strongly indicated that Appellant was feigning a severe mental illness. Appellant evinced knowledge of both mental illness and feigning during his impromptu discussion with Officer Brown in the jail. He did not appear to be hallucinating or suffering from delusions immediately after the offense. Multiple psychologists had come to the conclusion that Appellant was over-reporting or feigning mental illness. We are not persuaded that the neuro-imaging evidence would have been able to overcome the compelling evidence of Appellant's sanity.

We further find that Appellant has not shown prejudice from counsel's omission to present the proffered neuro-imaging evidence in the second stage of the trial. Reweighing the evidence in aggravation against both the mitigating evidence which was presented and the proffered neuro-imaging, we find that Appellant has not shown a reasonable probability that had counsel presented the neuro-imaging evidence the jury would have concluded that the balance of aggravating and mitigating circumstances did not warrant death.

The neuro-imaging evidence would not have contributed greatly to Appellant's case in mitigation. Counsel's omission to present the proffered evidence did not prevent the jury from considering any additional circumstance in mitigation because the neuro-imaging evidence was cumulative to Appellant's other mitigating evidence. The jury was instructed that they were able to consider Appellant's learning disability, the influence of his mental disturbance, his limitation in capacity to appreciate the criminality of his conduct, and his inability to conform his behavior to the requirements of the law among other potential mitigating circumstances. Since the proffered neuro-imaging evidence does not readily correlate to whether Appellant knew right from wrong, maintained criminal intent or suffered from schizophrenia we find that it did not corroborate Dr. Grundy's diagnosis of schizophrenia more adequately than the eyewitness accounts which defense counsel presented. Likewise, the proffered evidence would not have been sufficient to overcome the strong evidence that Appellant had feigned a severe mental illness. . . .

The proffered neuro-imaging evidence would not have been sufficient to overcome the State's evidence. As discussed above, the evidence establishing the aggravating circumstances of the murder was compelling. The great weight of the evidence showed that Henry endured conscious physical suffering and severe emotional trauma before dying. Appellant's behavior displayed a pattern of escalating criminal activity and violence. Coupled with the calloused nature of the offense, there was a clear probability that Appellant would continue to constitute a threat to society. Therefore, we conclude that Appellant has not shown clear and convincing evidence of a strong possibility that counsel was ineffective for failing to present neuro-imaging evidence. . . .

Hernandez v. State

180 So. 3d 978 (Fla. 2015)

PER CURIAM. Michael A. Hernandez, Jr., appeals an order of the circuit court denying his motion to vacate his conviction of first-degree murder and sentence of death. . . . He also petitions this Court for a writ of habeas corpus, alleging ineffective assistance of appellate counsel. . . . For the reasons explained below, we . . . deny his petition for a writ of habeas corpus.

BACKGROUND AND FACTS

Michael A. Hernandez, Jr., age twenty-three at the time of the crime, was convicted of the November 18, 2004, first-degree murder of Ruth Everett ("Everett") in Milton, Florida. Hernandez and a friend, Christopher Shawn Arnold, went to the home of Everett and her son David Everett, also known as "Snapper," from whom Arnold sometimes obtained drugs. Arnold and Hernandez went there looking for crack cocaine. When Everett answered the door and told them that her son was not home, Hernandez grabbed her and forced her into the house. Once Hernandez and Arnold were inside, Arnold demanded money and then went looking around the house for drugs. He returned, however, with a pillow, which he put over Everett's face in an attempt to smother her while Hernandez held her. During the struggle or thereafter she suffered a broken neck. Arnold left the house with the victim's purse and Hernandez then stabbed her in the neck. Hernandez returned to the car with blood on his clothes, and he and Arnold drove away. They used her ATM card several times to withdraw money which they used to buy crack cocaine. . . .

Trial Counsel's Performance Regarding Proof of Brain Damage

Hernandez . . . contends that trial counsel was ineffective in failing to obtain quantitative electroencephalography (qEEG) testing to determine if he had brain damage for the purpose of mitigation. When the qEEG testimony was offered at the evidentiary hearing, the State filed a "Motion to Prohibit the Use of Quantitative (qEEG) Testing," and the trial court conducted a *Frye* hearing during the evidentiary hearing to determine if the opinions based on qEEG testing would have been admissible in the 2007 trial of this case if trial counsel had obtained the testing and offered the opinions in mitigation. The postconviction court denied this claim, finding that the technology and opinions stemming from it would not have met the *Frye* test for admissibility at trial.

The postconviction court cited the testimony of the State's expert, Dr. Peter Kaplan, a medical doctor and neurologist who is board certified in psychiatry, neurology, and neurophysiology, and is a professor of neurology at Johns Hopkins University School of Medicine. He is an expert in the use of electroencephalogram (EEG) technology, and he explained that qEEG is a computer program that uses data provided by and chosen from the EEG test and compares that chosen EEG data to a database made up of an aggregate of subjects. Dr. Kaplan testified during the *Frye* portion of the evidentiary hearing that neurologists use EEG to help diagnose neurological conditions, although qEEG has been used in different settings to diagnose epilepsy. Dr. Kaplan testified that qEEG is not widely accepted by neurologists, who are the professionals who diagnose neurologic disease or brain damage. He testified that when qEEG is performed, it is often not done by a doctor or neurologist, and that "one doesn't reach a diagnosis by comparing to a clinical data base." Dr. Kaplan testified these flaws in qEEG were present in 2007 as well as currently.

On cross-examination, Dr. Kaplan agreed that the Veterans Administration has been using qEEG in relation to traumatic brain injury and some universities use the proprietary qEEG program, NeuroGuide, for some purpose. He explained, "You can use the [qEEG] technique to examine data. It's then how you apply the data to make a diagnosis" and "if you have other ways of interpreting those data to reach a clinical diagnosis, it could be, of course, completely valid." Dr. Kaplan also testified that if an individual did not cooperate or follow instructions during the EEG that is done to obtain the raw data, which is then fed into the qEEG software for quantification, the results could contain invalid data, although such lack of cooperation would be fairly obvious.

In denying relief on this claim, the postconviction court also cited testimony of Hernandez's witnesses. Dr. Gerald Gluck, a psychotherapist who testified that he has been using qEEG since the 1980's primarily for "neuro feedback" or "biofeedback," agreed that many neurologists do not use qEEG. He began using "NeuroGuide" software with its "normative data base" in 2001, and said qEEG was more common in the psychological community in 2001. Dr. Gluck performed a qEEG examination on Hernandez and concluded that Hernandez has "frontal, temporal, central deregulation, which is associated with brain injury and damage."

The postconviction court also cited the testimony of Hernandez's witness, Dr. J. Lucas Koberda, a neurologist who testified that he began using qEEG around 2010. The court cited Dr. Koberda's testimony that most neurologists do not use qEEG and that he did not use it in 2007. Dr. Koberda testified that he examined the EEG data collected by Dr. Gluck and the qEEG report he generated, and noted that the "regular EEG . . . showed abnormalities in the frontal and temporal lobes indicating potential brain damage there." In denying relief on this claim, the postconviction court also cited Dr. Koberda's testimony that there was not really any controversy in using qEEG to help diagnose memory problems, Alzheimer's disease, dementia, or epilepsy, but that there is controversy over use of it to diagnose brain damage.

Dr. Turner, one of Hernandez's trial experts, testified at the evidentiary hearing that he had difficulty in assessing whether Hernandez had brain damage at the time of trial primarily because Hernandez was uncooperative. He did not recommend qEEG testing to trial counsel, and he noted that, at that time, there was a dispute about the validity of qEEG testing. Penalty phase counsel Rollo testified at the evidentiary hearing that if he had presented qEEG testimony, and if it had been challenged as not being valid or efficacious, he would have been "injecting another level of uncertain nebulous evidence" in a case in which he was trying to maintain a coherent theme. . . .

The postconviction court held that Hernandez failed to establish that the qEEG analysis would have passed the *Frye* test at the time of trial by failing to demonstrate that qEEG was widely accepted by the relevant scientific community in 2007. Thus, the court held that trial counsel was not deficient in failing to pursue qEEG testing to show Hernandez suffered from brain damage.

Hernandez argues here that the proper test to apply for the admissibility of qEEG is *Daubert v. Merrell Dow Pharmaceuticals*, based on the Legislature's 2013 amendment to section 90.702, Florida Statutes. . . .

Section 90.702 was amended in 2013 to provide that testimony by an expert who is qualified by knowledge, skill, experience, training, or education may testify in the form of opinion if (1) the testimony is based upon sufficient facts or data; (2) the testimony is the product of reliable principles and methods; and (3) the witness has applied the principles and methods reliably to the facts of the case. The intent of the amendment, it has been said, is to tighten the rules for admissibility of any expert opinion. However, the Supreme Court in *Daubert* actually criticized *Frye* and its "exclusive test" imposing a "rigid 'general acceptance' requirement" as being at odds with the liberal thrust of the Federal Rules and their "general approach of relaxing the traditional barriers to 'opinion' testimony." Moreover, general acceptance in the relevant scientific community remains one factor among several even when the *Daubert* test is the applicable test.

Hernandez contends that the relevant scientific community is not limited to neurologists, as Dr. Kaplan testified and the trial court found. The postconviction court disagreed with this same contention, applied the *Frye* test to the expert testimony presented at the evidentiary hearing, and concluded that Hernandez failed to prove by a preponderance of evidence that qEEG was generally accepted in the relevant scientific community—that community being neurologists—at the time of trial. We agree. Dr. Kaplan testified that qEEG is not a reliable method for determining brain damage and is not widely accepted by those who diagnose neurologic disease or brain damage. His testimony provided competent, substantial evidence on which the court could conclude that the relevant scientific community was neurologists who generally diagnose brain damage and whose training and experience include conducting an EEG and reading and understanding the raw EEG data. Dr. Koberda also testified that most neurologists do not use qEEG and that he did not use it in 2007. Dr. Gluck testified that he has been using qEEG since the 1980's, primarily for "neuro feedback," but agreed that many neurologists do not use qEEG.

Furthermore, a number of judicial decisions in existence at the time of trial also held that qEEG testing was not admissible. . . .

Because the postconviction court had competent, substantial evidence on which to find that the relevant scientific community was neurologists whose job it is to diagnose brain damage, and because all the testifying experts agreed that qEEG was not generally accepted by that scientific community as a method of diagnosing brain damage, the court was correct in finding Hernandez's trial counsel was not deficient in failing to obtain qEEG testing on Hernandez as a way of demonstrating brain damage in 2007. . . .

NOTES AND QUESTIONS

1. For a lengthy opinion, including multiple graphics depicting basic brain science, see *Cone v. Carpenter*, No. 97-2312, 2016 WL 1274599 (W.D. Tenn. Mar. 31, 2016) (reviewing the neuroimaging testimony of one of the defendant's expert witnesses).

2. United States Supreme Court Justice Sonia Sotomayor has, in two separate cases, referenced brain evidence in dissenting from cert. denial. In *Elmore v. Holbrook*, 137 S. Ct. 3, 3-4 (2016), Justice Sotomayor observed in her dissent:

> A more experienced attorney encouraged Elmore's lawyer to investigate whether Elmore had suffered brain damage as a young man. . . . Experts who testified at Elmore's postconviction hearing agreed that this exposure placed him at serious risk of brain damage. They conducted neuropsychological tests that revealed mild to moderate cognitive impairments, including a marked inability to control his emotions and impulses. Elmore tested in the bottom one percent on tests measuring that characteristic. The experts concluded that damage to Elmore's frontal lobe had made him impulsive and susceptible to emotion. And they agreed that the murder Elmore later committed was linked to Elmore's cognitive deficits—for instance, by making him unable to "pu[t] on the brakes" when emotional. . . .

Similarly, in *Wessinger v. Vannoy*, 138 S. Ct. 952, 952 (2018), Justice Sotomayor wrote in her dissent:

> Petitioner Todd Wessinger was sentenced to death by a jury that was never presented with significant mitigation evidence that may have convinced its members to spare his life. For instance, Wessinger suffers from a major neurocognitive disorder that compromises his decision-making abilities. As a child, he experienced a stroke

in his left frontal lobe that affected how the left and right sides of his brain communicate. He also suffered from childhood seizures, and he has a hole in the area of his brain associated with executive functioning that resulted from some form of cerebrovascular illness. . . .

3. At present, fMRI is not utilized in the formal diagnosis of mental disorders in either the DSM-5 or the International Classification of Diseases (ICD-11). Vigorous research continues to seek such diagnostic measures. What if peer-reviewed research suggests the potential utility of fMRI to aid diagnosis, even if it is not recommended by the DSM-5 or ICD-11? Consider this argument:

> Functional MRI rests on a robust evidence-based, peer-reviewed literature when it comes to evaluating psychiatric conditions. . . . The ability of neuroimaging tools to help psychiatry correctly diagnose major mental illnesses may be of use to the legal system since the presence or absence of psychosis can be a critical issue in a number of different legal contexts. . . .

Lyn M. Gaudet, Julia R. Lushing & Kent A. Kiehl, *Functional Magnetic Resonance Imaging in Court*, 5 Am. J. Bioethics Neurosc. 43, 44 (2014).

G. ADMISSIBILTY OF NEUROSCIENCE EVIDENCE

In the ineffective assistance of counsel cases, the argument is typically that a lawyer was ineffective in failing to present brain evidence to the jury. But even when a lawyer wants to present neuroscientific evidence, the evidence may be excluded by a judge if it does not meet the jurisdiction's requirements for admissibility of expert evidence. The case excerpts below present judges making admissibility decisions for PET evidence in a criminal trial and for neuroscience testimony in a class action lawsuit.

People v. Bowman
2014 WL 718416 (Cal. Ct. App. Feb. 26, 2014) (not officially published)

KLEIN, P.J. James Bowman appeals the judgment entered following a trial in which the jury found him guilty of first degree willful, deliberate and premeditated murder with a finding he personally and intentionally discharged a firearm proximately causing death. . . .

CONTENTIONS
Appellant contends the trial court erred and denied him his constitutional right to present a defense by applying *People v. Kelly** to the PET scan results (positron

---

* In California, the admissibility of expert evidence is determined by the *Frye-Kelly* rule. "In *People v. Kelly*, 17 Cal. 3d 24, (1976), the state of California adopted a slightly modified version of the Frye test. The court held that the proper test for the admissibility of novel scientific evidence consisted of three parts. First, the reliability of the method must be established, usually by experts who can demonstrate that the method is generally accepted within the relevant community. Next, the testifying expert must be properly qualified. Finally, the proponent must show that the correct scientific procedures were used in the case before the court. This test became known as the Kelly/Frye test." 90 A.L.R.5th 453, 29 (comment, originally published in 2001).

emission tomography), and on the same grounds, excluding from evidence the related expert medical testimony from a neurologist, Dr. Arthur Kowell. . . .

DISCUSSION
1. The PET Scan Results and Dr. Kowell's Testimony.

Dr. Kowell had administered CT, MRI and PET scans to appellant and examined appellant personally prior to trial. At trial, the trial court ruled the PET scan results and Dr. Kowell's testimony concerning the PET scan results and his opinion concerning the results of his related examination of appellant were inadmissible on *Kelly* grounds. On appeal, appellant complains, if the doctor had been permitted to testify, he would have opined appellant's behavior during the shooting was "consistent with that of someone suffering from hypometabolism" in the temporal lobes, or with a decreased functioning of those lobes, and the condition would affect whether a person actually deliberated or premeditated as "it is associated with impulse control disorder." . . .

a. Dr. Kowell's Evidence Code Section 402 Testimony.

Prior to trial, in a written motion, the deputy district attorney raised objections to the doctor's testimony on grounds of *Kelly*. He argued the PET scan results are not generally accepted in the scientific medical community as disclosing anything about the elements of malice aforethought, including express malice (intent to kill), and deliberation and premeditation. Dr. Kowell's opinion was largely dependent on the PET scan results, and for that reason, it should be excluded. Insofar as Dr. Kowell's opinion was dependent on appellant's social and medical history, Dr. Kowell, a neurologist, was not qualified to testify as would a psychologist or psychiatrist as it was "out of his purview." The deputy district attorney urged the neurological opinion was irrelevant, or more prejudicial than probative, because the science does not permit anyone to draw a conclusion based on the PET scan or to know whether there was a biological sign five years previously when the shooting occurred that indicated an impulse control disorder.

The parties agreed Dr. Kowell was an experienced neurologist who frequently used PET scans. They agreed the PET scan was taken almost five years after the shooting through no fault of appellant or his trial counsel.

Dr. Kowell testified at the hearing. He said there were no abnormalities on the CT and MRI scans he ordered for appellant. (An MRI scan reveals structural abnormalities in the brain.) However, the PET scan demonstrated at the time of the scan, the nerve cells in the temporal lobes were less active than they should have been, which is an abnormality according to the study. The significance of the abnormality, however, had to be interpreted in light of other facts. A doctor cannot determine from a PET scan how long the abnormality has existed. He cannot tell the pathology responsible for the decrease in metabolism. A patient's history is then referenced to suggest "possibilities" for the decreased activity. Dr. Kowell could not say with any certainty what the cause of the abnormality was. But based on appellant's history, as appellant relates it, and the collateral documents provided to him, Dr. Kowell believed the causal factors for the decreased functioning probably were "chronic alcohol and/or marijuana abuse and/or cerebral trauma."

The doctor said the temporal lobes have a number of functions, one being it is "important in terms of impulse control." He claimed "a number of studies" indicate persons with hypometabolism have impaired impulse control. The "exact nature of this in terms of [brain] circuitry in the temporal lobe is not entirely well worked out." There is some relationship according to the studies, but to be fair, there are patients who have the decreased brain activity who do not have impaired impulse control. Dr. Kowell explained the scan tells you there is decreased activity; it does not indicate the cause of the decreased activity. The clinician must look to a patient's history to discern a cause for the condition. For appellant, Dr. Kowell opined a possible cause for the hypometabolism observed on the scan "would include chronic and/or marijuana abuse and cerebral trauma." He said, "I think that the hypometabolism would be consistent with his previous history as documented in the records of impulse control problems."

Trial counsel addressed Dr. Kowell with a hypothetical loosely based on appellant's postarrest statement to the police and his anticipated testimonial claims. She asked whether the shooting was a "type of behavior consistent with someone who suffers from hypometabolism in the temporal lobes?" Dr. Kowell replied, "It would be consistent with someone who has temporal lobe dysfunction of which hypometabolism provides at least a biological sign that there is a malfunction or dysfunction in the temporal lobe. In other words, hypometabolism itself doesn't mean he's going to pull out the gun and shoot someone, but hypometabolism indicates that there is a temporal lobe problem for which this patient may be at greater risk for a . . . impulsive behavior." Trial counsel asked whether given the "set of stressors" described in her hypothetical, would a person react in a more "violent fashion than someone without the hypometabolism?" Dr. Kowell, said, "In a statistical sense, yes."

Trial counsel asked whether a person with hypometabolism would necessarily take time to consider his actions beforehand? The doctor said, "Such a person would be at greater risk for not contemplating the consequences of their actions." He explained there is a condition causing the hypometabolism, and there could be several of them. It is that condition which results in the dysfunction seen on the scan, not the scan results, that creates the greater risk of a person not contemplating the consequences of their actions. Such a person with that condition would "react first and think later." The doctor agreed he could not say "definitively" that appellant had a "temporal lobe condition."

The doctor testified the PET scan itself produces reliable scan results. It is the interpretation of the abnormality disclosed by the test that presents problems not only in medicine but in a forensic context. "In other words, what does the abnormality mean." In appellant's case, the doctor had concluded likely candidates causing such an abnormality would be "chronic alcohol and/or marijuana abuse and cerebral trauma."

During the hearing, Dr. Kowell said he could not say to a high degree of certainty or probability that persons with the abnormality he saw on the PET scan have impulse control disorder. He could not diagnose a lack of impulse control or an impulse control disorder. The most he could say was that temporal lobe dysfunction is consistent with patients who have impulse control disorders. To be fair, however, the doctor pointed out that someone with hypometabolism may not have decreased impulse control, and a person with impulse control disorder may not have hypometabolism. The significance of the hypometabolism is unknown.

Dr. Kowell could not say what the condition of appellant's brain had been five years previously, much less the day before or the day after the scan. Such conditions as lack of sleep, depression, the taking of psychotropic medications, mood, brain activity taking place during the scan and other conditions could affect the level of the activity. Dr. Kowell could not quantify how the many variables might affect the scan nor could he control for them. The doctor acknowledged appellant was taking medication when the scan was taken. Also, appellant's circumstances — he was incarcerated and facing serious criminal charges — could cause depression. . . .

The deputy district attorney asked whether Dr. Kowell was familiar with *The Judge's Guide to Neuroscience, a Concise Introduction,* published in 2010 by Dr. Helen Mayberg. The doctor replied he was unaware of the publication, but aware of Dr. Mayberg, a specialist in nuclear medicine. The deputy district attorney read to Dr. Kowell from that publication: "'It is beyond the data generated from any currently published scanning protocol to make predictions about the rational capacity or lack thereof of a criminal defendant or to make inferences as to that defendant's intent at a specific moment in time before or during a specific criminal act. Time will tell if paradigms can be designed that meet the necessary criteria to make such inferences.'"

Dr. Kowell testified he agreed with Dr. Mayberg's claim — based on the results of the scan a doctor cannot state with certainty what a person's intent may have been at a specific moment in time during or before a specific criminal act as far as intent goes. The doctor clarified that the PET scan results can only be considered in combination with other information. He claimed where there is a biological basis for the patient's behavior, the PET scan can help reach a conclusion. By itself, the scan results cannot be used for a diagnosis.

The doctor acknowledged he knew of no literature indicating there was general acceptance in the medical scientific community of the use of PET scans to draw inferences about the "intent to do anything." He said he did not know whether there is a general consensus in the medical scientific community that a person with a modestly low metabolic problem, as disclosed by a PET scan, can be diagnosed as having poor impulse control. Nevertheless, Dr. Kowell said in his experience, the PET scan results were reliable in disclosing metabolic activity and in diagnosing conditions such as epilepsy, stroke and dementia. And, in his opinion, the scan results raise "a red flag" that there is a biological dysfunction, making it more likely the patient has an impulse control disorder. . . .

b. The Trial Court's Ruling.

The trial court commented it is undisputed that Dr. Kowell is an expert in neurology and in interpreting PET scans, that appellant had an abnormal PET scan revealing hypometabolism in his temporal lobes, and that the PET scan was performed correctly. The trial court concluded from the testimony that PET scans are legitimate tools for diagnosing medical disorders of the brain, particularly with regard to dementia, stroke and epilepsy.

The trial court said the issue raised is the reliability of the PET scan for use forensically in this case. It set out a number of problems with Dr. Kowell's testimony. The doctor could not date the onset of the abnormality nor the cause of the abnormality, and he cannot eliminate other contributing factors such as dementia, medication, depression, lack of sleep, etc. Nor can he predict whether the findings would be the same even one day before, or after, October 26, 2011, when the PET scan was taken. There are so many variables that affect the hypometabolism of the temporal lobes that the results can be almost transient depending on the variables.

Dr. Kowell could only interpret the results of the scan with the use of appellant's social, psychological, and medical history, taking that history from appellant and the other documents he was given to review.

What was most troubling is that even if a person has this abnormality in the temporal lobes, he might have reduced impulse control, but not necessarily. There is no consistent correlation between the PET scan finding and reduced impulse control. The PET scan is not a definitive test and not necessarily a predictor of behavior. There is no statistical correlation between abnormal PET scan results and the lack of impulse control. The doctor admitted there is no consensus in the medical scientific community that the interpretation of the PET scan results necessarily predicts reduced impulse control.

The trial court noted the radiologist, Dr. Susie Bash, said the following: " 'The significance of the temporal lobe hypometabolism is unknown at this point in time. Theoretically, the earliest beginning findings of a neuro dementia syndrome could potentially present like this; however, no formal neuro dementia diagnosis can be established on this initial examination, particularly since metabolism is within normal limits remote to the temporal lobes at this point in time.' "

There was no evidence of structural brain changes on the CT images or on the MRI. There was no suggestion of cerebral atrophy. No other tests document or corroborate that appellant has some type of brain malfunction or structural disorder that can more strongly be correlated to his behavior; that is, reduced impulse control.

The trial court further observed to conclude appellant had a loss of impulse control or an impulse control disorder is speculation. It is similar to saying a brain tumor one has today is responsible for a homicide five years previously. The defendant cannot prove the tumor existed five years previously, or that a brain tumor always results in homicidal behavior. Even if the PET scan had been taken immediately after the shooting, the same PET scan results would have been meaningless in terms of assisting appellant's defense.

The speculative nature of the abnormality here is the same. The opinion is not reliable in a forensic context, and the doctor seems to admit it.

The trial court found the foundation inadequate to comply with *Kelly*. If *Kelly* did not compel the exclusion, then the doctor's testimony and PET scan results should be excluded pursuant to Evidence Code section 352. The speculative nature of the results and the doctor's opinion would serve only to confuse the jury. The risk of possible confusion outweighs the probity of the testimony.

The trial court said it would not permit Dr. Kowell to testify "at least with regards to what he testified to here today." The trial court asked whether the parties wished to make any further record. Neither of the parties responded.

c. The Analysis.

In *Kelly*, the court held that evidence obtained through a new scientific technique may be admitted only after its reliability has been established under a three-pronged test. The first prong requires proof that the technique is generally accepted as reliable in the relevant scientific community. The second prong requires proof that the witness testifying about the technique and its application is a properly qualified expert on the subject. The third prong requires proof that the person performing the test in the particular case used correct scientific procedures. Here, we are concerned only with the first prong of the *Kelly* test.

Appellant argues the trial court improperly applied the *Kelly* rule to evaluate the admissibility of Dr. Kowell's testimony. He asserts the PET scan results were reliable for detecting brain dysfunction and were a proper basis for Dr. Kowell's opinion of possible brain dysfunction. . . .

The rule in *Kelly* applies to a limited class of expert testimony based in whole or in part on a technique, process, or theory which is new to science, and even more so to the law. Under *Kelly*, "the admissibility of evidence obtained by use of a scientific technique does not depend upon proof to the satisfaction of a court that the technique is scientifically reliable or valid. Because courts are ill suited to make such determinations, admissibility depends upon whether the technique is generally accepted as reliable in the relevant scientific community."

In his written motion objecting to the use of Dr. Kowell's testimony, the deputy district attorney listed a number of articles and publications indicating there is no consensus in the medical community as to whether the results of brain imaging tests are probative on the issue of drawing inferences concerning mental states in criminal cases. During the hearing, the deputy district attorney referred to Dr. Helen Mayberg's 2010 article in *The Judge's Guide to Neuroscience, a Concise Introduction,* which concluded a physician could not predict from any scanning protocol the rational capacity or lack thereof of a criminal defendant or draw inferences as to a defendant's intent at a specific moment in time before or during a criminal act. Dr. Kowell could not testify there was general agreement in the medical scientific community that someone with a modestly low metabolic problem, as disclosed by the PET scan, can be diagnosed as having poor impulse control. Nor could the doctor testify that science had advanced and the conclusions of the authorities no longer reflected the consensus of the medical community.

We acknowledge the medical scientific community may agree a PET scan is generally accepted for diagnosing tumors, epilepsy and dementia. However, the burden was on appellant as the proponent of the doctor's testimony, to show the *Kelly* test had been met. The evidence at the hearing was unequivocal in establishing the medical scientific community does *not* yet accept that PET scan results can provide information to the expert in a criminal case that may assist the jury in determining a defendant's mental state.

d. Conclusion.

After reviewing the relevant case law, we conclude the trial court properly applied the rationale in *Kelly* to exclude the results of the PET scan. Dr. Kowell's testimony made it appear the PET scan results were the cornerstone of the doctor's opinion with respect to whether appellant could be suffering a mental defect or brain dysfunction that affected his impulse control. Dr. Kowell's opinion belonged to "that limited class of expert testimony" which was "based, in whole or part, on a technique, process, or theory which is *new* to science and, even more so, the law."

The PET scan as used here is "scientific" as the "'unproven technique or procedure appears *in both name and description* to provide some definitive truth which the expert need only accurately recognize and relay to the jury.'" It is different from mere medical opinion, which jurors can temper with healthy skepticism "born of their knowledge all human beings are fallible." Dr. Kowell's opinion of possible brain dysfunction in large part was based on the results of a machine and its accompanying computer analysis. As lay persons, the jury may well have "ascribe[d] an inordinately high degree of certainty to proof derived from an apparently 'scientific' mechanism, instrument, or procedure[, when] aura of infallibility that often surrounds such evidence may well conceal the fact that [the methodology] remains experimental and tentative." . . .

DISPOSITION

The judgment is affirmed.

In re Horizon Organic Milk Plus DHA Omega-3 Mktg. & Sales Practice Litig.

No. 12–MD–02324, 2014 WL 1669930 (S.D. Fla. Apr. 28, 2014)

O'SULLIVAN, M.J. THIS MATTER is before the Court on the Defendant's Motion to Strike and/or Exclude the Testimony and Opinions of Richard P. Bazinet, Ph.D . . . [the Motion was granted and Dr. Bazinet's testimony was excluded. — EDS.]

INTRODUCTION

The defendant, WhiteWave Foods Company, is a wholly-owned subsidiary of Dean Foods Company which manufactures, distributes, markets and sells milk products fortified with algal-derived DHA Omega–3 ("DHA"). These DHA-fortified milk products are marketed as and packaged in cartons with labels that state "Supports Brain Health" and "Supports a Healthy Brain." The plaintiffs are consumers from six states who purchased the DHA-fortified milk. The plaintiffs claim that the defendant violated state laws by falsely representing on the milk cartons and in advertising that DHA "Supports Brain Health" and "Supports a Healthy Brain." The plaintiffs maintain that the defendant's representations about DHA in its products are false and that the competent, scientific evidence shows that these claims are false. The plaintiffs further maintain that they have suffered an economic injury because they all paid a premium price for the DHA-fortified milk products based on the defendant's false representations that DHA "Supports Brain Health" and "Supports a Healthy Brain."

On February 21, 2014, the defendant filed the instant motion seeking to strike or exclude the plaintiffs' expert, Richard P. Bazinet, Ph.D. . . .

STANDARD OF REVIEW

Under *Daubert v. Merrell Dow Pharms., Inc.,* and Rule 702 of the Federal Rules of Evidence, the Court serves as a gatekeeper to the admission of scientific evidence. . . . To determine the admissibility of expert testimony under Rule 702, the Court must undertake the following three-part inquiry:

(1) [T]he expert is qualified to testify competently regarding the matters he intends to address; (2) the methodology by which the expert reaches his conclusions is sufficiently reliable as determined by the sort of inquiry mandated by Daubert; and (3) the testimony assists the trier of fact, through the application of scientific, technical, or specialized expertise, to understand evidence or to determine a fact in issue. . . .

ANALYSIS

A. Dr. Bazinet's November 13, 2013 Report

Richard P. Bazinet, Ph.D. is an expert in the field of nutritional neuroscience. He was retained by the plaintiffs "to review and assess the 'Supports Brain Health' and 'Supports a Healthy Brain' representations on the labels of, and in advertisements for [the defendant's] organic milk and soy milk products with the algal oil derived DHA additive. . . ." Dr. Bazinet opines that the algal-derived DHA in defendant's milk products "is superfluous and provides no measurable brain health benefit or support." In his November 13, 2013 report, Dr. Bazinet states that he:

> reviewed several levels of evidence including randomized controlled trials using DHA and others using mixtures of omega–3 fatty acids from fish oil as well as observational studies of fish oil and meta-analyses of these studies. However, because there are sufficient randomized controlled trials assessing the algal DHA used in the Milk Products with added DHA on brain function, [he] did not need to consider studies examining fish oil, observational studies or other sources of lower quality evidence in forming [his] opinion. And, [he] limited [his] focus to healthy individuals as that is the target population for the Milk Products with added DHA. . . .

C. The Merits of the Instant Motion

The defendant seeks to strike or exclude the testimony of Dr. Bazinet on the grounds that it is not relevant and unreliable under Rule 702 of the Federal Rules of Evidence and Daubert. The defendant does not challenge Dr. Bazinet's qualifications as an expert. . . .

i. Relevance

. . . [T]he defendant maintains that the only labeling claims at issue are "Supports Brain Health" and "Supports a Healthy Brain." Thus, because the defendant did not make any representations that its "DHA Products would improve brain function or that people's brains would not be healthy if they did not drink the DHA Products" and because Dr. Bazinet testified that "brain function" is different from "brain health," Dr. Bazinet's testimony does not fit the case. At deposition, Dr. Bazinet testified as follows:

Q. Is brain function something different to you than brain health?
A. Yes.
Q. What's the distinction in your mind?
A. Brain function would include neurochemical reactions that we don't—that you can remove double and don't have any known impact on the brain.
Q. But a functioning—to have a healthy brain one has to have a functioning brain, correct?
A. Your brain must to function for it to be healthy. If it didn't function, it would not be healthy.

Deposition of Dr. Bazinet (DE# 146–4 at 26, 2/21/14) (emphasis added). In his March 28, 2014 declaration, Dr. Bazinet states "[b]rain health, in this context, can only mean one of two things: (1) contribution to brain structure or (2) contribution to brain function." Dr. Bazinet then explains that because the amount of DHA in the defendant's milk products is trivial and cannot contribute to brain structure, the only possible benefit of DHA in the defendant's milk products is to brain function. . . .

. . . The defendant's labeling claims state that its algal-derived DHA milk products "Support[ ] Brain Health" and "Support[ ] a Healthy Brain." Dr. Bazinet indicates that "brain function" is a measure of a healthy brain. Based on the foregoing, the undersigned concludes that Dr. Bazinet's testimony "fits" the instant case.

ii. Reliability

The defendant further argues that Dr. Bazinet's methodology is unreliable because: (1) Dr. Bazinet "cherry-picked" five randomized controlled trials ("RCTs") among "over a thousand scientific articles on DHA and the brain;" (2) the five "cherry-picked" RCTs do not support Dr. Bazinet's testimony and (3) Dr. Bazinet fails to explain how these 5 RCTs involving 49 women and 658 children (mostly in the United Kingdom) can be reliably extrapolated to all "healthy" people. . . .

a. Whether Dr. Bazinet "Cherry-picked" the Five RCTs

The defendant maintains that there are 1,375 scientific articles using the terms "DHA and brain," yet Dr. Bazinet "cherry-picked" the five RCTs to support his conclusion. . . .

The defendant's arguments go to the weight the trier of fact should give to Dr. Bazinet's testimony and not its admissibility. While the defendant is correct that an expert may not "cherry pick" the available data in order to manufacture a desired result, Dr. Bazinet has provided a reasonable, scientific explanation why he relied on some studies (the five RCTs involving algal derived DHA) and discounted other studies. Dr. Bazinet explained that RCTs are the "gold standard" when it comes to scientific studies and that observational studies are less reliable. . . .

b. Whether the Five RCTs Support Dr. Bazinet's Opinion

The defendant next argues that the 5 RCTs relied on by Dr. Bazinet do not support his testimony. The 5 RCTs relied on by Dr. Bazinet are the Johnson, Ryan, Kennedy, McNamara and Richardson RCTs. The defendant argues that the McNamara RCT does not support Dr. Bazinet's opinion because:

The **main finding** of the present study was that 8 wk of supplementation with either low- or high-dose DHA significantly increased functional activation in the DLPFC (BA9) [dorsolateral prefrontal cortex of the brain] during performance of an attention task compared with placebo. However, [t]his imaging trial had **important limitations**. . . . [T]he high level of performance [on the attention task] exhibited by all groups (80–90% accuracy) may have prevented the detection of potential performance-enhancing effects of DHA supplementation" and "the relatively small number of subjects randomly assigned to each treatment group may not be a representative sample of this age group. . . .

Similarly, the defendant argues that the remaining four RCTs do not support Dr. Bazinet's opinion that algal-derived DHA has no effect on brain function because they contain . . . contradictory conclusions. . . .

The defendant's criticisms of Dr. Bazinet's interpretation of the RCTs go to the weight and credibility of Dr. Bazinet's testimony. Dr. Bazinet did not simply ignore the portions of the RCT that did not support his opinion. He analyzed the RCTs and gave detailed reasons why these RCTs support his opinion. The defendant's critique that Dr. Bazinet should have interpreted the results of the RCTs differently is more appropriately left for cross-examination. . . .

c. Whether Dr. Bazinet can Extrapolate the 5 RCTs to the Purported Class of All–Purchasers

Finally, the defendant argues that Dr. Bazinet's testimony is unreliable under Daubert because he "failed to explain how he can extrapolate the results of five [ ]short studies in 49 women and 658 children to all 'healthy' people (let alone the 'all-purchaser' classes that [the p]laintiffs propose." The defendant notes that "well over half of the subjects in Dr. Bazinet's five studies were children living in the United Kingdom" and that "Dr. Bazinet makes no attempt to demonstrate that the results of studies conducted on U.K. children can be reliably extrapolated to U.S. children, let alone adults." The defendant further notes that "Dr. Bazinet's [March 28, 2014 declaration] is devoid of explanation as to how he can reliably extrapolate the studies he relies on to the facts of these cases, and [the p]laintiffs' opposition is likewise devoid of argument."

Neither the plaintiffs nor Dr. Bazinet address the defendant's extrapolation argument. "Determining the minimum sample size from which reliable extrapolations can be made to the sampled population is tricky." Here, Dr. Bazinet does not even attempt to argue that the sample size of the 5 RCTs of women and children (involving mostly subjects in the United Kingdom) are sufficient to make a reliable extrapolation to the putative classes of consumers of the defendant's milk products in the United States. The undersigned is not saying that the 5 RCTs cannot scientifically be extrapolated to apply to the putative classes through reliable expert testimony. Rather, Dr. Bazinet simply ignores the issue and makes no attempt to explain how this extrapolation can be made. . . . The party seeking to introduce the expert testimony has the burden of establishing reliability under Daubert. The plaintiffs have not shown that the RCTs underlying Dr. Bazinet's opinion can be reliably extrapolated to the putative classes. Based on this record, Dr. Bazinet's testimony is excluded as unreliable under Daubert.

CONCLUSION

In sum, the defendant does not dispute Dr. Bazinet's qualifications as an expert in his field of nutritional neuroscience. Dr. Bazinet's opinion "fits" the plaintiffs' case in that his opinion addresses the issue of whether the algal derived DHA in the defendant's milk products "Supports Brain Health" and/or "Supports a Healthy Brain." The methodology used by Dr. Bazinet to reach his conclusions, however, is not reliable under Daubert because Dr. Bazinet fails to explain how he can reliably extrapolate the 5 RCTs upon which he basis his opinion to the all-consumer putative classes in the instant case. . . .

NOTES AND QUESTIONS

1. The cases above reference both the *Frye* and the *Daubert* standards. Under what circumstances would it be likely to make a difference whether proffered neuroscientific evidence is being evaluated under one of these standards or the other?
2. Why, exactly, was the expert's testimony in the Horizon Organic Milk class action lawsuit excluded by the judge? Is this an appropriate application of *Daubert*?
3. Consider whether you agree with this view about how courts should treat neuroscientific evidence:

> In our view, at the present time, the use of brain images in the courtroom should be limited only to cases in which the images are to be admitted to show an association between a particular structural lesion (injury) or abnormality with a deficit of some kind, interpreted by a qualified neuroscientist. An example would be a plaintiff in a personal injury case who seeks to admit an image for the purpose of linking a brain

injury sustained in an accident to some kind of loss, such as paralysis of a limb. We disagree with the use of functional brain images for the purpose of linking secondary evidence of brain activity (such as blood flow or utilization of oxygen as evidence of neuronal function) to aberrations in human thought, will, motivation or propensity for culpable behavior, or to show an incapacity to inhibit that behavior, because such linkages assume that these complex functions of the brain are subserved by a modular brain that has "centers" for each one. The reason that those links cannot be made with presently available functional neuroimaging technologies (such as fMRI) is that these technologies are currently incapable of showing the multiple networks, each with multiple "centers" and connections creating different systems, which function in space and time. Even primary assessments such as QEEG still are unable to access all networks subserving such complex functions as truth-telling. For something like this ever to be possible would require many more technological developments and parallel developments in expertise and training of investigators and neuroscientists in administering the tests and interpreting them, none of which are available at this time or in the near future. To think otherwise is at best wishful thinking, and at worst, advocating pseudoscience.

Even in the case of evidence sought to be admitted for the limited purpose of linking a structural brain lesion or abnormality to a deficit, we suggest that medicine and neuroscience could provide specific guidance for judges who must make evidentiary determinations in the cases before them. Specifically, guidance on the clinical purposes for which respective imaging techniques have been validated, and the state of research on the validity and reliability of the theories and processes underlying the technologies would be important. . . .

Laura Stephens Khoshbin & Shahram Khoshbin, *Imaging the Mind, Minding the Image: An Historical Introduction to Brain Imaging and the Law*, 33 Am. J.L. & Med. 171, 186-87 (2007).

H. EFFECT OF BRAIN IMAGING EVIDENCE ON JUDGES AND JURORS

Conventional wisdom and anecdotal evidence such as that from the jurors in the Grady Nelson case suggest that courts are right to be concerned about the potentially prejudicial effects of brain imaging evidence on jurors. But do we know anything beyond these anecdotes about the effect of neuroscientific evidence on juror and judge decision-making? Over the past decade, scholars in law, psychology, neuroscience, and related disciplines have explored this question through a series of increasingly sophisticated experimental designs. Still, as the excerpts below suggest, the collective results are provocative, not dispositive.

As summarized by Shen et al.:

[T]he scholarly empirical literature on the effects of such evidence is decidedly mixed. Across nearly 30 previous studies, including over 50 unique experiments, the only result researchers can agree upon is that there are "conflicting results". At present, the "likely effect of neuroscientific evidence in legal settings is still unclear". Or, as Baker et al. (2015) describe it in a review, "empirical research into the neuroimage bias has produced what might appear to be a tangled mess of contradictory findings . . . [and a] research quagmire". . . . Amidst this quagmire of conflicting results, there is a growing appreciation that context matters. That is, research going forward is likely not to address "Does neuroscientific evidence affect outcomes?" (inviting a binary Yes/No answer), but rather "How much and under what circumstances does neuroscientific evidence affect outcomes?" . . .

Francis X. Shen et al., *The Limited Effect of Electroencephalography Memory Recognition Evidence on Assessments of Defendant Credibility*, 4 J.L. & Biosci. 330, 332 (2017).

We present a sampling of the findings from this literature, followed by two commentaries on the mix of results.

The Weisberg et al. study referred to in the articles below found evidence of the "seductive allure" of neuroscience explanations.

> Our most important finding concerns the effect that explanatorily irrelevant neuroscience information has on subject's judgments of the explanations. For novices and students, the addition of such neuroscience information encouraged them to judge the explanations more favorably, particularly the bad explanations. That is, extraneous neuroscience information makes explanations look more satisfying than they actually are, or at least more satisfying than they otherwise would be judged to be. . . .
>
> Because it is unlikely that the popularity of neuroscience findings in the public sphere will wane any time soon, we see in the current results more reasons for caution when applying neuroscientific findings to social issues. Even if expert practitioners can easily distinguish good neuroscience explanations from bad, they must not assume that those outside the discipline will be as discriminating.

Deena S. Weisberg et al., *The Seductive Allure of Neuroscience Explanations*, 20 J. Cogn. Neurosci. 470, 475-77 (2008). Weisberg et al. followed up their initial study with more experiments, confirming the seductive allure "effect is robust against changes to an explanation's length and to the terms in which the neuroscience information is described, [and] implying that preventing the seductive allure effect from happening may be difficult." Deena Skolnick Weisberg, Jordan C. V. Taylor & Emily J. Hopkins, *Deconstructing the Seductive Allure of Neuroscience Explanations*, 10 Judgment & Decision Making 429, 440 (2015).

Why is neuroscience alluring, and is there something unique about neuroscience? The consensus seems to be that it is *not* the image itself. Evidence from further experiments conducted by Weisberg's group suggests that it is the reductionist explanation that lay people find most appealing. In a series of experiments, the group tested the hypothesis that the seductive allure "is due to a general preference for reductive explanations, which means that it should manifest across different scientific domains." The "data support[ed] this hypothesis: Participants judged explanations containing irrelevant reductive information as bétter across a range of sciences. The seductive allure effect is thus not unique to the pairing of psychology and neuroscience." Deena Skolnick Weisberg, Jordan C. V. Taylor & Emily J. Hopkins, *The Seductive Allure is a Reductive Allure: People Prefer Scientific Explanations that Contain Logically Irrelevant Reductive Information*, 155 Cognition 67, 75 (2016).

Nicholas Scurich & Adam Shniderman
The Selective Allure of Neuroscientific Explanations
9 PLoS One e107529 (2014)

[W]e predict that, rather than a universal seductive allure, neuroscience will have a 'selective' allure depending on how it corresponds to one's predisposition about the issue for which it is proffered. Specifically, neuroscience will be appealing when it supports one's predisposition but not convincing when it is incongruent with one's predisposition. Such a finding would qualify claims that, in the eyes of the public, neuroscience will be able to definitively settle fundamental questions about human nature. It would also replicate the phenomenon of motivated reasoning in a new domain.

[The study included experiments on neuroscience and the death penalty, and on neuroscience and abortion. In the death penalty experiment, participants were assigned to either a group learning that fMRI studies show that neuroscience indicates the death penalty is a deterrent, or that neuroscience does not. Similarly, in the abortion experiment, participants were assigned either to a group that was told neuroscience suggests that fetuses experience pain, or to a group that did not. —EDS.]

> [In conclusion,] [t]wo independent experiments unequivocally supported the selective allure hypothesis. Whether neuroscience can provide the sort of objective truth that some commentators advert to, neuroscience is apparently not treated as objective by laypersons. Consistent with copious research from other domains, neuroscience is more likely to be accepted and credited when it confirms prior beliefs. Thus, while neuroscience might be viewed as more scientific in the abstract, it is unlikely to play a qualitatively different role in the way in which it shapes people's beliefs and informs issues of social policy. . . .

Martha J. Farah & Cayce J. Hook
The Seductive Allure of "Seductive Allure"
8 Perspect. Psychol. Sci. 88, 88-89 (2013)

As a tool for studying the human mind and brain, functional MRI has been subject to various criticisms. One often cited problem with fMRI is that the images are too dazzling, that is, that they cloud readers' judgment and mask the technology's limitations. As early as the 1990's neuroimaging has been described with the word "seductive." William Uttal (2011), a vocal critic of functional neuroimaging research in psychology, asserts, "Their charm, their novelty, and their pictorial splendor tend to overwhelm critical consideration. . . ." Whereas Roskies (2010) cautiously observes "Neuroimages are epistemically compelling: They invite us to believe," more pointed references to this problem come from Bloom (2006) who writes of "fMRI's seductive but deceptive grasp on our attentions" and Crawford (2008) who refers to neuroimaging as "that fast acting solvent of critical faculties" (p. 65). According to Poole (2012), "the [fMRI] pictures, like religious icons, inspire uncritical devotion."

What is the evidence for the seductive allure of brain imaging? The most frequently cited findings come from two articles published in 2008. McCabe and Castel (2008) assessed the effects of functional brain images on the perceived quality of cognitive neuroscience research. Using both fictional research descriptions and a real science news article, they documented higher ratings of credibility when the texts were accompanied by functional brain images compared to bar charts, topographical maps of scalp recorded EEG, or no image. . . . [Farah and Hook go on to critique the methodology of these two studies.—EDS.]

Despite their limitations, these two studies from 2008 have been cited hundreds of times in subsequent years as proof of brain images' power to overwhelm our judgment. Surprisingly little additional evidence has been published in support of the disproportionate persuasiveness of brain images. Specifically, to our knowledge only one subsequent published study has reported effects of functional brain images on ratings of scientific credibility, and this study did not compare ratings with and without images. . . .

Given the paucity of published support for the seductive allure hypothesis, the weaknesses in that support, and the recent null results, it is remarkable that the hypothesis has persisted. Why might this be? . . .

Adina L. Roskies, Nicholas J. Schweitzer & Michael J. Saks
Neuroimages in Court: Less Biasing Than Feared
17 Trends Cogn. Sci. 99, 99-100 (2013)

Because neuroimages have the potential to seem more "real" than other kinds of evidence and are a product of neuroscience—a field typically considered a "hard" science—brain images might have unusual impact as legal evidence. Brain images resemble photographs and laypersons might view them as simple and direct pictures of brain activity. Of course, brain imaging is not photography and is neither direct nor inferentially straightforward. The layperson is unaware of the many steps involved in producing a neuroimage and relating it to a particular cognitive process or capacity. . . .

Several studies tend to support the hypothesis that neuroscience information affects people's reasoning adversely. Weisberg et al. found that participants were able to distinguish good from bad scientific explanations when no neuroscientific information was included. However, when neuroscientific information was added, poor logic appeared sound. The authors interpreted their findings to suggest that laypeople are "dazzled by neurobabble." Although that study did not explicitly test the effect of neuroimages, another did. McCabe and Castel examined whether brain images affect people's judgments of scientific credibility. They found that, when neuroimages accompanied scientific summaries, the summaries were rated as more scientifically credible and sound than the summaries presented alone or paired with graphs.

These studies did not examine people's reasoning in legal contexts. However, a few studies do. Gurley and Marcus found that mock jurors were more likely to reach a verdict of not guilty by reason of insanity (NGRI) if psychiatric diagnoses were supplemented with anatomical brain images and McCabe et al. report a mock-trial experiment where functional MRI used for lie detection was significantly more persuasive than other technologies (e.g., polygraphs or thermal imaging lie-detection).

All these studies are consistent with the possibility that brain images are biasing or misleading, and many legal commentators have taken them as such. However, none of these studies isolate the effect of neuroimages *per se* while also setting the study in the context of a trial.

A different picture emerges from a series of new studies targeting the effects of neuroimages in the courtroom. Schweitzer et al. designed four experiments to isolate the effects of neuroimage evidence: laypersons were presented with mock trials containing various kinds of expert testimony. After being presented with the case, evidence, and legal instructions, participants were asked to evaluate the evidence and render a verdict and other judgments.

By using various control conditions, these experiments assessed the impact of neuroimages on juror decisions separately from the effects of other information in the trial. Various groups were presented with verbal expert testimony of psychologists, neuropsychologists, or neuroscientists, as well as a no-expert control. The neuroscience testimony was paired with brain images, graphs, or a neutral image (a courtroom). Expert testimony reflected what is typical in such cases. Among other measures, jurors provided judgments of criminal liability and punishment recommendations.

Neuroscientific evidence was introduced by the defense as exculpatory, supporting the claim that the defendant lacked necessary elements of criminal culpability. However, in experiments with crimes ranging from homicide to unintentional assault, the authors found no evidence that neuroimages influenced jurors' decisions about criminal liability or sentences. Convictions and punishments were, however, related to the level of perceived control by the defendant, and this was affected by the presence and kind of expert testimony—but not by neuroimages.

A subsequent experiment by Schweitzer and Saks examined the potential impact of brain images in insanity cases. Given the results from Gurley and Marcus, one might expect neuroimages to affect NGRI verdicts. However, Gurley and Marcus did not dissociate the effects of the neuroimage from those of the neurological expert testimony. Schweitzer and Saks did, and found no impact of neuroimages over and above the effects of verbal neuroscience testimony, while replicating the earlier findings that neuroscientific testimony was more effective in securing NGRI verdicts than psychological testimony. (Interestingly, mock jurors presented with no expert evidence rated neuroimages as the kind of evidence that they would have found most helpful.)

In summary, these recent studies asking whether neuroimages are biasing in trials where criminal liability is at issue found no inordinate effects—or any impact at all beyond that of conventional neuroscience expert testimony. . . .

The neuroimages used in the Schweitzer et al. experiments contained no information beyond that contained in the expert testimony, thus allowing assessment of whether images produced effects over and above the admissible verbal testimony. That is, the research asked whether images qua images affect jurors unduly. Contrary to expectation, no evidence emerged that neuroimages are biasing or misleading in forensic contexts. Indeed, the findings suggest that brain images have no special impact on juror decision-making beyond the neuroscientific testimony.

The studies described above were limited in scope, focusing on issues of exculpation in criminal cases. However, the issue of mitigation of punishment of convicted defendants is where neuroimages might have their greatest impact. Indeed, that is what was found in two studies of the penalty phase of capital cases, where neuroimages reduced the execution rate of psychopathic defendants.

These studies have an immediate practical implication. If neuroimages cannot be excluded as evidence and if neuroscience evidence is found to be mitigating in sentencing, neuroimages might come to be routinely offered as evidence in capital cases. Then, it will be increasingly important that judges and jurors be sufficiently educated to understand the ways in which neuroimaging evidence can be relevant to legal questions and to recognize when they are not. Devising effective ways of educating legal actors will be essential. Second, given the apparent impact of neuroscience testimony relative to non-neuroscientific testimony and the current costs of neuroimaging, as well as the importance of cross-examination to putting neuroscience in perspective, such evidence could exacerbate the effects of economic inequalities among defendants.

Moreover, some believe that neuroimaging will play a major role in civil law in the future, such as in tort and worker compensation cases. Research on the effects of imaging evidence in civil cases — where the threshold of proof for deciding liability is in closer balance — is needed.

The question of how probative neuroscience evidence is for the law remains an open one and the answer will depend on the precise techniques used and legal circumstances. . . .

There have been many additional experimental studies. A sampling of their findings includes:

- In a study of Swiss and French judges, judges were recruited to participate in an experiment that compared an expert report including neuroscientific data with a report that did not. The treatment group was told that "the neurobiological evaluation . . . [detected] . . . the presence of lesions in the frontal lobes of the brain which could have been produced by accidental traumas" and that "[a]n evaluation of the brain's structure . . . showed statistically significant differences . . . compared with a group of subjects of the same sex and same age group." The study found that "judges are more likely to criticize and to find shortcomings and omissions in expert reports when they do not contain neuroscience data," but also that "a minority of judges cited criticisms of brain imaging data, mentioning their unreliability, their hypothetical nature or the lack of a direct link between the brain and violent behavior." Valerie Moulin et al., *Judges' Perceptions of Expert Reports: The Effect of Neuroscience Evidence*, 61 Int'l J.L. & Psychiatry 22, 24-26 (2018).

- "Many authors initially cautioned that the glitzy brain images accompanying popular science news and neuroscientific expert testimony would be oversimplified, misinterpreted, and granted undeserved scientific credibility by those unfamiliar with the technology. While early research on the perception of neuroimages by the public substantiated this warning, the bulk of subsequent research has largely undermined these findings. Specifically, when neuroimages do sway judgments, it is only under specific conditions that are not yet well understood; as such, an overarching theory is still out of reach. This means the use of neuroimages to convey information to laypersons should continue to be scrutinized as the context and framing in which they are presented changes." Denise A. Baker et al., *Making Sense of Research on The Neuroimage Bias*, 26 Pub. Understanding Sci. 251, 256 (2015).

- Utilizing a contrastive vignette experiment involving the diagnosis of an impulse control disorder following a sexual assault, a study "observed three key findings: (1) Both brain evidence and psychological evidence had mitigating effects on prison sentences, but the mitigating effect of brain evidence was stronger. (2) Yet that same brain evidence evoked relative increases in involuntary hospitalization terms. (3) The variation in sentencing judgments was best explained by deontological considerations pertaining to moral culpability." Corey H. Allen et al., *Reconciling the Opposing Effects of Neurobiological Evidence on Criminal Sentencing Judgments*, 14 PLoS One e0210584 (2019).

• Examining the interactive effect of strength of case in a series of experiments, a study "found that although there is a statistically significant relationship between exposure to neuroscientific information and subjects' evaluations of the fictional defendant, the neuroscientific evidence was not as powerful a predictor as the overall strength of the case in determining outcomes. Our primary conclusion is that subjects are cognizant of, but not seduced by, brain-based memory recognition evidence. Subjects consider the evidence, and it has an effect in some contexts on their evaluations, but they generally weigh it as just one of many facts on the record." Francis X. Shen et al., *The Limited Effect of Electroencephalography Memory Recognition Evidence on Assessments of Defendant Credibility*, 4 J.L. & Biosci. 330, 333 (2017).

NOTES AND QUESTIONS

1. In a 2014 study, another experimental study led by Michael Saks *did* find an effect of neuroimages on jury-eligible subjects' decisions to assign life-in-prison or the death penalty to a hypothetical convicted murderer. What might explain the different findings across the different legal contexts? Michael J. Saks et al., *The Impact of Neuroimages in the Sentencing Phase of Capital Trials*, 11 J. Empirical Legal Stud. 105 (2014).

2. What should courts do in the face of contradictory research findings and interpretations, for instance between the Weisberg studies and others? If it is unknown whether there is such seductive allure, how should courts and legislatures respond? Concerns about the prejudicial effects of other types of evidence are also infrequently examined by empirical analysis. David A. Bright & Jane Goodman-Delahunty, *Gruesome Evidence and Emotion: Anger, Blame, and Jury Decision-Making*, 30 L. & Hum. Behav. 183 (2006). Should all judicial assumptions be empirically tested, or in some instances should common sense assumptions prevail?

3. In his 2009 Gifford Lecture neuroscientist Michael Gazzaniga asked: "Is there something about our culture that actually believes more about these scans than the scientists who produce them?" How would you answer this question?

4. How do you come out on your Rule 403 balancing? Consider this view:

> Because of the scientific uncertainties, our legal conclusion has to be conditional: If brain images are as confusing and misleading in trial contexts as they seem to be in reported experiments, and if they lack much probative value because they cannot overcome the problems listed above, then their moderate dangers "substantially outweigh" their minimal probative value, so brain images fail the balancing test of FRE 403 and should not be admitted into trials. That is a lot of "if," but it is all that we can conclude for now. . . .

Walter Sinnott-Armstrong et al., *Brain Images as Legal Evidence*, 5 Episteme 359, 371 (2008).

5. Would jury instructions help to reduce the so-called seductive allure of neuroscientific evidence? *See* E. Spencer Compton, *Not Guilty by Reason of Neuroimaging: The Need for Cautionary Jury Instructions for Neuroscience Evidence in Criminal Trials*, 12 Vand. J. Ent. & Tech. L. 333 (2010). What happens when jurors are instructed

to ignore evidence they have already heard? *See* Linda J. Demaine, *In Search of the Anti-Elephant: Confronting the Human Inability to Forget Inadmissible Evidence*, 16 Geo. Mason L. Rev. 99 (2008). Can you think of a law-relevant neuroscientific experiment to investigate this phenomenon?

6. Might there be an alternative, in which the judge improves jurors' "visual literacy"? Consider law professor Neal Feigenson's argument:

> In any given legal proceeding there may be real concerns about the reliability and relevance of fMRI-based expert testimony. Some of the fundamental questions raised by the contestable assumptions and varying methods underlying the creation and interpretation of fMRI data recommend a highly cautious approach to this evidence in general, at least given the present state of the science. Assuming, however, that the experts are qualified and that the testimony satisfies the basic criteria for admissibility, the law should not respond to the problems that the courtroom display of fMRIs may pose for good legal judgment by barring the images. Instead, the judges should admit the images (as appropriate) and seek to enhance everyone's visual literacy—that of the jurors, the lawyers and the judges themselves—so that legal judgments can, insofar as possible, be rendered consistently with the best available scientific knowledge.

Neal Feigenson, *Brain Imaging and Courtroom Evidence: On the Admissibility and Persuasiveness of fMRI*, 2 Int'l J.L. Context 233, 251 (2006).

7. In what other legal contexts might imaging evidence emerge? Researchers in 2009 reported success in performing "virtual autopsies"—using computed tomography (CT) to create images of dead bodies. *A Cut from CSI*, Economist (Dec. 12, 2009). Would such imagery, if deemed an accurate assessment of how the victim perished, be admissible? Why or why not?

FURTHER READING

Scientific Evidence:

David L. Faigman et al., *Modern Scientific Evidence: The Law and Science of Expert Testimony* (2019-2020 ed.).

Federal Judicial Center, *Reference Manual on Scientific Evidence* (3d ed. 2011).

Erin Murphy, *Neuroscience and the Civil/Criminal* Daubert *Divide*, 85 Fordham L. Rev. 619 (2016).

Neuroscience Evidence in the Courtroom:

Neuroimaging in Forensic Psychiatry: From the Clinic to the Courtroom (Joseph R. Simpson ed., 2012).

Teneille R. Brown & Emily R. Murphy, *Through a Scanner Darkly: Functional Neuroimaging as Evidence of a Criminal Defendant's Past Mental States*, 62 Stan. L. Rev. 1119 (2010).

Joseph H. Baskin, Judith G. Edersheim & Bruce H. Price, *Is a Picture Worth a Thousand Words? Neuroimaging in the Courtroom*, 33 Am. J. L. & Med. 239 (2007).

Stephen J. Morse, *Actions Speak Louder Than Images: The Use of Neuroscientific Evidence in Criminal Cases*, 3 J. L. & Biosciences 336 (2016).

Owen D. Jones et al., *Neuroscientists in Court*, 14 Nature Revs. Neurosci. 730 (2013).

Judith G. Edersheim et al., *Neuroimaging, Diminished Capacity, and Mitigation*, in *Neuroimaging in Forensic Psychiatry: From the Clinic to the Courtroom* 163 (Joseph Simpson ed., 2012).

Nat'l Acads. of Sci. et al., Engineering, and Med., *Neuroforensics: Exploring the Legal Implications of Emerging Neurotechnologies: Proceedings of a Workshop* (Nat'l Acads. Press 2018).

The Use and Abuse of Neuroimaging in the Courtroom (Special Issue), 5(2) Am. J. Neuro. (2014).

Joseph J. Avery, *Picking and Choosing: Inconsistent Use of Neuroscientific Legal Evidence*, 81 Alb. L. Rev. 941 (2018).

International Use of Neuroscience Evidence in Court:

Australia: Armin Alimardani & Jason Chin, *Neurolaw in Australia: The Use of Neuroscience in Australian Criminal Proceedings*, 12 Neuroethics 255 (2019).

Germany: Daniela Guillen Gonzalez et al., *Neuroscientific and Genetic Evidence in Criminal Cases: A Double-Edged Sword in Germany but Not in the United States?*, 10 Front. Psychol. 2343 (2019).

Iran: Armin Alimardani, *Neuroscience, Criminal Responsibility and Sentencing in an Islamic Country: Iran*, 5 J.L. & Biosci. 724 (2018).

Italy: Michele Farisco & Carlo Petrini, *On the Stand: Another Episode of Neuroscience and Law Discussion from Italy*, 7 Neuroethics 243 (2014).

Slovenia: Miha Hafner, *Judging Homicide Defendants by their Brains: An Empirical Study on the Use of Neuroscience in Homicide Trials in Slovenia*, 6 J.L. & Biosci. 226 (2019).

CORE THEMES IN LAW AND NEUROSCIENCE

Let's take stock. In Part 1 you were introduced to some of the main themes of Law and Neuroscience. In Part 2 you learned some brain basics—such as how brains are structured, how brains function, and what modern neuroscience techniques can—and cannot—do to measure that brain function in legally relevant ways. Part 3 considered the relationship of law, science, and behavior and witnessed the special advantages of, and corresponding challenges raised by, the use of scientific evidence in careful, accurate, and legally relevant ways.

We turn now, in Part 4, to examine the core themes for which you are now prepared. Many of these involve controversies that are currently percolating in courts and legislatures around the country. As you read and critically evaluate the materials and issues in these chapters, you will see how now-familiar themes of law and science are encountering brand new capabilities, opportunities, and challenges that arise when advances in neuroscience are heralded (for better or worse) as responses to the needs of the legal system—and the needs of clients and constituencies within it.

PART SUMMARY

This Part:
- Explores the legal implications of *The Injured Brain*—with chapters on Brain Death, Brain Injury, Pain and Distress, and Addicted Brains.
- Examines the ways in which legal outcomes are determined by *The Thinking and Feeling Brain*—with chapters on Memory, Emotions, Lie Detection, and Judging.
- Considers the unique response of law to *The Developing and Aging Brain*—with chapters on Adolescent Brains and Aging Brains.

CHAPTER 9

Brain Death

The boundaries which divide Life from Death are at best shadowy and vague.
Who shall say where the one ends, and where the other begins?
— Edgar Allan Poe, "The Premature Burial"†

It just so happens that your friend here is only mostly dead. There's a big
difference between mostly dead and all dead.
— Miracle Max in *The Princess Bride*

CHAPTER SUMMARY

This chapter:
- Introduces the statutory definitions of death in the United States and the role of brain function in defining death.
- Surveys current scientific understanding of disorders of consciousness, including coma, vegetative state, and minimally conscious state.
- Explores ethical issues related to brain death and organ transplantation.

INTRODUCTION

One of the best-known and most contentious right-to-die cases involved a state legislature, the U.S. Congress, and an emergency bill signed by the President at 1:00 A.M. It began in February 1990, when at the age of 26, Terri Schiavo suffered a full cardiac arrest. Paramedics found her unconscious, with no respiration or pulse. They attempted to resuscitate her, and she was intubated and ventilated upon arrival at the hospital.

Schiavo remained in the hospital in a coma, and after two and a half months her doctors issued a "vegetative state" diagnosis. She would remain this way for many years, despite a variety of methods employed to restore her to a state of awareness (including electrical stimulation of her thalamus). In light of the failure of these many efforts, in 1998, Schiavo's husband Michael petitioned the Florida courts to remove her feeding tube. Schiavo's parents, however, opposed the removal of the tube and argued that she was actually still conscious.

The Florida judiciary determined that Schiavo would not wish to continue life-prolonging measures. So, on April 24, 2001, her feeding tube was removed, only to

---

† Edgar Allan Poe, *The Premature Burial*, in *The Complete Short Stories* 719, 720 (MysteriousPress.com & Open Rd. Integrated Media 2014) (1844).

be reinserted several days later. The feeding tube was reinserted after a different judge granted an injunction and held the case should be reheard based on new evidence (the testimony of a former romantic interest of Michael Schiavo affirming that he had told her that he never discussed end-of-life wishes with Terri). On February 25, 2005, a Florida judge ordered the removal of Terri Schiavo's feeding tube once again—at which point the federal government intervened, with President George W. Bush signing legislation tailored to Schiavo's situation. All subsequent appeals through the federal court system upheld the original decision to remove the feeding tube. Consequently, it was removed for the last time on March 18, 2005. Schiavo was declared dead several days later, 15 years after she first collapsed.

Legal controversies about brain death continue to abound. One of the most legally and ethically complex cases is the story of 13-year-old Jahi McMath. Jahi was declared brain dead in Oakland, California on December 12, 2013 as a result of complications following a surgical procedure. Jahi's doctors communicated to her family that she was dead, but Jahi's mother, Lathasha Winkfield, insisted that her daughter was still alive.

With the hospital ready to suspend life support, Jahi's family went to court, where it asked for an independent second opinion regarding the brain death diagnosis. The court's ruling is indicative of the controversy around brain death. On one hand, the court ruled that Jahi was legally dead. But the judge also ordered the hospital to temporarily maintain mechanical ventilation until the McMath family was able to find another medical facility willing to continue treating Jahi.

On January 5, 2014, Jahi was transported from the hospital to the Alameda County coroner. The coroner pronounced her dead, and a death certificate was issued. Then, still on life support, Jahi's body was released to her mother and transported to a Catholic hospital in New Jersey. Therefore, Jahi was for a period dead in California but alive in New Jersey. (You will read later in this chapter about how the laws of brain death in New Jersey and New York differ from those in other states.) In New Jersey, Jahi continued receiving life-sustaining treatment until her liver eventually failed. On June 20, 2018, nearly five years after she had been declared dead in California, the McMath family attorney issued a statement explaining that Jahi had died as a result of liver failure complications.

These and other cases prompt many questions that are relevant to the issue of death determination. When did Jahi McMath and Terri Schaivo actually "die"? And how should the law answer that question? In light of new neuroscientific discoveries and techniques, this chapter explores the ancient question: What is death? The answer to this question is important because the legal consequences of the line between being dead or non-dead are quite broad and touch on one's tax liability, the status of contracts and property ownership, insurance policies, and criminal liability, among other things.

Yet drawing a line between life and death is difficult, even more so when the contested concept of "brain death" is introduced. Although the term "brain dead" is now regularly used in the legal, medical, and social lexicons, it is not without its critics. Moreover, defining brain death necessarily means exploring a gray area between life and death, namely the existence of disorders of consciousness that are now recognized by medicine and include a variety of distinctive categories, such as comatose, vegetative state (persistent and permanent), and minimally conscious state.

This chapter explores brain death and disorders of consciousness with an emphasis on their legal and policy implications, as well as the potential utility of neuroscientific methods for diagnosis of death and communication with patients thought to be in states of unconsciousness. Section A presents a brief history of how law has defined death and current statutory definitions. Section B explains how clinicians determine death. Section C introduces a variety of disorders of consciousness: comas, vegetative states, and minimally conscious states. Section D presents four cases, one criminal and three civil, in which brain death was at issue. Section E presents advances in neuroscience research that are raising new challenges to existing legal paradigms of consciousness disorders and brain death.

Before proceeding, we invite you to turn back to Chapter 3, on brain structure and brain function, to remind yourself of the respective roles of the brainstem and the cerebral cortex in the sustaining the body and the mind. And as you read the materials in this chapter, pay close attention to how legal systems define brain death at present, and consider what modifications, if any, you think are warranted in the future.

A. DEFINING DEATH

The excerpts in this section discuss and illustrate some of the key efforts to define death.

1. Historical Perspective

In her 2011 book, *The Law of Life and Death*, law professor Elizabeth Foley provides historical perspective on the legal definition of death. Death is a salient moment in many areas of law. At death one's last will and testament becomes effective. At death charges of murder or manslaughter become possible. At death life insurance contracts must be satisfied. However, when does the law recognize that someone is actually "dead"?

Certainly, decomposition of the body would be a sure sign of death, but the law has commonly preferred earlier measures related to cessation of particular vital functions. This raises the question of which vital functions to assess; possibilities include heartbeat, respiration, liver function, and brain function. Certainly, each is vital for sustaining normal life, so each signals a meaningful point of no return.

Common law defined death by the cessation of respiration. This was useful historically because anyone could observe when another stopped breathing. Also, cessation of respiration was for most of history irreversible, although this of course changed with the discovery of methods of cardiopulmonary resuscitation. In addition, cessation of respiration was associated with cessation of heart function. This was important historically because the heart was regarded as the source of thought and emotion. Still, cessation of respiration was not a certain sign of death. False positive diagnoses of death happened when the cessation was temporary due to various conditions.

In the 1850s the stethoscope gained common use, and physicians shifted the criteria for death to cessation of respiration and heartbeat combined. With two vital functions monitored, physicians avoided premature burials. Today, cardiopulmonary death is recognized as death in all states. (See the UDDA below.) In spite of the current legal recognition of brain death as an alternative vital sign to diagnose death, nearly all deaths are still diagnosed using the cardiopulmonary criteria.

Then, in the 1950s further advances in medical knowledge and technology created challenges for defining death that remain today. One major development was the ability to transplant healthy vital organs from donors who were defined dead according to the cardiopulmonary definition of death. By 1970 it became possible to save thousands of lives through such transplants. The only problem was acquiring enough fresh, oxygenated, healthy organs.

Meanwhile, methods and machines were developed that enabled hearts, lungs, and other vital organs to function even when the brain did not. Vital functions could be sustained by ventilators, heart-lung machines, pacemakers, dialysis, and stomach tubes. Consequently, cessation of cardiopulmonary function no longer necessarily meant cessation of other vital functions. The body could be saved from cardiopulmonary death.

Thus, for the law to insist on the traditional cardiopulmonary definition of death would have limited the benefits that could be reaped from organ transplantation. Therefore, to harvest the freshest organs possible, the legal definition of death needed to be expanded. This expansion was afforded by the concept of brain death.

2. Defining Brain Death

Robert D. Truog, Thaddeus Mason Pope & David S. Jones
The 50-year Legacy of the Harvard Report on Brain Death
320 JAMA 335, 335 (2018)

On August 5, 1968, an ad hoc committee at Harvard Medical School published a landmark report that laid the groundwork for a new definition of death, based on neurological criteria. The authors, under the leadership of anesthesiologist Henry Beecher, stated that their primary purpose was to "define irreversible coma as a new criterion for death." The concept of brain death has guided clinical practice for 50 years even though vigorous debate about its legitimacy has never ceased.

The Committee, Its Contexts, and Its Recommendations

The development of positive pressure ventilators in the 1950s enabled physicians to extend the lives of people who previously would have died. Some of these patients had no discernible cognitive function. Were these lives worth extending? . . .

In September 1967, Beecher convened a committee to consider the "ethical problems created by the hopelessly unconscious patient." Debate has been substantial ever since about whether the committee's primary motivation was to resolve controversy about withdrawal of life support or to increase access to transplantable organs. The final report named both issues: (1) the burden on patients, families, and hospitals, of a patient "whose brain is irreversibly damaged"; and (2) the concern that "obsolete criteria for the definition of death can lead to controversy in obtaining organs for transplantation." . . .

Beecher's committee produced . . . specific criteria. Coma could be considered irreversible and a patient declared dead if, over a 24-hour period, the patient did not respond to stimuli, had no spontaneous movement or breathing, and had no reflexes; a flat electroencephalogram provided valuable confirmation of the cessa-tion of brain function. These criteria clarified circumstances under which clinicians could withdraw life support. . . .

A Definition of Irreversible Coma: Report of the Ad Hoc Committee of the *Harvard Medical School to Examine the Definition of Brain Death*
205 JAMA 337, 337-38 (1968)

CHARACTERISTICS OF IRREVERSIBLE COMA

An organ, brain or other, that no longer functions and has no possibility of functioning again is for all practical purposes dead. . . . The condition [of a per-manently nonfunctioning brain] can be satisfactorily diagnosed by points 1, 2, and 3 to follow. The electroencephalogram (point 4) provides confirmatory data, and when available it should be utilized. In situations where for one reason or another electroencephalographic monitoring is not available, the absence of cerebral func-tion has to be determined by purely clinical signs, to be described, or by absence of circulation as judged by standstill of blood in the retinal vessels, or by absence of cardiac activity.

1. *Unreceptivity and Unresponsitivity.*—There is a total unawareness to externally applied stimuli and inner need and complete unresponsiveness—our defini-tion of irreversible coma. Even the most intensely painful stimuli evoke no vocal or other response, not even a groan, withdrawal of a limb, or quickening of respiration.

2. *No Movements or Breathing.*—Observations covering a period of at least one hour by physicians is adequate to satisfy the criteria of no spontaneous muscular move-ments or spontaneous respiration or response to stimuli such as pain, touch, sound, or light. After the patient is on a mechanical respirator, the total absence of spontaneous breathing may be established by turning off the respirator for three minutes and observing whether there is any effort on the part of the sub-ject to breathe spontaneously. . . .

3. *No Reflexes.*—Irreversible coma with abolition of central nervous system activity is evidenced in part by the absence of elicitable reflexes. The pupil will be fixed and dilated and will not respond to a direct source of bright light. . . .

4. *Flat Electroencephalogram.*—Of great confirmatory value is the flat or isoelectric EEG. . . .

All of the above tests shall be repeated at least 24 hours later with no change.

3. Uniform Determination of Death Act

Motivated by the disparity arising between common law definitions of death and medical advances that could support respiration and circulation after brain function ceased, in the early 1980s the Uniform Determination of Death Act (UDDA) was drafted and approved by the National Conference of Commissioners on Uniform State Laws, in cooperation with the American Medical Association, the American Bar Association, and the President's Commission for the Study of Ethical Problems in Medicine and Biomedical and Behavioral Research. All 50 states have recognized neurological criteria for determining death. New Jersey and New York, however, have laws or regulations to accommodate persons who object on religious grounds to declarations of death grounded only in neurological criteria. Below is the UDDA, followed by current New York and New Jersey law.

Uniform Determination of Death Act (1980)

Be it enacted. . .

§1. [**Determination of Death**]. An individual who has sustained either (1) irreversible cessation of circulatory and respiratory functions, or (2) irreversible cessation of all functions of the entire brain, including the brain stem, is dead. A determination of death must be made in accordance with accepted medical standards.

§2. [**Uniformity of Construction and Application**]. This Act shall be applied and construed to effectuate its general purpose to make uniform the law with respect to the subject of this Act among states enacting it.

§3. [**Short Title**]. This Act may be cited as the Uniform Determination of Death Act.

N.Y. Comp. Codes R. & Regs. tit. 10, §400.16 (2020)
Section 400.16 - Determination of Death

(a) An individual who has sustained either:

(1) irreversible cessation of circulatory and respiratory functions; or

(2) irreversible cessation of all functions of the entire brain, including the brain stem, is dead.

(b) A determination of death must be made in accordance with accepted medical standards.

(c) Death, as determined in accordance with paragraph (a)(2) of this section, shall be deemed to have occurred as of the time of the completion of the determination of death.

(d) Prior to the completion of a determination of death of an individual in accordance with paragraph (a)(2) of this section, the hospital shall make reasonable efforts to notify the individual's next of kin or other person closest to the individual that such determination will soon be completed.

(e) Each hospital shall establish and implement a written policy regarding determinations of death in accordance with paragraph (a)(2) of this section. Such policy shall include:

(1) a description of the tests to be employed in making the determination;

(2) a procedure for the notification of the individual's next of kin or other person closest to the individual in accordance with subdivision (d) of this section; and

(3) a procedure for the reasonable accommodation of the individual's religious or moral objection to the determination as expressed by the individual, or by the next of kin or other person closest to the individual.

N.J. Stat. Ann. §26:6A-1 et seq. (West 2020)
New Jersey Declaration of Death Act

Section 26:6A-2. Recognition of traditional cardio-respiratory criteria. An individual who has sustained irreversible cessation of all circulatory and respiratory functions, as determined in accordance with currently accepted medical standards, shall be declared dead.

Section 26:6A-3. Recognition of modern neurological criteria. Subject to the standards and procedures established in accordance with this act, an individual whose circulatory and respiratory functions can be maintained solely by artificial means, and who has sustained irreversible cessation of all functions of the entire brain, including the brain stem, shall be declared dead.

Section 26:6A-4. Standards and procedures for declaration of death based upon neurological criteria.

   a. A declaration of death upon the basis of neurological criteria pursuant to section 3 of this act shall be made by a licensed physician professionally qualified by specialty or expertise, based upon the exercise of the physician's best medical judgment and in accordance with currently accepted medical standards that are based upon nationally recognized sources of practice guidelines, including, but not limited to, those adopted by the American Academy of Neurology. . . .

Section 26:6A-5. Exemption to accommodate personal religious belief. The death of an individual shall not be declared upon the basis of neurological criteria pursuant to sections 3 and 4 of this act when the licensed physician authorized to declare death, has reason to believe, on the basis of information in the individual's available medical records, or information provided by a member of the individual's family or any other person knowledgeable about the individual's personal religious beliefs that such a declaration would violate the personal religious beliefs of the individual. In these cases, death shall be declared, and the time of death fixed, solely upon the basis of cardio-respiratory criteria pursuant to section 2 of this act.

4. Proposed Changes to the Current System of Determination of Death by Neurologic Criteria

Since its initial publication, many experts have weighed in on the Uniform Determination of Death Act's criteria. In 2019, an expert panel convened by the American Academy of Neurology (AAN) proposed a revised set of criteria. Of particular concern to the AAN was that brain death litigation could "undermine public trust in medical determination of death." The expert report critiqued the UDDA and argued that "developments have exposed unresolved ambiguities in the legal rules governing determination of death that must be addressed." Ariana Lewis et al., *Determination of Death by Neurologic Criteria in the United States: The Case for Revising the Uniform Determination of Death Act*, 47 J. L. Med. & Ethics 9, 9-10 (2019).

Ariane Lewis et al.

Determination of Death by Neurologic Criteria in the United States: The Case for Revising the Uniform Determination of Death Act
47 J.L. Med. & Ethics 9, 16-20 (2019)

To complement the actions being taken by the medical community, legal experts and policymakers should collaborate to promote clarity and uniformity in state laws on determination of death. This includes (1) addressing . . . variation in the statutory language governing the determination of death; (2) identifying the "accepted medical standards" for making brain death determinations; and (3) providing a clear plan for management of family objections to use of neurologic criteria to declare death. Accomplishing this requires a model for a Revised Uniform Determination of Death Act. . . .

STATUTORY LANGUAGE GOVERNING DETERMINATION
OF DEATH BY NEUROLOGIC CRITERIA

There appears to be conflict between the language of the UDDA (which includes the phrase "all functions of the entire brain") and accepted medical standards (which do not require demonstration of pituitary/hypothalamic dysfunction to declare death by neurologic criteria). . . .

In our view, the safest way forward is to amend the UDDA. There are two ways to do so. The first, . . . is to modify the text to clarify which functions matter and why. To be specific, this would involve removing the elusive term "all" and replacing it with "irreversible cessation of functions of the entire brain, including the brainstem, *leading to unresponsive coma with loss of capacity for consciousness, brainstem areflexia, and the inability to breathe independently.*" . . .

Another option to consider would be to modify the statutory criteria for declaring death to refer to "irreversible cessation of all functions of the entire brain, including the brainstem, *with the exception of hormonal function.*" This language would clarify the law and bring it in line with medical standards while requiring minimal changes to the UDDA. . . .

ACCEPTED MEDICAL STANDARD FOR DETERMINATION
OF DEATH BY NEUROLOGIC CRITERIA

The identity of "accepted medical standards" should be clearly stated in law and not be left to case-by-case trial court rulings. . . .

MANAGEMENT OF FAMILY OBJECTIONS <u>BEFORE</u> DETERMINATION
OF DEATH BY NEUROLOGIC CRITERIA

. . . [W]e recommend amending the UDDA to state that, "reasonable efforts should be made to notify a patient's legally authorized decision-maker before performing a determination of death by neurologic criteria, but consent is not required to initiate such an evaluation." This formulation emphasizes that family awareness about performance of a brain death determination is important, but that practitioners do not need permission to perform an assessment. . . .

NOTES AND QUESTIONS

1. Why do the definitions refer explicitly to the "brain stem"? Would the AAN's proposed statutory changes provide more clarity, or would ambiguity remain?
2. Consider *People v. Selwa*, in which the defendant crashed into a pregnant woman's car, leading to the delivery, via Caesarean section, of a six-and-a-half-month-old fetus. The question for the court was whether the baby was "born alive" such that a charge of negligent homicide could be brought. In defining life, the court wrote:

   > Because it is axiomatic that one who is not dead is alive and vice versa, we find that the definition of "death" becomes as equally helpful as the definition of "live birth" in determining whether a child was "born alive" and hence is a "person." If one is not born dead, one is born alive and vice versa. Although the definitions of "death" and its counterpart "life" do not include the term "birth," i.e., the extraction or expulsion of the fetus, Guthrie has held that an unborn fetus is not a person under

the negligent homicide statute. Thus, it is really the word "alive" that is the immediate subject of controversy.

People v. Selwa, 543 N.W.2d 321 (Mich. Ct. App. 1995). Do you agree with the court's analysis?

3. To what extent does and should "but for" reasoning play a role in the legal definition of death? For instance, if an individual would not be able to breathe *but for* a respirator, what effect (if any) should that have on the legal definition of death? What if an individual's heart will beat only with the help of a pacemaker? What if an individual can breathe only with the help of an oxygen tank? What distinctions should the law make between different types of mechanical aids in sustaining vital functions?

4. Determining time of death has important implications for property transfer at the time of death. *See* Restatement (Third) of Property: Wills & Donative Transfers) §1.2 (Am. Law Inst.1999). What problems of proof would be introduced in property law if brain death criteria were more routinely used? Could neuroscience provide the necessary proof?

5. Very early in the morning of August 5, 2013, 37-year-old Anthony Yahle had trouble breathing. Anthony's wife called 911, and he was taken to an Ohio hospital in cardiac arrest. That afternoon, his situation became grave. Anthony "had no electrical motion, no respiration . . . no heartbeat, and no blood pressure," and accordingly Dr. Raja Nazir, the treating cardiologist, declared him dead. Upon this pronouncement, Anthony's 17-year-old son came into the hospital room with the family's pastor. Lawrence told his father, "Dad you're not going to die today." A few minutes later, doctors noticed trace electrical electivity on the heart monitor and continued resuscitation efforts that ultimately proved successful. While rare, there are similar reported cases of air getting trapped, which prevents blood flow. Sustaining resuscitation efforts can eventually facilitate the flow. As Dr. Michael Sayre, spokesperson for the American Heart Association, said about the case, "You can be faked out." Barbara Mantel, *'Dead' Man's Recovery Shows Why Prolonged CPR Works*, NBC News (Aug. 22, 2013). Do stories such as this affect your thinking on brain death?

6. Maureen Condic proposes two criteria for the determination of death that are "stringent enough to avoid classifying the living as dead . . . but not so stringent that they require us to wait until every cell has died before declaring death." A human being will be alive so long as he shows either (1) "persistence of any form of brain function" or (2) "persistence of autonomous integration of vital functions." Under this theory, individuals in a persistent vegetative state, with high-level cervical spinal cord injury, or those who are unconscious and depend on artificial medical interventions but still have some kind of brain function, are deemed alive. On the contrary, an individual whose brain (including the brain stem) shows an irreversible cessation of all functions, is deemed dead. Maureen L. Condic, *Determination of Death: A Scientific Perspective on Biological Integration*, 41 J. Med. & Phil 257, 257-65 (2016). Do you agree with Condic's criteria for death determination? Is any form of brain function, no matter how deteriorated, enough to determine an individual is not dead? For a counter argument to Maureen Condic's theory, see E. Christian Brugger, *Are Brain Dead Individuals Dead? Grounds for Reasonable Doubt*, 41 J. Med. & Phil. 329 (2016).

7. Some religions understand death in a way that is incompatible with the current medical definition of brain death. For example, the Islamic scriptures describe in detail the signs that distinguish between life and death: Death is demarcated by the soul's departure from the body, and the soul will be considered to remain present in an individual so long as there is heart beating and breathing, regardless of whether these are aided by artificial ventilation. Therefore, in cases such as *Re A (A Child)* [2015] EWHC 443 (Fam) (in which a 19-month-old child was declared brain dead after choking on a small piece of fruit and going into cardiac arrest), a child that has been declared dead by a physician could still be considered alive by the Muslim community. For a further discussion regarding the discrepancies between the current medical and legal, neurological criteria for death and the Quranic definition of death, see Mohamed Y. Rady & Joseph L. Verheijde, *Legislative Enforcement of Nonconsensual Determination of Neurological (Brain) Death in Muslim Patients: A Violation of Religious Rights*, 57 J. Religion & Health 649 (2018).

8. The Roman Catholic church, through a statement made by Pope John Paul II, accepted the determination of death on the basis of "complete and irreversible cessation of all brain activity." However, such acceptance presupposed that total brain failure "inevitably marks the loss of human integration." A group of Catholic scholars participated in a Symposium on the Definition of Death and debated the validity of neurological criteria for the determination of death in light of evidence showing that "a higher degree of integration [than previously thought] can persist in the human body after total brain failure. . . ." For a discussion of Catholic points of unanimous and broad agreement regarding determination of brain by neurological criteria, see Melissa Moschella & Maureen L. Condic, *Symposium on the Definition of Death: Summary Statement*, 41 J. Med. & Phil. 351 (2016).

9. Some states are silent on the amount of deference that physicians should give to a patient's religious beliefs when choosing between the allowed methods to determine death. Other states, such as New Jersey (see excerpt above), provide a religious exception to the use of neurological criteria. Consider this review of how states might make religious accommodations:

> How much accommodation of these objections should be permissible by law? There are four options. . . . New Jersey . . . prohibits providers from declaring death until irreversible cessation of circulatory and respiratory function has occurred if a patient has religious or moral beliefs that death by neurologic criteria is not death. . . . California and New York['s approach] . . . does not impact the occurrence or time of death, yet encourages providers to "reasonably accommodate" religious objections. . . . [The] Illinois [approach] . . . [indicates] that religious and moral beliefs *should be taken into consideration* when determining time of death. Lastly, states could . . . declare that religious and moral beliefs *should not be taken into consideration* either when determining occurrence or time of death or when determining whether to continue organ support.

Ariana Lewis et al., *Determination of Death by Neurologic Criteria in the United States: The Case for Revising the Uniform Determination of Death Act*, 47 J. L. Med. & Ethics 9, 20 (2019). Which approach seems best, given the challenges in brain death determination discussed above?

10. The 2006 AAN Practice Parameters for neurological evaluation after cardiac arrest provide for prognostication at 72 hours in order to determine whether to withdraw life-sustaining treatment. However, these parameters were issued before therapeutic hypothermia was introduced as a neuroprotective intervention. Therapeutic hypothermia seems to decrease the proportion of patients who progress to brain death, and in certain cases, may result in awakening of patients beyond 72 hours. A study by Maximilian Mulder et al. shows that with the current guidelines, as many as 36% of post-cardiac arrest comatose patients are deprived of the opportunity to awake and have a good neurological outcome. Should current guidelines be updated to reflect changes in technology and treatment? Is it possible to create a set of guidelines flexible enough to withstand the passage of time? *See* Maximilian Mulder et al., *Awakening and Withdrawal of Life-Sustaining Treatment in Cardiac Arrest Survivors Treated with Therapeutic Hypothermia*, 42 Critical Care Med. J. 2493 (2014). For a discussion of other issues arising from the application of the current AAN Practice guidelines, see Natalie Gillson et al., *A Brain Death Dilemma: Apnea Testing While on High-Frequency Oscillatory Ventilation*, 135 Pediatrics e5 (2015); Eelco F.M. Wijdicks, *Who Improves from Coma, How Do They Improve, and Then What?*, 14 Nature Reviews Neurology 694 (2018).

11. How would we know if someone declared "brain dead" could be revived? The Reanima Project was a nonrandomized, open-labeled, interventional study initiated in India to document the feasibility of reversing brain death. This research study was quickly terminated due to claims that it was unethical and did not adhere to accepted scientific standards. Should researchers be allowed to study whether someone can be 'brought back from the dead'? *See* Mohamed Y. Rady & Joseph L. Verheijde, *Advancing Neuroscience Research in Brain Death: An Ethical Obligation to Society*, 39 J. Critical Care 293 (2017).

B. CLINICAL DETERMINATION OF BRAIN DEATH

The clinical diagnosis of brain death is rare, but when it is made the "overriding principle is that the diagnosis of brain death is a step-wise, systematic clinical process." Eelco F.M. Wijdicks, *Brain Death* 27 (2d ed., 2011). One of the standard tests is the *apnea test*, in which the ventilator is turned off and the physicians observe the patient's chest for spontaneous breathing. The Quality Standards Subcommittee of the American Academy of Neurology has issued standards for administering the apnea test, and when properly administered and evaluated, it can be used to make a determination of brain death in conjunction with other criteria.

There remains debate in the medical profession about which tests should be used to confirm brain death or whether these tests should be used at all. In the excerpt below, neurologist Eelco Wijdicks argues against the usage of confirmatory tests. As you read the excerpt, consider the relationship between clinical assessment (e.g., the physician observing the patient's response during the apnea test) and brain-based data (e.g., an EEG assessment).

Eelco Wijdicks
*The Case Against Confirmatory Tests for Determining Brain
Death in Adults*
75 Neurology 77, 81 (2010)

Truly, no reason exists for continuing confirmatory testing in brain death determination. For physicians to rely on these tests—or worse, to use the tests with the most
suitable results when multiple tests have been performed—is ill advised. . . .

The main reasons why confirmatory tests can be dismissed are as follows:

1. The "confirmatory" tests do not confirm anything. Brain death is synonymous
   with a certain clinical state and a certain set of findings (coma, apnea, and no
   brainstem reflexes in the absence of confounders) and no prototypical neuro-
   pathologic substrate exists.
2. There is no real need for confirmatory tests. Most countries do not demand
   confirmatory tests to declare brain death. The ones that do have no persuasive
   reason other than using it as "a safeguard."
3. The costs to the patient are substantial, particularly when multiple tests are performed. Confusion abounds when test results do not match.
4. A protocol for organ donation after cardiac death can be initiated for patients
   who have no brainstem reflexes but whose clinical condition is too unstable for
   them to undergo an apnea test.

The diagnosis of brain death has always been understood as an evaluation
that uses a set of clinical criteria. As it turns out, when neurologic examination
finds evidence of brain death, the findings are irrevocably true and no recovery
of function has ever been documented. Confirmatory tests for adults would not
be needed, especially if these tests are less than perfect. Also, neurologists are
unique in this respect. Imagine cardiologists being forced to confirm absence
of ventricular contractility with an echocardiogram in an apneic, cyanotic
patient, to attempt to perform an ECG-gated CT of the heart when uncertain,
and, despite that, to continue to search for a better test to exclude myocardial
contraction.

The central message is that a comprehensive clinical evaluation of brain death
is diagnostically accurate when done by skillful specialists, preferably in the neurosciences, who likely better appreciate potential confounders. This may include
a sufficient time of observation before starting the examination but one careful
clinical neurologic examination should suffice. (In some U.S. states and other countries, confirmation by a second physician may be required.) Clinical determination
of brain death is by no means simple. There are no "recoveries" on record other
than those highlighted in the media and in each instance were based on errors
and underappreciation of the careful stepwise process that starts with excluding
confounding factors. On the contrary, the diagnostic accuracy of cardiac death is
less than perfect, with well-documented cases of autoresuscitation after cardiopulmonary resuscitation.

One of my core tenets is that "confirmatory" tests for brain death are residua
from the earlier days of refining a clinical entity, now known as brain death. These
ancillary tests are not accurate, not conclusive, not pertinent, and not warranted.

To put it another way, a clinical neurologic examination is worthy all on its own and more than good enough.

NOTES AND QUESTIONS

1. A counter argument to the theory that confirmatory tests should be dismissed is that the clinical evaluation alone may produce human errors, particularly when physicians do not adhere to the established protocols and guidelines for brain death diagnosis. For example, Lionel Zuckier argues: "Radiographic testing before retrieval of organs from donors who meet clinical brain death criteria might provide conclusive evidence of permanent and irreversible loss of brain function, and more-routine use of ancillary brain flow analyses might reduce errors." Lionel S. Zuckier, *Radionuclide Evaluation of Brain Death in the Post-McMath Era*, 57(10) J. Nuclear Med. 1560, 1566 (2016). Is there a need of confirmatory tests? What is the right balance between achieving an accurate diagnosis and avoiding unnecessary or excessive medical costs?

2. If a physician suspects an individual might be brain dead, the physician proceeds to perform a neurological determination of death evaluation. If the results of the evaluation lead to the conclusion of brain death, then the patient is declared dead and appropriate decisions regarding withdrawal of life-sustaining care and donation of organs are made. Osamu Muramoto proposes an alternative to the current method via the introduction of more robust informed consent from the caregivers for the individual. The informed consent approach recognizes that some caregivers do not want their family members to be declared brain dead for religious, cultural, or other reasons. Under the informed consent proposal, family members could choose whether the death of their loved one would be assessed based on a cardio-pulmonary standard, or by a brain death standard. *See* Osamu Muramoto, *Informed Consent for the Diagnosis of Brain Death: A Conceptual Argument*, 11 Phil Ethics & Human. Med. 8 (2016).

C. COMA, VEGETATIVE STATE, AND MINIMALLY CONSCIOUS STATE

Brain injury can lead not only to brain death, but also to something short of brain death—a biological state in which an individual retains some, but not all, bodily and mental functioning. These "disorders of consciousness" are frequently portrayed in popular media and cinema: A character descends into a coma but recovers at a key moment in the plot. Such popular representations do not adequately capture the delineation of different types of states that clinicians now recognize.

The first excerpt of this section clarifies the different disorders of consciousness and raises some of the ethical questions related to them. The next two excerpts discuss neuroscientific advances in evaluating and communicating with patients who have these disorders. Although these diagnoses may bear on end-of-life decision-making (e.g., the Terri Schiavo case), no jurisdiction in the United States currently equates any of these disorders of consciousness with "death" itself. As you read the excerpts, consider whether there are any circumstances in which you would change the definition of death to include any of these other states of minimal (or no) consciousness.

Joseph J. Fins

Brain Injury: The Vegetative and Minimally Conscious States

in The Hastings Ctr., *From Birth to Death and Bench to Clinic: The Hastings Center Bioethics Briefing Book for Journalists, Policymakers, and Campaigns* 15-20 (Mary Crowley ed., 2008)

TERMINOLOGY: DEFINING DIFFERENT BRAIN STATES

Much to the confusion of lay readers, there are a host of newly defined brain states (and their acronyms, such as MCS and MCS-e) beyond the ubiquitous but still confusing PVS, or persistent vegetative state. These categories for different disorders of consciousness have both clinical and ethical implications.

The persistent vegetative state was first described in 1972 by the Scottish neurosurgeon Bryan Jennett and the American neurologist Fred Plum. In a landmark article in the British journal *The Lancet*, they described PVS as a state of "wakeful unresponsiveness" in which the eyes are open, but there is no awareness of self or others. Patients who are vegetative do not have cognitive or higher brain functions, such as the ability to think and reason. But they do have autonomic ones, such as the direction of cardiac and respiratory function and sleep-wake cycles, which originate in the brain stem—the lower part of the brain just above the spinal cord. Vegetative patients may also have a startle reflex, but this behavior is not intentional and involves only brain stem activity.

As was evident in the [Terri] Schiavo case, the vegetative state remains a disquieting one. It defies normal expectations about awareness and consciousness. Usually when the eyes are open there is awareness, but in the vegetative state a patient is stripped of ability to interact with others or the environment.

The vegetative state is often confused with a coma by nonclinicians. This is an important error to correct. Although comatose and vegetative patients are unresponsive and unarousable, there are important differences. Coma is an eyes-closed state, while the vegetative state is an eyes-open one. Moreover, coma is the initial presentation of severe brain injury and is self-limited, usually lasting a couple of weeks. A coma can progress in a number of ways, from brain death to complete recovery. The most ominous of comas progress to brain death, defined as the death of the whole brain, including brain stem and higher brain functions. Brain death is recognized as the equivalent of cardiopulmonary death in all states, although a couple of states allow for a religious or moral objection to this neurological definition of death.

Comatose states can also evolve into a vegetative state. A vegetative state is labeled as persistent once it lasts more than a month. It is considered permanent after three or 12 months, depending upon the nature of the initial injury. If the injury is from anoxia, or oxygen deprivation, as would be the case in a cardiac arrest or drowning accident, a vegetative state persisting for three months is considered permanent. In contrast, a vegetative state resulting from a traumatic brain injury, such as from a motor vehicle accident or a fall, would need to last for 12 months in order for it to be designated as permanent.

The different time courses to a permanent vegetative state relate to the nature of the injury. The potential for recovery for a traumatically injured brain exceeds that of the anoxically injured brain. This differential degree of recovery from anoxic injury helps explain why it takes longer for clinicians to conclude that a traumatic injury has resulted in a permanent vegetative state.

If a vegetative state has yet to become permanent, a patient may move into what has been described as minimally conscious state. MCS is a new clinical designation that has its origins in the Aspen Criteria published in the journal *Neurology* in 2002. Unlike the vegetative state—with which MCS may be confused—MCS is a state of consciousness. MCS patients demonstrate unequivocal but fluctuating evidence of awareness of self and the environment. They may say words or phrases and gesture. They also may show evidence of memory, attention, and intention. However, these behaviors may be fleeting. The inability to reproduce telltale signs of awareness is part of the biology of MCS and an expected and confounding part of the clinical picture.

A patient who reaches the minimally conscious state before becoming permanently vegetative is open to a degree of prognostic uncertainty about the possibility of further cognitive recovery. The prognosis can be fixed or open-ended, with rare occurrences of dramatic recoveries and emergence from MCS years and decades after injury.

Patients who have regained the ability to consistently engage with others and who reestablish functional communication are considered to have emerged from MCS. Emergence from MCS is taken to be the consistent and reproducible recovery of consciousness and an awareness of self, others, and the environment. In the last few years, there were two well-known cases of emergence from MCS in the United States.

Arkansan Terry Wallis emerged from MCS in 2003, bringing international media attention to this phenomenon against the backdrop of the evolving Schiavo saga. Wallis regained fluent speech after lingering for some 19 years in a nursing home after sustaining traumatic brain injury in a motor vehicle accident. During that time he had been labeled erroneously as being in a coma or vegetative state, although he was most certainly minimally conscious and recovered fluent speech from that prognostic milestone. In July 2003, he began to speak. His first words were "mom" and "Pepsi." In his mind it was still 1984, and Ronald Reagan was still president.

Another compelling case of emergence from MCS involved Don Herbert, a Buffalo firefighter. Herbert was injured in a 1995 fire, sustaining a mix of traumatic and hypoxic brain injury. For the first few months after his injury he met the criteria for MCS with occasional and episodic signs of awareness and verbalizations. For the next nine years he lingered, presumed to be vegetative, until he spontaneously regained fluent speech in 2005, emerging after a number of psychoactive drugs were given to him by a physiatrist.

DISTINGUISHING THE VEGETATIVE AND MINIMALLY CONSCIOUS STATES

Invariably, people asked how Terry Wallis or Don Herbert could recover when experts were so definitive in asserting that Terri Schiavo was permanently unconscious. The answer to these questions is found in the diagnostic categories just reviewed and in the important biological differences between the permanent vegetative state of Schiavo and the minimally conscious states of Wallis and Herbert. Unlike patients in the permanent vegetative state, patients who are in MCS have preserved brain networks that retain the potential for activation. Both Wallis and Herbert emerged from their long period of quiescence from the minimally conscious state, not from the vegetative state. They each had reached MCS before the vegetative state became permanent, thus retaining the potential for additional recovery. While such dramatic recoveries are uncommon and should not be overstated, they should not be entirely discounted.

Because of the biological and prognostic differences between the minimally conscious and the permanent vegetative states, it is critical that these patients be distinguished from each other. This is easier said than done because of the evolving nature of brain states after injury and because of discontinuity in care as patients are transferred from the hospital to chronic care facilities.

Patients may leave the hospital with a vegetative diagnosis that has yet to become permanent, and then over time migrate into MCS while in chronic care. If a clinician does not notice this change in status, the patient may be assumed to be in a permanent vegetative state. This potential for misdiagnosis is only compounded by the episodic nature of displays of consciousness in MCS. Typically, families will see behavioral evidence of awareness and seek to reproduce these signs for wary staff. But because these behaviors are only episodic in MCS, they are not reliably reproduced. Staff may conclude that family observations are the result of denial or wishful thinking. Perhaps a third of patients in nursing homes diagnosed as being in the vegetative state may in fact be in the minimally conscious state, according to estimates from small studies. Wallis and Herbert were among those who were misdiagnosed this way. Because of the diagnostic and prognostic importance of these brain states, greater precision in discussions about a patient's vegetative state is now recommended. Medical staff should avoid confusing terms like persistent or permanent and speak instead of the type of injury (anoxia or traumatic) and its duration. And an Institute of Medicine exploratory meeting on disorders of consciousness called for the establishment of registries to determine the number of patients in these brain states and to better delineate the natural history of these conditions.

VALUES, ETHICAL CONSIDERATIONS, AND LEGAL RAMIFICATIONS

. . . Disorders of consciousness highlight fundamental bioethical concerns. Modern American bioethics was founded on the centrality of patient self-determination and autonomy. These rights have coalesced in two discrete arenas: reproductive ethics and end-of-life care. The evolution of the right to die is centrally linked to disorders of consciousness, most notably through the case of Karen Ann Quinlan, a New Jersey woman who was in a vegetative state following a drug overdose and anoxic brain injury. Her parents sought to remove her ventilator and allow her to die.

In a landmark 1976 ruling, the New Jersey Supreme Court permitted the removal of Ms. Quinlan's life support, citing the irreversible nature of her vegetative state. As the court opined, based on testimony given by Dr. Fred Plum, Ms. Quinlan had forever and irretrievably lost the possibility of returning to a "cognitive sapient state." The irreversible nature of her injury, and its futility, became the ethical and legal justification for the removal of her ventilator. This case, in turn, launched the era of patients' rights at life's end.

This right to die was further codified in other cases involving the vegetative state, including those of Nancy Beth Cruzan and Terri Schiavo, both young women in the permanent vegetative state. In *Cruzan v. Director* in 1990, the U.S. Supreme Court recognized the constitutional right of a competent person to refuse life-sustaining therapy, equated artificial nutrition and hydration with other life-sustaining therapies, and ruled that each state could set evidentiary standards for the withdrawal of these therapies. *Cruzan* also led to the increased use of advance directives. Justice Sandra Day O'Connor's decision was the inspiration for the Patient Self-Determination Act, which was signed into law on December 1, 1991. With the passage of the PSDA, which requires many hospitals and other health care providers to inform patients of their rights under state laws governing advance directives, advance directives gained a central role in efforts to improve end-of-life care in the 1990's.

The advent of new brain states like MCS and their potential treatment has upset many of the presumptions that gave rise to modern bioethics and the right to die. Where it was once presumed that severe brain injury was invariably as dire as the vegetative state, we now know that prognostic outcomes can be variable. Therefore, it is increasingly inappropriate to view brain injured patients as untreatable.

To pursue therapeutic possibilities without engendering false hope, it is critically important to diagnose brain states as precisely as possible in order to balance burdens and benefits. . . . Clinicians and policymakers need to preserve the right to die, but also to affirm the right to care for those who might be helped. The purpose of this ethical imperative is to carefully distinguish the vegetative from minimally conscious states and to avoid the diagnostic shortfalls that stem from clinical ignorance or ideological intent.

An instructive figure showing the overlap among disorders and the level of cognitive and motor function loss present in a variety of disorders of consciousness can be found in Nicholas D. Schiff & Joseph J. Fins, *Brain Death and Disorders of Consciousness*, 26 Current Biology R543, R572-6 (2016).

David Fischer & Robert D. Truog
The Problems with Fixating on Consciousness in Disorders of Consciousness
8 Am. J. Bioethics Neuroscience 135, 138-40 (2017)

The ambiguity between the conscious and unconscious problematizes the decisions that have been framed as depending upon this distinction—decisions such as whether to withdraw [life-sustaining treatment] (LST), to allow access to intensive care unit (ICU) resources, or to grant rights. How then should we approach the families/surrogates of patients with disorders of consciousness about decision making for their loved ones?

WHERE DO WE GO FROM HERE?

We suggest a forthright approach, sharing with families and surrogates what we know and do not know about these patients. We . . . can share information about a patient's behaviors and brain injury . . . [and] discuss[] prognosis with families and surrogates, based on objective patient information and existing outcome data. In contrast, we must acknowledge and communicate that for patients who are awake but not interactive, their level of awareness is unknown. Thus, when making decisions about these patients, we suggest deemphasizing the question of whether they are conscious or unconscious, and instead recommend collaborating with families and surrogates to ask: What empirical characteristics (e.g., behaviors or physiological measures) would these patients have valued, and what prognoses would they have accepted, if they could make these decisions for themselves?

. . . Ultimately, which behaviors and functions will matter most to families/surrogates will depend on numerous factors, including preferences previously expressed by the patients . . . , the decision to be made . . . , considerations of quality of life . . . , religious considerations, social norms, and many others. . . .

[O]ne empirical function that will likely matter to many is interactive capacity, or a patient's ability to receive communicated information and generate a coherent response. . . . We have previously proposed that interactive capacity may serve as a useful marker for consciousness, in that it intuitively signifies consciousness . . . and it can be applied to both behavior and emerging technological assessments, and because it is commonly valued in considerations of whether to continue LST [life-sustaining support]. . . .

[In conclusion,] [w]e advocate for deemphasizing the conscious/unconscious distinction that, despite such intense scrutiny, is frequently unknown, and may be in principle unknowable. . . . For families/surrogates who insist upon using the presence/absence of consciousness as a guide for decisions, we suggest using interactive capacity as an indicator of consciousness, while acknowledging the uncertain consciousness of awake patients without interactive capacity.

Thaddeus Mason Pope

Brain Death Forsaken: Growing Conflict and New Legal Challenges

37 J. Legal Med. 265, 307-16 (2017)

U.S. law equates brain death with death of the human being. Brain death is legally defined as the "complete" cessation of "all" functions of the "entire" brain. But that is not what clinicians in U.S. hospitals are measuring. Instead, brain death tests measure only a small subset of brain functions. For example, they do not test hormonal balance salt/fluid or temperature control. There is a "mismatch" between the legal and medical standards for brain death.

. . . [I]t is no longer an option to conceal or ignore the mismatch. It must be remedied. And it must be remedied by amending the law. To make the medical criteria as rigorous as the UDDA demands would be expensive and time consuming. And it would probably adversely impact rates of organ procurement. Therefore, it is far more feasible to bring the law into line with current medical practice than bring medical practice into line with the law. But if we move away from legally requiring cessation of "all" functions, we must determine "which" functions are dispositive. In other words, we must determine when someone is "dead enough" to be legally dead. . . .

Given the legal status of brain death, clinicians typically have no duty to continue physiological support after brain death. But this rule presents a profound problem for patients with religious objections to brain death. For these individuals, the denial of physiological support after brain death violates fundamental values.

Indeed, hospitals often refuse to accommodate religious objections to brain death. I concede that granting a complete exemption to brain death may be problematic. Instead, I argue that all states should enact "reasonable accommodation" laws, requiring a brief period of continued ventilator support. . . .

NOTES AND QUESTIONS

1. Clinical best practices around disorders of consciousness are evolving. In 2018, new practice guidelines were released through a collaboration involving the American Academy of Neurology (AAN), the American Congress of Rehabilitation Medicine (ACRM), and the National Institute on Disability, Independent Living, and Rehabilitation Research (NIDILRR). Joe Giacino et al., *Practice Guideline Update Recommendations Summary: Disorders of Consciousness Report of the Guideline Development, Dissemination, and Implementation Subcommittee of the American Academy of Neurology; the American Congress of Rehabilitation Medicine; and the National Institute on Disability, Independent Living, and Rehabilitation Research*, 91 Neurology 10 (2018). The practice guidelines stressed the need for multidisciplinary expertise, improved communications with families, and the need for serial standardized evaluations. How should legal standards of care incorporate new guidelines such as these? How should legal standards account for the great variation in brain death policies across different hospitals? *See* David M. Greer et al., *Variability of Brain Death Policies in the United States*, 73 JAMA Neurology 213, 217 (2016) (finding that hospitals' "level of compliance with the 2010 practice parameters remains deficient, particularly for ensuring the absence of confounding conditions, some lower brainstem function testing, and some specifics of apnea testing, including PCo_2 goals. Last, the specifics of approved ancillary testing are often missing, and unapproved and/or nonvalidated ancillary tests are sometimes included.").

2. *The Terri Schiavo case.* The ethics of end-of-life care have rightly drawn increasing attention and have fueled legal devices such as advance directives. These decisions are particularly difficult when the patient is unable to communicate her/his wishes. Such was the case for Terri Schiavo. Ms. Schiavo had been in a vegetative state for many years, and when her husband obtained an order to direct withdrawal of food and water, her parents challenged the order, and a legal battle ensued, drawing national attention and both state and federal legislative action. The core issue for the trial court was this:

> In the final analysis, the difficult question that faced the trial court was whether Theresa Marie Schindler Schiavo, not after a few weeks in a coma, but after ten years in a persistent vegetative state that has robbed her of most of her cerebrum and all but the most instinctive of neurological functions, with no hope of a medical cure but with sufficient money and strength of body to live indefinitely, would choose to continue the constant nursing care and the supporting tubes in hopes that a miracle would somehow recreate her missing brain tissue, or whether she would wish to permit a natural death process to take its course and for her family members and loved ones to be free to continue their lives. After due consideration, we conclude that the trial judge had clear and convincing evidence to answer this question as he did.

Bush v. Schiavo, 885 So.2d 321 (Fla. 2004). An interesting question concerns what, if any, brain function Ms. Schiavo retained at the time her tubes were removed.

What, if any, tests would you want performed if your family member were in a similar position? What tests would you require if you were the court? Consider the view of law professor Steven Calabresi:

> First, state or federal courts did not order PET or brain scanning to be done on Mrs. Schiavo before her feeding and hydration tube was disconnected. . . . A subsequent autopsy suggested that Mrs. Schiavo had been brain-dead when feeding and hydration was discontinued, but this was not a known fact when the tube was disconnected. At a bare minimum, it ought to be presumed, until it can be scientifically shown otherwise, that a person—a person who was indisputably alive before a medical incident like the one Terri Schiavo experienced—has brain-functioning. . . . It seems cavalier and coarse to presume that Mrs. Schiavo was brain-dead without performing this basic and easily available medical procedure. Mrs. Schiavo was not terminally ill, and she was not in pain. She was in a vegetative state. Her parents, though, thought they had some ability to communicate with her, and the only way to establish whether this was the case and whether she was capable of regaining consciousness was to conduct a PET scan. For a state court to starve someone to death who was not terminally ill, was not in pain, did not need extraordinary life-preserving measures, and might have been able to regain consciousness is frankly immoral. In our society, where convicted murderers frequently receive extensive due process—with courts examining and reexamining evidence to ensure that the defendant is truly guilty beyond a reasonable doubt—federal courts could have at the very least ordered a PET scan in Terri Schiavo's case.
>
> Second, there was a real and contested disagreement between Michael Schiavo and Mrs. Schiavo's parents . . . over whether Terri Schiavo was responsive and over whether she would have wanted to die by starvation if she were ever in a vegetative state. The state courts early on appointed Michael Schiavo to be his wife's guardian, and they stuck by this appointment to the end, crediting his accounts of Mrs. Schiavo's wish to die by starvation over her parents' contrary wishes. This decision, too, seems to me to have been highly immoral. First, and to return to my initial point, absent a PET scan, I would not presume brain death and a loss of all consciousness in a person who was not terminally ill or in great pain, where the person's parents believe she was still mentally alive and interactive. Robert and Mary Schindler had known their daughter far longer than Michael had, and they felt that they had an ability to communicate with her. This feeling should have been honored and is another reason why the courts should have ordered a PET scan.

Steven G. Calabresi, *The Terri Schiavo Case: In Defense of the Special Law Enacted by Congress and President Bush*, 100 Nw. U.L. Rev. 151, 154-55 (2006).

3. How much variation should be allowed or encouraged in the procedures used by hospitals to assess brain death? How would you react if you found out that hospitals used different procedures in different states? In different counties or cities? On different floors? *See* David M. Greer et al., *Variability of Brain Death Determination Guidelines in Leading US Neurologic Institutions*, 71 Neurology 1125 (2008).

4. The Donation After Cardiac Death (DCD) protocol was employed at Denver Children's Hospital to procure hearts for transplantation from three neonates. Questions centered on whether DCD donors could be declared dead using cardiorespiratory criteria (irreversible cessation of circulation and respiration) when the intention is to restart the heart in living circulation after being transplanted into the recipient. If the heart is restarted in the transplant recipient, is it true that circulation had irreversibly stopped and thus that the donor was dead before the organs were removed? Or, was the cessation of circulation reversible,

as evidenced by the restarting of the heart in the transplant recipient? Robert M. Veatch, *Donating Hearts After Cardiac Death—Reversing the Irreversible*, 359 N. Eng. J. Med. 672 (2008).

5. Could brain stimulation be an effective treatment for patients with severe disorders of consciousness? At present the answer is not clear, but researchers are investigating the possibility. What legal and ethical considerations must be made when conducting such research? For a review and discussion, see Jonathan Vanhoecke & Marwan Hariz, *Deep Brain Stimulation for Disorders of Consciousness: Systematic Review of Cases and Ethics*, 10 Brain Stimulation 1013 (2017).

6. What terminology should be used? The AAN plays an active role in establishing diagnostic and prognostic guidelines and participated in the drafting and publication of the Practice Guideline Update Recommendations Summary: Disorders of Consciousness. In 2018, the AAN proposed replacing the term "*permanent* vegetative state" with "*chronic* vegetative state" (emphasis added). This new term seeks to acknowledge that at least some vegetative state patients will eventually evolve into a minimally conscious state. The new term is also intended to protect vegetative state patients from the stigmatizing effects of a nomenclature that implies that their condition is irreversible. Some experts, however, argue that this change is overly broad, and call instead for the addition of a number of disease classifications that properly describe the particular circumstances of different groups of patients generally considered to be in a vegetative state. From a legal perspective, what are the implications of these different terms? *See* Joseph J. Fins & James L. Bernat, *Ethical, Palliative, and Policy Considerations in Disorders of Consciousness*, 91 Neurology 471 (2018).

7. In England, decisions concerning withdrawal of life-sustaining treatment in patients with disorders of consciousness involve "best interests discussions." Best interests discussions are conversations between physicians and a patient's family members in which factors such as likely success of treatment, benefits, burdens and risks of treatments, as well as the patient's presumed wishes, are considered to determine whether a particular treatment is proportionate or not, and whether such treatment should be discontinued in case it is disproportionate or futile. Although the "best interests discussions" procedure applies to most decisions concerning discontinuance of treatment, there is an exception for the case of withdrawal of clinically assisted nutrition and hydration (CANH), which has to be submitted to a court for judicial approval. English and Welsh physicians, concerned by the ethical and medical implications of judicial scrutiny, which can extend for many months and consume significant resources, have proposed a "fast-track system" that would replace the current procedure of judicial approval and work alongside Advance Decisions/Directives and powers of attorney in all determinations regarding withdrawal of life-sustaining treatment. For a discussion of the legal framework surrounding discontinuance of medical care in disorder of consciousness' cases, see Jonathan Baker, Justice, Court of Appeal of Eng. and Wales, *Oxford Shrieval Lecture: A Matter of Life and Death* (Oct. 11, 2016). For a discussion of the aforementioned proposal, see Lynne Turner-Stokes, *A Matter of Life and Death: Controversy at the Interface Between Clinical and Legal Decision-making in Prolonged Disorders of Consciousness*, 45 J. Med. Ethics 469 (2016). For a discussion in favor of the current system of judicial scrutiny, see Mohamed Y. Rady & Joseph L. Verheijde, *Judicial Oversight of Life-ending Withdrawal of Assisted Nutrition and Hydration in Disorders of Consciousness in the United Kingdom: A Matter of Life and Death*, 85 Medico-Legal J. 148 (2017).

8. Organ-preserving cardiopulmonary resuscitation consists in the use of CPR following cardiac arrest to preserve organs for transplantation that is applied to brain-dead organ donors in order to avoid the spoilage of organs that could be used in other patients. Should a technique primarily aimed at keeping a patient alive be applied to patients that are legally dead? What are the ethical and psychological implications of such a practice for the physicians that perform it? For more information regarding organ-preserving cardiopulmonary resuscitation, see Anne L. Dalle Ave et al., *Cardio-pulmonary Resuscitation of Brain-Dead Organ Donors: A Literature Review and Suggestions for Practice*, 29 Transplant Int'l 12 (2015).

9. Is it time to revisit the "dead donor rule"? Some experts think so, arguing that "it is not obvious why certain living patients, such as those who are near death but on life support, should not be allowed to donate their organs, if doing so would benefit others and be consistent with their own interests." *See* Robert D. Truog et al., *The Dead-Donor Rule and the Future of Organ Donation*, 369 N. Engl. J. Med. 1287 (2013).

10. A 2019 study seeking to better understand the impact of cognitive-motor dissociation in disorder-of-consciousness cases determined that EEG testing can reveal the existence of covert consciousness in brain-injured patients who "appear behaviorally unresponsive on . . . standardized assessment instruments." These results raise ethical questions regarding whether current clinical management plans for patients with a disorder of consciousness are appropriate. Should EEG be offered as a complementary test for unresponsive patients? Should withdrawal of life support decisions be withheld until testing assessing covert consciousness has been performed? For a discussion of the study results and the ethical concerns underlying the discovery, see Joseph T. Giacino & Brian L. Edlow, *Covert Consciousness in the Intensive Care Unit*, 42 Trends Neurosci. 844 (2019).

D. BRAIN DEATH IN COURT

Next are three cases—two civil, one criminal—in which courts had to decide what "death" means and whether "brain death" fits within that definition. Consider whether the same definition of death should apply to all legal contexts. If not, what variables should sort them?

1. Civil Context

The case of 13-year-old Jahi McMath drew national attention and raised fundamental questions about the definition and determination of brain death. As you will read in the case below, McMath was declared dead in California. But her family challenged that determination and won a legal battle to transport Jahi's body to a hospital in New Jersey.

Both sides argued vigorously. In a motion for the defendant hospital, it was argued that "The court should not entertain plaintiffs' claim that Jahi has risen from the dead." One ethicist, critical of the family, "called the efforts to treat Jahi 'ghoulish' and said doctors and facilities treating her should be 'charged with desecrating a corpse.'" But the McMath family vehemently disagreed. The family posted video on YouTube that purported to show Jahi moving her foot in response to her mother's voice. Her mother posted on Facebook, "Our little sleeping beauty is doing great and progressing. She is moving more on her mother's command. As you can see, she is still alive and just as beautiful as ever. Flawless skin!"

Pediatric neurologist Dr. Alan Shewmon supported the family's argument and, based on neurological evaluation, concluded that "[h]er brain is alive in the neuropathological sense, and it is not necrotic. At this time, Jahi does not fulfill California's statutory definition of death, which requires the irreversible absence of all brain function, because she exhibits hypothalamic function and intermittent responsiveness to verbal command." Celeste McGovern, *Top Neurologist: Jahi McMath Is 'No Longer' Dead*, Nat'l Catholic Register (Nov. 30, 2015). Multiple lawsuits, in both state and federal court, were pursued. Below is the key California state opinion.

UCSF Benioff Children's Hosp. Oakland v. Superior Court of Cal., Cty. of Alameda

2016 WL 4495093 (Cal.) (July 22, 2016)

Under California's Uniform Determination of Death Act, when someone sustains irreversible cessation of all brain function, they are determined dead. The Health and Safety Code requires that when someone is pronounced dead, there shall be independent confirmation by a second physician. In this case, both criteria were met—McMath ceased all brain function, as was confirmed by an independent examination by another physician.

By means of a probate proceeding, McMath's mother, Latasha Nailah Spears Winkfield (Winkfield), contested this determination, petitioning to require UCSF Benioff Children's Hospital Oakland (Children's Hospital) to continue providing medical care to McMath. The probate court considered expert medical testimony, including that of a court appointed expert, applied the clear and convincing standard of proof, then confirmed that McMath was brain dead pursuant to California's Uniform Determination of Death Act. A final judgment was entered. A death certificate was issued and remains in effect.

The judgment was never appealed. However, the probate judgment has spawned a series of collateral and related actions, many of which seek to collaterally attack the previous brain death determination. For example, in this action McMath claims she is no longer dead and has standing to pursue a claim for personal injury—in addition to her claim for wrongful death.

No administrative agency or court has reversed the brain death determination from the probate proceeding. Defendants raised this issue by demurrer, arguing McMath is collaterally estopped to allege she is alive and lacks standing to pursue a claim for personal injury. Yet, the trial court, unsure of how to apply the probate judgment in subsequent civil litigation, overruled the demurrer, noted the difference of opinion, and certified two questions addressing the application of collateral estoppel and impact of finality of a death determination from a probate proceeding.

Unfortunately, the Court of Appeal summarily denied Children's Hospital's and Dr. Rosen's Petition for Writ of Mandate. Children's Hospital and Dr. Rosen will be irreparably harmed having to re-litigate issues that were previously litigated to finality. McMath's determination of death is final. What is more, since the publicity garnered by McMath's case, others are turning to the courts to challenge brain death determinations, adopting many of McMath's arguments and strategies.

This Court should grant review to resolve this unsettled issue and to clarify the scope of the collateral estoppel doctrine. . . .

A. FACTUAL BACKGROUND

1. Jahi McMath Was Pronounced Dead Using Accepted Medical Standards in Accordance with California's Uniform Determination of Death Act

McMath underwent a surgical procedure at Children's Hospital on December 9, 2013 to address her sleep apnea. Following the surgery, McMath went into cardiac arrest and was placed on a ventilator. When McMath's condition failed to improve, Children's Hospital physicians Robin Shanahan M.D., a board certified pediatric neurologist, and Scott Heidersbach, M.D., a board certified pediatric critical care physician, performed separate brain death examinations on McMath on December 11 and December 12, 2013, each independently concluding McMath was brain dead under accepted medical standards set forth in the Guidelines for Determination of Brain Death in Infants and Children: An Update of the 1987 Task Force Recommendation (the AAP Brain Death Guidelines). Based upon these two separate examinations, McMath was pronounced dead at Children's Hospital on December 12, 2013 under California's Uniform Determination of Death Act (UDDA), codified at Health and Safety Code sections 7180 and 7181. A death certificate was thereafter issued and remains in effect to date.

2. Probate Proceedings Were Initiated by Winkfield to Assert Her Position That McMath Was Alive

After McMath was pronounced dead under the UDDA, Winkfield filed a Petition for Temporary Restraining Order/Order Authorizing Medical Treatment and Authorizing Petitioner to Give Consent to Medical Treatment on December 20, 2013 . . . Children's Hospital opposed the petition, arguing that it could not be compelled to provide medical treatment to McMath because she was legally deceased.

The Probate Action would be the first in a series of at least six separate legal proceedings initiated by Winkfield to assert her position that McMath is alive.

Judge Evelio Grillo of the Alameda Superior Court appointed Paul Fisher, M.D., a board certified child neurologist, Chief of Child Neurology at Lucile Packard Children's Hospital and Professor of Child Neurology at Stanford University School of Medicine, to serve as the court's expert to independently evaluate and assess whether McMath met the criteria for irreversible brain death under Health and Safety Code Health section 7181. . . .

Dr. Fisher conducted an independent examination of McMath on December 23, 2013 at Children's Hospital and concluded McMath had suffered irreversible brain death under the AAP Brain Death Guidelines.

3. After an Evidentiary Hearing, Final Judgment Was Entered in the Probate Action Confirming McMath's Death

A comprehensive evidentiary hearing was held in the Probate Action on December 24, 2013 to decide whether McMath met the statutory criteria for brain death set forth in Health and Safety Code sections 7180 and 7181. At the hearing, the court heard live testimony from, and permitted cross-examination of, Dr. Fisher and Dr. Shanahan, both of whom confirmed McMath was legally deceased under the AAP Brain Death Guidelines. The court also considered evidence in the form of medical records, testimony and oral argument from counsel for Winkfield and Children's Hospital.

Following the hearing, Judge Grillo applied the heightened clear and convincing evidence standard to find McMath had suffered irreversible brain death on December 12, 2013 and was therefore legally deceased under the UDDA. Judge Grillo issued a comprehensive Final Order on January 2, 2014 confirming his findings made in open court on December 24, 2013 and thereafter entered judgment on January 17, 2014.

B. A DEATH CERTIFICATE WAS RECORDED AND REMAINS IN EFFECT

Subsequent to the court's finding that McMath met the criteria for brain death in the Probate Action, the Alameda County Coroner's Office issued a death certificate for McMath on January 3, 2014. On January 5, 2014, the Coroner transferred custody of McMath's body to her family who then removed it to an undisclosed facility in New Jersey, where it allegedly remains on ventilator support at the expense of the New Jersey Medicaid Program.

C. THE PROBATE JUDGMENT REMAINS UNCHALLENGED

Winkfield never appealed the Final Order and Judgment. Nor did she exhaust her administrative remedies to have the death certificate rescinded. Instead, she initiated multiple legal proceedings to collaterally challenge the Probate Court's brain death judgment. . . . In the Petition for Writ of Error, Winkfield sought to overturn the Probate Court's Final Order and Judgement based upon her newly proclaimed ability to "provide new, conclusive evidence" in the form of "new facts" showing "that Jahi McMath is not 'brain dead.'. . ." In response, the Court issued an order on October 8, 2014 appointing Dr. Fisher to again serve as the court's independent medical expert and attached a copy of a report by Dr. Fisher, stating that he had reviewed the evidence submitted by Winkfield in connection with the Petition for Writ of Error, and nothing in those submissions "provide[s] evidence that Jahi McMath is not brain dead." . . . The Final Order and Judgment entered in the Probate Action confirming McMath's death remains unchallenged.

D. PROCEDURAL BACKGROUND

After withdrawing her Petition for Writ of Error, . . . Plaintiffs filed a First Amended Complaint ("FAC") on November 4, 2015 alleging McMath is alive despite the valid Final Order, Judgment and death certificate confirming her death on December 12, 2013. Based on this erroneous and improper allegation, and despite the Final Order and Judgment confirming McMath is deceased under California law, the Alameda Superior Court has mistakenly permitted McMath to allege a cause of action to recover damages for personal injuries as though she is alive. The only valid cause of action is one for wrongful death, which McMath's purported next of kin have asserted as an alternative claim in this litigation. . . .

The trial court's certified questions remain unanswered and the important questions of whether collateral estoppel applies to probate court findings, and the scope of the changed circumstances exception, remain unanswered. Collateral estoppel is meant to protect litigants from relitigating an issue once it has been decided and confirmed through entry of final judgment. In this case, the lower courts have struggled with these doctrines' application because the facts alleged by plaintiffs challenge our personal philosophical framework for understanding how life and death are defined. Fortunately, the law is clear. The California legislature has defined death. Once the issue has been decided, whether in a probate proceeding or elsewhere, there is no changed circumstance—only different evidence—which, regardless of how it is viewed by the plaintiffs, does not merit reexamination of the issue.

The Supreme Court does not appear to have ever directly addressed the changed circumstances exception, and the appellate courts have created conflict and confusion regarding the exception's application. The Supreme Court has the opportunity to address the exception now, and should do so to provide much needed guidance.

REASONS REVIEW SHOULD BE GRANTED

II. WHETHER FINDINGS MADE IN CONNECTION WITH A PROBATE JUDGMENT COLLATERALLY ESTOP A SUBSEQUENT CIVIL ACTION IS AN OPEN QUESTION IN NEED OF RESOLUTION . . .

C. THE PROBATE ACTION PROCEEDINGS ADEQUATELY ADDRESSED ALL ISSUES PERTINENT TO CONFIRMING WHETHER MCMATH IS DECEASED UNDER THE UDDA

An individual is dead under California law if he or she has sustained "either (1) irreversible cessation of circulatory and respiratory functions, or (2) irreversible cessation of all functions of the entire brain, including the brain stem . . ." Health and Safety Code section 7180, which codifies the UDDA, goes on to provide that "[a] determination of death" under either cardiopulmonary criteria , or neurologic criteria , "must be made in accordance with accepted medical standards."

Section 7181 of the Health and Safety Code imposes an additional safeguard to individuals before they may be pronounced dead by neurologic criteria, mandating that "independent confirmation by another physician" is required "[w]hen an individual is pronounced dead by determining that the individual has sustained an irreversible cessation of all functions of the entire brain, including the brain stem." Nothing in the UDDA requires, or even suggests, that a court should be involved in deciding whether a person is legally dead. Instead, the plain language of the statute simply requires that a death determination made under neurologic criteria be made "in accordance with accepted medical standards," and independently confirmed by another physician.

Satisfied it had jurisdiction and authority to rule in the Probate Action, the probate court applied the heightened clear and convincing evidence standard to conclude there was sufficient evidence McMath had sustained brain death under section 7180 of the Health and Safety Code. The probate court's findings were based, in part, upon the declarations and live testimony given by a pediatric neurologist (Dr. Shanahan), a pediatric critical care specialist (Dr. Heidersbach) and a court appointed child neurology expert (Dr. Fisher), each of whose independent examinations of McMath confirmed she had sustained "irreversible cessation of all functions of the entire brain, including the brain stem" by "accepted medical standards." Finding all requirements for establishing brain death had been met under the Health and Safety Code, the probate court concluded McMath was dead under California law and entered the Final Order and Judgment to memorialize the finding.

. . . The Final Order and Judgment entered in the Probate Action should be given preclusive effect in this case even though, and perhaps even because, they were entered in the course of a probate proceeding before a court of competent jurisdiction. Collateral estoppel is meant to apply universally, even in those cases where the decision may be difficult to make in order to preserve the "integrity of the judicial system" and the rule of law. Stated even more directly, the collateral estoppel doctrine does not recognize an exception for probate proceedings, even when those proceedings address delicate issues of life and death. . . .

2. Plaintiffs Should Not Be Permitted to Raise the Changed Circumstances Exception Under the Correct Reading of the Law

McMath, through her guardian ad litem, claims new facts have occurred which materially alter the issue to be decided. They have not. The "new facts" cited by plaintiffs are in the form of expert analysis and results from testing performed after McMath's body was removed from Children's Hospital. Much like the lung biopsy results that could not have been obtained while the decedent was still alive in Evans, these "new facts"—consisting largely of expert opinion by practitioners who could not have performed examinations at Children's Hospital as they were without credentials necessary to examine McMath in California—would have done nothing more than alter the weight of evidence considered by the probate court when it decided McMath was deceased under California's UDDA. Winkfield did not challenge the proceedings held in the Probate Action by way of appeal, and has thus waived any challenge to the sufficiency of those proceedings. . . .

In the Jahi McMath case, the family did *not* want the hospital to end life-sustaining treatment. But in the Marlise Muñoz case below, the roles are flipped: It is the hospital that wants to maintain the life-sustaining treatment and a family member who does not.

Marlise Muñoz was pregnant when she suffered a blood clot in her lungs. The blood clot deprived her brain of oxygen for a prolonged period of time, causing significant damage. The Texas hospital to which she was admitted determined that she met the criteria for brain death. But the hospital refused to discontinue treatment, arguing that Texas Health and Safety Code § 166.049 required the hospital to maintain Marlise's organs in order to preserve the life of her fetus. Marlise's husband, Erick Muñoz, filed a complaint and a motion to discontinue life-sustaining treatment in a Texas state court. Muñoz argued that the Texas statute did not apply to Marlise. Muñoz also argued, though the court declined to rule on the issue, that the statute violated the Fourteenth Amendment.

Plaintiff's First Amended Motion to Compel Defendants to Remove *Marlise Muñoz from "Life Sustaining" Measures and Application for Unopposed Expedited Relief*

Muñoz v. John Peter Smith Hosp., 2014 WL 285054 (Trial Motion, Memorandum and Affidavit) (Tex. Dist. 2014)

[The Texas Health and Safety Code § 166.049 declares that "[a] person may not withdraw or withhold life-sustaining treatment . . . from a pregnant patient"].

INTRODUCTION

Erick Muñoz . . . vehemently opposes any further medical treatment be undertaken on the deceased body of his wife, Marlise Muñoz. . . . Erick requests this Court to issue an order requiring JPS [the hospital treating Marlise] to immediately cease conducting any further medical procedures on the body of Marlise, to remove Marlise from any respirators, ventilators or other "life support," and to release the body of Marlise Muñoz to her family for proper preservation and burial.

ARGUMENT

1. JPS Misinterprets Section 166.049 of the Texas Health and Safety Code.

In an effort to argue that Marlise must be subjected to "life sustaining" treatments, JPS argued that the Texas Health and Safety Code disallows it from withdrawing or withholding life-sustaining treatment from a pregnant patient. Tex. HS. Code 166.049. However, JPS entirely misconstrues Section 166.049, further failing to read this section in conjunction with the entirety of the Code. In fact, Marlise cannot possibly be a "pregnant patient"—Marlise is dead.

Section 671.001, also found in the Texas Health and Safety Code, provides medical and legal professional[s] with the definition of death in Texas.

> . . . (b) If artificial means of support preclude a determination that a person's spontaneous respiratory and circulatory functions have ceased, the person is dead when, in the announced opinion of a physician, according to ordinary standards of medical practice, *there is irreversible cessation of all spontaneous brain function. Death occurs when the relevant functions cease.*

Marlise has suffered clinical brain death. As a result, Marlise is legally dead—she has suffered "irreversible cessation of all spontaneous brain function." Thus, death for Marlise has occurred, and no further surgical procedures should be, or can be, undertaken on her deceased body. . . .

A. Life Sustaining Measures Cannot Apply to the Dead.

Consequently, as Marlise is deceased, she cannot possibly be a "pregnant patient" under Section 166.049 of the Texas Health and Safety Code, nor can Marlise be subject to any "life-sustaining" treatment pursuant to Chapter 166 of the Code. As defined by Section 166.002(10), "life-sustaining treatment" means treatment that "based on reasonable medical judgment, sustains the life of a patient and without which the patient will die. . ." However, in this case, Marlise Muñoz is already dead. No treatment can possibl[y] sustain the life of Marlise, and thus as JPS will not be "withdrawing or withholding life-sustaining treatment" from Marlise by removing her from the ventilator and all other associated machines, JPS will not be in violation of the Texas Health and Safety Code. Tex. HS. Code 166.049. As a result, JPS should be ordered to immediately remove Marlise from these devices. . . .

[A day after the motion was submitted, the Tarrant County District Court for the 96th Judicial District issued a judgment declaring Texas Health & Safety Code Section 169.0049 inapplicable to Marlise Muñoz and ordering the medical facility to declare Marlise's death and to remove the ventilator and all other "life sustaining" treatment. —EDS.]

2. Criminal Context

People v. Eulo

472 N.E.2d 286 (N.Y. 1984)

COOKE, C.J. These appeals involve a question of criminal responsibility in which defendants, charged with homicide, contend that their conduct did not cause death.

The term "death," as used in this State's statutes, may be construed to embrace a determination, made according to accepted medical standards, that a person has suffered an irreversible cessation of breathing and heartbeat or, when these functions are artificially maintained, an irreversible cessation of the functioning of the entire brain, including the brain stem. Therefore, a defendant will not necessarily be relieved of criminal liability for homicide by the removal of the victim's vital organs after the victim has been declared dead according to brain-based criteria, notwithstanding that, at that time, the victim's heartbeat and breathing were being continued by artificial means.

I

People v. Eulo

On the evening of July 19, 1981, defendant and his girlfriend attended a volunteer firemen's fair in Kings Park, Suffolk County. Not long after they arrived, the two began to argue, reportedly because defendant was jealous over one of her former suitors, whom they had seen at the fair. The argument continued through the evening; it became particularly heated as the two sat in defendant's pickup truck, parked in front of the home of the girlfriend's parents. Around midnight, defendant shot her in the head with his unregistered handgun.

The victim was rushed by ambulance to the emergency room of St. John's Hospital. A gunshot wound to the left temple causing extreme hemorrhaging was apparent. A tube was placed in her windpipe to enable artificial respiration and intravenous medication was applied to stabilize her blood pressure.

Shortly before 2:00 A.M., the victim was examined by a neurosurgeon, who undertook various tests to evaluate damage done to the brain. Painful stimuli were applied and yielded no reaction. Various reflexes were tested and, again, there was no response. A further test determined that the victim was incapable of spontaneously maintaining respiration. An electroencephalogram (EEG) resulted in "flat," or "isoelectric," readings indicating no activity in the part of the brain tested.

Over the next two days, the victim's breathing was maintained solely by a mechanical respirator. Her heartbeat was sustained and regulated through medication. Faced with what was believed to be an imminent cessation of these two bodily functions notwithstanding the artificial maintenance, the victim's parents consented to the use of certain of her organs for transplantation.

On the afternoon of July 23, a second neurosurgeon was called in to evaluate whether the victim's brain continued to function in any manner. A repetition of all of the previously conducted tests led to the same diagnosis: the victim's entire brain had irreversibly ceased to function. This diagnosis was reviewed and confirmed by the Deputy Medical Examiner for Suffolk County and another physician.

The victim was pronounced dead at 2:20 P.M. on July 23, although at that time she was still attached to a respirator and her heart was still beating. Her body was taken to a surgical room where her kidneys, spleen, and lymph nodes were removed. The mechanical respirator was then disconnected, and her breathing immediately stopped, followed shortly by a cessation of the heartbeat.

Defendant was indicted for second degree murder. After a jury trial, he was convicted of manslaughter. The Appellate Division, 97 A.D.2d 682, 467 N.Y.S.2d 464, unanimously affirmed the conviction, without opinion.

People v. Bonilla

At approximately 10:30 P.M. on February 6, 1979, a New York City police officer found a man lying faceup in a Brooklyn street with a bullet wound to the head. The officer transported the victim in his patrol car to the Brookdale Hospital, where he was placed in an intensive care unit. Shortly after arriving at the hospital, the victim became comatose and was unable to breathe spontaneously. He was placed on a respirator and medication was administered to maintain his blood pressure.

The next morning, the victim was examined by a neurologist. Due to the nature of the wound, routine tests were applied to determine the level, if any, of the victim's brain functions. The doctor found no reflex reactions and no response to painful stimuli. The mechanical respirator was disconnected to test for spontaneous breathing. There was none, and the respirator was reapplied. An EEG indicated an absence of activity in the part of the brain tested. In the physician's opinion, the bullet wound had caused the victim's entire brain to cease functioning.

The following day, the tests were repeated and the same diagnosis was reached. The victim's mother had been informed of her son's condition and had consented to a transfer of his kidneys and spleen. Death was pronounced following the second battery of tests and, commencing at 9:25 P.M., the victim's kidneys and spleen were removed for transplantation. The respirator was then disconnected, and the victim's breathing and heartbeat stopped.

An investigation led to defendant's arrest. While in police custody, defendant admitted to the shooting. He was indicted for second degree murder and criminal possession of a weapon. A jury convicted him of the weapons count and of first degree manslaughter. The conviction was affirmed by a divided Appellate Division.

II

Defendants' principal point in each of these appeals is that the respective Trial Judges failed to adequately instruct the juries as to what constitutes a person's death, the time at which criminal liability for a homicide would attach. It is claimed that in New York, the time of death has always been set by reference to the functioning of the heart and the lungs; that death does not occur until there has been an irreversible cessation of breathing and heartbeat.

There having been extensive testimony at both trials concerning each victim's diagnosis as "brain dead," defendants argue that, in the absence of clear instruction, the juries may have erroneously concluded that defendants would be guilty of homicide if their conduct was the legal cause of the victims' "brain death" rather than the victims' ultimate state of cardiorespiratory failure. In evaluating defendants' contentions, it is first necessary to review: how death has traditionally been determined by the law; how the principle of "brain death" is now sought to be infused into our jurisprudence; and, whether, if at all, this court may recognize a principle of "brain death" without infringing upon a legislative power or prerogative.

A person's passing from life has long been an event marked with a variety of legal consequences. A determination of death starts in motion the legal machinery governing the disposition of the deceased's property. It serves to terminate certain legal relationships, including marriage, and business partnerships. The period for initiation of legal actions brought against, by, or on behalf of the deceased is extended. And, in recent times, death marks the point at which certain of the deceased's organs, intended to be donated upon death, may be transferred. In the immediate context, pertinent here, determination of a person's "death" is relevant because our Penal Law defines homicide in terms of "conduct which causes the *death* of a person."

Death has been conceptualized by the law as, simply, the absence of life: "Death is the opposite of life; it is the termination of life." But, while erecting death as a critical milepost in a person's legal life, the law has had little occasion to consider the precise point at which a person ceases to live.

When the question arises as to when death occurs, it has been deemed one of fact, in which the fact finder may be called upon to evaluate expert medical testimony. . . .

Within the past two decades, machines that artificially maintain cardio-respiratory functions have come into widespread use. This technical accomplishment has called into question the universal applicability of the traditional legal and medical criteria for determining when a person has died.

These criteria were cast into flux as the medical community gained a better understanding of human physiology. It is widely understood that the human brain may be anatomically divided, generally, into three parts: the cerebrum, the cerebellum, and the brain stem. The cerebrum, known also as the "higher brain," is deemed largely to control cognitive functions such as thought, memory, and consciousness. The cerebellum primarily controls motor coordination. The brain stem, or "lower brain," which itself has three parts known as the midbrain, pons, and medulla, controls reflexive or spontaneous functions such as breathing, swallowing, and "sleep-wake" cycles.

In addition to injuries that directly and immediately destroy brain tissue, certain physical traumas may indirectly result in a complete and irreversible cessation of the brain's functions. For example, a direct trauma to the head can cause great swelling of the brain tissue, which, in turn, will stem the flow of blood to the brain. A respiratory arrest will similarly cut off the supply of oxygen to the blood and, hence, the brain. Within a relatively short period after being deprived of oxygen, the brain will irreversibly stop functioning. With the suffocation of the higher brain all cognitive powers are lost and a cessation of lower brain functions will ultimately end all spontaneous bodily functions.

Notwithstanding a total irreversible loss of the entire brain's functioning, contemporary medical techniques can maintain, for a limited period, the operation of the heart and the lungs. Respirators or ventilators can substitute for the lower brain's failure to maintain breathing. This artificial respiration, when combined with a chemical regimen, can support the continued operation of the heart. This is so because, unlike respiration, the physical contracting or "beating" of the heart occurs independently of impulses from the brain: so long as blood containing oxygen circulates to the heart, it may continue to beat and medication can take over the lower brain's limited role in regulating the rate and force of the heartbeat.

It became clear in medical practice that the traditional "vital signs"—breathing and heart beat—are not independent indicia of life, but are, instead, part of an integration of functions in which the brain is dominant. As a result, the medical community began to consider the cessation of brain activity as a measure of death.

The movement in law towards recognizing cessation of brain functions as criteria for death followed this medical trend. The immediate motive for adopting this position was to ease and make more efficient the transfer of donated organs. Organ transfers, to be successful, require a "viable, intact organ." Once all of a person's vital functions have ceased, transferable organs swiftly deteriorate and lose their transplant value. The technical ability to artificially maintain respiration and heartbeat after the entire brain has ceased to function was sought to be applied in cases of organ transplant to preserve the viability of donated organs. . . .

In New York, the term "death," although used in many statutes, has not been expressly defined by the Legislature. This raises the question of how this court may construe these expressions of the term "death" in the absence of clarification by the Legislature. . . .

We hold that a recognition of brain-based criteria for determining death is not unfaithful to prior judicial definitions of "death," as presumptively adopted in the many statutes using that term. Close examination of the common law conception of death and the traditional criteria used to determine when death has occurred leads inexorably to this conclusion.

Courts have not engaged in a metaphysical analysis of when life should be deemed to have passed from a person's body, leaving him or her dead. Rather, they have conceptualized death as the absence of life, unqualified and undefined. On a practical level, this broad conception of death as "the opposite of life" was substantially narrowed through recognition of the cardiorespiratory criteria for determining when death occurs. Under these criteria, the loci of life are the heart and the lungs: where there is no breath or heartbeat, there is no life. Cessation manifests death.

Considering death to have occurred when there is an irreversible and complete cessation of the functioning of the entire brain, including the brain stem, is consistent with the common law conception of death. Ordinarily, death will be determined according to the traditional criteria of irreversible cardiorespiratory repose. When, however, the respiratory and circulatory functions are maintained by mechanical means, their significance, as signs of life, is at best ambiguous. Under such circumstances, death may nevertheless be deemed to occur when, according to accepted medical practice, it is determined that the entire brain's function has irreversibly ceased.

Death remains the single phenomenon identified at common law; the supplemental criteria are merely adapted to account for the "changed conditions" that a dead body may be attached to a machine so as to exhibit demonstrably false indicia of life. It reflects an improved understanding that in the complete and irreversible absence of a functioning brain, the traditional loci of life—the heart and the lungs—function only as a result of stimuli originating from outside of the body and will never again function as part of an integrated organism. . . .

III

Each defendant correctly notes that the respective Trial Judges did not expressly instruct the juries concerning the criteria to be applied in determining when death occurred. Whether medically accepted brain-based criteria are legally cognizable became an issue in these cases when the respective juries heard testimony concerning the victims being pronounced medically dead while their hearts were beating and before artificial maintenance of the cardiorespiratory systems was discontinued. To properly evaluate whether these diagnoses of death were legally and medically premature and, therefore, whether the subsequent activities were possibly superseding causes of the deaths, the juries had to have been instructed as to the appropriate criteria for determining death: irreversible cessation of breathing and heartbeat or irreversible cessation of the entire brain's functioning.

The courts here adequately conveyed to the juries their obligation to determine the fact and causation of death. The courts defined the criteria of death in relation to the chain of causation. By specifically charging the juries that they might consider the surgical procedures as superseding causes of death, the courts made clear by ready implication that death should be deemed to have occurred after all medical procedures had ended.

The trial courts could have given express instructions that death may be deemed to have occurred when the victims' entire brain, including the brain stem, had irreversibly ceased to function. On the facts of these cases, that would have been the better practice. But, as mentioned, the brain-based criteria are supplemental to the traditional criteria, each describing the same phenomenon of death. In the context of a criminal case for homicide, there is no theoretical or practical impediment to the People's proceeding under a theory that the defendant "cause[d] the death" of a person, with death determined by either criteria. . . .

[T]here was sufficient evidence for both juries to have found beyond a reasonable doubt that the medical decisions did not break the causal chain linking defendants' conduct and the victims' deaths.

NOTES AND QUESTIONS

1. Is brain death legal "death"? How should courts handle the question of whether brain death constitutes death as used in homicide statutes? In 1989, the Minnesota Supreme Court declined to answer a certified question on this issue, holding that it was a question "best left to legislature." *State v. Olson*, 435 N.W.2d 530 (Minn. 1989). Do you agree?

2. The Jahi McMath case spurred significant critique and commentary about allowing families to pay for life-sustaining treatment even after a declaration of death. For a further discussion of the legal and ethical implications of the Jahi McMath holding, see Christopher M. Burkle et al., *Why Brain Death Is Considered Death and Why There Should Be No Confusion*, 83 Neurology 1464 (2014); Beverley Copnell, *Brain Death: Lessons from the McMath Case*, 23 Am. J. Critical Care 259 (2014). The *McMath* case also involved neuroimaging, as the family argued that Jahi's EEG "found evidence of electrical activity in her brain" and that MRI scans "found that her cerebrum[was] physically intact and receiving blood flow." R. Sam Barclay, *The Changing Definition of What Is 'Brain Dead'*, HealthLine (Aug 27, 2015).

3. In the wake of the *McMath* case, courts have seen a number of families challenging brain death determinations. David DeBolt, *More Families Now Challenging Doctors' Brain-Death Diagnoses*, Seattle Times (May 18, 2016). In Texas, one father

chose a different way to respond. George Pickering's son experienced a stroke and went into a coma. Concerned that his son was not getting proper care and that life-sustaining treatment would be removed, George Pickering brought a gun to his son's hospital room and threatened violence. He held his son's hand for hours and refused to leave. He eventually surrendered after he felt his son squeeze his hand.

> Pickering recounted that his son had had seizures in the past, so he knew the procedure. He also knew that contrary to what the hospital told him in January, his son wasn't "brain dead." . . . Something told Pickering that the hospital was wrong to order a "terminal wean," which would have slowly removed his son from life support. . . . [Pickering went on:] "They were moving too fast. The hospital, the nurses, the doctors, I knew if I had three or four hours that night that I would know whether George was brain dead.

After the event, the son's health improved, and he made a full recovery. Commenting on what his father did, the son reflected, "There was a law broken, but it was broken for all the right reasons. I'm here now because of it. It was love." Dallas Franklin, *Father Brings Gun to Hospital to Buy Time for His 'Brain Dead' Son*, KFOR (Dec. 22, 2015).

4. The *Muñoz* case complicates the ethical issues further because Muñoz was pregnant when she was declared brain dead. Would the court's analysis have changed if the pregnancy was further along? In 2014, a healthy baby was delivered from a woman declared brain dead. Ian Austen, *Canada: Healthy Baby Is Delivered by Woman Declared Brain-Dead*, N.Y. Times (Feb. 11, 2014). In 2019, the University Hospital in Brno, Czech Republic announced that a baby was born by Caesarean section to a mother who had been declared brain dead three months earlier and kept on life support. *Czech Doctors Deliver Baby Girl 117 Days After Mother's Brain-Death*, Reuters (Sept. 2, 2019). For a further discussion on the intersection of physician's ethical obligations, patients' rights, and the law, see Lawrence O. Gostin, *Legal and Ethical Responsibilities Following Brain Death: The* McMath *and* Muñoz *Cases*, 311 JAMA 903 (2015). For an interview with family members in the *Muñoz* case, see Manny Fernandez & Erik Eckholm, *Pregnant, and Forced to Stay on Life Support*, N.Y. Times (Jan. 7, 2014).

5. Some examples of "inexplicable" recoveries from a disorder of consciousness include those of Victoria Arlen, who became a Paralympic swimmer after spending close to four years in a locked-in state; Li Zhihua, who woke up five years after being declared in a permanent vegetative state; and Omar Salgado, who was able to communicate through blinking three months after a diffuse axonal shear injury that doctors believed had induced a permanent vegetative state. *See* Karen Weintraub, *Man Partly Wakes from 15-Year Vegetative State — What It Means*, Nat'l Geographic (Sept. 25, 2017). How should these types of miracle stories affect the law's analysis in cases involving disorders of consciousness?

6. The American Academy of Neurology Ethics, Law, and Humanities Committee convened a summit in October 2016 to discuss factors affecting the proliferation of brain death determination lawsuits and possible solutions to the issue. The attendants to the summit proposed a series of measures conducive to improving public trust regarding the legitimacy of determination of death by neurologic criteria, including: (1) uniform policies in health care institutions; (2) education initiatives on brain death determination for the health care and

legal communities, and the public; (3) brain death training and credentialing programs for physicians involved in brain death determination; (4) development of a singular standard for brain death determination for both adults and children; (5) country-wide consistent legal approach to brain death determination. For a further discussion of the results of the American Academy of Neurology's Summit, see Ariane Lewis et al., *An Interdisciplinary Response to Contemporary Concerns about Brain Death Determination*, 90 Neurology 423 (2018).

7. The evolution of state law on brain death, and the complex interplay between law and science, is illustrated by events in Nevada following the case of Aden Hailu. Hailu, a 20-year-old college student, failed to regain consciousness after a surgery in 2015. She was eventually declared brain dead. But when told by doctors that they intended to remove life support, Hailu's father sought a restraining order and the case eventually ended up in the Nevada Supreme Court. See Siobhan McAndrew, *The Contested Death of Aden Hailu*, Reno Gazette J. (Mar. 25, 2016). At issue was whether new AAN guidelines constituted "accepted medical standards" in the statutory requirement that a determination of death "must be made in accordance with accepted medical standards." NRS 451.007 (adopting the UDDA). The Court reviewed the legislative history of Nevada's adoption of the UDDA, and held that "[w]hile the Harvard criteria may not be the newest medical criteria involving brain death, we are not convinced with the record before us that the AAN guidelines have replaced the Harvard criteria as the accepted medical standard for states like Nevada that have enacted the UDDA." *In re Guardianship of Hailu*, 131 Nev. 892, 902 (2015). The Court went on to conclude, therefore, that a determination of brain death in Nevada still required "an 'irreversible cessation' of '[a]ll functions of the person's *entire* brain, including his or her brain stem." 11 NRS 451.007(1) (emphases added by the court). *In re Guardianship of Hailu*, 131 Nev. 892, 903 (2015). Hailu died in 2016, but the legal story continued in the Nevada legislature, where State Representative Michael Sprinkle proposed a new brain death statute. In describing the motivation for the bill, Rep. Sprinkle observed, "What we're trying to do here is make it very clear and also update how we do this, from relatively old and, if I might say, antiquated terms to what is current science and technology today. . .". Sandra Chereb, *Nevada Adopts National Brain Death Guidelines Under Bill*, Law Vegas Review-Journal (May 8, 2017).

The new Nevada brain death statute, NRS 451.007, now reads as follows:

1. For legal and medical purposes, a person is dead if the person has sustained an irreversible cessation of:

(a) Circulatory and respiratory functions; or

(b) All functions of the person's entire brain, including his or her brain stem.

2. A determination of death made under:

(a) Paragraph (a) of subsection 1 must be made in accordance with accepted medical standards.

(b) Paragraph (b) of subsection 1 must be made in accordance with the applicable guidelines set forth in:

(1) "Evidence-based Guideline Update: Determining Brain Death in Adults: Report of the Quality Standards Subcommittee of the American Academy of Neurology," published June 8, 2010, by the American Academy of Neurology, or any subsequent revisions approved by the American Academy of Neurology or its successor organization; or

(2) "Guidelines for the Determination of Brain Death in Infants and Children: An Update of the 1987 Task Force Recommendations," published January 27, 2012, by the Pediatric Section of the Society of Critical Care Medicine, or any subsequent revisions approved by the Pediatric Section of the Society of Critical Care Medicine or its successor organization.

E. NEUROSCIENCE PERSPECTIVES ON BRAIN DEATH

As you have read, the diagnosis of death often involves the use of electroencephalography (EEG), but how to assess EEG readings remains contested. To date, neuroscientific techniques have not allowed clinicians to reliably distinguish between disorders of consciousness, and reliably restore cognitive ability. But new neuroscience research excerpted below raises intriguing possibilities.

Steven Laureys & Nicholas D. Schiff

Coma and Consciousness: Paradigms (Re)Framed by Neuroimaging
61 Neuroimage 478, 488 (2012)

It is an exciting era for the field of brain injury and disorders of consciousness. The gray zones between the different clinical entities in the spectrum following coma are beginning to be better understood and defined by increasingly powerful neuroimaging technologies. . . . [A] yet to be determined minority of patients who are currently considered to be "vegetative" or unresponsive, show fMRI or EEG/ERP based signs of consciousness that are inaccessible to clinicians' motor-response dependent behavioral assessment. These ever improving technological means are changing the existing clinical boundaries and will permit some "non-communicative" and locked-in patients to communicate their thoughts and wishes and control their environment via non-motor pathways. . . . [O]ur understanding of consciousness and disorders of consciousness after coma is currently witnessing a significant paradigm shift.

For clinical medicine, the directions are fairly clear. The most important challenge now is to move from the above discussed single case reports and small cohort reports to large multi-centric studies further addressing the sensitivity and specificity of the discussed "high-tech" ancillary neuroimaging or electrophysiological tools. . . .

For the science of human consciousness the next steps are more likely to surprise than be strongly anticipated given the complexity of the problem. As more sophisticated measurements of brain function are applied to patients with near normal cognitive states who cannot speak or gesture our measurements will continue to confront our conceptual limitations of how such capacities are formed in the brain. . . .

In a not so far future, it is possible that real-time fMRI based communication or evoked potential brain computer interfaces will be used to address important clinical and ethical questions such as feeling of pain and discomfort. On the other hand, recent demonstrations that the injured brain may signal accurate communication with distinct patterns of basic brain responses compared to those of normal subjects (e.g. delayed hemodynamic signals; or EEG signals multiplexed in to novel frequency patterns, will challenge the easy translation of these techniques developed to communicate with cognitively intact subjects. Moreover, it is yet unclear whether in the absence of nuanced initiation of speech or gesture, the quality of such communications will ever reach a standard acceptable to adjudicate clinical and legal judgments.

Finally, this evolving field of work sets several broad and important challenges for medical ethics. As each discovery comes forward a marked ethical reframing continues to occur with the shifting models of recovery, diagnosis and prognosis. These frames will continue to change as these studies evolve and require that policies for patients with disorders of consciousness keep up with the times. Moreover, for the group of patients with a capacity to communicate these scientific discoveries bear on their fundamental rights for accurate diagnostic assessments and the basics of clinical care. . . .

Nicholas D. Schiff et al.
Behavioural Improvements with Thalamic Stimulation After Severe Traumatic Brain Injury
448 Nature 600, 600 (2007)

Disorders of consciousness that persist for longer than 12 months after severe traumatic brain injury are generally considered to be immutable; no treatment has been shown to accelerate recovery or improve functional outcome in such cases . . . [but] there might be residual functional capacity in some patients that could be supported by therapeutic interventions. . . . We hypothesize that further recovery in some patients in the MCS is limited by chronic underactivation of potentially recruitable large-scale networks. Here, in a 6-month double-blind alternating crossover study, we show that bilateral deep brain electrical stimulation (DBS) of the central thalamus modulates behavioural responsiveness in a patient who remained in MCS for 6 yr following traumatic brain injury before the intervention. . . .

[The patient was a 38-year-old man who suffered a closed head injury during an assault six years prior to the study. He was in a deep coma. Through the next two years during rehabilitation, the arousal level increased and occasional command-following was observed. This indicated a transition into the minimally conscious state. fMRI scans indicated that the patient could follow commands and had intact language networks. The stimulation elicited increased heart rate, sustained eye-opening, and head-turning in response to a voice. After stimulation, the patient responded to requests to name objects, but the speech was unintelligible, consisting only of brief periods of word-mouthing. Also, limb movements that were social gestures or use of objects were more common; however, complete action sequences were not produced. Continuous bilateral stimulation resulted in longer periods of eye-opening and increased responsiveness to command with some signs of object use and intelligible verbalization. — EDS.]

The frequency of specific cognitively mediated behaviors (primary outcome measures) and functional limb control and oral feeding (secondary outcome measures) increased during periods in which DBS was on as compared with periods in which it was off. . . . We interpret the DBS effects as compensating for a loss of arousal regulation that is normally controlled by the frontal lobe in the intact brain.

These findings provide evidence that DBS can promote significant late functional recovery from severe traumatic brain injury. Our observations, years after the injury occurred, challenge the existing practice of early treatment discontinuation for patients with only inconsistent interactive behaviors and motivate further research to develop therapeutic interventions. . . .

[After the formal study was completed, the patient showed more improvements when DBS was delivered continuously for 12 hours each day. Spontaneous speech remained rare, but prompted verbal responses became clearer. Speaking changed from silent utterances of single words to occasional audible multi-word sentences of as many as six words in length. Before the DBS the patient could not consume nutrition orally because of frequent choking. After the prolonged DBS, he received each meal orally and could consume thin liquids. Consequently, the cost of care became less, and he became better integrated with family members who could feed him. On the other hand, his ability to move his body worsened.—EDS.]

Glenn R. Butterton

How Neuroscience Technology Is Changing Our Understanding of Brain Injury, Vegetative States and the Law

20 N.C. J.L. & Tech. 331, 341-54 (2019)

Recent research sheds new light on the PVS phenomenon, and suggests the problem of misdiagnosis may be worse than previously thought. . . .

A. Imagery Tasks: Tennis and Navigation

[In a neuroscience study published in 2006] . . . researchers instructed a patient to perform certain imagery tasks while in an fMRI scanner. The patient, who had been unresponsive five months after a traffic accident, was verbally asked to *think about* playing tennis and also navigating or walking through rooms in her home. In healthy subjects, one finds that specific brain areas [such as the supplemental motor cortex, the para-hippocampal gyrus, and the visual cortex] are activated during the performance of these tasks. . . . The traffic accident victim showed exactly the same activations. In subsequent work with a large patient group of 54, the same verbal instructions were given, and five of those experimental patients, or roughly ten percent of the group, showed activation in exactly the same areas as the healthy subjects.

These results are of great interest since they appear to indicate that the patients in the subset were capable of following instructions. This is important because instructions fall within the linguistic category of commands, and the ability to carry out commands strongly suggests that the patients possess cognitive ability of some significant degree.

B. A Novel Way to Say "Yes" and "No"

A key follow-up experiment measurably advanced the conceptual ball. In that case, Patient No. 23 from the tennis and navigation group was asked to communicate . . . using a more complex signaling system. She was instructed to answer yes-no questions by making special use of the mental imagery exercise: when asked a question by a researcher, she could answer "Yes" by *thinking* of playing tennis, and "No" by *thinking* of navigating through the rooms of her home. . . . The researchers then asked a series of yes-no questions to which they knew the answers ("Do you have any brothers?" or "Is your father's name Alexander?" and so on). In this circumstance, the patient correctly answered five questions, but did not respond to a sixth.

C. Photographs & Sentences

Previously, experimenters had achieved promising results when using face and sentence recognition tasks. Kate Bainbridge was a 26-year-old school teacher who entered PVS after developing flu-like symptoms and then falling into a coma. The experimenter placed her in a PET scanner and projected in her visual field photographs of her family, which he alternated with images of faces that were so digitally-distorted as to be unrecognizable. Whenever the family faces appeared, her brain showed activation in the Fusiform Gyrus, which is used for the highly specialized task of face recognition, and her Fusiform activations were identical to those of healthy control subjects.

In other work, experimenters shifted from visual imagery to speech sounds, but using an analogous method, exposed patients to recordings of simple sentences alternating with nonsense sounds or "noise." In those cases, PVS patients showed the same fMRI activations in response to the recordings as healthy volunteers. Likewise, when ambiguous sentences were used, two PVS patients showed the very same fMRI activations—those of a brain struggling to interpret words—as those of healthy volunteers. . . .

V. CLINICAL AND LEGAL DESCRIPTIONS

A. Degradation, Indignity and Loss of Consciousness

Loss of consciousness is a key quality-of-life concern in PVS cases. We closely identify consciousness with our humanity, and if we are robbed of it by PVS, we may regard our quality of life as greatly degraded, so much so that words such as "undignified" are sometimes used to characterize it. For some, but not all, the adjective "vegetative" expresses that degradation and loss of dignity. . . .

Against the backdrop of this debate, it is worth noting that an expert assessment by a physician that the loss of consciousness is virtually permanent can be devastating and dispositive for family and friends. Indeed, it can play a key role in the decision to withdraw life support from the PVS patient, either by Advance Directive or through instructions given by a surrogate or clinicians in a default situation. . . .

Of course, one wants to avoid such catastrophic outcomes by ensuring to the extent practical that physicians, caregivers, family members, attorneys, and others potentially involved in crafting Advance Directives and shaping end-of-life protocols are adequately informed of the complexities of PVS diagnosis. . . .

B. Guidance for Advance Directives, Living Wills & End of Life Protocols

. . . Advance Directives are typically signed, and sometimes drafted, by persons of sound mind, whether healthy or ill, in anticipation of health problems that may render them unconscious or otherwise unable to make authoritative decisions concerning their own medical care. . . . PVS is a condition sometimes included among those that will trigger such an end-of-life instruction. Thus, an erroneous diagnosis or description of PVS, if not detected, may trigger an end-of-life instruction never intended by the author. . . .

C. Revisions and Reforms

In view of the research results presented above . . . we strongly recommend revisions that may benefit those whose lives are affected by PVS.

First, competent state authorities should be urged to revise or amend all PVS-relevant statutes and government-based regulations and guidelines, including all sample Advance Directives, "living wills," and associated literature, so that they reflect the current state of neuroscience research. Second, all PVS-relevant literature that may be distributed to patients and family members by physicians, hospitals, hospices, insurers and other participants in the healthcare delivery system should be similarly revised. Third, such revisions and amendments should be pursued in all jurisdictions, even though as a demographic matter, some jurisdictions — such as Sunbelt and other states that host substantial retirement communities — may have much greater numbers of at-risk residents than others. Fourth, given the pace of technological change, arrangements should be made for periodic updates, and for those updates to be communicated in a timely fashion through mass mailings and electronic distributions to hospitals and other facilities where administrators, physicians, nurses and other caregivers regularly work with prospective or actual PVS patients. . . .

NOTES AND QUESTIONS

1. What do you foresee as the impact on law of these new methods for communicating with people in states of minimal consciousness? *See* Dalia B. Taylor, *Communicating with Vegetative State Patients: The Role of Neuroimaging in American Disability Law*, 66 Stan. L. Rev. 1451 (2014).

2. Should an MCS patient who gains some speech ability due to DBS be deemed competent by the law to execute a contract? Change a will? Consent to experimental treatments?

3. Can neuroscience usefully aid clinicians (and thus the law) in differentiating between states of consciousness? In 2013 a group of researchers proposed a new method of assessing consciousness, building on the observation that subjective conscious experience requires "specialized areas of the thalamocortical system to interact rapidly and effectively to form an integrated whole." Thus, "consciousness requires an optimal balance between functional integration and functional differentiation in thalamocortical networks, otherwise defined as brain complexity." Taking advantage of these theoretical observations, the research team developed a method using transcranial magnetic stimulation to measure this brain complexity (and thus provide a new window into the consciousness of the patient). Adenauer G. Casali et al., *A Theoretically Based Index of Consciousness Independent of Sensory Processing and Behavior*, 5 Sci. Transl. Med. 198 (2013). Commenting on the findings, colleagues suggested that "the dream of such a quantitative 'consciousness-o-meter' may not be out of reach." Jacobo D. Sitt et al., *Ripples of Consciousness*, 17 Trends Cognitive Sci. 552, 553 (2013).

4. Research in the field of disorders of consciousness (DoC) is exploring multiple new modalities for assessing individual cognitive evaluations. For example, a 2017 study sought to determine the residual cognitive capacities of a group of patients with EEG by combining eight criteria (own name recognition, temporal

attention, spatial attention, detection of spatial incongruence, motor planning, and modulations of these effects by the global context). The researchers were able to successfully perform the protocol in a single one-and-a-half-hour EEG test and suggested that this test can help clinicians to determine the chances of recovery of patients in a minimally conscious state or vegetative state. Claire Sergent et al., *Multidimensional Cognitive Evaluation of Patients with Disorders of Consciousness Using EEG: A Proof of Concept Study*, 13 Neuroimage: Clinical 455 (2017).

5. New technologies employed to research disorders of consciousness give rise to ethical considerations regarding the adequacy of treatment received by patients suffering such disorders. When a patient has been diagnosed as being completely unconscious, the presence of pain or suffering is not discussed; however, fMRI technology has deemed some of these consciousness diagnoses erroneous, which means the patient might be suffering undetected pain without being able to communicate it. Should all patients suffering DoC receive pain medication as a measure to prevent unnecessary suffering? Would your answer change if the administration of such medications interacted negatively with a physician's ability to properly diagnose a patient's level of consciousness? *See* Kathinka Evers, *Neurotechnological Assessment of Consciousness Disorders: Five Ethical Imperatives*, 18 Dialogues Clin. Neurosci. 155 (2016). For a further discussion of the ethical obligations of physicians providing treatment to patients suffering a disorder of consciousness, see Joseph J. Fins, *Neuroethics and Disorders of Consciousness: Discerning Brain States in Clinical Practice and Research*, 18 AMA J. Ethics 1182 (2016).

6. Researchers are exploring the use of non-invasive brain imaging such as fMRI to determine a patient's "interactive capacity." Interactive capacity is defined as "the ability to receive communicated information and intentionally generate a coherent response. . . ." Interactive capacity may be a reliable measure of consciousness because it "builds on principles of the behavioral criteria, which also largely center around interactive behavior (e.g., following commands, answering yes-or-no questions), and in doing so appeals to intuitive conceptions of conscious behavior." For an argument for why interactive capacity has a lower potential for misdiagnosis than other diagnostic tools traditionally used in the field of disorders of consciousness, see David B. Fischer & Robert D. Truog, *What Is a Reflex? A Guide for Understanding Disorders of Consciousness*, 85 Neurology 543 (2015). How would the law respond to the new concept of "interactive capacity"?

7. As both EEG- and fMRI-based assessments of DoC remain relatively new, there are a host of methodological cautions to be considered. *See* Daniel Kondziella et al., *Preserved Consciousness in Vegetative and Minimal Conscious States: Systematic Review and Meta-analysis*, 87 J. Neurology Neurosurgery & Psychiatry 485 (2016).

FURTHER READING

Defining and Determining Death:

Elizabeth Price Foley, *The Law of Life and Death* (2011).
President's Council on Bioethics, *Controversies in the Determination of Death* (2008).
Eelco F.M. Wijdicks, *Brain Death* (3d ed. 2017).

Thaddeus Mason Pope, *Brain Death Forsaken: Growing Conflict and New Legal Challenges*, 37 J. Legal Med. 265 (2017).

Hilary H. Wang et al., *Improving Uniformity in Brain Death Determination Policies over Time*, 88 Neurology 562 (2017).

Sarah Wahlster et al., *Brain Death Declaration Practices and Perceptions Worldwide*, 84 Neurology 1870 (2015).

The Hastings Center Report: Defining Death: Organ Transplantation and the Fifty-Year Legacy of the Harvard Report on Brain Death (Special Issue) (2018).

Revisiting Death: Organ Donation and the Dead Donor Rule (Special Issue), 35(3) J. of Med. & Phil. (2010).

Special issue on brain death, 14(8) Am. J. of Bioethics (2014).

Neuroscience, Ethics, and Disorders of Consciousness:

Martin M. Monti et al., *Willful Modulation of Brain Activity in Disorders of Consciousness*, 362 New Eng. J. Med. 579 (2010).

Steven Laureys, *Death, Unconsciousness and the Brain*, 11 Nature Reviews Neurosci. 899 (2005).

Finding Consciousness: The Neuroscience, Ethics, and Law of Severe Brain Damage (Walter Sinnott-Armstrong ed., 2016).

Adrian M. Owen et al., *Detecting Awareness in the Vegetative State*, 313 Science 1402 (2006).

Laura Y. Cabrera & Judy Illes, *Balancing Ethics and Care in Disorders of Consciousness*, 17 Lancet Neurology 112 (2018).

Michael Nair-Collins & Franklin G. Miller, *Do the 'Brain Dead' Merely Appear to Be Alive?*, 43 J. Med. Ethics 747 (2017).

CHAPTER 10

Brain Injury

I will never be what I was.

—U.S. Soldier who experienced multiple bomb
blasts in combat in Afghanistan[†]

The human brain. Easily the most complex object in the known universe.
Consequently, litigation involving traumatic brain injury is highly demanding.
—Marketing material on a law firm website[††]

CHAPTER SUMMARY

This chapter:

- Introduces and illustrates a variety of legal issues that can arise from traumatic brain injuries.
- Explores the special challenges of defining and proving brain injuries in court, including malingering, causation, and assumption of risk, as they arise in brain injury litigation.
- Examines the unique legal and policy challenges associated with sport-related concussions.

INTRODUCTION

The human brain can be damaged in many ways, from before birth to late in life. Damage can come from strokes, toxins, certain viral infections, neurogenerative disorders, and even harmful emotional experiences. It can also originate from a single major impact (such as a car accident or a wartime blast) or from lesser but frequent impacts (such as football tackles or soccer headers). Worldwide, it is estimated that 69 million people experience a traumatic brain injury (TBI) each year, leading some to call TBI the "silent epidemic."[*] Brain injury can result in significant health, social, and economic consequences. TBI leads to an estimated $76 billion in direct and indirect medical expenses.[**]

[†] Sharon Weinberger, *Bomb's Hidden Impact: The Brain War*, 477 Nature 390, 393 (Sept. 21, 2011).

[††] BrainInjury.com, http://www.braininjury.com.

[*] Michael C. Dewan et al., *Estimating the Global Incidence of Traumatic Brain Injury*, 130 J. Neurosurgery 1080, 1080 (2018).

[**] National Institute of Neurological Disorders and Stroke, *Traumatic Brain Injury: Hope Through Research*, NIH Publication No. 16-158, at 1 (2015).

Because preventing, identifying, and treating brain injury have obvious medical and social implications, researchers are working to understand exactly how the brain is damaged and how it might be repaired. Researchers are also working to develop more objective methods of assessing TBI. Policymakers at the federal level, such as in the Department of Defense and the Department of Veterans Affairs, have increased investment in research and treatment for brain injury. At the state level, states have passed legislation and promulgated new regulations regarding, for example, concussions in high school sports. At the local level, school districts and youth sports organizations (such as youth football) have revised rules and regulations for participation. So, too, have some high-visibility professional sports organizations, such as the National Football League (which has revised its concussion policy, introduced more severe penalties for helmet-to-helmet hits, and changed rules of the game to minimize the incidence of hard collisions).

To be effective, the legal system's growing involvement in the brain injury arena—both through regulation at the front end and litigation at the back end—must be accompanied by up-to-date knowledge of the human brain's complex structure and operations. This is challenging when, as described later in this chapter, understanding of the neurobiology of brain injury is still incomplete.

In previous chapters, you have read about brain-based criminal defenses in which a defendant argues that a damaged brain (perhaps damaged through a traumatic event) should reduce culpability. Elsewhere in the legal system, decisions must be made about brain injury for purposes of disability benefits, veterans benefits claims, and the like. In this chapter, we focus on an especially prominent context in which brain injury meets law: civil litigation in which plaintiffs seek compensation for brain injury.

As you likely recall from your Torts class, the required elements for recovery of damages are: (1) duty; (2) breach of duty; (3) injury; and (4) proximate cause between the defendant's action (or inaction) and the injury. In the cases and commentaries that follow, you will see courts wrestle with complex questions regarding the nature and extent of the injury, and the extent to which the defendant is responsible for the traumatic event(s) that caused the injury. You will also see how neuroimaging evidence is proffered, and challenged, in these legal settings.

The chapter is organized into five sections. Section A examines how brain injury is defined and discusses efforts to create more reliable and objective measures of TBI. Section B illustrates some of the general principles—legal duties, assumptions of risk, and the impact of science on these—with illustrative examples from contact sports. Section C explores how lawyers prove brain injury in court, including how questions of plaintiff "malingering" (i.e., faking) are addressed, and how neuroimaging such as diffusion tensor imaging might be used to support a plaintiff's claim. Section D turns to the issue of causation, examining how law assesses the connection between a traumatic event and subsequent behavioral changes. Section E explores litigation and legislation related to youth sports concussions.

A. DEFINING BRAIN INJURY

Defining and diagnosing "brain injury" is difficult, and as noted in an excerpt below there are over 40 different definitions of "concussion." To date, clinicians have primarily relied on patient history, careful observation of patient behavior, and neuropsychological testing. But without more objective measures, diagnosis can be imprecise. For instance, patient history is instructive (e.g., it matters if a man falls down the stairs and hits his head). But patient history alone is not dispositive (e.g., the man who fell may get right up and show no immediate signs of behavioral deficit, despite damage that will manifest later). Similarly, observable behavior is instructive (e.g., if the man is slow to respond to certain questions it may be an indicator of injury), but also not in and of itself dispositive (since the man may have always been someone who is slow to respond to those types of questions). Neuropsychological testing, if available, may aid in diagnosis, but typically there is no baseline testing with which to compare the results. Amidst these challenges, clinicians have established a variety of methods for assessment of brain injury. Increasingly, researchers are proposing novel approaches to concussion diagnosis, utilizing eye tracking, blood tests, and brain scans. The following show some of the ways that clinicians currently categorize and evaluate TBI, as well as proposals for new diagnostic approaches.

Nat'l Inst. of Neurological Disorders & Stroke & Nat'l Insts. of Health
Traumatic Brain Injury: Hope Through Research
(2015)

Traumatic brain injury (TBI) is the leading cause of death and disability in children and young adults in the United States. TBI is also a major concern for elderly individuals, with a high rate of death and hospitalization due to falls among people age 75 and older. Depending on the severity of injury, TBI can have a lasting impact on quality of life for survivors of all ages—impairing thinking, decision making and reasoning, concentration, memory, movement, and/or sensation (e.g., vision or hearing), and causing emotional problems (personality changes, impulsivity, anxiety, and depression) and epilepsy. . . .

Not every TBI is alike. Each injury is unique and can cause changes that affect a person for a short period of time, or sometimes permanently.

The majority of people will completely recover from symptoms related to *concussion*, a mild type of TBI. However, persistent symptoms do occur for some people and may last for weeks or months. The long-term effects of TBI may vary depending on the number and nature of "hits" to the head, the age and gender of the individual, the speed with which the person received medical attention, and genetic and other factors. . . .

Many questions remain unanswered regarding the impact of TBIs, the best treatments, and the most effective methods for promoting recovery of brain function. . . .

WHAT IS A [TRAUMATIC BRAIN INJURY (TBI)]?

A TBI occurs when physical, external forces impact the brain either from a penetrating object or a bump, blow, or jolt to the head. Not all blows or jolts to the head result in a TBI. For the ones that do, TBIs can range from mild (a brief change in mental status or consciousness) to severe (an extended period of unconsciousness or amnesia after the injury). There are two broad types of head injuries: penetrating and non-penetrating.

Penetrating TBI (also known as *open TBI*) occurs when the skull is pierced by an object (for example, a bullet, shrapnel, bone fragment, or by a weapon such as hammer, knife, or baseball bat). With this injury, the object enters the brain tissue.

Non-penetrating TBI (also known as *closed head injury* or *blunt TBI*) is caused by an external force that produces movement of the brain within the skull. Causes include falls, motor vehicle crashes, sports injuries, or being struck by an object. Blast injury due to explosions is a focus of intense study but how it causes brain injury is not fully known. . . .

HOW DOES TBI AFFECT THE BRAIN?

TBI-related damage can be confined to one area of the brain, known as a *focal injury*, or it can occur over a more widespread area, known as a *diffuse injury*. The type of injury is another determinant of the effect on the brain. Some injuries are considered *primary*, meaning the damage is immediate. Other consequences of TBI can be *secondary*, meaning they can occur gradually over the course of hours, days, or weeks. These secondary brain injuries are the result of reactive processes that occur after the initial head trauma.

There are a variety of immediate effects on the brain, including various types of bleeding and tearing forces that injure nerve fibers and cause inflammation, metabolic changes, and brain swelling.

- *Diffuse axonal injury (DAI)* is one of the most common types of brain injuries. DAI refers to widespread damage to the brain's white matter. White matter is composed of bundles of axons (projections of nerve cells that carry electrical impulses). Like the wires in a computer, axons connect various areas of the brain to one another. DAI is the result of *shearing* forces, which stretch or tear these axon bundles. This damage commonly occurs in auto accidents, falls, or sports injuries. It usually results from rotational forces (twisting) or sudden deceleration. It can result in a disruption of neural circuits and a breakdown of overall communication among nerve cells, or neurons, in the brain. It also leads to the release of brain chemicals that can cause further damage. These injuries can cause temporary or permanent damage to the brain, and recovery can be prolonged.
- *Concussion*—a type of mild TBI that may be considered a temporary injury to the brain but could take minutes to several months to heal. Concussion can be caused by a number of things including a bump, blow, or jolt to the head, sports injury or fall, motor vehicle accident, weapons blast, or a rapid acceleration or deceleration of the brain within the skull (such as the person having been violently shaken). The individual either suddenly loses consciousness or has sudden altered state of consciousness or awareness, and is often called "dazed" or said to have his/her "bell rung." A second concussion closely following the first one causes further damage to the brain—the so-called "second hit" phenomenon—and can lead to permanent damage or even death in some instances.
- *Hematomas*—a pooling of blood in the tissues outside of the blood vessels. Hematomas can develop when major blood vessels in the head become damaged, causing severe bleeding in and around the brain. . . .

. . . Poor blood flow to the brain can also cause secondary damage. When the brain sustains a powerful blow, swelling occurs just as it would in other parts of the body. Because the skull cannot expand, the brain tissue swells and the pressure inside the skull rises; this is known as *intracranial pressure (ICP)*. When the intracranial pressure becomes too high it prevents blood from flowing to the brain, which deprives it of the oxygen it needs to function. This can permanently damage brain function.

Maya Elin O'Neil et al.
Complications of Mild Traumatic Brain Injury in Veterans and Military Personnel: A Systematic Review
(2013)

Classification of TBI Severity

Criteria	Mild	Moderate	Severe
Structural imaging	Normal	Normal or abnormal	Normal or abnormal
Loss of Consciousness (LOC)	0-30 min	>30 min and <24 hrs	>24 hrs
Alteration of consciousness/ mental state (AOC)	A moment up to 24 hrs	>24 hours. Severity based on other criteria	
Post-traumatic amnesia (PTA)	0-1 day	>1 and <7 days	>7 days
Glasgow Coma Scale (best available score in first 24 hours)	13-15	9-12	<9

NCAA Sports Science Institute
Interassociation Consensus: Diagnosis and Management of Sport-Related Concussion Best Practices
(2017)

There are more than 42 consensus-based definitions of concussion. The only evidence-based definition of concussion follows.

Concussion is:

- a change in brain function,
- following a force to the head, which
- may be accompanied by temporary loss of consciousness, but is
- identified in awake individuals, with
- measures of neurologic and cognitive dysfunction.

Diagnosis and management of sport-related concussion is a clinical diagnosis based on the judgment of the athlete's health care providers. The diagnosis and management of sport-related concussion is challenging for many reasons:

- The physical and cognitive examinations are often normal, and additional tests such as brain computerized tomography, brain MRI, electroencephalogram and blood tests are also commonly normal. Comprehensive neuropsychological tests may be a useful adjunctive tool supporting the diagnosis of sport-related concussion but the valid administration and interpretation of these tests is complex and requires appropriate training and/or supervisory oversight.

- The clinical effects of sport-related concussion are often subtle and difficult to detect with existing sport-related concussion assessment tools.
- The symptoms of sport-related concussion are not specific to concussion and it is challenging to evaluate a student-athlete who presents non-specific symptoms that may be related to other conditions.
- Sport-related concussion may manifest with immediate or delayed-onset symptoms. Symptom manifestation can vary between individuals and in the same individual who has suffered a repeat concussion.
- Modifying factors and co-morbidities—such as attention deficit hyperactivity disorder, migraine and other headache disorders, learning disabilities and mood disorders—should be considered in making the diagnosis, providing a management plan and making both return-to-play and return-to-learn recommendations. . . .
- Student-athletes may underreport symptoms and inflate their level of recovery in hopes of being rapidly cleared for return to competition.
- Clinical assessment of sport-related concussion is a surrogate index of recovery and not a direct measure of brain structure and functional integrity after concussion. . . .

In summary, the natural history of concussion remains poorly defined, diagnosis can be difficult, there are often few objective findings for diagnosis or physio-logical recovery that exist for clinical use, and there often remains a significant reliance on self-report of symptoms from the student-athlete. . . .

Danielle K. Sandsmark
Clinical Outcomes After Traumatic Brain Injury
16 Current Neurology & Neurosci. Rep. 52 (2016)

Heterogeneity in the mechanism of TBI, the mechanics of the applied force, and patient factors (including the use of protective gear and genetic factors) renders no two traumatic brain injuries exactly the same, though all are lumped under the TBI designation. As such, there is also huge variability in patient recovery after TBI, with some survivors regaining complete or near complete function while others remain severely disabled. This uncertainty can be incredibly unnerving for patients, families, and clinicians. . . .

One of the challenges in TBI outcomes and clinical research is the lack of a mechanistic, quantitative endpoint. If there was an objective metric that could be tracked over time, such as lactic acid in sepsis or the CA-125 cancer biomarker in ovarian cancer, that correlated with patient outcome, this would be a huge advance both for clinical practice and for research studies. In milder forms of traumatic brain injury, such as concussion, when imaging features of injury are typically lacking, biomarkers are being sought to diagnosis injury. In more severely injured patients, where diagnosis is generally readily made based on computed tomography imaging abnormalities, biomarkers in the acute, subacute, and chronic phases have the potential to lend insights into the timeline and biological mechanisms underlying brain injury, repair, and recovery after TBI.

Several candidate biomarkers have shown promise in their association with TBI outcomes when studied in cohorts of patients. These biomarkers include the glial protein S100-beta, neuron-specific enolase, and myelin basic protein, among others. However, each of these candidates has relatively low sensitivity and specificity when applied individually. . . .

————————————

Biomarkers for TBI.   The excerpts above make clear that there is a need for better diagnostic tools to initially diagnose and then track the trajectory of traumatic brain injury. In the following excerpts you will learn about a variety of efforts to develop biomarkers for brain injury. As you read, think about the legal implications of these new types of evidence.

Zoe Su Wen Gan et al.
Blood Biomarkers for Traumatic Brain Injury: A Quantitative Assessment of Diagnostic and Prognostic Accuracy
10 Frontiers Neurology 446 (2019)

Pathological responses to TBI in the CNS include structural and metabolic changes, as well as excitotoxicity, neuroinflammation, and cell death. Fluid biomarkers that may track these injury and inflammatory processes have been explored for their potential to provide objective measures in TBI assessment. . . .

[C]urrent practices in forming an opinion of concussion involve symptom reports, neurocognitive testing, and balance testing, all of which have elements of subjectivity and questionable reliability. . . . [Current assessment practice does] not identify any underlying processes that may have prognostic or therapeutic consequences. Furthermore, because patients with concussion typically present with negative head CT findings, there is a potential role for blood-based biomarkers to provide objective information regarding the presence of concussion, based on an underlying pathology. This information could inform management decisions regarding resumption of activities for both athletes and non-athletes alike.

Blood-based biomarkers have utility far beyond a simple detection of concussion by elucidating specific aspects of the injury that could drive individual patient management. . . .

Blood biomarkers also have the potential to help predict unfavorable outcomes across the spectrum of TBI severity. . . .

Blood biomarkers offer potentially valuable objective information that may augment rather than replace existing tools for clinical assessment and contribute to a holistic approach to management. . . .

Uzma Samadani
Will Eye Tracking Change the Way We Diagnose and Classify Concussion and Structural Brain Injury?
1 Concussion 2 (2015)

Potential modalities for more accurate assessment and classification of brain injury include quantitative EEG, serum and other bodily fluid biomarkers, infrared spectroscopy and other tests.

Recently, there has been a renewed interest in eye tracking as a potential diagnostic, biomarker and outcome measure for brain injury. . . .

The clinical basis for eye tracking as a diagnostic for brain injury has ancient roots. Some 3500 years ago, Egyptian physicians wrote the oldest known surviving surgical treatise stating that eyes that are askew may be evidence of brain injury. Prior to the invention of radiographic imaging, the assessment of eye movements was a major modality of diagnosis of neurologic impairment with entire textbooks dedicated to this topic.

Modern era optometrists can detect abnormal eye movements in up to 90% of patients with so-called mild traumatic brain injury or concussion. The most commonly detected abnormal eye movement associated with brain injury is a vergence problem. Vergence is the ability of the both eyes to focus together on a single point. If the point moves closer to the nose, the pupils converge. Following the point in space—or while watching TV—requires sustained vergence. Previous studies using eye tracking to assess patients with postconcussive symptoms suggest that these deficits may persist beyond the acute phase of injury. . . .

Nina Kraus & Travis White-Schwoch
Listen to the Brain to Suss Out Concussions
70 Hearing J. 56, 56-57 (2017)

We tested a new approach to identify concussions: the frequency-following response (FFR), an electrophysiological measure of sound-evoked synchronous neural activity. Making sense of sound is one of the brain's most difficult tasks, and an individual suffering from a concussion struggles to understand sound in complex listening environments. These observations motivated the hypothesis that measuring fine-grained neural processes could indicate the presence of a concussion.

To test this hypothesis, we measured the FFRs of adolescents diagnosed with a concussion in a sports medicine clinic. We found that neural responses to the fundamental frequency (F0) were disrupted after a concussion—they were about 30 percent lower and more sluggish than in healthy controls. The F0 is an important pitch-bearing cue for identifying sounds. . . .

We then tried to use the FFR to identify individuals with concussions, and found that the FFR accurately identified 90 percent of concussion patients and 95 percent of control patients. The FFR also tracked the symptom severity of a concussion; children, who reported the greatest symptom loads from injuries, had the lowest F0 responses. Additionally, we found that the FFR to the F0 improved as patients recovered, suggesting that FFR can be used to track recovery.

The FFR has many features that make it an attractive approach to augment concussion management. It is a fast and portable test, with available norms for patients of different ages. It also has a good test-to-test reliability. Perhaps the most useful feature of FFR for concussion management is that it does not require patients to do anything during the test—patients may sleep or watch a movie while the test is going on. . . .

While these results are promising, it is important to acknowledge that this study was just a proof of concept. . . .

NOTES AND QUESTIONS

1. Researchers and clinicians disagree about the terminology to be used in discussing concussion and brain injury. For instance, two specialists have proposed that "the term concussion should be retired because it has no clear and consistently understood definition, leads to diagnostic confusion and can limit the use of effective treatments of post-traumatic problems. Instead, neurologists should adopt a single classification system for all TBI based on injury severity and attempt a precise diagnosis of post-traumatic problems." David J. Sharp & Peter O. Jenkins, *Concussion Is Confusing Us All*, 15 Practical Neurology 172, 182 (2015). What are the legal implications of the uncertainty surrounding the terminology, definition, and classification of brain injury?

2. It is evident that biomarkers for brain injury are emerging but are not yet universally (or even widely) used. At what point should courts allow biomarker evidence of TBI to be shown to a jury. For instance, would a classification accuracy of 84% be sufficient? Consider this conclusion:

   > Previous studies have focused on finding abnormalities in white matter or functional connectivity group differences between mTBI [mild TBI] and HC [healthy control] subjects. The present work took a different approach where the classification of mTBIs and HCs (i.e., individual subjects via cross-validation) is the central point of the analysis. This methodology directly tests the use of dMRI [diffusion magnetic resonance imaging] and fMRI data as biomarkers for mTBI. . . . The present work intended to compare HC–mTBI classification power from proposed techniques to detect abnormalities in white matter with methods to assess abnormalities in functional connectivity.
   >
   > Looking side by side to results from dMRI versus fMRI, we can see that [resting state functional network connectivity] features deliver higher classification performance (84.1%) compared with FA [fractional anisotropy] (75.5%) after determining optimal [machine learning] parameters. . . .

   Victor M. Vergara et al., *Detection of Mild Traumatic Brain Injury by Machine Learning Classification Using Resting State Functional Network Connectivity and Fractional Anisotropy*, 34 J. Neurotrauma 1045, 1050 (2017).

3. Whatever the terminology or diagnostic criteria, at the core of brain injury is the recognition that the most powerful organ in the body has been damaged. When philosopher Megan Craig experienced a brain injury, she reflected on the profound effect it had on her life:

   > [A] concussion has a way of changing one's sense of the balance between mind and body. . . .
   >
   > The injury to my brain highlighted the degree to which my identity and my powers of identification have a specific seat in my brain. The concussed condition was an intimation of how terrifying dementia and other brain disorders must feel — the loss of a thread that has so far tied together one's life and tethered it to the lives of those one loves. In my case, the loss was temporary, but it was the first time that I have ever felt so distinctly the efforts of thinking, the brain as a muscle and the depression that accompanies the feeling of having lost oneself.

   Megan Craig, *A Philosopher on Brain Rest*, N.Y. Times (June 25, 2019).

4. Imagine that you were tasked with crafting your own legally relevant definitions of brain injuries. How would you approach this challenge?

5. The Brain Injury Association of America (BIAA) is an advocacy organization for plaintiffs' lawyers and their clients in brain injury litigation. In 2011, the BIAA announced that it had adopted a new definition of traumatic brain injury: "TBI is defined as an alteration in brain function, or other evidence of brain pathology, caused by an external force." The BIAA stated that "this updated definition will better capture the essence of the disease process and the many varying outcomes present in persons with TBI and will reflect more recent research conducted by experts across the country." *BIAA Adopts New TBI Definition*, BIAA (Feb. 6, 2011). Why would an advocacy organization proffer a definition of TBI? If you were representing a client seeking damages for brain injury, how would you evaluate this definition? If you were representing a defendant being sued for causing brain injury, would you adopt a different perspective on this definition?

6. The rise of mild TBI (mTBI) diagnoses have led some to challenge the use of mTBI as a diagnostic category. Evaluate this argument:

> [T]he diagnosis of traumatic brain injury (TBI), and in particular mild TBI (MTBI), is an example of what Ryle would have called a category mistake. A category mistake occurs when a property is associated to an object that cannot meaningfully possess that property or when a process is implemented in a context where it cannot be meaningfully implemented. For example, the statement "all asteroids are philosophers" is a category mistake. Similarly, a classification of asteroids according to philosophical school is a category mistake.
>
> Diagnosis is a process that can be meaningfully associated with a disease. A TBI is not a disease. It is an event. More precisely, TBI is an event or a sequence of events that can, in some instances, lead to a diagnosable neurological or psychiatric disorder. Although acute and chronic neurological and psychological deficits that follow brain injury can be assessed, the diagnosis of TBI as a discrete clinical entity is not a logical possibility.

Paul Rapp & Kenneth Curley, *Is a Diagnosis of "Mild Traumatic Brain Injury" a Category Mistake?*, 73 J. Trauma & Acute Care Surgery S13, S13 (2012).

B. LEGAL DUTIES, ASSUMPTION OF RISK, AND BRAIN INJURY

Much brain injury litigation involves claims of negligence on the part of the defendant. To win on a negligence claim, a plaintiff must establish that the defendant had a legal duty toward the plaintiff and that the defendant breached that legal duty. One defense to negligence is the assumption of risk. If the defendant can show that the plaintiff voluntarily and knowingly assumed the risk, recovery is generally barred. The cases that follow address these issues in the context of athletic activities, both amateur and professional.

1. Amateur Sports

Parker v. S. Broadway Athletic Club
230 S.W.3d 642 (Mo. Ct. App. 2007)

SHAW, J. W.C. Parker and Martha Parker ("the Parkers"), parents of Curtis Parker ("Curtis"), appeal from the trial court's judgment entered upon the jury's verdict in favor of The South Broadway Athletic Club ("Club") on their wrongful death claim. We affirm.

In 2002, Curtis, who was twenty-eight years old, mentioned his interest in professional wrestling to his friend Cecil Lowe ("Lowe"), who is a professional wrestler. Lowe recommended to Curtis that he train at the Club, which has all the facilities necessary to train as a wrestler. . . .

The first series of lessons Curtis received were devoted to teaching Curtis "bumps," or "how to . . . fall without injuring [himself]." After mastering bumps, a new wrestler learns how to perform holds and moves. The final set of lessons focus on teaching new wrestlers "how to put all these moves together for matches."

Curtis went to the Club for training several times that summer. During the fourth lesson, on July 16, 2002, Curtis said that "his head was hurting him pretty bad," and Harris told Curtis to "get out of the ring, sit down."

Curtis's fifth lesson was on Monday, July 22, 2002. When Curtis arrived at the Club, Harris asked him, "[H]ow are you feeling, kid[?]" Curtis replied, "Well, it took me forever to get rid of my headache. I took all kinds of Tylenols, Ibuprofens and everything. It finally went away after four or five days." Harris then asked him "[H]ow [are] you feeling now[?]", and Curtis responded, "I'm feeling great." Relying on Curtis's repeated assurances, and noting that Curtis "looked normal and . . . talked normal," Curtis was admitted back into the wrestling ring. Harris started the lesson by performing a bump on Curtis called a "six pack."

The final bump Curtis had to master was a "power bomb." To deliver a power bomb, a wrestler lifts his opponent to chest or shoulder height and drops him to the mat on his back. First, Harris showed Curtis the move with other wrestlers. Then, Harris performed the move on Curtis two times while cradling him the entire way down to the mat. The third power bomb involved a full release—Harris hoisted Curtis up and "just let him go." Curtis "free [fell] all the way down on his back." Harris noted that Curtis "landed perfectly."

Curtis sat up after striking the mat. Harris congratulated him and told Curtis that he was ready to advance to moves. Curtis turned around and "his eyes rolled up in his head." He went into a seizure and started "shaking ferociously" and foam and blood began to trickle out of his mouth. An ambulance transported Curtis to St. Louis University Hospital where he died nine days later.

The Parkers filed a wrongful death lawsuit . . . alleg[ing] that the Club failed to exercise reasonable care in not requiring Curtis to obtain medical clearance before allowing him to resume his wrestling lessons.

Dr. Mary Case, a board certified forensic pathologist and forensic neuropathologist, testified on behalf of the Parkers. Dr. Case reviewed the events preceding Curtis's injury and concluded that Curtis's death was caused by a subdural hemorrhage resulting from second-impact syndrome. Dr. Case testified that individuals who experience a second concussion before fully recovering from a prior concussion are susceptible to second-impact syndrome, which is characterized by very rapid brain swelling. . . .

On cross-examination, Dr. Case testified that there are many kinds of headaches, and that "you don't have to have a concussion to get a headache." She testified that while headaches are a symptom of a concussion, there are many others, including, dizziness, nausea, vomiting, lack of awareness of your surroundings, and being easily fatigued. In this case, other than complaining of a headache, Curtis did not have any other concussive symptoms. Dr. Case also testified that even if Curtis had gone to see a physician complaining of headaches and had a CT scan or an MRI of his brain, those procedures would not have revealed that Curtis had a concussion. On the other hand, Dr. Case testified that a PET scan would have shown this damage to his brain, but "[t]here would be no possibility that [Curtis] was going to get a PET scan." . . .

The jury returned a verdict in favor of the Club and the trial court entered a judgment on that verdict. After the trial court denied their motion for new trial, the Parkers appealed. . . .

[W]e affirm the trial court's judgment because the Parkers failed to make a submissible case.

In its brief, the Club specifically argues the Parkers failed to make a submissible case because they did not establish that the Club knew or should have known that Curtis sustained a concussion on July 16, 2002. We agree. . . .

As submitted in the trial court's verdict-directing instruction, the Parkers' claim depended on two essential issues. First, the Club knew or should have known that Curtis had sustained a concussion on July 16, 2002. Second, the Club had a duty to bar him from returning to wrestling activity absent an examination of his physical condition by a medical doctor. Because we find the Parkers did not satisfy the first essential element of their case, we hold they failed to make a submissible case and the trial court's judgment in favor of the Club should be affirmed.

The Parkers submitted their case on a theory that Curtis's death resulted from the second-impact syndrome. However, we do not find substantial evidence in the record to prove that the Club knew or should have known that Curtis had sustained a concussion on July 16, 2002.

Here, Harris was only aware that Curtis had a headache of unknown cause and origin that had resolved itself before Curtis returned to the Club for additional wrestling training on July 22, 2002. When Curtis returned to the Club to resume his wrestling activity on that day, Curtis looked and talked normally, and told Harris he was feeling great. . . .

Under these circumstances, we find the Parkers failed to prove that the Club knew or should have known that Curtis had sustained a concussion on July 16, 2002. If it would have been difficult for a doctor to diagnose an initial concussion without recourse to sophisticated diagnostic tests, the Club certainly could not have known that Curtis had sustained a prior, unhealed concussion solely based upon his complaint of having a headache. As such, the Parkers failed to make a submissible case against the Club.

The trial court's judgment in favor of the Club is affirmed.

NOTES AND QUESTIONS

1. An expert witness in the *Parker* case suggested that a structural brain scan such as MRI or CT would not have identified a concussion, but that had it been done, a PET scan might have revealed the injury. The expert also said, however, that there was no possibility that a PET scan would normally have been ordered in this type of case. What diagnostic duties should be required of those in the trainer's situation? More generally, what duties should coaches and training staff have for assessing brain injuries? Should every athlete who complains of a headache be sent to a brain imaging lab?

2. What assumptions does tort law make about the human person? Do challenges to the foundations of criminal responsibility also apply to tort law? Law professor

Peter Alces argues that the foundations of tort law must be re-examined in light of neuroscience:

> If *A* acts negligently and injures *B*, *A* is in no helpful sense morally responsible for the predicate negligent action. There is no essential *A* who could have that ultimate uncaused cause divinelike moral responsibility. . . .
>
>   Just as is the case with criminal law, the need for tort law does not evaporate once we identify the problems with the status quo. We would not loose the negligent to do what harm they will just because "they can't help it," and we would not excuse those whose behavior undermines general well-being. We would, though, rely on an authentic conception of human agency, a conception that makes no room for moral responsibility. . . .

Peter A. Alces, *The Moral Conflict of Law and Neuroscience* 160, 176 (2018).

3. Contact sports present unique challenges for tort law because the sanctioned athletic activity (e.g., body checking in hockey, tackling in football, sparring in boxing) would under other circumstances be considered tortious conduct. Although there are exceptions, many courts have adopted a "contact sports exception" that replaces the ordinary negligence rule with a requirement for greater malfeasance. In *Karas v. Strevell*, a minor was injured from a body check while playing youth hockey. Plaintiff alleged negligence on the part of the coaches and the league, but the court sided with the defendants and cited the contact sports exception in doing so.

> [P]laintiff's essential allegation against all three organizational defendants is that they failed to adequately enforce the rule against body-checking from behind. Yet, as noted earlier, rules violations are inevitable in contact sports and are generally considered an inherent risk of playing the game. Further, in an organized contact sport, such as the one at issue here, the enforcement of the rules directly affects the way in which the sport is played. Imposing too strict a standard of liability on the enforcement of those rules would have a chilling effect on vigorous participation in the sport. Finally, as the organizational defendants point out, coaching and officiating decisions involve subjective decision-making that often occurs in the middle of a fast moving game . . . Applying an ordinary negligence standard to these decisions would open the door to a surfeit of litigation and would impose an unfair burden on organizational defendants such as those in the case at bar. Accordingly, we conclude that, under the facts alleged here, the contact sports exception applies to the organizational defendants. To successfully plead a cause of action for failing to adequately enforce the rules in an organized full-contact sport, plaintiff must allege that the defendant acted with intent to cause the injury or that the defendant engaged in conduct "totally outside the range of the ordinary activity" involved with coaching or officiating the sport.

Karas v. Strevell, 227 Ill. 2d 440, 464-65 (2008).

   As a matter of policy, what types of rules, and what types of rule enforcement, are optimal for contact sports such as hockey and football? What are the benefits of encouraging vigorous participation in these sports, and how do you believe those benefits should be weighed against the risks of injury?

4. Rather than modify behavior through negligence-based tort lawsuits, should more dramatic action be taken? With regard to collision sports, such as football, some commentators and former players have argued that football should be prohibited because it is too dangerous. At the University of Colorado in 2019, the

issue arose when the University's Board of Regents was asked to approve a new multi-million-dollar contract for football coach Mel Tucker. Coach Tucker had described his approach to football as, "Our team, we will be physical. . . . My dad always told me the name of the game is hit, hit, H-I-T. There is always a place on the field for someone who will hit."

In response, Regent Linda Shoemaker, who is a journalist and attorney, voted against Coach Tucker's contract. She commented that, "I really thought at first that we could play football safely with better rules and better equipment; I drank the Kool-Aid . . . [but] I can't go there anymore. I don't believe it can be played safely anymore. I want these young men to leave C.U. with minds that have been strengthened, not damaged." Michael Powell, *At Colorado, a Breach in Football's Wall*, N.Y. Times (Apr. 18, 2019).

But others view things differently and emphasize allowing athletes to choose. Former NFL player Ray Lewis addressed the issue this way in an interview with David Greene in 2015.

> GREENE: Well, what do you tell people who today, in 2015, are increasingly seeing this game as too violent and too dangerous?
>
> LEWIS: You know, we want to make emphasis of this game being so brutal now. No, this game has been brutal. This game was brutal from the first time you told two men to take their bodies and run full speed into each other. The way you play the game is the way the game was designed. And I don't care what you do with helmets, what you do with shoulder pads, what you do with any of these things. It still comes down to a man running full speed into another man.
>
> GREENE: Well, what about a mom . . . whose son wants to play football desperately, and she says, I can't let you do that because I don't want you to have the risk of a brain injury. . . . [H]ow would you sit down with a family and talk to them about that decision?
>
> LEWIS: Because it's the same risk that somebody got to sit down and talk to a fireman, right? Somebody who wants to be a firemen — guess what the risk of that is. The risk of you going to save somebody else's life is you may lose your life. Policemen — you got the same risk. So everybody got risk. Like, so you choose what your risk is. I think my real argument is don't make this such a bad game because of the way the game was always played. And so when you sit down and talk to a child, just like I told my sons, you know what you need to do, right? There are people bigger. There's people stronger. And there's people faster. So if you're going to do what you need to do, you need to change your body. You need to look a different way. So it's a bunch of things that go into it. And then, at the end of the day, it's still a choice. If you think about it, nobody's really forcing us to do this. Nobody would ever have to force me to play the game. When I was in the schoolyards playing with no shoes on and every day I came home, nobody had to force me to do that. There was no referees. So when you got a busted lip and you got a busted nose, what you going to do? Say what, cry? OK, cry. Suck it up, and get back in there. . . .

National Public Radio, *In 'I Feel Like Going On,' Ray Lewis Doesn't Apologize for Hard Hits* (Nov. 4, 2015).

5. The issue of second-impact syndrome raises legal questions about what a coach's duty is to an athlete after complaint of an initial injury. Second Impact Syndrome refers to the damage that can occur when an individual experiences a second impact before the first injury is fully healed. Neurologist Robert Cantu describes a typical case:

> Typically, the athlete suffers post-concussion symptoms after the first head injury, which may include headache; labyrinthine dysfunction; visual, motor, or sensory

changes; or mental difficulty, especially cognitive and memory problems. Before these symptoms resolve, which may take days or weeks, the athlete returns to competition and receives a second blow to the head. The second blow may be remarkably minor, perhaps involving only a blow to the chest that indirectly injures the athlete's head by imparting accelerative forces to the brain. The affected athlete may appear stunned, but usually does not experience loss of consciousness (LOC) and in the case of football, he often completes the play. Indeed, the individual usually remains on their feet for 15 sec to 1 min or so, but appears dazed, like someone suffering from a grade 1 concussion without LOC. Frequently the affected athlete remains on the playing field or walks off under their own power. What happens in the next few seconds to several minutes, however, sets this syndrome apart from a concussion. During this period the athlete, who is conscious yet stunned, quite precipitously collapses to the ground, semi-comatose with rapidly dilating pupils, loss of eye movement, and respiratory failure. Although the vast majority of the second-impact syndrome (SIS) cases in the literature involve athletes under the age of 18, it can also be seen in college athletes. . . .

Robert C. Cantu & Alisa D. Gean, *Second-Impact Syndrome and a Small Subdural Hematoma: An Uncommon Catastrophic Result of Repetitive Head Injury with a Characteristic Imaging Appearance*, 27 J. Neurotrauma 1557, 1557 (2010).

2. Professional Football

A series of high-profile suicides, including those of All-Pro linebacker Junior Seau (at age 43) All-Pro tight end Aaron Hernandez (at age 27), and All-Pro safety Dave Duerson (at age 50), have sparked tremendous interest in the debilitating effects of football concussions. Autopsies of many of these brains have revealed the frequent presence of Chronic Traumatic Encephalopathy (CTE), a brain degeneration associated with such things as memory loss, aggression, confusion, and depression.

Over 5,000 former NFL players, more than 1/3 of the 12,000 living former players, sued the league. As described below, in 2015 the players and the NFL reached a settlement agreement, which was finalized on appeal in 2016. The settlement agreement included $765 million to fund medical exams and offer compensation for player injuries (though subsequent litigation has involved disputes over who deserves compensation). What follows in this section are first the two original briefs—the Master Complaint on behalf of the retired players, and the NFL's reply—followed by the ruling that gave final approval of the settlement terms, on appeal in the United States Court of Appeals, Third Circuit. As you read these materials, focus in particular on the legal theories motivating these (and similar) claims, as well as defenses to those claims. In light of the science and the law, would you have agreed to the settlement if you were representing the players? The NFL?

Plaintiff's Amended Master Admin. Long-Form Complaint at 4–19
In re National Football League Players' Concussion Injury Litigation
No. 2:12-md-02323-AB, MDL No. 2323 (E.D. Pa. July 17, 2012)

INTRODUCTION

1. This case seeks a declaration of liability, injunctive relief, medical monitoring, and financial compensation for the long-term chronic injuries, financial losses, expenses, and intangible losses suffered by the Plaintiffs and Plaintiffs' Spouses as a result of the Defendants' intentional tortious misconduct, including fraud, intentional misrepresentation, and negligence.

2. This action arises from the pathological and debilitating effects of mild traumatic brain injuries (referenced herein as "MTBI") caused by the concussive and sub-concussive impacts that have afflicted former professional football players in the NFL. For many decades, evidence has linked repetitive MTBI to long-term neurological problems in many sports, including football. The NFL, as the organizer, marketer, and face of the most popular sport in the United States, in which MTBI is a regular occurrence and in which players are at risk for MTBI, was aware of the evidence and the risks associated with repetitive traumatic brain injuries virtually at the inception, but deliberately ignored and actively concealed the information from the Plaintiffs and all others who participated in organized football at all levels.

3. The published medical literature, as detailed later in this Complaint, contains studies of athletes dating back as far as 1928 demonstrating a scientifically observed link between repetitive blows to the head and neuro-cognitive problems. The earliest studies focused on boxers, but by the 1950s and 1960s, a substantial body of medical and scientific evidence had been developed specifically relating to neuro-cognitive injuries in the sport of football. . . .

22. The NFL caused or contributed to the injuries and increased risks to Plaintiffs through its acts and omissions by, among other things: (a) historically ignoring the true risks of MTBI in NFL football; (b) failing to disclose the true risks of repetitive MTBI to NFL players; and (c) since 1994, deliberately spreading misinformation concerning the cause and effect relationship between MTBI in NFL football and latent neurodegenerative disorders and diseases. . . .

HEAD INJURIES, CONCUSSIONS, AND NEUROLOGICAL DAMAGE

67. Medical science has known for many decades that repetitive and violent jarring of the head or impact to the head can cause MTBI with a heightened risk of long term, chronic neuro-cognitive sequelae.

68. The NFL Defendants have known or should have known for many years that the American Association of Neurological Surgeons (the "AANS") has defined a concussion as "a clinical syndrome characterized by an immediate and transient alteration in brain function, including an alteration of mental status and level of consciousness, resulting from mechanical force or trauma." The AANS defines traumatic brain injury ("TBI") as:

> a blow or jolt to the head, or a penetrating head injury that disrupts the normal function of the brain. TBI can result when the head suddenly and violently hits an object, or when an object pierces the skull and enters brain tissue. Symptoms of a TBI can be mild, moderate or severe, depending on the extent of damage to the brain. Mild cases may result in a brief change in mental state or consciousness, while severe cases may result in extended periods of unconsciousness, coma or even death.

69. The NFL Defendants have known or should have known for many years that MTBI generally occurs when the head either accelerates rapidly and then is stopped, or is rotated rapidly. The results frequently include, among other things, confusion, blurred vision, memory loss, nausea, and sometimes unconsciousness.

70. that medical evidence has shown that symptoms of MTBI can appear hours or days after the injury, indicating that the injured party has not healed from the initial blow.

71. that once a person suffers an MTBI, he is up to four times more likely to sustain a second one. Additionally, after suffering even a single sub-concussive or concussive blow, a lesser blow may cause MTBI, and the injured person requires more time to recover. . . .

72 that clinical and neuro-pathological studies by some of the nation's foremost experts demonstrate that multiple head injuries or concussions sustained during an NFL player's career can cause severe neuro-cognitive problems such as depression and early-onset of dementia.

74. that neuropathology studies, brain imaging tests, and neuropsychological tests on many former football players, including former NFL players, have established that football players who sustain repetitive head impacts while playing the game have suffered and continue to suffer brain injuries that result in any one or more of the following conditions: early-onset of Alzheimer's Disease, dementia, depression, deficits in cognitive functioning, reduced processing speed, attention and reasoning, loss of memory, sleeplessness, mood swings, personality changes, and the debilitating and latent disease known as Chronic Traumatic Encephalopathy ("CTE"). The latter condition involves the slow build-up of the Tau protein within the brain tissue that causes diminished brain function, progressive cognitive decline, and many of the symptoms listed above. CTE is also is associated with an increased risk of suicide. . . .

76. The NFL Defendants have known for many years of the reported papers and studies documenting autopsies on over twenty-five former NFL players. The papers and studies show that over ninety percent of the players suffered from CTE.

[The Complaint goes on to provide support for its claims about CTE. — EDS.]

Reply Memorandum of Defendant at 1–12
In re National Football League Players' Concussion Injury Litigation
No. 2:12-md-02323-AB, MDL No. 2323 (E.D. Pa. Dec. 17, 2012)

Defendants National Football League ("NFL") and NFL Properties LLC ("NFLP," and together with the NFL, the "NFL Defendants") respectfully submit this reply memorandum in support of their motion to dismiss, on preemption grounds, the Amended Master Administrative Long-Form Complaint. . . .

As described in detail in the NFL's moving brief, since 1968, CBAs [Collective Bargaining Agreements] and the NFL Constitution and Bylaws (the "Constitution") have set forth the terms and conditions of employment of NFL players and the rules that govern professional football. The CBAs, for example, provide that the NFL's Member Clubs and their medical staffs have the responsibility for treating player injuries, including determining injury recovery times, deciding when players may return to play, and advising the players of the risks of continued performance. Such provisions reflect the complicated reality of player safety in professional sports leagues where both players and Clubs have incentives—sometimes parallel, sometimes conflicting—for healthy players to play and injured players to heal. These issues are thus natural subjects of bargaining as reflected in the CBAs. The CBAs also set forth procedures governing the NFL's promulgation and review of rules and regulations relating to player safety and the basic rules of the game, which also obviously impact player safety.

In light of these provisions, to determine whether the NFL breached a purported duty "to exercise reasonable care in safeguarding Players from neurological injuries," the Court would need to interpret the CBA provisions setting forth the player safety responsibilities of the Member Clubs and their physicians. As numerous courts have already held, any duty owed by the NFL . . . could not be defined or considered without also taking into account the "physician provisions" of the CBAs. That is because "determining the degree of care owed by the NFL and how it relates to the NFL's alleged failure to establish guidelines or policies to protect the mental health and safety of its players" cannot be ascertained without a consideration of the nature and scope of the duties that these provisions impose. . . .

[T]he CBAs, in comprehensively assigning roles and responsibilities for regulating player safety, create a scheme in which the duties of any single actor, including the NFL, can be defined only by assessing the overall allocation of duties. Moreover, in contractually defining the roles of various actors, the CBA effectively authorized the NFL to rely on the Member Clubs. . . .

As the NFL's moving brief demonstrated . . . resolution of Plaintiffs' negligence-based claims requires interpretation of the CBAs' numerous medical care provisions. A court cannot assess the scope of the NFL's duty without first interpreting the scope of the duties imposed on the Clubs and their medical staff by the CBAs. . . .

For example, assessing the existence or scope of the NFL's duty "to warn Players about neurological risks" will require the Court to interpret the CBAs to determine the scope of the duties placed on the Clubs' medical staffs. Thus, if Plaintiffs' alleged medical conditions were ones that "could be significantly aggravated by continued performance," the Clubs' medical staffs may have had a duty to warn players before returning to play, which "would be one factor tending to show that the NFL's alleged failure to take action to protect [them] from concussive brain trauma was reasonable." . . .

Similarly, to assess whether the NFL acted reasonably by failing to establish return-to-play guidelines, the Court would first need to interpret the scope of the duty imposed by the CBA provisions providing that "[a]ll determinations of recovery time for . . . injuries" are to be made "by the Club's medical staff and in accordance with the Club's medical standards." . . .

[T]he duties of the parties would obviously be very different were collective bargaining and the resulting agreements not involved. That is why numerous courts—in this and other contexts—have properly concluded that the NFL's conduct concerning player health and safety "cannot be considered in a vacuum," but "must be considered in light of pre-existing contractual duties imposed by the CBA on the individual NFL clubs concerning the general health and safety of the NFL players." . . .

In re Nat'l Football League Players Concussion Injury Litig.

821 F.3d 410 (3d Cir. 2016), as amended (May 2, 2016)

AMBRO, C.J.

I. INTRODUCTION

The National Football League ("NFL") has agreed to resolve lawsuits brought by former players who alleged that the NFL failed to inform them of and protect them from the risks of concussions in football. The District Court approved a class action settlement that covered over 20,000 retired players and released all concussion-related claims against the NFL. Objectors have appealed that decision, arguing that class certification was improper and that the settlement was unfair. But after thorough review, we conclude that the District Court was right to certify the class and approve the settlement. Thus we affirm its decision in full.

II. BACKGROUND

A. Concussion Suits Are Brought Against the NFL

In July 2011, 73 former professional football players sued the NFL and Riddell, Inc. in the Superior Court of California. The retired players alleged that the NFL failed to take reasonable actions to protect them from the chronic risks of head injuries in football. The players also claimed that Riddell, a manufacturer of sports equipment, should be liable for the defective design of helmets.

The NFL removed the case to federal court on the ground that the players' claims under state law were preempted by federal labor law. More lawsuits by retired players followed and the NFL moved under 28 U.S.C. §1407 to consolidate the pending suits before a single judge for pretrial proceedings. In January 2012, the Judicial Panel on Multidistrict Litigation consolidated these cases before Judge Anita B. Brody in the Eastern District of Pennsylvania as a multidistrict litigation ("MDL"). Since consolidation, 5,000 players have filed over 300 similar lawsuits against the NFL and Riddell. Our appeal only concerns the claims against the NFL. . . .

The Master Complaints tracked many of the allegations from the first lawsuits. Football puts players at risk of repetitive brain trauma and injury because they suffer concussive and sub-concussive hits during the game and at practice (sub-concussive hits fall below the threshold for a concussion but are still associated with brain damage). Plaintiffs alleged that the NFL had a duty to provide players with rules and information to protect them from the health risks — both short and long-term — of brain injury, including Alzheimer's disease, dementia, depression, deficits in cognitive functioning, reduced processing speed, loss of memory, sleeplessness, mood swings, personality changes, and a recently identified degenerative disease called chronic traumatic encephalopathy (commonly referred to as "CTE").

Because CTE figures prominently in this appeal, some background on this condition is in order. It was first identified in 2002 based on analysis of the brain tissue of deceased NFL players, including Mike Webster, Terry Long, Andre Waters, and Justin Strzelczyk. CTE involves the build-up of "tau protein" in the brain, a result associated with repetitive head trauma. Medical personnel have examined approximately 200 brains with CTE as of 2015, in large part because it is only diagnosable post-mortem. That diagnosis requires examining sections of a person's brain under a microscope to see if abnormal tau proteins are present and, if so, whether they occur in the unique pattern associated with CTE. Plaintiffs alleged that CTE affects mood and behavior, causing headaches, aggression, depression, and an increased risk of suicide. They also stated that memory loss, dementia, loss of attention and concentration, and impairment of language are associated with CTE.

The theme of the allegations was that, despite the NFL's awareness of the risks of repetitive head trauma, the League ignored, minimized, or outright suppressed information concerning the link between that trauma and cognitive damage. For example, in 1994 the NFL created the Mild Traumatic Brain Injury Committee to

study the effects of head injuries. Per the plaintiffs, the Committee was at the forefront of a disinformation campaign that disseminated "junk science" denying the
link between head injuries and cognitive disorders. Based on the allegations against
the NFL, plaintiffs asserted claims for negligence, medical monitoring, fraudulent
concealment, fraud, negligent misrepresentation, negligent hiring, negligent retention, wrongful death and survival, civil conspiracy, and loss of consortium.

After plaintiffs filed the Master Complaints, the NFL moved to dismiss, arguing
that federal labor law preempted the state law claims. Indeed, §301 of the Labor
Management Relations Act preempts state law claims that are "substantially dependent" on the terms of a labor agreement. The NFL claimed that resolution of plaintiffs' claims depended upon the interpretation of Collective Bargaining Agreements
("CBAs") in place between the retired players and the NFL. If the CBAs do preempt
plaintiffs' claims, they must arbitrate those claims per mandatory arbitration provisions in the CBAs. Plaintiffs responded that their negligence and fraud claims would
not require federal courts to interpret the CBAs and in any event the CBAs did not
cover all retired players.

B. The Parties Reach a Settlement

On July 8, 2013, while the NFL's motion to dismiss was pending, the District
Court ordered the parties to mediate and appointed a mediator. On August 29,
2013, after two months of negotiations and more than twelve full days of formal
mediation, the parties agreed to a settlement in principle and signed a term sheet.
It provided $765 million to fund medical exams and offer compensation for player
injuries. The proposed settlement would resolve the claims of all retired players
against the NFL related to head injuries.

In January 2014, after more negotiations, class counsel filed in the District Court
a class action complaint and sought preliminary class certification and preliminary
approval of the settlement. The Court denied the motion because it had doubts that
the capped fund for paying claims would be sufficient. It appointed a Special Master
to assist with making financial forecasts and, five months later, the parties reached a
revised settlement that uncapped the fund for compensating retired players.

Class counsel filed a second motion for preliminary class certification and preliminary approval in June 2014. The District Court granted the motion, preliminarily approved the settlement, conditionally certified the class, approved classwide
notice, and scheduled a final fairness hearing. . . .

Following preliminary certification, potential class members had 90 days to
object or opt out of the settlement. Class counsel then moved for final class certification and settlement approval. On November 19, 2014, the District Court held a day-
long fairness hearing and heard argument from class counsel, the NFL, and several
objectors who voiced concerns against the settlement. After the hearing, the Court
proposed several changes to benefit class members. The parties agreed to the proposed changes and submitted an amended settlement in February 2015. On April 22,
2015, the Court granted the motion for class certification and final approval of the
amended settlement, that grant explained in a 123-page opinion. Objectors filed 12
separate appeals that were consolidated into this single appeal before us now.

C. The Proposed Settlement

The settlement has three components: (1) an uncapped Monetary Award
Fund that provides compensation for retired players who submit proof of certain

diagnoses; (2) a $75 million Baseline Assessment Program that provides eligible retired players with free baseline assessment examinations of their objective neurological functioning; and (3) a $10 million Education Fund to instruct football players about injury prevention.

1. Monetary Award Fund

Under the settlement, retired players or their beneficiaries are compensated for developing one of several neurocognitive and neuromuscular impairments or "Qualifying Diagnoses." By "retired players," we mean players who retired from playing NFL football before the preliminary approval of the class settlement on July 7, 2014. The settlement recognizes six Qualifying Diagnoses: (1) Level 1.5 Neurocognitive Impairment; (2) Level 2 Neurocognitive Impairment; (3) Alzheimer's Disease; (4) Parkinson's Disease; (5) Amyotrophic Lateral Sclerosis ("ALS"); and (6) Death with CTE provided the player died before final approval of the settlement on April 22, 2015. A retired player does not need to show that his time in the NFL caused the onset of the Qualifying Diagnosis.

A Qualifying Diagnosis entitles a retired player to a maximum monetary award:

Qualifying Diagnosis	Maximum Award
Level 1.5 Neurocognitive Impairment	$1.5 Million
Level 2 Neurocognitive Impairment	$3 Million
Parkinson's Disease	$3.5 Million
Alzheimer's Disease	$3.5 Million
Death with CTE	$4 Million
ALS	$5 Million

This award is subject to several offsets, that is, awards decrease: (1) as the age at which a retired player is diagnosed increases; (2) if the retired player played fewer than five eligible seasons; (3) if the player did not have a baseline assessment examination; and (4) if the player suffered a severe traumatic brain injury or stroke unrelated to NFL play.

To collect from the Fund, a class member must register with the claims administrator within 180 days of receiving notice that the settlement has been approved. This deadline can be excused for good cause. The class member then must submit a claims package to the administrator no later than two years after the date of the Qualifying Diagnosis or within two years after the supplemental notice is posted on the settlement website, whichever is later. This deadline can be excused for substantial hardship. The claims package must include a certification by the diagnosing physician and supporting medical records. The claims administrator will notify the class member within 60 days if he is entitled to an award. The class member, class counsel, and the NFL have the right to appeal an award determination. To do so, a class member must submit a $1,000 fee, which is refunded if the appeal is successful and can be waived for financial hardship. A fee is not required for the NFL and class counsel to appeal, though the NFL must act in good faith when appealing award determinations.

The Monetary Award Fund is uncapped and will remain in place for 65 years. Every retired player who timely registers and qualifies during the lifespan of the settlement will receive an award. If, after receiving an initial award, a retired player receives a more serious Qualifying Diagnosis, he may receive a supplemental award.

2. Baseline Assessment Program

Any retired player who has played at least half of an eligible season can receive a baseline assessment examination. It consists of a neurological examination performed by credentialed and licensed physicians selected by a court-appointed administrator. Qualified providers may diagnose retired players with Level 1, 1.5, or 2 Neurocognitive Impairment. The results of the examinations can also be compared with any future tests to determine whether a retired player's cognitive abilities have deteriorated.

Baseline Assessment Program funds will also provide Baseline Assessment Program Supplemental Benefits. Retired players diagnosed with Level 1 Neurocognitive Impairment—evidencing some objective decline in cognitive function but not yet early dementia—are eligible to receive medical benefits, including further testing, treatment, counseling, and pharmaceutical coverage.

The Baseline Assessment Program lasts for 10 years. All retired players who seek and are eligible for a baseline assessment examination receive one notwithstanding the $75 million cap. Every eligible retired player age 43 or over must take a baseline assessment examination within two years of the Program's start-up. Every eligible retired player younger than age 43 must do so before the end of the program or by his 45th birthday, whichever comes first.

3. Education Fund

The Education Fund is a $10 million fund to promote safety and injury prevention in football. The purpose is to promote safety-related initiatives in youth football and educate retired players about their medical and disability benefits under the CBA. Class counsel and the NFL, with input from the retired players, will propose specific educational initiatives for the District Court's approval.

4. The Proposed Class

All living NFL football players who retired from playing professional football before July 7, 2014, as well as their representative claimants and derivative claimants, comprise the proposed class. Representative claimants are those duly authorized by law to assert the claims of deceased, legally incapacitated, or incompetent retired players. Derivative claimants are those, such as parents, spouses, or dependent children, who have some legal right to the income of retired players. Even though the proposed class consists of more than just retired players, we use the terms "class members" and "retired players" interchangeably.

The proposed class contains two subclasses based on a retired players' injuries as of the preliminary approval date. Subclass 1 consists of retired players who were not diagnosed with a Qualifying Diagnosis prior to July 7, 2014, and their representative and derivative claimants. Put another way, subclass 1 includes retired players who have no currently known injuries that would be compensated under the settlement. Subclass 2 consists of retired players who were diagnosed with a Qualifying Diagnosis prior to July 7, 2014, and their representative claimants and derivative claimants. Translated, subclass 2 includes retired players who are currently injured and will receive an immediate monetary award under the settlement. The NFL estimates that the total population of retired players is 21,070. Of this, 28% are expected to be diagnosed with a compensable disease. The remaining 72% are not expected to develop a compensable disease during their lifetime.

Class members release all claims and actions against the NFL "arising out of, or relating to, head, brain and/or cognitive injury, as well as any injuries arising out of, or relating to, concussions and/or sub-concussive events," including claims relating to CTE. The releases do not compromise the benefits that retired players are entitled to receive under the CBAs, nor do they compromise their retirement benefits, disability benefits, and health insurance.

Of the over 20,000 estimated class members (the NFL states that the number exceeds 21,000), 234 initially asked to opt out from the settlement and 205 class members joined 83 written objections submitted to the District Court. Before the fairness hearing, 26 of the 234 opt-outs sought readmission to the class. After the District Court granted final approval, another 6 opt-outs sought readmission. This leaves 202 current opt-outs, of which class counsel notes only 169 were timely filed. . . .

NOTES AND QUESTIONS

1. Look over the Complaint point-by-point. Which salient points are most difficult for the players to prove? Least difficult? Why do you think the parties settled?
2. Examine the settlement carefully. What challenges do you anticipate in its administration? What modifications would you have made to the settlement?
3. *New York Times* reporter Alan Schwarz is credited with bringing much of this research on football and brain injury to light through a series of investigative articles. In an interview discussing this work, Schwarz summarized his findings as follows:

   Interviewer: Many of your early stories dealt with the prevalence of brain damage among former NFL players. Why do you think many players from that era have brain damage today?

   Schwarz: I can't say. I don't know how many players from that era have this damage. Nobody knows. All I and The Times have ever emphasized is that there are two things that we do know. One is that some players have it — or had it before they died — and the only way you can get it is through repetitive brain trauma. These guys did not get it from banging their heads on a wall. They got it from banging their heads on the football field. Maybe it was in the NFL, maybe it was in college, maybe it was in high school, maybe it was in youth football. We don't know when it happened.

   The other thing we know is that the prevalence of a medical diagnosis of dementia has been made in NFL players at rates vastly higher than that of the national population by age. The rates are high enough, among a group large enough, that it is impossible for it to be a fluke. It happened because of something they did in their lives, and the common things that they share is that they're male and that they played professional and amateur football for x number of years.

   Those two things, in combination, showed that football was more dangerous than many people either understood or wanted to admit. . . .

   SportsLetter, *SL Interview: Alan Schwarz of the New York Times Chronicles Concussions in Football,* LA84 Foundation (Dec. 1, 2010).
4. The NFL created a poster on concussions, to be displayed in team locker rooms and practice facilities. The top of the poster reads "A Must Read for NFL Players" and "Let's Take Brain Injuries Out Of Play." If such a poster had existed and been posted earlier, would it affect your legal analysis in the cases mentioned above?

5. In a 2012 interview Chicago Bears All-Pro linebacker Brian Urlacher said that he would lie about his concussion status to team trainers:

> If I have a concussion these days, I'm going to say something happened to my toe or knee just to get my bearings for a few plays . . . I'm not going to sit in there and say I got a concussion. (Then) I can't go in there the rest of the game. [Urlacher also said in the interview] . . . we love football . . . We want to be on the field as much as we can be. If we can be out there, it may be stupid, it may be dumb, call me dumb and stupid then because I want to be on the football field.

Chuck Sudo, *Brian Urlacher Would Lie About a Concussion to Stay on the Field, Admits to Toradol Use*, Chicagoist (Jan. 24, 2012).

In a poll of 103 NFL players taken in 2012, the question was asked: Would you try to hide concussion symptoms to keep playing? Fifty-six percent of players said Yes, and 44% replied No. Said one player, "If I don't play, I feel like I'm letting my team down. I'm not going to put myself at serious risk. But if I can play through it, I'm going to play through it." But said another: "I've seen too many concussions and what they can do, and I'd never try to hide the symptoms. I've seen the long-term ramifications, and it's scary. With the knowledge, information and treatment we have now, you'd be crazy to try to hide symptoms." One player explicitly made reference to new information when he observed: "Before all the new info . . . yes. Not worth it now. So no." Sporting News, *NFL Concussion Poll: 56 Percent of Players Would Hide Symptoms to Stay on Field*, SportingNews (Nov. 12, 2012). Do comments and survey results such as these affect your legal analysis? Why or why not? How do you think legal duties with regards to player safety have changed across the last four decades? How do you predict they are likely to change across the next four?

6. In your view, what amount and kinds of brain evidence would warrant legislation prohibiting certain kinds of previously common activities, such as football? On that basis, or some other you can articulate, should boxing be outlawed? How do you think the legal system, if not prohibiting such activities outright, should (if at all) regulate them differently?

C. PROVING BRAIN INJURY

Once a duty, and a breach of that duty, are established, a plaintiff must show that there is a resulting harm. That is, the plaintiff must show that he/she actually has sustained a brain injury and must establish a monetary value to compensate for the loss. Making such a showing is not always a straightforward task. This is for a similar reason that it is difficult to assess *mens rea*: We can't see into the head of the (possibly) injured plaintiff. Or, at least we couldn't until the advent of neuroimaging. As the readings in this section suggest, neuroimaging provides the possibility of helping law better assess the nature and extent of brain injuries. Some attorneys are even now marketing their firms by emphasizing that they are neuroscience-focused. But, as the readings also suggest, it's not yet clear how or when neuroimaging will add meaningfully to more just resolution of brain injury litigation. In particular, courts are wrestling with whether or not to admit diffusion tensor imaging (DTI) evidence in brain injury cases. For a review of DTI methods, refer back to Chapter 4.

1. Neuroimaging Evidence and Brain Injury

J. Sherrod Taylor

Neurolaw and Traumatic Brain Injury: Principles for Trial Lawyers

84 UMKC L. Rev. 397, 400-08 (2015)

The main purpose of the civil justice system, in meritorious TBI cases, is to provide money to secure monetary awards that maybe [sic] utilized for medical and rehabilitation treatment programs. In this way, better legal outcomes promote better clinical outcomes. . . .

The second principle of neurolaw holds that success in neurolitigation is dependent largely upon the quality and quantity of expert evidence adduced at trial. Testifying experts are often part of a multidisciplinary TBI team that may include neurologists, orthopedic surgeons, psychiatrists, psychologists, neuropsychologists, physical rehabilitation specialists, occupational therapists, nurses, social workers, and case managers. . . .

The third principle of neurolaw states that mutual cooperation among concerned professionals enhances the probability of successful neurolitigation. Thus, neurolaw encourages specialists from many disciplines to work together in harmony. . . .

The fourth principle observes that, to be successful, clinical and legal professionals require litigation literacy. To participate fully in neurolitigation, clinical and legal professionals need to understand that *litigation literacy* simply means: a basic awareness of the intricacies of the civil justice system. . . .

Proving the *cause* of mTBI, therefore, has always been a challenge during neurolitigation. Many brain injuries are not revealed during standard medical testing procedures—e.g., X-rays. For this reason, neurolawyers tend to employ clinical neuropsychologists, who have developed various test instruments to explore brain-behavior relationships following injury. . . .

The fifth principle of neurolaw provides that persuasive evidence presented by lay witnesses contributes heavily to successful neurolitigation. Lay witnesses constitute a necessary bridge—linking the testimony of plaintiffs to the evidence supplied by their experts—to present a clear picture of how TBI affects life for brain injury survivors in the real world. . . .

[N]euroimaging of mTBI may be ready to take its place in TBI trials. . . .

Judges, like umpires calling balls and strikes, face a plethora of challenges in the twenty-first century—especially as they discover that neuroscience cases, like baseball pitches, often present intricate questions of first impression. . . .

[W]e may conclude that neurolaw is unique among the various areas of trial practice. It is now clear that the conjoining of law and neuroscience, as it is presently unfolding, embodies, not only the substance of neurolitigation, but also the tools necessary to pursue this endeavor. As to substance, in the future, neuroimaging probably will be regularly admitted into evidence to confirm subjective reports of pain, prove the white matter injuries associated with mTBI, and furnish evidence of physical bases for emotional distress. . . .

Shana De Caro & Michael V. Kaplen

Current Issues in Neurolaw

33 Psychiatric Clinics N. Am. 915, 917-25 (2010)

PRELIMINARY LEGAL CONSIDERATIONS FOR ADMISSIBILITY OF EXPERT TESTIMONY

There are a multitude of medical professionals whose opinions are typically used by attorneys litigating TBI cases, including neurologists, psychiatrists, rehabilitation medicine specialists, and radiologists. The opinions of professionals without a medical degree, such as neuropsychologists, are also frequently relied upon. Experts possessing medical degrees have traditionally been given wide latitude to render opinions, by virtue of their training and experience, concerning both the existence and cause of an injury, often referred to in legal parlance as the proximate or competent producing cause. Neurologists, psychiatrists, and rehabilitation specialists are often called on to render expert opinions based on their examination and treatment of injured claimants. Because of the interest of the legal profession in establishing "objective" evidence of brain damage, the assistance of neuroradiologists will become more prevalent and necessary as more objective tests of brain function are improved and developed. . . .

Clinical neuropsychology has been defined as "an applied science concerned with the behavioral expression of brain dysfunction." Neuropsychologists are often called on to provide neuropsychological evaluations in legal proceedings based on their interpretation of neuropsychological test results. . . .

Experts often encounter challenges to their opinions on the very existence of brain injury, based on questions concerning the reliability of neuropsychological testing and functional neuroimaging studies on which they rely. These objections often result in protracted court hearings with expert testimony elicited by both sides, and the introduction into evidence of conflicting scientific literature. . . .

Reliance on neuropsychological testing alone is insufficient to completely resolve the questions of whether an individual has sustained a TBI and the extent of that injury. Research supports the proposition that many individuals may perform satisfactorily on traditional neuropsychological testing and yet have difficulty with everyday decision-making, and fail to do well in an unstructured environment or situation. Moreover, this testing fails to address the important day-to-day dilemmas facing victims of brain injury. It is imperative that the testimony of the individual, friends, workers, and often disinterested coworkers be elicited to establish the day-to-day struggles and predicaments with which these individuals are confronted.

Imaging studies, such as positron emission tomography (PET) scans, diffusion tensor magnetic resonance imaging (DTI) studies, and functional MRI studies, have been subject to judicial scrutiny, with inconsistent rulings on their admissibility. The judicial hearings held to determine the admissibility of these studies typically focus on: (1) the presence or absence of acceptable norms or control groups, (2) evidence tending to establish whether the particular study has achieved general scientific acceptance in the field of TBI, (3) whether the test can validly detect brain damage in an individual, and (4) whether an expert can opine that an impairment can be linked to a specific outside event. As these imaging studies continue to gain acceptance in the scientific community, it can be anticipated that favorable court rulings will continue to proliferate.

WHAT IS MILD TRAUMATIC BRAIN INJURY?

Questions surrounding mild TBI generate the most attention and controversy in the legal realm. The debate concerning this condition finds origin in the dissonance in the medical profession concerning both the definition and diagnosis. There is friction regarding the assessment of behavioral and psychiatric issues, and disputes as to the long-term consequences. A jury's acceptance of mild TBI in a contested legal proceeding has the potential to result in substantial compensation of the victim, and therefore has particular significance to the legal profession.

The evidentiary issues facing victim and counsel in a mild TBI case are magnified, due to the "invisible" aspects of this injury to the unenlightened observer. The defense in many of these cases seems plausible because the individual appears normal, was not rendered unconscious, did not sustain any physical injuries, had a normal ED examination including a gross neurological evaluation, and had normal standard imaging studies.

Although many professional organizations have attempted to construct a working definition of mild TBI, these endeavors have been thwarted by the ongoing controversy concerning the relative importance of loss of consciousness and amnesia. Most current definitions of mild TBI include periods of observed or self-reported confusion or disorientation; however, the precise definition of these components is also subject to much conflict. The event that gives rise to the injury is often unwitnessed, resulting in the absence of credible, immediate, on the scene observations regarding transient loss of consciousness, disorientation, and confusion. When emergency personnel arrive, the victim is often found walking and talking, and therefore the emergency responder may erroneously mistake such conduct for the absence of confusion, disorientation, or loss of consciousness. . . .

Inherent in any definition of mild TBI is trauma of some sort. However, the amount, direction, or type of force required to produce this injury has not been settled. . . .

The search for objective evidence to substantiate the mild TBI often turns into a courtroom battle over the presence or absence of positive imaging studies. There is almost complete unanimity of medical opinion that the absence of positive imaging findings in CT studies and MRI studies is inconclusive as to the existence of brain injury. However, this offers little assistance to jurors who are searching for positive proof of injury, or to attorneys seeking positive confirmation of their client's symptoms and complaints. Newer imaging modalities such as PET scans, diffusion tensor imaging studies, and functional MRI studies have intensified attention on neuroradiological detection and objective confirmation of mild TBI, and may offer further guidance to both the court and jurors. . . .

MALINGERING

Individuals claiming disability as a result of TBI are frequently confronted with accusations of malingering, exaggeration, and secondary gain, which must be addressed by the forensic evaluation. These issues are most frequently seen in cases of mild TBI. . . .

Malingering has been defined by the APA as the "intentional production of false or grossly exaggerated physical or psychological symptoms motivated by external incentives." . . .

While there are several malingering tests in existence, there is no single test that has achieved universal acceptance as the "gold standard" in determining whether an individual is malingering. . . .

THE FAKE BAD SCALE AND ITS ROLE IN FORENSIC EVALUATIONS

Perhaps no area in the forensic evaluation of brain injury survivors provokes more controversy than the administration and analysis of the Fake Bad Scale (FBS), as part of the Minnesota Multiphasic Personality Inventory (MMPI-2). Although the MMPI is reportedly the most widely administered psychological test in the world, its inclusion of the FBS scale in 2006 has provoked contentious debate in brain injury litigation. The test has recently been renamed the symptom validity scale, to avoid the negative connotation that the former name aroused. The scale requires an individual to respond "true" or "false" to 43 subjective statements concerning his or her health, and emotional and physical status. On the basis of a scaled score, Lees-Hailey and English opine that symptom exaggeration and falsification can be detected. Critics of the scale, including James Butcher, one of the principal coinvestigators of the revised MMPI-2 norms, contend that "the scale is likely to classify an unacceptably large number of individuals who are experiencing genuine psychological distress as malingerers. It is recommended that the FBS not be used in clinical settings nor should it be used during disability evaluations."

A brief review of the 43 true-false questions, quoted in a front-page Wall Street Journal story, such as "My sleep is fitful and disturbed," "I have nightmares every few nights," "I have very few headaches," "I have few or no pains," "There seems to be a lump in my throat much of the time," "Once a week or oftener, I suddenly feel hot all over, for no reason," "I have a great deal of stomach trouble," are statements that one might expect a person with brain damage, sleep disorders, headaches, posttraumatic stress disorder, depression, and/or anxiety to endorse. The patient accumulates points for confirming the very symptoms characteristic of his or her condition. Critics further contend that the test has a bias against women. Lees-Hailey and Fox have set a cutoff score of 20 for men and 24 for women. The criticism leveled against the FBS has been characterized by test proponents as being "naïve and inaccurate" and "absurd." While the publishers of the MMPI-2, University of Minnesota Press, still use and score the FBS, reportedly the APA Committee on Disability Issues in Psychology (CDIP), in a letter dated May 31, 2007, strongly recommended that an independent empirical evaluation of the FBS be conducted to determine the scale's validity. . . .

Marsh v. Celebrity Cruises, Inc.

2017 WL 6987718 (S.D. Fla. Dec. 15, 2017)

UNGARO, D.J. This cause is before the Court upon Defendant's *Daubert* Motion to Strike or Exclude the Unreliable Opinion Testimony of Plaintiff's Expert Dr. Gerald York, M.D., Derived from Diffusion Tensor Imaging. . . .

For reasons set forth below, the Motion is DENIED.

BACKGROUND

. . . Plaintiff filed her Complaint against Defendant, Celebrity Cruises, Inc. ("Celebrity"). The Complaint alleged a singular claim for negligence based on

Plaintiff's slip and fall on a puddle of water on the Solarium floor of the Celebrity cruise ship, Celebrity Solstice (the "Solstice"). Plaintiff alleges that Celebrity created a dangerous condition by failing to: (i) properly maintain the Solarium in the area where she slipped; and (ii) warn passengers of the danger. Plaintiff claims to have sustained physical injuries as a result of her accident, including a mild traumatic brain injury ("TBI"). . . .

LEGAL STANDARD

Federal Rule of Evidence 702 states: "A witness who is qualified as an expert by knowledge, skill, experience, training, or education may testify in the form of an opinion or otherwise if: (a) the expert's scientific, technical, or other specialized knowledge will help the trier of fact to understand the evidence or to determine a fact in issue; (b) the testimony is based on sufficient facts or data; (c) the testimony is the product of reliable principles and methods; and (d) the expert has reliably applied the principles and methods to the facts of the case." Under Rule 702, the trial judge acts as a gatekeeper to ensure that expert evidence is both reliable and relevant.

The Supreme Court set forth the criteria for the admissibility of scientific expert testimony under Rule 702 in *Daubert* by instructing trial judges to "determine at the outset, pursuant to Rule 104(a), whether the expert is proposing to testify to (1) scientific knowledge that (2) will assist the trier of fact to understand or determine a fact in issue," which includes "a preliminary assessment of whether the reasoning or methodology underlying the testimony is scientifically valid and of whether that reasoning or methodology properly can be applied to the facts in issue." . . .

In *Rink v. Cheminova, Inc.*, the U.S. Court of Appeals for the Eleventh Circuit established a three-part test to determine whether expert testimony should be admitted under *Daubert*, explaining that all of the following elements must be established prior to the presentation of expert testimony to the jury:

> (1) the expert is qualified to testify competently regarding the matters he intends to address; (2) the methodology by which the expert reaches conclusions is sufficiently reliable as determined by the sort of inquiry mandated in Daubert; and (3) the testimony assists the trier of fact, through the application of scientific, technical, or specialized expertise, to understand the evidence or to determine a fact in issue. . . .

DISCUSSION

Plaintiff has designated Dr. Gerald York, M.D., a board-certified neuroradiologist and radiologist, as an expert witness. . . . Dr. York has extensive education, training, and experience in interpreting and analyzing MRI diagnostic scans for the purpose of clinical neuroradiology diagnosis of mild, moderate, and severe TBIs. Dr. York has also participated in the development of approved protocols for neuroimaging of the brain and contributed to the American College of Radiology's Guidelines for Neuroimaging.

Plaintiff retained Dr. York to provide his expert opinion on whether Plaintiff suffered a mild TBI as a result of her accident aboard the Solstice. After reviewing Plaintiff's diffusion tensor imaging ("DTI"), in conjunction with a multitude of other tests and records, Dr. York concluded that Plaintiff suffered a mild TBI as a result of her slip and fall. In its Motion, Celebrity seeks to exclude Dr. York's testimony solely because of his reliance on DTI. "DTI is a more sensitive, three-dimensional type of

MRI that examines the microstructure of the white matter in the brain. DTI can show reduction in fractional anisotrophy ("FA") meaning that the white matter in the brain has been damaged." *Ruppel v. Kucanin*, 2011 WL 2470621, at *5 (N.D. Ind. June 20, 2011). DTI is used because while "a traditional MRI shows the structure of the brain . . . the majority of people with mild brain injury will have a normal MRI even if they have significant impairment." Id.

i. Parties' Arguments

In the instant Motion, Celebrity does not attack Dr. York's qualifications. Instead, Celebrity argues that Dr. York's opinions are unreliable and will not assist the trier of fact. Celebrity's arguments are based mainly on its claim that DTI is nothing more than "junk science" and that "Dr. York's DTI-based opinions that Plaintiff sustained a mild TBI amount to unsubstantiated speculation." However, DTI findings and testimony have been deemed reliable and admitted by courts across the country for almost a decade. E.g. . . . *White v. Deere, & Co.*, 2016 WL 462960, at *4 (D. Colo. Feb. 8, 2016); *Andrew v. Patterson Motor Frieght, Inc.*, 2014 WL 5449732, at *8 (W.D. La. Oct. 23, 2014) (citations omitted) ("In sum, the evidence submitted shows DTI has been tested and has a low error rate; DTI has been subject to peer review and publication; and DTI is a generally accepted method for detecting TBI."); *Ruppel v. Kucanin*, 2011 WL 2470621, at *6-12 (N.D. Ind. June 20, 2011) (finding DTI to be a reliable method); . . . *Hammar v. Sentinel Ins. Co., Ltd.*, No. 08–019984 at *2 (Fla. Cir. Ct. 2010) (allowing DTI evidence to be admitted under the Frye standard); . . . Celebrity further asserts that Dr. York's opinions are inadmissible because DTI "'on its own' cannot serve as a valid and reliable diagnostic tool of mild TBI." However, Dr. York's opinions are not exclusively based on his review of Plaintiff's DTI scans. Dr. York specifically stated in his deposition testimony that his opinions are based not only on his review of Plaintiff's DTI scans, but also of her volumetrics, FLAIR imaging, T2 imaging, susceptibility weighted images, and T1 anatomic imaging, as well as Plaintiff's neurology and neuropsychology records.

Celebrity also asserts that "[t]he DTI's acquisition of data is . . . affected by the field strength of the magnet", and that there is "a lack of a standardized protocol for the acquisition and interpretation of DTI results." However, these issues do not make DTI technology "junk science" nor render Dr. York's opinions unreliable. Dr. York has "provided all the relevant information necessary for [Celebrity] to explore th[ese] topic[s] on cross examination." Furthermore, Plaintiff points out that Dr. York "is aware of the error potential and uses his best medical judgment in collating the objective abnormalities shown by the diagnostic procedures to clinical findings." In doing so, Dr. York "arrived at medical conclusions regarding the meaning of the findings of [Plaintiff's] MRI scan, and the likely cause of those findings, all to a reasonable degree of medical probability."

Finally, Celebrity argues that "permitting Dr. York to testify to the results of the DTI and the opinions he derived therefrom may confuse the jury as to the accuracy of any perceived connection between the DTI results and Plaintiff's alleged mild TBI". However, Celebrity oversimplifies the basis of Dr. York's opinions by focusing solely on his review of Plaintiff's DTI scans. As explained *supra*, Dr. York's expert opinion is not derived exclusively from his review of Plaintiff's DTI scans, but also his review of a number of other imaging sequences and medical records. . . .

Dr. York's expert determination would certainly assist the jury in determining injury and causation in this case.

ii. The Court's Ruling

The Court will admit Dr. York's testimony as his opinions meet the Eleventh Circuit's three-part test for admission under *Daubert*. Celebrity does not question the fact that Dr. York is qualified to testify regarding the matters he intends to address. Accordingly, the first *Rink* prong is met. As to the second *Rink* prong, the Court must determine whether DTI is sufficiently reliable under *Daubert*. In making this assessment, a "pertinent consideration" is whether the technique has gained general acceptance. "DTI of the brain is a proven and well-established imaging modality in the evaluation and assessment of normal and abnormal conditions of the brain." *Roach v. Hughes*, 2016 WL 9460306, at * 3 (W.D. Ky. March 9, 2016) (quoting Hammar v. Sentinel Ins. Co., No. 08-019984 (Fla. Cir. Ct. 2010) [DN 133-22] ¶ 3). DTI is regularly used as a diagnostic tool at the Detroit Medical Center, Cedars-Sinai, Brooke Army Medical Center, Duke University Medical Center, and at other locations throughout the country. *Ruppel v. Kucanin*, 2011 WL 2470621, at *7; D.E. 57-1 at *28; D.E. 67 at *16. Furthermore, the United States Army Telemedicine and Advanced Technology Research Command sponsored a Diffusion MRI TBI Roadmap Development Workshop "at which it was acknowledged that 'DTI has detected abnormalities associated with brain trauma.'" Ruppel, 2011 WL 2470621, at *7 (internal citation omitted). Additionally, the United States Food and Drug Administration has approved the use of DTI technology. Id.; D.E. 57-1 at *28. . . . The Court therefore concludes that DTI is a generally accepted method for analyzing and diagnosing TBIs.

Another key question under *Daubert's* reliability inquiry is whether the technique at issue has been subjected to peer review and publication. 509 U.S. at 594. "As of early 2010, there were 3,472 papers on DTI published in peer review journals. Eighty-three of these articles involved DTI in relation to TBI." *Ruppel*, 2011 WL 2470621 at *8. Furthermore, in 2013, the "American Journal of Neuroradiology . . . published 'A Decade of DTI in Traumatic Brain Injury: 10 years and 100 Articles Later,' comprehensively show[ing] that the use of DTI in the evaluation of TBI has been tested, validated, [and] peer reviewed." M.B. Hulkhower et al., A Decade of DTI in Traumatic Brain Injury: 10 Years and 100 Articles Later, 34 Am. J. Neuroradiology 2064, 2071 (2013) ("A unifying theme can be deduced from this large body of research: DTI is an extremely useful and robust tool for the detection of TBI-related brain abnormalities."); Thus, there are extensive peer-reviewed articles on the effectiveness of DTI.

Another consideration under *Daubert's* reliability analysis is whether a known error rate exists for the technique in question. 509 U.S. at 594. "DTI scan[s] and resulting FA quantification analysis can be tested and replicated and [ ] the error rate is not higher than other methods commonly relied upon such as MRIs." *Ruppel*, 2011 WL 2470621, at *9 (internal citation omitted). Furthermore, "Dr. York indicates that the DTI makes no error in obtaining data per the FDA approved protocol, he estimates a 1-2% error in interpreting the data in his own career. . . . This testimony gives this [C]ourt a 98% certainty error free rate in Dr. York's analysis." Taken together, it is the conclusion of the Court that the methodology by which Dr. York reaches his conclusions is sufficiently reliable.

As to the final *Rink* prong, the Court finds that Dr. York's testimony regarding the tests and records he reviewed in conjunction with Plaintiff's DTI scans, and the conclusions he derived therefrom, will assist the jury in determining whether Plaintiff sustained a mild TBI as a result of her accident aboard the Solstice.

CONCLUSION

Celebrity's primary argument for exclusion of Dr. York's testimony is his reliance on DTI to reach his conclusions. As discussed above, DTI is a reliable method, especially when used in conjunction with the other medical tests and assessments relied upon by Dr. York. The Court, therefore, finds that Dr. York's testimony meets the requirements for admissibility under Rule 702 and *Daubert.* . . .

Brouard v. Convery
70 N.Y.S.3d 820 (N.Y. Sup. Ct. 2018)

HUDSON, J. The matter at hand is an action for damages sounding in negligence. It arises from an automobile accident. . . . Plaintiffs Denise Brouard and Gerard Brouard, (hereinafter referred to as "the Brouards") allege . . . that the Defendant, James Convery, was making a left-hand turn with his vehicle when he struck the front of Plaintiff Denise Brouard's car, causing mild traumatic brain injury ("MTBI"), as well as neck, back, shoulder and knee injuries.

Plaintiffs now move for an order from this Court for various relief: (1) to take judicial notice of the general acceptance and acceptability of technology known as Diffusion Tensor Imaging ("DTI") pursuant to *Frye v. United States*, 293 F. 1013 (D.C. Cir. 1923); and (2) to preclude Defendant from contesting any expert testimony put forth by Plaintiffs in this regard.

Defendants oppose the motion and cross-move pursuant to CPLR §4532—a for relief which consists of the following: (1) an order precluding certain neuroradiological studies including DTI to diagnose minor traumatic brain injury ("TBI") based upon the *Frye* standard; or (2) to conduct a *Frye* hearing to determine the admissibility of methods, technologies and theories for determining minor traumatic brain injury allegations. . . .

The facts which have prompted the Plaintiffs to make the above referenced motion are that methodology and technology utilizing DTI was used to examine Plaintiff in 2008 and 2014. Plaintiffs claim that this specific technology enjoys general acceptance by the scientific and medical community and therefore passes the long-recognized rule contained in *Frye v. United States*. Given the status of DTI, Plaintiffs contend that the Defense must be precluded from adducing any expert testimony claiming that any MRI using DTI technology is not generally accepted by the scientific/medical community to investigate mild TBI's. . . .

The march of science is inexorable. This has created a challenge for trial courts in deciding what "scientific" evidence is truly worthy of the name. How is a Judge, a presumed expert in jurisprudence, but a lay person in science, to make such a determination? It is the Court's solemn duty to winnow the proof, finding and separating the modern day alchemy from chemistry as a metallurgist would remove dross from gold. In the ninety-five years since Frye was handed down to us, case law and medicine have both developed. Other jurisdictions have abandoned the Frye analysis and embraced the reasoning in *Daubert v. Merrell Dow Pharmaceuticals*. New York, however has continued to follow the *Frye* rule, wisely leaving innovation to scientists and legislators. . . .

As *Frye* evolved, its progeny added the refinement that the term "general acceptance" did not refer to a mere head-count of experts. Instead, it became clear that there should be a clinical (not just scientific) consensus, and that the proper foundation be laid as well as acceptable methods employed in each particular case. This is the analysis we apply to the instant controversy.

This case began in 2005 and in the intervening passage of time, DTI technology and the scientific/medical literature discussing it has proceeded apace. Early indications of approbation, however, have given way to doubt regarding acceptance of DTI technology to evaluate mild brain trauma injuries.

A significant case cited by Plaintiffs is *LaMasa v. Bachman*, 56 A.D.3d 340 [1st Dept. 2008]. The Appellate Court found that DTI technology met the *Frye* standard. At first glance this would seem to end the inquiry. On the contrary, La Massa was followed by a "white paper" in 2014 which cast the First Department holding into doubt (M. Wintermark, P.C. Sanelli, Y. Anzai, A.J. Tsiouris and C.T. Whitlow on behalf of the American College of Radiology Head Injury Institute, Imaging Evidence and Recommendations for Traumatic Brain Injury: Advanced Neuro- and Neurovascular Imaging Techniques, American Journal of Neuroradiology, November 2014). Immediately after its publication, it gained notoriety among the Neuroradiology community. This white paper (supported and endorsed by members of the scientific/clinical medical community) holds that new advances in neuro-imaging techniques are showing promising results in group comparison analyses (DTI, PET, QEEG, etc.). Nevertheless, the article concludes that there is insufficient evidence supporting the routine clinical use of advanced neural imaging for diagnoses and/or prognostications at the individual patient level.

In deciding the significance of the white paper (whose authenticity is not questioned), the Court is guided by the recent holding in *Dovberg v. Laubach*, 63 N.Y.S.3d 417 [2d Dept. 2017].

Dovberg emphasized that the burden of proving general acceptance of scientific principles or procedures for the admissibility of expert testimony rests upon the party offering the disputed expert testimony. That general acceptance of scientific principles or procedures which are required for admissibility of expert testimony can be demonstrated through scientific or legal writings, judicial opinions, or expert opinions other than the proffered expert. In addition to the requirement that the technology be generally accepted (and supported by adequate documentation), the movant must meet the standards of *Parker v. Mobil Oil Corp*.

Applying the prior precedents in *Dovberg*, the Second Department found the proposed "expert testimony" to be inadmissible based on the Defendant not meeting his burden of proof. Specifically, the Second Department found that the expert testimony did not meet generally accepted scientific principles (*Frye*). The Court noted that the proffered evidence failed to make reference to any empirical data or any peer-reviewed journals, and did not provide the names of the authors and years of publication (*Parker*).

The parallels between this case and *Dovberg* are clear and dispositive. The white paper by M. Wintermark et al. makes it clear that DTI technology is not generally accepted as yet in the field of neurology for use in the clinical treatment of individ-ual patients. The rule in *LaMasa v. Bachman, supra*, though superbly researched and written, has been outpaced by current scientific knowledge. Accordingly, evidence of DTI technology must be shielded from the jury's review.

Consequently, based on the issue of general acceptability in a given field, the Court finds that DTI does not (at the time of this writing) have a general acceptance to be used as the standard in clinical/medical treatment of individual patients who are being treated for TBI's.

. . . All of the foregoing obliges the Court to the following conclusion: Under the circumstances presented, the Court denies Plaintiff's motion in its entirety. The Defendants' cross-motion to preclude Plaintiff from using DTI technology by their expert is granted. . . .

NOTES AND QUESTIONS

1. Re-read the application of *Daubert* to the facts in *Marsh*. Note that the proposition that "DTI of the brain is a proven and well-established imaging modality in the evaluation and assessment of normal and abnormal conditions of the brain" is supported by citation to previous legal cases (as opposed to citing directly to sci-entific literature.) If the previous case law conducted extensive, accurate reviews of the relevant science, relying on the case law seems an efficient mechanism for assessing the validity of the scientific evidence. But what if the scientific analysis in the earlier case law was incomplete or mistaken?

2. State and federal courts are arriving at differing conclusions about the admis-sibility of DTI evidence in brain injury cases. In *Marsh v. Celebrity Cruises, Inc.*, decided in *2017*, the court concluded that "DTI is a generally accepted method for analyzing and diagnosing TBIs." But a year later, in *2018*, the court in *Brouard v. Convery* concluded that "DTI does not (at the time of this writing) have a gen-eral acceptance to be used as the standard in clinical/medical treatment of indi-vidual patients who are being treated for TBIs". How do you reconcile these two cases?

3. *Brouard* makes reference to a scientific publication that references the G2i Group to individual inference problem, which you have seen in previous chapters:

> Currently, there is evidence from group analyses that DTI can identify TBI-associated changes in the brain across a range of injury severity, from mild to severe TBI. Evidence also suggests that DTI has the sensitivity necessary to detect acute and chronic TBI-associated changes in the brain, some of which correlate with injury outcomes. These data, however, are based primarily upon group analyses, and there is insufficient evidence at the time of writing this article that DTI can be used for routine clinical diagnosis and/or prognostication at the individual patient level. Even though a few studies have reported z score methods for individual patient TBI evaluation, there remains insufficient evidence at the time of writing to suggest that these methods are valid, sensitive, and specific for routine clinical evaluation of TBI at the individual patient level. . . .

Max Wintermark et al., *Imaging Evidence and Recommendations for Traumatic Brain Injury: Advanced Neuro- and Neurovascular Imaging Techniques*, 12 J. Am. C. Radiology E1, E3 (2015).

4. Commentators are not in agreement about the appropriateness of DTI for courtroom use. For instance, consider this critical perspective from Martha E. Shenton et al.:

> Over the past 15 years, the courts' initially cautious approach to the use of DTI in personal injury litigation has given way to more liberal patterns of admission. This has occurred despite continuing lack of standardization with respect to the methods for acquiring and analyzing DTI data, and its uncertainty as a clinical metric in cases of mTBI. This has also occurred despite sound neurologic and medicolegal critiques that legal inferences from group DTI data to individual diagnosis and prognosis would rarely withstand a Daubert analysis. Further, an analysis of the small number of published traumatic brain injury litigations involving the use of DTI indicates that the courts have thus far failed to understand the distinction between the use of DTI in more well-established diagnostic domains (i.e., moderate to severe TBI) and less established domains. The courts have, as noted previously, also struggled to understand the importance of control group data for the interpretation of individual scans, and are also unclear regarding which experts are technically qualified to interpret the data derived from these scans. . . .
>
> . . . The cases summarized above reveal a concerning pattern. The courts appear to be making blanket endorsements of the use of DTI in mTBI by analogizing from the use of this modality in the diagnosis of moderate and severe brain injury. This facile analogy overlooks the challenges of using DTI to diagnose individual cases of mTBI, and the pitfalls of failing to examine the appropriateness of the underlying imaging data and control groups, as well as the appropriateness of the methods of analysis, and the variability in post processing and interpretation of the data. . . .
>
> DTI, with its great promise as a tool to detect objective signs of neuronal injury, is an attractive modality for the legal arena. It promises to solve many of the pitfalls surrounding mTBI litigation, including an over-reliance on subjective symptom reporting, in the context of secondary monetary gain. Conventional brain imaging modalities such as CT and MRI also often miss subtle diffuse axonal injuries, raising the specter of false negative findings. It is, consequently, highly tempting to bring a novel technology such as DTI into the courtroom, even in its infancy. . . .
>
> We . . . caution against the premature use of new advances in imaging such as DTI, before standards are established in the clinical arena, which are well informed and validated in the research arena. Judges, who are now gatekeepers with respect to evaluating the admissibility of evidence, need also to be informed with respect to the sensitivity and specificity of scientific measures, to issues of standardization, to appropriate methods of analyses, etc. in the use of DTI as evidence of mTBI in the courtroom.
>
> Further, while DTI is the most promising technique available today for detecting diffuse axonal injury, and is beginning to be used clinically, it remains largely within the purview of research. Its probative value is also not clear as it may be both prejudicial and misleading given that standardization is not yet established in either the clinic or in the courtroom, and thus it may be premature for use in either. . . .
>
> Finally, we also caution against the use of neuroimaging techniques such as DTI in the courtroom as we are not yet at the tipping point where these advances provide important and meaningful data with respect to their probative value. There is much to be learned and much to support evidence of subtle brain injury that will move from the purview of research in the near future. Additionally, we note that while it may be premature now to bring new imaging tools into the courtroom, we should remain hopeful that such tools will be ready in the very near future. At

this time, however, the gold standard remains the clinical interpretation by the neuroradiologist. . . .

Martha E. Shenton et al., *Mild Traumatic Brain Injury: Is DTI Ready for the Courtroom?*, 61 Int'l J.L. & Psychiatry 50, 59-61 (2018).

5. If a new neuroimaging technique is shown to be significantly better at detecting concussions, could this also change the reasonable standard of care? Would someone who does not utilize this diagnostic technology be considered negligent? Is your view influenced by factors such as cost? Distance to diagnostic facility? Consider this perspective:

> The availability of biomarkers of effect may expand the concussive management duties of schools or other sponsors of youth sports teams to include periodic testing of their players for biomarker indications of concussive injury. These duties may include testing players before play, during the season, and after the season. Pre-play screening will establish an individual player's baseline, while monitoring will help determine whether the player has suffered concussive injury and whether the concussion is resolved, making it safe to return to play. This duty may arise even if a player does not manifest outward symptoms of brain injury.

Betsy J. Grey & Gary E. Marchant, *Biomarkers, Concussions, and the Duty of Care,* 2015 Mich. St. L. Rev. 1911, 1955 (2015).

D. PROVING CAUSATION

A plaintiff must show that the defendant's breach of duty was the actual and proximate cause of the plaintiff's injuries. As the cases and commentary in this section demonstrate, establishing causation can be difficult.

Hendrix ex rel. G.P. v. Evenflo Co.
609 F.3d 1183 (11th Cir. 2010)

ANDERSON, C.J. Plaintiff-Appellant Rhonda Hendrix alleges that her son, G.P., sustained traumatic brain injuries when a child restraint system manufactured by Defendant-Appellee Evenflo Company, Inc., ("Evenflo"), malfunctioned during a minor traffic accident. Hendrix further alleges that those brain injuries caused G.P. to develop autism spectrum disorder ("ASD") and a spinal cord defect known as syringomyelia. The district court excluded testimony from two of Hendrix's expert witnesses that the accident caused G.P.'s ASD. The district court concluded that the methods used by Hendrix's experts were not sufficiently reliable under *Daubert v. Merrell Dow Pharmaceuticals, Inc.* The district court then granted partial summary judgment to Evenflo on Hendrix's compensatory damages claim, determining that without the excluded testimony there was no reliable evidence to support Hendrix's theory that the accident caused G.P.'s ASD. . . .

It is undisputed that the carrier fractured during the accident. While it is also undisputed that G.P. suffered a closed-head injury as a result of the accident, the parties do dispute the severity of the injury and whether G.P. suffered brain damage. G.P.'s medical records reveal that he suffered, at the very least, a contusion on his forehead and bleeding in his brain. G.P.'s injuries do not appear to have caused immediate neurologic impairment, as G.P. exhibited no developmental problems at his 2, 4, or 10-month check-ups.

Nearly eighteen months after the accident, G.P. began to exhibit developmental problems. When occupational therapy failed to cause improvement, G.P. was referred to Dr. Suhrbier, a pediatric neurologist. Dr. Suhrbier administered a neurologic evaluation to address G.P.'s severe neurodevelopmental delay, impaired social interactions, and history of seizures.

Approximately three years after the accident, Dr. Suhrbier diagnosed G.P. with an asymptomatic spinal cord cyst. Hendrix argues that the cyst is a syringomyelia, which can be caused by trauma but may not appear for several years following the causative trauma. . . .

B. EXCLUSION OF EXPERT TESTIMONY ON CAUSAL LINK BETWEEN TRAUMATIC BRAIN INJURY AND ASD

1. Legal Standards for Admitting Scientific Evidence of Causation

Hendrix seeks to admit expert testimony that the traumatic brain injury G.P. sustained in the accident caused his ASD. Because this is a diversity case, we apply Florida's substantive law regarding a plaintiff's burden of proof on causation. Under Florida law, Hendrix may recover damages upon showing that the trauma was a "substantial factor" causing G.P.'s ASD. A purported cause is a substantial factor if it operates in combination with another cause, such as the negligent act of another or the plaintiff's pre-existing physical condition, to cause an injury.

Although the standards for finding causation are governed by Florida law, we apply federal law to determine whether the expert testimony proffered to prove causation is sufficiently reliable to submit it to the jury. . . . [The Court next performed a *Daubert* analysis.]

Hendrix's experts rely primarily on the differential etiology method to link G.P.'s traumatic brain injury to his ASD diagnosis. Differential etiology is a medical process of elimination whereby the possible causes of a condition are considered and ruled out one-by-one, leaving only one cause remaining. Hendrix argues that the experts' opinions were reliable because differential etiology is a well-recognized scientific method that has been accepted by many courts as a valid basis for expert testimony. We have previously noted that, when applied under circumstances that ensure reliability, the differential etiology method can provide a valid basis for medical causation opinions. Here, the reliability of the method must be judged by considering the reasonableness of applying the differential etiology approach to the facts of this case and the validity of the experts' particular method of analyzing the data and drawing conclusions therefrom.

A reliable differential etiology analysis is performed in two steps. First, the expert must compile a "comprehensive list of hypotheses that might explain the set of salient clinical findings under consideration. . . . The issue at this point in the process is which of the competing causes are *generally* capable of causing the patient's symptoms." Second, the expert must eliminate all causes but one.

With regard to the first step, the district court must ensure that, for each possible cause the expert "rules in" at the first stage of the analysis, the expert's opinion on general causation is "derived from scientifically valid methodology." This is because "a fundamental assumption underlying [differential etiology] is that the final, suspected 'cause' . . . must actually be capable of causing the injury." Thus, the experts' purported use of the differential etiology method "will not overcome a fundamental failure to lay the scientific groundwork" for the theory that traumatic brain injury can, in general, cause autism.

Some specific principles arise in the context of establishing general causation in cases dealing with medical injuries. In *McClain*, we distinguished cases in which the medical community generally recognizes that a certain chemical can cause the injury the plaintiff alleges from those in which the medical community has not reached such a consensus. We stated that in the second category of cases, the district court must apply the *Daubert* analysis not only to the expert's methodology for figuring out whether the chemical caused the plaintiff's *specific* injury, but also to the question of whether the drug or chemical can, in general, cause the harm plaintiff alleges. Thus, the district court must assess the reliability of the expert's opinion on *general*, as well as specific, causation. . . .

In the second step of the differential etiology analysis, the expert must eliminate all causes but one. While the first step focuses on general causation, in the second step the expert applies the facts of the patient's case to the list created in the first step in order to form an opinion about the actual cause of the patient's symptoms, i.e., to determine specific causation. In *Clausen*, the Ninth Circuit stated that an "expert must provide reasons for rejecting alternative hypotheses using scientific methods and procedures and the elimination of those hypotheses must be founded on more than subjective beliefs or unsupported speculation." Thus, "[a] district court is justified in excluding evidence if an expert 'utterly fails . . . to offer an explanation for why the proffered alternative cause' was ruled out." . . .

We have carefully and exhaustively reviewed the literature cited by Dr. Hoffman and conclude that the district court's conclusion with regard to each piece of literature was reasonable. We hold that the district court reasonably concluded that none of the literature supported the reliability of Dr. Hoffman's proffered physiological process, and that none of the literature supported Dr. Hoffman's opinion that a traumatic brain injury like GP's could have caused or contributed to the development of ASD. . . .

We found the most direct statement supporting the theory that traumatic brain injury can cause ASD in a textbook submitted by Dr. Hoffman that was not brought to our attention on appeal. That textbook states:

> Considerable precedent for deleterious effects of various perinatal insults on organizational events is provided by studies with experimental animals. Initial studies of later cortical neuronal development in "undamaged" areas adjacent to ischemic cortical injury in human infants show dendritic aberrations that could contribute importantly to subsequent cognitive deficits and epilepsy. It is a clinical truism that some children affected by one or more perinatal insults may exhibit neurological sequalae that are more severe than might be predicted from the extent of injury recognized by the usual brain imaging or neuropathological techniques.

Volpe, *Human Brain Development in Neurology of the Newborn* at 82.

In other words, this textbook provides some support for the idea that even minor injuries sustained by newborn brains can result in more severe neurologic impairments than one would expect from the initial extent of the injury. The textbook does not, however, link such injuries to ASD, or provide any support for Dr. Hoffman's theory of ASD causation involving abnormal cerebral spinal fluid pressure. . . .

The medical literature indicates that there are a dizzying array of other factors that have been mentioned as possible causes, including as many as 90 gene mutations that could play a role in the development of autism. Dr. Hoffman conceded in his deposition testimony that, unless one of the genetic chromosome anomalies that is known to cause autism is identified, medical science simply does not know what causes autism. Obviously, in such a situation, the task of "ruling out" other plausible causes is extremely complex. In light of our decision that Dr. Hoffman failed to reliably "rule in" his theory of ASD causation, we need not in this case venture into the quagmire of attempting to define the parameters of a reliable process of "ruling out" other possible causes of autism. . . .

NOTES AND QUESTIONS

1. The court uses an approach to first rule in, and then rule out, the plaintiff's theory about causation. What certainty is required for each step of this analysis in order to admit expert testimony? For more on differential etiology in law, see David Faigman et al., *Modern Scientific Evidence* §20-1.1 (2019-2020 ed.).
2. One of the reasons that concussions in professional football have received so much attention is the high-profile suicides of former NFL players. How would you describe the causal relationship between concussions experienced from playing football and these suicides? David Hovda, director of the UCLA Brain Injury Research Center, observes, "There are a lot of reasons people commit suicide and commit murder. . . . I'm not sure we can tag CTE [Chronic Traumatic Encephalopathy] onto this." Stephanie Smith, *More Cases of Brain Disease Found in Football Players*, CNN (Dec. 4, 2012). If you applied the approach taken in the *Hendrix* case, how would you analyze the issue?
3. Some athletes who have experienced brain injury playing football have sued the manufacturers of the football helmets they were wearing. Consider this case: A sixteen-year-old high school football player "was severely injured by a blow to the head during football practice. Through his guardian ad litem, he sued the designer and manufacturer of the football helmet that he was wearing, alleging that its defective design was the cause of his injury." If you were representing this individual, what argument would you make about the causal relationship between the manufacture of the helmet and the injury? What if you were representing the defendant manufacturer? *See Austria v. Bike Athletic Co.*, 107 Or. App. 57, 59-61 (Or. Ct. App. 1991).
4. Litigants frequently argue over what types of experts should be allowed to testify about causation, and courts must adjudicate these disputes. Courts are split on how to handle this issue of testifying about causation:

> There seems little dispute that a psychologist may testify as to the existence of a brain injury, or at least the condition of the brain in general.
>
> The courts have split, however, over the question involved in this case: whether a psychologist may give expert testimony regarding the causation of brain injury. The majority of the states that have passed on the issue have permitted such testimony. . . .
>
> Other jurisdictions, however, have barred psychologists from testifying about causation of physical injuries. In addition to the basic theory that a psychologist lacks proper training to testify competently as to medical causation, some courts

have looked to their respective statutory definitions of the practice of psychology as a basis for the restriction of such testimony.

Some courts have espoused intermediate rules. Although Florida generally bars psychologists from testifying as to the cause of organic brain injury, two courts have allowed such testimony on harmless error grounds. . . .

Hutchison v. Am. Family Mut. Ins. Co., 514 N.W.2d 882 (Iowa 1994).

5. In *Bennett v. Richmond*, 960 N.E.2d 782 (Ind. 2012), the driver (and eventual plaintiff) in a rear-end collision auto accident claimed to have experienced whiplash, resulting in brain injury, and further resulting in a variety of symptoms, including memory loss. His neuropsychologist's testimony did not reach the mechanics of the accident (such as speed of impact, amount of force, etc.). Should that failure render the neuropsychologist's testimony inadmissible?

6. A 2017 study reported that 178 of 179 deceased professional football players had CTE. How, if at all, is this likely to affect future litigation and legal policy? Jesse Mez et al., *Clinicopathological Evaluation of Chronic Traumatic Encephalopathy in Players of American Football*, 318 JAMA 360 (2017). Would it affect your analysis to learn that the pathology of CTE has also been reported in individuals who have never played contact sports and who have not experienced a concussion? Grant L. Iverson et al., *Chronic Traumatic Encephalopathy Neuropathology Might Not Be Inexorably Progressive or Unique to Repetitive Neurotrauma*, 142 Brain 3672 (2019). *See also* Douglas H. Smith et al., *Chronic Traumatic Encephalopathy—Confusion and Controversies*, 15 Nature Reviews Neurology 179 (2019).

E. YOUTH SPORTS CONCUSSION LITIGATION AND LEGISLATION

In addition to professional sports leagues and the NCAA, youth sports teams and school-sponsored sports are also now ripe for litigation and legislation. In the 2010s all 50 states passed a youth sports concussion law, multiple lawsuits were brought against youth sports organizations, and scholarship began to explore the possibilities and limits of these responses to sports concussion. In this section we begin with some contextualizing data on the incidence of youth sports concussion. We then present an example of sports concussion litigation and conclude by reviewing state concussion statutes.

1. The Landscape of Youth Sports Concussions

Carly Rasmussen et al.

How Dangerous Are Youth Sports for the Brain? A Review of the Evidence

7 Berkeley J. Ent. & Sports L. 67, 86-88 (2018)

WHAT WE KNOW: DETAILED REVIEW OF RESEARCH ON YOUTH SPORTS CONCUSSION INCIDENCE

[W]e review the peer-reviewed studies . . . of youth sports concussion incidence . . . [and the] review suggests the following conclusions.

1. *First*, precisely estimating the actual incidence of youth sports concussions is difficult because different research methodologies lead to markedly different

conclusions. For instance, estimating the number of sports-related concussions amongst youth athletes using emergency department data likely underestimates incidence.

2. *Second*, and recognizing many caveats about methodology, it appears that across all high school sports for which data has been collected, the incidence rate of sports concussion is roughly between 0.4 to 0.5 concussions per 1,000 athlete encounters ("AEs"). Athlete encounters include both practices and games.

3. *Third*, there is great variation from sport-to-sport in concussion rates, ranging from 0 to 0.92 concussions per 1,000 AEs. Sports with the consistently highest concussion rates are football, wrestling, ice hockey, soccer, and lacrosse. To illustrate, if a youth football league has 10 teams, with 25 athletes per team, playing 4 days a week for 15 weeks, that league will have 15,000 athlete exposures and should, on average, expect about 8-10 concussions for the season. A high school league of 10 teams, with more athletes and more practices per week, will have 45,000 athlete exposures and should expect between 20-40 concussions per season.

4. *Fourth*, in the past 15 years, reported concussion incidence, and associated concussion incidence rates, have approximately doubled in youth sports.

5. *Fifth*, this increase in reported concussions is likely due to improved reporting, rather than an increase in concussions.

6. *Sixth*, although the data is not robust, it is very likely the case that most concussions are not "severe" concussions. That is, post-concussion symptoms resolve on their own, within 2-3 weeks, for roughly 90% of youth athletes.

7. *Seventh*, concussion risk and severity is increased by a history of prior concussion, and several studies have shown high rates of recurrent concussions in youth populations.

8. *Eighth*, symptom recovery is slower in youth and high school athletes than collegiate athletes.

9. *Ninth*, female athletes appear to experience as high as double the rate of concussions as their male athlete counterparts in comparable sports. This finding, as well as additional demographic variation in concussion incidence, remains in need of further research.

10. *Tenth*, in the past 15 years, return to play within 24 hours has significantly decreased; today, less than 1% of concussed athletes return to play within a day. This is a marked change from previous decades, when up to 50% of athletes returned to play on the same day.

2. Litigation

Mayall ex rel. H.C. v. USA Water Polo, Inc.
909 F.3d 1055 (9th Cir. 2018)

FLETCHER, C.J. Alice Mayall brought this putative class action against USA Water Polo as a representative of her minor daughter, alleging negligence, breach of voluntary undertaking, and gross negligence. The gravamen of Mayall's complaint is that USA Water Polo failed to implement concussion-management and return-to-play protocols for its youth water polo league. The Second Amended Complaint ("SAC") alleges that H.C., Mayall's daughter, was returned to play as a goalie in a youth water polo tournament after being hit in the face by the ball and while manifesting concussion symptoms. After she was returned to play, H.C. received additional hits to the head. As a result, she suffered from severely debilitating post-concussion syndrome. The district court dismissed the suit under Federal Rule of Civil Procedure 12(b)(6) for failure to state a claim under California law.

We have jurisdiction under 28 U.S.C. §1291. We reverse and remand.

I. BACKGROUND

According to the SAC, H.C. was a "healthy, high-achieving, straight-A honors student and multi-sport athlete" who played for a water polo team under the governance of USA Water Polo. On February 15, 2014, when H.C. was either fifteen or sixteen, she was injured while playing goalie during an annual three-day "WinterFest" tournament organized and managed by USA Water Polo. H.C. "was hit hard in the face by a shot which led to a concussion." The game continued while "H.C. swam to the side of the goal and spoke with her coach. . . ." The coach, who was "lacking any concussion management training, qualifications, and education from USA Water Polo," asked "a couple questions." Even though she was "dazed," H.C. was returned to play for the remainder of the game. Later that day, H.C. played in more games and took more shots to the head, exacerbating her initial injury. The additional shots to the head were witnessed by the referee and by H.C.'s coach. H.C. was never evaluated by a medical professional during the tournament.

Two days later, H.C. suffered from headaches, sleepiness, and fatigue so severe that she was unable to attend school. For the next two weeks, H.C. experienced excessive sleeping, dizziness, intolerance to movement, extreme sensitivity to light, headaches, decreased appetite, and nausea. On March 4, 2014, Mayall took H.C. to a doctor, who diagnosed her with post-concussion syndrome. On March 12, the doctor recommended a consultation with a neurologist. The neurologist confirmed the diagnosis.

H.C.'s symptoms persisted, and she was unable to return to school. H.C. took part in a "home-and-hospital instructional program" for the remainder of the 2013-2014 school year. H.C.'s academic ability was severely degraded. Her neuropsychologist noted that H.C. demonstrated "a deficit in her ability to hold information in her mind or complete tasks, and was functioning in a low-average range in memory and controlled attention." At the time of filing the SAC, H.C. continued to suffer from persistent post-concussion syndrome, characterized by excessive sleeping, chronic headaches, and limited physical stamina. Because of her symptoms, H.C. was unable to attend public school.

The SAC alleges that USA Water Polo is the " 'national governing body for the sport of water polo in the United States' " (quoting from USA Water Polo bylaws). "USA Water Polo is the sanctioning authority for more than 500 Member Clubs and more than 400 tournaments are conducted nationwide each year[.]" "USA Water Polo requires all players and participants to follow the policies, bylaws, rules of conduct, and regulations it has enacted." USA Water Polo's "Policies and Guidelines" state that USA Water Polo is "committed to creating a healthy and safe environment for all of our members." "[A]s acknowledged by USA Water Polo's CEO, Christopher Ramsey, USA Water Polo's corporate documents support the obligation that USA Water Polo is responsible for health and safety issues."

The SAC alleges that scientific studies show that there are substantial neurological risks in allowing athletes to return to play before they have completely recovered from a concussion. One study cited by the SAC concludes that "returning an athlete to participation before complete recovery may greatly increase the risk of lingering, long-term, or even catastrophic neurologic sequelae." The SAC alleges, "As of 2002, consensus had been reached in the medical and scientific community for the cornerstones of the management and treatment of concussions." Reflecting this consensus, an international group of experts has agreed on post-concussion "return-to-play" protocols, the most recent of which is the "Zurich II Protocol," published in 2012. With respect to children and adolescents, the Zurich II Protocol provides:

> Because of the different physiological response and longer recovery after concussion and specific risks (e.g., diffuse cerebral swelling) related to head impact during childhood and adolescence, a more conservative RTP [return-to-play] approach is recommended. It is appropriate to extend the amount of time of asymptomatic rest and/or length of the graded exertion in children and adolescents. It is not appropriate for a child or adolescent athlete with concussion to RTP on the same day as the injury, regardless of the level of athletic performance.

In 2011, three years prior to H.C.'s injury, USA Water Polo had developed a detailed "USA Water Polo Concussion Policy" for athletic trainers for USA Water Polo's national team. However, USA Water Polo did not require, or even recommend, that its Concussion Policy be followed by other water polo teams under its governance. The SAC alleges it ignored repeated requests—even pleas—to implement a concussion protocol for its other teams.

Between 2011 and 2014, USA Water Polo received numerous emails reporting incidents in which young athletes suffered concussions and requesting implementation of a concussion policy for all water polo events. For example, in August 2011, officials at Fullerton College "alerted USA Water Polo about a player who was injured during a USA Water Polo-sanctioned game" and "requested any USA Water Polo concussion guidelines[.]" USA Water Polo's Director of Club and Member Programs, Claudia Dodson, acknowledged that there was no concussion policy applicable to the college. Professor Peter Snyder, the Head Swim Coach at Fullerton, then sent another email regarding the incident, encouraging USA Water Polo to implement a concussion-management and return-to-play protocol. After USA Water Polo responded by sending Snyder the national team's policy, Snyder pointed out that the policy "was only applicable to an extremely small portion of the USA Water Polo membership," and "implored" USA Water Polo to implement a protocol for all levels of play. But USA Water Polo took no action.

The SAC alleges that at the time of H.C.'s injury in 2014 and during the class period, USA Water Polo had no concussion-management policy or return-to-play protocol for its youth water polo teams. However, USA Water Polo did have "Rules Governing Conduct" applicable to all coaches, referees and athletes, not limited to those associated with the national team. "[B]uried in the fine print" of the Rules was a provision stating that USA Water Polo coaches were "expected to demonstrate good sportsmanship," including "avoiding . . . encouraging or permitting an athlete to return to play pre-maturely following a serious injury (e.g., a concussion) and without the clearance of a medical professional."

The SAC alleges three causes of action under California law: negligence; breach of voluntary undertaking; and gross negligence. The district court granted a motion to dismiss under Rule 12(b)(6), holding that (1) the SAC fails to allege a duty owed to H.C. by USA Water Polo and therefore fails to allege actionable negligence; (2) the SAC insufficiently alleges that a task or duty was "specifically" undertaken by USA Water Polo, and that USA Water Polo had increased the risk of harm to H.C.; and (3) the SAC fails to allege gross negligence because it fails to allege a duty owed to H.C. by USA Water Polo, and it fails to allege an "extreme departure from ordinary standards of conduct."

We reverse and remand for further proceedings. . . .

1. "Primary Assumption of Risk" Doctrine . . .

"Although defendants generally have no legal duty to eliminate (or protect a plaintiff against) risks inherent in the sport itself, it is well established that defendants generally do have a duty to use due care not to increase the risks to a participant over and above those inherent in the sport."

Mayall does not argue that USA Water Polo is liable under §1714(a) for the injury incurred when H.C. was hit in the head the first time. Rather, she argues that USA Water Polo is liable for injuries suffered when H.C. was hit in the head *again*, after she was returned to play. USA Water Polo argues that such secondary head injuries are inherent in the sport of water polo and that it is therefore not liable under §1714(a). The question before us is thus whether, under California law, secondary head injuries such as those suffered by H.C. are "inherent in the sport" of water polo. The district court held that they are inherent, and that USA Water Polo therefore did not owe a duty of care to H.C. We disagree . . . [the Court then reviewed California case law.]

2. Fulfilling the Duty of Care

USA Water Polo argues in its brief that if it did owe a duty of care to H.C., the "existence" of its "Rules Governing Coaches' Conduct," applicable to all USA Water Polo teams, fulfilled that duty. We disagree. . . .

The USA Water Polo Concussion Policy applicable to the national team, as well as the Zurich II Protocol, are substantially different from the Rules of Conduct. The Concussion Policy is a one-page single-spaced document, promulgated and applied to the national team in 2011, three years before H.C.'s injury. The Policy addresses only head injuries. It provides:

Once a player has been identified as suffering a concussion or mild traumatic brain injury (MTBI) by a medical professional or a coach or team manager recognizes the following:

Any injury that may result in a bad headache, altered levels of alertness, or unconsciousness and/or affecting memory, judgment, reflexes, speech, balance, coordination, and sleep patterns.

The following Protocol should be followed:

1. Initial evaluation by an ATC, EMT, DC, D.O., or MD following the SCAT 2 protocol (see attached).

2. The team physician should be notified immediately and <u>return to play is prohibited</u> on the same day and will be determined by the team physician or physician responsible for the athlete. Protocol is as per SCAT 2

> recommendations as well. The athlete will be followed periodically by the physician to access [sic] return to play.
>
>   3. The physician will notify the coach after each evaluation as to athlete's condition pending the athlete's consent to share medical information.

(Italics and underlining in original.) "SCAT 2" is shorthand for Sport Concussion Assessment Tool 2. SCAT 2 is a detailed four-page questionnaire designed to assess the seriousness of a head injury. On its first page are twenty-two criteria such as "headache," "dizziness," and "confusion," with assessments rated on a scale of 0 to 6 for each of the criteria. SCAT 2 at 1. At the bottom of the first page, SCAT 2 states in bold print: "**Any athlete with a suspected concussion should be REMOVED FROM PLAY, medically assessed, monitored for deterioration (i.e., should not be left alone) and should not drive a motor vehicle.**" *Id.*

The Zurich II Protocol was published in 2012, one year after USA Water Polo promulgated its Water Polo Concussion Policy and applied it to the national team. The Protocol is a twelve-page single-spaced document devoted entirely to concussions in sporting activities. Among other things, the Protocol provides detailed guidance for detecting and treating concussions. It provides:

> **On-field or sideline evaluation of acute concussion**
>
> When a player shows ANY features of a concussion:
>
>   A. The player should be evaluated by a physician or other licensed healthcare provider onsite using standard emergency management principles and particular attention should be given to excluding a cervical spine injury.
>
>   B. The appropriate disposition of the player must be determined by the treating healthcare provider in a timely manner. If no healthcare provider is available, the player should be safely removed from practice or play and urgent referral to a physician arranged.
>
>   C. Once the first aid issues are addressed, an assessment of the concussive injury should be made using the SCAT3 or other sideline assessment tools.
>
>   D. The player should not be left alone following the injury and serial monitoring for deterioration is essential over the initial few hours following injury.
>
>   E. A player with diagnosed concussion should not be allowed to RTP [Return to Play] on the day of injury.

(Bolding in original.) The Protocol attaches copies of SCAT 2, SCAT 3 and Child SCAT 3, as appendices.

The differences between the Rules Governing Coaches' Conduct, on the one hand, and the Water Polo Concussion Policy and the Zurich II Protocol, on the other, are striking. First, the Rules cover a large variety of topics, ranging far beyond concussions. Second, the Rules are merely hortatory, saying what the coaches are "expected" to do. Third, the language in the Rules referring to concussions is, as stated in the SAC, "buried in the fine print." Fourth, the language referring to concussions comes under the misleading heading of "sportsmanship." Fifth, the language comes under the additionally misleading heading of "physical abuse," defined as "(i) contact or non-contact conduct that results in, or reasonably threaten[s] to, cause physical harm . . . or (ii) any act or conduct . . . [such as] child abuse, child neglect, assault." Sixth, the language is provided only as the seventh example of such "physical abuse." Finally, the language is vague, advising coaches against allowing an athlete to return to play following a "serious injury," and providing a concussion only as an example of such an injury.

In stark contrast, the USA Water Polo Concussion Policy and the Zurich II Protocol are single-topic documents addressing only head injuries. They are mandatory rather than hortatory. Their instructions are detailed and clear, instructing coaches and others precisely what to do to in order to assess the seriousness of a blow to the head, and in order to protect athletes who may have suffered a concussion. Finally, they make clear the seriousness of a suspected concussion, with SCAT 2 telling coaches in bold print, "Any athlete with a suspected concussion should be REMOVED FROM PLAY, medically assessed, monitored for deterioration[.]" . . .

3. Statutes

State of Washington
Wash. Rev. Code §28A.600.190 (2009)
(The "Lystedt Law")

Youth Sports — Concussion and Head Injury Guidelines — Injured Athlete Restrictions — Short Title

(1)(a) Concussions are one of the most commonly reported injuries in children and adolescents who participate in sports and recreational activities. The centers for disease control and prevention estimates that as many as three million nine hundred thousand sports-related and recreation-related concussions occur in the United States each year. A concussion is caused by a blow or motion to the head or body that causes the brain to move rapidly inside the skull. The risk of catastrophic injuries or death are significant when a concussion or head injury is not properly evaluated and managed.

(b) Concussions are a type of brain injury that can range from mild to severe and can disrupt the way the brain normally works. Concussions can occur in any organized or unorganized sport or recreational activity and can result from a fall or from players colliding with each other, the ground, or with obstacles. Concussions occur with or without loss of consciousness, but the vast majority occurs without loss of consciousness.

(c) Continuing to play with a concussion or symptoms of head injury leaves the young athlete especially vulnerable to greater injury and even death. The legislature recognizes that, despite having generally recognized return to play standards for concussion and head injury, some affected youth athletes are prematurely returned to play resulting in actual or potential physical injury or death to youth athletes in the state of Washington.

(2) Each school district's board of directors shall work in concert with the Washington interscholastic activities association to develop the guidelines and other pertinent information and forms to inform and educate coaches, youth athletes, and their parents and/or guardians of the nature and risk of concussion and head injury including continuing to play after concussion or head injury. On a yearly basis, a concussion and head injury information sheet shall be signed and returned by the youth athlete and the athlete's parent and/or guardian prior to the youth athlete's initiating practice or competition.

(3) A youth athlete who is suspected of sustaining a concussion or head injury in a practice or game shall be removed from competition at that time.

(4) A youth athlete who has been removed from play may not return to play until the athlete is evaluated by a licensed health care provider trained in the evaluation

and management of concussion and receives written clearance to return to play from that health care provider. The health care provider may be a volunteer. A volunteer who authorizes a youth athlete to return to play is not liable for civil damages resulting from any act or omission in the rendering of such care, other than acts or omissions constituting gross negligence or willful or wanton misconduct.

(5) This section may be known and cited as the Zackery Lystedt law.

Minnesota
Minn. Stat. §121A.37 (2011)

Youth Sports Programs

(a) Consistent with section 121A.38, any municipality, business, or nonprofit organization that organizes a youth athletic activity for which an activity fee is charged shall:

(1) make information accessible to all participating coaches, officials, and youth athletes and their parents or guardians about the nature and risks of concussions, including the effects and risks of continuing to play after receiving a concussion, and the protocols and content, consistent with current medical knowledge from the Centers for Disease Control and Prevention, related to:

(i) the nature and risks of concussions associated with athletic activity;

(ii) the signs, symptoms, and behaviors consistent with a concussion;

(iii) the need to alert appropriate medical professionals for urgent diagnosis and treatment when a youth athlete is suspected or observed to have received a concussion; and

(iv) the need for a youth athlete who sustains a concussion to follow proper medical direction and protocols for treatment and returning to play; and

(2) require all participating coaches and officials to receive initial online training and online training at least once every three calendar years thereafter, consistent with clause (1) and the Concussion in Youth Sports online training program available on the Centers for Disease Control and Prevention website.

(b) A coach or official shall remove a youth athlete from participating in any youth athletic activity when the youth athlete:

(1) exhibits signs, symptoms, or behaviors consistent with a concussion; or

(2) is suspected of sustaining a concussion.

(c) When a coach or official removes a youth athlete from participating in a youth athletic activity because of a concussion, the youth athlete may not again participate in the activity until the youth athlete:

(1) no longer exhibits signs, symptoms, or behaviors consistent with a concussion; and

(2) is evaluated by a provider trained and experienced in evaluating and managing concussions and the provider gives the youth athlete written permission to again participate in the activity.

(d) Failing to remove a youth athlete from an activity under this section does not violate section 604A.11, subdivision 2, clause (6), consistent with paragraph (e).

(e) This section does not create any additional liability for, or create any new cause of legal action against, a municipality, business, or nonprofit organization or any officer, employee, or volunteer of a municipality, business, or nonprofit organization.

(f) For the purposes of this section, a municipality means a home rule charter city, a statutory city, or a town.

Francis X. Shen
Are Youth Sports Concussion Statutes Working?
56 Duq. L. Rev. 7, 10-11 (2018)

The evolution of state youth sports concussion laws, which began with a Washington state statute passed in 2009, has been well documented. All fifty states have now enacted youth sports concussion statutes, and most of these laws are based on the initial Washington statute (nicknamed the "Lystedt Law" in honor of Zackery Lystedt, a high school football player from Spokane who was seriously injured after being returned to play despite having a concussion).

There is variation in the laws, but in general, the existing state laws "are organized around three central provisions: education of athletes, parents, and coaches; immediate removal of play of concussed athletes; and medical clearance before returning to play."

Following this "first wave" of concussion legislation, states are beginning to revisit the issue. Since initial passage, 22 states have amended their laws. The "amendments generally fall into three types: (1) expanding coverage of the law (e.g., to include younger grades or recreational sports leagues), (2) tightening or clarifying existing requirements, and (3) efforts to prevent concussions from occurring in the first place (primary prevention) and improve early detection (secondary prevention)."

Even with these amendments, scholars have pointed out a variety of flaws in the statutes. Law professor Hosea Harvey, for instance, has shown that these laws were influenced by the NFL, and that they fail to adequately address relevant public health concerns. Law professor Douglas Abrams (who starred in college as a hockey goalie and has been a youth hockey coach for decades) has criticized both the scope and implementation of the laws. Others have suggested that the laws could improve: scope of coverage, enforcement mechanisms, providing resources for implementation, greater emphasis on prevention, reporting mechanisms, and evaluation and definition of concussion. . . .

NOTES AND QUESTIONS

1. Although there are many similarities across state statutes, each state's youth sports concussion law is different. Compare the Washington State and Minnesota statutes. What are noticeable differences? What challenges do you see in the administration of each statute?

2. State concussion laws have been criticized for not going far enough. Law professor Hosea Harvey identifies several key weaknesses:

> The aforementioned interventionist public health law approaches to concussions have many common features, a few innovations, and a high degree of uniformity. All but a few suffer from three critical shortcomings. First, they fail to include evaluative metrics to determine whether the law's reforms are helping to solve the problem. Second, existing youth sports TBI laws have a singular focus on reducing the secondary efforts of concussions rather than attacking their root causes. Finally, existing youth sports TBI laws fail to track individual athletes and the rise in risk associated with athletes who suffer multiple concussions. These factors may undermine the efficacy of existing youth sports TBI laws; solutions are proposed here to remedy that effectiveness gap and potentially address root causes. These are just

some of an array of potential policy innovations, but their efficacy can only fully be valued by policymakers with a more robust and consistent research agenda and use of data—which at the moment all but a few states do not collect or analyze for trends.

Hosea H. Harvey, *Refereeing the Public Health*, 14 Yale J. Health Pol'y L. & Ethics 66, 104-05 (2014).

3. With knowledge about youth sports concussions improving rapidly, how should courts assess the standard of care? *See* Steven Pachman & Adria Lamba, *Legal Aspects of Concussion: The Ever-Evolving Standard of Care*, 52 J. Athletic Training 186 (2017).

FURTHER READING

Biomarkers and Assessment of Brain Injury:

Biomarkers for Traumatic Brain Injury (Svetlana Dambinova, Ronald L. Hayes & Kevin K.W. Wang eds., 2012).

Christopher C. Giza & David A. Hovda, *The New Neurometabolic Cascade of Concussion*, 75 Neurosurgery S24 (2014).

Textbook of Traumatic Brain Injury, (Jonathan M. Silver, Thomas W. McAllister & David B. Arciniegas eds., 3d ed. 2018).

CTE:

Ann C. McKee et al., *The First NINDS/NIBIB Consensus Meeting to Define Neuropathological Criteria for the Diagnosis of Chronic Traumatic Encephalopathy*, 131 Acta Neuropathologica 75 (2016).

Grant L. Iverson et al., *A Critical Review of Chronic Traumatic Encephalopathy*, 56 Neurosci. & Biobehav. Reviews 276 (2015).

Litigating Brain Injury:

Richard W. Petrocelli, Thomas J. Guilmette & M.D.M. Eileen McNamara, *Traumatic Brain Injury: Evaluation and Litigation* (2019).

Valerie Gray Hardcastle, *Traumatic Brain Injury, Neuroscience, and the Legal System*, 8 Neuroethics 55 (2014).

Sport-Related Brain Injuries:

Paul McCrory et al., *Consensus Statement on Concussion in Sport—The 5th International Conference on Concussion in Sport Held in Berlin, October 2016*, 51 Brit. J. Sports Med. 838 (2017).

Christopher C. Giza, Mayumi L. Prins & David A. Hovda, *It's Not All Fun and Games: Sports, Concussions, and Neuroscience*, 94 Neuron 1051 (2017).

Steven P. Broglio et al. and CARE Consortium Investigators, *A National Study on the Effects of Concussion in Collegiate Athletes and US Military Service Academy Members: The NCAA–DoD Concussion Assessment, Research and Education (CARE) Consortium Structure and Methods*, 47 Sports Med. 1437 (2017).

Jessica L. Roberts et al., *Evaluating NFL Player Health and Performance: Legal and Ethical Issues*, 165 U. Pa. L. Rev. 227 (2016).

CHAPTER *11*

Pain and Distress

A robust, accurate way to determine whether someone is in pain or not would be a godsend for the legal system.
    —Henry Greely[†]

No one can measure another's pain and suffering; only the person suffering knows how much he or she is suffering, and even this person cannot accurately say what would be reasonable compensation for it.
    —Judge Lewis R. Sutin, *Grammer v. Kohlhaas Tank & Equip. Co.* (writing for the majority)[††]

CHAPTER SUMMARY

This chapter:

- Introduces legal and scientific conceptions of pain, including new insights on pain from neuroscience.
- Explores the future of neuroscience pain detection and its implications for law and policy.
- Discusses the law's distinctions between mental injury and physical injury, and how some of these distinctions are being challenged with new neuroscientific evidence.

INTRODUCTION

In the previous two chapters, you read about the law's treatment of dead or classically injured brains. This chapter focuses on a particular and important but also subtle kind of brain injury: pain (or *nociception*) and distress. As Professor Hank Greely has noted:

> Hundreds of thousands of legal proceedings each year in the United States turn on the existence of someone's (usually a plaintiff's or claimant's) pain. Sometimes those are personal injury cases, in which plaintiffs seek damages for their "pain and suffering" for the past, present, and predictably future in the aftermath of accidents. Most of them are actually disability cases, brought under federal or state disability schemes, or against private disability insurers. Although the technical question in those cases is not pain per se, it is quite often a question as to whether the claimants' pains are so great as to prevent them from working.

[†] Tracie White, *Does That Hurt? Objective Way to Measure Pain Being Developed at Stanford*, Stan. U. Med. Ctr. (Sept. 13, 2011).
[††] *Grammer v. Kohlhaas Tank & Equip. Co.*, 604 P.2d 823, 833 (N.M. Ct. App. 1979).

Henry T. Greely, *Neuroscience, Mindreading, and the Courts: The Example of Pain*, 18 J. Health Care L. & Pol'y 171, 178 (2015).

Professor Greely notes that the vast sums at issue ensure that defendants, disability programs, and insurers are not going to be satisfied with only the claimant's self-report. The legal system therefore looks for plausible causes of the reported pain, behavioral evidence consistent with reported pain, and, sometimes, expert testimony regarding the causes and levels of pain.

Reliable and objective measures of pain and mental anguish remain elusive to scientists and the law. Nevertheless, the legal system cannot avoid deciding cases in which pain and distress are crucial. And neuroscience may be improving our understanding and measurement of both, though it remains to be seen if and how the legal system will best operationalize that new knowledge.

The readings in the first half of this chapter, Sections A and B: discuss historical and current legal definitions of pain; survey neuroscience evidence on pain; and raise questions about whether this new science of pain should change the law. The chapter then turns in Section C to a related issue: Should bodies of law distinguish between mental and physical injury or illness? As the cases will illustrate, the distinction between the "merely" mental and the physical has implications in a variety of legal arenas, including civil liability, insurance coverage, and criminal sentencing. The chapter explores whether these traditional dividing lines are challenged by neuroscientific understandings of mental phenomena as being physically instantiated in the brain. The chapter ends by examining, in Section D, recent invocations of neuroscience in support of abortion-reform legislation.

A. PAIN IN LAW

As you read the following case excerpts, try to characterize and compare the perspectives on when and how pain is legally relevant. What does this suggest to you about the variables that make law's treatment of pain so complex? Will neuroscience have something valuable to contribute to law's engagement with pain? Consider, for example: What if the plaintiff or claimant in these pain cases had been evaluated with neuroimaging techniques? What factors would likely govern whether that is more likely to help or to hurt one's case?

Luchansky v. J.V. Parish, Inc.
157 N.E.2d 388 (Ohio Ct. App. 1957)

PHILLIPS, J. Crossing from the northerly to the southerly side of Indianola Avenue at the crosswalk on the westerly side of Market Street in Youngstown, at 10:30 on a snowy December morning in 1954, plaintiff was struck by defendant's truck . . . and injured resulting in an action for damages in the court of common pleas.

The jury returned a verdict for the plaintiff for $25,000. The trial judge overruled defendant's motions for judgment non obstante veredicto and for a new trial, and entered judgment on the verdict. From that judgment defendant appealed to this court on questions of law. . . .

The trial judge charged the jury in writing before argument, erroneously defendant claims, the following propositions of law submitted by plaintiff separately and not as a series: . . .

'4. Ladies and gentlemen of the jury, the court charges you that the term "pain" means a disturbed sensation causing suffering or distress.' . . .

Defendant claims charge number four is objectionable because it defines pain, which is a commonly understood word requiring no definition.

The definition of the word "pain" as submitted by the plaintiff and charged by the trial judge is that contained in Blakiston's New Gould Medical Dictionary, which word the author thereof thought was sufficiently uncommon to define in his highly rated work. . . .

In our opinion the trial judge committed no error prejudicial to the defendant in charging the jury as requested by plaintiff in request to charge before argument numbered four. . . .

Wiltz v. Barnhart
484 F. Supp. 2d 524 (W.D. La. 2006)

METHVIN, M.J. Before the court is an appeal of the Commissioner's finding of non-disability. . . . [I]t is recommended that the Commissioner's decision be REVERSED.

Background. . . . [Twenty-year-old] Wiltz applied for childhood supplemental security income benefits alleging disability as of May 12, 1999 due to migraine headaches, learning problems, sinusitis, and adjustment disorder. Wiltz's application was denied on initial review, and an administrative hearing was held on September 24, 2003. Because Wiltz had turned eighteen on February 25, 2003, the ALJ's opinion, issued on May 27, 2004, considered Wiltz's eligibility for benefits under both the child's standards and the adult standards. The ALJ determined that Wiltz was not disabled because his impairments do not meet or equal a listing, and there are jobs which exist in significant numbers in the economy which Wiltz could perform. A request for review was denied by the Appeals Council. . . .

Assignment of Errors Wiltz alleges the . . . ALJ erred in not finding that his migraine headaches, sinusitis, and adjustment disorder result in extreme limitations which satisfy the requirements of a Listed impairment. . . .

Standard of Review. The court's review is restricted [by statute] to two inquiries: (1) whether the Commissioner's decision is supported by substantial evidence in the record; and (2) whether the decision comports with relevant legal standards. . . . A finding of no substantial evidence is appropriate only if no credible evidentiary choices or medical findings exist to support the decision. . . .

ALJ's Decision: Adult Disability Benefits. A person applying for disability and/or SSI benefits bears the burden of proving that he is disabled within the meaning of the Social Security Act, 43 U.S.C. §423(d). Initially, the burden is on the claimant to show that he cannot perform his previous work. Once the claimant satisfies his initial burden, the Secretary then bears the burden of establishing that the claimant is capable of performing substantial gainful activity and is therefore not disabled. In determining whether a claimant is capable of performing substantial gainful activity, the Secretary uses a five-step sequential procedure set forth in 20 C.F.R. §404.1520(b)-(f) (1992):

1. If a person is engaged in substantial gainful activity, he will not be found disabled regardless of the medical findings.
2. A person who does not have a "severe impairment" will not be found to be disabled.
3. A person who meets the criteria in the list of impairments in Appendix 1 of the regulations will be considered disabled without consideration of vocational factors.
4. If a person can still perform his past work, he is not disabled.
5. If a person's impairment prevents him from performing his past work, other factors including age, education, past work experience, and residual functional capacity must be considered to determine if other work can be performed.

When a mental disability claim is made, the Commissioner utilizes a corollary sequential procedure [that] substitutes specialized rules at Step 2 for determining whether a mental impairment is severe, and also provides detailed guidelines for making the Step 3 determination as to whether the mental impairment meets or exceeds the Listings. The Regulations require:

> [T]he ALJ to identify specifically the claimant's mental impairments, rate the degree of functional limitation resulting from each in four broad functional areas, and determine the severity of each impairment. Furthermore. . . . the ALJ must document his application of this technique to the claimant's mental impairments.

In the instant case, the ALJ determined that Wiltz's borderline intelligence and adjustment disorder were severe impairments. The ALJ assessed Wiltz's residual functional capacity. . . . and concluded that Wiltz could perform the exertional demands of work at all exertional levels with the following non-exertional limitations: work must be limited to one-step to three-step operations under general supervision with limited interaction with the public. Relying on the testimony of a vocational expert, the ALJ concluded that Wiltz is capable of making an adjustment to work that exists in significant numbers in the national economy, and is therefore not disabled.

Findings and Conclusions. . . . [T]he undersigned concludes that the ALJ's findings and conclusions are not supported by substantial evidence in the record.

I. ADMINISTRATIVE RECORD

Medical Records.   . . . [Wiltz's medical records showed that he began receiving treatment for his migraines in 1998. Since then, Wiltz had also been seen by a neurologist, who prescribed pain and migraine medication. As a result of the migraines, Wiltz's primary care physician had excused him from over 24 days of school at first and had eventually placed him on homebound educational status. In 2002 Wilts complained of decreased energy, feelings of guilt, and suicidal thoughts. In 2003 his physician described his illness as activity-limiting and incapacitating. Wiltz was also examined by a medical consultant who performed several disability assessments and concluded that Wiltz had "mild restrictions" in daily living activities, "moderate" comprehension and memory limitations, and "less-than-marked" limitations in the acquisition and use of information. Additionally, an examining internist concluded that Wiltz had no exertional limitation but should nonetheless avoid exposure to loud noises. — EDS.]

Administrative Hearing. Wiltz was unrepresented during the administrative hearing. Wiltz testified that his headaches start between his eyes and he becomes dizzy. Once he gets a migraine, he takes his medication and stays in a dark room. Wiltz estimated that some weeks he may have headaches every other day that require him to stay in a dark room. He testified that smoke and dust aggravate his condition. . . .

II. FINDING OF NON-DISABILITY: CHILDHOOD BENEFITS

Wiltz does not dispute the ALJ's finding that his impairments do not meet a Listed impairment, however, Wiltz argues that the ALJ erred in not finding that he functionally equals a Listed impairment due to the extreme limitations posed by his impairments.

Once it is determined that an impairment does not meet the requirements of a listed impairment, the impairment is evaluated to determine whether it functionally equals an Appendix 1 listing. A medically determinable impairment or combination of impairments functionally equals a listed impairment if it results in marked limitations in two of the following six domains, or an extreme limitation in one domain:

(i) Acquiring and using information;
(ii) Attending and completing tasks;
(iii) Interacting and relating with others;
(iv) Moving about and manipulating objects;
(v) Caring for yourself; and
(vi) Health and physical well-being.

A "marked" limitation in a domain means an impairment "interferes seriously with [the] ability to independently initiate, sustain, or complete activities." A "marked" limitation is "more than moderate" but "less than extreme." An "extreme" limitation will be found when an impairment "interferes very seriously with [the] ability to independently initiate, sustain, or complete activities" within a domain. An extreme limitation is "more than marked," but "does not necessarily mean a total lack or loss of ability to function." Day-to-day functioning is considered to be seriously limited regardless of whether the impairment limits only one activity within a domain, or several.

The ALJ concluded that Wiltz's impairments did not functionally equal a listed impairment: . . .

> In the domain of Health and Well-Being, the undersigned finds that the claimant has a marked limitation. He complains of continuing headaches and received homebound education per doctor's orders. However, there are no records of tests, hospitalizations, MRI's, brain scans, etc. to provide a basis for the complaints of headaches. The undersigned concludes that the doctor appears to rely heavily on the claimant's subjective complaints in reaching his conclusions.
>
> The claimant has no limitations in any of the following areas: Attending and Completing Tasks, Interacting and Relating with Others, Moving About and Manipulating Objects, and Caring for yourself.

Thus, the ALJ's determination ultimately centered around credibility determinations. Since [Wiltz's physician] relied "heavily on the claimant's subjective complaints," and the record does not contain objective findings establishing the basis for the headaches, the ALJ determined that the fact that Wiltz's headaches resulted in homebound education was insufficient to establish an extreme limitation.

The ALJ is entitled to determine the credibility of the examining physicians and medical experts and to weigh their opinions accordingly. Although the opinion and diagnosis of a treating physician should be afforded considerable weight in determining disability, "the ALJ has sole responsibility for determining a claimant's disability status [and can] reject the opinion of any physician when the evidence supports a contrary conclusion." The ALJ is certainly able to decrease reliance on treating physician testimony for good cause. "Good cause for abandoning the treating physician rule includes 'disregarding statements [by the treating physician] that are brief and conclusory, not supported by medically acceptable clinical laboratory diagnostic techniques, or otherwise unsupported by evidence.'"

The ALJ's insistence upon objective medical evidence of Wiltz's migraine headaches was error. Migraine headaches are particularly unsusceptible to diagnostic testing. . . . [W]hile laboratory tests cannot prove the existence of migraine headaches, there are [recognized medical signs and symptoms, sufficient to justify the diagnosis and treatment of migraine headaches] which should be viewed as "objective evidence" [of migraines, given that these signs are often the only means available to prove their existence]. . . .

Thus, in cases involving complaints of disabling pain due to migraine headaches, courts look to other objective medical signs to determine whether the claimant's complaints are consistent with the existence of disabling migraine pain. . . .

The record shows that Wiltz has consistently sought treatment for migraines. The record further shows that he was prescribed medication for this condition. Additionally, Wiltz told Dr. Snatic that his migraines sometimes result in vomiting, and he testified that once he gets a migraine he becomes dizzy and must stay in a dark room until the headaches is gone.

Thus, the undersigned concludes that the ALJ erred in disregarding the diagnosis of Dr. Matis on grounds that there were no "tests, hospitalizations, MRI's, brain scans, etc." to support it. It is clear that Wiltz's headaches rendered him incapacitated and prevented him from attending school on a regular basis. Since his headaches limited him from day-to-day functioning in a school environment, the undersigned concludes that Wiltz's had an extreme limitation in the domain of "health and well-being." Accordingly, the ALJ erred in not finding that Wiltz was entitled to . . . disability benefits because his impairments functionally equaled a Listed impairment.

III. FINDING OF NON-DISABILITY: ADULT BENEFITS . . .

The overwhelming evidence of record shows that Wiltz's condition is of a chronic and severe nature, which prohibited him from attending school and would likewise cause him to be frequently absent from work. Considering this, and the fact that the vocational expert testified that employers would not tolerate an employee's frequent absences, the undersigned finds that the ALJ's determination that Wiltz could perform work that exists in significant numbers is not supported by substantial evidence.

Conclusion. Considering the foregoing, it is recommended that case be REVERSED and that plaintiff be awarded childhood benefits from March 20, 2002 through February 25, 2003 (the date he attained the age of eighteen) and adult benefits consistent with an onset date of February 25, 2003. . . .

[The Court subsequently adopted these recommendations from the Magistrate Judge, and reversed, awarding Wiltz childhood benefits for the period of March 20, 2002 through February 25, 2003 (the date he attained the age of eighteen) and adult benefits consistent with an onset date of February 25, 2003. —EDS.]

In 2018 the Social Security Administration requested public comment on whether—and if so how—to propose revisions to its current policy regarding the evaluation of pain in connection with claims for disability benefits. Public comment closed in 2019, and the matter remains pending. Before we begin in Section B to look more closely at the neuroscience of pain, consider the following excerpt from one public comment submitted, which helps to frame one possible intersection of law and neuroscience, and which highlights the potentially important distinction between "acute pain" (caused by immediate trauma, and usually dissipating as injured tissues heal) and "chronic pain" (which is often long-lasting and may be dissociated from injured tissue).

Amanda C. Pustilnik et al.
Comment on the Social Security Administration's Consideration of Pain in the Disability Determination Process, 83 FR 64493
(Dec. 17, 2018)

INTRODUCTION AND SUMMARY

Chronic pain disorders are simultaneously the most common yet most difficult conditions to evaluate. The opportunity exists to substantially improve accuracy, efficiency, and fairness within the disability adjudication process by revising the regulations to comport with contemporary biomedical models of chronic pain disorders.

The last two decades have seen a revolution in the understanding of chronic pain disorders. . . .

The Social Security Disability Regulations relating to the evaluation of pain, drafted in 1984,were consistent with the biomedical understanding of pain at the time, primarily an understanding of pain as a symptom of other injuries or anatomical abnormalities. We now know that this describes a subset of pain conditions yet affirmatively misdescribes a majority of chronic pain conditions. This creates inadvertent inefficiencies and inaccuracies, as examiners search for an elusive correspondence between anatomical findings and degree of pain, and endeavor, with little contemporary guidance, to evaluate the legitimacy of all other types of claimed pain. . . .

COMMENTS

1. The Regulations' requirement that pain arise from an "injury or condition expected to produce the pain" should be revised to account for the contemporary biomedical understanding of many chronic pain disorders as independent medical entities.

Chronic pain disorders exist as well-described, independent medical entities. By contrast, current regulations, and the interpretation thereof by disability examiners, conceive of pain primarily as a symptom of a distinct, non-pain condition, usually an injury or tissue damage. . . .

(a) Bring regulations and review practices in line with contemporary pain science. Chronic pain disorders constitute a set of medical conditions in themselves that may arise spontaneously, with incidental relationships to anatomical findings, be precipitated by relatively trivial injuries, or persist after the apparent resolution of the injury or condition that initially gave rise to the pain. Research in neuroscience, immunology, and medicine establishes that these severe chronic pain disorders generally occur without relationship to a gross, anatomical "smoking gun." . . .

(b) Streamline and enhance accuracy of the review process. Currently, disability examiners attempt to reconcile apparently conflicting medical evidence of substantial pain and of insignificant or absent anatomical findings. In doing so, they are attempting to match two factors that often have no relationship, which is frustrating, time-consuming, and orthogonal to achieving accurate results.

A simpler, more accurate approach would be to direct examiners to evaluate applications involving chronic pain conditions against the known, clinical features of the pain condition alleged. Unlike in decades past, pain conditions are increasingly well-described clinical entities, with their own signs, symptoms, and diagnostic tests. Evaluating pain as a symptom of a chronic pain condition is neither circular nor does it mean taking claims on faith: It means matching claims of pain against a pattern of known clinical presentation and testing.

2. The regulations' requirement that pain be proportionate to the injury or disease claimed to produce the pain contravenes the weight of scientific and medical authority; "disproportionate pain" is a misleading term that should be discarded.

The current Regulations define pain greater than would be expected for a particular injury or pathology to be "disproportionate" pain. Such "disproportionate pain" is defined as a "subjective complaint." . . .

A legal expectation that pain should be proportionate to injury or distinct disease state, while seemingly intuitive, is misplaced in evaluating non-nociceptive chronic pain. Indeed, all pain experiences are sculpted by a complex mosaic of factors, which in addition to injury or disease include multiple biological, psychological and social influences that vary widely across individuals and over time. This "renders the pain experienced completely individualized." The concept of "'disproportionate" pain should be discarded as to the evaluation of chronic pain disorders, and the use of "subjective," if retained, should be revised to conform to the accepted medical definition of pain subjectivity.

Chronic pain disorders represent a category of pathological phenomena in which pain is inherently, definitionally out of proportion to identifiable causal factors and that frequently arise in the absence of currently-identifiable causal factors. It is characterized by a broken relationship between stimulus and perception. Chronic pain disorders may arise in the absence of any apparent injury, persist after apparent healing, or be triggered by a seemingly slight initial injury. . . .

Second, the current definition of disproportionate pain as "subjective" is misaligned with the meaning of "subjective" in scientific and medical definitions of pain. The International Association for the Study of Pain (IASP) defines all pain as "subjective," as all human sensory perception is subjective. . . . [The term subjective is being used to describe] the degree of credibility we might accord to a person reporting the pain: For pain experiences that match general cultural expectations, we require comparatively less evidence, while for pain that defies the general cultural perception of pain as a relationship between stimulus and response, we require more evidence, although not always of the relevant kinds. . . .

3. Examiners should be discouraged from over-reliance on structural imaging: Imaging is often misleading in chronic pain disorders and favors unnecessary medical procedures.

The Agency's emphasis on imaging tests such as CT, MRI, and X-ray misleads examiners, creates unpredictably in adjudication and can encourage unnecessary medical procedures. This is because chronic neuropathic pain and other centralized pain disorders often have no known relationship to anatomical abnormalities in the location where the pain is felt. The presence of a local finding does not prove pain, and the absence of a local finding does not disprove pain. . . .

4. The Agency can improve accuracy and reduce waste by promulgating guidance on the expected features of chronic pain conditions, with particular attention to revising a federal judicial standard that inadvertently promotes fraud.

Federal district and appellate courts play an important role in implementing the disability regulations by adjudicating disability denial appeals. In the absence of clear guidance on evaluating claims of pain alleged by applicants, courts in federal circuits across the United States have developed their own standards. In certain federal circuits, the judicially developed standard systematically disfavors legitimate applications and rewards fraud. . . .

In the Fifth Circuit, and in some cases in the Second, Third, Fifth, Sixth, Seventh, and Eight Circuits, courts hold that chronic pain rises to the level of disability if and only if it is "constant, unremitting, and wholly unresponsive to therapeutic treatment." However, pain is intrinsically variable. It is the absence of variability that should be a red flag. Thus, this standard contravenes medical descriptions of chronic pain disorders and favors only those claims that are malingered or fabricated.

To remedy this problem, the Agency should promulgate guidance in which it identifies the hallmarks of well-described chronic pain conditions versus those of simulated pain conditions. . . .

5. The Agency should remove disincentives to recovery built into the current evaluation process. . . .

6. For technical, efficiency-related, and ethical reasons, the Agency should not adopt fMRI- or EEG-based pain measurement devices as standard practice in evaluations nor promote them in clinical settings.

The authors of this Comment, and the [International Association for the Study of Pain] Task Force on pain measurement devices, recommend that, if a reliable technology or technique is developed for the measurement of chronic pain and is validated across relevant populations and pain conditions, it should be employed only in particularly complex or disputed cases. Reliance on fMRI- or EEG-based pain measurement devices should not become standard in clinical or legal practice for reasons relating to accuracy, efficiency, and fairness. . . .

(a) Accurate detection is not yet possible. Pain-detection technologies currently only are reliable as to the detection of acute pain, not chronic pain and its related impairments. Under ideal laboratory conditions, fMRI- and EEG-based systems can determine with substantial accuracy whether a healthy subject is experiencing pain acute from an experimentally applied stimulus. No equivalent technology exists for chronic pain. Chronic pain, particularly centralized pain, does not appear to present with a distinct "signature" like acute, nociceptive pain. . . .

NOTES AND QUESTIONS

1. Do you think there are contexts in which the legal system should define what pain is and how it might best be calculated, for the purposes of tort actions or claims for disability benefits? Or are you persuaded by the plaintiff's argument in *Luchansky* that terms such as these are commonly understood? With respect to that common understanding, how do you think most of your non-law peers would define "pain" in the *colloquial* sense?

2. A person can be eligible for social security disability benefits even when their sole disability is pain. I. J. Schiffres, Annotation, *Pain as "Disability" Entitling Insured to Disability Benefits Under §103 of The Social Security Act (42 U.S.C. §423)*, 23 A.L.R.3d 1034 (2020). And one of the fastest-growing bases for disability claims is back pain. Chana Joffe-Walt, *Unfit for Work: The Startling Rise of Disability in America*, NPR (2011). Given the need to separate the deserving claimant from the faking one, how would you try to distinguish the two if you were an administrative law judge? What, specifically, would you want to know, and why? Given your answers, what kinds of evidence should attorneys aim to present?

B. PAIN IN NEUROSCIENCE

So, what is pain, exactly? And what does neuroscience have to say about the subject?

1. Defining Pain

From the perspective of neuroscience, pain is a distinct feeling from the body that has multiple aspects, including: location, feeling, and intensity; associated emotion; and the body's autonomic and muscular reactions. Thus, touching a hot tea kettle could involve the burning sensation on the fingers, irritation with oneself at perceived carelessness, elevated heart rate, rapid withdrawal of the hand, and so forth. The ability to sense pain is of course crucial for well-being, so that the body can sense departures from normalcy and initiate behaviors that, by avoiding pain, avoid injury.

Usually, the behavioral drive that we call pain matches the intensity of the sensory stimulus causing the signal to the brain. However, it can vary under different conditions, becoming intolerable or, alternatively, disappearing, similar to hunger or thirst. Neuroscientists have described the pain pathways from nerve sensors in the body, in the skins and joints, as well as around internal organs, through the spinal cord to the brainstem. The brain senses and represents pain through pathways that are distinct from the standard somatosensory system that is responsible for our sense of touch and limb positions. In humans, unlike rats, cats, and dogs, the pain pathway reaches the cerebral cortex in the insula and anterior cingulate cortex. The insula is believed to "represent," mentally, the state of the body. This affords the capacity for conscious awareness of painful and uncomfortable states of the body. The anterior cingulate cortex is believed to regulate the response to a painful stimulus. This affords the capacity to attenuate the reaction to a painful stimulus based on, for example, social context. Thus, if the hot tea kettle is both very expensive and a family heirloom, then the reflex to drop it may be overcome.

Nat'l Inst. of Neurological Disorders & Stroke & Nat'l Insts. of Health
Pain: Hope Through Research
(2001)

Introduction: The Universal Disorder.   You know it at once. It may be the fiery sensation of a burn moments after your finger touches the stove. Or it's a dull ache above your brow after a day of stress and tension. Or you may recognize it as a sharp pierce in your back after you lift something heavy.

It is pain. In its most benign form, it warns us that something isn't quite right, that we should take medicine or see a doctor. At its worst, however, pain robs us of our productivity, our well-being, and, for many of us suffering from extended illness, our very lives. Pain is a complex perception that differs enormously among individual patients, even those who appear to have identical injuries or illnesses. . . .

A Brief History of Pain.   Ancient civilizations recorded on stone tablets accounts of pain and the treatments used: pressure, heat, water, and sun. Early humans related pain to evil, magic, and demons. Relief of pain was the responsibility of sorcerers, shamans, priests, and priestesses, who used herbs, rites, and ceremonies as their treatments.

The Greeks and Romans were the first to advance a theory of sensation, the idea that the brain and nervous system have a role in producing the perception of pain. But it was not until the Middle Ages and well into the Renaissance—the 1400s and 1500s—that evidence began to accumulate in support of these theories. Leonardo da Vinci and his contemporaries came to believe that the brain was the central organ responsible for sensation. Da Vinci also developed the idea that the spinal cord transmits sensations to the brain.

In the 17th and 18th centuries, the study of the body—and the senses—continued to be a source of wonder for the world's philosophers. In 1664, the French philosopher René Descartes described what to this day is still called a "pain pathway." Descartes illustrated how particles of fire, in contact with the foot, travel to the brain and he compared pain sensation to the ringing of a bell.

In the 19th century, pain came under more rigorous scientific study, paving the way for advances in pain therapy. Physician-scientists discovered that opium, morphine, codeine, and cocaine could be used to treat pain. These drugs led to the development of aspirin, to this day the most commonly used pain reliever. Before long, anesthesia—both general and regional—was refined and applied during surgery. . . .

The Two Faces of Pain: Acute and Chronic.   What is pain? The International Association for the Study of Pain defines it as:

> An unpleasant sensory and emotional experience associated with actual or potential tissue damage or described in terms of such damage.

It is useful to distinguish between two basic types of pain, acute and chronic, and they differ greatly.

Editor's Note To understand how pain relievers (known technically as *analgesics*) work, it is necessary to understand the origin of pain. When you are injured, by a paper cut for example, the body begins both to protect and to heal the wound. A natural component of this healing process is inflammation. The five signs of inflammation are pain, redness, immobility, swelling, and heat. Simply put, pain relievers reduce or eliminate the signals sent to the brain that signal pain.

There are several types of analgesics. Aspirin, derived from a substance in willow bark, reduces inflammation and stops the pain message travelling to the brain. It is known as a non-steroidal anti-inflammatory drug (NSAID). Ibuprofen (Advil) is a synthetic NSAID that has fewer side-effects. An alternative analgesic, acetaminophen (Tylenol), is understood to act in the central nervous system by preventing the formation of a substance associated with pain perception. The most potent (and dangerous) analgesics are the opioids such as morphine. This class of drug acts by mimicking the natural endorphins in the brain; they are agonists for these neurotransmitters. Morphine-like drugs reduce pain but also increase drowsiness, cloud thinking, and change mood most commonly to a sense of euphoria.

- **Acute pain**, for the most part, results from disease, inflammation, or injury to tissues. This type of pain generally comes on suddenly, for example, after trauma or surgery, and may be accompanied by anxiety or emotional distress. The cause of acute pain can usually be diagnosed and treated, and the pain is self-limiting, that is, it is confined to a given period of time and severity. In some rare instances, it can become chronic.
- **Chronic pain** is widely believed to represent disease itself. It can be made much worse by environmental and psychological factors. Chronic pain persists over a longer period of time than acute pain and is resistant to most medical treatments. It can—and often does—cause severe problems for patients. . . .

How Is Pain Diagnosed? There is no way to tell how much pain a person has. No test can measure the intensity of pain, no imaging device can show pain, and no instrument can locate pain precisely. Sometimes, as in the case of headaches, physicians find that the best aid to diagnosis is the patient's own description of the type, duration, and location of pain. Defining pain as sharp or dull, constant or intermittent, burning or aching may give the best clues to the cause of pain. These descriptions are part of what is called the pain history, taken by the physician during the preliminary examination of a patient with pain.

Physicians, however, do have a number of technologies they use to find the cause of pain. Primarily these include:

- *Electrodiagnostic* procedures include *electromyography (EMG), nerve conduction studies*, and *evoked potential (EP)* studies. . . .
- Imaging, especially *magnetic resonance imaging* or *MRI*, provides physicians with pictures of the body's structures and tissues. MRI uses magnetic fields and radio waves to differentiate between healthy and diseased tissue.
- In a *neurological examination* the physician tests movement, reflexes, sensation, balance, and coordination.
- *X-rays* produce pictures of the body's structures, such as bones and joints. . . .

2. Detecting and Measuring Pain

From 2012 through 2014 two teams of neuroscientists achieved breakthroughs in imaging pain. In one experiment, for instance, the researchers applied a (mildly) painful heat stimulus to the left forearm of subjects while those subjects were in the fMRI scanner. By varying the intensity of the heat (and correlating it with self-reported pain sensation by subjects), the research team identified a neural signature of pain. The other experiment described structural differences that distinguished individuals suffering lower back pain from healthy controls with 76% accuracy. While cautioning that the generalizability of the findings needed to be further studied, the authors concluded that "brain-based signatures could be useful in confirming pain in situations in which patients are unable to communicate pain effectively or when self-reports are otherwise suspect." The following excerpt provides an update on this line of experiments and reasoning. *See* Tor D. Wager et al., *An fMRI-Based Neurologic Signature of Physical Pain*, 368 New Eng. J. Med. 1388, 1396 (2013); Hoameng Ung et al., *Multivariate Classification of Structural MRI Data Detects Chronic Low Back Pain*, 24 Cerebral Cortex 1037 (2014).

Maite M. van der Miesen, Martin A. Lindquist & Tor D. Wager

Neuroimaging-based Biomarkers for Pain: State of the Field and Current Directions

4 Pain Rep. e751 (2019)

Accordingly, a number of recent funding initiatives are directed at development of biomarkers for pain. Some, like the U.S. National Institutes of Health's "Helping to End Addiction LongTerm" (HEAL) initiative, take a multipronged approach. Some HEAL funding programs focus on preclinical pain markers. Others, like the Acute to Chronic Pain Signatures program, focus on human prognostic biomarkers. . . .

. . . Hundreds of studies have contributed to our understanding of the brain bases of pain, but we restrict our review to studies that develop brain models suitable for diagnosing the presence of pain, predict its intensity in individual people, or predict treatment outcomes. In addition, the studies we review attempt to validate their predictions on new, out-of-sample individuals from the same or different populations. These models generally use multiple brain features to form a prediction of pain incidence or intensity, based on the idea that pain encoding is distributed across multiple brain systems.

... [W]e restrict the scope of the review to ... [structural magnetic resonance imaging] (sMRI) and functional MRI (fMRI) and electroencephalography (EEG). . . . These methods are complementary, and each has its unique strengths and use cases. Structural MRI relies on relatively standardized acquisition methods available at virtually every major hospital and can identify stable changes that confer risk of chronic pain or result from pain-inducing injuries. Functional MRI can track within-person fluctuations in pain over time, yielding insights into the brain systems most closely associated with the experience of pain itself or associated behaviors. Electroencephalography is the most cost-effective measure of the 3 and can yield millisecond-level information about the timing of pain-related signals. . . . Both [resting state fMRI (rs-fMRI)] and EEG can yield measures of stable person-level characteristics. . . .

[The authors next discuss types of biomarkers, criteria for evaluating biomarkers, and the use of multivariate pattern analysis, coupled with machine learning analysis.—EDS.]

3. PAIN BIOMARKERS: STATE OF THE FIELD . . .

[The authors next discuss the parameters of the literature search that they employed, which resulted in 47 peer-reviewed publications. They also observe that machine learning techniques are used progressively more often to identify brain signatures of pain.—EDS.]

3.1. Functional Magnetic Resonance Imaging

3.1.1. Evoked Pain

... [D]ecoding in fMRI was [developed] in vision research, [and in] 2010 . . . the first article was published predicting pain. [Researchers] demonstrated the feasibility of predicting subjective heat pain intensity from whole-brain fMRI . . . a relatively rare example of the use of machine learning. . . . A second study predicted pain intensities. . . . Further developments . . . used a . . . a form of prospective validation. They first measured fMRI activity during painful and nonpainful thermal stimulation and trained [a machine learning algorithm] that was used to classify pain . . . with accuracy of 86.6%. . . . The . . . model included . . . regions known to receive nociceptive input—chiefly the mid-insula, anterior cingulate cortex, and somatosensory cortex—which is an important neuroanatomical validation. . . .

. . . [Another study combined a] machine learning with a dynamic nonlinear psychophysical model . . . [that] captured the transformation of noxious input into pain. . . . This study illustrates the advantages of combining machine learning and dynamic psychophysical models.

. . . [Most previous] studies . . . focused on within-person prediction—which means that the brain model differed across individuals—without attempting to develop a biomarker tracking pain intensity that could be applied to new individuals. . . . In 2013, [researchers] developed a . . . model that predicted pain intensity across individuals. . . . The model . . . showed high sensitivity and specificity (94% or more) for discriminating pain from nonpainful warmth, pain anticipation, and pain recall when applied to new individuals. It also discriminated pain from the "social pain" induced by viewing stimuli related to romantic rejection, which had previously been found to activate many "pain-processing" areas, including the insula, anterior cingulate cortex, and secondary somatosensory cortex. Finally, the [model] response was suppressed by [an] opiate . . . but unaffected by a placebo manipulation . . . showing differential responses to pharmacological and psychological interventions.

A later modeling effort [captured] additional variability related to psychological influences and decision-making processes. . . . This model was positively associated with pain in 98% of the participants and mediated influences of expectancy cues and perceived control. . . .

Further studies have [tested] the specificity of [pain models] across different conditions, showing no responses to aversive pictures, observations of others in pain, and pain anticipation. Studies have also shown generalization to multiple types of evoked pain, including thermal, mechanical, laser, electrical, and visceral (rectal distension). The [pain brain signature model] . . . shows moderately high test–retest reliability, comparable with, but somewhat lower than the reliability for self-reported pain. . . .

3.1.2. Chronic Pain

A recurring theme in chronic pain research is the idea that patients exhibit long-term brain reorganization that makes them react differently to evoked pain. Several early studies used evoked responses to predict whether individuals experienced chronic pain. For example, [one study] found that patients with chronic low back pain . . . showed reduced responses to painful stimulus offset in the nucleus accumbens. . . . [Another study] used fMRI during evoked electrical stimulation on the back to classify patients with [chronic low back pain] vs healthy controls with 92.3% accuracy. . . .

. . . Using fMRI data . . . , researchers were able to distinguish between patients with fibromyalgia and healthy controls with 82% accuracy. Increased visual sensitivity in patients was also correlated with their pain intensity. . . . [Another] study, [discriminated] patients with fibromyalgia . . . from matched controls with 93% cross-validated accuracy.

3.2. Evaluation

. . . fMRI has been used primarily for diagnostic purposes, and a priority for the future is the development of prognostic and predictive biomarkers. In addition, models have focused on pain but neglected other outcomes, including functionality, resistance to distraction under pain, and other pain-relevant outcomes.

Most models show good classification performance, and some have been validated . . . Some models predicting evoked pain, . . . have been extensively validated across samples, but evoked pain models predicting clinical pain have not been validated in independent samples. This is a priority for future work. In terms of interpretability, activation of the insula, anterior cingulate, secondary somatosensory cortex, and thalamus are recurring themes, demonstrating some convergence. However, whether the models produce consistent or divergent brain patterns is difficult to ascertain, and more direct model comparisons are needed. In summary, a range of evoked pain models exist, and the most promising models should be tested further, particularly for utility across clinical pain conditions. . . .

[The authors then survey biomarkers for pain using the techniques of resting-state functional magnetic resonance imaging, structural magnetic resonance imaging, electroencephalography, and multimodal neuroimaging. —EDS.]

4. DISCUSSION

In this review, we described a variety of pain-predictive models using fMRI, rs-fMRI, sMRI, and EEG. . . . Although many of these models show great promise, further steps need to be taken to improve biomarkers. High-accuracy models must be tested across research groups. . . . Cross-validation is only a partial solution because it is still possible to inadvertently overfit models and capitalize on chance. Overfitting is a substantial problem in decoding models. There are many possible steps and manipulations in the analysis pipeline, which could result in [unreliable results]. Some of the discussed results might also be guilty of this. There are very few tests of specificity or attempts to train models with high specificity and generalizability. Developing prognostic and predictive biomarkers in particular will also require larger samples.

Increasing sample size and testing sensitivity and specificity across disorders will be greatly facilitated by data-sharing initiatives. . . . Open data platforms will also aid in the problem of overfitting, making reproducibility, validation, and generalization easier to investigate. In addition, it is important to share models, so that their performance can be evaluated across contexts and samples. . . .

Furthermore, it is important to actively assess the convergent validity of biomarkers. Models are often not directly comparable, and it is unclear how results and models from different studies fit together, and how they form a coherent, cumulative understanding. The gap between animal and human studies is large (and growing), and models should increasingly use results and concepts from animal neuroscience to constrain and corroborate human predictive models.

The field will likely develop many more biomarkers the coming years. . . . Important points to evaluate in new studies could include (1) sample size; (2) use of validated or standardized methodology; (3) adequate analysis and correction for potential movement and clinical confounds; (4) transparent and shareable models; (5) neuroscientific explanation and external validation; (6) independent cohort(s) for validation and/or generalization; and (7) data/tool open availability at the time of publication, among others. Attention to these criteria will help the field to curate and promote state-of-the-art approaches and move the field towards biomarkers useful both in understanding the neural bases of pain and in translational applications.

NOTES AND QUESTIONS

1. In 2005, while on the job, Carl Koch was badly burned on his face, ear, and arm by some-300-degree molten tar at an asphalt plant. A year later he reported that he was still in pain, and sued his former employer, Western Emulsions. Joy Hirsch, a neuroscientist then at Columbia University, brain scanned Koch and noted that actions with his affected arm yielded brain activity in areas associated with pain, while the same actions with the opposite arm did not. Sean Mackey, a neurologist at Stanford, served as an expert witness for the defense, in support of the effort to exclude the brain imaging evidence from trial. He argued that it wasn't possible to draw a strong inference about subjective pain from the activity Hirsch recorded. The judge ultimately decided to admit the evidence, which prompted settlement for $800,000, more than ten times what the defense had originally offered. As of 2015, Hirsch (then at Yale) was conducting two to three

pain-related scans per month, many of them relating to lawsuits. Sara Reardon, *The Painful Truth*, 518 Nature 474 (2015). For more on this story and on the use of brain imaging for cases concerning back pain, see Kevin Davis, *Personal Injury Lawyers Turn to Neuroscience to Back Claims of Chronic Pain*, ABA J. (Mar. 1, 2016). What does this case suggest to you about the potential of brain imaging to affect pain-based litigation?

2. As law professor Amanda Pustilnik has noted, American law tends to incorporate concepts of pain that are appropriate to acute but not chronic pain (even though some jurisdictions have begun to treat them differently). Amanda C. Pustilnik, *Legal Evidence of Subjective States: A Brain-Based Model of Chronic Pain Increases Accuracy and Fairness in Law*, 25 Harv. Rev. Psychiatry 279 (2017). Would it be a good idea for courts or legislators to develop explicitly distinct legal definitions, with correspondingly different standards of proof and implications for damages/benefits, for acute and chronic pain? Why or why not? Does it matter whether or not legal definitions mirror neuroscientific definitions?

3. Consider the extent to which pain neuroimaging evidence might be admissible for some purposes, but not others. Would you recommend variable admissibility depending on whether the evidence was offered for purposes of: a) establishing the general biology of chronic pain; b) the cognitive and emotional effects of chronic pain; c) general debiasing of decision-maker assumptions about pain; d) proving that a claimant is in pain; or e) proving that a claimant is in a lot of pain? For an exploration of these issues, see Amanda C. Pustilnik, *Imaging Brains, Changing Minds: How Pain Neuroimaging Can Inform the Law*, 66 Ala. L. Rev. 1099 (2015).

4. How confident can the law be that neuroimaging is accurately measuring a litigant's pain? Consider this scientific critique:

> One important question challenges the use of functional neuroimaging to derive 'biomarkers' of pain perception: does the brain activity sampled by these techniques when an individual experiences pain correspond to the neuronal activity causing the emergence of the painful percept? . . . [W]e and others have expressed concern regarding the specificity for pain of the brain responses classically observed when experiencing transient pain, i.e. the so-called 'pain matrix', a label covertly implying some specificity for pain. The concern is based on the observation that largely the same functional neuroimaging responses can be elicited by non-painful stimuli, provided that they are salient enough. More recently it was also shown that a virtually identical 'pain matrix' response can be observed in patients with congenital insensitivity to pain, thus providing further evidence that these brain responses are largely non-specific for pain. (This statement does not imply that neural activities specific for pain do not exist. Instead, it implies that the neural activities captured by current EEG or functional MRI techniques, which reflect synchronous activity within large populations of neurons, are—at the very least—largely unspecific for pain.) To escape from these controversies, many researchers now refrain from using the term 'pain matrix', and opt instead for terms like 'pain network', 'pain signature' or 'neural circuits'. Such labels are equally suggestive of the idea that the brain responses that are being measured reflect neural activity somehow unique for pain. To elaborate on only one of these examples, the term 'signature' denotes a distinctive pattern, product or characteristic by which something can be unequivocally identified. . . . [W]e argue that the attempts to falsify the hypothesis that the brain responses being measured are specific for pain using appropriate

control stimuli have been insufficient, and the liberal use of terms implying specificity has biased the interpretation of several pain neuroimaging results. . . .

André Mouraux & Gian Domenico Iannetti, *The Search for Pain Biomarkers in the Human Brain*, 141 Brain 3290, 3291 (2018).

C. EMOTIONAL HARM AND MENTAL INJURY

In insurance, tort, and criminal law, courts typically distinguish between bodily and non-bodily injury for purposes of liability and culpability. In the cases and commentary that follow, these distinctions are identified and at times challenged. Following the cases are commentaries from legal scholars describing the status of mind-body dualism in neuroscience and critiquing law's reliance on that dualism.

1. Distinguishing "Bodily" and "Mental" Injuries

Garrison v. Bickford

377 S.W.3d 659 (Tenn. 2012)

CLARK, C.J. On June 9, 2006, a car driven by Andy Bickford struck and killed eighteen-year-old Michael Garrison, who was riding a minibike on a road near his home. Garrison's parents, Jerry and Martha Garrison, and younger brother, Daniel Garrison, heard, but did not see, the collision. Jerry and Daniel Garrison, the first people to arrive at the scene, observed the deceased's injuries. Mr. Garrison testified that the deceased was "barely breathing [and] blood [was] flowing everywhere." Mr. Garrison waited with his critically injured son more than an hour for an ambulance to arrive. Mrs. Garrison testified that when she arrived at the scene a crowd had already gathered and she "was screaming for [Michael], to tell him I was there. I just was calling to him the whole time . . . telling him that I was there and to hang on." The young man was airlifted to a hospital in Chattanooga where he died from his injuries.

The Garrisons filed claims for wrongful death and negligent infliction of emotional distress against Andy Bickford and the owner of the car, Rita Bickford. . . . According to the complaint, the Garrisons, upon hearing the collision, went to render aid when they saw the deceased's "mangled body" face down in a ditch beside the road. As a result of what they saw, the Garrisons "suffered grief, fright, shock, depression, loss of sleep and other problems" for which they sought compensatory damages.

In addition to filing suit against the Bickfords, the Garrisons served a copy of the complaint upon their own insurance company, State Farm Mutual Automobile Insurance Company ("State Farm"), pursuant to the uninsured motorist provisions of their policy. The Garrisons' policy with State Farm covered "damages for bodily injury an insured is legally entitled to collect from the owner or driver of an uninsured motor vehicle." The policy defined "bodily injury" as "bodily injury to a person and sickness, disease, or death that results from it." The uninsured motorist coverage of the policy included a $100,000 limit for "Each Person" and a $300,000 limit for "Each Accident."

As the litigation progressed, the Garrisons settled their wrongful death claim against Andy Bickford for $25,000, plus $25,000 for the negligent infliction of emotional distress claim. The Garrisons . . . settled their wrongful death claim with State Farm for $75,000, which State Farm asserted was the amount remaining under the "Each Person" limit of the policy. However, State Farm refused to pay damages for the Garrisons' emotional distress claim on the basis that emotional harm was not a "bodily injury" as defined in the policy. . . .

. . . In ruling in favor of coverage, the trial court found that the "bodily injury" provision of the uninsured motorist statute, Tennessee Code Annotated section 56-7-1201, was broader than the definition of "bodily injury" contained in the policy. Accordingly, the trial court found that the policy provided, by operation of law, coverage for the Garrisons' emotional distress claim. . . . [State Farm successfully appealed.]

We granted the Garrisons' application for permission to appeal to determine whether "bodily injury" as defined in the policy includes mental injuries standing alone. For the reasons explained below, we conclude that it does not.

Our analysis of this case is guided by several well-established principles. First, Tennessee law is clear that questions regarding the extent of insurance coverage present issues of law involving the interpretation of contractual language. . . . Equally well-established is the principle that "[i]nsurance policies are, at their core, contracts." As such, courts interpret insurance policies using the same tenets that guide the construction of any other contract. Thus, the terms of an insurance policy "'should be given their plain and ordinary meaning, for the primary rule of contract interpretation is to ascertain and give effect to the intent of the parties.'" . . . In addition, contracts of insurance are strictly construed in favor of the insured, and if the disputed provision is susceptible to more than one plausible meaning, the meaning favorable to the insured controls. . . .

. . . [T]he crux of this appeal is whether, as a matter of insurance and contract law, the Garrisons' mental injuries constitute "bodily injury" under the policy. . . .

The legislature has established the minimum standard of protection acceptable for uninsured motorist coverage in Tennessee as follows:

> Every automobile liability insurance policy delivered, issued for delivery or renewed in this state, covering liability arising out of the ownership, maintenance, or use of any motor vehicle designed for use primarily on public roads and registered or principally garaged in this state, shall include uninsured motorist coverage, subject to provisions filed with and approved by the commissioner, for the protection of persons insured under the policy who are legally entitled to recover compensatory damages from owners or operators of uninsured motor vehicles *because of bodily injury, sickness or disease, including death, resulting from injury, sickness or disease.*

. . . The statutory language at the core of this case is "bodily injury, sickness or disease, including death." The policy issued to the Garrisons by State Farm provides coverage for "bodily injury to a person and sickness, disease, or death that results from it." . . . State Farm asserts that the words "injury, sickness or disease" as used in section 56-7-1201(a) are restricted by the word "bodily," and that the plain meaning of "bodily injury" excludes an emotional or mental injury in both the statute and the policy. . . . The Garrisons respond that if the legislature had intended to exclude mental injury claims from the reach of uninsured motorist coverage, it would have omitted "sickness or disease" from section 56-7-1201(a). . . .

Although the meaning of "bodily injury" for purposes of uninsured motorist coverage is an issue of first impression in Tennessee, there has been no shortage

416 Chapter 11. Pain and Distress

of litigation in other jurisdictions addressing this issue. The majority of courts facing the question in various contexts have concluded that "bodily injury" does not include mental or emotional harm absent a physical injury to the insured. . . . While some cases . . . find no coverage on the basis that the term "bodily" modifies or restricts the words that follow, namely "sickness or disease", other cases place no significance on which words "bodily" modifies because "[n]either sickness nor disease arguably includes emotional distress." . . .

Still other cases focus on typical dictionary definitions to find the meaning of "bodily injury." For instance, in concluding that "the common meaning of the phrase 'bodily harm, sickness or disease' as used to define 'bodily injury' is not ambiguous," one court has observed that "[i]n dictionary definitions, 'bodily' is equated with 'physical' . . . as contrasted with 'mental.'" Thus, "'bodily injury' . . . refers to physical conditions of the body and excludes mental suffering or emotional distress." Moreover, "in insurance law 'bodily injury' is considered to be a narrower concept than 'personal injury' which covers mental or emotional injury."

As this discussion illustrates, most courts "conclusively exclud[e] emotional distress from the insurance definition [of] 'bodily injury, sickness or disease.'" While these cases represent the clear majority view, other cases considering the issue have been decided in favor of coverage. . . . See . . . *Pekin Ins. Co. v. Hugh*, 501 N.W.2d 508, 512 (Iowa 1993) (holding that emotional distress arising from "a bystander claim is a bodily injury for purposes of insurance coverage" because "[a]ny attempt to distinguish between 'physical' and 'psychological' injuries just clouds the issue").

After considering the approaches of other jurisdictions, we are persuaded that the phrase "bodily injury," as used in both section 56-7-1201(a) and the policy before us, does not include damages for a mental or emotional injury by itself. The commonly understood meaning of the words "bodily injury to a person and sickness, disease, or death that results from it" as used in the policy, or the words "bodily injury, sickness or disease, including death" as used in the statute, are unambiguous. These words, when used to define "bodily injury," refer to physical, not emotional, conditions of the body. . . .

The majority view, which we adopt, is consistent with older, analogous Tennessee cases. . . . [T]he Court of Appeals concluded that "bodily injury," defined in a commercial general liability policy as "bodily injury, sickness or disease," did not include "embarrassment, humiliation, mental anguish, [and] emotional pain and suffering." . . .

The result we have reached in this case is also consistent with the nature of the tort of negligent infliction of emotional distress itself. At one time, some form of physical harm was required to successfully pursue such a claim. That is no longer the case, however, as emotional harm alone forms the basis of the tort, apart from a claim for personal injury. Indeed, it is now generally accepted that "[e]motional harm is distinct from bodily harm and means harm to a person's emotional tranquility." See Restatement (Third) of Torts §4 cmt. a (2010). On the other hand, physical or bodily harm "means the physical impairment of the human body," namely, "physical injury, illness, disease, impairment of bodily function, and death." *Id.* at §4. This definition "is meant to preserve the ordinary distinction between bodily harm and emotional harm." *Id.* at cmt. b. . . . Our decision today is in accord with these established principles. A contrary decision would blur the distinction between physical and mental injuries and merely serve to confuse matters.

In sum, a bystander claim for negligent infliction of emotional distress, such as that asserted by the Garrisons, is not a claim for bodily harm. Accordingly, we conclude that in the context of purely emotional injuries, the phrase "bodily injury," as defined in the policy before us, is unambiguous. Its ordinary meaning connotes a physical injury. Thus, we hold that, as applied to this case, "bodily injury" does not include damages for emotional harm alone. We further conclude that the definition of "bodily injury" in the policy does not conflict with the uninsured motorist statute, section 56-7-1201(a). Consequently, we reject the Garrisons' argument that the statute supersedes the policy language. [Affirmed.]

Allen v. Bloomfield Hills Sch. Dist.
760 N.W.2d 811 (Mich. Ct. App. 2008)

MARKEY, J. In this suit alleging negligent operation of a governmentally owned and operated school bus, plaintiffs, Charles and Lisa Allen, appeal by right the trial court's order granting defendant's motion for summary disposition . . . based on governmental immunity because Charles had not suffered a "bodily injury." We agree with the trial court that a plaintiff seeking to avoid governmental immunity from tort liability through the motor vehicle exception,. . . must establish a "bodily injury." Here, however, plaintiffs presented objective medical evidence that Charles Allen suffered a brain injury, specifically post traumatic stress disorder as a result of the accident. If believed, we conclude that this evidence would establish a "bodily injury" . . .; consequently, the trial court erred in granting defendants summary disposition on this issue. Therefore, we reverse.

Plaintiff Charles Allen (Allen) was operating a train . . . when he observed a Bloomfield Hills School District (the district) school bus enter the railroad-grade crossing . . . and attempt to proceed across the grade by maneuvering around the lowered gate. The train, which was traveling at a speed of approximately 65 miles an hour, was unable to stop and collided with the school bus. After stopping the train and running approximately one-half mile back to the accident scene, Allen was informed that there were no children on the bus at the time of the accident, but that the bus driver was severely injured. Allen was subsequently diagnosed with post traumatic stress disorder (PTSD) stemming from the accident. Allen and his wife filed this suit for recovery of noneconomic and excess economic damages alleging Allen had suffered a serious impairment of body function. But the trial court concluded that Allen did not suffer a "bodily injury" within the meaning of the motor vehicle exception to governmental immunity and granted defendant summary disposition. . . .

A governmental agency is generally immune from tort liability arising out of the exercise or discharge of its governmental functions. This would include a public school district's operation of a bus system. But the broad immunity afforded by the statute is limited by several narrowly drawn exceptions. One of these exceptions, at issue here, is that for motor vehicles: "Governmental agencies shall be liable for bodily injury and property damage resulting from the negligent operation by any officer, agent, or employee of the governmental agency, of a motor vehicle of which the governmental agency is owner. . . ."

. . . Because the statute does not define the term "bodily injury," we resort to dictionary definitions and accord the term its plain and ordinary meaning. Random

House Webster's College Dictionary (2001) defines "bodily" as "of or pertaining to the body" and "corporeal or material, as contrasted with spiritual or mental." It defines "injury" as "harm or damage done or sustained, esp. bodily harm." Black's Law Dictionary (7th ed.), p. 789, also defines "bodily injury" as "[p]hysical damage to a person's body." Our Supreme Court in *Wesche* . . . applied a similar analysis to the words "bodily injury." . . . The Court held that " 'bodily injury' simply means a physical or corporeal injury to the body." Consequently, the Court held that "because loss of consortium is a nonphysical injury, it does not fall within the categories of damage for which the motor-vehicle exception waives immunity."

Plaintiff argues that he suffered a "bodily injury" because the accident caused physical damage to his body as evidenced by a positron emission tomography (PET) scan of his brain. He relies on the affidavit of Dr. Joseph C. Wu, who reviewed plaintiff's PET scan and opined that it depicted "decreases in frontal and subcortical activity consistent with depression and post traumatic stress disorder." Dr. Wu further opined that "the abnormalities in Mr. Allen's brain as depicted on the September 8, 2006, PET scan are quite pronounced and are clearly different in brain pattern from any of the normal controls. They are also consistent with an injury to Mr. Allen's brain." Dr. Wu related the abnormalities to the January 13, 2004, accident. Plaintiff also relies on the report of Dr. Gerald A. Shiener, who opined that PTSD "causes significant changes in brain chemistry, brain function, and brain structure."

The brain is a part of the human body, so "harm or damage done or sustained" is injury to the brain and within the common meaning of "bodily injury" in MCL 691.1405, as elucidated in *Wesche*. The question on appeal then becomes, for purposes of reviewing the trial court's grant of summary disposition to defendant, whether plaintiff produced sufficient evidence to create a material question of fact that he suffered a "bodily injury" as so defined. In doing so, we must still adhere to the court rules and follow the law. We must review any evidence of a claimed "bodily injury" in a light most favorable to the nonmoving party. Also, we must conduct our review with common sense, and with cognizance of modern medical science and the human body. Here, plaintiff presented objective medical evidence that a mental or emotional trauma can indeed result in physical changes to the brain.

Although the brain is the organ responsible for our thoughts and emotions, it is also the organ that controls all our physical functions. The fact that it serves more than one function hardly detracts from the fact that it is one of our major organs. It can be injured. It can be injured directly and indirectly. It can be injured by direct and indirect trauma. What matters for a legal analysis is the existence of a manifest, objectively measured injury to the brain. Consequently, to survive a motion for summary disposition, we must determine whether plaintiff produced sufficient evidence that Allen suffered from an objectively manifested physical injury to his brain.

Plaintiff Allen underwent a PET scan of his brain. When Dr. Wu reviewed plaintiff's PET scan, he concluded that it demonstrated "decreases in frontal and subcortical activity consistent with depression and post traumatic stress disorder" and that "the abnormalities in . . . Allen's brain as depicted on the . . . PET scan are quite pronounced and are clearly different in brain pattern from any of the normal controls. They are also consistent with an injury to Mr. Allen's brain." (Emphasis added.) Plaintiff's other expert doctor, Dr. Shiener, essentially corroborated Dr. Wu's conclusion and indicated that PTSD "causes significant changes in brain chemistry, brain function and brain structure. The brain becomes 'rewired' to overrespond to circumstances that are similar to the traumatic experience." So, two separate medical doctors provided evidence that Allen suffered an injury to his brain.

We must view this evidence in the light most favorable to the nonmoving party to assess whether reasonable minds could not differ. It is evident that with this proffered evidence reasonable minds could most certainly differ about whether plaintiff suffered a "bodily injury." We therefore conclude that this evidence is adequate, at least, to preclude summary disposition because there exists a genuine issue of material fact. In the instant case, Dr. Wu's affidavit testimony along with Dr. Shiener's report was sufficient to create a genuine issue of material fact regarding whether plaintiff suffered a "bodily injury."

We find unpersuasive the dissent's reliance on the rationale of Bobian v. CSA Czech Airlines. . . that because all thoughts and emotions are connected to brain activity, accepting plaintiff's injury as a "bodily injury" would require completely breaking down the barrier between emotional and physical harms. First of all, the *Bobian* court did not interpret our Michigan statute; it analyzed the term "bodily injury" with respect to air carrier liability under Article 17 of the Warsaw Convention. Moreover, lower federal court decisions are not binding precedent in this Court. But just as important, we find the analysis in *Bobian* profoundly superficial and contrived.

The Legislature has not defined the words "bodily injury" as used in MCL 691.1405. That is why this Court and our Supreme Court in *Wesche* looked to dictionary definitions for guidance in ascertaining their plain and ordinary meanings. And, unless one reads into both the ruling in *Wesche* and the term "bodily injury" in the statute the requirement that an injury ensue solely from direct trauma, the dissent significantly alters the definition of "bodily injury" in a manner inconsistent with both the plain wording of the statute and our Supreme Court's interpretation of that term in *Wesche*.

We also note that the dissent appears to concede that indeed plaintiff has an objectively verified brain injury. Its problem seems to be that plaintiff suffered no direct blow to the head, as the cause of the brain injury. Ironically, just a few years ago, the courts in this state had a difficult time understanding and accepting what is now also a universally recognized medical phenomenon and one suffered by thousands of our soldiers: closed head injuries. As we on the bench struggled with how long or whether one had to be rendered unconscious or what tests were sufficient to demonstrate the nature and severity of a closed head injury—including whether MRIs were legally cognizable evidence—the medical community was already a long way down the road in developing treatments and strategies for coping with these mere "mental, emotional," or "psychiatric" injuries. But as a matter of medicine and law, there should be no difference medically or legally between an objectively demonstrated brain injury, whether the medical diagnosis is a closed head injury, PTSD, Alzheimer's, brain tumor, epilepsy, etc. A brain injury is a "bodily injury." If there were adequate evidence of a brain injury to meet the requisite evidentiary standards, i.e., objective medical proof of the injury, summary disposition was improper.

In sum, plaintiff here presented sufficient objective medical evidence to raise a material question of fact regarding whether he suffered a brain injury from the accident and whether such brain injury is an injury to the body. Consequently, the trial court erred by granting defendants summary disposition on this issue.

We reverse and remand to the trial court for further proceedings consistent with this opinion.

HOEKSTRA, J. (concurring in part and dissenting in part). I agree with the majority's conclusion that a plaintiff seeking to avoid governmental immunity and recover third-party no-fault damages from a governmental agency must establish a "bodily injury." . . . I disagree that post traumatic stress disorder (PTSD) can be such an injury. . . .

Plaintiffs argue that plaintiff Charles Allen suffered a "bodily injury" because the accident caused physical damage to his body, as evidenced by a positron emission tomography (PET) scan of his brain. In making this argument, plaintiffs rely on the affidavit of Joseph Wu, M.D., who reviewed Allen's PET scan and opined that it depicted "decreases in frontal and subcortical activity consistent with depression and post traumatic stress disorder." Wu further opined that "the abnormalities in . . . Allen's brain as depicted on the . . . PET scan are quite pronounced and are clearly different in brain pattern from any of the normal controls. They are also consistent with an injury to Mr. Allen's brain." Wu related the abnormalities to the train-bus accident. Plaintiffs also rely on the report of Gerald Shiener, M.D., who opined that PTSD "causes significant changes in brain chemistry, brain function, and brain structure." Allen's PTSD is alleged to have been caused by the emotional upset resulting from his belief, as the accident was occurring, that his operation of the train was "about to maim or kill numerous school children," rather than a physical impact on his body during the collision.

In my opinion, plaintiffs' evidence concerning Allen's brain abnormalities does not satisfy the definition of "bodily injury" discussed above. Rather, plaintiffs' evidence demonstrates, at most, mental or psychiatric abnormalities or changes. Although not binding on this Court, I find persuasive the analysis in Bobian . . . , regarding whether PTSD constitutes a "bodily injury" compensable under Article 17 of the Warsaw Convention. There, in addressing the plaintiffs' claim that PTSD constitutes a bodily injury by virtue of the physical effects of PTSD on the brain, the court stated, "Given that all human thoughts and emotions are in some fashion connected to brain activity, and therefore at some level 'physical,' to accept Plaintiffs' argument would be to break down entirely the barrier between emotional and physical harms. . . ." Following this reasoning, any change to Allen's brain functions resulting from the accident is properly characterized as a mental, emotional, or psychiatric injury rather than a bodily injury. Because the term "bodily injury" in MCL 691.1405 does not encompass these types of changes, defendant was immune from suit, including Allen's claim for economic damages and plaintiff Lisa Allen's claim for loss of consortium. As such, I would hold the trial court properly granted summary disposition for defendant.

Francis X. Shen

Sentencing Enhancement and the Crime Victim's Brain
46 Loy. U. Chi. L.J. 405, 417-20 (2014)

For centuries, thinkers have debated the relationship between mind and body, a relationship known in academic circles as the "mind-body" problem. The theory that "mental" substance is something wholly different from "bodily" substance is known as "substance dualism," because it posits that there are dual types of substances in the universe. The French mathematician and philosopher René Descartes famously made the case for substance dualism, also known as "Cartesian dualism." Descartes's theory was held in high regard for many years.

Today, however, this is no longer the case. . . . Consider these snippets:

- "The modern science of mind proceeds on the assumption that the mind is simply what the brain does. . . . We scientists take the mind's physical basis for granted."—Neuroscientist Joshua Greene
- "The idea of mind as distinct in this way from the brain, composed not of ordinary matter but of some other, special kind of stuff, is dualism, and it is deservedly in disrepute today. . . . [D]ualism is to be avoided at all costs."— Philosopher Daniel Dennett
- "[T]he theory that mind and brain are separable is untenable . . ."— Neuroscientist David Redish
- "Dualistic views on human nature, often associated with Descartes, rarely gain proponents among brain scientists."—Neuroscientists Jacek Debiec & Joseph E. LeDoux
- "[M]ost neuroscientists are not terribly interested in the old mind-body debates. Most thinkers are satisfied to believe that mind is simply the brain in action . . . mind emerges as naturally from brain functions as digestion emerges from normal gastric processes."—Neuroscientist Jaak Panksepp
- "Substance dualism is no longer considered a respectable philosophical position today."—Philosopher Neil Levy50
- "[W]e must admit that dualism is dead."—Professor of Law and Biology Owen Jones

These quotations could go on for some time, but the point is clear: in the scientific community, substance dualism has been thoroughly rejected.

[But] . . . in contrast to the scholarly consensus, much of the general public retains a dualist view of the world. Scholars also continue to explore why we are intuitive dualists, why we behave like dualists, and whether this is a problem. . . .

Dov Fox & Alex Stein
Dualism and Doctrine
90 Ind. L.J. 975, 975-1010 (2015)

What kinds of harm among those that tortfeasors inflict are worthy of compensation? Which forms of self-incriminating evidence are privileged against government compulsion? What sorts of facts constitute a criminal defendant's intent? Existing doctrine pins the answer to all of these questions on whether the injury, facts, or evidence at stake are "mental" or "physical." The assumption that operations of the mind are meaningfully distinct from those of the body animates fundamental rules in our law.

A tort victim cannot recover for mental harm on its own because the law presumes that he is able to unfeel any suffering arising from his mind, in contrast to his bodily injuries over which he exercises no control. The Fifth Amendment forbids the government from forcing a suspect to reveal self-incriminating thoughts as a purportedly more egregious form of compulsion than is compelling no less incriminating evidence that comes from his body. Criminal law treats intentionality as a function of a defendant's thoughts altogether separate from the bodily movements that they drive into action. . . .

. . . [N]euroscience, psychology, and psychiatry . . . expose dualism as empirically flawed and conceptually bankrupt. . . . the fiction of dualism distorts the law and . . . the most plausible reasons for dualism's persistence cannot save it. . . .

Contemporary neuroscience, psychology, and psychiatry make plain that our mental and physical lives interact with each other (and our environment). A person cannot be reduced to his mind or separated from his body. He is, inescapably, both at once. We have called on courts and legislatures to expel dualism from our doctrine in favor of this integrated vision of the ways in which people think and act. It is this vision that must guide the formation of our legal policies and rules. . . .

NOTES AND QUESTIONS

1. The Restatement (Third) of Torts: Liability for Physical and Emotional Harm (2005) (referenced in the *Garrison* case above) draws a distinction, even in its title, between physical and emotional harm. Section 4, Physical Harm, provides that:

   "Physical harm" means the physical impairment of the human body ("bodily harm") [or harms to real or tangible personal property]. Bodily harm included physical injury, illness, diseases, impairment of bodily function, and death.

   Comment b to Section 4 adds:

   Bodily harm and emotional harm. The definition of bodily harm is meant to preserve the ordinary distinction between bodily harm and emotional harm. Accordingly, if the defendant's negligent conduct (for example, negligent driving) frightens the plaintiff (for example, a pedestrian crossing the street), the harm to the plaintiffs nerve centers caused by this fear does not constitute bodily harm. This distinction is not precise and may be difficult to make in certain cases, but the more restrictive rules for recovery for emotional harm . . . require that such determinations be made. The essential difference is that bodily harm usually provides objective evidence of its existence and extent while the existence and severity of emotional harm is usually dependent upon the report of the person suffering it or symptoms that are capable of manipulation or multiple explanations. Whether a specific injury constitutes bodily harm and therefore supports a claim for liability under . . . this Restatement is a question of law for the court to decide.

   Section 45, Emotional Harm, provides that:

   "Emotional harm" means impairment or injury to a person's emotional tranquility.

   And comment a to Section 45, which also has language echoing comment b of Section 4, adds:

   Most physical harm, with the exception of disease, results from traumatic impact with the human body, while emotional harm can occur without such trauma, indeed without any event that resembles a physical-harm tort.

   Do you think that the objective-versus-subjective evidence distinction is alone sufficient to justify the distinction the Restatement draws between physical and emotional harm? What sort of changes to the Restatement, if any, do you think would be advisable if neuroscience were able to provide objective evidence of pain?

2. Assume for the moment that you are counsel to an insurance company that seeks to amend its statement of coverage to clarify coverage for "physical" and "emotional" injuries. What approaches and what language might you recommend? What, if anything, would you do differently from the Restatement (Third) of Torts?

3. These two cases represent only some of the many ways in which the distinction between mental and physical injury can be legally relevant. In what other contexts might the distinction arise? In a 2009 statement supporting mental health parity legislation, former Representative Patrick Kennedy (D-RI) argued that insurance companies must "acknowledge that the brain is part of the body," for purposes of insurance coverage. 55 Cong. Rec. H8188 (daily ed. July 16, 2009). That is, there should be parity between how these companies treat mental illness and physical ailments. Should there be similar parity in other bodies of law?

4. Fox and Stein argue that dualism is "conceptually bankrupt" and "distorts the law." Dov Fox & Alex Stein, *Dualism and Doctrine*, 90 Ind. L.J. 975, 975 (2015). Is the law's embrace of dualism any more problematic than its adoption of other legal fictions? If so, what is so pernicious? If not, does this limit the relevance of neuroscience in legal approaches to pain?

5. In criminal sentencing, the criminal law implicitly makes an assumption about the relative harms of physical versus mental pain. In general, sentencing schemes tend to punish offenders who cause great "bodily" harm more harshly than those who cause great "mental" harm. Is this distinction between physical and mental pain more or less acceptable because it is being made in the context of criminal sentencing? For a further discussion of these questions, see Francis X. Shen, *Sentencing Enhancement and the Crime Victim's Brain*, 46 Loy. U. Chi. L.J. 405, 407 (2014) (arguing that to "the extent that neuroscience better illuminates—and eventually can measure . . . [mental harm]—it can contribute to more precise, just, and evidence-based enhancements for harms to others.")

6. Some courts suggest that the definition of bodily injury is intuitive—a matter of common sense, and clear on its face to the lay juror. One court has asserted, "Clearly the term 'bodily injury' is not a phrase which requires an elaborate explanation in order to be understood." *Messer v. Kemp*, 760 F.2d 1080, 1093 (11th Cir. 1985). And another writes, "We can think of no phenomenon of more common experience and understanding than the concepts of 'bodily injury' and 'physical pain.'" *Rogers v. State*, 396 N.E.2d 348, 352 (Ind. 1979). Do you agree? If you asked 100 people on the street to define or describe bodily injury, would they give you the same basic answer? See if your intuition matches up to the data by looking at Francis X. Shen, *Mind, Body, and the Criminal Law*, 97 Minn. L. Rev. 2036 (2013) (reporting on experimental studies assessing lay understanding of bodily injury in law).

7. To what extent do you think that emotional pain (such as from a breakup with lover) differs from physical pain (such as that from a broken arm)? *See* Eric Jaffe, *Why Love Literally Hurts*, Ass'n Psychol. Sci. (Jan. 30, 2013). Is it even coherent to think of these two types of pains as the same? Or is it incoherent to think of them as any different, given that both are experienced in the brain?

8. Legal scholars Jean Macchiaroli Eggen and Eric J. Laury have proposed a new model of tort law, informed by neuroscience, that includes recognizing the "neural bonds between mental and physical conditions." Do you agree with their approach, summarized below?

> In negligence law, the neuroscience model we propose would abandon the distinction between the treatment of mental and physical disabilities upon the introduction of reliable and relevant neuroscience evidence. Where the neuroscience evidence shows an organic basis in the brain for a party's mental illness, evidence satisfying the rules of admissibility would effectively transform a mental disability into a physical disability, and would allow the mental disability to be considered as one of the circumstances the jury may assess when determining breach of duty. Arguably, transforming this rule would undermine the public policy bases of the rule ignoring mental disabilities in negligence actions. Assuming those policies ever had or continue to have validity, the distinction is not justified when an organic basis for the mental disability can be demonstrated.
>
> Why not simply abandon the rule for mental disabilities altogether and treat all mental disabilities the same as physical disabilities, whether or not the mental disabilities have a demonstrable organic basis? It may well be that the rule will move in that direction as the organic bases of all mental illnesses and disabilities are eventually discovered. For the present, however, in situations in which no organic cause is demonstrable, retaining the traditional rule ignoring the mental disability is not unreasonable. At the least, in those cases the rule serves the concern for objectively verifiable claims of mental disability.

Jean Macchiaroli Eggen & Eric J. Laury, *Toward a Neuroscience Model of Tort Law: How Functional Neuroimaging Will Transform Tort Doctrine*, 13 Colum. Sci. & Tech. L. Rev. 235, 289-90 (2012). For an argument to the contrary, see Erica Rachel Goldberg, *Emotional Duties*, 47 Conn. L. Rev. 809 (2014).

9. Govind Persad notes that even if technology calls into question whether the traditional distinction between physical and emotional injuries has a basis in fact, there still might be moral reasons to treat the two differently, in tort law. However, he argues we should move beyond the debate pitting the preservationists (those who would keep the distinction) against the assimilationists (who would abolish it). We should, in his view, determine the compensability of all harms on a more nuanced case-by-case basis, with courts and juries focusing on the details of particular injuries and the characteristics of the actors involved. *See* Govind Persad, *Law, Science, and the Injured Mind*, 67 Ala. L. Rev. 1179 (2016). Do you agree with Persad's approach? What are some of the factors or circumstances that you would consider relevant in deciding whether a given emotional injury was or was not compensable in a tort action?

10. Post-Traumatic Stress Disorder (PTSD) has been both influential and controversial in a variety of legal contexts, both criminal and civil, since its recognition by the APA in the *DSM-III*. In charting the history of PTSD in law, legal scholar Deirdre Smith concludes that "[t]he line between law and medicine is not merely blurred in PTSD; it is absent." She writes that "[i]f the law decides to address problems of justice by looking to psychiatry or other branches of medicine and science for solutions, it must only do so with a full appreciation and understanding of the origins and limitations of the concepts it seeks to adopt. Absent such acknowledgement, together with a determination that

such concepts are in fact appropriate to import into law, the legal system simply delegates juridical authority to those fields." Deirdre M. Smith, *Diagnosing Liability: The Legal History of Posttraumatic Stress Disorder*, 84 Temp. L. Rev. 1, 66, 69 (2011). Do you agree with this view? To what extent should or shouldn't legal categories map onto medical ones?

2. Damages and Mitigation

If wider recovery were allowed for mental and emotional injuries, tort law would, even more than at present, need to confront the challenge of placing dollar values on such injuries. Could neuroscience aid in this valuation process? In addition, if emotional pain and distress are considered brain injuries, and if the brain is as much a part of the body as the arm or leg, should brain mitigation be required in ways that we require treatment for injuries to other parts of the body? Such questions are, at present, not yet in courts. The commentaries below speculate on possible futures of damages and mitigation in tort law.

Professor Shen considers the possibility that PTSD could be recast as a bodily injury, instead of a mental one. Professor Kolber discusses the ability of an existing drug (about which more will be said in Chapter 13, the chapter on memory) to ease emotional pain by softening the instantiation, recollection, and experience of the memory of an unpleasant event, if the drug is taken shortly after the event. In some instances, the drug may interfere with the release of stress hormones that otherwise strengthen memories. This raises the question: To what extent could a person recover emotional distress damages for distress that could have been avoided by taking a drug?

Francis X. Shen
Monetizing Memory Science: Neuroscience and the Future of PTSD Litigation
in *Memory and the Law* 325, 333-48 (Lynn Nadel & Walter Sinnott-Armstrong eds., 2013)

A plaintiff's lawyer is hired, in part, to creative search for legal avenues of recovery. And civil defense lawyers, in turn, attempt to counteract those searches and limit liability and exposure for their clients. . . .

One possible new avenue for recovery would be to open up liability that had previously been restricted solely for what the law deems *bodily* as distinct from *mental*, injuries. . . .

The potential of cognitive neuroscience to either expand or contract the PTSD personal injury litigation market rests in part . . . on (1) whether or not neuroscience information will make individuals more likely to view PTSD as a bodily injury, and (2) whether neuroscience information will affect the valuation of PTSD claims. [Behavioral experiments were conducted to test these propositions.]. . .

Taken together, the experiments take some of the wind out of the neuro sails in the PTSD civil litigation context. In terms of putting a price on PTSD damages, it seems that neuroscience evidence, so long as it is contested (as it surely will be), is not likely to persuade individuals to change their valuation strategy. The traditional factors that make for a "good case"—a sympathetic plaintiff, a deep pockets defendant, and so forth—are likely to outweigh the neuroscience evidence. Even if a PTSD biomarker were to survive scrutiny by the scientific community, it is unlikely it could survive a good cross-examination. To conduct a good cross-examination, of course, as well as to develop a strong case, will require both the plaintiff and defense bar to remain up to date on the fast-moving memory and neuroscience fields. . . .

Adam J. Kolber

Therapeutic Forgetting: The Legal and Ethical Implications of Memory Dampening

59 Vand. L. Rev. 1561, 1592-95 (2006)

3. MITIGATION OF EMOTIONAL DISTRESS DAMAGES.

Many share the intuition that the government should not limit our freedom to control something as deeply personal as our own minds and, hence, that the government should not be in the business of regulating our control over our memories. While this intuition may provide answers to many public policy questions, even if it is correct, it does not resolve all of the wide-ranging legal issues that could arise in a world with memory dampening. Even if the government allows people to make dampening decisions for themselves, the law would still need to establish background expectations about the reasonableness of decisions to dampen or to refuse to do so.

The tort doctrine of damage mitigation illustrates how expectations as to the reasonableness of dampening could seep into the law. Consider an easy case first. Suppose that a defendant negligently drives his car into the plaintiff such that the plaintiff is hospitalized with both physical and emotional damages. Suppose further that when the plaintiff enters the hospital, for whatever reason, he refuses to allow the medical staff to set his leg in a cast for a week. As a result, the plaintiff needs more medical attention prior to the setting of his leg and more physical therapy afterward. These additional costs, however, need not be compensated by the defendant. Under longstanding principles of damage mitigation, the defendant need not compensate the plaintiff for damages that could have been prevented had the plaintiff taken reasonable steps after the commission of the tort to avoid them.

A more difficult case would arise if the plaintiff failed to mitigate the emotional, rather than the physical, aspect of his injuries. Thus, suppose that the plaintiff promptly attended to his physical injuries but declined a psychiatrist's reasonable advice to dampen his memories. In such a case, the defendant could assert that, according to general principles of mitigation, the plaintiff's recovery for emotional damages should be reduced by whatever portion of those damages is attributable to the plaintiff's failure to dampen his memories.

The plaintiff might argue in response that he has a deeply-held interest in not altering his memory. In an arguably related context, however, such arguments have largely failed to persuade courts. In cases where plaintiffs have refused medical treatment on religious grounds, where, for example, a Jehovah's Witness refuses to undergo surgery to correct an injury caused by the defendant, the prevailing approach refuses to compensate the religious plaintiff for damages that would have been avoided by a reasonable person who lacked those religious beliefs. Even though the religious plaintiff has a deeply-held interest in following his religious tradition—the free exercise of which is constitutionally protected—the damage mitigation doctrine does not consider his idiosyncratic interests, deeply held as they may be. Thus, the plaintiff in our example is not likely to get much help for his argument by appealing to the mitigation doctrine in the context of plaintiffs who refuse medical care on religious grounds.

Fortunately for our hypothetical plaintiff, courts are disinclined to require plaintiffs to treat their emotional injuries. While courts have not categorically held that emotional damages need not be mitigated, most courts do not reduce plaintiffs' emotional distress damages when plaintiffs fail to adequately treat them. Only on rare occasions have courts mitigated emotional damages where plaintiffs fail to undergo psychotherapy or refuse to take recommended antidepressants. As mental health treatments become more effective, however, a plaintiff's failure to use them may appear more unreasonable, and courts may become more willing to penalize plaintiffs who fail to mitigate emotional damages.

Assuming that memory dampeners were part of mainstream medical practice, courts would be asked to decide whether and under what circumstances a plaintiff could be put to the choice of either dampening painful memories or else forgoing compensation for the pain attached to those memories that could have been dampened. Whatever the best solution may be, the issue cannot be resolved simply by saying that individuals should be free to decide whether or not to dampen memories. For even if they were free to choose, we would still have to make societal determinations (or, at least, court and jury determinations) as to the reasonableness of such decisions.

Of course, the issue of damage mitigation in the memory-dampening context is largely mooted if plaintiffs must maintain their memories in order to effectively prepare and pursue their claims. Some jurisdictions help amnesic plaintiffs by creating a presumption that they were exercising due care at the time of an accident; it is doubtful, however, that courts would apply such a presumption to a plaintiff who intentionally dampened memories. Therefore, as a practical matter, the mitigation issue might only arise if plaintiffs can dampen emotional aspects of their memories without affecting their evidentiary content. Alternatively, plaintiffs may dampen memories when those memories are not needed to prove a cause of action or when plaintiffs are able to adequately record their memories prior to dampening for purposes of future litigation. Such wrinkles demonstrate, however, that the principal roles that memory plays in the law—an evidentiary role and an affective role—may be hard to separate if some plaintiffs are effectively forced to preserve a memory's emotional pain in order to preserve its evidentiary value. . . .

3. Comparative Perspectives

The American approach to recovery for emotional harm in tort law varies from that of Britain. Law professor Betsy Grey explores these differences and raises the question: Ought the American model shift in light of neuroscientific research?

Betsy J. Grey

Neuroscience and Emotional Harm in Tort Law: Rethinking the American Approach to Free-Standing Emotional Distress Claims

in *Law and Neuroscience: Current Legal Issues* 203, 203-28 (M. Freeman ed., 2011)

American tort law traditionally distinguishes between "physical" and "emotional" harm for purposes of liability, with emotional harm treated as a second-class citizen. The customary view is that physical injury is more entitled to compensation because it is considered a more trustworthy harm and perhaps more important. The current draft of the Restatement of the Law (Third) of Torts . . . explain[s] the reasoning behind the distinction by noting that "emotional distress is less objectively verifiable than physical harm and therefore easier for an individual to feign, to exaggerate or to engage in self deception about the existence or extent of the harm." Advances in neuroscience suggest that this concern over verification may no longer be valid, and that the phenomena we call "emotional" harm has a physiological basis. Because of these early scientific advances, this may be an appropriate time to re-examine our assumptions with regard to tort recovery for emotional harm.

Emotional harm is a legal, not a scientific, concept, but one that relates closely to cognitive or mental disorders identified by the medical community. The medical field recognizes the physiological aspect of mental disorders. The Diagnostic and Statistical Manual of Mental Disorders ("DSM-IV"), the leading guide to clinical practice in psychiatry, puts it most succinctly: [In 2013, the *DSM-5* was published.]

> Although this volume is titled the Diagnostic and Statistical Manual of Mental Disorders, the term mental disorder unfortunately implies a distinction between "mental" disorders and "physical" disorders that is a reductionistic anachronism of mind/body dualism. A compelling literature documents that there is much "physical" in "mental" disorders and much "mental" in "physical" disorders. The problem raised by the term "mental" disorders has been much clearer than its solution, and unfortunately, the term persists in the title of DSM-IV because we have not found an appropriate substitute.

The DSM-IV further explains that the terms "mental disorder" and "general medical condition," used throughout the manual, are not intended to "to imply that there is any fundamental distinction between mental disorders and general medical conditions, that mental disorders are unrelated to physical or biological factors or processes, or that general medical conditions are unrelated to behavioral or psycho-social factors or processes."

Studies in neuroscience have begun to document the physiological basis of cognitive disorders. . . . As we continue to discover the physiological origins of emotional harm, the distinction between emotional and physical harm may become outmoded. This would argue in favor of including emotional harm under the rubric of bodily or personal injury, instead of treating it as a separate (and separable) harm.

The approach in English law to tort recovery for emotional harm accommodates this unitary view. Although the English approach developed long before these advances in neuroscience occurred, English courts have consistently treated mental illnesses as an aspect of bodily harm. Letting medicine rather than law assume the lead in cases of emotional harm, English law requires the plaintiff to show a recognizable or diagnosable psychiatric illness before the plaintiff can proceed with the tort claim. English decisions express concerns similar to those cited by American courts, such as floodgates and the need for bright lines, but do not draw a sharp distinction between the physical and emotional. Instead, the decisions treat psychiatric illness as a part of personal injury. . . .

ENGLISH APPROACH: RECOGNIZABLE PSYCHIATRIC ILLNESS

The English courts approach the issue of emotional harm differently from American courts. Instead of drawing a sharp distinction between emotional and physical harm, English courts impose a threshold requirement on the plaintiff to prove a diagnosable psychiatric illness as an aspect of bodily harm. . . .

. . . For primary victims, absent a claim of physical harm, the plaintiff must satisfy an absolute threshold requirement that he or she is suffering from a recognizable psychiatric illness, or "nervous shock" as it is referred to in common legal terminology. Specific illnesses are not required, as long as it is a recognized psychiatric disorder. Damages have been awarded for wide-ranging illnesses, including morbid depression, hysterical personality disorder, post-traumatic stress disorder, pathological grief disorder, and chronic fatigue syndrome.

Courts distinguish between "mere feelings" and "injury." Anxiety, fear, or even short term symptoms of shock are not compensable conditions, if they are not a diagnosed psychiatric illness. . . . Thus, under English law, the plaintiff must affirmatively prove the appearance of a psychiatric illness, rather than simply arguing the absence of mental well being. . . .

There are three major stumbling blocks with regard to practical applications of neuroimaging to the area of emotional harm specifically: (1) establishing the "before" picture, or the plaintiff's baseline; (2) extrapolating information gleaned in generalized studies to a specific instance, or "individuation"; and (3) dealing with the different paces at which science will document different disorders.

Establishing a baseline goes to the issue of causation, that is, whether plaintiff's emotional harm is really due to the events plaintiff has experienced as opposed to his or her prior history or some other event. We must continue to emphasize the distinction between correlation and causation in using neuroimaging data in court. Finding a correlation often misleads us into believing that a causative effect exists, but discovering the neural correlates of cognitive phenomena does not tell us that the defendant's negligence caused the dysfunction. Without some evidence of the plaintiff's condition prior to the accident, it is hard to evaluate whether it was the negligence that actually caused the plaintiff's psychological harm or aggravated it further, or whether it was a pre-existing condition.

It is unlikely that the plaintiff will have had previous brain scans to compare to the current scan. We have other measures, however, to help give us a "before" picture. . . .

Even assuming that we can establish a baseline through relatively trustworthy evidence, however, another related problem remains—that of individuation. . . . At best, the brain scans show us the average brain states of individuals who suffer from, say, PTSD usually exhibit. It will be difficult to extrapolate from those neural correlations to prove injury in an individual case. This also requires us to determine the boundaries of the tort. Since the use of brain scan evidence is so new, we have yet to define the level of correlation we will require—i.e., how many different brain states must the plaintiff's scan correlate to before we qualify it as a recognized harm under the law?

Further, it is likely that neuroscience evidence will develop at different paces for different disorders. And it is likely that there will be disorders that we will not be able to measure pending years of scientific development. If we have neuroscientific support for some disorders, like PTSD, but not yet (or ever) for others, should we disallow the claim for the scientific laggards? Presumably, we do not want to limit compensable injury to emotional harm that is measurable by neuroimaging if other forms of reliable proof exist. Similarly, it is unlikely that we would preclude evidence we currently use to verify emotional harm, such as insomnia, nightmares and nausea. How will this evidence relate to brain scan evidence—will it be considered prerequisite, superfluous, or corroborative evidence? . . .

NOTES AND QUESTIONS

1. When a victim suffers tremendous pain from an acute event, so much pain that she forgets the event (and the pain), is the pain still compensable? That is, what is the law really compensating for when it compensates for "past pain": past pain or the *present memory* of past pain?

2. Should courts require that mental injuries be mitigated in the same ways that physical injuries are? *See* Eugene Kontorovich, *The Mitigation of Emotional Distress Damages*, 68 U. Chi. L. Rev. 491 (2001); Lars Noah, *Comfortably Numb: Medicalizing and Mitigating Pain and Suffering Damages*, 42 U. Mich. J.L. Reform 431 (2009); Kevin C. Klein & G. Nicole Hininger, *Mitigation of Psychological Damages: An Economic Analysis of the Avoidable Consequences Doctrine and its Applicability to Emotional Distress Injuries*, 29 Okla. City U. L. Rev. 405 (2004).

3. In 2013, the *DSM-5* was released, sparking renewed debate and discussion about the diagnosis of psychiatric disorders. One critic has been Allen Frances, a psychiatrist who led the task force that produced the *DSM-IV*. Dr. Frances observes that the *DSM* "is accorded the authority of a bible in areas well beyond its competence. It has become the arbiter of who is ill and who is not—and often the primary determinant of treatment decisions, insurance eligibility, disability payments and who gets special school services. D.S.M. drives the direction of research and the approval of new drugs. It is widely used (and misused) in the courts." He further argues that "[p]sychiatric diagnosis is simply too important to be left exclusively in the hands of psychiatrists. They will always be an essential part of the mix but should no longer be permitted to call all the shots." Allen Frances, *Diagnosing the D.S.M.*, N.Y. Times (May 11, 2012).

4. The then-Director of the National Institutes of Mental Health (NIMH) also commented on the *DSM*:

> While DSM has been described as a "Bible" for the field, it is, at best, a dictionary, creating a set of labels and defining each. The strength of each of the editions of DSM has been "reliability"—each edition has ensured that clinicians use the same terms in the same ways. The weakness is its lack of validity. Unlike our definitions of ischemic heart disease, lymphoma, or AIDS, the DSM diagnoses are based on a consensus about clusters of clinical symptoms, not any objective laboratory measure. In the rest of medicine, this would be equivalent to creating diagnostic systems based on the nature of chest pain or the quality of fever. Indeed, symptom-based diagnosis, once common in other areas of medicine, has been largely replaced in

the past half century as we have understood that symptoms alone rarely indicate the best choice of treatment.

Patients with mental disorders deserve better. NIMH has launched the Research Domain Criteria (RDoC) project to transform diagnosis by incorporating genetics, imaging, cognitive science, and other levels of information to lay the foundation for a new classification system. . . . This approach began with several assumptions:

- A diagnostic approach based on the biology as well as the symptoms must not be constrained by the current DSM categories,
- Mental disorders are biological disorders involving brain circuits that implicate specific domains of cognition, emotion, or behavior,
- Each level of analysis needs to be understood across a dimension of function,
- Mapping the cognitive, circuit, and genetic aspects of mental disorders will yield new and better targets for treatment.

It became immediately clear that we cannot design a system based on biomarkers or cognitive performance because we lack the data. In this sense, RDoC is a framework for collecting the data needed for a new nosology. But it is critical to realize that we cannot succeed if we use DSM categories as the "gold standard." The diagnostic system has to be based on the emerging research data, not on the current symptom-based categories. Imagine deciding that EKGs were not useful because many patients with chest pain did not have EKG changes. That is what we have been doing for decades when we reject a biomarker because it does not detect a DSM category. We need to begin collecting the genetic, imaging, physiologic, and cognitive data to see how all the data—not just the symptoms—cluster and how these clusters relate to treatment response.

. . . We are committed to new and better treatments, but we feel this will only happen by developing a more precise diagnostic system. The best reason to develop RDoC is to seek better outcomes.

. . . [P]atients and families should welcome this change as a first step towards "precision medicine," the movement that has transformed cancer diagnosis and treatment. RDoC is nothing less than a plan to transform clinical practice by bringing a new generation of research to inform how we diagnose and treat mental disorders. . . .

Thomas Insel, *Post by Former NIMH Director Thomas Insel: Transforming Diagnosis*, Nat'l Inst. Mental Health (Apr. 29, 2013).

D. THE SPECIAL CASE OF FETAL PAIN

For some time, the neuroscience of fetal pain has been an issue in government regulation of abortion, with many arguing that abortions should be prohibited or otherwise limited (by, for instance, denial of federal funding) past the moment when fetuses can experience pain. Although it appears that most chemical and behavioral studies of fetal pain agree that the fetus can experience pain in the third trimester, whether or not the fetus can do so in the second trimester remains controversial.*

---

* Carlo V. Bellieni & Giuseppe Buonocore, *Is Fetal Pain a Real Evidence?*, 25 J. Maternal-Fetal & Neonatal Med. 1203 (2012).

A 2019 article summarizing evidence increasing and decreasing the probability that second trimester fetuses experience pain listed the following factors as increasing that probability: presence of thalamus and subplate; adequate nociceptive pathways; periods of wakefulness; arousability; and hormonal and behavioral signs of pain. It listed the following as decreasing that probability: immature cortex; scarce myelination; continuous sleep state; presence of neuroinhibitors; fetal non-verbality.* One semantic yet crucial issue is whether reacting to and avoiding a painful stimulus is evidence of "feeling" or "experiencing" pain, or whether sufficient conscious awareness of the stimulus and one's reaction to it is necessary for a fetus to feel or experience pain. A Kansas law currently requires physicians who will be performing an abortion to inform the woman in writing that, "By no later than 20 weeks from fertilization, the unborn child has the physical structures necessary to *experience* pain." Kan. Stat. Ann. §65-6709 (2017) (emphasis added).

To stimulate your thinking on the potential relationship between neuroscience and law, in this important domain, this section presents views from both sides. First, reference to a "pain-capable unborn child protection act," from Louisiana, and related commentary. Then, one of a growing number of court cases to grapple with the constitutionality of fetal pain provisions.

Susan J. Lee et al.

Fetal Pain: A Systematic Multidisciplinary Review of the Evidence

294 JAMA 947, 947-52 (2005)

Over the last several years, many states, including California, Kentucky, Minnesota, Montana, New York, Oregon, and Virginia, have considered legislation requiring physicians to inform women seeking abortions that the fetus feels pain and to offer fetal anesthesia. . . . Although this legislation would not affect most US abortions because only 1.4% are performed at or after 21 weeks' gestational age, this legislation raises important scientific, clinical, ethical, and policy issues. When does a fetus have the functional capacity to feel pain? If that capacity exists, what forms of anesthesia or analgesia are safe and effective for treating fetal pain? As a first step in answering these questions, we reviewed the literature on fetal pain and fetal anesthesia and analgesia. . . .

Pain is an emotional and psychological experience that requires conscious recognition of a noxious stimulus. Consequently, the capacity for conscious perception of pain can arise only after thalamocortical pathways begin to function, which may occur in the third trimester around 29 to 30 weeks' gestational age, based on the limited data available. . . .

While the presence of thalamocortical fibers is necessary for pain perception, their mere presence is insufficient—this pathway must also be functional. . . . Tests of cortical function suggest that conscious perception of pain does not begin before the third trimester. . . .

A variety of anesthetic and analgesic techniques have been used for fetal surgery, including maternal general anesthesia, regional anesthesia, and administration of medications for placental transfer to the fetus. However, these techniques are not

---

* Carlo V. Bellieni, *New Insights into Fetal Pain*, 24 Seminars Fetal & Neonatal Med. 101001 (2019).

necessarily applicable to abortions. Surgical procedures undertaken for fetal benefit use anesthesia to achieve objectives unrelated to pain control, such as uterine relaxation, fetal immobilization, and possible prevention of neuroendocrine stress responses associated with poor surgical outcomes. Thus, fetal anesthesia may be medically indicated for fetal surgery regardless of whether fetal pain exists. . . .

Testimony Before the United States Congress

—Testimony of Jean Wright, Professor and Chair of Pediatrics, Mercer School of Medicine, Pain of the Unborn Hearing Before the Subcommittee on the Constitution of the Committee on the Judiciary House of Representatives 109th Cong., 1st Sess. (2005):

> It was in the mid-'90's when I was here and we were discussing that legislation and we began to talk about pain in the third trimester, but now we know that it is not just the third trimester, but it is as early as 20 weeks, and there is data that shows 16 weeks and even earlier, many of these infants feel pain and have negative outcomes from it.

—Testimony of Dr. Sunny Anand, Director, Pain Neurobiology Laboratory, Arkansas Children's Hospital Research Institute, and Professor of Pediatrics, Anesthesiology, Pharmacology, and Neurobiology, University of Arkansas College of Medicine, Hearing Before the Subcommittee on the Constitution of the Committee on the Judiciary House of Representatives 109th Cong., 1st Sess. (2005):

> Many years of careful research in which I have participated has shown that the neonate, or the fetus, is not a little adult; that the mechanisms and structures used for pain processing are very different at different stages of development. Indeed the nervous system will use the elements available at that time, at a particular stage of development, to transduce external and internal stimuli, and pain is an inherent, innate part of this system. . . . My opinion is, based on evidence suggesting that the types of stimulation that will occur during abortion procedures, very likely most fetuses at 20 weeks after conception will be able to perceive that as painful, unpleasant, noxious stimulation.

—Testimony of Robert J. White, MD, Ph.D., Professor of Neurosurgery, Case Western Reserve University, Hearing on Partial-Birth Abortion Before the Subcomm. on the Constitution of the House Comm. on the Judiciary, 105th Cong., 1st Sess. (1995):

> An unborn child at 20 weeks gestation "is fully capable of experiencing pain. . . . Without question, [abortion] is a dreadfully painful experience for any infant subjected to such a surgical procedure."

Pain-Capable Unborn Child Protection Act, 2015 La. Rev. Stat., ch. 40, art. 1061, §1 (codified at La. Stat. Ann. §40:1061.1).

Pain-Capable Unborn Child Protection Act

. . . *B. Legislative intent.* The legislature makes the following findings:

(a) Pain receptors (nociceptors) are present throughout the unborn child's entire body and nerves link these receptors to the brain's thalamus and subcortical plate by no later than twenty weeks.

(b) By eight weeks after fertilization, the unborn child reacts to touch. After twenty weeks, the unborn child reacts to stimuli that would be recognized as painful if applied to an adult human, for example, by recoiling.

(c) In the unborn child, application of such painful stimuli is associated with significant increases in stress hormones known as the stress response.

(d) Subjection to such painful stimuli is associated with long-term harmful neuro-developmental effects, such as altered pain sensitivity and, possibly, emotional, behavioral, and learning disabilities later in life.

(e) For the purposes of surgery on unborn children, fetal anesthesia is routinely administered and is associated with a decrease in stress hormones compared to their level when painful stimuli are applied without such anesthesia.

(f) The position, asserted by some medical experts, that the unborn child is incapable of experiencing pain until a point later in pregnancy than twenty weeks after fertilization predominately rests on the assumption that the ability to experience pain depends on the cerebral cortex and requires nerve connections between the thalamus and the cortex. However, recent medical research and analysis, especially since 2007, provides strong evidence for the conclusion that a functioning cortex is not necessary to experience pain.

(g) Substantial evidence indicates that children born missing the bulk of the cerebral cortex, those with hydranencephaly, nevertheless experience pain.

(h) In adults, stimulation or ablation of the cerebral cortex does not alter pain perception, while stimulation or ablation of the thalamus does.

(i) Substantial evidence indicates that structures used for pain processing in early development differ from those of adults, using different neural elements available at specific times during development, such as the subcortical plate, to fulfill the role of pain processing.

(j) The position, asserted by some medical experts, that the unborn child remains in a coma-like sleep state that precludes the unborn child's experiencing pain is inconsistent with the documented reaction of unborn children to painful stimuli and with the experience of fetal surgeons who have found it necessary to sedate the unborn child with anesthesia to prevent the unborn child from thrashing about in reaction to invasive surgery.

(k) Consequently, there is substantial medical evidence that an unborn child is capable of experiencing pain by twenty weeks after fertilization.

(2)(a) It is the purpose of the state to assert a compelling state interest in protecting the lives of unborn children from the stage at which substantial medical evidence indicates that they are capable of feeling pain.

(b) Louisiana's compelling state interest in protecting the lives of unborn children from the stage at which substantial medical evidence indicates that they are capable of feeling pain is intended to be separate from and independent of Louisiana's compelling state interest in protecting the lives of unborn children from the stage of viability, and neither state interest is intended to replace the other. . . .

E. Abortion of unborn child of twenty or more weeks postfertilization age prohibited.

(1) No person shall perform or induce or attempt to perform or induce an abortion upon a woman when it has been determined, by the physician performing or inducing or attempting to perform or induce the abortion or by another physician upon whose determination that physician relies, that the probable postfertilization age of the woman's unborn child is twenty or more weeks, unless the pregnancy is diagnosed as medically futile or, in reasonable medical judgment, she has a condition which so complicates her medical condition as to necessitate the abortion of her pregnancy to avert her death or to avert serious risk of substantial and irreversible

physical impairment of a major bodily function, not including psychological or emotional conditions. . . .

Planned Parenthood of Indiana, Inc. v. Comm'r of Indiana State Dep't of Health

794 F. Supp. 2d 892 (S.D. Ind. 2011)*

PRATT, D.J. Following a vigorous and often contentious legislative debate, Governor Mitch Daniels signed House Enrolled Act 1210 ("HEA 1210") into law on May 10, 2011. The new law accomplishes two objectives. First, HEA 1210 prohibits certain entities that perform abortions from receiving any state funding for health services unrelated to abortion—including for cervical PAP smears, cancer screenings, sexually transmitted disease testing and notification, and family planning services (the "defunding provision"). This portion of the law—codified at Ind. Code §5-22-17-5.5(b) through (d)—went into effect immediately. Second, HEA 1210 modifies the informed consent information that abortion providers must give patients prior to receiving abortion services (the "informed consent provision"). This portion of the law—codified at Ind. Code §16-34-2-1.1(a)(1)—goes into effect July 1, 2011.

Within minutes of HEA 1210 being signed into law, Plaintiffs—Planned Parenthood of Indiana, Inc. ("PPIN"), Michael King, M.D., Carla Cleary, C.N.M., Letitia Clemons, and Dejiona Jackson (collectively, "Plaintiffs")—filed a lawsuit against the Commissioner of the Indiana State Department of Health, et al. (collectively, "Commissioner"), challenging the legality of both the defunding provision and the informed consent provision. That same day, this Court heard oral arguments on Plaintiffs' Motion for a Temporary Restraining Order ("TRO"), which related only to the defunding provision. The next day, on May 11, 2011, the Court denied Plaintiffs' Motion. In doing so, the Court cited the exacting standard required for a TRO, PPIN's limited evidence supporting immediate and irreparable harm, and the fact that the Commissioner had not yet had the opportunity to brief the relevant issues.

Now, this matter is before the Court on Plaintiffs Motion for Preliminary Injunction. . . .

Ind. Code §16-34-2-1.1(a)(1)(G) relates to the fetus and its potential ability to feel pain. Specifically, this provision requires the Practitioner to inform the woman seeking an abortion that "objective scientific information"—a term statutorily defined as "data that have been reasonably derived from scientific literature and verified or supported by research in compliance with scientific methods"—shows that a fetus can feel pain at or before twenty (20) weeks of postfertilization age. This section's mandated statement is based upon the following legislative findings, enacted as part of the bill:

1) There is substantial medical evidence that a fetus at twenty (20) weeks of postfertilization age has the physical structures necessary to experience pain.

---

* [This case was aff'd in part, rev'd in part sub nom. in *Planned Parenthood of Indiana, Inc. v. Comm'r of Indiana State Dep't of Health*, 699 F.3d 962 (7th Cir. 2012), cert. denied, 133 S. Ct. 2736, 186 L. Ed. 2d 193 (U.S. 2013), and cert. denied, 133 S. Ct. 2738, 186 L. Ed. 2d 193 (U.S. 2013). The issues related to pain science were not part of the appeal. — EDS.]

2) There is substantial medical evidence that a fetus of at least twenty (20) weeks of postfertilization age seeks to evade certain stimuli in a manner similar to an infant's or adult's response to pain.

3) Anesthesia is routinely administered to a fetus of at least twenty (20) weeks of postfertilization age when prenatal surgery is performed.

4) A fetus has been observed to exhibit hormonal stress responses to painful stimuli earlier than at twenty (20) weeks of postfertilization age. 2011 Ind. Legis. Serv. P.L. 193-2011, Sec. 6.

The Commissioner contends that based upon the statutory definition of "objective scientific information" and the legislative findings enacted as part of the bill, Ind. Code §16-34-2-1.1(a)(1)(G)'s statement is truthful, non-misleading, and relevant. In the context of Plaintiffs' as-applied challenge, however, the Court respectfully disagrees.

The Commissioner presents evidence in the form of articles, affidavits, declarations, and reports relating to the present research and growing science of fetal pain perception. The Commissioner principally argues that in order to be "objective scientific information" as defined by the statute and therefore truthful and non-misleading, the statement need not be the "majority" view within the scientific community. Instead, it need only be reasonably derived or supported by research in compliance with scientific methods. . . .

Although this argument has merit, the Court has been given no evidence to support the finding that within the scientific community even a minority view exists that contends pain perception is possible during the first trimester of pregnancy—the time during which PPIN exclusively performs its abortion services. The Commissioner's evidence posits only preliminary evidence that may support the inference that pain is felt by a fetus at as early as sixteen (16) weeks postfertilization.

Evidentiary documents that contain statements such as "the substrate and mechanisms for conscious pain perception are developed in a fetus well before the third trimester of human gestation," "by twenty weeks, perhaps even earlier, all the essential components of anatomy, physiology, and neurobiology exist to transmit painful sensations from the skin to the spinal cord and to the brain," "therapeutic response in pain receptors of fetuses at 16-21 weeks," and "we cannot dismiss the high likelihood of fetal pain perception before the third trimester," do not show that a fetus at twelve weeks or earlier of postfertilization can feel pain. Nor do they support a view that has been reasonably derived from scientific literature and verified or supported by research in compliance with scientific methods. Even in its own statement of facts, the Commissioner admits only that "[m]ultiple lines of scientific evidence converge to support the conclusion that the human fetus can experience pain from 20 weeks of gestation, and possibly as early as 16 weeks of gestation." Importantly, the Commissioner conceded at oral arguments that to his knowledge, there is no objective scientific information that a fetus can feel pain at 12 weeks.

Because PPIN exclusively performs abortion services on patients in their first trimester, this Court finds that Plaintiffs have provided sufficient evidence demonstrating that requiring PPIN Practitioners to state that "objective scientific information shows that a fetus can feel pain at or before twenty week of postfertilization age" may be false, misleading, and irrelevant. In this as-applied challenge, PPIN has demonstrated likelihood of success on the merits. When a party seeks a preliminary injunction on the basis of a potential First Amendment violation, the likelihood of success on the merits will often be the determinative factor. Here, the Court has found that Plaintiffs' possess the requisite likelihood of success on the merits that the mandated statement found in §16-34-2-1.1(a)(1)(G) would constitute impermissible compelled speech. The loss of First Amendment freedoms, for even minimal periods of time, constitutes irreparable injury.

In its briefing, the Commissioner addressed the possibility that the Court might find it misleading to tell a first-trimester patient that her fetus would feel pain at or before twenty weeks postfertilization. Relying on *Ayotte*, . . . the Commissioner argues that facial invalidation is disfavored, even in abortion-regulation cases, and that the Court may not enjoin application of the provision in its entirety. The Court is persuaded. The enjoining of §16-34-2-1.1(a)(1)(G), as applied only to Plaintiffs, cannot be shown to inflict irreparable harm to Defendants when the injunction prevents the enforcement of a potentially unconstitutional statute. It is always in the public interest to protect First Amendment liberties. Although a preliminary injunction is an "extraordinary remedy," based upon the aforementioned analysis, the Court finds that Plaintiffs have made the requisite showing. Accordingly, the Court GRANTS Plaintiffs' Motion and enjoins the enforcement of Ind. Code §16-34-2-1.1(a)(1)(G) as applied to Plaintiffs' performance of first-trimester abortions. . . .

NOTES AND QUESTIONS

1. Fetal pain legislation often cites scientific findings from some neuroscientists and medical professionals. A key question is: How representative and widely accepted are those findings? The American Congress of Obstetricians and Gynecologists, for instance, released a statement in June 2013 called "Facts Are Important." The statement reads:

   > A rigorous 2005 scientific review of evidence published in the Journal of the American Medical Association (JAMA) concluded that fetal perception of pain is unlikely before the third trimester.
   >
   > Although ultrasound monitoring can show intrauterine fetal movement, no studies since 2005 demonstrate fetal recognition of pain. . . .
   >
   > The American Congress of Obstetricians and Gynecologists (ACOG), representing more than 58,000 ob-gyns and partners in women's health, supports robust, factual debate on issues of importance to the American people.

   Gov't Relations & Outreach Dep't, Am. Coll. of Obstetricians & Gynecologists, *Facts Are Important: Fetal Pain*, Am. College of Obstetricians and Gynecologists (June 2013). What policies should govern legislative use of neuroscience? If a legislative committee has a hearing that includes competing scientific views, each voiced by a qualified individual, is that sufficient? What if a strong majority of a legislator's constituents agree with one view of the science over another?

2. Does the neuroscience of pain have implications for the constitutionality of these laws? Consider law professor Glenn Cohen's argument against the constitutionality of such laws:

   > The legislatures passing these laws say that preventing this pain is a compelling state interest that justifies prohibiting abortion. Hence, the loophole: Although

the Supreme Court has identified preserving fetal life after viability as a compelling interest, the justices have never said it is the only one. These statutes might be thought of as asking the courts to find that preventing pain to fetuses is also a compelling state interest. Alternatively, states may argue that, although preventing pain is not compelling on its own, it becomes so when combined with the state's interest in preserving fetal life before viability.

I. Glenn Cohen, *The Flawed Basis Behind Fetal-Pain Abortion Laws*, Wash. Post (Aug. 1, 2012). Is this a convincing argument? Why or why not? What role, if any, does the science of pain research have on your conclusions?

FURTHER READING

Legal Perspectives:

Amanda C. Pustilnik, *Legal Evidence of Subjective States: A Brain-Based Model of Chronic Pain Increases Accuracy and Fairness in Law*, 25 Harv. Rev. Psychiatry 279 (2015).

Amanda C. Pustilnik, *Imaging Brains, Changing Minds: How Pain Neuroimaging Can Inform the Law*, 66 Ala. L. Rev. 1099 (2015).

Amanda C. Pustilnik, *Pain as Fact and Heuristic: How Pain Neuroimaging Illuminates Moral Dimensions of Law*, 97 Cornell L. Rev. 801 (2012).

Adam J. Kolber, *Pain Detection and the Privacy of Subjective Experience*, 33 Am. J.L. & Med. 433 (2007).

Adam J. Kolber, *The Experiential Future of the Law*, 60 Emory L.J. 585 (2011).

Brady Somers, *Neuroimaging Evidence: A Solution to the Problem of Proving Pain and Suffering?* 39 Seattle U. L. Rev. 1391 (2015).

Defining and Assessing Pain:

International Association for the Study of Pain, *http://www.iasp-pain.org*.

M. Catherine Bushnell et al., *Cognitive and Emotional Control of Pain and Its Disruption in Chronic Pain*, 14 Nature Reviews Neurosci. 502 (2013).

Neuroscience of Pain and Pain Detection:

Maite M. van der Miesen, Martin A. Lindquist & Tor D. Wager, *Neuroimaging-based Biomarkers for Pain: State of the Field and Current Directions*, 4 Pain Rep. e751 (2019).

Sean Mackey, Henry T. Greely & Katherine T. Martucci, *Neuroimaging-based Pain Biomarkers: Definitions, Clinical and Research Applications, and Evaluation Frameworks to Achieve Personalized Pain Medicine*, 4 Pain Rep. e762 (2019).

Pain Rep., Special Issue on *Innovations and Controversies in Brain Imaging of Pain-Methods and Interpretations* (Karen D. Davis ed., 2019).

Karen D. Davis et al., *Brain Imaging Tests for Chronic Pain: Medical, Legal and Ethical Issues and Recommendations*, 13 Nature 624 (2017).

Joyce T. Da Silva & David A. Seminowicz, *Neuroimaging of Pain in Animal Models: A Review of Recent Literature*, 4 Pain Rep. e732 (2019).

Irene I. Tracey & Anthony A. Dickenson, *SnapShot: Pain and Perception*, 148 Cell 1308 (2012).

Anthony Wagner, Steven Laken & Irene I. Tracey, Panel at the Second Raymond & Beverly Sackler USA-UK Scientific Forum: Neuroscience and the Law Under the Auspices of The National Academy of Sciences: Mind Reading (Including Lie Detection, Pain, and False Memory) (Mar. 2-3, 2011).

Naomi I. Eisenberger, *The Pain of Social Disconnection: Examining the Shared Neural Underpinnings of Physical and Social Pain*, 3 Nature Reviews Neurosci. 421 (2012).

Roland Peyron et al., *Functional Imaging of Brain Responses to Pain: A Review and Meta-Analysis*, 30 Neurophysiology Clinics 263 (2000).

Justin E. Brown et al., *Towards a Physiology-Based Measure of Pain: Patterns of Human Brain Activity Distinguish Painful from Non-Painful Thermal Stimulation*, 6 PLoS ONE e24124 (2011).

Massieh Moayedi et al., *Pain Neuroimaging in Humans: A Primer for Beginners and Non-Imagers*, 19 J. Pain 961-e1 (2018).

Neuroethics of Pain and Pain Detection:

Pain Neuroethics and Bioethics (Daniel Z. Buchman & Karen Davis eds., 2018)

James Giordano et al., *Pain Assessment: Subjectivity, Objectivity, and the Use of Neurotechnology Part One: Practical and Ethical Issues*, 13 Pain Physician 305 (2010).

Fetal Pain:

Carlo V. Bellieni, *New Insights into Fetal Pain*, 24 Seminars Fetal & Neonatal Med. 101001 (2019).

Greg Miller, *Pioneering Study Images Activity in Fetal Brains*, 355 Science 117 (2017).

E. Christian Brugger, *The Problem of Fetal Pain and Abortion: Toward an Ethical Consensus for Appropriate Behavior*, 22 Kennedy Instit. Ethics J. 263 (2012).

CHAPTER 12

Addicted Brains

If addicts can be punished for their addiction, then the insane can also be punished for their insanity. Each has a disease and each must be treated as a sick person.

—Justice William O. Douglas, *Robinson v. California*
(concurring)[†]

To say that addiction is a brain disease is useful as a rhetorical tool in a debate about public policy; but, scientifically, it is both incomplete and premature.
—Richard J. Bonnie[††]

CHAPTER SUMMARY

This chapter:
- Introduces clinical definitions of addiction and substance abuse.
- Examines relevant neuroscience research on addiction and substance abuse.
- Explores the legal implications of addiction in a variety of criminal and civil contexts.

INTRODUCTION

Drug addiction and substance abuse are costly to individuals and to society, and they present special challenges to the legal system. For instance, it is estimated that substance-involved inmates account for 85% of all incarcerated offenders.[*] More than 20% of inmates for violent crimes were under the influence of alcohol when acting violently, more than 40% of first-time offenders have a history of drug use, and more than 80% of those with five or more convictions have a history of drug use.[**]

Economic ramifications are significant. The National Institute on Drug Abuse (NIDA) estimates that drug abuse and addiction cost over $740 billion a year in the United States alone. The National Institutes of Health (NIH) estimates that worldwide, hundreds of millions of people are facing drug addiction and the potentially harmful consequences that follow. In light of these concerns, there is extensive neuroscience research on addiction. For instance, NIDA, whose mission is to "lead the Nation in bringing the power of science to bear on drug abuse and addiction,"

[†] *Robinson v. California*, 370 U.S. 660, 674 (1962) (Douglas, J., concurring).
[††] Richard J. Bonnie, *Responsibility for Addiction*, 30 J. Am. Acad. Psychiatry L. 405, 406 (2002).
[*] Nat'l Ctr. on Addiction and Substance Abuse at Columbia Univ., *Behind Bars II: Substance Abuse and America's Prison Population* 2 (2010).
[**] Joan Petersilia, *When Prisoners Come Home: Parole and Prisoner Reentry* 48 (2003).

has an annual budget over $1 billion. Much of the research funded by NIDA is conducted by neuroscientists who view addiction as a brain disease. In a provocative and widely cited piece, neuroscientist and former director of NIDA Alan Leshner wrote in 1997:

> Dramatic advances over the past two decades in both the neurosciences and the behavioral sciences have revolutionized our understanding of drug abuse and addiction. Scientists have identified neural circuits that subsume the actions of every known drug of abuse, and they have specified common pathways that are affected by almost all such drugs. . . . Research has also begun to reveal major differences between the brains of addicted and nonaddicted individuals and to indicate some common elements of addiction, regardless of the substance.
>
> That is the good news. The bad news is the dramatic lag between these advances in science and their appreciation by the general public or their application in either practice or public policy settings. . . . One major barrier is the tremendous stigma attached to being a drug user or, worse, an addict. . . . [A] common view is that drug addicts are weak or bad people, unwilling to lead moral lives and to control their behavior and gratifications. To the contrary, addiction is actually a chronic, relapsing illness, characterized by compulsive drug seeking and use. The gulf in implications between the "bad person" view and the "chronic illness sufferer" view is tremendous. . . .*

One of the ways in which law interfaces with addiction is through criminal responsibility doctrine related to intoxication.** Criminal responsibility is established if the prosecution can prove all of the requisite elements beyond a reasonable doubt and no affirmative defense succeeds. This typically requires the prosecution to prove that the defendant acted voluntarily and with a culpable state of mind. In general, the law does not permit an intoxicated defendant to deny the existence of an act if the defendant initially became intoxicated *voluntarily*. If the agent was *involuntarily intoxicated* — the intoxication was not the agent's fault because, say, someone slipped a substance in his or her drink without the agent's knowledge — then the law is more likely to permit the agent to claim that she did not *act*.

Voluntary and involuntary intoxication can clearly affect the formation of legally relevant mental states. One may be so drunk at a restaurant, for example, that one forgets to pay the bill rather than intentionally not paying it. Or, one may be so drunk that one is not aware of a substantial risk that one would be aware of when sober. For example, one may be so drunk while driving that the driver will not consciously realize the obvious risk that his dangerous driving is risking the death of other motorists or pedestrians.

Criminal law is conflicted about whether or not a defendant should be permitted to introduce evidence of voluntary intoxication for the purpose of casting doubt on the formation of a requisite mental state. The Supreme Court has held that, for various reasons, the Constitution does not require states to permit defendants this right. Nevertheless, a large number of states do permit the defendant to introduce

---

* Alan I. Leshner, *Addiction Is a Brain Disease, and It Matters*, 278 Science 45, 45 (1997).

** [The rest of this paragraph, and the three paragraphs that follow, are drawn with permission from *Criminal Law and Related Doctrines Pertaining to Addictions*, MacArthur Foundation Law & Neuroscience Project Law/Philosophy Working Group (May 2008) (unpublished manuscript) (on file with authors) —EDS.]

voluntary intoxication evidence to negate the presence of mental states, but all place substantial limitations on when the defendant may do so. Jurisdictions tend to be more permissive about introducing evidence of involuntary intoxication to negate a required mental state. Whether the intoxicated defendant is an addict does not affect the outcome. The same rules apply to intoxicated addicts and non-addicts.

Addiction per se is not an excuse in criminal law, even when it may play a causal role in producing the criminal's behavior. There have been attempts to persuade appellate courts to establish an addiction excuse, and as you will read in this chapter, there have been constitutional challenges to certain probation requirements for addicts. But to date these legal arguments have failed. Many have argued that the excuse of legal insanity should encompass some cases involving addiction. However, although substance use disorder is a *DSM* diagnosis, addiction is routinely not accepted as a sufficient mental disorder on which to base an insanity defense and it is specifically excluded in some jurisdictions.

Whether the criminal law, or any other part of law, will change (or should change) in light of neuroscientific research on addiction is the focus of this chapter. The chapter presents views of addiction from neuroscience, contrasts those with views of addiction from law, and asks you to assess what differences emerge, whether those differences are well-founded, and whether they matter for legal adjudication. Should advances in the science of addiction be readily transferred to the legal domain? Or do the goals of law require it to take a different approach to addiction? We begin in Section A by introducing the concepts of addiction and dependence as they are defined and debated by medical professionals and research scientists. Section B considers the legal implications of addiction. Section C briefly reviews the neurobiology of addiction. Finally, Section D concludes with consideration of policy issues that may be informed by addiction science, giving special attention to how the opioid epidemic has shaped drug policy.

A. DEFINING ADDICTION AND DEPENDENCE

The diagnosis of psychological and behavioral disorders is complex not only because the line between normal and disordered is very blurry but also because the diagnostic criteria can be both vague and arbitrary. The American Psychiatric Association ratifies particular definitions and criteria for diagnosis of mental disorders in the *Diagnostic and Statistical Manual of Mental Disorders*. The fifth edition, *DSM-5*, was published in May of 2013. Planning for *DSM-5*, begun in 1999, involved 13 working groups as well as a *DSM-5* Task Force, a Scientific Review Committee, and a Clinical and Public Health Committee. The *DSM-5* is used broadly, but not uniformly. For example, the National Institute of Mental Health (NIMH) has stated that while *DSM-5* may be effective for practitioners, it is inadequate for researchers. NIMH's goal is to establish a diagnostic system that more directly reflects neuroscience, even if this entails reconsidering traditional *DSM* categories. To that end, NIMH has developed the Research Domain Criteria (RDoC) project as an alternative taxonomy for mental disorders based on genetics, neuroscience, and behavioral science. While *DSM-5* and RDoC can be regarded as complementary, not competing, frameworks, you will learn below that the two perspectives are also at times in tension with one another. It should also be noted that classification schemes beyond the DSM and RDoC are also in use, most importantly the International Classification of Diseases, Eleventh Revision (ICD-11). ICD-11 is published by the World Health Organization (WHO) and is utilized by clinicians across the globe. World Health Org., *International Classification of Diseases and Health Related Problems* (11th rev. 2019).

DSM-IV defined substance-related problems under two diagnoses: substance abuse and substance dependence. In recognition of the artificial distinction between substance abuse and dependence, *DSM-5* combined these categories into a single "substance use" disorder, diagnosed along a continuum from mild to severe based on the number and severity of the symptoms. The goal was to combine and strengthen the diagnostic criteria. For example, drug craving was added to the list of symptoms. Also, recurrent legal problems were eliminated because of the cultural differences that make this criterion challenging to apply across international and regional jurisdictions.

Sara Gordon

The Use and Abuse of Mutual-Support Programs in Drug Courts

2017 U. Ill. L. Rev. 1503, 1514-17 (2017)

B. DIAGNOSING ADDICTION

. . . whether we characterize addiction as a brain disease, or a biopsychosocial disorder, or "somewhere in [the] middle ground," the DSM-5 requires clinicians to diagnose addiction based on behavioral criteria, not biological criteria. By this standard, individuals can be diagnosed with a "substance use disorder" on a continuum from mild to severe.[77] Unlike its predecessor, the new edition of the DSM does not distinguish among substances, and almost all substances are diagnosed using the same set of behavioral criteria.[78] Moreover, the DSM-5 does not use the word "addiction"; although the word "addiction" is often used to describe "severe problems related to compulsive and habitual use of substances," the DSM-5 uses the "more neutral term substance use disorder . . . to describe the wide range of the disorder, from a mild form to a severe state of chronically relapsing, compulsive drug taking." The DSM-5 chose to eliminate "addiction . . . because of its uncertain definition and its potentially negative connotation."

To be diagnosed with Substance Use Disorder, the individual must meet two of the eleven criteria listed in the DSM-5. If the individual meets two or three criteria, this indicates a mild substance use disorder; meeting four or five factors indicates a moderate disorder; and meeting six or more indicates a severe substance use disorder. The eleven criteria in the DSM-5 can be further broken down into four different categories: impaired control, social impairment, risky use, and physiological effects.

---

[77] [Am. Psychiatric Ass'n. Diagnostic and Statistical Manual of Mental Disorders (5th ed. 2013)] at 484 ("Substance use disorders occur in a broad range of severity, from mild to severe, with severity based on the number of symptom criteria endorsed.").

[78] As the DSM-5 notes, "the diagnosis of a substance use disorder can be applied to all 10 classes included in this chapter except caffeine. For certain classes some symptoms are less salient, and in a few instances not all symptoms apply . . . ." *Id.* at 483. The ten classes of addictive substances referenced in the DSM include alcohol, caffeine, cannabis, hallucinogens, inhalants, opioids, sedatives, stimulants, and tobacco. *Id.* at 482.

Criterion A, Impaired Control (DSM Criterion 1-4), relates to the individual's loss of control over her substance use. This category includes situations in which the person takes the substance in larger amounts or over a longer period of time than she originally intended; the person tries to cut down or regulate her substance use and is unsuccessful; the person spends large amounts of time obtaining, using, or recovering from the substance; and the person has intense cravings for the substance, especially in environments where she previously used or obtained the substance.

Criterion B, Social Impairment (DSM Criterion 5-7), includes social impairment, which arises when the person's substance use results in a failure to fulfill obligations at work, school, or home; the person continues use despite social or other interpersonal problems; or the person withdraws from important social, work, and recreational activities because of her substance use. Criteria C, Risky Use (DSM Criterion 8-9), pertains to risky use of a particular substance, and involves the use of the substance in dangerous situations, or continued use of a substance despite knowledge that the substance is likely to affect the person's physical or psychological well-being. Finally, Criteria D, Physiological Effects (DSM Criterion 10-11), includes pharmacological criteria, and are met when the person develops a tolerance to the substance and must use greater amounts to achieve the desired effect, and when an individual develops withdrawal symptoms upon discontinued use of the substance.

Furthermore, there is a growing literature examining "behavioral addictions," or nonsubstance addictions, which are "analogous to substance addiction, but with a behavioral focus other than ingestion of a psychoactive substance." Apart from gambling disorder, which the most recent version of the DSM has moved to a new section entitled "Non-Substance-Related Disorders,"89 these types of behaviors are typically classified as impulse-control disorders, and include things like kleptomania and pyromania. Other behaviors were considered for inclusion in the DSM, including compulsive buying, pathologic skin picking, sexual addiction, excessive tanning, computer/video game playing, and Internet addiction. Of these, only Internet Gaming Disorder found a place in the DSM-5 as a condition that should receive further study. . . .

Am. Psychiatric Ass'n
Substance-Related and Addictive Disorders
in *Diagnostic and Statistical Manual of Mental Disorders* (5th ed. 2013)

The substance-related disorders are divided into two groups: substance use disorders and substance-induced disorders. The following conditions may be classified as substance-induced: intoxication, withdrawal, and other substance/medication-induced mental disorders (psychotic disorders, bipolar and related disorders, depressive disorders, anxiety disorders, obsessive-compulsive and related disorders, sleep disorders, sexual dysfunctions, delirium, and neurocognitive disorders).

SUBSTANCE USE DISORDERS: FEATURES

The essential feature of a substance use disorder is a cluster of cognitive, behavioral, and physiological symptoms indicating that the individual continues using the substance despite significant substance-related problems. . . . For certain classes some symptoms are less salient, and in a few instances not all symptoms apply. . . .

An important characteristic of substance use disorders is an underlying change in brain circuits that may persist beyond detoxification, particularly in individuals with severe disorders. The behavioral effects of these brain changes may be exhibited in the repeated relapses and intense drug craving when the individuals are exposed to drug-related stimuli. These persistent drug effects may benefit from long-term approaches to treatment. . . .

SUBSTANCE USE DISORDERS: SEVERITY AND SPECIFIERS

Substance use disorders occur in a broad range of severity, from mild to severe, with severity based on the number of symptom criteria endorsed. As a general estimate of severity, a mild substance use disorder is suggested by the presence of two to three symptoms, moderate by four to five symptoms, and severe by six or more symptoms. . . .

The *DSM-5* makes references to the brain's reward system. Research on this reward system and how it is related to addiction has been ongoing for several decades. The following excerpts summarize some of the key findings from this research literature and make clear that our understanding of the addicted brain is still emerging.

Nora D. Volkow et al.
Addiction Circuitry in the Human Brain
52 Ann. Rev. Pharmacology & Toxicology 321, 322-32 (2012)

The rewarding effect of drugs of abuse is the main reason why humans use them and laboratory animals self-administer them. However, most individuals using drugs never escalate to uncontrollable levels of drug use and only a relatively small percentage does (approximately 10–20%). . . . Who becomes addicted (term used in lieu of the dependence term used by DSM IV to avoid confusion with physical dependence) and who does not are strongly influenced by genetic (50% of risk), developmental (risk is higher in adolescence than adulthood), and environmental factors (drug access, stress), as well as the type of drug (some drugs produce addiction faster than others, e.g., methamphetamine versus marijuana).

It is generally accepted that the rewarding effects of drugs are due to their ability to increase dopamine (DA) particularly in the nucleus accumbens (NAc). The potency of drugs as well as the mechanism by which they increase DA differs for the various drug classes. Interestingly, DA's role in drug reward (as well as reward in general) does not seem to equate with hedonic pleasure (mediated in part by endogenous opioids and cannabinoids), but instead DA appears to encode prediction of reward, imprinting incentive value to reinforcers (energizing approach behavior) and facilitating learning of reward associations (conditioning) through its modulation of subcortical (including the NAc) and cortical brain regions. . . .

Neurotransmitters other than DA (e.g., cannabinoids, opioids) are also involved with drug reward, and their relative contribution to a drug's rewarding effects is determined in part by their pharmacological effects (e.g., endogenous opioids for heroin, alcohol, nicotine). Similarly, several neurotransmitters are also involved in the neuroadaptations associated with addiction (e.g., decreases in endogenous opioid signaling in cocaine addiction), including the central role of glutamate in the neuroplastic changes associated with chronic drug exposures.

Clinical studies have used positron emission tomography (PET) to evaluate DA's role in drug reward and addiction (and, to a lesser extent, the role of endogenous opioids), whereas fMRI studies have concentrated on delineating the neuronal pathways affected by drugs in addicted subjects. These findings show that addiction affects not only the reward circuit, but also circuits involved with memory (conditioning/habits), motivation (energy, drive), executive function (inhibitory control, salience attribution, decision-making), mood (stress reactivity and hedonic state), and interoception (internal awareness). . . .

[In summary] several brain circuits are relevant in the neurobiology of addiction and result in an enhanced motivational value of the drug (secondary to learned associations through conditioning and habits) at the expense of other reinforcers (secondary to decreased sensitivity of the reward circuit) and an impaired ability to inhibit the intentional actions associated with the strong desires to take the drug (secondary to impaired executive function) that result in compulsive drug taking in addiction. In addition, disrupted executive function contributes to impaired insight in addiction, which interferes with the recognition of disease and the need for treatment. Because these neuronal systems also play fundamental roles in social behaviors, understanding their disruption in addiction is providing insight into why drugs can be so disruptive to social relationships and why the typical positive reinforcers used to promote positive behaviors (e.g., pay increases, promotion) or the typical negative reinforcers used to deter negative behaviors (e.g., incarceration, fines) are by themselves ineffective in stopping drug use in addicted subjects. This model suggests a multipronged therapeutic approach to addiction designed to strengthen the neuronal systems that become disrupted in addiction.

Substance abuse is a challenging health and social problem because the brain mechanisms resulting in the dependence seem to take over the will of the individual. Thus, the question becomes: Is addiction a disease, a personal weakness, or both? The following excerpts explore debates about the utility of the "brain disease" model of addiction and alternative views of addiction.

Nora D. Volkow, George F. Koob & A. Thomas McLellan
Neurobiologic Advances from the Brain Disease Model of Addiction
374 New Eng. J. Med. 363, 363-67 (2016)

In the past two decades, research has increasingly supported the view that addiction is a disease of the brain. Although the brain disease model of addiction has yielded effective preventive measures, treatment interventions, and public health policies to address substance-use disorders, the underlying concept of substance abuse as a brain disease continues to be questioned, perhaps because the aberrant, impulsive, and compulsive behaviors that are characteristic of addiction have not been clearly tied to neurobiology. . . .

 . . . After centuries of efforts to reduce addiction and its related costs by punishing addictive behaviors failed to produce adequate results, recent basic and clinical research has provided clear evidence that addiction might be better considered and treated as an acquired disease of the brain. . . . Research guided by the brain disease model of addiction has led to the development of more effective methods of prevention and treatment and to more informed public health policies. . . .

Nonetheless, despite the scientific evidence and the resulting advances in treatment and changes in policy, the concept of addiction as a disease of the brain is still being questioned. The concept of addiction as a disease of the brain challenges deeply ingrained values about self-determination and personal responsibility that frame drug use as a voluntary, hedonistic act. In this view, addiction results from the repetition of voluntary behaviors. How, then, can it be the result of a disease process? The concept of addiction as a brain disease has even more disconcerting implications for public attitudes and policies toward the addict. This concept of addiction appears to some to excuse personal irresponsibility and criminal acts instead of punishing harmful and often illegal behaviors. Additional criticisms of the concept of addiction as a brain disease include the failure of this model to identify genetic aberrations or brain abnormalities that consistently apply to persons with addiction and the failure to explain the many instances in which recovery occurs without treatment.

Advances in neurobiology have begun to clarify the mechanisms underlying the profound disruptions in decision-making ability and emotional balance displayed by persons with drug addiction. These advances also provide insight into the ways in which fundamental biologic processes, when disrupted, can alter voluntary behavioral control, not just in drug addiction but also in other, related disorders of self-regulation, such as obesity and pathologic gambling and video-gaming—the so-called behavioral addictions. . . .

. . . In persons with addiction, the impaired signaling of dopamine and glutamate in the prefrontal regions of the brain weakens their ability to resist strong urges or to follow through on decisions to stop taking the drug. These effects explain why persons with addiction can be sincere in their desire and intention to stop using a drug and yet simultaneously impulsive and unable to follow through on their resolve. Thus, altered signaling in prefrontal regulatory circuits, paired with changes in the circuitry involved in reward and emotional response, creates an imbalance that is crucial to both the gradual development of compulsive behavior in the addicted disease state and the associated inability to voluntarily reduce drugtaking behavior, despite the potentially catastrophic consequences. . . .

Wayne Hall, Adrian Carter & Cynthia Forlini

The Brain Disease Model of Addiction: Is It Supported by the Evidence and Has It Delivered on Its Promises?

2 Lancet Psychiatry 105, 108-09 (2015)

Considerable scientific value exists in the research into the neurobiology and genetics of addiction, but this research does not justify the simplified BDMA [brain disease model of addiction] that dominates discourse about addiction in the USA, and, increasingly, elsewhere. . . . Understanding of addiction, and the policies adopted to treat and prevent problem drug use, should give biology its due, but no more than it is due. . . . Economic, epidemiological, and social scientific evidence shows that the neurobiology of addiction should not be the over-riding factor when formulating policies toward drug use and addiction.

The BDMA has not helped to deliver the effective treatments for addiction that were originally promised . . . and its effect on public health policies toward drug addiction has been modest. Arguably, the advocacy of the BDMA led to overinvestment by US research agencies in biological interventions to cure addiction that will have little effect on drug addiction as a public health issue. Increased access to more effective treatment for addiction is a worthy aim that we support but this aim should not be pursued at the expense of simple, cost effective, and efficient population-based policies to discourage the whole population from smoking tobacco and drinking heavily. . . .

Our rejection of the BDMA is not intended as a defense of the moral model of addiction. We share many of the aspirations of those who advocate the BDMA, especially the delivery of more effective treatment and less punitive responses to people with addiction issues. Addiction is a complex biological, psychological, and social disorder that needs to be addressed by various clinical and public health approaches. Research into the neuroscience of addiction has provided insights into the neurobiology of decision-making, motivation, and behavioral control in addiction. Chronic use of addictive drugs can impair cognitive and motivational processes and might partly explain why some people are more susceptible than others to developing an addiction. The challenge for all addiction researchers — including neurobiologists — is to integrate emerging insights from neuroscience research with those from economics, epidemiology, sociology, psychology, and political science to decrease the harms caused by drug misuse and all forms of addiction.

Sally Satel & Scott O. Lilienfeld
Addiction and the Brain-Disease Fallacy
in *Brainwashed: The Seductive Appeal of Mindless Neuroscience* 49, 49-57 (2013)

In 1970, high-grade heroin and opium flooded Southeast Asia. . . . [N]early half of all U.S. Army enlisted men . . . had tried opium or heroin, and between 10 and 25 percent of them were addicted. . . . Fearful that the newly discharged veterans would join the ranks of junkies already bedeviling inner cities, President Richard Nixon commanded the military to begin drug testing. No one could board a plane home until he had passed a urine test. Those who failed could attend an army-sponsored detoxification program.

Operation Golden Flow . . . succeeded. As word of the new directive spread, most GIs stopped using narcotics. . . . Once they were home, heroin lost its appeal. Opiates may have helped them endure a war's alternating bouts of boredom and terror, but stateside, civilian life took precedence. The sordid drug culture, the high price of heroin, and fears of arrest discouraged use, veterans told Lee Robins, the Washington University sociologist who evaluated the testing program from 1972 to 1974. Robins' findings were startling. Only 5 percent of the men who became addicted in Vietnam relapsed within ten months after return, and just 12 percent relapsed briefly within three years. . . . The fact that addicts could quit heroin and remain drug free overturned the belief that "once an addict, always an addict."

Unfortunately, that lesson has faded into the past. By the mid-1990s, the truism "once an addict, always an addict" was back, repackaged with a new neurocentric twist: "Addiction is a chronic and relapsing brain disease." It was promoted tirelessly by . . . Alan I. Leshner, then the director of the National Institute on Drug Abuse (NIDA) . . . and is now the dominant view of addiction in the field. The brain-disease model is a staple of medical school education and drug counselor training and even appears in the antidrug lectures given to high-school students.

That may be good public relations, but it is bad public education. . . . The brain-disease model of addiction is not a trivial rebranding of an age-old human problem. It plays to the assumption that if biological roots can be identified, then a person has a "disease." And being afflicted means that the person cannot choose, control his or her life, or be held accountable. [T]raining the spotlight too intently on the workings of the addicted brain leaves the addicted person in the shadows, distracting clinicians, policy makers, and sometimes patients themselves from other powerful psychological and environmental forces that exert strong influence on them.

As one psychiatrist put it memorably, "The war on drugs is a war between the hijacked reward pathways that push the person to want to use, and the frontal lobes, which try to keep the beast at bay." Note the word "hijacked."

The familiar late-1980s slogan "This is your brain on drugs" is still with us, but now with the brain itself substituting for the fried egg. But that egg is not always sizzling. There is a surprising amount of lucid time in the daily life of addicts. In their classic 1969 study "Taking Care of Business: The Heroin User's Life on the Street," criminologists Edward Preble and John J. Casey found that addicts spend only a small fraction of their days getting high. Most of their time is spent either working or hustling. The same is true for many cocaine addicts. . . .

The paradox at the heart of addiction is this: How can the capacity for choice coexist with self-destructiveness? . . . Addicts find themselves torn between the reasons to use and reasons not to. . . . And it turns out that quitting is the rule, not the exception—a fact worth acknowledging, given that the official NIDA formulation is that "addiction is a chronic and relapsing brain disease."

. . . Researchers and medical professionals err in generalizing from the sickest subset of people to the overall population of patients. . . .

Psychiatrist Jerome Jaffe, an eminent figure in the field and the first White House adviser on drugs (the precursor of the "drug czar"), sees the adoption of the brain-disease model as both a tactical triumph and a scientific setback. "It was a useful way for particular agencies to convince Congress to raise the budgets, [and] it has been very successful," he said. . . . But Jaffe argues that the brain-disease paradigm presents "a Faustian bargain—the price that one pays is that you don't see all the other factors that interact [in addiction]." . . .

You have learned that the neurotransmitter dopamine is a central player in discussions of addiction. When the role of dopamine in reward was first conceived, only six neurotransmitters were known. Today we recognize more than 100 neurotransmitters. In spite of this and many other discovered complexities, the basic theory has not changed. You will now learn that it offers an incomplete and not completely correct explanation of addictive behaviors.

David J. Nutt et al.

The Dopamine Theory of Addiction: 40 Years of Highs and Lows

16 Nature Revs. Neurosci. 305, 306-10 (2015)

[A] prevailing view developed that that the dopamine system had a central role in addiction that was applicable to all addictive drugs. Dopamine became characterized as the 'pleasure' neurotransmitter in the human brain—that is, the one that produces reward. This model of addiction even made the cover of Time magazine and is widely quoted as a fact in current textbooks and by Wikipedia . . . .

From the beginning there were doubts about whether this theory applied to drugs other than stimulants and even whether dopamine release was central to the rewarding effects of stimulants in humans. Studies in rats showed that dopamine receptor blockade did not dampen the rewarding actions of opiates . . . . , and subsequent clinical trials revealed that blocking dopamine receptors was generally ineffective in blocking the rewarding effects of stimulants in humans or in treating human addiction (even stimulant addiction). Moreover, several studies found that opiate administration was not associated with striatal dopamine release in opiate dependence. For example, a study in individuals addicted to heroin revealed that an intravenous dose of 50 mg heroin had no effect on striatal dopamine levels, despite producing a pronounced euphoric high. . . .

Increased dopamine release has also been reported in rewarding activities such as playing computer games, practicing meditation and eating. . . . These findings have been used to 'prove' the dopamine theory of addiction because they associate rewarding activities with dopamine release and thereby generalize the model to one that proposes all rewarding activities must be mediated by dopamine release. However, these studies imaged small numbers of participants and have rarely been replicated. . . .

The dopamine theory of reward and addiction, which states that dopamine release mediates reward and thus leads to addiction, has had huge traction. However, it became accepted as a 'universal' theory without properly accounting for findings from studies in different drug addictions that did not support the theory. Tellingly, the dopamine theory has not led to any new treatments for addiction. We suggest that the role of dopamine in addiction is more complicated than the role proposed in the dopamine theory of reward. We propose that dopamine has a central role in addiction to stimulant drugs, which act directly via the dopamine system, but that it has a less important role, if any, in mediating addiction to other drugs, particularly opiates and cannabis. . . .

[T]his account of the rise and fall of the universal dopamine theory of addiction serves as a lesson in neuroscience research. Unifying theories, although intrinsically appealing, should be subject to careful scrutiny just like other theories—and perhaps even more so because they can lead the field into directions that ultimately prove to be unfruitful.

———————————

One prominent critic of the brain disease model of addiction is Dr. Carl Hart, who argues that "[t]he notion that drug addiction is a brain disease is catchy but empty: there are virtually no data in humans indicating that addiction is a disease of the brain, in the way that, for instance, Huntington's or Parkinson's are diseases of the brain." Carl L. Hart, *Viewing Addiction as a Brain Disease Promotes Social Injustice*, 1 Nature Hum. Behav. 1, 1 (2017). Hart, a professor of neuroscience and psychology at Columbia University, takes a different view on what addiction is and how it affects the brain. The excerpt below is taken from Hart's personal memoir. Hart's research provides empirical support for an alternative approach to addressing addiction known as contingency management, in which desired behaviors are rewarded and undesired behaviors are extinguished.

Carl L. Hart

High Price: A Neuroscientist's Journey of Self-Discovery That Challenges Everything You Know About Drugs and Society
322-30 (2013)

"So, are you saying that we should legalize hard drugs like cocaine, heroin, and methamphetamine?" The question was in response to the presentation that I had just given to a group of white, aging New York City hipsters. They were fairly well educated; you know, the NPR type. Some were even professionals such as neurologists, psychologists, and social workers. All had come to a basement bar in Brooklyn to hear me speak at their monthly "secret science club" meeting. . . .

And to be fair, I had just told this audience, many of whom took great pride in their critical thinking skills, that they had been hoodwinked and miseducated for much of their lives about what drugs do and don't do. I used a mountain of scientific data to call into question some of the purported damaging effects of the "hard drugs" on brain functioning. I explained that there has been an ongoing concerted effort to overstate the dangers of drugs like cocaine, heroin, and methamphetamine. The primary players in this effort are scientists, law enforcement officials, politicians, and the media.

While I acknowledged the potential for abuse and harm caused by these drugs, I emphasized that there had been extensive misinterpretation of the scientific evidence and considerable hyping of anecdotal reports. This situation, I explained, has not only wrongly stigmatized drug users and abusers; it has also led to misguided policy making. . . . Briefly, we're too afraid of these drugs and of what we think they do. Our current drug policies are based largely on fiction and misinformation. Pharmacology—or actual drug effects—plays less of a role when policies are devised. . . .

[T]o begin a serious national discussion about decriminalization, first, the public will have to be reeducated about drugs, separating the real potential dangers from monstrous or salacious fable. . . . And given how entrenched some drug myths are, one should not expect change to occur within a short period. . . .

Both the scientists who study toxicity in animals and the police who arrest users and sellers often have a limited view of the complexity of the ideas I have presented to you. No one [who] focuses only on one aspect of illicit drug use can . . . imagine all the intended and unintended consequences of continuing our current policy of treating illicit drug use primarily as a criminal issue.

The media . . . is another major source of drug misinformation . . . [that has] fanned the flames of drug hysteria. It seems as though there's a "new deadly drug" nearly every year. And invariably some police officer or politician is interviewed, warning parents about the dangers this drug poses to their children. (Of course, neither cop nor elected official should be the professional educating the public about the potential effects of drugs.) Usually, after the hysteria has subsided, we discover that the drug in question wasn't as dangerous as we were initially told. In fact, it wasn't even new. But by then the new laws have been passed and they require stiff penalties for possession and distribution of the so-called new, dangerous drug. I am not optimistic that the media will change its reporting on drugs anytime soon. . . .

Nonetheless, you should know that scientists have studied nearly all of the popular recreational drugs in people. We have learned a great deal about the conditions under which either positive or negative effects are more likely to occur. Unfortunately, this knowledge is rarely disseminated to the public, primarily because of the irrational belief that it might lead [to more] drug use. In light of the fact that there are already more than 20 million Americans[3] who use illegal drugs regularly, it seems that a rational approach—one that aims to reduce drug-related harms—would be to share what we've learned with drug users and those in positions to help keep them safe. . . .

Richard J. Bonnie
Responsibility for Addiction
30 J. Am. Acad. Psychiatry & L. 405, 406-11 (2002)

IS ADDICTION A "BRAIN DISEASE"?

The scientific leadership of the addiction field is waging a broad dissemination campaign to bring these advances to professional and public attention, within medicine, among opinion-makers, and in the general public. This campaign has a motto: "Addiction is a Brain Disease." . . .

The characterization of addiction as a brain disease has been contested. At the present time, I think this claim has to be understood more as a political statement than as a scientific proposition. To say that addiction is a brain disease is useful as a rhetorical tool in a debate about public policy; but, scientifically, it is both incomplete and premature. It is incomplete because it fails to communicate the whole story about the behavioral and contextual components of addiction. (In his standard presentation, Dr. Leshner was always careful to note that addiction is "not just a brain disease.") Behavioral components are much more substantial in addiction than in Alzheimer's disease, Parkinson's disease, or epilepsy or even in schizophrenia. It is premature, because research has not connected the observed changes in the brain to behavior. . . .

---

3. Current numbers are available through the National Survey on Drug Use and Health. According to the 2018 survey of the use of marijuana, cocaine (including crack), heroin, hallucinogens, inhalants, and methamphetamine, plus misuse of prescription stimulants, tranquilizers or sedatives, pain relievers, among those aged 12 or older, an estimated 53.2 million used illicit drugs. In other words, 1 in 5 Americans aged 12 or older used illicit drugs in the past year. The most commonly used illicit drug was marijuana (43.5M). The second most common was the misuse of prescription pain relievers (9.9M), and third was misuse of prescription tranquilizers or sedatives (6.4M). Meanwhile, 5.5M used cocaine, 1.9M used methamphetamine, and around 800,000 used heroin.

Notwithstanding its scientific shortcomings, I embrace the characterization of addiction as a brain disease because of its value as a political statement. Medicalization of addiction (as a policy choice) will have salutary effects on the lives of people enmeshed in drug use and on society, whether or not this term captures the full complexity of the condition. Addiction is amenable to treatment, although outcome evaluations of treatment must take into account the high probability of relapse, and our society should be investing more resources in treatment while reducing its expenditures on incarceration. Moreover, continued investment in research is likely to pay off in therapeutic advances (although there is likely to be no biological "fix" for addiction). . . .

The emphasis on involuntariness bristles with implication for responsibility. Medicalizing addiction and emphasizing its neurobiological underpinnings is meant to negate the common belief that addiction manifests a moral weakness or a flaw of character and thereby to counteract stigmatization and punishment. Presumably, people should not be held morally and legally accountable for behavior that is involuntary. But we should take a much closer look at these assertions. What is meant by involuntariness in this context? Is an addict's drug use involuntary after the switch is flipped? In what sense? Is relapse involuntary? In what sense? Do people voluntarily take the risk of becoming an addict when they begin to use drugs? Should this matter? These are very difficult questions, and the answers have a direct bearing on legal issues of responsibility. . . .

Addiction.   What is meant when it is said that drug use becomes involuntary after "the switch is flipped"? Does the disease cause drug use in the way that a brain lesion causes epileptic seizures or loss of cerebral blood flow causes loss of consciousness? This is the language of mechanism, and the language of choice, or voluntariness, has no place in it. Clearly, however, something more is involved with addiction than mechanism. Addiction is not just a brain disease. The link between brain and behavior is mediated through consciousness. Thus, when we say that the addict's drug use is "involuntary" and symptomatic of disease, we mean something different from what is meant when we say that having a seizure is involuntary. In terms of responsibility, this is a very important distinction. . . .

Addiction and Legal Responsibility.   . . . The law reflects a fairly strong commitment to the rule of personal responsibility for becoming addicted when one knowingly uses addictive substances; and medical use of drugs whose addictive properties are unknown can give rise to manufacturer liability. . . . There is but one possible deviation from this rule—the prospect of an industry's having liability for addicting adolescents to tobacco and alcohol. This would be the exception that reaffirms the rule—by marketing alcohol and tobacco to children and adolescents, who are unable to appreciate the consequences of their behavior (especially the grip of addiction), the manufacturers could be held liable for causing their addiction.

Responsibility for Behavior Symptomatic of Addiction.   According to the standard vocabulary, the hallmark of addiction is loss of control over drug use. I have no doubt that prolonged use of drugs is accompanied by many changes in brain function that are correlated with the experience of loss of control, but what are the implications of this phenomenon for personal responsibility, whether moral or legal? Are addicts responsible for using drugs after the switch has been flipped? If not, are they responsible for other conduct prerequisite to drug use (e.g., theft) or consequent to use (e.g., public drunkenness)? Does the brain disease formulation have a bearing on these questions? . . .

Responsibility for Relapse.   To incarcerate a severely addicted person for using drugs before detoxification and short-term withdrawal is inhumane and unwise, but what about revoking a defendant's pretrial release for failing a periodic urine screen? Or revoking an offender's probation for failing to remain dry or clean after agreeing to do so or after signing a so-called last chance agreement (LCA)? Is requiring abstinence as a condition of probation for an addict reasonable? Courts have held that it is, at least when the offender's drug use was connected to the offense. Using probation as a tool for keeping the addict engaged in treatment and for prolonging the period of abstinence seems ethically permissible because it is intended to help the addict achieve personal responsibility for managing his or her condition. To put it another way, it eschews punishment for addiction while holding the offender responsible for relapse. . . .

NOTES AND QUESTIONS

1. The concept of addiction as a brain disease was adopted by the U.S. Surgeon General in the 2016 report *Facing Addiction in America: The Surgeon General's Report on Alcohol, Drugs, and Health* ("Well-supported scientific evidence shows that addiction to alcohol or drugs is a chronic brain disease that has potential for recurrence and recovery."). But is it possible that the basic premise of the brain disease model of addiction debate itself is flawed — that framing the question in the mutually exclusive terms of *either* choice *or* disease is a fallacy? Consider the following perspective:

   > [T]he term "the hijacked brain" often appears [in recent scientific studies], along with other language that emphasizes the addict's lack of choice in the matter. Sometimes the pleasure-reward system has been "commandeered." Other times it "goes rogue." These expressions are often accompanied by the conclusion that there are "addicted brains." . . . In a hijacking situation, it is very easy to assign blame and responsibility. The villain is easy to identify. So are the victims, people who have had the bad luck to be in the wrong place at the wrong time. Hijacked people are given no choice in the matter. . . . The complexity of each person's experience with addiction should caution us to avoid false quandaries, like the one that requires us to define addiction as either disease or choice, and to adopt more nuanced conceptions. Addicts are neither hijackers nor victims. It is time to retire this analogy.

   Peg O'Connor, *The Fallacy of the "Hijacked Brain"*, N.Y. Times (June 10, 2012).
2. How would *you* define "addiction"? Would you distinguish it from "dependence"?
3. Some research suggests that addicted individuals pursue substances of abuse even in the clear presence of positive outcomes that may be foregone and negative outcomes that may occur. For human neuroimaging support for computational models of addiction, see Pearl H. Chiu, Terry M. Lohrenz & P. Read Montague, *Smokers' Brains Compute, but Ignore, a Fictive Error Signal in a Sequential Investment Task*, 11 Nature Neurosci. 514 (2008).

4. One of the changes in *DSM-5* was new labeling and categorization for substance use disorders. How do you think the words used to define a particular mental disorder matter? Consider this historical perspective on the history of *DSM:*

> During the mid-1980s a group of addiction experts organized by the American Psychiatric Association, with representation from the World Health Organization, met to revise the Diagnostic and Statistical Manual version III (DSM-III) of the substance-related disorders section. . . . [T]he committee agreed that the disorder in question was compulsive, uncontrolled, drug-seeking behaviour, and defined it by a set of criteria that produced excellent inter-rater reliability. . . . There was a significant disagreement, however, among members of the committee with respect to the label that should be used. The clinicians on the committee were in favor of calling the disorder "addiction" or "addictive disorder," but the non-clinicians argued that the word "addiction" was pejorative and would lead to alienation of the patients whom we want to help. They argued in favor of the more neutral term "dependence." . . .
>
> Clinicians, however, pointed out that the word "dependence" was already in use to mean something completely different and normal. They pointed out that "tolerance," consisting of reduced effect of a drug with repeated use, and "withdrawal symptoms" that occurred with medications given to treat pain, depression or anxiety were already labeled "dependence" and were in no way similar to the disorder of uncontrolled drug-seeking as defined in the proposed DSM-III-R. After much discussion and debate, the word "dependence" was chosen by the margin of a single vote.

Charles O'Brien, *Addiction and Dependence in DSM-V*, 106 Addiction 866, 866 (2011). How would you have voted and why?

5. *DSM-5* has been criticized by the chairman of the team that produced *DSM-IV:*

> DSM-5 has just been published—not a happy moment in the history of psychiatry or for me personally. It risks turning diagnostic inflation into hyperinflation—further cheapening the currency of psychiatric diagnosis and unleashing a wave of new false epidemics. The bad news is that . . . DMS-5 . . . will significantly add to, not correct, the already existing problems of overdiagnosis and overtreatment.
>
> The excessive DSM-5 ambition to effect a paradigm shift in psychiatric diagnosis expressed itself in three initiatives. First was the unrealistic goal of transforming psychiatric diagnosis by somehow basing it on the exciting findings of neuroscience. [B]ut the effort failed for the obvious reason that it is still a bridge too far.

Allen Frances, *Saving Normal: An Insider's Revolt Against Out-of-Control Psychiatric Diagnosis, DSM-5, Big Pharma, and the Medicalization of Ordinary Life* 170-71 (2013).

B. ADDICTION, RESPONSIBILITY, AND THE LAW

Robinson v. California
370 U.S. 660 (1962)

Justice STEWART delivered the opinion of the Court. A California statute makes it a criminal offense for a person to "be addicted to the use of narcotics." This appeal draws into question the constitutionality of that provision of the state law, as construed by the California courts in the present case.

The appellant was convicted after a jury trial in the Municipal Court of Los Angeles. The evidence against him was given by two Los Angeles police officers. Officer Brown testified that he had had occasion to examine the appellant's arms one evening on a street in Los Angeles some four months before the trial. The officer testified that at that time he had observed "scar tissue and discoloration on the inside" of the appellant's right arm, and "what appeared to be numerous needle marks and a scab which was approximately three inches below the crook of the elbow" on the appellant's left arm. The officer also testified that the appellant under questioning had admitted to the occasional use of narcotics. . . .

The appellant testified in his own behalf, denying the alleged conversations with the police officers and denying that he had ever used narcotics or been addicted to their use. He explained the marks on his arms as resulting from an allergic condition contracted during his military service. His testimony was corroborated by two witnesses.

The trial judge instructed the jury that the statute made it a misdemeanor for a person "either to use narcotics, or to be addicted to the use of narcotics. That portion of the statute referring to the 'use' of narcotics is based upon the 'act' of using. That portion of the statute referring to 'addicted to the use' of narcotics is based upon a condition or status. They are not identical. To be addicted to the use of narcotics is said to be a status or condition and not an act. It is a continuing offense and differs from most other offenses in the fact that (it) is chronic rather than acute; that it continues after it is complete and subjects the offender to arrest at any time before he reforms. The existence of such a chronic condition may be ascertained from a single examination, if the characteristic reactions of that condition be found present."

The judge further instructed the jury that the appellant could be convicted under a general verdict if the jury agreed either that he was of the "status" or had committed the "act" denounced by the statute. . . .

It would be possible to construe the statute under which the appellant was convicted as one which is operative only upon proof of the actual use of narcotics within the State's jurisdiction. But the California courts have not so construed this law. Although there was evidence in the present case that the appellant had used narcotics in Los Angeles, the jury were instructed that they could convict him even if they disbelieved that evidence. The appellant could be convicted, they were told, if they found simply that the appellant's "status" or "chronic condition" was that of being "addicted to the use of narcotics." And it is impossible to know from the jury's verdict that the defendant was not convicted upon precisely such a finding. . . .

This statute, therefore, is not one which punishes a person for the use of narcotics, for their purchase, sale or possession, or for antisocial or disorderly behavior resulting from their administration. It is not a law which even purports to provide or require medical treatment. Rather, we deal with a statute which makes the "status" of narcotic addiction a criminal offense, for which the offender may be prosecuted "at any time before he reforms." California has said that a person can be continuously guilty of this offense, whether or not he has ever used or possessed any narcotics within the State, and whether or not he has been guilty of any antisocial behavior there.

It is unlikely that any State at this moment in history would attempt to make it a criminal offense for a person to be mentally ill, or a leper, or to be afflicted with a venereal disease. A State might determine that the general health and welfare require that the victims of these and other human afflictions be dealt with by compulsory treatment, involving quarantine, confinement, or sequestration. But, in the light of contemporary human knowledge, a law which made a criminal offense of such a disease would doubtless be universally thought to be an infliction of cruel and unusual punishment in violation of the Eighth and Fourteenth Amendments.

We cannot but consider the statute before us as of the same category. In this Court counsel for the State recognized that narcotic addiction is an illness. Indeed, it is apparently an illness which may be contracted innocently or involuntarily. We hold that a state law which imprisons a person thus afflicted as a criminal, even though he has never touched any narcotic drug within the State or been guilty of any irregular behavior there, inflicts a cruel and unusual punishment in violation of the Fourteenth Amendment. To be sure, imprisonment for ninety days is not, in the abstract, a punishment which is either cruel or unusual. But the question cannot be considered in the abstract. Even one day in prison would be a cruel and unusual punishment for the "crime" of having a common cold.

We are not unmindful that the vicious evils of the narcotics traffic have occasioned the grave concern of government. There are, as we have said, countless fronts on which those evils may be legitimately attacked. We deal in this case only with an individual provision of a particularized local law as it has so far been interpreted by the California courts.

Reversed.

Justice DOUGLAS, concurring. While I join the Court's opinion, I wish to make more explicit the reasons why I think it is "cruel and unusual" punishment in the sense of the Eighth Amendment to treat as a criminal a person who is a drug addict.

In Sixteenth Century England one prescription for insanity was to beat the subject "until he had regained his reason." In America "the violently insane went to the whipping post and into prison dungeons or, as sometimes happened, were burned at the stake or hanged"; and "the pauper insane often roamed the countryside as wild men and from time to time were pilloried, whipped, and jailed."

As stated by Dr. Isaac Ray many years ago:

> "Nothing can more strongly illustrate the popular ignorance respecting insanity than the proposition, equally objectionable in its humanity and its logic, that the insane should be punished for criminal acts, in order to deter other insane persons from doing the same thing." Treatise on the Medical Jurisprudence of Insanity (5th ed. 1871), p. 56.

Today we have our differences over the legal definition of insanity. But however insanity is defined, it is in end effect treated as a disease. While afflicted people may be confined either for treatment or for the protection of society, they are not branded as criminals. . . .

The impact that an addict has on a community causes alarm and often leads to punitive measures. Those measures are justified when they relate to acts of transgression. But I do not see how under our system being an addict can be punished as a crime. If addicts can be punished for their addiction, then the insane can also be punished for their insanity. Each has a disease and each must be treated as a sick person. . . .

[The addict] may, of course, be confined for treatment or for the protection of society. Cruel and unusual punishment results not from confinement, but from convicting the addict of a crime. . . . A prosecution for addiction, with its resulting stigma and irreparable damage to the good name of the accused, cannot be justified as a means of protecting society, where a civil commitment would do as well. . . . This prosecution has no relationship to the curing of an illness. Indeed, it cannot, for the prosecution is aimed at penalizing an illness, rather than at providing medical care for it. We would forget the teachings of the Eighth Amendment if we allowed sickness to be made a crime and permitted sick people to be punished for being sick. This age of enlightenment cannot tolerate such barbarous action.

Powell v. Texas
392 U.S. 514 (1968)

Justice MARSHALL announced the judgment of the Court and delivered an opinion in which THE CHIEF JUSTICE, Justice BLACK, and Justice HARLAN join. In late December 1966, appellant was arrested and charged with being found in a state of intoxication in a public place, in violation of Vernon's Ann. Texas Penal Code, Art. 477 (1952), which reads as follows:

"Whoever shall get drunk or be found in a state of intoxication in any public place, or at any private house except his own, shall be fined not exceeding one hundred dollars."

Appellant was tried in the Corporation Court of Austin, Texas, found guilty, and fined $20. . . .

Appellant testified concerning the history of his drinking problem. He reviewed his many arrests for drunkenness; testified that he was unable to stop drinking; stated that when he was intoxicated he had no control over his actions and could not remember them later, but that he did not become violent; and admitted that he did not remember his arrest on the occasion for which he was being tried. On cross-examination, appellant admitted that he had had one drink on the morning of the trial and had been able to discontinue drinking. In relevant part, the cross-examination went as follows:

Q: You took that one at eight o'clock because you wanted to drink?
A: Yes, sir.
Q: And you knew that if you drank it, you could keep on drinking and get drunk?
A: Well, I was supposed to be here on trial, and I didn't take but that one drink.
Q: You knew you had to be here this afternoon, but this morning you took one drink and then you knew that you couldn't afford to drink any more and come to court; is that right?
A: Yes, sir, that's right.
Q: So you exercised your will power and kept from drinking anything today except that one drink?
A: Yes, sir, that's right.
Q: Because you knew what you would do if you kept drinking that you would finally pass out or be picked up?
A: Yes, sir.
Q: And you didn't want that to happen to you today?

A: No, sir.
Q: Not today?
A: No, sir.
Q: So you only had one drink today?
A: Yes, sir.

On redirect examination, appellant's lawyer elicited the following:

Q: Leroy, isn't the real reason why you just had one drink today because you just had enough money to buy one drink?
A: Well, that was just give to me.
Q: In other words, you didn't have any money with which you could buy any drinks yourself?
A: No, sir, that was give to me.
Q: And that's really what controlled the amount you drank this morning, isn't it?
A: Yes, sir.
Q: Leroy, when you start drinking, do you have any control over how many drinks you can take?
A: No, sir.

. . . [T]here is no agreement among members of the medical profession about what it means to say that "alcoholism" is a "disease." One of the principal works in this field states that the major difficulty in articulating a "disease concept of alcoholism" is that "alcoholism has too many definitions and disease has practically none." This same author concludes that "a disease is what the medical profession recognizes as such." In other words, there is widespread agreement today that "alcoholism" is a "disease," for the simple reason that the medical profession has concluded that it should attempt to treat those who have drinking problems. There the agreement stops. Debate rages within the medical profession as to whether "alcoholism" is a separate "disease" in any meaningful biochemical, physiological or psychological sense, or whether it represents one peculiar manifestation in some individuals of underlying psychiatric disorder.

Nor is there any substantial consensus as to the "manifestations of alcoholism." . . . .

Dr. Wade did testify that once appellant began drinking he appeared to have no control over the amount of alcohol he finally ingested. Appellant's own testimony concerning his drinking on the day of the trial would certainly appear, however, to cast doubt upon the conclusion that he was without control over his consumption of alcohol when he had sufficiently important reasons to exercise such control. However that may be, there are more serious factual and conceptual difficulties with reading this record to show that appellant was unable to abstain from drinking. Dr. Wade testified that when appellant was sober, the act of taking the first drink was a "voluntary exercise of his will," but that this exercise of will was undertaken under the "exceedingly strong influence" of a "compulsion" which was "not completely overpowering." Such concepts, when juxtaposed in this fashion, have little meaning. . . .

There is as yet no known generally effective method for treating the vast number of alcoholics in our society. Some individual alcoholics have responded to particular forms of therapy with remissions of their symptomatic dependence upon the drug.

But just as there is no agreement among doctors and social workers with respect to the causes of alcoholism, there is no consensus as to why particular treatments have been effective in particular cases and there is no generally agreed-upon approach to the problem of treatment on a large scale. Most psychiatrists are apparently of the opinion that alcoholism is far more difficult to treat than other forms of behavioral disorders, and some believe it is impossible to cure by means of psychotherapy; indeed, the medical profession as a whole, and psychiatrists in particular, have been severely criticized for the prevailing reluctance to undertake the treatment of drinking problems. Thus it is entirely possible that, even were the manpower and facilities available for a full-scale attack upon chronic alcoholism, we would find ourselves unable to help the vast bulk of our "visible"—let alone our "invisible"-alcoholic population.

However, facilities for the attempted treatment of indigent alcoholics are woefully lacking throughout the country. It would be tragic to return large numbers of helpless, sometimes dangerous and frequently unsanitary inebriates to the streets of our cities without even the opportunity to sober up adequately which a brief jail term provides. Presumably no State or city will tolerate such a state of affairs. Yet the medical profession cannot, and does not, tell us with any assurance that, even if the buildings, equipment and trained personnel were made available, it could provide anything more than slightly higher-class jails for our indigent habitual inebriates. Thus we run the grave risk that nothing will be accomplished beyond the hanging of a new sign-reading "hospital"—over one wing of the jailhouse. . . .

Appellant claims that his conviction on the facts of this case would violate the Cruel and Unusual Punishment Clause of the Eighth Amendment as applied to the States through the Fourteenth Amendment. The primary purpose of that clause has always been considered, and properly so, to be directed at the method or kind of punishment imposed for the violation of criminal statutes; the nature of the conduct made criminal is ordinarily relevant only to the fitness of the punishment imposed.

Appellant, however, seeks to come within the application of the Cruel and Unusual Punishment Clause announced in *Robinson v. State of California* (1962), which involved a state statute making it a crime to "be addicted to the use of narcotics." This Court held there that "a state law which imprisons a person thus afflicted (with narcotic addiction) as a criminal, even though he has never touched any narcotic drug within the State or been guilty of any irregular behavior there, inflicts a cruel and unusual punishment."

On its face the present case does not fall within that holding, since appellant was convicted, not for being a chronic alcoholic, but for being in public while drunk on a particular occasion. The State of Texas thus has not sought to punish a mere status, as California did in *Robinson*; nor has it attempted to regulate appellant's behavior in the privacy of his own home. Rather, it has imposed upon appellant a criminal sanction for public behavior which may create substantial health and safety hazards, both for appellant and for members of the general public, and which offends the moral and esthetic sensibilities of a large segment of the community. This seems a far cry from convicting one for being an addict, being a chronic alcoholic, being "mentally ill, or a leper."

Robinson so viewed brings this Court but a very small way into the substantive criminal law. And unless *Robinson* is so viewed it is difficult to see any limiting principle that would serve to prevent this Court from becoming, under the aegis of the Cruel and Unusual Punishment Clause, the ultimate arbiter of the standards of criminal responsibility, in diverse areas of the criminal law, throughout the country.

It is suggested in dissent that *Robinson* stands for the "simple" but "subtle" principle that "[c]riminal penalties may not be inflicted upon a person for being in a condition he is powerless to change." In that view, appellant's "condition" of public intoxication was "occasioned by a compulsion symptomatic of the disease" of chronic alcoholism, and thus, apparently, his behavior lacked the critical element of mens rea. Whatever may be the merits of such a doctrine of criminal responsibility, it surely cannot be said to follow from *Robinson*. The entire thrust of *Robinson*'s interpretation of the Cruel and Unusual Punishment Clause is that criminal penalties may be inflicted only if the accused has committed some act, has engaged in some behavior, which society has an interest in preventing, or perhaps in historical common law terms, has committed some *actus reus*. It thus does not deal with the question of whether certain conduct cannot constitutionally be punished because it is, in some sense, "involuntary" or "occasioned by a compulsion." . . .

Ultimately, then, the most troubling aspects of this case, were *Robinson* to be extended to meet it, would be the scope and content of what could only be a constitutional doctrine of criminal responsibility. In dissent it is urged that the decision could be limited to conduct which is "a characteristic and involuntary part of the pattern of the disease as it afflicts" the particular individual, and that "(i)t is not foreseeable" that it would be applied "in the case of offenses such as driving a car while intoxicated, assault, theft, or robbery." That is limitation by fiat. In the first place, nothing in the logic of the dissent would limit its application to chronic alcoholics. If Leroy Powell cannot be convicted of public intoxication, it is difficult to see how a State can convict an individual for murder, if that individual, while exhibiting normal behavior in all other respects, suffers from a "compulsion" to kill, which is an "exceedingly strong influence," but "not completely overpowering." Even if we limit our consideration to chronic alcoholics, it would seem impossible to confine the principle within the arbitrary bounds which the dissent seems to envision.

It is not difficult to imagine a case involving psychiatric testimony to the effect that an individual suffers from some aggressive neurosis which he is able to control when sober; that very little alcohol suffices to remove the inhibitions which normally contain these aggressions, with the result that the individual engages in assaultive behavior without becoming actually intoxicated; and that the individual suffers from a very strong desire to drink, which is an "exceedingly strong influence" but "not completely overpowering." Without being untrue to the rationale of this case, should the principles advanced in dissent be accepted here, the Court could not avoid holding such an individual constitutionally unaccountable for his assaultive behavior.

Traditional common-law concepts of personal accountability and essential considerations of federalism lead us to disagree with appellant. We are unable to conclude, on the state of this record or on the current state of medical knowledge, that chronic alcoholics in general, and Leroy Powell in particular, suffer from such an irresistible compulsion to drink and to get drunk in public that they are utterly unable to control their performance of either or both of these acts and thus cannot be deterred at all from public intoxication. And in any event this Court has never articulated a general constitutional doctrine of mens rea.

We cannot cast aside the centuries-long evolution of the collection of inter-
locking and overlapping concepts which the common law has utilized to assess the
moral accountability of an individual for his antisocial deeds. The doctrines of *actus
reus*, *mens rea*, insanity, mistake, justification, and duress have historically provided
the tools for a constantly shifting adjustment of the tension between the evolving
aims of the criminal law and changing religious, moral, philosophical, and medical
views of the nature of man. This process of adjustment has always been thought to
be the province of the States. . . .

Affirmed.

Justice FORTAS, with whom Justice DOUGLAS, Justice BRENNAN, and Justice STEWART
join, dissenting. . . . The issue posed in this case is a narrow one. There is no challenge here to the validity of public intoxication statutes in general or to the Texas
public intoxication statute in particular. This case does not concern the infliction
of punishment upon the "social" drinker—or upon anyone other than a "chronic
alcoholic" who, as the trier of fact here found, cannot "resist the constant, excessive
consumption of alcohol." Nor does it relate to any offense other than the crime of
public intoxication.

The sole question presented is whether a criminal penalty may be imposed upon
a person suffering the disease of "chronic alcoholism" for a condition—being "in
a state of intoxication" in public-which is a characteristic part of the pattern of his
disease and which, the trial court found, was not the consequence of appellant's
volition but of "a compulsion symptomatic of the disease of chronic alcoholism."
We must consider whether the Eighth Amendment, made applicable to the States
through the Fourteenth Amendment, prohibits the imposition of this penalty in
these rather special circumstances as "cruel and unusual punishment." This case
does not raise any question as to the right of the police to stop and detain those who
are intoxicated in public, whether as a result of the disease or otherwise; or as to the
State's power to commit chronic alcoholics for treatment. Nor does it concern the
responsibility of an alcoholic for criminal acts. We deal here with the mere condition of being intoxicated in public. . . .

Robinson stands upon a principle which, despite its subtlety, must be simply
stated and respectfully applied because it is the foundation of individual liberty and
the cornerstone of the relations between a civilized state and its citizens: Criminal
penalties may not be inflicted upon a person for being in a condition he is powerless to change. In all probability, Robinson at some time before his conviction
elected to take narcotics. But the crime as defined did not punish this conduct.
The statute imposed a penalty for the offense of "addiction"—a condition which
Robinson could not control. Once Robinson had become an addict, he was utterly
powerless to avoid criminal guilt. He was powerless to choose not to violate the
law. . . .

NOTES AND QUESTIONS

1. Would it be fair, or not, to say that the effect of the statute in *Robinson* was to
   authorize criminal punishment for a bare desire to commit a criminal act? See
   Justice Harlan's concurrence.

2. In *Robinson*, the U.S. Supreme Court evaluated the constitutionality of a statute that criminalized the "status of narcotic addiction." In *Powell*, the court evaluated the constitutionality of a statute that criminalized the "state of intoxication." How can these two cases be best distinguished?

3. If *Powell* had been decided differently, would it necessarily mean that addiction would serve as an excuse for all crimes? Philosopher Gideon Yaffe argues that addicts "deserve a bigger break for crimes like Leroy Powell's than they do for crimes like stealing to gain money to buy drugs. . . . [This] should provide solace to some who fear that were the law to give a break to addicts for crimes such as public intoxication, they would also need to be given breaks for crimes such as theft and assault, which seems to some a bridge too far." For discussion of how Yaffe draws the line, see Gideon Yaffe, *Compromised Addicts*, in *Oxford Studies in Agency and Responsibility Volume 5: Themes from the Philosophy of Gary Watson* 191 (D. Justin Coates & Neal A. Tognazzini eds., 2019). Would you draw a line as Yaffe suggests, and if so, how?

4. A petitioner before an immigration judge may apply for cancellation of removal, which requires that a person be "of good moral character." Under relevant immigration laws, "[n]o person shall be regarded as . . . a person of good moral character who . . . is, or was . . . a habitual drunkard[.]" 8 U.S.C. §1101(f)(1) (2018). Can you think of any constitutional challenges to this statute? In *Ledezma-Cosino v. Sessions*, the Ninth Circuit held that the "habitual drunkard" provision does not violate equal protection rights. 857 F.3d 1042 (9th Cir. 2017). The petitioner, a construction worker who entered the United States from Mexico in 1987, argued that it was irrational to classify habitual drunks as lacking good moral character. The court disagreed: "Because the denial of cancellation of removal to habitual drunkards is rationally related to the legitimate governmental interest in public safety, Petitioner's equal protection argument fails." *Id.* at 1049.

5. In his dissent in *Powell*, Justice Fortas articulated that "[c]riminal penalties may not be inflicted upon a person for being in a condition he is powerless to change." Part of Justice Fortas's view touches on impulse control — the ability for a person to prevent himself from acting on a desire. How should courts treat someone with *impaired* impulse control? Consider that researchers investigating the effects of long-term drug addiction have shown that chronic drug abuse can lead to impaired executive functioning. *See* Robert D. Rogers & Trevor W. Robbins, *Investigating the Neurocognitive Deficits Associated with Chronic Drug Misuse*, 11 Current Opinion Neurobiology 250 (2001). In one research paradigm, the "IOWA gambling task," participants with chronic substance disorders frequently make more risky and maladaptive choices than do control participants. Danielle Barry & Nancy M. Petry, *Predictors of Decision-Making on the Iowa Gambling Task: Independent Effects of Lifetime History of Substance Use Disorders and Performance on the Trail Making Test*, 66 Brain & Cognition 243 (2008). In the task, participants are presented with four decks of cards and asked to select a card. Each card provides an award or punishment value. Importantly, each deck of cards has a different reward schedule. Some decks offer high initial rewards but also high punishments, and thus they are disadvantageous over the long run. Other decks offer small initial rewards but also small punishments, and thus they are advantageous over the long run. The experiment is generally stopped after the participant has selected 100 cards. Researchers found that while healthy

control participants are good at navigating to the low risk, "good" decks, participants with substance use disorders are not. Rather, they more frequently choose cards from high-risk, "bad" decks. They thereby incur greater losses over time than control participants. What implications, if any, should this research have on responsibility in law? If individuals with substance abuse disorder frequently make riskier decisions, should the law treat them differently?

6. Should courts recognize addiction as a factor in reducing criminal culpability? Here's one court's response:

> [W]e decline to adopt a general rule of law which absolves one from responsibility for criminal conduct based solely on the consequences of the voluntary use of drugs. Consequently, even if medical experts may undertake to characterize drug addiction in medical terms as a mental disease or defect, we reject drug addiction alone as qualifying as a mental disease or defect for the purpose of applying the [Massachusetts insanity test].
>
> The essential consideration is not whether the medical profession characterizes drug addiction as a mental disease or defect but rather whether our society should relieve from criminal responsibility a drug addict who at the time of the commission of the crime was unable to conform his conduct to the requirements of law because of his addiction. . . .
>
> . . . If the defendant's lack of substantial capacity to appreciate the wrongfulness of his conduct or to conform his conduct to the requirements of law is solely the product of his voluntary consumption of drugs, he does not meet the [insanity] test, even if he has a mental disease or defect. . . .
>
> . . . In addition, we reject drug addiction alone as an adequate justification for finding that a defendant's consumption of drugs was involuntary and thus his conduct somehow excusable. . . . We suspect that knowledge of the consequences of drug consumption on human behavior has not yet reached its full potential, and it is clear that, in many aspects, medical views differ. . . .

Commonwealth v. Sheehan, 376 Mass. 765, 767-771 (1978). Based on the reasoning in this decision, what—if any—new medical knowledge would or should change its approach to addiction and criminal responsibility?

Robinson and *Powell* remain the most important Supreme Court statements on addiction and responsibility in American law. But new constitutional challenges, invoking neuroscience, are beginning to appear. The first set of excerpts below follow the case of Julie Eldred, who made such an argument in 2018 in Massachusetts. You will first read two opposing amicus briefs, followed by the decision of the Massachusetts Supreme Judicial Court. We then consider *sentencing* and addiction. Should addiction always (or ever) be grounds for a reduced sentence? And what role does neuroscience play in answering that question? *United States v. Hendrickson* (2014) explores these questions.

Amicus Curiae Brief of the American Civil Liberties Union of Massachusetts, Inc. et al. in Support of the Petitioner at 1-3
Commonwealth v. Eldred, 101 N.E.3d 911 (Mass. 2018) (No. SJC-12279)

The question in this case is whether to allow the judiciary's power over probation to be used to jail addicted individuals on the grounds that they have relapsed. . . .

[A] probation officer requested and a judge ordered Julie Eldred to be sent to jail after she tested positive for fentanyl. It is undisputed that Ms. Eldred suffers from substance use disorder. And it is equally undisputed that countless others who suffer from this disease will continue to face the threat of imprisonment if trial courts are permitted to impose a condition of probation that requires them to remain drug free.

For two reasons, this Court should disallow that condition in cases involving addiction. First, it is contrary to this Court's precedents, which protect probationers from being saddled with conditions that they cannot reasonably be expected to achieve. This Court held in Commonwealth v. Henry that an individual cannot be required to pay a restitution amount that she cannot afford. It has also held that a homeless person who lacked access to the necessary electrical outlet could not therefore be found to have violated a condition of his probation requiring electronic monitoring.

The reasoning of those cases controls here. Because addicted individuals cannot reasonably be expected to remain drug free, they may not be required to do so as a condition of probation.

Second, even if precedent did not resolve this case, this Court should use its superintendence power to prohibit requiring addicted probationers to remain drug free, because imposing that condition is dangerous and unjust. Probation is a judicial function, and this Court may exercise its supervisory power to ensure that it is not used unjustly.

That intervention is warranted here because allowing courts to require that individuals suffering from addiction remain drug free—however well-intentioned—harms both probationers and the integrity of the justice system. It predictably leads to the imprisonment of untold numbers of addicted individuals simply because they stumble on their road to recovery. It interrupts their treatment and imperils lives. It also creates disparate impacts on poor communities and people of color, and contributes to the worst excesses of the ill-fated War on Drugs.

The Commonwealth seeks a contrary result. It argues that courts may require Ms. Eldred and other individuals who suffer from addiction to remain drug free as a condition of their probation, and may revoke their probation and imprison them if they relapse. It reasons that addiction does not "completely eliminate[]" someone's ability to choose not to use drugs. Two amicus briefs supporting the Commonwealth's position also contend that people with addiction retain the ability to make choices, and may be punished with a revocation of probation when they use drugs. But the existence of some degree of "choice" does not make it just for the courts to create and administer a regime that routinely cages people for failing to resoundingly defeat a disease.

More fundamentally, the metaphysics of the free will and choices made by people suffering from addiction is not the issue here. The primary question here is what choice this Court will make about the lives of addicted individuals. It can choose the path that will incarcerate many of them, interrupt their treatment, and endanger their lives. It is the path the compounds inequality and makes probation an instrument of the War on Drugs. Or it can strike a different course, preventing probation from being used to imprison addicted individuals for drug use. That is the path that will prevent injustice and save lives.

Brief of Amici Curiae of 11 Addiction Experts in Support of Appellee at 30-39

Commonwealth v. Eldred, 101 N.E.3d 911 (Mass. 2018) (No. SJC-12279)

The basis of the probationer's claim is that she cannot fairly be expected to refrain from using drugs as a condition of probation because she cannot control her drug use and therefore is not responsible for it. . . . [W]e consider the implications of the view that the addict is not responsible for her use of drugs.

Let us begin with the effect on probation and parole. Staying drug-free is a universal condition of criminal justice supervision. Not only is possession of controlled substances a crime in itself in all jurisdictions, it is well-known that for many reasons, including feeding their habit, addicts often commit other crimes related to the addiction. If addicts cannot be sanctioned for violating this condition of probation and parole, the state will lose this powerful contingency management technique for assisting addicts to remain free of drugs and for protecting society. The threat of being incarcerated or re-incarcerated or sanctioned in some way gives the addict an extremely powerful incentive to stay clean. It will not always be successful, but. . . . it decreases the rate of violations markedly, an outcome the elasticity of demand for addictive substances predicts. . . .

What would be the effect of losing this tool on sentencing judges and parole authorities? The inability to impose sanctions will almost certainly increase recidivism substantially. Many judges and parole authorities who are conscious of their duty to protect society would hesitate before granting probation or parole that might otherwise give people a chance to live a productive life in freedom. In an age in which our society is criticized for too much incarceration, this would be an unfortunate outcome. Paradoxically, if judges no longer granted probation or parole and incarceration took its place, this might serve as a deterrent to possession because the "cost" of this crime would increase, but we doubt it. In any case, arguing against probation or parole without the condition of staying drug-free (and, indirectly for incarceration as a deterrent) would be an odd position for supporters of the probationer to take because their argument in her favor currently rests on the claim, in effect, that addicts cannot be deterred. Diversion programs would be imperiled, if not crippled. Various types of diversion programs for nonviolent crimes, including specialty drug or mental health courts, depend for their success on the contingency management tool of making staying clean a condition of successfully completing the program with all the benefits that accrue. If the probationer's petition is granted, it entails that virtually no diverted addict could succeed. The rationale for these worthy programs would evaporate. Can the effect of holding that probationers are not responsible for violating the condition of drug abstinence be limited to the context of probation and parole? There is no principled argument for so cabining the holding. . . .

This case raises important questions about principles of behavior, criminal responsibility, and the sound and fair administration of criminal justice. The probationer claims that she should not be held accountable for her failure to "remain drug free" as a condition of her probation because she suffers from addiction, or substance use disorder [SUD], wherein her continued use of substances despite negative consequences is a sign of that disorder. Her claim is flawed in a number of ways. As a straightforward matter of definition, we note that nowhere in the Diagnostic and Statistical Manual of the American Psychiatric Association, the most widely used taxonomy of psychiatric disorders, is drug use in the context of SUD regarded as a behavior completely beyond the control of the addicted user. More substantively, the core of her argument, which depends largely on the implications of the brain-disease model of addiction—namely, that the brain changes associated with addiction render the addict incapable of behavioral control—is demonstrably untrue. The mere association of drug taking with expected neurobiological changes in the brain is not evidence that drug use is beyond control. This is abundantly evident from the large volume of data demonstrating that addiction is a set of behaviors whose course can be altered by foreseeable consequences. The same cannot be said of conventional brain diseases such as Alzheimer's or multiple sclerosis.

In sum, the best scientific and clinical data are strongly at odds with the view that addicts are unable to choose not to use substances. We believe that a decision in favor of the probationer could have significant, even devastating, implications for the future of treatment-based approaches to criminal justice as well as for criminal responsibility more generally. We conclude that the probationer's claim should be denied because it is based on erroneous, refuted scientific premises and will have negative consequences if it is accepted.

Commonwealth v. Eldred
101 N.E.3d 911 (Mass. 2018)

LOWY, J. Following a probation violation hearing, a judge in the District Court found that the defendant, Julie A. Eldred, had tested positive for fentanyl, in violation of a condition of her probation requiring her to abstain from using illegal drugs. The judge ordered that the conditions of her probation be modified to require her to submit to inpatient treatment for drug addiction. The defendant appeals from that finding and disposition. The judge also reported a question drafted by the defendant concerning whether the imposition of a "drug free" condition of probation, such as appeared in the original terms of defendant's probation, is permissible for an individual who is addicted to drugs and whether that person can be subject to probation violation proceedings for subsequently testing positive for illegal drugs.

We conclude that, in appropriate circumstances, a judge may order a defendant who is addicted to drugs to remain drug free as a condition of probation, and that a defendant may be found to be in violation of his or her probation by subsequently testing positive for an illegal drug. Accordingly, we affirm the finding that the defendant violated her probation and the order requiring her to submit to inpatient treatment for her addiction.

BACKGROUND AND PRIOR PROCEEDINGS

On July 18, 2016, the defendant was arraigned on a felony charge of larceny for stealing jewelry valued over $250. . . . The defendant admitted to the police that she had stolen the jewelry and had sold it to obtain money to support her heroin addiction. . . . A judge in the District Court continued the defendant's case without a finding, and imposed a one-year term of probation with special conditions related to her substance abuse that included requiring her to remain drug free, submit to random drug screens, and attend outpatient substance abuse treatment three times each week. Prior to accepting the terms of her probation, the defendant did not object to the condition that she remain drug free, or otherwise express that her diagnosis of substance use disorder (SUD) rendered her incapable of remaining drug free.

On August 29, 2016, the defendant began outpatient addiction treatment at a hospital. As a component of her treatment, an addiction specialist prescribed the defendant a medication that is used to treat symptoms of withdrawal and addiction to opiates.

On September 2, 2016, only eleven days after the case had been continued without a finding and the probation had been imposed, the defendant tested positive for fentanyl, following a random drug test administered by her probation officer. . . . Despite conceding [at her probation violation hearing] that she had used fentanyl, the defendant contested that she had violated the terms of her probation. The defendant argued, for the first time, that she had been diagnosed with SUD, which rendered her incapable of remaining drug free. In the defendant's view, her use of drugs could not constitute a wilful violation of her probationary condition to remain drug free. She submitted several affidavits from experts in support of her claim; however, no expert testimony was offered at the hearing to opine on SUD or its potential effects on the brain. . . .

The judge determined that the defendant had violated the drug free condition of her probation by testing positive for fentanyl. The defendant filed a motion to vacate the condition of probation requiring her to stay drug free, arguing that the condition violated various State and Federal constitutional rights. That motion was denied. . . . We granted the defendant's motion for direct appellate review.

DISCUSSION

1. The Reported Question

. . . "Where a person who committed a crime is addicted to illegal drugs, may a judge require that person to abstain from using illegal drugs as a condition of probation? If that person violates the 'drug free' condition by using illegal drugs while on probation, can that person be subject to probation revocation proceedings? Additionally, at a detention hearing, if there is probable cause to believe that a person with a 'drug free' condition of probation has violated that condition by using an illegal drug, may that person be held in custody while awaiting admission into an inpatient treatment facility, pending a probation violation hearing?"

. . . [G]iven relevant statutes, and court rules and policies, coupled with the goals of probation, we answer each portion of the . . . question in the affirmative.

The circumstances of the defendant's case exemplify why the imposition of a drug free condition of probation and the enforcement of such a condition are permissible within the confines of the probation process. From crafting special conditions of probation to determining the appropriate disposition for a defendant who has violated one of those conditions, judges should act with flexibility, sensitivity, and compassion when dealing with people who suffer from drug addiction. The rehabilitative goals of probation, coupled with the judge's dispositional flexibility at each stage of the process, enable and require judges to consider the unique circumstances facing each person they encounter—including whether that person suffers from drug addiction. This individualized approach to probation fosters an environment that enables and encourages recovery, while recognizing that relapse is part of recovery.

2. Probation

a. Disposition

As an alternative or supplement to incarceration, probation is "a legal disposition which allows a criminal offender to remain in the community subject to certain conditions and under the supervision of the court." *Commonwealth v. Durling*, 407 Mass. 108, 111, 551 N.E.2d 1193 (1990). The primary goals of probation are two-fold: rehabilitation of the defendant and protection of the public from the defendant's potential recidivism. . . .

Here, the defendant pleaded guilty to larceny and admitted that her drug use motivated her to commit the crime. The sentencing judge imposed the special conditions that the defendant remain drug free, continue outpatient drug treatment, and submit to random drug screens. The conditions directly addressed the defendant's personal circumstances and, significantly, her stated motivation for committing the crime — purchasing illegal drugs. Not only were these conditions tailored to the characteristics of the defendant and the underlying crime, they furthered the rehabilitative goal of probation by facilitating treatment for the defendant's drug addiction. These conditions also furthered the goal of protecting the public, because each condition addressed the fact that the defendant's drug use motivated her to commit the crime. . . .

The defendant argues that because she suffers from SUD, requiring her to remain drug free sets her up for unconstitutional cruel and unusual punishment when the inevitable relapse occurs. As discussed, revoking or modifying conditions of probation is not a punishment for drug use but for the underlying crime. We also agree with the Commonwealth that the defendant's claim of SUD rests on science that was not tested below. Nor do we agree with the defendant that the requirement of remaining drug free is an outdated moral judgment about an individual's addiction. Rather, . . . the requirement is based on the judge's consideration of the defendant's circumstances and that she committed the underlying crime to support her drug use.

The judge here did not abuse her discretion by imposing the special condition of probation requiring the defendant to remain drug free.

b. Probation Violation Proceedings.

i. Detention hearing. . . .

Trial court judges, particularly judges in the drug courts, stand on the front lines of the opioid epidemic. . . . [J]udges must have the authority to detain a defendant facing a probation violation based on illicit drug use pending a final violation hearing for the safety of the defendant and the community. Such decisions should be made thoughtfully and carefully, recognizing that addiction is a status that may not be criminalized. But judges cannot ignore the fact that relapse is dangerous for the person who may be in the throes of addiction and, often times, for the community in which that person lives.

Here, on the Friday before the Labor Day weekend, the defendant tested positive for fentanyl. After the defendant rejected inpatient treatment, and with her home support network unavailable, the defendant's probation officer initiated the probation violation proceedings and moved for a detention hearing that day. At that hearing, the judge determined that there was probable cause to believe the defendant had violated the drug free condition of her probation, based on the results of the drug test. The judge first sought to have the defendant admitted to an inpatient treatment facility pending her final violation hearing; however, a placement was not immediately available. To stabilize the defendant's situation, the judge held her in custody until a placement at an inpatient treatment facility became available. . . . The judge was faced with either releasing the defendant and risking that she would suffer an overdose and die, or holding her in custody until a placement at an inpatient treatment facility became available.

The defendant claims that the judge's decision to detain her constituted a punishment for her relapse and positive drug test. We do not agree. . . .

ii. Probation violation hearing. . . .

The defendant contends that the District Court judge erred in finding that she violated the drug free condition of her probation because the violation was not wilful. In the defendant's view, her purported inability to refrain from using drugs is tantamount to a homeless probationer not being able to comply with a condition of probation because of the circumstances inherent in that homelessness. In *Canadyan*, we concluded that the defendant did not commit a wilful violation of probation for failing to wear an operable global positioning system (GPS) monitoring device because the evidence conclusively established that the defendant was homeless and that the homeless shelter he was staying at could not accommodate the technological requirements of the GPS equipment. Therefore, "there was no evidence of wilful noncompliance." Although the appellate record before this court is inadequate to determine whether SUD affects the brain in such a way that certain individuals cannot control their drug use, based on the evidence presented to the judge who conducted the violation hearing, that judge did not abuse her discretion in concluding that there was a wilful violation of the defendant's drug free probationary condition. . . .

CONCLUSION

We conclude that, based on the evidence presented at each stage of the probation process and for the reasons described above, the judge did not abuse her discretion in concluding the defendant violated her probation. We further answer the reported question, as we have reframed it, in the affirmative: (1) where a person who commits a crime is addicted to illegal drugs, a judge may require that person to remain drug free as a condition of probation; (2) a person may be subject to probation violation proceedings for violating the drug free condition of probation by subsequently testing positive for illegal drugs; and (3) in the appropriate circumstances, a judge has discretion at a detention hearing to hold the defendant, who has tested positive for illegal drugs in violation of the drug free condition of probation, pending a probation violation hearing. . . .

You've been primed on several perspectives on the brain disease model of addiction. Consider how those authors might respond to the next excerpt, which touches on the implications that the brain disease model might have regarding legal responsibility.

United States v. Hendrickson

25 F. Supp. 3d 1166 (N.D. Iowa 2014)

When science began to study addictive behavior in the 1930s, people addicted to drugs were thought to be morally flawed and lacking in willpower. Those views shaped society's responses to drug abuse, treating it as a moral failing rather than a health problem, which led to an emphasis on punitive rather than preventative and therapeutic actions. Today, thanks to science, our views and our responses to drug abuse have changed dramatically.[1]

BENNETT, D.J. As a federal judge with two decades of experience sentencing drug-addicted criminal defendants, the quote above, from the director of the National Institute on Drug Abuse, evokes both optimism and dismay. On one hand, it reflects society's progress in understanding addiction as a public-health problem. On the other hand, it is a sobering reminder that advances in science continue to outpace advances in law. While science may have changed our views on drug abuse, the law still responds to drug abusers with punitive force, rather than preventative or therapeutic treatment. It is therefore unsurprising that, since 1980, the number of federal prisoners serving drug-related sentences has skyrocketed. In short, the quote above speaks to how far we've come, and how far we've yet to go.

Just as science and the law treat addiction differently, so too do federal judges. In particular, judges disagree about whether a defendant's addiction mitigates his or her culpability, and whether a defendant's addiction may support a downward variance under 18 U.S.C. § 3553(a). I recently attended a seminar for federal district court judges where I was reminded that some judges believe that addiction cannot be mitigating because it is so common among defendants, especially those being sentenced for drug crimes. In defending this view, one judge commented: "Addiction in drug cases is not outside the heartland." The "heartland" refers to the "set of typical cases embodying the conduct that [a particular sentencing] guideline describes." U.S.S.G. Ch. 1, Pt. A, intro. comment. 4(b). I respectfully disagree with the view that addiction can be mitigating only if it is outside the heartland or extraordinary. I write to explain my view that drug addiction is generally mitigating, especially in cases, like this one, where the defendant is both young and has been addicted to drugs throughout adolescence and most of his early adulthood.

I. INTRODUCTION

Defendant Kailab Hendrickson (Hendrickson) is before me for sentencing. On February 4, 2014, Hendrickson pleaded guilty to one count of possessing stolen firearms . . . Hendrickson stole 15 firearms . . . Hendrickson told the agents that, before the burglary, he had been drinking at a bar, where he got into an altercation with another man. Hendrickson then left the bar and broke into a house looking for drugs. He found 15 guns and a bow instead. He stole the weapons, hid the guns at his relatives' home, and gave the bow to someone else to settle a $400 methamphetamine debt.

---

1. Nora D. Volkow, *Preface* to *National Institute on Drug Abuse, Drugs, Brains, and Behavior: The Science of Addiction* 1 (2010).

Hendrickson is a 23-year-old young man with an unfortunate history of abusing multiple drugs and making impulsive decisions. He began using alcohol, marijuana, and methamphetamine when he was just 14 years old. He admits that he is addicted to both marijuana and methamphetamine. Before his arrest in this case, Hendrickson used marijuana as often as he could, and used methamphetamine daily since 2012. Hendrickson also suffers from ADHD. These facts are uncontroverted.

Along with Hendrickson's drug addictions came criminal behavior. At age 14 and 15, Hendrickson was adjudicated for Burglary 3rd Degree and Possession of Marijuana. At ages 16 and 17, he participated in two outpatient substance abuse programs, but continued abusing drugs. Hendrickson was then placed in a residential substance abuse program where he attempted to deliver methamphetamine to the other participants. Hendrickson was adjudicated for Possession of Methamphetamine with Intent to Deliver, and was committed to a state training school for boys. The training school discharged him one month before his 18th birthday. Hendrickson's poor decision-making continued as a young adult. At ages 21 and 22, he was convicted once for Trespass, three times for Theft in the 5th Degree, and once for Theft in the 3rd Degree — all in addition to his possession-of-stolen-firearms conviction currently before me.

In light of these facts, I must now determine what sentence is appropriate for Hendrickson.

II. ANALYSIS

[Judge Bennett discussed sentencing methodology under the federal sentencing guidelines and then determined that Hendrickson's Guidelines range was 37 to 46 months. Neither party requested a variance, i.e. a sentence below or above the guidelines range. Judge Bennett independently considered whether addiction should be a mitigating factor under §3553(a).] . . .

Under § 3553(a), I must "impose a sentence sufficient, but not greater than necessary, to comply with the purposes set forth in [18 U.S.C. § 3553(a)(2)]." Section 3553(a)(2) provides: The court, in determining the particular sentence to be imposed, shall consider . . . the need for the sentence imposed . . . to reflect the seriousness of the offense, to promote respect for the law, and to provide just punishment for the offense; . . . to afford adequate deterrence to criminal conduct; . . . to protect the public from further crimes of the defendant; and . . . to provide the defendant with needed educational or vocational training, medical care, or other correctional treatment in the most effective manner[.]

In determining whether a sentence is "sufficient, but not greater than necessary," I must consider, among other factors, "the nature and circumstances of the offense and the history and characteristics of the defendant[.]" 18 U.S.C. § 3553(a)(1).

As I discussed above, Hendrickson's history and characteristics reveal that he has struggled with drug abuse and addiction since age. This addiction continued through Hendrickson's young adulthood, as he abused marijuana frequently and methamphetamine daily. Under § 3553(a), I must consider what effect, if any, Hendrickson's addiction should have on his sentence.

1. Addiction and Culpability

. . . I begin where this opinion began, recognizing that science offers important insights into how addiction affects people. "As a result of scientific research, we know that addiction is a disease that affects both brain and behavior." The fact that addiction is a disease is something that the United States Supreme Court has recognized, at least implicitly, since 1925. . . . Compulsive drug seeking and use despite harmful consequences certainly characterizes Hendrickson's conduct. Thus, while addiction was once thought of as merely a moral failure, it is now rightly identified as a serious medical condition.

"[Drug addiction] is considered a brain disease because drugs change the brain—they change its structure and how it works." These changes are physical, rather than merely psychological:

> Brain imaging studies from drug-addicted individuals show physical changes in areas of the brain that are critical to judgment, decisionmaking, learning and memory, and behavior control. Scientists believe that these changes alter the way the brain works, and may help explain the compulsive and destructive behaviors of addiction.

A recent study suggests that drug abuse damages a person's orbitofrontal cortex (OFC)—the brain region responsible for evaluating hasty decisions—impairing the person's judgment, especially regarding a decision's long-term consequences. Damage to the OFC is particularly harmful because "the OFC contributes to a variety of behavioral states and functions, including the processing or reward, emotion and decision making, which are essential components of motivational-directed behavior."

By changing the brain, addiction affects a person's thinking and behavior. While "[t]he initial decision to take drugs is mostly voluntary . . . when drug abuse takes over, a person's ability to exert self control can become seriously impaired." "[D]rugs of abuse are characterized as 'hijacking' the neuro-biological mechanisms by which the brain responds to reward. . . ." "When faced with a choice that brings immediate reward, even at the risk of incurring future negative outcomes, including loss of reputation, job, and family, [addicts] appear oblivious to the consequences of their actions." Stated plainly, addiction biologically robs drug abusers of their judgment, causing them to act impulsively and ignore the future consequences of their actions. . . . Hendrickson's criminal conduct clearly reflects his lack of judgment and impulse control.

Taken together, this scientific evidence speaks to a fundamental issue at sentencing: culpability. One of the goals of sentencing is retribution—the notion that one's punishment should be proportional to his or her offense. . . . Section 3553(a) promotes this goal, requiring that each sentence "reflect the seriousness of the offense . . . [and] provide just punishment for the offense. . . ." 18 U.S.C. § 3553(a)(2)(A). "The heart of the retribution rationale is that a criminal sentence must be directly related to the personal culpability of the criminal offender." And, in evaluating a defendant's personal culpability, I must consider the history and characteristics of the defendant. When addiction appears in a defendant's history and characteristics, the question becomes: How does addiction affect culpability?

The answer, at least in most cases, is that addiction mitigates a defendant's culpability. By physically hijacking the brain, addiction diminishes the addict's capacity to evaluate and control his or her behaviors. Rather than rationally assessing the costs of their actions, addicts are prone to act impulsively, without accurately weighing future consequences. This is certainly true for Hendrickson, whose criminal history coincides with, and directly relates to, periods of drug abuse. During allocution, in a moment of self-reflection, Hendrickson noted that "drugs clouded my mind and motivated me to do things I would never do had I been sober." Hendrickson, therefore, acknowledges that drugs diminished his capacity to make good decisions—something both defense counsel and the AUSA acknowledge, too.

The capacity to evaluate the consequences of one's actions is central to one's culpability. This is why we consider the defendant who commits a crime during a momentary lapse in judgment less blameworthy than the defendant who commits a crime after a period of sober calculation. Even the United States Sentencing Guidelines recognize that a defendant's reduced mental capacity may warrant a lesser sentence. . . . But the idea that capacity affects culpability is not limited to sentencing; it echoes throughout the criminal law. The first-degree murderer is more culpable than the second-degree murderer. The defendant acting on free will is more culpable than the defendant acting under coercion. The adult is more culpable than the child. Simply put, we expect those with a better capacity for decision-making to make better decisions.

Additionally, addiction is mitigating for much the same reasons that the United States Supreme Court has recognized youth is mitigating. . . . Just as there are fundamental differences between the juvenile and adult brain, so too are there fundamental differences between the addict and non-addict brain. Because of these differences, addicts, like juveniles, tend to make "impetuous and ill-considered" decisions. Thus, for the same reasons juveniles are generally less culpable, so too are addicts.

This is not to say, however, that addiction is limitlessly mitigating. For example, addiction may not be mitigating, or may be less mitigating, where there is no nexus between the defendant's addiction and offense; or where the defendant has had numerous opportunities for treatment and has either declined drug treatment or failed to meaningfully attempt to complete drug treatment. Also, there may be some point at which a defendant no longer gets the "benefit" of addiction-based mitigation—like the defendant who, after sentencing, repeatedly violates his or her terms of supervised release by using drugs or alcohol. Addiction could even be aggravating in certain situations. Each case must be carefully considered on its own and all of the § 3553(a) factors must be balanced.

In balancing the § 3553(a) factors here, I find that Hendrickson's addiction is mitigating, especially when considered together with Hendrickson's youth. Hendrickson has been addicted to drugs since he was 14 years old. He is now only 23 years old. Hendrickson has abused brain-altering drugs through most of the years during which his adolescent brain was still physically developing. As a result, Hendrickson has sadly, but predictably, made poor decisions based on impulse and immaturity. Letters from Hendrickson's family members . . . confirm this. For example, Hendrickson's mother observed that Hendrickson is "young and immature," that he "has struggled with drugs off and on ever[ ] since he [ ] first started using them," and that "drugs had a huge influence on his decision making." Hendrickson's aunt commented that Hendrickson "has always been mentally younger than he looks" and that "he doesn't stop to think about his actions before he does them." These observations are consistent with the scientific evidence discussed above, and they support the conclusion that Hendrickson's addition is mitigating.

. . . [I]n my view, the § 3553(a) factors justify a variance of 6 months below the low end of Hendrickson's Guidelines range.

In sum, because addiction is a serious brain disease that diminishes one's capacity to evaluate decisions and regulate behavior, I consider addiction to be a generally and substantially mitigating factor under § 3553(a)(1), weighing in favor of a downward variance here. I next consider, more specifically, district courts' discretion to consider a defendant's addiction in varying below a Guidelines sentence.

NOTES AND QUESTIONS

1. *Eldred* held that a court may require a person to remain drug-free as a condition of her probation. May a statute prohibit a person suffering from alcohol use disorder from simply possessing alcohol, despite having no alcohol-related convictions? What arguments could you make using *Robinson, Powell,* and *Eldred?* In *Manning v. Caldwell,* a group of homeless individuals brought a class action suit challenging the constitutionality of a Virginia statute that made it a criminal offense for "habitual drunkards" to possess, consume, or purchase alcohol. The Fourth Circuit Court of Appeals first held that the term "habitual drunkard" was unconstitutionally vague, then went on to consider the plaintiffs' Eighth Amendment arguments:

> Each of the named Plaintiffs in this case, Bryan Manning, Ryan Williams, Richard Deckerhoff, and Richard Eugene Walls, alleges that he has been interdicted as an "habitual drunkard" pursuant to this statutory scheme. Each alleges that he suffers from alcohol use disorder, commonly called alcoholism, which causes him a "profound drive or craving to use alcohol" that is "compulsive or non-volitional." Each further alleges that he is homeless and that his homelessness exacerbates his addiction, "mak[ing] it nearly impossible . . . to cease or mitigate alcohol consumption." Notably, however, nothing in the complaint or elsewhere in the record indicates that any Plaintiff was convicted of any alcohol-related offenses before being interdicted. . . .
>
> As we have explained, the term "habitual drunkard" as used in Virginia law is so vague as to offer no meaningful standard of conduct. But even if this term could be narrowed to apply only to those individuals who, like Plaintiffs, suffer from alcoholism, such a construction would raise independent Eighth Amendment concerns. We now turn to those concerns.
>
> **A.**
> The Eighth Amendment's Cruel and Unusual Punishments Clause "circumscribes the criminal process in three ways." *Ingraham v. Wright,* 430 U.S. 651, 667, 97 S.Ct. 1401, 51 L.Ed.2d 711 (1977). The Clause operates to (1) "limit[ ] the kinds of punishment that can be imposed on those convicted of crimes," (2) "proscribe[ ] punishment grossly disproportionate to the severity of the crime," and (3) "impose[ ] substantive limits on what can be made criminal and punished as such." *Id.* . . .
>
> Applying the teachings of *Robinson* and *Powell* to the factual allegations in Plaintiffs' complaint, we can only conclude that—even assuming the term "habitual drunkard," as used in Virginia law, could be limited to alcoholics—Plaintiffs have alleged a viable claim for relief under the Eighth Amendment. Plaintiffs allege they are addicted to alcohol and that this addiction, like narcotics addiction, is an illness. They allege that their addiction causes them to "pathologically pursue alcohol use," without any volitional control over their drinking.

Plaintiffs thus allege that the challenged Virginia scheme targets them for special punishment for conduct that is both *compelled by their illness* and is *otherwise lawful* for all those of legal drinking age. If true, the challenged scheme indeed violates the Eighth Amendment as applied to Plaintiffs. . . .

Virginia's two-pronged statutory scheme may be less direct than the statute at issue in *Robinson*, but it yields the same result: it effectively criminalizes an illness. If the statute challenged in *Robinson* had instead allowed California to "interdict" prescription drug addicts and then arrest interdicted addicts for filling those prescriptions, the statute *effectively* would also have criminalized "being addicted to narcotics" even if it *nominally* punished only filling prescriptions. Such a statute would surely be just as unconstitutional as the statute in *Robinson*, and for precisely the same reasons.

Similarly, although Virginia's statutory scheme may nominally penalize "possession" or "consumption," even a sufficiently definite construction limited to alcoholics effectively targets and punishes Plaintiffs based on their illness, which *Robinson* holds violates the Eighth Amendment. As Justice White explained, the thin distinction between "hav[ing] an irresistible compulsion" and "yield[ing] to such a compulsion" is not one of constitutional magnitude under *Robinson. See Powell*, 392 U.S. at 548, 88 S.Ct. 2145 (White, J., concurring in the result). That the Commonwealth civilly brands alcoholics as "habitual drunkards" before prosecuting them for involuntary manifestations of their illness does nothing to cure the unconstitutionality of this statutory scheme.

We therefore conclude that, even if the term "habitual drunkard" could be construed to apply only to those who suffer from alcoholism, Plaintiffs have stated an independent claim that the challenged statute violates the Eighth Amendment.

Manning v. Caldwell, 930 F.3d 264 (4th Cir. 2019). Did the court reach the correct result?

2. How far could a court go in mandating that a person remains sober? Would it be constitutional to force someone to receive an anti-intoxicant vaccine? Though not yet on the market, such vaccines may soon be a reality: vaccines that prevent the highs from heroin, cocaine, and methamphetamine, among others, are currently undergoing human clinical trials. As Kellen Russoniello explains, these vaccines would trigger the immune system to stop certain chemical compounds from producing pleasurable effects in the brain. Supreme Court precedent suggests that mandatory vaccines are not unconstitutional. *Jacobson v. Massachusetts*, 197 U.S. 11 (1905). For a rebuttal to the presumed constitutionality of anti-intoxicant vaccines, see Kellen Russoniello, *The End of* Jacobson*'s Spread: Five Arguments Why an Anti-Intoxicant Vaccine Would Be Unconstitutional*, 43 Am. J.L. & Med. 57 (2017).

3. Should there be a "reasonable addict" standard in criminal law or other bodies of law? Consider law professor Gideon Yaffe's argument:

> [A]ddicts should be given some kind of break, but not excused entirely. . . . What will be argued here, in short, is that an addict is not responsible for violating a norm if he could comply with it only by giving up control of his behavior to someone or something that is independent of his own decision-making capacities. We cannot expect people, that is, to give up their autonomy in order to comply with norms. However, it is also argued that in virtually every case of a norm violation by an addict, if not all, there is a less stringent norm that the addict can be held responsible for violating, precisely because he would not have to give up his autonomy in order to comply with it. . . . [Yaffe reviews relevant neuroscience of addiction studies.]

Imagine . . . that the addict can pursue drugs zealously or pursue them weakly; he can, for instance, kill people for them, or he can merely deceive and manipulate his relatives in order to get them. He should not do either. But imagine, further, that to avoid even weakly pursuing drugs he would need to give up control of his behavior; he would need to rely entirely on someone or something else to make his decisions for him. But he knows enough to see the reasons against zealous pursuit and is capable of guiding his behavior in accordance with such reasons; he thus need not give up his autonomy in order to comply with the norm against zealous pursuit. If what has been said here is correct, it follows, as in the earlier example, that the addict cannot be expected to comply with the norm against weak pursuit, but can be expected to comply with the norm against zealous pursuit. There are thus some things that we can hold the addict responsible for doing in service of his addiction, and others we cannot. The line between these two is determined by the burdens of compensation involved in performance. Where the addict would have to compensate for his learning deficit by giving up his autonomy, we cannot expect compliance, and so cannot hold the addict responsible for failure; but where he would not, we have no reason to believe that we cannot and so we should.

Gideon Yaffe, *Lowering the Bar for Addicts*, in *Addiction & Responsibility* 113, 113, 135 (George Graham & Jeffrey Poland eds., 2011).

4. If addicts are different from non-addicts, does the size and nature of that difference matter? Legal scholars Douglas Husak and Emily Murphy have pointed out that:

[T]he vast majority of research [in addiction neuroscience] looks for statistically significant differences between two groups—in this case, addicts and non-addicts. A statistically significant difference, however, need not be a dramatic difference. It merely indicates that the measurable difference (in behavior, brain activation, neurotransmitter or receptor quantity, etc.) is highly unlikely to be due to chance. By contrast, effect size studies quantify the magnitude of the effect, which is more significant for assessing the seriousness of the impairment and its impact on the activities of the user in his real life. Unfortunately, for purposes of understanding the relevance of the neuroscience of addiction to the criminal law, few effect-size studies have been done. Thus a dearth of evidence addresses the issue of how bad an addiction really is in either groups or individuals. For the neuroscience of addiction to be helpful to the criminal law, explanations and data would have to include quantification, and possibly ranking, of the severity of drug effects.

Douglas Husak & Emily Murphy, *The Relevance of the Neuroscience of Addiction to Criminal Law*, in *A Primer on Criminal Law and Neuroscience* 216, 223 (Stephen J. Morse & Adina L. Roskies eds., 2013). What effect size—that is, the size of the difference between an addict and a non-addict—should be required for the law to respond? For instance, what if a brain imaging scan could demonstrate that the defendant in *Powell* or the defendant in *Robinson* suffered from a 4% reduction in an ability to control his behavior as a result of his addiction? What if it were 74%? Could the law account for this partial impairment? Could different bodies of law respond differently?

C. THE NEUROBIOLOGY OF ADDICTION

In Section A we introduced differing points of view about the degree to which addiction is a biological predisposition as compared to a responsible choice. We now present more detailed consideration of the two sides of the debate by leaders in their respective fields of neuroscience and legal scholarship.

Steven E. Hyman
The Neurobiology of Addiction: Implications for Voluntary Control of Behavior
7 Am. J. Bioethics 8, 8-10 (2007)

The question of whether and to what extent an addicted individual is responsible for his or her actions remains a matter of unsettled debate. One proxy (albeit imperfect) for this question is disagreement as to whether addiction is best conceptualized as a brain disease, as a moral condition, or as some combination of the two. Those who argue for the disease model not only believe it is justified by empirical data, but also see virtue in the possibility that a disease model decreases the stigmatization of addicted people and increases their access to medical treatments. Those who argue that addiction is best conceptualized as a moral condition are struck by the observation that drug seeking and drug taking involve a series of voluntary acts that often require planning and flexible responses to changing conditions—not simply impulsive or robotic acts. They worry that medicalization will lead addicted people to fatalism about their condition and to excuses for their actions rather than full engagement with treatment and rehabilitation and an effort to conform to basic societal expectations.

Current definitions of addiction come from medical texts and thus, not surprisingly, favor a disease model. Indeed, addiction looks very much like a disease (admittedly definitions of "disease" remain somewhat fuzzy). Addiction has known risk factors (family history, male sex) and a typical course and outcome: often a chronic course punctuated by periods of abstinence followed by relapse. . . .

What is more interesting is that modern definitions of addiction focus squarely on the issue of voluntary control. The current medical consensus is that the cardinal feature of addiction is compulsive drug use despite significant negative consequences. The term *compulsion* is imprecise, but at a minimum implies diminished ability to control drug use, even in the face of factors (e.g., illness, failure in life roles, loss of job, arrest) that should motivate cessation of drug use in a rational agent willing and able to exert control over behavior. The focus on "loss of control" is not derived primarily from a theory, but from extensive observation of the behavior of addicted individuals and indeed recognition of the failure of previous definitions to capture clinical realities. The current focus on compulsive use as the defining features of addiction superseded previous views that focused on dependence and withdrawal. These previous views implied that addicted individuals take drugs to seek pleasure and avoid aversive withdrawal symptoms. Although the avoidance of withdrawal might create strong motivation to take drugs, this view does not imply a loss of voluntary control. This previous view failed on several counts. First, some highly addictive drugs such as cocaine and amphetamine may produce mild withdrawal symptoms and lack a physical withdrawal syndrome entirely. Moreover, the previous view does not explain the stubborn persistence of relapse risk long after detoxification, long after the last withdrawal symptom, if any, has passed, and despite incentives to avoid a resumption of drug use.

... [T]he science is in its early stages and ... there is not yet a fully convincing theory of how addiction results from the interaction of risk factors, drugs, and the brain. Moreover, there are still disagreements at the theoretical level of what the existing data signifies for the mechanisms of addiction. This state of affairs invites skepticism from those wary of a disease model. Nonetheless, we cannot select models of human behavior based on desired social implications, but must rely on the scientific evidence we have. Despite somewhat different views of mechanism, all current mainstream formulations agree that addiction diminishes voluntary behavioral control. At the same time, none of the current views conceives of the addicted person to be devoid of all voluntary control and thus absolved of all responsibility for self-control.

Short of being harshly coerced, severely psychotic, or significantly demented, what can it mean to say that a person cannot control his or her actions? An alcoholic must obtain money, go to the liquor store or otherwise obtain alcohol (perhaps carefully hidden from a spouse) and consume drinks. A heroin user may have to go to great lengths to obtain the drug, perhaps committing one of more crimes, before beginning the ritual that ends in self-injection. How can these extended chains of apparently voluntary acts be the result of compulsion? In my view, addictive drugs tap into and, in vulnerable individuals, usurp powerful mechanisms by which survival-relevant goals shape behavior.

Diverse organisms, including humans, pursue goals with positive survival value such as food, safety, and opportunities for mating; such goals act as "rewards." Rewards are experienced as pleasurable and as motivating (they are desired). Environmental cues that predict their availability (e.g., the smell of baking bread) are rapidly learned and are imbued with incentive properties: they activate "wanting" and initiate behaviors aimed at obtaining the desired goal. Such goal-directed behaviors tend to increase in frequency over time (reinforcement) and to become highly efficient. Of course rewarding goals for humans can vary enormously in immediacy, complexity, and motivational power, ranging from a well-liked food to seeing a favorite painting in a museum.

The brain has evolved several specialized mechanisms to maximize the ability of an organism to obtain rewards. There are mechanisms to provide internal representations of rewards and to assign them relative values compared with pursuing other possible goals; these mechanisms depend primarily on the orbital prefrontal cortex. There are mechanisms that permit an organism to learn and to make relatively efficient and automatic, sequences of actions to obtain specific rewards; these depend primarily on the dorsal striatum. Mechanisms of cognitive control support successful completion of goal-directed behaviors by maintaining the goal representation over time, suppressing distractions, and inhibiting impulsive actions that redirect the organism. Cognitive control is dependent on the prefrontal cortex and its connections to the striatum and thalamus. In humans, the capacity for cognitive control appears to be a relatively stable trait that is an important predictor of life success. Deficits in cognitive control play an important role in attention deficit hyperactivity disorder and may increase vulnerability to later substance misuse.

These circuits respond in a coordinated fashion to new information about rewards through the action of the neurotransmitter dopamine. Dopamine is released from neurons with cell bodies in the ventral tegmental area (VTA) and substantia nigra within the midbrain. These neurons project widely through the forebrain and can influence all of the circuits involved in reward-related learning, as well as in other aspects of cognition and emotion. Dopamine projections from the VTA to the nucleus accumbens bind the pleasurable (hedonic) response to a reward to desire and to goal-directed behavior. Dopamine projections from the VTA to the prefrontal cortex play a critical role in the assignment of value and in updating goal representations in response to the state of the organism. Dopamine projections from the substantia nigra to the dorsal striatum are critical for consolidating new behavioral responses so that reward-related cues come to activate efficient strategies to reach the relevant goal.

Addictive drugs are Trojan horses. Unlike natural rewards, addictive drugs have no nutritional, reproductive, or other survival value. However, all addictive drugs exert pharmacologic effects that cause release of dopamine. Moreover, the effects of addictive drugs on dopamine release are quantitatively greater than that produced by natural rewards under almost all circumstances.

Normally dopamine serves as a "learning signal" in the brain. Dopamine is released when a reward is new, better than expected, or unpredicted in a particular. When the world is exactly as expected, there is nothing new to learn; no new circumstances to connect either to desire or to action—and no increase in dopamine release. Because addictive drugs increase synaptic dopamine by direct pharmacologic action, they short circuit the normal controls over dopamine release that compare the current circumstance with prior experience. Thus, unlike natural rewards, addictive drugs always signal "better than expected." Neural circuits "overlearn" on an excessive and grossly distorted dopamine signal. Cues that predict drug availability such as persons, places, or certain bodily sensations gain profound incentive salience and the ability to motivate drug seeking. Because of the excessive dopamine signal in the prefrontal cortex drugs become overvalued compared with all other goals. Rational goals such as self-care, working, parenting, and obeying the law are devalued. In addition, normal aspects of cognitive control weaken; even if the addicted person wants to "cut down," prepotent cue-initiated drug-seeking responses are extremely difficult to suppress. If the person is successful in delaying drug seeking (or is, for external reasons unable to seek drugs), intense craving may result. Because the changes in synaptic weight and synaptic structure that underlie memory are among the longest-lived alterations in biology, the ability of drug-related cues to cause relapses may persist for many years, even a lifetime. . . .

Our current models help explain why recovery is difficult and why relapses occur even long after detoxification and rehabilitation. The long experience of humanity with addiction does not counsel fatalism, but implacable efforts to overcome the behavioral effects of neural circuits hijacked by drugs. Finally, views based on cognitive neuroscience and studies of addiction pathogenesis suggest that some apparently voluntary behaviors may not be as freely planned and executed as they first appear. . . .

Stephen J. Morse

Voluntary Control of Behavior and Responsibility

7 Am. J. Bioethics 12, 12-13 (2007)

Before we can reach any conclusion about moral or legal implications, we need to know the criteria for free and unfree, or for control and loss of control. Whether addiction's causal mechanism is primarily genetic, neurobiological, psychological, sociological, or some combination of these—as is almost certainly the case—involuntariness is a conclusion we reach about behavior. Consequently, we must have behavioral criteria for the conclusion that the addict's seeking and using behavior is unfree or beyond his or her control.

Let us begin with the behavioral phenomenology of addiction. Here, in brief, is what we knew before we had a neuroscientific foundation for causal hypotheses. Some people who use drugs over time develop a powerful, insistent desire to take drugs, often termed a craving, a desire that is stimulated and enhanced by the environmental cues that are associated with the activity. They engage in repetitive seeking and using behavior that is termed compulsive because the addict reports that he or she subjectively feels compelled to use drugs and the activity continues despite markedly and often disastrously negative life effects. Even if they are able to quit, addicts are in substantial danger of re-engaging in drug use. . . .

What can we infer from this description? It is reasonable to conclude that drug use causes some type of change in the person that increases desire to extremely high levels. Viewed objectively, most addiction is not rational in the sense that few people would on reflection choose to be in a position that caused them so much misery. For the same reason, we can infer that addiction undermines the addict's rational capacities and that avoiding the behavior is very difficult, making use appear compulsive. Finally, the risk of relapse among quitters suggests that the predisposing causal mechanisms persist, even if the former addict is not using at a given time. Note, that we could draw these inferences prior to any neurobiological understanding of the addict's brain.

These inferences raise two familiar excusing conditions: lack of rational capacity and compulsion. Of the two . . . lack of rational capacity is the better explanation of why addiction might excuse or mitigate responsibility and in fact explains perceived loss of control. In brief, the argument is that the addict's strong desires—the "go" mechanism—make it very difficult for the addict to think straight about what he or she has good reason to do—the "stop" mechanism. If the go mechanism is sufficiently strong, it will make it very difficult for the stop mechanism to work properly. If the stop mechanism is independently weakened, then the go mechanism gains increased motivational advantage.

It is just this loss of capacity to bring good reason to bear that makes it so difficult to control oneself. After all, most of our self-control measures use our capacity for rationality directly or indirectly. A picture of a pig on the refrigerator door, for example, is meant to remind the overeater of the good reasons not to eat at just the moment he or she is about to indulge. When the craving is greatest, the addict can scarcely think about anything except using drugs despite the many rational incentives not to do so and constructs self-defeating rationalizations if necessary. Anyone who has ever been in a state of strong desire for something that they know is not good for them will find this account all too familiar.

Diminished capacity to bring reason to bear rationally to evaluate and to control one's conduct can be caused by a large number of variables in addition to craving. Consider rage, for example. Whatever causal mechanism is at work, there is a common final behavioral pathway. What is doing the potential work of mitigation or excuse is the final pathway, diminished rationality, rather than any particular brain mechanism. This, I suggest, is the best interpretation of the behavioral criteria for lack of cognitive control, for the inability to "freely plan and execute" behavior. Lack of voluntariness really means lack of rational capacity. . . .

The question for morality and law, then, is always how much loss of rational capacity justifies mitigation and excuse. This is a normative question, a matter of practical reason that science cannot resolve. Science can, however, help determine how much loss of rational capacity has occurred. But, ultimately, the question for the law and morals is behavioral, not brain states. People, not brains, are held responsible, are praised and blamed, rewarded and punished. If the brain findings and behavior are inconsistent, the behavior must be our guide. . . .

Michael S. Moore
Addiction, Responsibility, and Neuroscience
2020 U. Ill. L. Rev. 375, 378-466 (2020)

My question is whether addicts who commit crimes deserve to be punished for those crimes, or whether instead they should be fully or partly excused whenever their crimes were the result of their addiction. In short, my question is whether addiction is an excuse, both for moral responsibility and from liability to criminal punishment. . . .

[A]s a matter of statutory, common, and constitutional law, addiction does not presently serve as any kind of defense in Anglo-American criminal law. But that doesn't answer the normative question of whether the law is not mistaken in this regard. Does doing some wrongful and illegal act in order to satisfy a desperate craving for the drug to which one is addicted, reduce or eliminate one's moral blameworthiness for doing that act? If so, then by standard theories of punishment there should be some legal defense. . . .

[W]ill the neuroscientific explanation of addiction . . . help us with the moral question of when if ever addicts are excused by their addiction? Take the "imbalance" explanation proffered by [neuroscientist Kent] Berridge. . . . According to Berridge, the brains of addicts have been rewired such that the drugs that initially gave them pleasure (in their hedonic hot spots) no longer do so, yet the wanting for drugs that that pleasure once brought on carries on despite the absence of much or any reinforcement of that wanting by a liking for drugs; further, that a potential for such liking-independent wanting persists so that confronting drug related cues can trigger such cravings long after all drug use has ceased. The findings in neuroscience on which Berridge relies in the giving of this account were not the source of this explanation; phenomenology and behavioral psychology made this plausible before we knew that the mechanisms of pleasure were different in anatomical region and in neurotransmitter usage than the mechanisms of wanting and motivation. Still, the neuroscience helps to validate and refine these initial deliverances of phenomenology and behavioral observation, and it thereby gives us grounds to prefer this explanation to the many competing accounts we earlier explored based just of phenomenology and behavioral observation. It thus makes us more confident in the truth of the explanation vis-à-vis its competitors and this makes us consider more seriously the possibility of excuse lurking in such explanation (although, again, discovering the "mechanical filling" by itself does nothing to increase the excusing potential of such explanation).

What are the moral implications of a desire (that motivates a wrongful action) being cut off from the normally controlling feedback of the reward circuit? I earlier opined that morality is indifferent to the sources of our desires, that responsibility rests on our abilities to choose to act or not to act on such desires, not on our ability to create or change those desires themselves. In a recent paper Richard Holton appears to dissent from this conclusion, urging that addicts have less responsibility for their choices than non-addicts because Berridge's incentive salience explanation shows that addicts have "little control, once they encounter a cue, over their cravings."[4] The incentive salience account does indeed seem to show this. The account shows that one of the resources that we can use to tame our desires, bequeathed to us by natural selection, is absent from the tool kits of addicts. That resource was the dislike or at least absence of liking that normally feeds back to dampen the desire for the thing not liked. Addicts who wish to choose not to take drugs are deprived of this resource for dampening the opposing input to that wish in making that choice, according to the incentive salience theory. Yet my original point survives this thought. To be responsible for choosing to act on a desire does not require that we be responsible for the desire or its strength; the abilities relevant to responsibility are the abilities to choose otherwise and to act otherwise, not the ability to desire otherwise.

These same considerations militate against thinking that the alternative account of addicts' motivation to use drugs—the desires to avoid the "dark side" effects of not using drugs that George Koob believes motivated addicts—also have any potential to enlarge the category of those excused because of their addiction. Indeed, these desires have even less potential for excuse because, unlike the desires of the incentive salience theory, the dark side desires: are not intrinsic desires but rather, instrumental desires in the service of avoidance various forms of dysphoria; are not unmoored from the liking system; are not experienced as cravings. The only feature of these desires inclining towards excuse would be their strength, and strength of desire, as we have seen, is no grounds for excusing choices and actions satisfying of that desire.

Richard Holton seeks to supplement the positive motivational account of drug use by adverting to another feature of addicted drug use (in addition to the separation of wanting from liking Holton uses to ground his conclusion about the undampenability of drug cravings). What Holton adverts to here is certainly a well-established feature suggested by the phenomenology of addicts. This is the fact that the choice to use drugs not only goes against what the addict likes but also against what the addict values. As Holton puts it, there is for addicts a "conflict between beliefs—beliefs broadly about what is valuable—and desires. . . . The crucial feature is that the unwilling addict judges that taking the drug is not the best course. . . ."[5] On this picture, addicts' decisions to take drugs flies in the face not

4. Richard Holton, "Addiction, Desire, Pleasure, Pollution," draft, 2019, p. 13 (quoted with permission of the author).
5. Holton, "Addiction, Desire, Pleasure, Pollution," p. 17. As was noted earlier, Holton's conclusion here is disputed by Gideon Yaffe (Yaffe, "Are Addicts Akratic?"). Yet Yaffe's criticism here is no more than an amendment to the thesis that addicts choose against their own values, amending the thesis to be diachronic rather than synchronic—addicts choose against the values they hold both before and after they choose to take drugs even though at the exact moment that they take drugs they most value doing just that.

only of what they like but also of what they value ("value" here being a shorthand reference to their evaluative beliefs about what is desirable and worth pursuing).

In my view the neuroscience that backs up this claim for phenomenology is both poorly developed (and incidentally, not distinctive of the incentive salience theory proper). For we do not know the anatomical locations or neurotransmitters distinctive of evaluative beliefs the way we know both of those things for both the reward and the wanting systems. All we have are fMRI studies showing the areas of the PFC activated when such evaluative beliefs are in play to control desires. Still, it is plausible enough to suppose that there are such mechanisms and that one day neuroscience will discover what they are. It is also plausible to speculate that such discoveries will verify the deliverance of phenomenology here, namely, that addicts often choose against their own values when they choose to take drugs.

Suppose that all of this is well-established fact. Does it make for excuse? I see three routes by which one might think so. One is to go the route of the habit and learning theorists of addiction. One might reason that wants that are (1) intrinsic in the sense that they are not in the service of any further goals; (2) not in accord with what one likes (takes pleasure in); (3) not in accord with what one judges to be worthwhile and desirable; and (4) nonetheless win out in determining behavior, must be by-passing choice and causing drug-seeking behavior directly. The idea would be that a "choice" dictated by a craving with these features must not really be a choice at all, that it couldn't be since it is so irrational in its behavioral conclusion. Yet the unyielding barrier here is the same one against which the habit and learning theories generally come to grief: drug use by addicts just does not get experienced like nibbling on cake or other habits. Drug use is chosen; there is choice, and the machinery of choosing is not by-passed.

The second route is . . . that addicts' cravings have the four features above mentioned might also tempt one to think that they are properly regarded as "ego-alien," i.e., not part of the self. If a want doesn't bring us pleasure when it is satisfied and we know that it will not, if that want is for something we don't think to be valuable and worth wanting, and yet that want is the one that determines our behavior, this might be taken to blunt the earlier objection I inherited from Freud, viz, that the size of our agency for responsibility purposes is not up to us to fix by our self-identifications. We might then justify feeling like there was indeed one "bad-ass demon"[6] inside of us doing the choosing of behavior satisfying such a want. Yet we know that there really is no such demon in possession of our choosing faculties. There is just each of us as whole persons doing battle with a craving that is admittedly hard to resist. But unless the strength of such a craving, together with its content going against what we like and value, are enough to excuse, our choice cannot be excused either. The decision is ours, and the craving is ours, howevermuch we beat ourselves up about both having it and yielding to it.

The third route to excuse is more promising. What if the anatomical and chemical mechanisms that neuroscience may discover to underlie evaluative beliefs and the means by which those beliefs exert their influence over decisions, are of such a nature that long term drug abuse destroys the brain pathway by which such beliefs influence decisions about drug usage by addicts? That would seem to cut into the

---

6. A paraphrase of the cocaine addict quoted before in the *National Geographic*.

addict's ability to choose other than he did when he chose to use drugs. Applying the counterfactual test for free will: the addict could very strongly value all the things dependent on his not using drugs and thus strongly value abstinence over use, and yet those evaluative beliefs would be without causal effect on his choice because he would still choose to use drugs. That he *would* do so in such possible worlds means that *could* not do so in the actual world.

If such pathways of control are damaged such that, at least for choices in the face of drug related cues, evaluative beliefs cannot get any purchase in determining decisions, then such equipment failure would constitute incapacity, the kind of incapacity that should excuse. Indeed, one might imagine that some future neuroscience could likewise discover the pathways by virtue of which desires opposed to drug use — desires for non-drug rewards that seek things that give pleasure if attained and are therefore liked as well as desired — influence choices about drug use. If that science also discovered that such pathways were damaged such that such desires too, along with evaluative beliefs, were incapable of influencing decision, one would have additional grounds for concluding that the addict lacked the ability to choose not to use drugs. For in such a circumstance, no matter how strongly the addict wanted all the things dependent upon his not using drugs, he would still choose to use drugs because those contrary wants were without causal effect.

I conclude that the potential for neuroscience to expand the category of those excused by addiction rests mostly on the discoveries of a neuroscience not yet done. Indeed, such discoveries may depend on facts that do not exist, in which case such discoveries will never be made. The facts about the brain having the most potential for excuse are thus, unfortunately, the least known by the contemporary neuroscience of addiction. Still, that should be grounds motivating future research, not grounds for despair. Neuroscience may yet show us that more addicts are excused by the effects of their addiction than we had thought.

Apart from expanding the categories of offenders excused by addiction, neuroscience also has the potential to verify when those conditions we currently think excuse offenders, are actually present in individual cases. If we had definitive brain markers for the presence or absence of the mental states on which responsibility depends — intentions, factual beliefs, desires, likings, evaluative beliefs — and if we had such markers for the intensity and content of such mental states, together with the interrelationships between them, then we would have a larger and more precise evidential base from which to infer conclusions in individual cases. Such evidence could supplement or even supplant the phenomenological and behavioral evidence on which we now rely. Such a neuroscience may well be a long way off, but we shouldn't lose sight of this potential for neuroscience to be the handmaiden to the law.[7] It needn't always be revolutionary or even reformist of the law to be useful to the law.

---

7. The "handmaiden" characterization I take from the late John Cacioppo, my co-chair of the MacArthur Foundation's Law and Neuroscience Project's Intentions and Decisions Working Group, who at one point expressed his exasperation at my continued harping on the need for legal relevance of our work, "I didn't sign on to this to be your damned handmaiden."

NOTES AND QUESTIONS

1. If the *Robinson* and *Powell* cases discussed earlier were decided today, would an amicus brief from a scientist or a scientific community be appropriate? What might it say?

2. In some child custody hearings, a parent's fitness for parenting is an issue. How should courts view addiction to drugs or alcohol in such cases? Consider this analysis from such a case:

   > The task before the trial court was to determine whether clear and convincing evidence showed that the appellant is presently unfit as a parent and thus not entitled to custody. . . . [Appellant] testified: "I am an alcoholic. I have a disease of alcoholism." (Some experts who regard it a disease claim that the addict has an inborn instinctive "genetic predisposition. . . . The diseased individual undergoes molecular depletion of the endorphin-enkephalin metabolism with the ancient, reptilian-derived survival hypothalamic brain . . . derived for survival of the species." Our courts have rejected this speculative notion of its being a disease and have held that it is a product of the free will and it is the drinker's choice to drink. Drinking a six-pack of beer every day for almost six weeks is a substantial addiction. The children said that the appellant had a Coors Lite in his hand most of the time when they were with him. Appellant claims that, although he admits to being an alcoholic, his treatment may have caused abatement of the addiction. . . .

   In re R.L.L., 386 S.E.2d 852, 853 (Ga. Ct. App. 1989).

3. Courts have formulated theories of addiction for many years. Consider this case from 1872, in which a court had to determine whether a life insurance policy was voided due to a provision stipulating that "if the insured should die 'by reason of intemperance from the use of intoxicating liquors, . . . this policy shall be void, null, and of no effect.'" The court reasoned as follows:

   > The defense was that the insured, at the time of effecting the insurance and until his death, was addicted to intemperance and died from the excessive use of intoxicating liquors. Now, those who use intoxicating liquors at all within the purview of such insurance policies, may be divided into three classes.
   >
   > The first drink sometimes, and upon occasions, as it were more by accident than otherwise, even to intoxication, but in so exceptional a manner that no one can say that they have any habit in regard to such use. They can stop at any time, even take the glass from their lips in the midst of the banquet, and whether such drinking injures the health of those who do it or not, no one can tell with certainty—some think it does, others not. It is obvious that this class would not be embraced in the terms of a policy such as that in this case.
   >
   > A second class acquire a constant appetite for the use of intoxicating liquors, and a regular habit of using them, so that the whole system is kept under the immediate influence of alcoholic stimulants. They are known as constant, habitual drunkards. This class would be within the prohibition of this policy.
   >
   > A third class acquire a constitutionally nervous appetite for alcoholic liquors. It really amounts to a disease. A case is easily recognized by all who are well acquainted with the person. Such persons may remain sober for a month, three, or six months, or even a year at a time, and refuse to taste any intoxicating drinks (they must refuse if they would not get drunk), and then go upon what is called "a spree" of great intensity and lasting for a longer or a shorter period, usually until prostration and sickness, and often delirium, compel a cessation and terminate the "spree." When beginning, or in the midst of such periodical debauch, no earthly

considerations or persuasions can arrest the course of the subject or induce him to stop drinking. In this he is strikingly different from the first class above named who use intoxicating liquors. And there are two varieties of "spreers." The one is boisterous, is seen everywhere, and seeks out and talks to everybody. The other is conscious of his self-degradation and disgrace, and hides himself from observation at his home or room so as not to be seen and not to have his condition and habit known. And few except his family, intimates or neighbors may know or suspect him. I have not mentioned a class of persons, who use intoxicating liquors prescribed as medicine, or who use them at meals, as part of their food, without any observable mental or physical effects. They do not come within the purview of legal consideration in connection with life insurance. The classes within such policies are not those whose wills completely regulate and control their use of intoxicating liquors, but those in which the use and habit daily or periodically control and master the will—where desire and appetite contend with and master the wish and judgment to refrain.

Mut. Benefit Life Ins. Co. v. Holterhoff, 13 Ohio Dec. Reprint 961, 963 (Super. Ct. Ohio 1872). In what ways is this classification of addicts similar to or different from the definitions provided in the *DSM*? To what extent should legal views on addiction be informed by medical views?

4. Whatever the implications for responsibility, advances in neuroscience and genetics may aid personalized clinical treatment of addiction. *See* Markus Heilig et al., *Pharmacogenetic Approaches to the Treatment of Alcohol Addiction*, 12 Nature Revs. Neurosci. 670 (2011). Some pilot research even suggests that opioid-dependent criminal offenders may be successfully treated with extended-release injectable naltrexone. Donna M. Coviello et al., *A Multisite Pilot Study of Extended-Release Injectable Naltrexone Treatment for Previously Opioid-Dependent Parolees and Probationers*, 33 Substance Abuse 48 (2012). If pharmacological interventions proved safe and reliable, should they be a mandatory condition of parole?

5. How does addiction vary by sex and gender? Ongoing research is beginning to shed some light on this question. *See* Jill B. Becker, Michele L. McClellan & Beth Glover Reed, *Sex Differences, Gender and Addiction*, 95 J. Neurosci. Res. 136, 136-47 (2017). Studies have shown that, among those vulnerable to addiction, women progress much quicker through the addiction phases than men, i.e., women move from casual drug usage to drug addiction faster than their male counterparts. This is accompanied by higher relapse rates in women. It remains unclear why these differences exist, but Becker et al. advance several theories, discussing both neurobiological and sociocultural factors.

6. How might new discoveries in the neuroscience of addiction change criminal law doctrine? Philosopher and legal theorist Michael Moore argues:

Neuroscientific research has the potential to advance our understanding of addiction in two dimensions. One, it can change our explanation of addiction. This it can do in a variety of ways: (1) it can *deepen* our folk psychological explanations by showing how the variables in such explanations are underlain by the mechanisms of brain function; (2) it can *precisify* the folk explanations by making the folk psychological states more precise in their boundaries or more precise in the modes of their combination; (3) it can *correct* mistakes in the folk psychological explanation; and/or (4) it can *broaden* those explanations by supplementing them with explanations couched in the terms and variables of cognitive psychology, genetics, and neuroscience. Secondly, such research has the potential to change how we evaluate the behavior of addicts. It might show that we should excuse where currently we do not or that we should not excuse when currently we do. Alternatively, our present evaluations of excuse could remain unchanged but they could be supported and justified by neuroscientific explanations, showing us that addicts are incapacitated to the point of excuse just where and to the extent that we currently think that they are.

Michael S. Moore, *Addiction, Responsibility, and Neuroscience*, 2020 U. Ill. L. Rev. 375, 434 (2020).

D. POLICY PERSPECTIVES

This section reviews policy challenges related to addiction, beginning with the opioid epidemic, and how neuroscience research may inform policy response. Since 2010, the topic at the forefront of the drug policy discussion has been the opioid epidemic. According to the U.S. Department of Health and Human Services, an estimated 130 Americans die every day from opioid-related overdoses, and approximately 2 million people suffer from opioid use disorders.

1. Opioid Epidemic

United States v. Walker
423 F. Supp. 3d 281 (S.D.W. Va. 2017)

GOODWIN, J.

I. INTRODUCTION

The court must decide whether, under Rule 11 of the Federal Rules of Criminal Procedure, to accept or reject the plea agreement between the defendant, Mr. Charles York Walker, and the government. While Rule 11 gives defendants and prosecutors the ability to enter into plea agreements, it also obligates judges to accept or reject those agreements. Rule 11 is silent on what the court should or may consider in its decision.

It is the court's function to prevent the transfer of criminal adjudications from the public arena to the prosecutor's office for the purpose of expediency at the price of confidence in and effectiveness of the criminal justice system. The community of the Southern District of West Virginia must not be systemically excluded from its proper place in this participatory democracy, especially with regard to the heroin and opioid crisis. Because I FIND that the plea agreement proffered in this case is not in the public interest, I REJECT it.

II. BACKGROUND

a. Factual Background

On September 13, 2016, the grand jury in the Southern District of West Virginia returned an indictment against the defendant in case number 2:16-cr-174-1. The indictment charged the defendant with three counts of distributing a quantity of heroin in violation of 21 U.S.C. § 841(a)(1); two counts of distributing a quantity of fentanyl in violation of 21 U.S.C. § 841(a)(1); and one count of being a felon in possession of a firearm in violation of 18 U.S.C. §§ 922(g)(1) and 924(a)(2). The charged conduct occurred between April 14, 2016, and July 14, 2016.

The defendant and the government later entered into a plea agreement. The defendant agreed to plead guilty to a separate, single-count information, and the government agreed to move this court to dismiss the grand jury indictment. On January 23, 2017, the single-count information was filed against the defendant in case number 2:17-cr-10. The information charged Mr. Walker with a single count of possession with intent to distribute a quantity of heroin on July 14, 2016, in violation of 21 U.S.C. § 841(a)(1). On January 26, 2017, the defendant pled guilty to that information. Although I accepted the defendant's guilty plea, I deferred acceptance of the parties' plea agreement until I reviewed the presentence investigation report. I have done so.

During the presentence investigation, a number of troubling facts regarding Mr. Walker's criminal history and the criminal conduct at issue emerged. First, Mr. Walker is intimately familiar with the criminal justice system. At age thirteen, Mr. Walker broke into an apartment and stole jewelry, a radio, and a Nintendo gaming set. . . . From ages fourteen to seventeen, Mr. Walker was convicted of six more theft-related crimes. As an adult, Mr. Walker has been convicted eighteen additional times. His convictions include: possession of a controlled substance, carrying a concealed weapon without a permit, wanton endangerment, possession of cocaine base with intent to distribute, possession of crack cocaine, felon in possession of a firearm, disorderly conduct, three no operator's license convictions, reckless operation of a vehicle, speeding, seatbelt violation, three driving under suspension convictions, and driving under the influence. . . . Additionally, forty-seven other charges against Mr. Walker since the time he was thirteen were either dismissed, dropped, or have an unknown disposition. Despite his very lengthy criminal history, courts and prosecutors have repeatedly given him leniency. . . .

For most of his life, Mr. Walker has been involved with illicit drugs. He began using marijuana at age twelve, cocaine at age thirteen, alcohol at age twenty, PCP at age twenty-six, pills such as Subutex, Roxicodone, and Xanax around age twenty-six, and heroin at age thirty. He admitted that he continued to use marijuana, cocaine, alcohol, pills, and heroin through the time of his arrest for this matter. . . .

c. Cultural Context

The plea agreement proffered by the parties in this case was made in the context of a clear, present, and deadly heroin and opioid crisis in this community. West Virginia is ground zero.

i. The Heroin & Opioid Crisis

The heroin and opioid crisis is a cancer that has grown and metastasized in the body politic of the United States. Heroin and opioids are different from other addictive substances. The principal difference lies in the fact that recreational use is too often deadly. The questionable level of potency in each dose of heroin frequently causes overdose. All too often news stories emerge of "bad batches" that cause a deluge of fatal overdoses. Furthermore, users develop a tolerance over time and, as a result, seek out the highest potency possible without regard to the related risk of death. The Centers for Disease Control and Prevention ("CDC") found that between 2012 and 2014, heroin caused the most overdose deaths of any drug.

Heroin use has increased across the United States in all genders, in most age groups, and in all income levels. "Some of the greatest increases [have] occurred in demographic groups with historically low rates of heroin use: women, the privately insured, and people with higher incomes." It is estimated that 580 people initiate heroin use each day. This rapid increase in heroin use has had deadly consequences. Between 2002 and 2013, the rate of heroin-related overdose deaths per 100,000 people increased 286%. The number of drug overdoses involving heroin tripled from 2010 to 2014. In 2015, heroin caused 12,989 deaths. Heroin arrests by the Drug Enforcement Administration ("DEA") increased at the fastest annual average rate from 2002 to 2014.

In addition to heroin, there is a surge in the popularity of fentanyl and other powerful synthetic opioids. The DEA estimates that "[a]bout two milligrams of fentanyl—about what comes out with a single jiggle of a salt shaker—is considered lethal." Fentanyl and synthetic opioids are particularly dangerous because they can be—and often are—mixed with other drugs without the consumer's knowledge. The national overdose death rate from synthetic opioids increased 72.2% from 2014 to 2015. Illegally made fentanyl is likely the driving force of this increase. According to the National Forensic Laboratory Information System, state and local labs reported 942 fentanyl submissions from law enforcement in 2013 and 3,344 fentanyl submissions in 2014. From 2013 to 2014, the CDC reported significant increases in overdose deaths involving fentanyl in several states.

More dangerous opioids are being developed in order to meet growing demand. An example is furanyl fentanyl, a synthetic designer opioid, commonly referred to as "China White." Furanyl fentanyl can be up to 100 times more potent than heroin. Its effects last longer, and an overdose is more difficult to treat than one caused by heroin alone. Traditional naloxone treatment is often not enough. Laboratory analysis confirmed furanyl fentanyl in Mr. Walker's July 12, 2016 controlled buy.

Another synthetic opioid on the rise is carfentanil, a drug lawfully used to sedate elephants and other large animals. It is an even more potent version of fentanyl often used to "lace" heroin. Carfentanil is 10,000 times more potent than morphine. Because of carfentanil's tremendous potency, it poses a tremendous risk to users and first responders who inadvertently come into contact with the drug in the course of their duties.

The heroin and opioid epidemic is one of the great public health problems of our time. The CDC found that opioids, primarily prescription pain relievers and heroin, are the chief drugs associated with overdose deaths. In 2015, the most recent year for which data is available, opioids were involved in 33,091 deaths, which is more than 63% of all drug overdose deaths. On average, ninety-one Americans die from an opioid overdose every day. Preliminary numbers for 2016 suggest that overdose deaths are growing at a rate comparable to the rate of H.I.V.-related deaths at the height of the H.I.V. epidemic.

In a November 2016 report, the DEA referred to opioid prescription drugs, heroin, and fentanyl as the most significant drug-related threats to the United States. Indeed, opioid overdoses have quadrupled nationally since 1999. According to the CDC, the significant increase in overdose death rates is attributable to synthetic opioids such as heroin and fentanyl.

These drugs are far more dangerous and far more available for abuse. Opioids are in the medicine cabinets of homes all over America and are available at every hospital and doctor's office. With the rise of prescription opioid abuse, heroin, which up until recently had been a tiny fraction of the illicit drug trade, came roaring back. The return of that pale horse may prove to be the event horizon of drug abuse and addiction.

ii. West Virginia's Epidemic

West Virginia has the highest rate of fatal drug overdoses in the nation—and that rate continues to rise. This past year, 86% of overdose deaths involved at least one opioid. From 2001 to 2016, the number of people in the state who died from a drug overdose increased 400%. Our state's fatal drug overdose rate was 41.5 per 100,000 people in 2015, far above the national average of 16.3 per 100,000 people. The West Virginia Health Statistics Center released information that showed that at least 844 people in the state died of drug overdoses in 2016, an increase of 16.9% from 2015 to 2016.

The rate of drug overdose deaths involving synthetic opioids in West Virginia increased 76.4% from 2014 to 2015. In just the last three years, fentanyl use has increased tenfold in West Virginia. The vast majority of patients at the Addiction Program at West Virginia University Hospitals are treated for heroin. Along with Massachusetts, New Hampshire, Ohio, and Rhode Island, West Virginia experienced the largest absolute rate change in death from synthetic opioids.

The Southern District of West Virginia has been hit especially hard. Last August, twenty-six people overdosed during a four-hour span in Huntington. National press reporters quote local health officials as estimating that one in four Huntington residents abuses heroin or some other opioid, meaning that approximately 12,000 people are dealing with opioid addiction in a town of 50,000 people. In April, a pregnant mother in Charleston overdosed at ten o'clock on a Wednesday morning, killing both herself and her unborn baby. No one is immune from the epidemic.

West Virginia leads the nation in the incidence of babies born exposed to drugs and has the highest rate of babies born dependent on opioids. In Huntington, for example, one in ten babies born at the hospital suffers withdrawal from substances such as heroin, opiates, cocaine, or alcohol. That is about fifteen times the national average.

The heroin and opioid crisis in our state implicates the general welfare in a preeminent way. Public safety is the purpose of the criminal justice system. The seriousness of this crisis in West Virginia convinces me that I should carefully scrutinize plea agreements that bargain away multi-count grand jury indictments. Grand jurors are members of our community who have, under their oaths, investigated, and determined that there is probable cause that certain crimes have been committed by the defendant named in the indictment. . . .

III. DISCUSSION

The United States Constitution makes plain that the United States is a participatory democracy. This is a government of the people and by the people. Each of the three branches of government depend upon and require the active participation of the people in the exercise of power.

The exigencies of a changing world have required acceptance of processes that are more streamlined than those contemplated by our Founding Fathers. Plea bargaining is one such process that we have come to embrace. Plea bargaining eliminates the jury and conflates the judge's and prosecutor's roles, creating an administrative system of criminal justice. A species of trial does indeed occur, but it occurs in "the shadow of guilty pleas" rather than in open court.

Without question, resolution of criminal charges by plea bargaining has replaced resolution by jury trial. I concede that plea bargaining is an efficient and convenient system and that public participation in government is inherently inconvenient. Governance by decree is expedient. However, the Founding Fathers intended the wheels of justice to grind slowly and exceedingly fine in order to discern the truth. . . .

. . . I FIND that the plea agreement is not in the public interest, and I REJECT the plea agreement.

IV. CONCLUSION

My twenty-two years of imposing long prison sentences for drug crimes persuades me that the effect of law enforcement on the supply side of the illegal drug market is insufficient to solve the heroin and opioid crisis at hand. I also see scant evidence that prohibition is preventing the growth of the demand side of the drug market. Nevertheless, policy reform, coordinated education efforts, and expansion of treatment programs are not within my bailiwick. I may only enforce the laws of illicit drug prohibition.

The law is the law, and I am satisfied that enforcing the law through public adjudications focuses attention on the heroin and opioid crisis. The jury trial reveals the dark details of drug distribution and abuse to the community in a way that a plea bargained guilty plea cannot. A jury trial tells a story. The jury members listening to the evidence come away with personally impactful information about the deadly and desperate heroin and opioid crisis existing in their community. They are educated in the process of performing their civic duty and are likely to communicate their experience in the courtroom to family members and friends. Moreover, the attendant media attention that a jury trial occasions communicates to the community that such conduct is unlawful and that the law is upheld and enforced. The communication of a threat of severe punishment acts as an effective deterrent. As with other criminalized conduct, the shame of a public conviction and prison sentence specifically deters the sentenced convict from committing the crime again — at least for so long as he is imprisoned.

Over time, jury verdicts involving the distribution of heroin and opioids reinforce condemnation of the conduct by the public at large. In turn, respect for the law propagates. This respect for the law may eventually reduce such criminal conduct.

The secrecy surrounding plea bargains in heroin and opioid cases frequently undermines respect for the law and deterrence of crime. The bright light of the jury trial deters crime, enhances respect for the law, educates the public, and reinforces their sense of safety much more than a contract entered into in the shadows of a private meeting in the prosecutor's office.

For the reasons stated, I REJECT the plea agreement.

NOTES AND QUESTIONS

1. Should a court be permitted to consider the effects of the opioid epidemic during sentencing? In *United States v. Robinson*, the defendant accused the district court of improperly considering the local community's increase in opioid-related

deaths without also considering that his own illegal behavior was compelled by addiction. For his crimes related to drug trafficking activity, the district court sentenced Robinson to 118 months in prison, varying upward by 40 months from the advisory Guidelines imprisonment range of 63 to 78 months. The Sixth Circuit affirmed the district court's sentence, finding no abuse of discretion in the district court's consideration of the devastating effects on the community of dealing "death drugs." Does this result seem fair? *United States v. Robinson*, 892 F.3d 209 (6th Cir. 2018). Compare *Robinson* with *United States v. Hendrickson* (excerpted earlier in the chapter). In *Hendrickson*, the defendant—a 23-year-old man who began using marijuana and methamphetamine when he was 14—was convicted of possessing stolen firearms. Noting that the defendant's "addiction . . . appears to be extraordinary given how young he was when he started abusing marijuana and methamphetamine, and how directly his criminal history is related to, and influenced by, his addiction," the judge issued a sentence that was six months below the low end of the sentencing guidelines range. Which approach do you think is better? What legal and policy considerations should be most important for judges when making this determination?

2. Are there any individuals or entities that can be held liable for the opioid epidemic's widespread destruction? Until recently, the answer seemed to be no, as lawsuits brought by addicts against opioid manufacturers were regularly unsuccessful. More recently, however, suits filed by state and local governments have shown more promise, as pharmaceutical companies have chosen to pay large settlements rather than litigate. As tracked by the organization Good Jobs First, since 2000 pharmaceutical companies have paid a total of $38,272,710,449 in penalties.

  The first case to go to trial over opioid-manufacturer liability was decided in August of 2019, when an Oklahoma District Court held that drug maker Johnson & Johnson owed $572 million in damages (later reduced to $465 million after the judge acknowledged an error in calculation) on a public nuisance theory of liability that stemmed from Johnson & Johnson's misleading marketing efforts. Sara Randazzo & Jared S. Hopkins, *Judge Rules Johnson & Johnson Helped Fuel Opioid Epidemic*, Wall St. J., Aug. 27, 2019, at A1. Whether or not the district court's holding will survive Johnson & Johnson's appeal, filed in December of 2019, remains to be seen.

  In addition to public nuisance, other potential theories to hold opioid manufacturers and distributors liable include negligence, negligent marketing, fraudulent misrepresentation and fraudulent concealment claims, and statutory violation claims. *See* Richard C. Ausness, *The Current State of Opioid Litigation*, 70 S.C. L. Rev. 565 (2019).

3. How should the law respond to medically assisted treatment options for addiction? Consider this contrast:

> For Shawn Schneider, a carpenter and rock musician, the descent into addiction began one Wisconsin winter with a fall from a rooftop construction site onto the frozen ground below. As the potent pain pills prescribed for his injuries became his obsessive focus, he lost everything: his band, his job, his wife, his will to live. Mr. Schneider was staying in his parents' basement when he washed down 40 sleeping pills with NyQuil and beer. His father heard him gasping and intervened, a reprieve that led Mr. Schneider into rehab, not his first program, but the one where

he discovered buprenorphine, a substitute opioid used to treat opioid addiction. In the two years since, by taking his "bupe" twice daily and meeting periodically with the prescribing psychiatrist, Mr. Schneider, 38, has rebounded. He is sober, remarried, employed building houses, half of a new acoustic duo and one of the many addicts who credit buprenorphine, sold mostly in a compound called Suboxone, with saving their lives.

Suboxone did not save Miles Malone, 20; it killed him. In 2010, a friend texted Mr. Malone an invitation to use the drug recreationally—"we can do the suboxins as soon as I give them to u, iight, dude?"—and he died that night in South Berwick, Me., of buprenorphine poisoning. The friend, Shawn Verrill, was sentenced this summer to 71 months in prison. "I didn't know you could overdose on Suboxone," Mr. Verrill said in an interview at a federal prison in Otisville, N.Y. "We were just a bunch of friends getting high and hanging out, doing what 20-year-olds do. Then we went to sleep, and Miles never woke up." . . . Mr. Verrill pleaded guilty to the distribution of buprenorphine resulting in death. "I feel guilty," he said in the recent interview, wearing prison khaki, his arms inked with the saying, "What goes around comes around."

Deborah Sontag, *Addiction Treatment with a Dark Side*, N.Y. Times, Nov. 16, 2013, at A1.

Buprenorphine is regularly used to treat addiction, and courts are now often asked to incorporate it as part of an offender's treatment plan. What questions should judges and attorneys ask when considering such treatment plans?

4. Before the wave of litigation against opioid manufacturers and distributors, there was a similar wave of litigation against cigarette manufacturers. In 1998 a Tobacco Master Settlement Agreement was reached between the attorneys general of 46 states and the four largest tobacco companies in the United States. However, before and even since the settlement agreement, the addictiveness of nicotine has not always persuaded juries to allow recovery. The legal doctrines at the center of these cases are assumption of risk (by the smoker) and duty of care (by the manufacturer). Describing such litigation, Professor Richard Cupp writes:

> Classic assumption of risk doctrine completely precluded recovery when a plaintiff subjectively appreciated a risk and voluntarily encountered it. With the rise of comparative fault principles, however, many courts have become reluctant to require that a plaintiff's claim be eliminated altogether by assumption of risk. . . . But if the defendant owes a duty of care and the plaintiff impliedly assumes a risk, courts are increasingly treating the plaintiff's choice as equivalent to comparative fault. Indeed, many jurisdictions have held that assumption of risk no longer exists as a legal doctrine in such situations; it is subsumed by the doctrine of comparative fault. . . . Whether viewed as a potential complete bar to recovery or as equivalent to comparative fault, the assumption of risk doctrine's requirements of subjective appreciation of risk and voluntariness are highly flexible. Because of this flexibility, moral judgments by courts and juries may significantly influence how the requirements are interpreted. . . .
>
> The moral drama invited by assumption of risk's flexible nature has special significance in tobacco litigation. Because most jurors have found the specter of smokers suing over cigarettes morally offensive, the jurors have had little difficulty interpreting the voluntariness and knowledge requirements in a manner that denied plaintiffs recovery. . . . Unlike cases involving employees injured by products used at work, courts and jurors have seen no compelling reason to rescue tobacco plaintiffs from the consequences of their choices.

Richard L. Cupp, Jr., *A Morality Play's Third Act: Revisiting Addiction, Fraud and Consumer Choice in "Third Wave" Tobacco Litigation*, 46 U. Kan. L. Rev. 465, 477-81 (1998). How might these doctrines be invoked today with respect to opioid litigation?

2. Drug Policy, Treatment, and Rehabilitation

David M. Eagleman, Mark A. Correro & Jyotpal Singh
Why Neuroscience Matters for Rational Drug Policy
11 Minn. J.L. Sci. & Tech. 7, 10-26 (2010)

In the twentieth century, American drug policy vacillated between punishment and rehabilitation. . . . [A]t the dawn of the twenty-first century, the decades-long demand for punishment is straining the criminal justice system. . . . We suggest that the most fruitful path is to forego the arguments of responsibility in favor of concentrating neuroscientific efforts on rehabilitation.

III. NEUROSCIENTIFIC STRATEGIES FOR REHABILITATION

Cutting-edge ideas on the horizon offer new hope for directly treating drug addiction rather than focusing on punishment. We briefly outline the evidence-based strategies currently in use. We then turn to two innovative strategies—cocaine vaccines and real-time feedback in neuroimaging—which offer fresh approaches and new opportunities for dialogue in the problem of drug addiction. Such neurally-based treatments can equip policy-makers with tools to treat additions with maximal efficacy and minimum cost. . . .

B. Real-Time Feedback Using Neuroimaging

. . . [C]raving reduction—already a prime target of cognitive-behavioral, psychotherapeutic, and pharmaceutical approaches—is one of the prime objectives for new technologies. Dozens of functional neuroimaging studies, mostly in nicotine and cocaine-dependent individuals, have highlighted a distributed network of brain regions that show increased activity in response to drug-related cues. . . . [D]ata point to the distributed neural network involved in craving (and the insula in particular) as prime targets for craving-reduction.

. . . [T]here is another half to drug addiction besides craving: deficits in impulse control. Neuroimaging has revealed a related network of areas involved in cognitive control, involving areas known as the orbitofrontal cortex (OFC), anterior cingulate cortex (ACC), and dorsolateral prefrontal cortex (DLPFC). . . . These data suggest direct therapeutic interventions should be used to enhance cognitive control in drug addicts.

How can we hope to directly affect specific brain networks? A new technology on the horizon—real-time neurofeedback—suggests one possibility. Neuroimaging known as functional magnetic resonance imaging (fMRI) allows the viewing of neural activity. In a new development owing to the introduction of fast computation and efficient algorithms, raw data from the imaging can be reconstructed on-the-fly (in close to "real-time") and visually displayed in the scanner. In this way, neural activity can be shown directly to an individual and that person can attempt to modify it. This technique is known as real-time fMRI, or rt-fMRI, or simply as neurofeedback.

The approach is similar to the biofeedback strategies of previous decades, except that it allows a view inside the skull, giving a level of precision never before possible. . . . It puts the individual in the driver's seat of his own neural circuitry. To date, this technology has been used to address pain and depression. Neuroscience is leveraging this technology for a novel approach to addiction. Specifically, rt-fMRI is being used to decrease neural activations associated with craving and increase neural activations associated with cognitive control. This strategy may allow the overcoming of habitual responses to drug-cues in addicts. . . . This technology, together with other new developments, may reinvigorate the discussion of possibilities for customized rehabilitation.

C. The Cocaine Vaccine

Another complementary approach circumvents the continued reinforcement generated by the drug high. This possibility is a drug vaccine, an intervention that renders the individual unable to become high since the immune system will "fight" the drug before it reaches the brain.

A drug vaccination is accomplished in the traditional biological manner of all inoculations: a foreign substance is injected into the blood stream, and the immune system then raises antibodies against the invader. In this case, the cocaine molecule, which is attached to a large protein molecule, is injected. The new antibodies come to recognize not only the cocaine-protein complex, but also the naked cocaine molecule. Now that the body has hosted an immune response, new injections of cocaine into the bloodstream will be surrounded by the body's natural antibodies. In this way, the vaccination prevents—or at minimum slows down—the crossing of the cocaine molecules across the blood-brain barrier. The high is thus eliminated or at least attenuated. Currently, the cocaine vaccine is in clinical trials and shows early promise.

Dr. Tom Kosten, one of the lead developers of the vaccine, sees the vaccine as most useful for addicts who desire to stop using cocaine, but continue to be stymied by relapses. The strategy is simple (if yet unproven): if an individual vaccinates and then relapses, she will not find the expected high, and her craving will eventually recalibrate. In other words, she will lose interest.

If the vaccine works well, it could shift treatment from counseling and rehabilitation programs to a mandatory vaccination. There are, of course, some potential problems with the notion of a drug vaccine. One is that addicts inoculated against cocaine may well turn to another drug for satisfaction, and this highlights the importance of addressing the craving and impulse control issues surrounding drug taking. As Robert Julien notes: "Just as focus cannot be solely on the drug of dependence and its rewarding and withdrawal effects . . . neither can it be only on pharmacotherapy for treatment. . . . [A]ddicts will have to be able to handle later exposure to craving-eliciting cues in the environment." Vaccines in combination with neurofeedback may well prove to be a fruitful combination. . . .

NOTES AND QUESTIONS

1. The challenges of addiction are not unique to the United States. A report from the European Monitoring Centre for Drugs and Drug Addiction recommended a series of responses, including:

> The autonomy of addicts is variable so care is required in using medical, paternalistic and criminal measures to control and treat addiction. If an addict is conceptualized as being wholly without autonomy, which is not the case in lucid periods, then human rights and appropriate ethical values are likely to take a back seat to the public interest. When autonomy is seriously impaired, it may be appropriate to take paternalistic measures to protect addicts from harming themselves or others. Responses to addiction need to include both punitive measures (i.e., in response to the autonomy and responsibilities of drug users) and improved access to addiction treatment.
>
> . . . The autonomy of addicts is impaired by their addiction but not usually sufficiently so to warrant strong paternalistic interventions that override their wishes. Treatment of addiction should aim to build on and support addicts' autonomy and ensure that their consent to treatment is as informed and given as freely as possible.

   Benjamin Capps et al., *Conclusions and Possible Implications of Advances in Addiction Neurobiology for Future Drug Policies*, in *Addiction Neurobiology: Ethical and Social Implications* 125 (European Monitoring Ctr. for Drugs and Drug Addiction 2009). How should public policy account for the autonomy of addicts? What balance should be struck between paternalistic policies and policies that allow for more individual choice?

2. Some research suggests that when given the choice, users will prefer money over cocaine or methamphetamine. *See* C.L. Hart et al., *Alternative Reinforcers Differentially Modify Cocaine Self-Administration by Humans*, 11 Behav. Pharmacology 87 (2000); William W. Stoops et al., *Alternative Reinforcer Response Cost Impacts Cocaine Choice in Humans*, 36 Progress Neuro-Psychopharmacology & Biological Psychiatry 189 (2012); J. Adam Bennett et al., *Alternative Reinforcer Response Cost Impacts Methamphetamine Choice in Humans*, 103 Pharmacology Biochemistry & Behav. 481 (2013). If cocaine and methamphetamine users prefer money to drugs, would a more intelligent drug policy simply pay them to stop instead of incarcerating them? How would this research affect your views on the wisdom of pursuing vaccines against various drug addictions?

3. Even with a growing body of research on addiction and its neurobiology, public policy has struggled to find effective ways to respond. As Keith Humphreys et al. explain, many aspects of public policy are seemingly inconsistent with the neuroscience of addiction. For example, health insurance typically only covers short-term detoxification, even though research suggests that long-term contingency management programs, such as sober living and enhanced case management, are significantly more effective. Keith Humphreys et al., *Brains, Environments, and Policy Responses to Addiction*, 356 Science 1237 (2017). Even where insurance companies do cover medication to treat opioid addiction, many doctors find the unique "prior-authorization" process required by insurers too burdensome and opt out of prescribing those medications. Brian Barnett, Opinion, *Insurers Are Making It Harder for Me to Treat My Opioid-Addicted Patients*, Wall St. J. (Apr. 24, 2018).

   As the opioid epidemic's death toll grows more and more alarming, calls for changes in public policy are mounting. In response, Congress added an additional $500 million to the National Institutes of Health's budget, effective 2018, to a new initiative called Helping to End Addiction Long-term (HEAL). HEAL will focus its efforts on two primary areas: "improving treatments for opioid misuse and addiction as well as enhancing strategies for pain management." Francis S. Collins, Walter J. Koroshetz & Nora D. Volkow, *Helping to End Addiction over the Long-Term: The Research Plan for the NIH HEAL Initiative*, 320 J. Am. Med. Ass'n 129, 129 (2018). If you were in charge of HEAL, what research opportunities would you fund to accomplish these goals? How would you change the criminal justice system in light of emerging research on addiction?

4. Not all agree that the solution requires more basic science research. Consider the perspective of psychiatrist Dr. Allen Frances:

> The human brain is the most complicated thing in the known universe and keeps its secrets well hidden. Genetics and neuroimaging have shown how remarkably complex and interacting are the biopsychosocial causes of mental illness and that there will likely never be magic bullets. . . . We need a moon-shot mentality—and it doesn't require rocket science or new research. We have known for 50 years how to provide good care for severe mental illness. There is nothing mysterious or complicated about it. Decent housing. Easily accessible treatment. Social clubs. Vocational rehab. Positive regard, respect, and empathy. Family support.

Allen Frances, *Dungeons and Back Alleys: The Fate of the Mentally Ill in America*, Psychiatric Times (Oct. 4, 2019).

5. Some in law and public health argue that "[p]overty and substance use problems operate synergistically, at the extreme reinforced by psychiatric disorders and unstable housing." Nabarun Dasgupta, Leo Beletsky & Daniel Ciccarone, *Opioid Crisis: No Easy Fix to Its Social and Economic Determinants*, 108 Am. J. Pub. Health 182, 183 (2018). What other factors beyond brain science should be considered when addressing the legal consequences of addiction?

6. Despite studies suggesting that methadone is the most effective treatment for opioid use disorder, methadone remains difficult to obtain in the United States. James Bell & John Strang, *Medication Treatment of Opioid Use Disorder*, 87 Biological Psychiatry 82 (2020). Currently, methadone is only available through "methadone clinics," where patients visit a clinic site for daily treatment. The last time Congress enacted legislation addressing opioid use treatment medication was in 2000. Is it time for Congress to enact a new law expanding access to the drug? What might explain congressional hesitation to relax access to the medication? *See* Jeffrey H. Samet, Michael Botticelli & Monica Bharel, *Methadone in Primary Care—One Small Step for Congress, One Giant Leap for Addiction Treatment*, 379 New Eng. J. Med. 7 (2018).

   Researchers are now looking beyond traditional prescription medications to alternative treatments for substance use disorder, though more research is necessary to determine efficacy. As one example, transcranial direct current stimulation has been shown to temporarily reduce alcohol cravings, although relapse remains high; electroconvulsive therapy and transcranial magnetic stimulation show more promise. Celeste A. Azevedo & Antonios Mammis, *Neuromodulation Therapies for Alcohol Addiction: A Literature Review*, 21 Neuromodulation 144 (2017); Mailu Enokibara et al., *Establishing an Effective TMS Protocol for Craving in Substance Addiction: Is It Possible?*, 25 Am. J. on Addictions 28 (2016).

7. Humans regularly become addicted to more than just substances. Many, for instance, are addicted to gambling. A prominent example is the former Mayor of

San Diego, Maureen O'Connor. Once worth more than $50 million, O'Connor became addicted to video gambling and over a period of ten years won and lost in over $1 billion worth of transactions. Madison Gray, *Maureen O'Connor: Former San Diego Mayor Bet More than $1 Billion as a Result of Gambling Addiction*, Time (Feb. 15, 2013). She was charged with a crime when it was discovered that she had stolen $2.1 million from her late husband's charitable foundation. She stole the money to fuel her gambling. Should addiction to gambling be recognized as a criminal defense and mitigating factor at sentencing? To what extent should companies that create and promote gambling technology be held liable? *See* Natasha Dow Schüll, *Addiction by Design: Machine Gambling in Las Vegas* (2012). For a review of the neurobiology of addiction to gambling, see Mira Fauth-Bühler, Karl Mann & Marc N. Potenza, *Pathological Gambling: A Review of the Neurobiological Evidence Relevant for its Classification as an Addictive Disorder*, 22 Addiction Biology 885 (2017).

3. Drug Courts

State v. Little
66 P.3d 1099 (Wash. Ct. App. 2003)

HUNT, C.J. Seth C. Little appeals the trial court's denial of his motion to dismiss an information charging him with unlawful possession of a controlled substance. He argues that the lack of a drug court in Grays Harbor County denied him equal protection of the law. We disagree and affirm.

Having been charged with unlawful possession of a controlled substance (methamphetamine), Little asked the Grays Harbor Superior Court either (1) to provide him with access to a drug court program, which Grays Harbor County does not have; or (2) to dismiss the information with prejudice because the lack of a drug court program violated his right to equal protection. The trial court denied Little's motion and, following a bench trial on stipulated facts, convicted him as charged.

In 1999, the Legislature enacted RCW 2.28.170, which enables counties to establish drug courts. It provides in pertinent part as follows:

> (1) Counties *may* establish and operate drug courts.
> (2) For the purposes of this section, "drug court" means a court that has special calendars or dockets designed to achieve a reduction in recidivism and substance abuse among nonviolent, substance abusing offenders by increasing their likelihood for successful rehabilitation through early, continuous, and intense judicially supervised treatment; mandatory periodic drug testing; and the use of appropriate sanctions and other rehabilitation services.

RCW 2.28.170 (emphasis added). At the time of Little's trial and sentencing, Grays Harbor County had not established a drug court.

Little argues that the lack of a drug court program in Grays Harbor County deprived him of his right to equal protection of the law because similarly situated drug offenders in other counties have access to drug courts. He further contends that we should apply the strict scrutiny standard of review because felony convictions result in a loss of fundamental civil rights. . . .

. . . Little has not shown that he is part of a similarly situated class being treated differently so as to trigger equal protection analysis here. There is no suspect class at issue here such as race, alienage, or national origin. Committing a drug crime in a smaller county or one with limited financial resources, as compared to committing a drug crime in a large or resource-rich county, is not such a suspect classification; rather, it is not a classification for equal protection purposes at all.

Little is correct that drug defendants in counties with drug court diversion programs have the opportunity to avoid a felony post-conviction loss of fundamental rights by successfully completing such a program, an opportunity that he does not have in Grays Harbor County. The goal of drug courts, however, is treatment. But there is no fundamental right to treatment, in lieu of prosecution, once a person has violated the law. Thus, equal protection analysis is more appropriate under the rational relationship standard.

Under the rational relationship test, "the legislative classification will be upheld unless it rests on grounds wholly irrelevant to achievement of legitimate state objectives." The challenger must also do more than challenge the wisdom of the legislative classification; he must "show conclusively that the classification is purely arbitrary."

In passing RCW 2.28.170, the "legislature recognize[d] the utility of drug court programs in reducing recidivism and assisting the courts by diverting potential offenders from the normal course of criminal trial proceedings." Little does not dispute that this purpose is a legitimate state objective. Rather, he contends that by failing to require all counties to establish drug courts, the statute has created two classifications: counties with drug counties and counties without. Thus, the alleged equal protection issue is whether this so-called legislative classification is rationally related to the legislation's purpose.

First, as we noted earlier, RCW 2.28.170 does not create classifications. Thus, our inquiry could end here. . . .

Moreover, "equal protection does not require that a state choose between attacking every aspect of a problem and not attacking the problem at all." . . .

Little has failed to carry his heavy burden of establishing an equal protection violation. The Legislature acted rationally in approaching the pervasive illegal drug use problem in a piecemeal fashion, rather than not acting at all, and in learning from the experience of counties that choose to implement drug courts. . . .

Morris B. Hoffman
Problem-Solving Courts and the Psycholegal Error
160 U. Pa. L. Rev. PENNumbra 129, 129-38 (2011)

Every two-stoplight town now has a drug court. . . . Most of these courts still do not "work" . . . ; they often make things worse. . . . Their therapeutic subset relies on a whole addiction industry that is more snake oil than science . . . , populated largely by recovering addicts rather than trained . . . professionals. These courts have changed parts of the judiciary from a coequal branch of government to a bureaucratic thirteenth step along a road to social recovery. . . .

. . . Drug courts . . . are popular with judges and . . . bureaucrats because [they] typically drive case numbers up [that improve chief judge budgets]. Filings go up because . . . the existence of the drug court itself stimulates more case filings. The mechanisms of [so-called] net-widening are not always clear. . . . But the effects can be significant. In Denver, where I preside, drug filings almost tripled one year after the institution of our drug court . . . [because] police and prosecutors are no longer [detecting] crime; they are trolling for patients. Arrests that might never be made in the shadow of a truth-finding system get regularly made when guilt and truth are irrelevant. Cases that prosecutors would never have filed if they actually had to be proved beyond a reasonable doubt are regularly filed in therapeutic systems, where a not guilty plea is called denial, and proof is all back-loaded to the question of whether a defendant complied with required therapy. . . .

Treatment courts do not admit that they are "excusing" their "clients," but . . . the treatment component is enforced by way of conditions to a deferred judgment. . . .

Which brings us to the puzzle of addiction. . . . [V]ery little is really known about the neurology of addiction. . . .

Somehow, most of [us] are able to maintain a satisfying level of pleasure without having to overindulge. But others of us . . . need more and more indulgence to maintain the same level of dopamine-driven satisfaction. . . . At the extreme, addicts are not getting any pleasure at all from their drug of choice. . . . Their pleasure circuits have become dopamine-starved pain circuits.

But because we know so little about [the difference between] cocaine [and] sex or potato chips, we . . . know very little about when [a] behavior should be treated as a "choice" for purposes of responsibility [or as] the product of an excused cause — the excuse of addiction. . . .

So when it comes to the criminal decisions of addicted minds, the law has remained . . . unimpressed with the therapeutic movement, and . . . resistant to the lure of the psycholegal error. When an addict rapes . . . , his addiction is not the "cause" of the rape . . . and it is almost never an excuse. And yet, when that same addict is charged with the crime of possessing the drug to which he is addicted, the addiction suddenly becomes the cause of his possession, and in therapeutic courts a complete excuse. . . . But if the addict in both cases does not "choose" to use, then how can the addict-rapist's use be ignored under the rubric of voluntary intoxication? In both cases, under the therapeutic model, the addict had no choice but to use. Yet our . . . courts excuse the crime of continued use but not the crime of drug-induced rape. Why? . . .

Morris B. Hoffman
Drug Courts and the Myth of the Addict's Diseased Brain
29 Fed. Sent'g Rep. 207, 207-09 (2017)

All I can say . . . based on my [understanding of] the discipline, neuroscience can currently shed almost no light on how healthy brains make decisions, and therefore almost no light on how addicted brains make decisions, let alone with the degree of confidence justifying national and international norms by which drug use is being forgiven but the failure to be cured is being punished. . . .

Addiction isn't . . . a "brain disease." . . . Psychiatrists have long understood that behaviors, as opposed to pathologies of the body, are almost always products of profoundly complicated relationships between intention, will, choice, consequence, psychology, emotion, social setting, and culture. As a result, virtually no behaviors, whether benign, prosocial, self-destructive, or antisocial, have any identifiable mechanism of causation. That's why . . . why not a single psychiatric diagnosis in the DSM-V is described as a "disease." These diagnoses are instead labelled "disorders" or syndromes" to emphasize the fact that their etiology is unknown.

What's the harm in a little medical or neuroscientific exaggeration in the cause of the greater good of getting the public interested in trying to help addicts? The answer is that the disease model of addiction [has] sent some in the therapeutic community on a dangerously illusive hunt for addiction's "cause." Now brains are being treated instead of people. . . .

The very fact that, when treatment push comes to shove, drug courts end up sending their uncured patients to prison suggests that we all recognize . . . that like all behaviors, addictions are a complex mix of many ingredients, including that old-fashioned one now held in such disrepute: will. . . . By continuing the myth that addiction is a brain disease, we continue to ignore the critical role of will and its messy constituents of choice, consequence, social milieu, and culture. We do so at our peril.

NOTES AND QUESTIONS

1. Drug court programs may involve urine testing, therapy, and court appearances. Some research into the success rates of these programs suggests that individuals routed to drug courts have reduced rates of recidivism compared to those who enter the traditional criminal system. Ojmarrh Mitchell et al., *Assessing the Effectiveness of Drug Courts on Recidivism: A Meta-Analytic Review of Traditional and Non-Traditional Drug Courts*, 40 J. Crim. Just. 60 (2012). But other assessments are less favorable. Josh Bowers, *Contraindicated Drug Courts*, 55 UCLA L. Rev. 783 (2008). What would you want to know about a drug court before implementation? How expansive would the court be?

2. Law professor and neuroscientist Emily Murphy writes: "Rather than only asking how neuroscience technologies could be effectively integrated into drug courts—indeed a complex question in and of itself—the potential risks and benefits promised by new technologies should shift the essential question to: are drug courts the right way to tackle the problem?" How might neuroscience shift this more fundamental debate? Emily R. Murphy, *Paved with Good Intentions: Sentencing Alternatives from Neuroscience and the Policy of Problem-Solving Courts*, 37 L. & Psychol. Rev. 83, 111 (2013).

FURTHER READING

Addiction Science:

Carlton K. Erickson, *The Science of Addiction: From Neurobiology to Treatment* (2007).

Deborah S. Hasin et al., *DSM-5 Criteria for Substance Use Disorders: Recommendations and Rationale*, 170 Am. J. Psychiatry 834 (2013).

Gene M. Heyman, *Addiction: A Disorder of Choice* (2009).

P. Read Montague, *The Freedom to Choose and Drug Addiction*, in *4 Moral Psychology: Free Will and Moral Responsibility* 279 (Walter Sinnott-Armstrong ed., 2014).

Nat'l Inst. on Drug Abuse, *Drugs, Brains, and Behavior: The Science of Addiction* (2018).

Charles P. O'Brien, *Drug Use Disorders and Addiction*, in *Goodman & Gilman's The Pharmacological Basis of Therapeutics* (Laurence Brunton et al. eds., 13th ed. 2018).

Antonio Rangel et al., *A Framework for Studying the Neurobiology of Value-Based Decision Making*, 9 Nature Revs. Neurosci. 545 (2008).

A. David Redish et al., *A Unified Framework for Addiction: Vulnerabilities in the Decision Process*, 31 Behav. & Brain Sci. 415 (2008).

U.S. Dep't of Health & Human Servs., Substance Abuse and Mental Health Servs. Admin., https://www.samhsa.gov.

Antonio Verdejo-Garcia et al., *A Roadmap for Integrating Neuroscience into Addiction Treatment: A Consensus of the Neuroscience Interest Group of the International Society of Addiction Medicine*, 10 Frontiers Psychiatry 877 (2019).

Addiction and Legal Responsibility:

Addiction and Self-Control: Perspectives from Philosophy, Psychology, and Neuroscience (Neil Levy ed., 2014).

Michael S. Moore, *Addiction and Responsibility*, in *The Palgrave Handbook of Applied Ethics and the Criminal Law* (2019).

Stephen J. Morse, *Addiction, Genetics and Criminal Responsibility*, 69 L. & Contemp. Probs. 165 (2006).

Gideon Yaffe, *Are Addicts Akratic?: Interpreting the Neuroscience of Reward*, in *Addiction and Self-Control: Perspectives from Philosophy, Psychology, and Neuroscience* (Neil Levy ed., 2014).

Addiction and Public Policy:

Charles Dackis & Charles O'Brien, *Neurobiology of Addiction: Treatment and Public Policy Ramifications*, 8 Nature Neurosci. 1431 (2005).

Richard A. Millstein & Alan I. Leshner, *The Science of Addiction: Research and Public Health Perspectives*, 3 J. Health Care L. & Pol'y 151 (1999).

David F. Musto, *The American Disease: Origins of Narcotic Control* (1999).

CHAPTER 13

Memory

Memory is a biological process that can be manipulated by modern biology like anything else. Not only can you disrupt it, you can improve it.
— Dr. Timothy Tully, Founder of Helicon Therapeutics[†]

It took me a very, very long time to get that out of my memory. Why would I want to talk about that? Would you?
— Sexual Assault "Victim 7" (2012)[††]

CHAPTER SUMMARY

This chapter:
- Introduces what is currently understood about how humans remember and forget.
- Explores how memory is linked to law through eyewitness testimony, false memories, cross-race identification, amnesia, and the like.
- Introduces current psychological and brain science research on our ability, and inability, to detect false memories in ourselves and others.

INTRODUCTION

The waking hours of every day are filled with unceasing floods of events, facts, and feelings. We remember some better than others. And rarely do facts relevant to the legal system arrive with the advance notice: *Warning: Pay special attention — Someday you will be asked to testify about the events that are about to happen.*

But we at least remember *important* things. Or do we? On September 11th, 2001, the most devastating attack on American soil since Pearl Harbor happened. A study of people's recollections of the traumatic events of the terrorist attacks in New York, Washington, D.C., and Pennsylvania — both immediately after and years later — suggests that people more accurately remember some kinds of details better than they accurately remember other kinds.[*] For example, subjects tended to misremember the intensity with which they felt sadness, anger, fear, confusion, frustration,

---

† O. Carter Snead, *Memory and Punishment*, 64 Vand. L. Rev. 1195, 1213 (2011).

†† Associated Press, *Grilling Leaves Base Sex Scandal Accuser in Tears* (July 19, 2012). The witness responded to allegations of inconsistencies in her testimony, during a court martial case against a staff sergeant at Lackland Airforce Base. The defendant was found guilty of rape and sexual assault.

* William Hirst et al., *Long-Term Memory for the Terrorist Attack of September 11: Flashbulb Memories, Event Memories, and the Factors that Influence Their Retention*, 138 J. Experimental Psychol. 161 (2009).

and shock more than they misremembered the logistical details of where and from whom they learned of the attacks.

As the science excerpts in this chapter will make clear, we know that human memory does not function like a video recorder. Moreover, there are tremendous individual differences in memory ability. You probably know people who never forget a face and always remember your birthday. But you probably also know people who always forget their keys and can never remember where they parked. What explains our differing abilities to remember and forget? Scientists do not have wholly satisfying answers, but memory science has advanced greatly and already influences law in a number of ways.

In this chapter we consider some of the special problems the science of memory poses for the legal system. Evidence in the form of recollected and described memories is so widespread in both criminal and civil legal proceedings that it is hard to step back to ask: How much of a difference is there between what we believe to be true about memories and what science shows to be true? Yet, given the enormity of what is often at stake in litigation, ensuring a minimally just legal system may require us to confront that difference and to assess its magnitude.

This chapter opens in Section A with a brief survey of the current state of knowledge about the organization and function of human memory. Section B excerpts material from two cases, *State v. Henderson* and *Perry v. New Hampshire*, that grappled directly with the uneven accuracy of eyewitness testimony, and that illustrate the extent to which this area of law is in flux. Section C focuses on the thorny problems surrounding so-called "false memories," which, if actually false, can inspire the legal system to errors that may ruin multiple lives. Section D examines legal responses to research on the difficulties of cross-racial identification. In addition to the material covered in this chapter, memory enhancement and memory dampening are covered in Chapter 19 on Cognitive Enhancement.

A. ORGANIZATION AND FUNCTION OF HUMAN MEMORY

Memory is central to legal doctrine, legal practice, and to legal studies. In the two excerpts to follow law professor O. Carter Snead and psychologist Daniel Schacter provide a brief summary of the current state of psychological knowledge about legally relevant memory science and detail the specific limitations of human memory.

O. Carter Snead
Memory and Punishment
64 Vand. L. Rev. 1195, 1199-1212 (2011)

I. WHAT IS MEMORY? A COGNITIVE AND SCIENTIFIC ACCOUNT

[This section surveys] the cognitive and biological dimensions of memory. The science of memory is obviously a vast and contested domain. . . . The following will be a necessarily cursory treatment. . . .

Though memory has long been the focus of philosophical reflection, the first empirical study of memory and its function was done by Hermann Ebbinghaus in 1885, who conducted an experiment . . . to measure the temporal relationship between encoding, retrieving, and forgetting information. He memorized long sequences of nonsense syllables, and tested his own memory, varying the length of time between learning the lists and trying to recall them. He found that the longer the delay, the less he could recall. He also learned that memories are strengthened by repetition. Later . . . evolutionary biologist Richard Semon published a monograph . . . in which he tried to unite the biological analysis of heredity with the psychological analysis of memory. . . . One of Semon's lasting contributions . . . was his term "engram" denoting the "enduring change in the nervous system ('memory trace') that conserves effects of experience over time." . . . [T]his notion of a "memory trace" closely tracks the modern view that a new pattern of neural connections in the brain, strengthened over time, is the "brain's record of the event."

Many important early developments in the science of memory in human subjects emerged from research involving amnesiacs. The famous case of Henry Molaison ("H.M.") . . . shed light on the distinctive systems of memory and their reliance on different regions of the brain. As a treatment for seizures, H.M. had a number of structures in his medial temporal lobes removed, including much of his hippocampus, his amygdala, and some adjacent portions of the temporal cortex. This erased his memories of personal experiences shortly before the operation, though he could still retain . . . memories predating that event. He was incapable, however, of forming new memories of personal experiences, though he could learn new skills. The case of H.M. revealed that the [medial temporal lobe] plays a time-limited role in encoding certain kinds of memories, memory and cognition are separate and distinct, short-term (working) memory does not rely on the same structures in the [medial temporal lobe], and some types of long-term memory (motor skills, etc.) do not rely on the [medial temporal lobes].

[Building on the earlier work] . . . an interdisciplinary synthesis of clinicians (including psychologists, neurologists, and psychiatrists), cognitive psychologists, and neuroscientists revolutionized the science of memory. This has opened the possibility of a cognitive neuroscience of memory integrated with a molecular biology of cognition. As a result, memory can now be explored in terms of cognition, cellular and molecular mechanisms, and the neural systems of the brain.

A. The Cognitive "Systems" of Memory

Modern [researchers] have long suspected that memory is a multifaceted faculty, composed of distinctive divisions. . . . The current understanding is that memory includes an array of distinctive processes and systems, involving different neural structures. [The current understanding of the organization of human memory is illustrated in Figure 13.1, which also identifies the major brain structures responsible for the different kinds of memories. —EDS.] It has been suggested that various memory systems evolved because they serve starkly different purposes. Nevertheless, the systems of memory do not operate in isolation—one experience can produce many forms of memory, and different kinds of memory may recruit overlapping regions of the brain.

The term "declarative" memory was introduced to capture one system, and "nondeclarative" memory to capture . . . various motor and perceptual skills, habits, and emotional learning, as well as . . . habituation, sensitization, and classical and operant conditioning. Nondeclarative memory is unconscious. . . . It is not true or false. Examples include . . . riding a bicycle. . . .

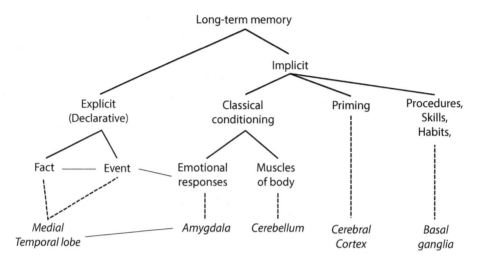

Figure 13.1 Organization of human memory. Thick lines indicate hierarchical organization. Dotted lines highlight the neural substrates for the different kinds of memories. Thin lines draw attention to functional linkages across kinds of memories. Explicit (also known as declarative) memory about facts and events requires the medial temporal lobe. This is what most people consider as memory. Implicit memory is not experienced consciously but represents enduring changes of behavior derived from different kinds of experiences. Classical conditioning refers to the associations of general stimuli like sights or sounds with primary stimuli like food or pain. These associations, linked to emotional responses, require the amygdala. Anatomical pathways between the medial temporal lobe and amygdala (indicated by the thin lines) mediate the coloring of memory for events by emotional context. Other forms of classical conditioning can influence body movements, but these are unlikely to have much legal relevance. Priming refers to changes in responses to stimuli that happen after repeated exposures to an item; the item can be perceptual (e.g., sensory stimuli) or conceptual (e.g., word lists or pictures). Although priming is not experienced consciously, it can influence decisions. Priming depends on the cerebral cortex. Finally, memory of procedures, skills and habits (e.g., riding a bicycle) are acquired through practice and depend on the basal ganglia.—EDS.

By contrast, "declarative" memory . . . is present in the individual's [consciousness] and can be intentionally called to mind. It is memory of "knowledge that can potentially be declared, that is, brought to mind as a verbal proposition or as a mental image." Declarative memory can be further divided into what is sometimes called "short-term" and "long-term" memory. Short-term memory denotes the cognitive faculty that retains information only temporarily until it is forgotten or consolidated into a more long-term form of storage. Short-term memory . . . captures information that is the object of current attention . . . such as a . . . phone number. Immediate memory can be retained for several minutes if it [is] rehearsed actively (for example, repeating a phone number to oneself prior to dialing).

Long-term declarative memory can be divided into "semantic" and "episodic." Semantic memory is . . . factual knowledge that does not require remembering any particular past event. . . . By contrast, episodic memory . . . is autobiographical—it pertains to personal, . . . information gathered directly by the individual through experience, at a particular place and time. Remembering a trip to Paris requires the exercise of episodic memory; remembering that Paris is the capital of France requires semantic memory. Episodic memory . . . allows one to re-experience past events in one's life, and has been likened to a form of time travel. It is arguably the richest form of memory and is certainly most directly relevant to the relationship between memory and punishment.

B. Biological Mechanisms of Memory

There is a vast and rich scientific literature on the biology of memory. For present purposes, however, it is necessary only to review briefly the scientific findings most relevant to memory (and its modification). . . . Thus, the following discussion will focus primarily on the basic biological mechanisms of long-term declarative memory (with special emphasis on episodic memory), and will briefly touch on how emotion augments such memory. By necessity, the discussion to follow will be brief and stated in the simplest possible terms.

1. Systems Neuroscience of Long-Term Declarative Memory

Stimuli encountered through the senses activate networks of neurons throughout the brain. . . . "In each of the relevant areas, persistent changes are thought to occur in the strengths of connections among neurons, and as a result neurons respond differently after learning. It is thought that the aggregate activity in the collection of altered neurons comprises the long-term memory of what is perceived." The strength of connections among neurons is increased through a process called "*Long-Term Potentiation.*"

Neither memory in general, nor long-term declarative memory in particular, is "stored" in any one particular region of the brain. . . . Moreover, declarative memory of objects appears to be stored in a distributed manner across those brain regions that are activated while visually perceiving attributes of such objects in the first instance, including size, color, shape, and the like. Retrieving declarative memory thus seems to involve the reconstruction of information (reactivation of the original network) distributed across these brain regions in response to a cue. But it is not simply the activation of the original network. The network likewise incorporates new information from the present environment. Thus, "when we remember, we complete a pattern with the best match available in memory; we do not shine a spotlight on a stored picture." Retrieval is likewise affected by emotion, mood, and state of mind.

A key region of the brain for storing long-term declarative memory is the *medial temporal lobe*. The [medial temporal lobe (MTL)] is necessary for the initial encoding of new information, and remains essential for the consolidation of the memory and its ultimate establishment in the cortex. . . . Thus, the [medial temporal lobe] plays a temporary but crucial role in the transition of declarative memory from short-term to long-term memory. The observation of patients such as H.M., whose MTL had become disabled, has confirmed this. H.M. and others like him lost those memories that had not yet been consolidated into long-term storage in networks across the cortex, and were unable to form new long-term memories. . . . Nevertheless, those memories that had undergone consolidation and relocated to the cortex (distributed across various networks), or did not otherwise depend on the [medial temporal lobe] (for example, procedural or skills memory) remained intact.

The foregoing account applies to long-term declarative memory, including semantic memory. It is thought that episodic memory is encoded and consolidated in similar fashion, but that it additionally requires the work of the frontal lobes to store information about where and when the memory was acquired.

Additional support for the notion that the frontal lobes are required for episodic memory to a greater degree than semantic memory comes from functional neuroimaging studies (PET and fMRI) of healthy adults. . . .

2. Molecular Mechanisms of Long-Term Declarative Memory

The transition of short-term memory to long-term memory, described above, requires anatomical changes in the neurons themselves. Beginning in the early 1960s, several research scientists found that the formation of long-term memory in mice . . . requires the synthesis of new proteins. They discovered that interference with protein synthesis shortly after training severely impaired long-term memory formation. . . . Subsequent discoveries as to which proteins were required and how they were formed came later from study of other animal models, including Aplysia (a marine slug).

Genes encode the information necessary to produce proteins on which all biological processes (including memory) depend. . . . Gene expression—activation (turning on) and repression (turning off)—is most commonly regulated by "*transcriptional control mechanisms*."

Regulation of gene expression . . . is crucial to consolidation of memory from short-term to long-term. Eric Kandel* and colleagues discovered a transcription factor, CREB-1 (cAMP-response element binding protein-1), that activates some of the genes necessary to build proteins that support long-term memory. Kandel likewise discovered an inhibitory transcription factor, CREB-2, that constrains the actions of CREB-1, and hinders the formation of long-term memory. . . .

What are the . . . mechanisms for long-term declarative memory? This is a complex question, but for present purposes it is sufficient to note a key finding of Kandel and others regarding *long-term potentiation*—modification of the synaptic connections in the network of neurons that comprise memory. In the brain regions necessary for consolidation of long-term declarative memory . . . , [long-term potentiation] depends on mechanisms of gene transcription that increase the number of synaptic contacts in a manner similar to the process for consolidation of nondeclarative long-term memory. . . .

Thus, in both declarative and nondeclarative memory, it appears that consolidation into long-term storage requires anatomical changes that depend on new protein synthesis—which, of course, depends on specific genetic and epigenetic mechanisms. For present purposes, this is an important insight, as many of the novel interventions for modifying memory make use of this new knowledge.

C. Role of Emotion in Memory

[Research in psychology and neuroscience has studied how we remember emotions and the many ways in which emotions influences remembering. One of the research approaches, neuroscience research with mice and rats, has used a procedure known as *fear conditioning.*—EDS.]

---

* [In 2000 Kandel shared a Nobel Prize in Physiology or Medicine for this work.—EDS.]

"Emotional Memory" acquired by fear conditioning is not a form of declarative memory, and relies on different structures of the brain (for example, the amygdala). Nevertheless, the emotions (and the brain function that subserves them) play a crucial role in understanding declarative memory, and, by extension, efforts to modify it by neurobiological means. As pioneer in the science of memory and emotion, Joseph LeDoux has noted, "Emotional and declarative memories are stored and retrieved in parallel, and their activities are joined seamlessly in our conscious experience."

A surfeit of emotions can directly affect the clarity and durability of declarative memory. The amygdala, a region of the brain crucial to emotion, plays "an essential part in modulating the storage and strength of memories." LeDoux explains: "Emotion is not just unconscious memory; it exerts a powerful influence on declaratory memory and other thought processes." In some instances, increased stress and emotion can enhance declarative memory—the memories are longer-lived, clearer, and suffused with emotional content. Mysteriously, stress and emotion can likewise (and sometimes at the same time) induce retrograde amnesia.

. . . [T]hese insights about the relationship between emotion and long-term declarative memory have been an important foundation for efforts at developing neurobiological techniques of memory modification.

D. Conclusions

The foregoing (necessarily compressed and basic) discussion of the biology of memory reveals a number of important conclusions. . . . First, there are multiple neurocognitive "systems" of memory, defined according to function. Second, different regions of the brain play distinctive roles in encoding, consolidating, and retrieving memory. Third, memory is encoded and distributed across networks of neurons. Fourth, the strength of memory, and its consolidation from short-term to long-term storage, depends on the strength of connections between neurons in the distributed network. Converting short-term memory into long-term memory requires changes in synaptic connections that depend on anatomical changes in the neuron itself. Fifth, these anatomical changes occur through genetic and epigenetic mechanisms involving the synthesis of proteins. Sixth, and finally, the neurobiological processes that subserve emotion, though distinct from those that support and sustain long-term declarative memory, nevertheless exert a strong effect on this latter faculty.

NOTES AND QUESTIONS

1. The initials H.M. are well known to anyone who has studied neuroscience or psychology of memory. They were used to protect the anonymity of a surgical patient who became a pathbreaking subject for research on human memory. With his death of natural causes in 2008, his identity could be revealed. Henry Molaison, born in 1926, suffered from epilepsy. In 1953, at the age of 27, to treat the incapacitating seizures, a neurosurgeon removed the medial temporal lobe on both sides of his brain. His epilepsy became manageable, but he could create no new memories. The nature of his deficit and retained abilities were investigated scientifically from 1957 until his death. The anatomical details of his brain were described by slicing it into thin sections. You can learn more about

it here: https://www.thebrainobservatory.org/project-hm. Further details about his life, the scientists, and this unusual case are detailed in books by Suzanne Corkin, the investigator who studied Molaison most, and by Luke Dittrich, a grandson of Molaison's neurosurgeon. *See* Suzanne Corkin, *Permanent Present Tense: The Unforgettable Life of the Amnesic Patient, H.M.* (2013); Luke Dittrich, *Patient H.M.: A Story of Memory, Madness, and Family Secrets* (2016). In 1953, drugs to treat epilepsy were not as effective as today, and the brain circuits supporting memory were not understood. Today, no one receives such radical surgery.

Daniel L. Schacter
The Seven Sins of Memory: Insights from Psychology and Cognitive Neuroscience
54 Am. Psychologist 182, 182-98 (1999)

[President Bill Clinton testifying before a federal grand jury in 1998.]

Question: If Vernon Jordan has told us that you have an extraordinary memory, one of the greatest memories he has ever seen in a politician, would that be something you would care to dispute?

Clinton: No. I do have a good memory. At least I have had a good memory in my life. . . . It's also—if I could say one thing about my memory—I have been blessed and advantaged in my life with a good memory. I have been shocked and so have members of my family and friends of mine at how many things that I have forgotten in the last six years—I think because of the pressure and the pace and the volume of events in a president's life, compounded by the pressure of your four-year inquiry, and all the other things that have happened.

When President Clinton testified before Kenneth Starr's grand jury, his numerous lapses of memory prompted investigators to query him about his reputation for prodigious recall. The logic implicit in their question . . . seems clear: How could someone with such a seemingly exceptional memory forget as much as Clinton did about the details of his encounters with Monica Lewinsky? Starr's lawyers were, to put it mildly, suspicious about the self-serving aspects of Clinton's failures to recall potentially damning incidents and statements. Although their skepticism may indeed be warranted, the contrast between Clinton's reputation for extraordinary memory on the one hand, and his claims of sketchy recollections for his encounters with Lewinsky on the other, also illustrates a fundamental duality of memory.

I have previously referred to this duality as memory's "fragile power." The power of memory is evident when one contemplates what the various forms of memory make possible in our everyday lives: a sense of personal history, knowledge of facts and concepts, and learning of complex skills. Because of memory's importance in everyday life, it is easy to see why Vernon Jordan would be struck by Clinton's "extraordinary memory" and how that ability would enhance Clinton's prospects as a politician. But, as Clinton professed to have learned during his term as President, memory also has a darker, more fragile side. People may forget events rapidly or gradually, distort the past in surprising ways, and sometimes experience intrusive recollections of events that they wish they could forget.

This darker side of memory has occupied center stage in recent scientific, clinical, and popular discussions. As most psychologists are acutely aware, a bitter controversy has raged throughout the 1990s concerning the accuracy of recovered memories of childhood sexual abuse. Some recovered memories have been corroborated and appear to be accurate, but there are also good reasons to believe that many such memories are inaccurate. False memories of childhood sexual abuse are associated with devastating psychological consequences for accusers and their families. As the debate concerning recovered memories has raged, memory researchers have focused increasingly on developing experimental paradigms to explore illusory or false memories in which people confidently claim to recollect events that never happened. . . .

We are all affected by memory's shortcomings in our everyday lives, and scientists have studied them for decades. But there have been few attempts to systematically organize or classify the various ways in which memory can lead us astray and to assess the state of the scientific evidence concerning them. Given the scientific attention paid recently to the fallibility of memory, and the important real-world consequences that are sometimes associated with forgetting and distortion, such an undertaking would appear to be both timely and potentially useful.

I suggest that memory's transgressions can be divided into seven basic "sins." I call them transience, absent-mindedness, blocking, misattribution, suggestibility, bias, and persistence. The first three sins reflect different types of forgetting. *Transience* involves decreasing accessibility of information over time, *absent-mindedness* entails inattentive or shallow processing that contributes to weak memories of ongoing events or forgetting to do things in the future, and *blocking* refers to the temporary inaccessibility of information that is stored in memory. The next three sins all involve distortion or inaccuracy. *Misattribution* involves attributing a recollection or idea to the wrong source, *suggestibility* refers to memories that are implanted as a result of leading questions or comments during attempts to recall past experiences, and *bias* involves retrospective distortions and unconscious influences that are related to current knowledge and beliefs. The seventh and final sin, *persistence*, refers to pathological remembrances: information or events that we cannot forget, even though we wish we could.

Like the biblical seven deadly sins—pride, anger, envy, greed, gluttony, lust, and sloth—the seven sins of memory occur frequently in human affairs. The biblical sins, however, can also be seen as exaggerations of human traits that are in many respects useful and even necessary for survival. So, too, is the case for the seven sins of memory. As annoying and occasionally dangerous as they may be, I suggest later in this article that memory's sins should not be viewed as flaws in system design or unfortunate errors made by Mother Nature during the course of evolution. Instead, the seven sins are more usefully conceptualized as by-products of otherwise desirable features of human memory. Perhaps paradoxically, then, the seven sins can provide insights into the very operations of memory that make it such a valuable resource in numerous aspects of our everyday lives.

In the body of this article, I summarize two major types of evidence and ideas concerning each of the seven sins. First, much of what is known about the seven sins comes from work in cognitive, social, and clinical psychology; I summarize recent research from each of these domains. Second, I consider what we have learned about the seven sins from the perspective of contemporary cognitive neuroscience. . . .

THE SEVEN SINS: COSTS OF AN ADAPTIVE SYSTEM?

Considering together the seven sins of memory could easily lead one to question the wisdom of Mother Nature in building such a seemingly flawed system: It is sobering—and perhaps even depressing—to contemplate all the ways in which memory can land us in trouble. J. R. Anderson and Milson summarized the prevailing perception that memory's sins reflect poorly on its fundamental design:

> Human memory is typically viewed by lay people as quite a defective system. For instance, over the years we have participated in many talks with artificial intelligence researchers about the prospects of using human models to guide the development of artificial intelligence programs. Invariably, the remark is made, "Well, of course, we would not want our system to have something so unreliable as human memory."

. . . As tempting as such views may be, I suggest that it is a mistake to view the seven sins as flaws in system design that ought to have been corrected during the course of evolution. Instead, . . . the seven sins can be usefully viewed as by-products of otherwise adaptive features of memory. [For example, in considering] transience (i.e., forgetting over time) . . . it is often useful and even necessary to forget information that is no longer current, such as old phone numbers or where we parked the car yesterday. Information that is no longer needed will tend not to be retrieved and rehearsed, thereby losing out on the strengthening effects of postevent retrieval and becoming gradually less accessible over time. . . . [A]n adapted system retains the kind of information that is most likely to be needed in the environment in which the system operates. . . . [T]races of more recent and more frequently retrieved events are more likely to be needed than are traces of less recent and less frequently retrieved events. Thus, a system that exhibits gradual forgetting of the kind documented for human memory is adapted to the demands of its informational environment.

A similar analysis can be applied to blocking. As noted earlier, blocking reflects the operation of inhibitory processes in memory. Consider what might result without the operation of inhibition: A system in which all information that is potentially relevant to a retrieval cue invariably and rapidly springs to mind. Although such a system might be free of the occasionally annoying episodes of blocking that plague human rememberers, it would likely result in mass confusion produced by an incessant coming to mind of numerous competing traces.

The third of the forgetting-related sins—absent-mindedness—involves similar considerations on the "front end" of memory. Absent-minded errors occur in part because establishment of a rich memory representation that can later be recollected voluntarily requires attentive, elaborate encoding; events that receive minimal attention have little chance of being recollected subsequently. But what if all events were registered in elaborate detail, regardless of the level or type of processing to which they were subjected? The result would be a potentially overwhelming clutter of useless details, as happened in the famous case of Shereshevski, the mnemonist studied by Luria. Shereshevski was unable to function at an abstract level because he was inundated with unimportant details of his experiences—details that are best denied entry to the system in the first place. An elaboration-dependent system ensures that only those events that are important enough to warrant extensive encoding have a high likelihood of subsequent recollection. Such a system allows us to enjoy the considerable benefits of operating on "automatic pilot," without having memory cluttered by unnecessary information about routine activities.

Similar ideas can be applied to the three sins that involve distortion of prior experiences: misattribution, suggestibility, and bias. These sins are rooted, to a large extent, in three fundamental features of memory. First, many instances of misattribution, and at least some instances of suggestibility, reflect poor memory for the source of an experience—the precise details of who told us a particular fact, where we saw a familiar face, or whether we witnessed an event ourselves or only heard about it later. When such details are not initially well-encoded, or become inaccessible over time, individuals become quite vulnerable to making the kinds of misattributions associated with false recognition or cryptomnesia, and may also be vulnerable to incorporating postevent suggestions regarding the nature of specific details that are remembered only vaguely. But what would be the consequences and costs of retaining the myriad of contextual details that define our numerous daily experiences? Consider again [the] notion that memory is adapted to retain information that is most likely to be needed in the environment in which it operates. How often do we need to remember all the precise, source-specifying details of our experiences? Would an adapted system routinely record all such details as a default option, or would it record such details only when circumstances dictate?

A second and related factor that contributes to misattributions involving false recall and recognition concerns the distinction between memory for gist and verbatim or specific information. False recall and recognition often occur when people remember the semantic or perceptual gist of an experience but do not recall specific details. However, memory for gist may also be fundamental to such abilities as categorization and comprehension and may facilitate the development of transfer and generalization across tasks. . . .

A third factor that is particularly relevant to many instances of bias concerns the influences of preexisting knowledge and schemas. Although they can sometimes contribute to distorted recollections of past events, schemas also perform important organizing functions in our cognitive lives. Schemas are especially important in guiding memory retrieval, promoting memory for schema-relevant information, and allowing us to develop accurate expectations of events that are likely to unfold in familiar settings on the basis of past experiences in those settings. In a somewhat different vein, as discussed earlier, retrospective biases frequently involve memory distortions that exaggerate consistency or change between present and past attitudes and beliefs. [Some] have argued that such distortions often serve to enhance appraisals of one's current self and thus in some sense contribute to life satisfaction.

Of all the seven sins, it is perhaps easiest to see the positive or adaptive side of persistence. Although intrusive recollections of trauma can be disabling, it is critically important that emotionally arousing experiences, which may occur in response to dangers that can be life threatening, persist over time and provide a basis for long-lasting memories. The fact that the amygdala and related structures help to increase the persistence of such experiences by modulating memory formation may sometimes result in memories we wish we could forget. But it also provides us with a mechanism that increases the likelihood that we will retain information about arousing or traumatic events whose recollection may be crucial for survival.

The idea that the seven sins of memory are byproducts of otherwise adaptive features of memory requires some cautions and clarifications. . . . [P]sychologists use the term "adaptation" or "adaptive features" in at least two different ways. One comes from evolutionary theory and involves a highly specific, technical definition of an adaptation as a feature of a species that came into existence though the operation of natural selection because it in some way increased reproductive fitness. The other is a more colloquial, nontechnical sense of the term that refers to a feature of an organism that has generally beneficial consequences, whether or not it arose directly in response to natural selection during the course of evolution. . . . [M]any generally useful or "adaptive" features of humans and other animals are not, strictly speaking, adaptations. Sometimes termed "exaptations," these useful functions arise as a consequence of other related features that are adaptations in the technical sense. Such adaptations are sometimes co-opted to perform functions other than the one for which they were originally selected. In an evolutionary analysis of memory systems, [I have] emphasized the possible role of exaptations in human memory:

> few of the current functions that memory serves can be genuine adaptations of memory. Human memory is clearly not an adaptation for remembering telephone numbers, though it performs these functions fairly well, nor it is an adaptation for learning to drive a car, though it handles this rather different function effectively, too. The idea of exaptation emphasizes the difference between the current functions memory systems perform and their evolutionary histories.

In view of these considerations, we must be cautious about making any strong claims for the evolutionary status of the adaptive features of memory considered here; they might be adaptations, exaptations, or both. As far as the sevens sins go, it seems possible that some are genuine adaptations, whereas others are clearly by-products of adaptations or exaptations. For example, [an] analysis of forgetting would lead us to view transience as a genuine adaptation to the structure of the environment. By contrast, misattributions involved in source memory confusions are clearly not adaptations, but are more likely by-products of adaptations and exaptations that have yielded a memory system that does not routinely preserve all the details required to specify the exact source of an experience. Similarly, false recall and recognition may be by-products of gist-based memory processes that themselves could have arisen either as adaptations or exaptations.

These kinds of by-products resemble what Gould and Lewontin called "spandrels." A spandrel is a type of exaptation that is a side consequence of a particular function. The term spandrel is used in architecture to designate the left-over spaces between structural elements in a building. As an example, Gould and Lewontin described the four spandrels in the central dome of Venice's Cathedral of San Marco: leftover spaces between arches and walls that were subsequently decorated with four evangelists and four Biblical rivers. The spandrels were not built in order to house these paintings, although they do so very well. Architectural spandrels generally have benign consequences. Perhaps some of the seven sins discussed here can be thought of as spandrels gone awry—side consequences of a generally adaptive architecture that sometimes get us into trouble. Future research in psychology and cognitive neuroscience that incorporates an evolutionary perspective should help to increase our understanding of the nature and source of the seven sins of memory.

NOTES AND QUESTIONS

1. Given the "sins" of memory, lawyers have sometimes tried to counter eyewitness memory evidence harmful to their client by introducing a memory scientist to testify about the weaknesses of eyewitness memory. Courts, both in the U.S. and the U.K., are not always receptive to this strategy, as discussed by the British Psychological Society in *Guidelines on Memory and the Law: Recommendations from the Scientific Study of Human Memory*:

> In legal cases memory may feature prominently as the main or as the only source of evidence. In such cases, evaluating accounts put forward as memories is nearly always critical to the course and outcome of the case or litigation.
>
> The law generally is unaware of the findings from the scientific study of human memory. Consequently, courts and hearings typically cannot take advantage of these findings and use them to inform their decision-making. Most importantly, courts/hearings cannot draw upon a scientifically informed understanding of human memory during the process of evaluating an account that claims to derive from a memory of an experienced event.
>
> Currently the main way to deal with this problem, when a court/hearing acknowledges it as a problem, is to seek the advice of an expert. But this is often especially unsatisfactory, as many professionals are willing to act as memory expert witnesses, when this is not their area of expertise.
>
> Another, even more problematic solution is to deny that the court/hearing needs any expert advice on issues relating to memory. The argument here is that as the jurors all have memories, they know enough about memory from the experience of their own memories to make reliable evaluations of accounts put forward as memories. Thus, the argument goes, evaluating a memory is a "jury matter."

British Psychology Soc'y Research Bd. Working Grp., *Guidelines on Memory and the Law: Recommendations from the Scientific Study of Human Memory* 2-4 (2008).

2. How would you fashion a rule to govern the admissibility of expert testimony on eyewitness memory? Consider the rule espoused in *United States v. Rodriguez-Berrios* (in which the defendant was charged with killing his ex-wife, and the eyewitness testimony at issue was what placed him in the car with the victim shortly before her disappearance).

> *Exclusion of an Expert Witness on Eyewitness Identification.* . . . Although appellant urges us to adopt a rule that would categorically allow expert testimony on the flaws inherent in eyewitness identification, we have consistently maintained that the admission of such testimony is a matter of case-by-case discretion and have refused to adopt such a blanket rule for its admission or exclusion. We adhere to that position. While such testimony will sometimes comply with the strictures of Federal Rule of Evidence 702 (the rule that governs expert testimony) because it "will assist the trier of fact to understand the evidence or to determine a fact in issue," Fed. R. Evid. 702, other times it will not. . . .

573 F.3d 55 (1st Cir. 2009). The court (in affirming the conviction, resulting in a sentence of life in prison) suggests that sometimes expert memory testimony will help, and other times it will not. If you agree, how would you determine whether a case should involve expert testimony on memory? If you disagree, would you never allow, always allow, or always require a memory expert?

3. Memory is not static, and our capacity to remember information can be improved (or fall into disrepair). Consider the case of London taxi drivers, who, in order to become licensed, must pass the famous "Knowledge of London" examination. Known simply as "The Knowledge," the series of exams is notoriously difficult and typically takes over three years to complete. Neuroscientists at University College London published a study in 2011 that examined brain structure in a group of taxi drivers studying for The Knowledge. Katherine Woollett & Eleanor A. Maguire, *Acquiring "the Knowledge" of London's Layout Drives Structural Brain Changes*, 21 Current Biology 2109 (2011). A press release described the study:

> Previous studies of qualified London taxi drivers, led by Professor Eleanor Maguire from the Wellcome Trust Centre for Neuroimaging at UCL (University College London), have shown a greater volume of grey matter—the nerve cells in the brain where processing takes place—in an area known as the posterior hippocampus and less in the anterior hippocampus relative to non-taxi drivers.
>
> The studies also showed that although taxi drivers displayed better memory for London-based information, they showed poorer learning and memory on other memory tasks involving visual information, suggesting that there might be a price to pay for acquiring the Knowledge. The research suggested that structural brain differences may have been acquired through the experience of navigating and to accommodate the internal representation of London.
>
> To test whether this was the case, Professor Maguire and colleague Dr Katherine Woollett followed a group of 79 trainee taxi drivers and 31 controls (non-taxi drivers), taking snapshots of their brain structure over time using magnetic resonance imaging (MRI) and studying their performance on certain memory tasks. Only 39 of the group passed the tests and went on to qualify as taxi drivers, giving the researchers the opportunity to divide the volunteers into three groups for comparison: those that passed, those that trained but did not pass, and the controls who never trained.
>
> The researchers examined the structure of the volunteers' brains at the start of the study, before any of the trainees had begun their training. They found no discernible differences in the structures of either the posterior hippocampus or the anterior hippocampus between the groups, and all groups performed equally well on the memory tasks.
>
> Three to four years later—when the trainees had either passed the test or had failed to acquire the Knowledge—the researchers again looked at the brain structures of the volunteers and tested their performance on the memory tasks. This time, they found significant differences in the posterior hippocampus—those trainees that qualified as taxi drivers had a greater volume of grey matter in the region than they had before they started their training. . . .
>
> "The human brain remains 'plastic,' even in adult life, allowing it to adapt when we learn new tasks," explains Professor Maguire, a Wellcome Trust Senior Research Fellow. "By following the trainee taxi drivers over time as they acquired—or failed to acquire—the Knowledge, a uniquely challenging spatial memory task, we have seen directly and within individuals how the structure of the hippocampus can change with external stimulation. This offers encouragement for adults who want to learn new skills later in life.
>
> "What is not clear is whether those trainees who became fully fledged taxi drivers had some biological advantage over those who failed. Could it be, for example, that they have a genetic predisposition towards having a more adaptable, 'plastic' brain? In other words, the perennial question of 'nature versus nurture' is still open."

Press Release, Wellcome Trust, *Changes in London Taxi Drivers' Brains Driven by Acquiring 'The Knowledge,' Study Shows* (Dec. 9, 2011).

4. In the 2000 movie *Memento* the main character Leonard Shelby suffers from anterograde amnesia and cannot form new explicit memories. The movie chronicles the challenges that this presents and serves as a reminder that without memories life is fundamentally altered. Writing about real life extreme cases in which individuals either remember everything or nothing, Joshua Foer observes that these "cases say more than any brain scan about the extent to which our memories make us who we are. . . . Those three pounds or so of wrinkled flesh balanced atop our spines can retain the most trivial details about childhood experiences for a lifetime but often can't hold on to even the most important telephone number for just two minutes. Memory is strange like that." Joshua Foer, *Remember This: In the Archives of the Brain, Our Lives Linger or Disappear*, Nat'l Geographic (Nov. 2007). In a review of decades of research on long-term memory, psychologist Henry Roediger concluded that "one central lesson to be gained from thousands of experimental studies is that no general laws of memory exist. All statements about memory must be qualified." Henry L. Roediger, *Relativity of Remembering: Why the Laws of Memory Vanished*, 59 Ann. Rev. Psychol. 225, 227 (2008). If it's true that human memory is strange and that it is difficult to state general laws, what implications does this have for legal doctrine and practice?

5. Consider these implications in one discrete situation. Following several highly-publicized police killings of unarmed citizens, activists have demanded that police wear body cameras while on active duty. One controversial issue discussed by criminologists Michael White and Henry Fradella is whether officers should be allowed to review the body camera recordings of high-stress "critical incidents" prior to filing their own reports. On the one hand, allowing officers to review the footage, which may have perceptual distortions, could alter their recollection of the event. Alternatively, disparities between an officer's memory and the events as depicted on film could destroy credibility. Michael D. White & Henry F. Fradella, *The Intersection of Law, Policy, and Police Body-Worn Cameras: An Exploration of Critical Issues*, 96 N.C. L. Rev. 1579 (2018).

B. EYEWITNESS MEMORY IN COURT

In 2011 and 2012 two significant cases brought about notable developments in the legal status of eyewitness memory evidence in U.S. courts. First, the New Jersey Supreme Court in *State v. Henderson* (2011) revisited its legal standard for analyzing the reliability of eyewitness identifications. Second, the U.S. Supreme Court in *Perry v. New Hampshire* (2012) revisited the issue of eyewitness memory for the first time in decades. As you read these cases, consider whether the respective courts went too far, not far enough, or in the wrong direction in responding to advances in the science of memory. Shortly after *Henderson* and *Perry* were decided, a National Academy of Sciences report reviewed all available information on eyewitness identification and developed recommendations that could be implemented to "increase the accuracy and utility of eyewitness identifications." Nat'l Research Council, *Identifying the Culprit: Assessing Eyewitness Identification* (2014). We summarize that report to begin this section.

The scientific co-chair of the Committee, Thomas D. Albright, summarized the report in *Why Eyewitnesses Fail*, 114 Proc. Nat'l Acad. Sci. U.S. 7758, 7758-7763 (2017). The Committee surveyed applied research on the challenge of eyewitness identification. This research has investigated how different kinds of variables influence the accuracy of identification by eyewitnesses. Researchers distinguish between different types of variables that affect eyewitness identification.

One category of variables depend on the circumstances in which the event was witnessed. These variables include things like viewing conditions, the presence of other simultaneous events and objects that would be distracting, the race and gender of the witness and of the suspect, and the cognitive state of the witness at that moment, e.g., was she alert or distracted. These variables cannot be controlled by law enforcement.

A second category of variables depends on what happens after the event takes place: the conditions under which the witness's memory is examined. These variables include how a lineup of suspects is presented to the eyewitness, the instructions and feedback given to the witness during the identification procedures, and whether the official administering the lineup knows who among the participants in the lineup the actual suspect is. The latter set of variables can be controlled by law enforcement.

Research studies have found that the accuracy and reliability of eyewitness identifications can vary according to how the possible suspects are presented to the witness. The following elements are important: whether the possible suspects are presented simultaneously or sequentially, the number of non-suspect lineup participants, how similar to the suspect the non-suspect lineup participants are, and the suspect's location in the presentation. Studies indicate that the frequency of incorrect identifications is reduced when the lineup participants are presented sequentially rather than simultaneously. Other studies, though, report that witnesses can discriminate better among lineup participants when they are presented simultaneously.

The Committee considered why eyewitness testimony can be erroneous. Errors can arise in the perception of the suspect and events. Errors can also arise in the recall of the person and events. The accuracy of a visual (or any other) experience can be limited by three things. First, uncertainty about perception can arise from poor visibility due to the quality of light, angle of view, and presence of other distracting objects. Second, bias can arise in the recall of the perception based on predispositions or knowledge that the witness may have. Third, in spite of these two factors, witnesses can express over-confidence in their report of what they observed. Indeed, the degree of confidence in a report actually does not predict the accuracy of that report. Perceptions must be stored in memory to be recalled. As we have seen, recall of memories is also error-prone. In fact, recollections of perceptions are also subject to uncertainty, bias, and over-confidence.

The Committee developed a number of detailed recommendations to address these challenges. Briefly, the problem of uncertainty inherent in perception and memory can be at least partially neutralized by quantifying aspects of the viewing conditions that may limit perception. The problem of bias in framing perceptions and recalling memories can be addressed through identification of factors that would contribute to such bias, and by introducing procedures to minimize its effects on the eyewitness report. The problem of over-confidence by the witness can be neutralized by obtaining a measure of confidence at the time of the initial report, such as at a lineup identification. This measure of confidence will be obtained before the witness can have access to other sources of information, which might encourage inappropriate levels of confidence in their reported perception. Recent research has shown that statements of confidence made at the time of the initial identification correlate well with identification accuracy.

The Committee also drew attention to the disparity between old legal standards for eyewitness evidence and current scientific understanding of human vision and memory. Consequently, they offered several recommendations, including using pretrial judicial inquiries and scientific expert testimony to characterize the degree of uncertainty, bias, and overconfidence that an eyewitness might bring to the proceedings. They also suggested that juries should be informed about when eyewitness identifications were conducted, and instructed that identification accuracy should be judged higher if the confidence was expressed at the time of the initial identification.

State v. Henderson

27 A.3d 872 (N.J. 2011)

Chief Justice RABNER delivered the opinion of the Court.

I. INTRODUCTION

In the thirty-four years since the United States Supreme Court announced a test for the admission of eyewitness identification evidence, which New Jersey adopted soon after, a vast body of scientific research about human memory has emerged. That body of work casts doubt on some commonly held views relating to memory. It also calls into question the vitality of the current legal framework for analyzing the reliability of eyewitness identifications.

In this case, defendant claims that an eyewitness mistakenly identified him as an accomplice to a murder. Defendant argues that the identification was not reliable because the officers investigating the case intervened during the identification process and unduly influenced the eyewitness. After a pretrial hearing, the trial court found that the officers' behavior was not impermissibly suggestive and admitted the evidence. The Appellate Division reversed. It held that the officers' actions were presumptively suggestive because they violated guidelines issued by the Attorney General in 2001 for conducting identification procedures.

After granting certification and hearing oral argument, we remanded the case and appointed a Special Master to evaluate scientific and other evidence about eyewitness identifications. The Special Master presided over a hearing that probed testimony by seven experts and produced more than 2,000 pages of transcripts along with hundreds of scientific studies. He later issued an extensive and very fine report, much of which we adopt.

We find that the scientific evidence considered at the remand hearing is reliable. That evidence offers convincing proof that the current test for evaluating the trustworthiness of eyewitness identifications should be revised. Study after study revealed a troubling lack of reliability in eyewitness identifications. From social science research to the review of actual police lineups, from laboratory experiments to

DNA exonerations, the record proves that the possibility of mistaken identification is real. Indeed, it is now widely known that eyewitness misidentification is the leading cause of wrongful convictions across the country.

We are convinced from the scientific evidence in the record that memory is malleable, and that an array of variables can affect and dilute memory and lead to misidentifications. Those factors include system variables like lineup procedures,* which are within the control of the criminal justice system, and estimator variables like lighting conditions or the presence of a weapon,** over which the legal system has no control. To its credit, the Attorney General's Office incorporated scientific research on system variables into the guidelines it issued in 2001 to improve eyewitness identification procedures. We now review both sets of variables in detail to evaluate the current *Manson/Madison* test.

In the end, we conclude that the current standard for assessing eyewitness identification evidence does not fully meet its goals. It does not offer an adequate measure for reliability or sufficiently deter inappropriate police conduct. It also overstates the jury's inherent ability to evaluate evidence offered by eyewitnesses who honestly believe their testimony is accurate.

Two principal steps are needed to remedy those concerns. First, when defendants can show some evidence of suggestiveness, all relevant system and estimator variables should be explored at pretrial hearings. A trial court can end the hearing at any time, however, if the court concludes from the testimony that defendant's threshold allegation of suggestiveness is groundless. Otherwise, the trial judge should weigh both sets of variables to decide if the evidence is admissible.

Up until now, courts have only considered estimator variables if there was a finding of impermissibly suggestive police conduct. In adopting this broader approach, we decline to order pretrial hearings in every case, as opposed to cases in which there is some evidence of suggestiveness. We also reject a bright-line rule that would require suppression of reliable evidence any time a law enforcement officer missteps.

Second, the court system should develop enhanced jury charges on eyewitness identification for trial judges to use. We anticipate that identification evidence will continue to be admitted in the vast majority of cases. To help jurors weigh that evidence, they must be told about relevant factors and their effect on reliability. To that end, we have asked the Criminal Practice Committee and the Committee on Model Criminal Jury Charges to draft proposed revisions to the current model charge on eyewitness identification and address various system and estimator variables. With the use of more focused jury charges on those issues, there will be less need to call expert witnesses at trial. Trial courts will still have discretion to admit expert testimony when warranted.

The factors that both judges and juries will consider are not etched in stone. We expect that the scientific research underlying them will continue to evolve, as it has in the more than thirty years since *Manson*. For the same reason, police departments are not prevented from improving their practices as we learn more about variables

---

* [System variables also include such things as: double-blind administration of identification procedures; sequential versus simultaneous presentation; and feedback by investigators during identification procedures. — EDS.]

** [Estimator variables also include such things as the effects on identification accuracy of stress, cross-racial effects, and the like. — EDS.]

that affect memory. New approaches, though, must be based on reliable scientific evidence that experts generally accept.

The changes outlined in this decision are significant because eyewitness identifications bear directly on guilt or innocence. At stake is the very integrity of the criminal justice system and the courts' ability to conduct fair trials. Ultimately, we believe that the framework described below will both protect the rights of defendants, by minimizing the risk of misidentification, and enable the State to introduce vital evidence.

The revised principles in this decision will apply purely prospectively except for defendant Larry Henderson and defendant Cecilia Chen, the subject of a companion case also decided today. . . .

A. Facts

In the early morning hours of January 1, 2003, Rodney Harper was shot to death in an apartment in Camden. James Womble witnessed the murder but did not speak with the police until they approached him ten days later.

Womble and Harper were acquaintances who occasionally socialized at the apartment of Womble's girlfriend, Vivian Williams. On the night of the murder, Womble and Williams brought in the New Year in Williams' apartment by drinking wine and champagne and smoking crack cocaine. Harper had started the evening with them but left at around 10:15 P.M. Williams also left roughly three hours later, leaving Womble alone in the apartment until Harper rejoined him at 2:00 to 2:30 A.M.

Soon after Harper returned, two men forcefully entered the apartment. Womble knew one of them, co-defendant George Clark, who had come to collect $160 from Harper. The other man was a stranger to Womble.

While Harper and Clark went to a different room, the stranger pointed a gun at Womble and told him, "Don't move, stay right here, you're not involved in this." He remained with the stranger in a small, narrow, dark hallway. Womble testified that he "got a look at" the stranger, but not "a real good look." . . .

Meanwhile, Womble overheard Clark and Harper argue over money in the other room. At one point, Harper said, "do what you got to do," after which Womble heard a gunshot. Womble then walked into the room, saw Clark holding a handgun, offered to get Clark the $160, and urged him not to shoot Harper again. As Clark left, he warned Womble, "Don't rat me out, I know where you live."

Harper died from the gunshot wound to his chest on January 10, 2003. Camden County Detective Luis Ruiz and Investigator Randall MacNair were assigned to investigate the homicide, and they interviewed Womble the next day. Initially, Womble told the police that he was in the apartment when he heard two gunshots outside, that he left to look for Harper, and that he found Harper slumped over in his car in a nearby parking lot, where Harper said he had been shot by two men he did not know.

The next day, the officers confronted Womble about inconsistencies in his story. Womble claimed that they also threatened to charge him in connection with the murder. Womble then decided to "come clean." He admitted that he lied at first because he did not want to "rat" out anyone and "didn't want to get involved" out of fear of retaliation against his elderly father. Womble led the investigators to Clark, who eventually gave a statement about his involvement and identified the person who accompanied him as defendant Larry Henderson.

The officers had Womble view a photographic array on January 14, 2003. That event lies at the heart of this decision and is discussed in greater detail below. [Womble was first given a photographic array by an officer (Weber) not involved in the investigation. Womble narrowed the array down to two photographs but could not make a positive identification. The two officers in charge of the investigation then intervened. Apparently believing Womble was still afraid of retaliation, they told him he would be protected, and that he should simply relax and make the identification if he saw the perpetrator. Those officers left and Weber reshuffled the photos, showing them to Womble again. Womble then identified Henderson as having participated in the shooting.] Ultimately, Womble identified defendant from the array, and Investigator MacNair prepared a warrant for his arrest. Upon arrest, defendant admitted to the police that he had accompanied Clark to the apartment where Harper was killed, and heard a gunshot while waiting in the hallway. But defendant denied witnessing or participating in the shooting. . . .

At the close of trial on July 20, 2004, the court relied on the existing model jury charge on eyewitness identification and instructed the jury as follows:

> [Y]ou should consider the observations and perceptions on which the identification is based, and Womble's ability to make those observations and perceptions. If you determine that his out-of-court identification is not reliable, you may still consider Womble's in-court identification of Gregory Clark and Larry Henderson if you find that to be reliable. However, unless the identification here in court resulted from Womble's observations or perceptions of a perpetrator during the commission of an offense rather than being the product of an impression gained at an out-of-court identification procedure such as a photo lineup, it should be afforded no weight. The ultimate issues of the trustworthiness of both in-court and out-of-court identifications are for you, the jury to decide.
>
> To decide whether the identification testimony is sufficiently reliable evidence . . . you may consider the following factors:
>
> First of all, Womble's opportunity to view the person or persons who allegedly committed the offense at the time of the offense; second, Womble's degree of attention on the alleged perpetrator when he allegedly observed the crime being committed; third, the accuracy of any prior description of the perpetrator given [b]y Womble; fourth, you should consider the fact that in Womble's sworn taped statement of January 11th, 2003 to the police. . . . Womble did not identify anyone as the person or persons involved in the shooting of Rodney Harper. . . .
>
> Next, you should consider the degree of certainty, if any, expressed by Womble in making the identification. . . .
>
> You should also consider the length of time between Womble's observation of the alleged offense and his identification. . . . You should consider any discrepancies or inconsistencies between identifications. . . .
>
> Next, the circumstances under which any out-of-court identification was made including in this case the evidence that during the showing to him of eight photos by Detective Weber he did not identify Larry Henderson when he first looked at them and later identified Larry Henderson from one of those photos.
>
> . . . You may also consider any other factor based on the evidence or lack of evidence in the case which you consider relevant to your determination whether the identification made by Womble is reliable or not.

. . . On July 20, 2004, the jury acquitted defendant of murder and aggravated manslaughter, and convicted him of reckless manslaughter, N.J.S.A. 2C:11-4(b)(1), aggravated assault, and two weapons charges. In a bifurcated trial the next day, the jury convicted defendant of the remaining firearms offense: possession by a previously convicted person. The court sentenced him to an aggregate eleven-year term of imprisonment, with a period of parole ineligibility of almost six years under the No Early Release Act, N.J.S.A. 2C:43-7.2. Defendant appealed his conviction and sentence.

[The court reviewed in detail the science of memory, leading it to conclude that the State's framework for evaluating eyewitness identification evidence needed to be revised.]

C. Revised Framework

Remedying the problems with the current *Manson/Madison* test requires an approach that addresses its shortcomings: one that allows judges to consider all relevant factors that affect reliability in deciding whether an identification is admissible; that is not heavily weighted by factors that can be corrupted by suggestiveness; that promotes deterrence in a meaningful way; and that focuses on helping jurors both understand and evaluate the effects that various factors have on memory—because we recognize that most identifications will be admitted in evidence.

Two principal changes to the current system are needed to accomplish that: first, the revised framework should allow all relevant system *and* estimator variables to be explored and weighed at pretrial hearings when there is some actual evidence of suggestiveness; and second, courts should develop and use enhanced jury charges to help jurors evaluate eyewitness identification evidence.

The new framework also needs to be flexible enough to serve twin aims: to guarantee fair trials to defendants, who must have the tools necessary to defend themselves, and to protect the State's interest in presenting critical evidence at trial. With that in mind, we first outline the revised approach for evaluating identification evidence and then explain its details and the reasoning behind it.

First, to obtain a pretrial hearing, a defendant has the initial burden of showing some evidence of suggestiveness that could lead to a mistaken identification. That evidence, in general, must be tied to a system—and not an estimator—variable. . . .

Second, the State must then offer proof to show that the proffered eyewitness identification is reliable—accounting for system and estimator variables—subject to the following: the court can end the hearing at any time if it finds from the testimony that defendant's threshold allegation of suggestiveness is groundless. . . .

Third, the ultimate burden remains on the defendant to prove a very substantial likelihood of irreparable misidentification. To do so, a defendant can cross-examine eyewitnesses and police officials and present witnesses and other relevant evidence linked to system and estimator variables.

Fourth, if after weighing the evidence presented a court finds from the totality of the circumstances that defendant has demonstrated a very substantial likelihood of irreparable misidentification, the court should suppress the identification evidence. If the evidence is admitted, the court should provide appropriate, tailored jury instructions. . . .

We adopt this approach over the initial recommendation of defendant and the ACDL that any violation of the Attorney General Guidelines should require per se exclusion of the resulting eyewitness identification. Although that approach might yield greater deterrence, it could also lead to the loss of a substantial amount of reliable evidence. We believe that the more flexible framework outlined above protects defendants' right to a fair trial at the same time it enables the State to meet its responsibility to ensure public safety. . . .

E. Trial

As is true today, juries will continue to hear about all relevant system and estimator variables at trial, through direct and cross-examination and arguments by counsel. In addition, when identification is at issue in a case, trial courts will continue to "provide[ ] appropriate guidelines to focus the jury's attention on how to analyze and consider the trustworthiness of eyewitness identification." Based on the record developed on remand, we direct that enhanced instructions be given to guide juries about the various factors that may affect the reliability of an identification in a particular case.

Those instructions are to be included in the court's comprehensive jury charge at the close of evidence. In addition, instructions may be given during trial if warranted. For example, if evidence of heightened stress emerges during important testimony, a party may ask the court to instruct the jury midtrial about that variable and its effect on memory. Trial courts retain discretion to decide when to offer instructions.

As discussed earlier, the State maintains that many jurors, through their life experiences and intuition, generally understand how memory works. To the extent some jurors do not, the State argues that cross-examination, defense summations, the current jury charge, fellow jurors, and other safeguards can help correct misconceptions.

But we do not rely on jurors to divine rules themselves or glean them from cross-examination or summation. Even with matters that may be considered intuitive, courts provide focused jury instructions. For example, we remind jurors to scrutinize the testimony of a cooperating witness with care. A simple reason underlies that approach: it is the court's obligation to help jurors evaluate evidence critically and objectively to ensure a fair trial.

Moreover, science reveals that memory and eyewitness identification evidence present certain complicated issues. In the past, we have responded by developing jury instructions consistent with accepted scientific findings. We acted similarly in response to social science evidence about Battered Women's Syndrome and Child Sexual Abuse Accommodation Syndrome. Ultimately, as the Special Master found, "[w]hether the science confirms commonsense views or dispels preconceived but not necessarily valid intuitions, it can properly and usefully be considered by both judges and jurors in making their assessments of eyewitness reliability."

Expert testimony may also be introduced at trial, but only if otherwise appropriate. . . .

We anticipate, however, that with enhanced jury instructions, there will be less need for expert testimony. Jury charges offer a number of advantages: they are focused and concise, authoritative (in that juries hear them from the trial judge, not a witness called by one side), and cost-free; they avoid possible confusion to jurors created by dueling experts; and they eliminate the risk of an expert invading the jury's role or opining on an eyewitness' credibility. That said, there will be times when expert testimony will benefit the trier of fact. We leave to the trial court the decision whether to allow expert testimony in an individual case.

Finally, in rare cases, judges may use their discretion to redact parts of identification testimony, consistent with *Rule* 403. For example, if an eyewitness' confidence was not properly recorded soon after an identification procedure, and evidence revealed that the witness received confirmatory feedback from the police or a co-witness, the court can bar potentially distorted and unduly prejudicial statements about the witness' level of confidence from being introduced at trial. . . .

[The case was remanded for retrial.]

Perry v. New Hampshire
565 U.S. 228 (2012)

Justice GINSBURG delivered the opinion of the Court. In our system of justice, fair trial for persons charged with criminal offenses is secured by the Sixth Amendment, which guarantees to defendants the right to counsel, compulsory process to obtain defense witnesses, and the opportunity to cross-examine witnesses for the prosecution. Those safeguards apart, admission of evidence in state trials is ordinarily governed by state law, and the reliability of relevant testimony typically falls within the province of the jury to determine. This Court has recognized, in addition, a due process check on the admission of eyewitness identification, applicable when the police have arranged suggestive circumstances leading the witness to identify a particular person as the perpetrator of a crime.

An identification infected by improper police influence, our case law holds, is not automatically excluded. Instead, the trial judge must screen the evidence for reliability pretrial. If there is "a very substantial likelihood of irreparable misidentification," Simmons v. United States, 390 U.S. 377, 384 (1968), the judge must disallow presentation of the evidence at trial. But if the indicia of reliability are strong enough to outweigh the corrupting effect of the police-arranged suggestive circumstances, the identification evidence ordinarily will be admitted, and the jury will ultimately determine its worth.

We have not extended pretrial screening for reliability to cases in which the suggestive circumstances were not arranged by law enforcement officers. Petitioner requests that we do so because of the grave risk that mistaken identification will yield a miscarriage of justice. Our decisions, however, turn on the presence of state action and aim to deter police from rigging identification procedures, for example, at a lineup, showup, or photograph array. When no improper law enforcement activity is involved, we hold, it suffices to test reliability through the rights and opportunities generally designed for that purpose, notably, the presence of counsel at post-indictment lineups, vigorous cross-examination, protective rules of evidence, and jury instructions on both the fallibility of eyewitness identification and the requirement that guilt be proved beyond a reasonable doubt.

I

A

Around 3 A.M. on August 15, 2008, Joffre Ullon called the Nashua, New Hampshire, Police Department and reported that an African-American male was trying to break into cars parked in the lot of Ullon's apartment building. Officer Nicole Clay responded to the call. Upon arriving at the parking lot, Clay heard what "sounded like a metal bat hitting the ground." She then saw petitioner Barion Perry standing between two cars. Perry walked toward Clay, holding two car-stereo amplifiers in his hands. A metal bat lay on the ground behind him. Clay asked Perry where the amplifiers came from. "[I] found them on the ground," Perry responded.

Meanwhile, Ullon's wife, Nubia Blandon, woke her neighbor, Alex Clavijo, and told him she had just seen someone break into his car. Clavijo immediately went downstairs to the parking lot to inspect the car. He first observed that one of the rear windows had been shattered. On further inspection, he discovered that the speakers and amplifiers from his car stereo were missing, as were his bat and wrench. Clavijo then approached Clay and told her about Blandon's alert and his own subsequent observations.

By this time, another officer had arrived at the scene. Clay asked Perry to stay in the parking lot with that officer, while she and Clavijo went to talk to Blandon. Clay and Clavijo then entered the apartment building and took the stairs to the fourth floor, where Blandon's and Clavijo's apartments were located. They met Blandon in the hallway just outside the open door to her apartment.

Asked to describe what she had seen, Blandon stated that, around 2:30 A.M., she saw from her kitchen window a tall, African-American man roaming the parking lot and looking into cars. Eventually, the man circled Clavijo's car, opened the trunk, and removed a large box.

Clay asked Blandon for a more specific description of the man. Blandon pointed to her kitchen window and said the person she saw breaking into Clavijo's car was standing in the parking lot, next to the police officer. Perry's arrest followed this identification.

About a month later, the police showed Blandon a photographic array that included a picture of Perry and asked her to point out the man who had broken into Clavijo's car. Blandon was unable to identify Perry.

B

Perry was charged in New Hampshire state court with one count of theft by unauthorized taking and one count of criminal mischief. Before trial, he moved to suppress Blandon's identification on the ground that admitting it at trial would violate due process. Blandon witnessed what amounted to a one-person showup in the parking lot, Perry asserted, which all but guaranteed that she would identify him as the culprit.

The New Hampshire Superior Court denied the motion. To determine whether due process prohibits the introduction of an out-of-court identification at trial, the Superior Court said, this Court's decisions instruct a two-step inquiry. First, the trial court must decide whether the police used an unnecessarily suggestive identification procedure. If they did, the court must next consider whether the improper identification procedure so tainted the resulting identification as to render it unreliable and therefore inadmissible.

Perry's challenge, the Superior Court concluded, failed at step one: Blandon's identification of Perry on the night of the crime did not result from an unnecessarily suggestive procedure "manufacture[d] . . . by the police." Blandon pointed to Perry "spontaneously," the court noted, "without any inducement from the police." Clay did not ask Blandon whether the man standing in the parking lot was the man Blandon had seen breaking into Clavijo's car. Nor did Clay ask Blandon to move to the window from which she had observed the break-in.

The Superior Court recognized that there were reasons to question the accuracy of Blandon's identification: the parking lot was dark in some locations; Perry was standing next to a police officer; Perry was the only African-American man in the vicinity; and Blandon was unable, later, to pick Perry out of a photographic array. But "[b]ecause the police procedures were not unnecessarily suggestive," the court ruled that the reliability of Blandon's testimony was for the jury to consider.

At the ensuing trial, Blandon and Clay testified to Blandon's out-of-court identification. The jury found Perry guilty of theft and not guilty of criminal mischief.

On appeal, Perry repeated his challenge to the admissibility of Blandon's out-of-court identification. The trial court erred, Perry contended, in requiring an initial showing that the police arranged the suggestive identification procedure. Suggestive circumstances alone, Perry argued, suffice to trigger the court's duty to evaluate the reliability of the resulting identification before allowing presentation of the evidence to the jury.

The New Hampshire Supreme Court rejected Perry's argument and affirmed his conviction. Only where the police employ suggestive identification techniques, that court held, does the Due Process Clause require a trial court to assess the reliability of identification evidence before permitting a jury to consider it.

We granted certiorari to resolve a division of opinion on the question whether the Due Process Clause requires a trial judge to conduct a preliminary assessment of the reliability of an eyewitness identification made under suggestive circumstances not arranged by the police.

II

A

The Constitution, our decisions indicate, protects a defendant against a conviction based on evidence of questionable reliability, not by prohibiting introduction of the evidence, but by affording the defendant means to persuade the jury that the evidence should be discounted as unworthy of credit. Constitutional safeguards available to defendants to counter the State's evidence include the Sixth Amendment rights to counsel, compulsory process, and confrontation plus cross-examination of witnesses. Apart from these guarantees, we have recognized, state and federal statutes and rules ordinarily govern the admissibility of evidence, and juries are assigned the task of determining the reliability of the evidence presented at trial.

Contending that the Due Process Clause is implicated here, Perry relies on a series of decisions involving police-arranged identification procedures. . . .

B

Perry concedes that, in contrast to every case in the *Stovall* line, law enforcement officials did not arrange the suggestive circumstances surrounding Blandon's identification. He contends, however, that it was mere happenstance that each of the *Stovall* cases involved improper police action. The rationale underlying our decisions, Perry asserts, supports a rule requiring trial judges to prescreen eyewitness evidence for reliability any time an identification is made under suggestive circumstances. We disagree.

Perry's argument depends, in large part, on the Court's statement in *Brathwaite* that "reliability is the linchpin in determining the admissibility of identification testimony." 432 U.S., at 114, 97 S. Ct. 2243. If reliability is the linchpin of admissibility under the Due Process Clause, Perry maintains, it should make no difference whether law enforcement was responsible for creating the suggestive circumstances that marred the identification.

Perry has removed our statement in *Brathwaite* from its mooring, and thereby attributes to the statement a meaning a fair reading of our opinion does not bear. [T]he *Brathwaite* Court's reference to reliability appears in a portion of the opinion concerning the appropriate remedy *when the police use an unnecessarily suggestive identification procedure.* The Court adopted a judicial screen for reliability as a course preferable to a per se rule requiring exclusion of identification evidence whenever law enforcement officers employ an improper procedure. The due process check for reliability, *Brathwaite* made plain, comes into play only after the defendant establishes improper police conduct. The very purpose of the check, the Court noted, was to avoid depriving the jury of identification evidence that is reliable, notwithstanding improper police conduct. . . .

Perry's argument, reiterated by the dissent, thus lacks support in the case law he cites. Moreover, his position would open the door to judicial preview, under the banner of due process, of most, if not all, eyewitness identifications. External suggestion is hardly the only factor that casts doubt on the trustworthiness of an eyewitness' testimony. As one of Perry's *amici* points out, many other factors bear on "the likelihood of misidentification," — for example, the passage of time between exposure to and identification of the defendant, whether the witness was under stress when he first encountered the suspect, how much time the witness had to observe the suspect, how far the witness was from the suspect, whether the suspect carried a weapon, and the race of the suspect and the witness. There is no reason why an identification made by an eyewitness with poor vision, for example, or one who harbors a grudge against the defendant, should be regarded as inherently more reliable, less of a "threat to the fairness of trial," than the identification Blandon made in this case. To embrace Perry's view would thus entail a vast enlargement of the reach of due process as a constraint on the admission of evidence. . . .

C

In urging a broadly applicable due process check on eyewitness identifications, Perry maintains that eyewitness identifications are a uniquely unreliable form of evidence. . . . We do not doubt either the importance or the fallibility of eyewitness identifications. Indeed, in recognizing that defendants have a constitutional right to counsel at postindictment police lineups, we observed that "the annals of criminal law are rife with instances of mistaken identification." Wade, 388 U.S., at 228, 87 S. Ct. 1926.

We have concluded in other contexts, however, that the potential unreliability of a type of evidence does not alone render its introduction at the defendant's trial fundamentally unfair. We reach a similar conclusion here: The fallibility of eyewitness evidence does not, without the taint of improper state conduct, warrant a due process rule requiring a trial court to screen such evidence for reliability before allowing the jury to assess its creditworthiness.

Our unwillingness to enlarge the domain of due process as Perry and the dissent urge rests, in large part, on our recognition that the jury, not the judge, traditionally determines the reliability of evidence. We also take account of other safeguards built into our adversary system that caution juries against placing undue weight on eyewitness testimony of questionable reliability. These protections include the defendant's Sixth Amendment right to confront the eyewitness. Another is the defendant's right to the effective assistance of an attorney, who can expose the flaws in the eyewitness' testimony during cross-examination and focus the jury's attention on the fallibility of such testimony during opening and closing arguments. Eyewitness-specific jury instructions, which many federal and state courts have adopted, likewise warn the jury to take care in appraising identification evidence. The constitutional requirement that the government prove the defendant's guilt beyond a reasonable doubt also impedes convictions based on dubious identification evidence. . . .

Given the safeguards generally applicable in criminal trials, protections availed of by the defense in Perry's case, we hold that the introduction of Blandon's eyewitness testimony, without a preliminary judicial assessment of its reliability, did not render Perry's trial fundamentally unfair.

* * *

For the foregoing reasons, we agree with the New Hampshire courts' appraisal of our decisions. Finding no convincing reason to alter our precedent, we hold that the Due Process Clause does not require a preliminary judicial inquiry into the reliability of an eyewitness identification when the identification was not procured under unnecessarily suggestive circumstances arranged by law enforcement. Accordingly, the judgment of the New Hampshire Supreme Court is *Affirmed*.

NOTES AND QUESTIONS

1. In dissent, Justice Sotomayor wrote:

> This Court has long recognized that eyewitness identifications' unique confluence of features—their unreliability, susceptibility to suggestion, powerful impact on the jury, and resistance to the ordinary tests of the adversarial process—can undermine the fairness of a trial. Our cases thus establish a clear rule: The admission at trial of out-of-court eyewitness identifications derived from impermissibly suggestive circumstances that pose a very substantial likelihood of misidentification violates due process. . . .
>
> Our due process concern, however, arises not from the act of suggestion, but rather from the corrosive effects of suggestion on the reliability of the resulting identification. By rendering protection contingent on improper police arrangement of the suggestive circumstances, the Court effectively grafts a *mens rea* inquiry onto our rule. The Court's holding enshrines a murky distinction—between suggestive confrontations intentionally orchestrated by the police and, as here, those inadvertently caused by police actions—that will sow confusion. It ignores our precedents' acute sensitivity to the hazards of intentional and unintentional suggestion alike and unmoors our rule from the very interest it protects, inviting arbitrary results. And it recasts the driving force of our decisions as an interest in police deterrence, rather than reliability. Because I see no warrant for declining to assess the circumstances of this case under our ordinary approach, I respectfully dissent.

Justice Ginsburg and Justice Sotomayor disagree on the role that suggestiveness should play in delineating constitutional due process protections. Who has the better argument and why?

2. The New Jersey Supreme Court extended the protections in *Henderson* even further in 2019, holding that if law enforcement officers fail to prepare an "electronic, or contemporaneous, verbatim written recording" of the identification process, the defendant is "entitled to a pretrial hearing on the admissibility of identification evidence," with or without evidence of suggestiveness. *State v. Anthony*, 204 A.3d 229 (N.J. 2019).

Did the holdings in *Henderson, Perry*, and *Anthony* go far enough, in your view? Assuming you'd agree that eyewitness testimony should not be excluded wholesale, according to what factors would you ideally have courts draw lines to determine the admissibility of eyewitness testimony?

3. *Henderson* illustrates how state supreme courts can initiate comprehensive reform to eyewitness identification procedures. It is not just courts, however, that bring about this type of change. As of 2019, over 20 states have adopted legislation to address this issue. Given this trend, should other states follow suit? Are courts or legislators better equipped to define the contours of reform?

4. Here are the recommendations of the National Research Council:

RECOMMENDATIONS TO ESTABLISH BEST PRACTICES FOR THE LAW ENFORCEMENT COMMUNITY

The committee's review of law enforcement practices and procedures, coupled with its consideration of the scientific literature, has identified a number of areas where eyewitness identification procedures could be strengthened. The practices and procedures considered here involve acquisition of data that reflect a witness' identification and the contextual factors that bear on that identification. A recurrent theme underlying the committee's recommendations is development of and adherence to guidelines that are consistent with scientific standards for data collection and reporting.

Recommendation #1: Train All Law Enforcement Officers in Eyewitness Identification

The committee recommends that all law enforcement agencies provide their officers and agents with training on vision and memory and the variables that affect them, on practices for minimizing contamination, and on effective eyewitness identification protocols.

Recommendation #2: Implement Double-Blind Lineup and Photo Array Procedures

The committee recommends blind (double-blind or blinded) administration of both photo arrays and live lineups and the adoption of clear, written policies and training on photo array and live lineup administration.

Recommendation #3: Develop and Use Standardized Witness Instructions

The committee recommends the development of a standard set of easily understood instructions to use when engaging a witness in an identification procedure.

Recommendation #4: Document Witness Confidence Judgments

The committee recommends that law enforcement document the witness' level of confidence verbatim at the time when she or he first identifies a suspect.

Recommendation #5: Videotape the Witness Identification Process

The committee recommends that the video recording of eyewitness identification procedures become standard practice.

RECOMMENDATIONS TO STRENGTHEN THE VALUE OF
EYEWITNESS IDENTIFICATION EVIDENCE IN COURT

The best guidance for legal regulation of eyewitness identification evidence comes not from constitutional rulings, but from the careful use and understanding of scientific evidence to guide fact-finders and decisionmakers. The Manson v. Brathwaite test under the Due Process Clause of the U.S. Constitution for assessing eyewitness identification evidence was established in 1977, before much applied research on eyewitness identification had been conducted. This test evaluates the "reliability" of eyewitness identifications using factors derived from prior rulings and not from empirically validated sources. As critics have pointed out, the Manson v. Brathwaite test includes factors that are not diagnostic of reliability. Moreover, the test treats factors such as the confidence of a witness as independent markers of reliability when, in fact, it is now well established that confidence judgments may vary over time and can be powerfully swayed by many factors. While some states have made minor changes to the due process framework, wholesale reconsideration of this framework is only a recent development.

Recommendation #6: Conduct Pretrial Judicial Inquiry

The committee recommends that, as appropriate, a judge make basic inquiries when eyewitness identification evidence is offered.

Recommendation #7: Make Juries Aware of Prior Identifications

The committee recommends that judges take all necessary steps to make juries aware of prior identifications, the manner and time frame in which they were conducted, and the confidence level expressed by the eyewitness at the time.

Recommendation #8: Use Scientific Framework Expert Testimony

The committee recommends that judges have the discretion to allow expert testimony on relevant precepts of eyewitness memory and identifications.

Recommendation #9: Use Jury Instructions as an Alternative Means to Convey Information

The committee recommends the use of clear and concise jury instructions as an alternative means of conveying information regarding the factors that the jury should consider.

RECOMMENDATIONS TO IMPROVE THE SCIENTIFIC FOUNDATION
UNDERPINNING EYEWITNESS IDENTIFICATION RESEARCH

Basic scientific research on visual perception and memory provides important insight into the factors that can limit the fidelity of eyewitness identification. Research targeting the specific problem of eyewitness identification complements basic scientific research. However, this strong scientific foundation remains insufficient for understanding the strengths and limitations of eyewitness identification procedures in the field. Many of the applied studies on key factors that directly affect eyewitness performance in the laboratory are not readily applicable to actual practice and policy. Applied research falls short because of a lack of reliable or standardized data from the field, a failure to include a range of practitioners in the establishment of research agendas, the use of disparate research methodologies, failure to use transparent and reproducible research procedures, and inadequate reporting of research data. The task of guiding eyewitness identification research toward the goal of evidence-based policy and practice will require collaboration in the setting of research agendas and agreement on methods for acquiring, handling, and sharing data.

Recommendation #10: Establish a National Research Initiative on Eyewitness Identification

The committee recommends the establishment of a National Research Initiative on Eyewitness Identification.

Recommendation #11: Conduct Additional Research on System and Estimator Variables

The committee recommends broad use of statistical tools that can render a discriminability measure to evaluate eyewitness performance and a rigorous exploration of methods that can lead to more conservative responding. The committee further recommends that caution and care be used when considering changes to any existing lineup procedure, until such time as there is clear evidence for the advantages of doing so."

Nat'l Research Council, *Identifying the Culprit: Assessing Eyewitness Identification* (2014).

5. Does reducing the incidence of false positives also lead to a decrease in the number of *correct* identifications? That is, are the optimal procedures for obtaining eyewitness identifications necessarily those that minimize false positives? Experts in psychology have debated this question. *See* Steven E. Clark, *Cost and Benefits of Eyewitness Identification Reform*, 7 Persp. Psychol. Sci. 238 (2012); Eryn J. Newman & Elizabeth F. Loftus, *Clarkian Logic on Trial*, 7 Persp. Psychol. Sci. 260 (2012); John T. Wixted & Laura Mickes, *The Field of Eyewitness Memory Should Abandon Probative Value and Embrace Receiver Operating Characteristic Analysis*, 7 Persp. Psychol. Sci. 275 (2012); Gary L. Wells et al., *Eyewitness Identification Reforms: Are Suggestiveness-Induced Hits and Guesses True Hits?*, 7 Persp. Psychol. Sci. 264 (2012).

   One study found that the post-*Henderson* jury instruction in New Jersey resulted in reduced juror reliance on both weak and strong evidentiary testimony. Athan P. Papailiou et al., *The Novel New Jersey Eyewitness Instruction Induces Skepticism but Not Sensitivity*, 10 PLoS ONE 0142695 (2015). Is this type of trade-off desireable?

   Some courts say no. In *State v. Pettiford*, the Court of Appeals of Ohio declined to require jury instructions like those used in New Jersey, noting that "the memory science pertaining to witness identification is the proper subject for expert testimony rather than the use of additional or disputed jury instructions." *State v. Pettiford*, No. 27490, 2019-Ohio-892 (Ohio Ct. App. filed March 15, 2019). *See also Corbin v. United States*, 120 A.3d 588 (D.C. Cir. 2015).

6. What role could and should neuroscience play in future cases that resemble *Henderson* and *Perry*? Consider this view from psychologists Daniel L. Schacter and Elizabeth Loftus:

   [G]iven the relatively short life of scientific explorations of neuroimaging and complex memories that might be true and might be false, we believe that it is wise to be skeptical now of efforts to introduce neuroimaging data into the courtroom arena as evidence in individual cases where memory accuracy is at issue. . . . [N]euroscientific evidence concerning memory, together with evidence from cognitive psychology, could help in educating jurors and other participants in the legal system generally about the nature of memory. However, we draw a distinction between such a general educational role and the application of neuroimaging data to individual cases. . . .

Daniel L. Schacter & Elizabeth Loftus, *Memory and Law: What Can Cognitive Neuroscience Contribute?*, 16 Nature Neurosci. 119 (2013). Do you agree with the distinction they draw?

7. Carefully consider the following list of "key points" from a report of the British Psychological Society, which was referenced earlier in this chapter. Assess each point for its potential relevance to the legal system. If you had the authority to pick only three that would form the core of a day-long training for all trial judges, which would you pick and why? On what bases did you choose?

   i. *Memories are records of people's experiences of events and are not a record of the events themselves.* In this respect, they are unlike other recording media such as videos or audio recordings, to which they should not be compared.

   ii. *Memory is not only of experienced events but it is also of the knowledge of a person's life, i.e. schools, occupations, holidays, friends, homes, achievements, failures, etc.* As a general rule memory is more likely to be accurate when it is of the knowledge of a person's life than when it is of specific experienced events.

   iii. *Remembering is a constructive process.* Memories are mental constructions that bring together different types of knowledge in an act of remembering. As a consequence, memory is prone to error and is easily influenced by the recall environment, including police interviews and cross-examination in court.

   iv. *Memories for experienced events are always incomplete.* Memories are time compressed fragmentary records of experience. Any account of a memory will feature forgotten details and gaps, and this must not be taken as any sort of indicator of accuracy. Accounts of memories that do not feature forgetting and gaps are highly unusual.

   v. *Memories typically contain only a few highly specific details.* Detailed recollection of the specific time and date of experiences is normally poor, as is highly specific information such as the precise recall of spoken conversations. As a general rule, a high degree of very specific detail in a long-term memory is unusual.

   vi. *Recall of a single or several highly specific details does not guarantee that a memory is accurate or even that it actually occurred.* In general, the only way to establish the truth of a memory is with independent corroborating evidence.

   vii. *The content of memories arises from an individual's comprehension of an experience, both conscious and non-conscious.* This content can be further modified and changed by subsequent recall.

   viii. *People can remember events that they have not in reality experienced.* This does not necessarily entail deliberate deception. For example, an event that was imagined, was a blend of a number of different events, or that makes personal sense for some other reason, can come to be genuinely experienced as a memory (these are often referred to as "confabulations").

   ix. *Memories for traumatic experiences, childhood events, interview and identification practices, memory in younger children and older adults and other vulnerable groups all have special features.* These are features that are unlikely to be commonly known by a non-expert, but about which an appropriate memory expert will be able to advise a court.

   x. *A memory expert is a person who is recognized by the memory research community to be a memory researcher.* It is recommended that, in addition to current requirements, those acting as memory expert witnesses be required to submit their full curriculum vitae to the court as evidence of their expertise.

British Psychology Soc'y Research Bd. Working Grp., *Guidelines on Memory and the Law: Recommendations from the Scientific Study of Human Memory* 2-4 (2008).

9. Is it possible that the legal community's distrust of eyewitness memory is misplaced? Contemplate the position advanced by John T. Wixted et al.:

> "From this perspective, eyewitness memory has been wrongfully convicted of mistakes that are better construed as having been committed by other actors in the legal system, not by the eyewitnesses themselves. Eyewitnesses typically provide reliable evidence on an initial, uncontaminated memory test, and this is true even for most of the wrongful convictions that were later reversed by DNA evidence."

John T. Wixted et al., *Rethinking the Reliability of Eyewitness Memory*, 13 Persp. Psychol. Sci. 324, 324 (2018).

10. Consider, separate from eyewitness contexts, issues surrounding juror memory. Sometimes courts will offer jury instructions that admonish the jury to completely disregard offered evidence or to limit the way jurors consider that evidence. Do you think such instructions are more likely to be effective, or counter-productive? On the other hand, in what ways should courts encourage jurors to remember what they hear? Some courts do not allow jurors to take written notes. What would the rationale for such a policy be, and do you agree?

11. One complication of eyewitness testimony is the effect of stress on the accuracy of memory. Although the effect of stress on the creation of the memory has long been a topic of study, research suggests that stress during the time of remembering can also interfere with retrieving memories, by disrupting hippocampal and cortical responses. Stephanie A. Gagnon et al., *Stress Impairs Episodic Retrieval by Disrupting Hippocampal and Cortical Mechanisms of Remembering*, 29 Cerebral Cortex 2947 (2019).

C. CROSS-RACIAL IDENTIFICATION

A wide body of behavioral research has discovered that we are better at recognizing same-race as compared to other-race faces. And analysis of fMRI measured during memory of same- or other-race faces suggests that group-based face memory biases arise, in part, because people tend to pay more attention to same-race faces, compared to other-race faces.* All this has potential implications for the accuracy of cross-race identification in legal settings, especially criminal trials. In this section we review two cases that deal with the issue of whether to allow jurors to hear about this type of research.

Smith v. State
880 A.2d 288 (Md. 2005)

BATTAGLIA, J. This case involves an attempted robbery in which a cross-racial identification was made by the victim of two defendants, Jason Mack and James Smith, as the perpetrators. The trial court denied defense counsel's request to argue the difficulties

---

* Thackery I. Brown et al., *Cognitive Control, Attention, and the Other Race Effect in Memory*, 12 PLoS ONE 0173579 (2017).

of cross-racial identification in closing argument and to have the jury instructed concerning the cross-racial nature of the identifications. Based upon the circumstances of this case, we hold that the trial court erred in prohibiting defense counsel from commenting on cross-racial identification in their closing arguments and reverse the defendants' convictions. We do not reach the jury instruction question.

FACTS

On May 8, 2002, at approximately 10:30 P.M., Christine Crandall, a white female, parked her car in front of her residence in the Fells Point neighborhood of Baltimore City, when she noticed two black males walking toward her on the other side of the street. Ms. Crandall said "hey guys" to the two men, after which one of the men pointed a gun at her and stated "give me your keys, bitch. I'll shoot you." Shortly thereafter, the second man attempted to grab the keys from Ms. Crandall's hand, but she maintained a tight fist around them, repeatedly stating "you don't want to do this," to the men.

During the altercation, one of Ms. Crandall's neighbors, Mary Jo Slowey, looked out a nearby second-floor window and asked Ms. Crandall if she was okay. In response, Ms. Crandall yelled, "call 911, they have a gun." At that point, the two men started to walk away, but the gunman allegedly turned and again pointed his weapon at Ms. Crandall, before leaving the scene.

Police officers responded to Ms. Slowey's call but were unable to locate the two men. Ms. Crandall provided a general description of them and stated that the man with the gun had "dreds." Two days after the incident, Detective Randolph Wynn, an officer with the Baltimore City Police Department assigned to the case, met with Ms. Crandall at the police station and showed her an array of photographs based upon her description of the perpetrators. After viewing the photo arrays, Ms. Crandall wrote on the back of the last photo, "Out of these 6 photos, I do not recognize the ones who attempted to car jack me."

Thereafter, Detective Wynn continued to investigate and prepared two additional photo arrays, which included pictures of the petitioners, Mr. Smith and Mr. Mack. On May 23, 2002, about two weeks after the incident, Ms. Crandall was shown the photos, and she identified Mr. Mack as the man who held the gun, although she noted that his hair was different because the man in the picture appeared to have his hair in "cornrows" rather than "dreds." Ms. Crandall then wrote on the back of Mr. Mack's photo, "He looks very much like the man who had the gun and attempted to rob me. The hair is changed but still looks like the man." Ms. Crandall also chose Mr. Smith's photo and wrote on the back, "This looks like the man wearing the hat that attempted to rob me. He tried to take the keys from my hand while the other man held the gun to me." Based upon Ms. Crandall's identification of Mr. Smith and Mr. Mack, both men were arrested on June 5 and 6, 2002, respectively.

PROCEDURAL HISTORY

[Mack and Smith were charged with Attempted Armed Robbery, among other things.] Prior to the jury trial . . . [defendants] submitted a motion *in limine* . . . requesting that the jury be instructed on cross-racial eyewitness identification to enable the parties to raise the issue in opening statements. After hearing arguments by the parties, the judge denied the motion and stated that the issue of cross-racial identification could not be argued during opening statements. . . .

[T]he State produced three witnesses to testify in support of its case-in-chief. Detective Wynn testified that he had been assigned to investigate an attempted robbery of Ms. Crandall and that she had provided a general description of the suspects. He explained that he had prepared several photo arrays for review by Ms. Crandall, who upon seeing the photos, had stated with certainty that Mr. Smith and Mr. Mack were the two people who had pointed the gun at her and tried to take her keys, respectively. . . .

Finally, counsel for the State asked Ms. Crandall why she was so sure that the defendants were the two individuals who had attempted to rob her, to which she replied that she was "extremely good with faces." . . .

On cross-examination, defense counsel questioned Ms. Crandall about the sequence of events and her ability to identify the defendants, but did not ask specific questions relating to cross-racial identification.

During a recess of the proceedings, defense counsel requested permission to comment on the difficulty of the cross-racial identifications during closing arguments. [The Court denied the request, indicating there was "not evidence in the case to that effect."]

Prior to closing arguments, counsel for Mr. Mack renewed his request to argue cross-racial identification in his closing. The trial judge again denied the request [indicating that counsel was only permitted to say that the client is black and the victim is white].

During closing arguments neither defense counsel raised the cross-racial identification issue, nor did either counsel mention the races of the defendants or the victim.

[Both defendants were found guilty of some crimes, and not guilty of others. Both were sentenced and both appealed, arguing that the trial court abused its discretion in denying the requested jury instruction, and in denying the opportunity to argue the difficulty of cross-racial identification in closing.] [The intermediate appellate court affirmed, on the basis], that there was no evidence presented during the trial to show that race played a part in the identification of the defendants or that cross-racial identification was an issue. [Defendants petitioned for, and were granted, review.]

Because we hold that under the circumstances of this case, the trial judge erred in precluding the defendants from discussing cross-racial identification in their closing arguments and reverse the defendants' convictions, we do not reach the jury instruction question.

CROSS-RACIAL IDENTIFICATION

In general, a cross-racial identification occurs when an eyewitness of one race is asked to identify a particular individual of another race. Over the past half-century, a growing body of scientific laboratory and field research concerning eyewitness cross-racial identifications has emerged suggesting that some witnesses are better able to identify members of their own race, but are significantly impaired when attempting to identify individuals of another race or ethnicity. This "phenomenon" has been termed the "own-race" or "other-race" effect, or "own-race" bias. . . .

Numerous of these studies have shown that the own-race effect is strongest when white participants attempt to recognize black faces. In one study, white subjects misidentified black faces two-to-three times more often than they misidentified white faces. [The court discussed the findings of three published field studies, each of which provides some support for the cross-race effect.]

Overall, there is strong consensus among researchers conducting both laboratory and field studies on cross-racial identification that some witnesses are more likely to misidentify members of other races than their own. Although many scientists and researchers conducting these studies agree that some witnesses exhibit own-race bias, they disagree on the extent to which such bias affects eyewitness identification due to the variations in the statistical data showing a cross-race effect.

[The court discussed three theories that have been proposed to explain the existence of the cross-race effect, noting multiple points of contention in the literature.]

Because there is debate concerning the results of the studies on cross-racial identification, researchers and other professionals have questioned whether courts should recognize the own-race effect in cases involving cross-racial identification of a defendant by a victim or witness.

Some courts, however, when addressing the issue of a cross-racial identification of a criminal defendant, without crediting the studies themselves, have permitted jury instruction or closing argument on cross-racial identification.

CLOSING ARGUMENT

In this instance, the gist of the issue before us is whether the trial court should have allowed defense counsel to argue the difficulties of cross-racial identification in closing argument. . . .

[D]uring closing argument, counsel may "state and discuss the evidence and all reasonable and legitimate inferences which may be drawn from the facts in evidence," *Henry v. State*, 324 Md. 204, 230, (1991), in addition to argue matters of common knowledge. "Subject to the trial court's discretion, both the State's Attorney and defense counsel are given wide latitude in the conduct of closing argument, including the right to explain or to attack all the evidence in the case." *Trimble v. State*, 300 Md. 387, 405, (1984). Closing argument, however, is not without limitation, in that the court should not permit counsel to state and comment upon facts not in evidence or to state what he or she would have proven. What exceeds the limits of permissible comment or argument by counsel depends on the facts of each case.

The case *sub judice* involves the victim's eyewitness cross-racial identification of the defendants, which was the sole piece of significant evidence. During her testimony, Ms. Crandall described the physical characteristics of the defendants and opined on her ability to identify them. She stated that she was "extremely good with faces," looked for distinctive features, and was "obsessed with people's postures," as the basis for identifying the defendants. Ms. Crandall further qualified her experience in recognizing people by stating that she was a teacher and had been studying art and painting people since childhood.

Defense counsel clearly was entitled to challenge Ms. Crandall's "educated" identification of the defendants by arguing to the jury that her identification should not be accorded the weight that she credited to her own ability to identify them. At this juncture the extent to which own-race bias affects eyewitness identification is unclear based on the available studies addressing this issue, so that we cannot state with certainty that difficulty in cross-racial identification is an established matter of common knowledge. Here, however, the victim's identification of the defendants was anchored in her enhanced ability to identify faces. Under these circumstances, defense counsel should have been allowed to argue the difficulties of cross-racial identification in closing argument. . . .

[Reversed and remanded for a new trial.]

Dissenting Opinion by HARRELL, J. which WILNER and GREENE, JJ., join. . . . Although, as the majority painstakingly demonstrates, there may be social science research and theories in academia on the topic of own-race bias and associated cross-racial identification difficulties, the "jury," so to speak, is still "out" on the reliability of that research and conclusions. This healthy skepticism appears not only in some of the cases cited by the majority, but also in the majority opinion itself. . . . Where does that leave the majority with respect to proper legal analysis in deciding this case? . . .

The majority opinion, in a scant two paragraphs of actual legal analysis, concludes that the defendants were entitled to offer argument regarding the difficulties of cross-racial identification to challenge the eyewitness's/victim's actual testimony concerning her "enhanced ability to identify faces." It is unclear to me, under any analysis (social science or law), how or why arguments related to cross-racial identifications are relevant or legitimate in impeaching the witness with regard to her self-assessed abilities and her background in the study of art. . . .

The science behind the concept of own-race bias and its effects on cross-racial identification has not been vetted sufficiently on this record or generally in the social science or legal fields. The question also exists of how one defines race for purposes of the context of what the majority opinion appears to recognize as new Maryland common law. The majority opinion, as do most of the cases cited by the majority, treat race as a well-defined issue. It is not always so clear. . . .

This Court should not let the Genie from the bottle without considering and giving guidance to Bench and Bar as to how its holding should be applied. . . .

People v. Boone
30 N.Y.3d 521 (N.Y. 2017)

FAHEY, J. In light of the near consensus among cognitive and social psychologists that people have significantly greater difficulty in accurately identifying members of a different race than in accurately identifying members of their own race, the risk of wrongful convictions involving cross-racial identifications demands a new approach. We hold that when identification is an issue in a criminal case and the identifying witness and defendant appear to be of different races, upon request, a party is entitled to a charge on cross-racial identification.

I.

On February 16, 2011, a white man in his 20s was walking in Brooklyn when he was approached by a stranger, a short-haired black man. The stranger asked to know the time, and the young man retrieved his cell phone. The stranger snatched the cell phone and fled. The victim gave chase, until the robber pulled out a knife and told him to stay where he was. The victim described his attacker as an African-American man, about six feet tall, weighing about 170 pounds, and wearing a baseball cap and a hooded sweatshirt.

Ten days later, a white teenager was walking in the same neighborhood of Brooklyn, sending a text message from his cell phone, when a man behind him asked the time. The teenager looked back over his shoulder and observed a stranger, a black man, wearing a winter coat and a hat with flaps that covered his ears and the top of his head. The teenager looked at his cell phone and told the stranger the time. The stranger then grabbed the phone. The teenager did not immediately let go, and the robber stabbed him. The robber then took the phone and fled. Before the victim was taken to the hospital, he described the perpetrator to the police as an African-American man, about 18 years old and approximately six feet, two inches tall, and he gave an estimated weight.

Defendant Otis Boone, a black man who was short-haired, 19 years old, and 6 feet tall, and weighed about 170 pounds, was suspected of committing the crimes. On March 14, 2011, defendant was placed in two six-person lineups and the victims separately identified him. The teenager was initially unsure whether defendant was his attacker, but identified him after he spoke the words "What time is it?" Defendant and the fillers in the lineups all wore hats.

Neither cell phone was recovered, and no physical evidence linked defendant to the crimes.

II.

Defendant was charged with two counts of robbery in the first degree and other crimes.

At defendant's jury trial in July 2012, during the charge conference, defense counsel requested that the jury be instructed on cross-racial identification. Supreme Court denied the request, on the basis that there had been no expert testimony or cross-examination concerning "a lack of reliability of cross-racial identification." The trial court gave the jury an expanded charge on eyewitness identification, based on the pertinent Criminal Jury Instruction omitting the part of the pattern instruction addressing cross-racial identification.

The jury found defendant guilty of both robbery counts. On appeal from the judgment of conviction and sentence, defendant argued that Supreme Court denied him a fair trial by refusing to charge the jury on the inaccuracy of cross-racial identification.

The Appellate Division modified the judgment, as to the sentence, and affirmed as modified, holding that Supreme Court had not erred in declining to instruct the jury on cross-racial identification. The Appellate Division reasoned that defendant had not "placed the issue in evidence during the trial."

A Judge of this Court granted defendant leave to appeal from the Appellate Division order, and we now reverse.

III.

Mistaken eyewitness identifications are "the single greatest cause of wrongful convictions in this country" (*State v Delgado*, 188 NJ 48, 60 [2006]). Inaccurate identifications, especially misidentifications by a single eyewitness, play a role in the vast majority of post-conviction DNA-based exonerations in the United States. Indeed, a recent report by the National Academy of Sciences concluded that "at least one mistaken eyewitness identification was present in almost three-quarters" of DNA exonerations (Identifying the Culprit: Assessing Eyewitness

Identification 11 [2014]). According to amicus The Innocence Project, about 70% of DNA exonerations nationally involve eyewitness misidentification. This Court has noted in recent years the prevalence of eyewitness misidentifications in wrongful convictions and the danger they pose to the truth-seeking function and integrity of our justice system.

Social scientists have found that the likelihood of misidentification is higher when an identification is cross-racial. Generally, people have significantly greater difficulty accurately identifying members of other races than members of their own race. According to a meta-analysis of 39 psychological studies of the phenomenon, participants were "1.56 times more likely to falsely identify a novel other-race face when compared with performance on own-race faces" (Christian A. Meissner & John C. Brigham, *Thirty Years of Investigating the Own-Race Bias in Memory for Faces: A Meta-Analytic Review*, 7 Psychol. Pub Pol'y. & L 3, 15 [2001]). The phenomenon is known as the cross-race effect or own-race bias. . . .

The cross-race effect is "generally accepted" by experts in the fields of cognitive and social psychology (Identifying the Culprit at 96), a point that the People do not dispute. Indeed, in a survey of psychologists with expertise in eyewitness identification, 90% of the experts believed that empirical evidence of the cross-race effect was sufficiently reliable to be presented in court. The phenomenon has been described as "[o]ne of the best documented examples of face recognition errors" (Steven G. Young et al., *Perception and Motivation in Face Recognition: A Critical Review of Theories of the Cross-Race Effect*, 16 Personality & Soc. Psychol. Rev. 116, 116 [2012]).

There is, however, a significant disparity between what the psychological research shows and what uninstructed jurors believe. . . . These findings demonstrate that, while the cross-race effect is a matter of common sense and experience for some jurors, it is by no means a universal belief shared by all. The need for a charge on the cross-race effect is evident. The question becomes how this instruction is best given.

IV.

As to each crime of which he was convicted, defendant, who is black, was found guilty entirely on the basis of the testimony of a single white witness identifying defendant as the person who had robbed him. Nevertheless, Supreme Court refused to give the requested charge instructing the jury on the relative inaccuracy of cross-racial identifications. One of Supreme Court's reasons for refusing to give the charge was that such an instruction should not be given if there has been no expert testimony on the subject. We reject this rationale and hold that Supreme Court erred in relying on it. For this reason and because the error was not harmless, we reverse.

Expert testimony on the cross-race effect is not a precondition of a jury charge on the subject. Indeed, the People do not contend that it is, but instead insist, at least in this appeal, that expert testimony on the cross-race effect is a preferable substitute for a jury charge and one that renders the charge superfluous. We disagree.

The decision to grant a request for expert testimony on the subject of cross-racial identification remains within the trial court's discretion. However, expert testimony is not necessary to establish the right to the charge.

A psychological principle such as the cross-race effect may lend itself to expert testimony. "Despite the fact that jurors may be familiar from their own experience with factors relevant to the reliability of eyewitness observation and identification, it cannot be said that psychological studies regarding the accuracy of an identification are within the ken of the typical juror" (*Lee*, 96 N.Y.2d at 162; *see also Santiago*, 17 N.Y.3d at 672; *Abney*, 13 N.Y.3d at 268; *LeGrand*, 8 N.Y.3d at 458). Contrary to the People's position, this does not mean that the cross-race effect cannot be expressed in a jury charge.

We have recognized that the same psychological principle may be the subject of expert testimony and a jury charge. For example, the pattern jury instructions ask jurors to consider "[f]or what period of time . . . the witness actually observe[d] the perpetrator", because exposure time, the amount of time a witness has to view a perpetrator, affects that person's ability to identify someone accurately as the perpetrator. Yet, we have held that a trial court abused its discretion in refusing to hold a *Frye* hearing with regard to an expert's proposed testimony on the effect of exposure time, among other factors.

Similarly, as noted above, a juror may have a tentative belief, based on his or her ordinary experiences, that cross-racial identifications are often inaccurate, but most jurors will have no knowledge of the research demonstrating the cross-race effect. Expert testimony explaining the studies to the jury is admissible, because "it would help to clarify an issue calling for professional or technical knowledge, possessed by the expert and beyond the ken of the typical juror" (*De Long v County of Erie*, 60 N.Y.2d 296, 307 [1983]), with the decision to admit subject to the trial court's discretion. Such expert testimony does not render a charge regarding the cross-race effect superfluous.

In short, the absence of expert testimony on cross-racial identification does not preclude the charge.

V.

Supreme Court also erred in assuming that a cross-racial identification charge should be predicated on whether defense counsel cross-examined the People's witnesses about their identifications. An eyewitness is often utterly confident about an identification, expressing the identification or recollection of identification with subjective certainty, and hence entirely unshakable on cross-examination. . . .

Honesty and accuracy are entirely different categories by which jurors evaluate testimony. It is the fact of a cross-racial identification that should be the basis of the court's charge, not the nature of the questions asked on the examination.

Amici former judges and prosecutors observe that cross-examination that is "aimed at establishing that a witness may have difficulty identifying members of another race may offend the witness and the jury, without any benefit to the examiner" (brief of former judges and prosecutors as amici curiae at 8, citing Epstein at 775). The amici note that

> "[a]s a society, we do not discuss racial issues easily. Some jurors may deny the existence of the cross-race effect in the misguided belief that it is merely a racist myth . . . while others may believe in the reality of this effect but be reluctant to discuss it in deliberations for fear of being seen as bigots. That, however, makes an instruction all the more essential" (brief of former judges and prosecutors at 15 [internal quotation marks, citations and brackets omitted]).

As with whether to seek expert testimony, cross-examination should be a decision that counsel makes within the context of an individual case.

VI.

High courts in other states have recently considered the significance of the cross-race effect and three have required that trial courts, in appropriate cases, instruct juries regarding the phenomenon. . . .

In *Commonwealth v Bastaldo*, the Supreme Judicial Court of Massachusetts, relying on the Report and Recommendations of the Supreme Judicial Court Study Group on Eyewitness Evidence, held that in light of the fact that "[t]he existence of the 'cross-race effect' . . . has reached a near consensus in the relevant scientific community and has been recognized by courts and scholars alike" (472 Mass. at 23), an instruction on the inaccuracy of cross-racial identification must be given, unless the parties agree that there was no cross-racial identification.

> "[I]n criminal trials that commence after the issuance of this opinion, the following instruction should be included when giving the model eyewitness identification instruction, unless all parties agree to its omission:
> "'If the witness and the person identified appear to be of different races, you should consider that people may have greater difficulty in accurately identifying someone of a different race than someone of their own race'" (472 Mass. at 27).

Defendant urges this Court to require that a jury charge on the cross-race effect be given in all cases unless both parties agree that no cross-racial identification has occurred, or, alternatively, when requested by defense counsel. . . .

VIII.

In light of our discussion of the cross-race effect, which has been accepted by a near consensus in the relevant scientific community of cognitive and social psychologists, and recognizing the very significant part that inaccurate identifications play in wrongful convictions, we reach the following holding: in a case in which a witness's identification of the defendant is at issue, and the identifying witness and defendant appear to be of different races, a trial court is required to give, upon request, during final instructions, a jury charge on the cross-race effect, instructing (1) that the jury should consider whether there is a difference in race between the defendant and the witness who identified the defendant, and (2) that, if so, the jury should consider (a) that some people have greater difficulty in accurately identifying members of a different race than in accurately identifying members of their own race and (b) whether the difference in race affected the accuracy of the witness's identification. The instruction would not be required when there is no dispute about the identity of the perpetrator nor would it be obligatory when no party asks for the charge. . . .

X.

The People's remaining arguments, including that defendant did not preserve or abandoned his request for a cross-racial identification charge and that any error was harmless, are without merit.

Accordingly, the order of the Appellate Division should be reversed and a new trial ordered.

NOTES AND QUESTIONS

1. For over 100 years experimental psychologists have consistently found that people recognize cross-race faces less accurately than same-race faces. It was widely believed that this happens because people simply have less experience recognizing cross-race faces, so they do not encode subtle variations of facial features in cross-race faces. However, other research has found that when people place too much emphasis on whether someone is a particular race, then they overlook facial characteristics that distinguish individuals. Daniel T. Levin, *Race as a Visual Feature: Using Visual Search and Perceptual Discrimination Tasks to Understand Face Categories and the Cross-Race Recognition Deficit*, 129 J. Experimental Psychol. 559 (2000). The cross-race effect is reduced or eliminated by educating people about the effect and motivating them to focus on individual facial characteristics. Kurt Hugenberg et al., *The Categorization-Individuation Model: An Integrative Account of the Other-Race Recognition Deficit*, 117 Psychol. Rev. 1168 (2010). Not surprisingly, neural correlates of this variation in perceptual quality have been found, and activation in face-selective brain areas, such as the fusiform face area, is weaker for cross-race faces. Grit Herzmann et al., *The Neural Correlates of Memory Encoding and Recognition for Own-Race and Other-Race Faces*, 49 Neuropsychologia 3103 (2011); Alexandra J. Golby et al., *Differential Responses in the Fusiform Region to Same-Race and Other-Race Faces*, 4 Nature Neurosci. 845 (2001).

2. The *Smith* majority opinion and dissent disagree about the state of the science on cross-race identification. When *Boone* was decided 12 years later, the New York Court of Appeals, the highest court in New York, approached the science of cross-race identification as nearly universally accepted. Do you think the introduction of further neuroscientific studies on race and recognition of faces clears up this disagreement or exacerbates it?

3. In the *Boone* decision, the court cites a study finding that regarding the veracity of memory, eyewitness and memory experts disagreed with the average juror on nearly 87% of the issues, while they disagreed with judges and law enforcement officials on around 60% of the issues presented. Tanja Rapus Benton et al., *Eyewitness Memory Is Still Not Common Sense: Comparing Jurors, Judges and Law Enforcement to Eyewitness Experts*, 20 Applied Cognitive Psychol. 115 (2006). Another investigation of the United States population found many misconceptions about memory and how it functions. Daniel J. Simons & Christopher F. Chabris, *What People Believe About How Memory Works: A Representative Survey of the U.S. Population*, 6 PLoS ONE 22757 (2011). In their survey, Simons and Chabris found that 55% of Americans believed that memory could be enhanced through hypnosis, 48% believed memory to be permanent, 63% believed that memory worked like a camera, and 37% believed that a single eyewitness would be sufficient to convict a criminal defendant. What should be done to improve these discrepancies? Would requiring eyewitness experts at every trial undermine the value of all eyewitness testimony? What alternative solution would refine the process without devaluing eyewitness testimony entirely?

4. Research suggests that in addition to a racial bias in remembering faces, there is also an age bias; we recognize faces closer rather than further from our own age.

Matthew G. Rhodes & Jeffrey S. Anastasi, *The Own-Age Bias in Face Recognition: A Meta-Analytic and Theoretical Review*, 138 Psychol. Bull. 146 (2012). Would you adopt the same evidentiary rules regarding the admissibility of expert testimony or instructions on age-related recognition biases as you would for race-related biases?

D. FALSE MEMORIES

Perhaps nowhere else in the legal system are false memories more problematic than in cases involving alleged childhood abuse. Such cases typically rely heavily, or entirely, on the memory of the alleged victim. If the memories of abuse are accurate, dismissing them would be a grave injustice. Similarly, if the memories of abuse are not accurate, relying on them for a conviction or monetary judgment would be equally unjust. In the case that follows we see one example of how courts try to meet this difficult challenge. The excerpt includes an Appendix in which the Court reproduced some of the interview transcripts with the alleged child victims. Following the case is an excerpt from a psychology review article that summarizes our current knowledge on how to discriminate between true and false memories.

State v. Michaels
642 A.2d 1372 (N.J. 1994)

HANDLER, J. In this case a nursery school teacher was convicted of bizarre acts of sexual abuse against many of the children who had been entrusted to her care. She was sentenced to a long prison term with a substantial period of parole ineligibility. . . .

In September 1984, Margaret Kelly Michaels was hired by Wee Care Day Nursery ("Wee Care") as a teacher's aide for preschoolers. Located in St. George's Episcopal Church, in Maplewood, Wee Care served approximately fifty families, with an enrollment of about sixty children, ages three to five.

Michaels, a college senior from Pittsburgh, Pennsylvania, came to New Jersey to pursue an acting career. She responded to an advertisement and was hired by Wee Care, initially as a teacher's aide for preschoolers, then, at the beginning of October, as a teacher. Michaels had no prior experience as a teacher at any level.

Wee Care had staff consisting of eight teachers, numerous aides, and two administrators. The nursery classes for the three-year-old children were housed in the basement, and the kindergarten class was located on the third floor. During nap time, Michaels, under the supervision of the head teacher and the director, was responsible for about twelve children in one of the basement classrooms. The classroom assigned to Michaels was separated from an adjacent occupied classroom by a vinyl curtain.

During the seven-month period that Michaels worked at Wee Care, she apparently performed satisfactorily. Wee Care never received a complaint about her from staff, children, or parents. According to the State, however, between October 8, 1984, and the date of Michaels's resignation on April 26, 1985, parents and teachers began observing behavioral changes in the children.

On April 26, 1985, the mother of M.P., a four-year old in Michaels's nap class, noticed while awakening him for school, that he was covered with spots. She took the child to his pediatrician and had him examined. During the examination, a pediatric nurse took M.P.'s temperature rectally. In the presence of the nurse and his mother, M.P. stated, "this is what my teacher does to me at nap time at school." M.P. indicated to the nurse that his teacher, Kelly (the name by which Michaels was known to the children), was the one who took his temperature. M.P. added that Kelly undressed him and took his temperature daily. On further questioning by his mother, M.P. said that Kelly did the same thing to S.R.

The pediatrician, Dr. Delfino, then examined M.P. He informed Mrs. P. that the spots were caused by a rash. Mrs. P. did not tell Dr. Delfino about M.P.'s remarks; consequently, he did not examine M.P.'s rectum. In response to further questioning from his mother after they had returned home, M.P., while rubbing his genitals, stated that "[Kelly] uses the white jean stuff." Although M.P. was unable to tell his mother what the "white jean stuff" was, investigators later found vaseline in Wee Care's bathroom and white cream in the first-aid kit. During the same conversation, M.P. indicated that Kelly had "hurt" two of his classmates, S.R. and E.N.

M.P.'s mother contacted the New Jersey Division of Youth and Family Services ("DYFS") and Ms. Spector, Director of Wee Care, to inform them of her son's disclosures. On May 1, 1985, the Essex County Prosecutor's office received information from DYFS about the alleged sexual abuse at Wee Care. The Prosecutor's office assumed investigation of the complaint.

The Prosecutor's office interviewed several Wee Care children and their parents, concluding their initial investigation on May 8, 1985. During that period of investigation, Michaels submitted to approximately nine hours of questioning. Additionally, Michaels consented to taking a lie detector test, which she passed. Extensive additional interviews and examinations of the Wee Care children by the prosecutor's office and DYFS then followed.

Michaels was charged on June 6, 1985, in a three count indictment involving the alleged sexual abuse of three Wee Care boys. . . .

The bulk of the State's evidence consisted of the testimony of the children. That testimony referred extensively to the pretrial statements that had been elicited from the children during the course of the State's investigations. The State introduced limited physical evidence to support the contention that the Wee Care children had been molested. . . .

[A]fter twelve days of deliberation, the jury returned guilty verdicts on 115 counts, including aggravated sexual assault (thirty-eight counts), sexual assault (thirty-one counts), endangering the welfare of children (forty-four counts), and terroristic threats (two counts). . . .

The focus of this case is on the manner in which the State conducted its investigatory interviews of the children. In particular, the Court is asked to consider whether the interview techniques employed by the state could have undermined the reliability of the children's statements and subsequent testimony. . . .

The Appellate Division carefully examined the record concerning the investigatory interviews. It concluded that the interrogations that had been conducted were highly improper. The court determined from the record that the children's accusations were founded "upon unreliable perceptions, or memory caused by improper investigative procedures." . . .

As the Appellate Division noted, a constantly broadening body of scholarly authority exists on the question of children's susceptibility to improper interrogation. . . . Among the varying perspectives, however, the Appellate Division found a consistent and recurrent concern over the capacity of the interviewer and the interview process to distort a child's recollection through unduly slanted interrogation techniques. The Appellate Division concluded that certain interview practices are sufficiently coercive or suggestive to alter irremediably the perceptions of the child victims. . . .

We . . . determine that a sufficient consensus exists within the academic, professional, and law enforcement communities, confirmed in varying degrees by courts, to warrant the conclusion that the use of coercive or highly suggestive interrogation techniques can create a significant risk that the interrogation itself will distort the child's recollection of events, thereby undermining the reliability of the statements and subsequent testimony concerning such events. . . .

. . . The interrogations undertaken in the course of this case utilized most, if not all, of the practices that are disfavored or condemned by experts, law enforcement authorities and government agencies. . . .

. . . The record is replete with instances in which children were asked blatantly leading questions that furnished information the children themselves had not mentioned. All but five of the thirty-four children interviewed were asked questions that indicated or strongly suggested that perverse sexual acts had in fact occurred. . . . In addition, many of the children, some over the course of nearly two years leading up to trial, were subjected to repeated, almost incessant, interrogation. Some children were re-interviewed at the urgings of their parents.

The record of the investigative interviews discloses the use of mild threats, cajoling, and bribing. Positive reinforcement was given when children made inculpatory statements, whereas negative reinforcement was expressed when children denied being abused or made exculpatory statements. . . .

Seventeen of the thirty-four children were actually told that other children had told investigators that Kelly had done bad things to children. . . .

We thus agree with the Appellate Division that the interviews of the children were highly improper and employed coercive and unduly suggestive methods. As a result, a substantial likelihood exists that the children's recollection of past events was both stimulated and materially influenced by that course of questioning. Accordingly, we conclude that a hearing must be held to determine whether those clearly improper interrogations so infected the ability of the children to recall the alleged abusive events that their pretrial statements and in-court testimony based on that recollection are unreliable and should not be admitted into evidence. . . .

In conclusion, we find that the interrogations that occurred in this case were improper and there is a substantial likelihood that the evidence derived from them is unreliable. We therefore hold that in the event the State seeks to re-prosecute this defendant, a pretrial hearing must be held in which the State must prove by clear and convincing evidence that the statements and testimony elicited by the improper interview techniques nonetheless retains a sufficient degree of reliability to warrant admission at trial. Given the egregious prosecutorial abuses evidenced in this record, the challenge that the State faces is formidable. If the statements and proffered testimony of any of the children survive the pretrial hearing, the jury will have to determine the credibility and probative worth of such testimony in light of all the surrounding circumstances. . . .

[Affirmed and remanded for retrial.]

APPENDIX

This Appendix presents a detailed summary of several interviews.

1. *R.F.*

R.F., a three-year-old girl, was interviewed on June 21, 1985, by the Essex County Prosecutor's Office at the Wee Care facility. After several minutes of small talk, R.F. told the investigator that Kelly sometimes sings in school. In response to her inquiry, R.F. indicated that the school owned a piano and that she would show the investigators where it was. At that point, the interview went off the record and R.F. apparently took the interviewers to the piano room. On their return to the interview room, the following colloquy took place between the investigator and R.F.

The investigator asked, "Do you remember what you were saying to me? You said,—you said Kelly did a lot of bad things to the children."

R.F. responded, "No, she's in jail. . . . Because she did a lot of bad things.

R.F. was unable to identify any of the "bad things" that Kelly did because, according to R.F., "she only did them to D.A." Then, after several minutes of trying to get R.F. to draw pictures, including one of Kelly, the investigators returned to the alleged abuse. An investigator asked if Kelly or Brenda (another teacher at Wee Care) had ever hurt her. R.F. was clear and unambiguous with her response. R.F. was absolutely certain that they had done nothing to her. The investigators continued to press the questioning. R.F. continually stressed that she had not been hurt or touched. R.F. did say, however, that "they (Kelly and Brenda) did hurt D.A." The interview continued uneventfully, ending with R.F. telling the interviewers that she would like to come back to the school.

A detective from the Prosecutor's office interviewed R.F. again on July 3, 1985. The detective approached his questioning of R.F. somewhat differently than had the previous investigators in that he appeared not to have any warm up period with the child. Prior to engaging in any small talk or even introducing himself to R.F., he asked her "where's Kelly?" In an effort to find out what relationship R.F. had with Kelly the investigator asked the following questions:

Detective:	Do you know Kelly?
R.F.:	Yes.
Detective:	Was Kelly your teacher?
R.F.:	Yeah, but she did a lot of bad things to me.
Detective:	[W]hat did she do to you that was bad?
R.F.:	Yesterday she did something. But I don't know what it is.
Detective:	Sure you do, would you like to show me instead of tell me?

R.F. then drew a picture of Kelly, giving her a "mad" face. She indicated to him that she drew a mad face simply because she wanted Kelly to have a mad face. The detective continued the interview asking pointed questions:

Detective:	Do you think Kelly can hurt you?
R.F.:	No.
Detective:	Did Kelly say she can hurt you? Did Kelly ever tell you she can turn into a monster?
R.F.:	Yes.
Detective:	What did she tell you?
R.F.:	She was gonna turn into a monster.

* * *

Detective:	What did Kelly,—was Kelly a good girl or a bad girl?
R.F.:	She was a bad girl.
Detective:	She was a bad girl, were there any other teachers that were bad?
R.F.:	No.
Detective:	No, O.K. Kelly was the only bad girl? What did Kelly do that made her a bad girl?
R.F.:	She readed [sic].
Detective:	She what?
R.F.:	She um, she readed [sic] and she came to me and I said no, no, no.
Detective:	Did she hurt you?
R.F.:	I hurted [sic] her.
Detective:	How did you hurt her?
R.F.:	Because she, I didn't want to write, and she write and I said no, no, no, no, and I hit her.

* * *

The Detective then questioned R.F. using anatomically correct dolls in an apparent attempt to elicit from R.F. the level of understanding she had concerning certain body parts.

Detective:	What are these?
R.F.:	Dolls.
Detective:	O.K. But what am I pointing to? What's that?
R.F.:	An eye, mouth, nose arm.
Detective:	What do you call this right here?
R.F.:	Vagina.
Detective:	What's this right here?
R.F.:	Tooshie.
Detective:	Tooshie. O.K. What do you call these right up here?
R.F.:	I don't know.
Detective:	O.K. what do you want to name them? Do you want to name them breasts?
R.F.:	Yeah.
Detective:	Now we are going to pretend that this is a little boy.
R.F.:	Let me see the little boy.
Detective:	It has no arms or legs or anything, but we are going to pretend that it's a little boy doll, O.K.? What do you call the little thing between the little boy's legs?
R.F.:	Um, feet.
Detective:	No, up farther between the legs. Right here.
R.F.:	Vagina.
Detective:	No, it's a vagina on a little girl, what is it on a little boy?
R.F.:	Penis.
Detective:	Penis, very good. O.K. Now did you ever see a little boy's penis in the school?
R.F.:	Yes, M.Z.'s.
Detective:	O.K. Who else was there?
R.F.:	That's it, only one.
Detective:	Just M.Z. and you? Was Kelly there?
R.F.:	She was at jail.

The questioning of R.F. continued; the detective sought to uncover any "bad things" Kelly might have done to R.F. or to anyone else. The following sequence of questions and answers was the first time the use of utensils entered the discussion:

Detective:	Now, did Kelly ever do any bad things to you?
R.F.:	No.
Detective:	Not at all?
R.F.:	No.
Detective:	Did Kelly ever hurt you?
R.F.:	No.
Detective:	Do these look familiar?
R.F.:	What are them [sic]?
Detective:	You tell me what they are?
R.F.:	Knife.
Detective:	Knife.
R.F.:	Do you have anything to eat in here?
Detective:	We're going to pretend that this is a spoon, O.K.?
R.F.:	O.K., and this is a knife.
Detective:	Did Kelly ever do anything to you with a knife that hurt you? Or bad things to you with a knife?
R.F.:	No.
Detective:	No. O.K. Do [sic] she ever do bad things or hurt you with a spoon?—No. Did she ever do bad things or hurt you with a knife—I mean fork? OK. What about a wooden spoon? Did you ever see her do bad things or hurt anybody?
R.F.:	Um, no.

After concluding the discussion of utensils, and whether Kelly had used utensils on R.F. or any other child, the discussion once again focused on Kelly's alleged mistreatment of R.F. The questioning of this child continued for several more transcript pages. In an attempt to obtain additional information from R.F., the detective told her that he had spoken to several of her friends already and that the information she could provide would help her friends. . . .

Daniel M. Bernstein & Elizabeth F. Loftus
How to Tell if a Particular Memory Is True or False
4 Persp. Psychol. Sci. 370, 370-73 (2009)

Consider the following situation. Mary X sits on the witness stand in court, recounting an emotionally charged memory involving childhood sexual abuse. Her report is both detailed and emotional. She explains how her grandfather molested her and how she had repressed the event for many years before recovering the memory in therapy. Is Mary's report the result of a real memory or a product of suggestion or imagination or some other process?

This hypothetical example has many real-world parallels: Individuals claim that they have recovered memories of events long forgotten. Lacking corroborative evidence or a confession that can be trusted, what are we to make of these claims? Although the field of memory research has demonstrated repeatedly that memory is fallible and prone to distortion, often we are faced with a difficult question: How do we tell if a particular memory is true or false? We regard this as one of the biggest challenges in human memory research.

Cognitive scientists have developed several techniques to measure groups of memories. Also, police, lawyers, and researchers have developed techniques to help them judge whether a person can be believed or not. These two approaches — focusing on the memories reported or the person reporting the memories — represent two very different ways of answering the thorny question we have posed. Unfortunately, neither approach presently can assess whether a particular memory is true or false. . . .

FOCUSING ON A PARTICULAR MEMORY

[R]esearchers can focus on groups of memories or on the individual reporting the memory to determine whether a particular memory is true or false. One approach to determining if an individual memory report is authentic is to analyze the contents of the memory report. Investigators have developed several procedures for assessing the validity of written and verbal statements concerning events. In the laboratory, we have the advantage of knowing who is reporting accurately and who is reporting falsely as we have control over the materials and methods. We can control which events the person experiences and which events are new. The challenge, though, is to apply what we have learned from the laboratory to the real world, where experiences can be highly emotional and even traumatic. Also, in the real world, we do not know who is telling the truth and who is lying or which memories are true and which are false.

After a suggestion-free memory report has been obtained from someone, how do we determine if it is true or false? One popular technique used by researchers is criteria-based content analysis. Originally developed for children, this technique also applies to adults. The idea behind criteria-based content analysis is that false statements are inherently different from and differentiable from true statements. This assumption applies both to lies and false beliefs and memories. . . .

Consistent with other work, true memory reports tend to contain more detail — especially sensory detail like sight, sound, touch, taste, and smell — than do false memories. Criteria-based content analysis appears to be most useful as a first step in helping police investigators form rough ideas about the truthfulness of witness statements.

Many cases of allegedly recovered memories have turned out to be false memories implanted by well-meaning therapists who use suggestion and imagination to guide the search for memories. The more elaborate and detailed the implanted false memory is, the more real and authentic it will seem to the individual, and the harder it will be to determine whether it is true or false. What techniques can be used to determine whether the unintentional liar holds a false belief?

Recently, we have moved from planting event details in people's minds to planting entirely false memories. Our methods involve strong suggestion and imagination of event details, combined with painstaking efforts to ensure that the memory that we are suggesting is, in fact, a false memory for the individual. . . .

[In one study] subjects who viewed a suggestive advertisement for Disney came to believe that, as children, they had met and shook hands with Bugs Bunny at Disneyland. For anyone who knows anything about Disney, you will realize that such an event is impossible. Bugs Bunny is a Warner Brothers character, and Disney does not have Warner Brothers' characters in its theme parks. Even with impossible events, a substantial minority of subjects come to believe that the false event occurred in their past. This work tells us much about the formation of what we call rich false memories—detailed memories for individual events that never occurred. However, like the focus on groups of memories and on the individual reporting the memory, the focus on single rich memories presently does not tell us whether a particular memory is true or false. . . .

CONCLUSION

Let's return to Mary X in the courtroom. She has finished recounting the details of her childhood abuse. Without independent corroboration from another person or hard evidence that the abuse occurred (e.g., a recently discovered medical report verifying and detailing the abuse), how can we determine whether Mary's memory is real? On average, real memories have more sensory and conceptual information, including visual, auditory, and olfactory details and spatial and temporal details. So, we might closely examine Mary's memory report to see if it has sensory detail. But even if we find such detail, how can we be sure that the memory is real and not the product of suggestion? We now know that suggestion and imagination can make a false memory feel and appear real.

In essence, all memory is false to some degree. Memory is inherently a reconstructive process, whereby we piece together the past to form a coherent narrative that becomes our autobiography. In the process of reconstructing the past, we color and shape our life's experiences based on what we know about the world. Our job as memory researchers and as human beings is to determine the portion of memory that reflects reality and the portion that reflects inference and bias. This is no simple feat, but one worthy of our continued investigation.

NOTES AND QUESTIONS

1. If you were a juror listening to testimony in the *Michaels* case, how would you decide whether the defendant was guilty? In the case the prosecution relied almost entirely on the testimony of the preschool-aged children. One child testified that Michaels had briefly turned him into a mouse. Another said she made him insert a sword into her own rectum. The only physical evidence admitted was a jar of peanut butter and a page of Michaels' journal, on which she had written down lyrics to a Bob Dylan song, which the prosecution argued were suggestive. Dorothy Rabinowitz, *From the Mouths of Babes to a Jail Cell*, Harper's Mag. (May 1990) at 52.

2. In December of 1994, after Michaels won her appeal and earned a new trial, prosecutors formally dropped all charges against her. The county prosecutor stated the requirement that the reliability of the children's testimony be proven by clear and convincing evidence unduly burdened the case, especially given the young age of the children at the time, the age of the case, and the fact many of the children were no longer available to testify. If you were the prosecutor for a case such as this, and you had to speak with preschool or young school-aged children, what types of questions and interview techniques would you use? How would you decide whether to pursue the case?

3. What strategy should Michaels' defense attorney have used at trial? Note, for example, that a comparison of the interview transcripts in the *Michaels* case with a comparison group of Child Protection Service (CPS) interviews found the interviewers of Michaels' alleged victims were more likely to: introduce new suggestive and sexual information into the interview; provide praise, promises, and positive reinforcement for declarations of abuse; express that they disapproved of, disagreed with, or disbelieved denials of abuse; exert pressure to conform; and ask the children to "pretend or speculate about supposed events." Nadja Schreiber et al., *Suggestive Interviewing in the* McMartin *Preschool and* Kelly Michaels *Daycare Abuse Cases: A Case Study*, 1 Soc. Influence 16, 16 (2006).

4. Is there, in your view, any age that is categorically too young to provide witness or victim testimony? If so, according to what factors would you—if you could—structure the legal relationships between increasing age and testimony over time?

5. What if an adult victim recovers a memory from infancy and toddlerhood? Consider the approach adopted by New South Wales in Australia for applicants seeking compensation under the Victims Rights and Support Act. In *CDK v. Commissioner of Victims Rights*, the victim claimed to have recovered memories of ritualistic sexual abuse through therapy that began when she was nine months old and continued until she was twelve. The tribunal strictly applied the *Guidelines on Memory and the Law* (discussed earlier in this chapter), which cautioned that "[a]ll memories dating to the age of three years and below should be viewed with great caution and should not be accepted as memories without independent corroborating evidence." The tribunal, after hearing the victim's oral submissions, noted that while "[the victim] clearly believes that her memories . . . are accurate," the lack of both corroborating evidence and evidence from a memory expert for an event that occurred when she was "a very young child" simply didn't satisfy the *Guidelines*. Should the tribunal have considered the memories recovered from her later childhood years separately? *CDK v. Comm'r of Victims Rights* [2016] NSWCATAD 300 (Dec. 20, 2016) (Austl.).

6. In 2013 neuroscientists reported that they had been able to implant false memories in laboratory mice. Steve Ramirez et al., *Creating a False Memory in the Hippocampus*, 341 Science 387 (2013). Outside the lab, researchers have been able to implant false memories into adults. Suppose you were a member of the bar tasked with making recommendations about how the legal system could best confront the existence of implanted memories. How would you outline the challenges involved in this task?

   Should courts consider implementing systems to stimulate repressed or forgotten memories, particularly in cases from decades prior? What if the witness or victim objected to the intrusion? *See* Adam J. Kolber, *The Limited Right to Alter Memory*, 40 J. Med. Ethics 658 (2014) (arguing that the victim should have the choice in medication or limitations on memory, and that the prosecution should not be permitted to override those wishes to preserve the memories for purposes of testifying).

7. One study partnered fMRI with machine learning algorithms to train up an algorithm to distinguish between when a subject was viewing images from a camera that had been worn around her own neck (and had been taking photos automatically) and when that subject was seeing images from some other subject's

camera. Jesse Rissman et al., *Decoding fMRI Signatures of Real-World Autobiographical Memory Retrieval*, 28 J. Cognitive Neurosci. 604 (2016). The whole-brain multi-voxel pattern classifier achieved near-perfect accuracy at this task. The work has been extended to distinguish memories of personal experience from memories of second-hand descriptions, by others. Tiffany E. Chow, Andrew J. Westphal & Jesse Rissman, *Multi-voxel Pattern Classification Differentiates Personally Experienced Event Memories from Secondhand Event Knowledge*, 176 NeuroImage 110 (2018). And additional studies have connected false memories with fMRI scans and activity in the temporal pole region of the brain. Martin J. Chadwick, *Semantic Representations in the Temporal Pole Predict False Memories*, 113 Proc. Nat'l Acad. Sci. U.S. 10180 (2016). Given this progress, what possible legal implications do you see?

8. For legal proceedings that rely on a witness to recollect past events, the accuracy and reliability of that witness's memories are critical. But what if the witness, especially a victim, prefers to forget a painful memory? In the 2004 movie *Eternal Sunshine of the Spotless Mind* a fictional company called Lacuna, Inc. offers clients a procedure that can erase specific memories. The movie's main character seeks out the firm's services to erase memories of a past relationship. Although it is currently farfetched with respect to humans, researchers have reported progress in selectively eliminating specific memories in mice. *See* Emily Singer, *The Maestro of Memory Manipulation*, Quanta Mag. (June 23, 2016). Supposing the technique could someday be used in humans, do you see any circumstances in which the legal system should discourage the use of memory removal or memory-dampening? On these subjects, see Adam J. Kolber, *Therapeutic Forgetting: The Legal and Ethical Implications of Memory Dampening*, 59 Vand. L. Rev. 1561 (2006); and Katrina Hui & Carl E. Fisher, *The Ethics of Molecular Memory Modification*, 41 J. Med. Ethics 515 (2015).

   Note that as human brain science advances, the development of such procedures seems increasingly probable. Although scientists have not yet uncovered techniques to completely erase specific memories, several memory-modifying techniques have been described in research laboratories. The most successful techniques target memory reconsolidation by attempting to modify or disrupt the restorage of a memory after it has been initially encoded. Such modification has been observed through both pharmacological and behavioral intervention, though it is still largely unknown how to apply these techniques in clinical or legal settings. *See* Elizabeth A. Phelps & Stefan G. Hofmann, *Memory Editing from Science Fiction to Clinical Practice*, 572 Nature 43 (2019).

9. What if the defendant, rather than the victim, has no recollection of the event? Consider the Supreme Court case of *Madison v. Alabama*, in which the defendant, after sitting on death row for nearly 30 years, suffered from several strokes that left him with vascular dementia. He claimed to have no memory of his crime and argued that he was mentally incompetent for execution. Under the *Panetti v. Quarterman* standard the Court applied, the Eighth Amendment ban on cruel and unusual punishment prohibits an execution when the prisoner's mental illness leaves him incapable of reaching "a rational understanding of the reason for the execution." 551 U.S. 930, 958. In holding that it is possible for a prisoner with no memory of the crime to nevertheless rationally understand the reason to execute him, the Court wrote:

What matters is whether a person has the "rational understanding" *Panetti* requires—not whether he has any particular memory or any particular mental illness. . . . Do you recall your first day of school? Probably not. But if your mother told you years later that you were sent home for hitting a classmate, you would have no trouble grasping the story. And similarly, if you somehow blacked out a crime you committed, but later learned what you had done, you could well appreciate the State's desire to impose a penalty. Assuming, that is, no other cognitive impairment, loss of memory of a crime does not prevent rational understanding of the State's reasons for resorting to punishment. . . .

Madison v. Alabama, 139 S. Ct. 718, 727 (2019). In an amicus brief opposing the execution, the American Psychological Association and American Psychiatric Association stated that "execution serves no purposes . . . because madness is its own punishment." What purpose does this execution serve? Does it offend humanitarian principles to execute an elderly prisoner with dementia?

FURTHER READING

Attention and Memory Mechanisms:

Daniel J. Simons & Ronald A. Rensink, *Change Blindness: Past, Present, and Future*, 9 Trends Cognitive Sci. 16 (2005).

Howard Eichenbaum, *The Cognitive Neuroscience of Memory: An Introduction* (2d ed. 2011).

Eric R. Kandel, *In Search of Memory: The Emergence of a New Science of Mind* (2007).

Ueli Rutishauser, *Testing Models of Human Declarative Memory at the Single-Neuron Level*, 23 Trends Cognitive Sci. 510 (2019).

Forgetting and Emotional Arousal:

Tali Sharot et al., *How Personal Experience Modulates the Neural Circuitry of Memories of September 11*, 104 Proc. Nat'l Acad. Sci. U.S. 389 (2007).

Elizabeth A. Kensinger & Daniel L. Schacter, *When the Red Sox Shocked the Yankees: Comparing Negative and Positive Memories*, 13 Psychonomic Bull. & Rev. 757 (2006).

John T. Wixted, *The Psychology and Neuroscience of Forgetting*, 55 Ann. Rev. Psychol. 235 (2004).

Brian H. Bornstein & Timothy R. Robicheaux, *Methodological Issues in the Study of Eyewitness Memory and Arousal*, 42 Creighton L. Rev. 525 (2009).

Memory and Law:

Memory and Law (Lynn Nadel & Walter P. Sinnott-Armstrong eds., Oxford Univ. Press 2012).

Daniel L. Schacter & Elizabeth F. Loftus, *Memory and Law: What Can Cognitive Neuroscience Contribute?*, 16 Nature Neurosci. 119 (2013).

Joyce W. Lacy & Craig E.L. Stark, *The Neuroscience of Memory: Implications for the Courtroom*, 14 Nature Reviews Neurosci. 649 (2013).

Tanja Rapus Benton et al., *Eyewitness Memory Is Still Not Common Sense: Comparing Jurors, Judges and Law Enforcement to Eyewitness Experts*, 20 Applied Cognitive Psychol. 115 (2006).

Elin M. Skagerberg & Daniel B. Wright, *Manipulating Power Can Affect Memory Conformity*, 22 Applied Cognitive Psychol. 207 (2008).

U.S. Dep't of Justice, *Eyewitness Evidence: A Guide for Law Enforcement* (1999).

Nat'l Research Council, *Identifying the Culprit: Assessing Eyewitness Identification* (2014).

Mark L. Howe, Lauren M. Knott & Martin A. Conway, *Memory and Miscarriages of Justice* (2018).

Elizabeth F. Loftus, *Eyewitness Science and the Legal System*, 14 Ann. Rev. L. & Soc. Sci. 1 (2018).

False Memories:

Elizabeth F. Loftus, *Planting Misinformation in the Human Mind: A 30-Year Investigation of the Malleability of Memory*, 12 Learning & Memory 361 (2005).

CHAPTER **14**

Emotions

Detached reflection cannot be demanded in the presence of an uplifted knife.
　　　　　—Justice Oliver Wendell Holmes, *Brown v. United States*
　　　　　　　　　　　　　　　　　　(writing for the majority)[†]

My dear fellow—let's not forget that small emotions are the great captains of our lives, and that these we obey without knowing it.
　　　　　—Vincent van Gogh[††]

CHAPTER SUMMARY

This chapter:

- Introduces neuroscientific perspectives on emotion.
- Explores criminal and civil contexts in which emotions play important roles, and considers the extent to which the influence of emotions can or should be regulated.
- Examines the roles of emotions in defendants, jurors, judges, and legislators.

INTRODUCTION

James Thornton, a law student, found his estranged wife, Lavinia, having sex in their home with a man named Mark McConkey, whom he shot. Within two weeks, McConkey had died of complications from his wound, leading to Thornton's conviction for first degree murder. On appeal, the Tennessee Supreme Court set aside the murder conviction and remanded the case with instructions to sentence Thornton for voluntary manslaughter. It reasoned as follows:

> Appellant actually discovered his wife *in flagrante delicto* with a man who was a total stranger to him, and at a time when appellant was trying to save his marriage and was deeply concerned about both his wife and his young child. He did not fire a shot or in any way harm the victim until he actually discovered the victim and his wife engaged in sexual intercourse in appellant's own home. In our opinion the passions of any reasonable person would have been inflamed and intensely aroused by this sort of discovery, given the factual background of this case. Even though he was not legally insane so as to relieve him of all criminal responsibility for the tragic death which occurred, in our opinion this was a classic case of voluntary manslaughter and no more. . . .

　[†] *Brown v. United States*, 256 U.S. 335, 343 (1921).
　[††] Letter from Vincent van Gogh to Theo van Gogh (July 14 or 15, 1889), *in Ever Yours: The Essential Letters* 683 (Hans Luijten, Leo Jansen & Nienke Bakker eds., 2014).

State v. Thornton, 730 S.W.2d 309, 315 (Tenn. 1987). This case, involving so-called "heat of passion," illustrates the complicated—even tumultuous—relationship between human emotions and law. As you are undoubtedly aware, emotions are powerful and imperfectly controllable aspects of every person's experience—despite the pride we as a species take in our capacities for cool contemplation, analysis, and decisions. Throughout history, emotions have often been viewed as clouding sound judgment, the antithesis of rationality. On the other hand, evolutionary biologists consider emotions and analytic deliberation to be but two different evolved pathways to reaching context-appropriate actions. What we call "emotions" are, from this perspective, evolved and speedy shortcuts to actions that, on average, led their bearers in ancestral conditions to better survival outcomes and to greater reproductive success. As you'll see below, neuroscientists (whose perspectives focus on the biophysical processes that mediate the brain's evolved capabilities) are uncovering neural circuits—some more distinct, some more broadly integrated—that underlie human emotions.

In this chapter we explore some of the many intersections of law and emotion, repeatedly asking whether—and if so, how—the emerging neuroscientific understandings of emotion can or should influence the legal system's approaches. The chapter proceeds in five sections. Section A provides some background on the neuroscientific perspectives on emotions. Section B considers law's encounters with defendants' emotions, through the lens of heat of passion cases. Sections C, D, and E consider the roles of emotions in jurors, judges, and legislators, respectively.

A. THE EMOTIONAL BRAIN

From the perspective of behavioral biology, the brain is an information processor that evolutionary processes, including *natural selection*,* have left far better at solving certain kinds of problems than others. Some evolved capacities, such as our ability to self-consciously analyze options, are quite deliberative. Other evolved capacities are less deliberative pathways to action. From this perspective, what we call "emotions" are body states that, on average, led to adaptive behavior for our ancestors in the environments they faced. That is, emotions increased the probability that certain kinds of stimuli (e.g., a large predator) would very reliably elicit certain categories of response (e.g., high physical alert and running away) instead of other possible responses (e.g., nap-taking or continued foraging).

Emotions are not recent products of human culture, although culture both reflects human emotions and reciprocally affects how and when we express and act on them. Emotions are part of our evolutionary heritage. It is important to add, however, that we should not automatically privilege (or automatically devalue) emotions based on that fact alone. Every emotion reflects the internal state of an evolved

---

* There is more to this than can be covered here. But the core thing you should know is that natural selection is the inevitable result of any system combining three factors: (1) replication; (2) variation, however slight, during replication; and (3) differential replication as a consequence of variation. Put another way, the variations in an organism's genes that increase that organism's chances of survival and reproduction (compared to the chances of other contemporaneously living organisms of that species) are preserved and multiplied from generation to generation, at the expense of less advantageous variations. The ongoing results of this process tend to yield organisms that are, on average, better adapted to thriving in the environments their ancestors inhabited.

nervous system. And emotions can be understood as mechanisms that set and aid pursuit of our brain's most basic goals.

It is important to remember that people living today are roughly 37,000 times further from their first primate ancestor than they are from the year 1 A.D. Our ancestors were primates for approximately 45 million years before they began to diverge into what later became gorillas, orangutans, chimpanzees, bonobos, and early hominids. Creatures that you would recognize as *Homo sapiens* like you have been present during only the last 100,000 years (i.e., less than two hundredths of our history as primates). Throughout that long time our pre-sentient ancestors were motivated by the same impulses that most powerfully motivate us today. These impulses determined when, where, and what to approach or avoid, to persist or retreat.

Think, for example, of these basic perceptions, impulses, and desires: thirst (to satisfy bodily fluid balance), hunger (to obtain necessary nutrition), fatigue (to rest), disgust (to avoid fluids and substances that would make you sick), pain (to alert to damaged bodily tissue), fear (to avoid dangerous actors and threatening situations), anger (to react aggressively to dangerous actors or threatening situations), motivation (to continue a rewarding action or avoid an unrewarding action), disappointment (to recognize less than expected reward), frustration (to change unrewarding behaviors), regret (to appreciate the value of alternative actions), sexual desire (to procreate).

All animals survive only by and through the appropriate expression of these basic emotions. While social creatures like us necessarily express these basic emotions, other kinds or levels of emotions are also expressed. These include despair, grief, and sadness (soliciting affection when expected reward is not obtained or may no longer be obtained), rumination and worry (soliciting compassion when pain or threat is expected), greed (soliciting contribution to avoid or prevent inequity), happiness or joy (soliciting affiliation when pain ceases, threat is removed, bad situation ends, or good situation begins), affection or love (soliciting companionship with family and extended group). Some impulses are complex combinations of the foregoing. Jealousy, for example, combines affection, greed, and rumination.

Having said that, the concept and scientific formulation of emotions remains less certain than many other terms and concepts in human experience. The word "emotion" entered the English language only in the early 17th century through translation of a French philosophical manuscript, denoting a physical disturbance and bodily movement. In the 18th century the term "emotion" referred to the mental feelings accompanying bodily stirrings or to the body movements associated with passions and affections. In the 19th century the term began to refer more to the internal state causing the observed body movement, like the grimace or the smile.*

Although many different views remain, concerning the categories, origins, and relations of emotions,** there are signs of increasing consensus. For instance, a recent survey assessed the amount of agreement among a sample of 150 scientists.*** When asked which emotion labels can be considered empirically established, they agreed about anger, fear, disgust, sadness, and happiness. Half

---

* Thomas Dixon, *"Emotion": The History of a Keyword in Crisis*, 4 Emotion Rev. 338, 340 (2012).
** *See, e.g.,* Julie Beck, *Hard Feelings: Science's Struggle to Define Emotions*, The Atlantic (Feb. 24, 2015).
*** Paul Ekman, *What Scientists Who Study Emotion Agree About*, 11 Persps. on Psychol. Sci. 31 (2016).

agreed about embarrassment, shame, and surprise. One-third agreed about awe, contempt, envy, guilt, love, and pain. And only 5-10% agreed about compassion, gratitude, and pride. Still, that level of agreement far exceeds the amount measured in a similar survey in 1994.

In spite of areas of scientific uncertainty, we all know that emotions fundamentally and unavoidably energize life and are not fully optional. What implications might this have in the legal arena?

In this chapter we explore this question in five sections. Section A provides some background on psychological and neuroscientific perspectives on emotions. Section B considers law's encounters with defendants' emotions, through the lens of heat-of-passion cases. Sections C, D, and E consider the roles of emotions in jurors, judges, and legislators respectively.

Eric A. Posner
Law and the Emotions
89 Geo. L.J. 1977, 1979-83 (2001)

THE EMOTIONS

Although psychology lacks a widely accepted theory of emotion and many fundamental issues about the nature of emotion remain unresolved, much progress has been made in the last thirty years, and agreement on some important issues has been achieved. An emotion is a psychological phenomenon with the following distinctive characteristics: Emotions are usually stimulated by the world, either via the mediation of cognition or through a more primitive stimulus-response-like neurological mechanism. They have a certain feel or affect characterized, usually, by a focus on a particular stimulus with the result that the rest of the environment "fades" (a little or a lot, depending on the strength of the emotion) though does not disappear altogether. An angry person feels a kind of warmth and agitation, which is directed usually at another person, the result of a slight or offense. A person who is disgusted feels a kind of nausea, which is directed at the object that provokes the disgust. The rest of the world remains, but at a remove: An angry person might restrain himself because he does not want to be arrested for assault; a disgusted person might overcome the urge to withdraw because he wants to help a person with a disgusting wound or he knows that the disgusting substance is medicine. Although emotions are usually accompanied by physiological changes, there does not appear to be a one-to-one correspondence between the different emotions and physiological states; emotion has an irreducibly mental component. . . .

From a normative perspective, the bare fact that a person has acted under the influence of emotion does not excuse his conduct. In fact, while some emotions mitigate guilt, others enhance guilt. Anger provoked by betrayal mitigates guilt, but anger provoked by unacceptable moral beliefs may increase guilt. Hate rarely excuses murder, but real fear, even if not fully justified, might mitigate culpability.

Both of these observations assume that people remain rational while under the influence of emotion; emotion is rarely a mere reflex to some external stimulus. An angry, disgusted, fearful, or sad person usually can deliberate about his behavior and does not (with the possible exception of certain kinds of fear) engage in reflexive action. This suggests that people continue to act rationally while in an emotion state, even though they act differently from the way they do in the calm state. One can capture this point by positing that during the emotion state people experience temporary variations in their preferences, abilities, and beliefs.

Their preferences change so that what psychologists call the "action tendency" of an emotion becomes relatively attractive. The action tendency of anger is to strike out. We can say that a person, while angry, develops a temporary preference to strike the person who offends him. The action tendency of disgust is to withdraw. A person, while disgusted, develops a temporary preference to withdraw from the disgusting object. Grief produces withdrawal from other people and preoccupation with the lost person or thing; fear produces flight from a threat; pity produces aid. But before—and usually after—the emotion state, the person's preferences are constant (the "calm preferences"), so he might disapprove of what he expects to do, or did, in the emotion state. It is this inconsistency over time that makes emotional behavior seem irrational, but it is important to see that a person in an emotion state does not act irrationally given his temporary preferences.

Abilities may also change in the grip of an emotion. When the emotion state occurs, the agent may find himself more alert and vigorous, perhaps stronger, or simply less reliant on slow-moving deliberation. The angry person is aroused; he feels less pain, tires less quickly, responds more rapidly to movement. The anxious or fearful person becomes more alert to the environment and flees quickly from danger. A grief-stricken person may experience a decline in abilities; everything becomes more difficult to do. Evidence of physiological changes—hormonal changes, increase in the heart rate, and so forth—supports the view that abilities change during some emotion states.

Finally, beliefs may change during emotion states. An angry person overestimates the probability that the offender will attack him, or that the provocation was not an accident but the result of intent to harm or humiliate. A fearful person overestimates the probability of harm associated with the threat that causes his fear. Joyful people underestimate risks of harm, while pessimistic people overestimate the same risks.

Thus, my claim is that during the emotion state, a person acts rationally, that is, internally consistently, given the new and usually temporary preferences, abilities, and beliefs that the person has in that emotion state. The actions taken during the emotion state will, of course, affect the agent's endowments, and this may have consequences for the person's behavior after the emotion state is over. Aside from that, I assume that preferences, abilities, and emotions during the calm state are the same before and after the emotion state.

My final point is that agents anticipate their emotion states and take actions in anticipation of them. "Emotional disposition" refers to a person's tendency to feel an emotion. An irascible person is more likely to become angry; a fearful person is more likely to become scared. People usually know their emotional dispositions and can take steps to modify them or to avoid conditions that activate them. Suppose, for example, that a person knows that if he goes to a rowdy bar, he may be insulted, and further he knows that he is irascible. Upon being insulted, he might strike the person who insulted him. To avoid this, he can (1) knowing about his emotional disposition avoid the bar, or (2) earlier on try to overcome his irascibility through meditation or other behavior modification techniques.

One can unify these ideas about the emotions using the metaphor of emotional capacities as information-processing mechanisms. To understand this metaphor, consider the instinctive withdrawal of the hand from a hot surface. One does not deliberate before withdrawing the hand; one just does it. Yet it is possible to resist the impulse and sometimes desirable to do so — for example, in order to withdraw a valuable object from a fire. Evolution explains the instinct as a cognitive shortcut; on average, the individual does better by withdrawing quickly than by deliberating, but in certain cases it is better not to withdraw. There is a kind of psychological compromise. The pain drives the individual to withdraw, but with special effort he can overcome the pain and engage in the desirable action. On average, the individual submits to the pain and withdraws; in special circumstances, he resists the pain.

So with emotions. The best response to a stimulus may be rapid reaction even before enough information is available to make a correct decision. On average, fleeing from a tiger, withdrawing from a smelly substance, striking someone who insults you, and so forth, may be the best thing to do; but in particular cases it may be better to resist the emotional reaction. By supplying the optimal average reaction, the emotional capacities economize on information-processing, but sometimes produce outcomes different from those that would be chosen if there were enough time to deliberate. When a person deliberates in a calm state, he is less likely to deviate from his optimal behavior, but he will spend more time before making the choice. The affect accompanying the emotion — the sense of fear, of nausea — must be overcome as a pain must be overcome, and it will be overcome only when the offsetting considerations are significant.

Emotional capacities in humans evolved in a primitive environment and so are not always attuned to modern needs. But individuals (and their parents) "invest" in these assets in order to bring them closer in line with the requirements of modern living. That means being able to avoid being angered by stimuli when anger will lead to retaliation, jail, or other injuries, or being able to control one's anger after it is stimulated. It means being able to control pity or greed when they are stimulated by conditions for which these emotions are unsuited. The con man exploits these emotions and is particularly successful with businessmen who are alone in strange cities, without friends or associates to reason with them. The doctor, servant, and soldier invest in different kinds of thick skin: the doctor, against disgust; the servant, against envy; and the soldier, against fear. Those who make good investments obtain high returns in their interactions with other people.

The metaphor of emotional capacity as information-processing mechanism helps one see that emotional capacities are a form of human capital, and thus appropriate objects for legal concern. . . .

Paul Gewirtz
On "I Know It When I See It"
105 Yale L.J. 1023, 1029-36 (1996)

All too often judges and scholars who write about law assert an inappropriately sharp distinction between the rational and the nonrational, especially between reason and emotion — invoking an overly narrow concept of reason and contrasting reason and emotion in an overly simplified manner. These discussions usually arise in the context of a traditional normative argument that judging is a realm of reason, not emotion. Thus, to characterize some judicial or jury behavior as not "reason" but "emotion" is to say it is illegitimate. The Supreme Court, for example, has often said that the decision whether to impose the death penalty must turn on a "reasoned moral response . . . and not an emotional response." This has led the Court to conclude that feelings of "sympathy" have no place in the decision whether or not to impose the death penalty. Until recently, it led the Court to hold victim-impact evidence inadmissible at capital sentencing because of its tendency to produce an emotional, rather than reasoned, response. In each case, I think, the Supreme Court has been led astray by not recognizing the relevance of what it calls an "emotional response," largely because it does not appreciate how compassion, mercy, and sympathy for both defendants and victims can be elements of a rational punishment decision.

The glib distinction between "reasoned" and "emotional" responses is far too simplistic. At least since Plato, philosophers have recognized that emotions come in many varieties: Some are like physical drives, such as hunger, and others are closely related to what we usually call rationality. More recently, a chorus of scholars from fields as diverse as philosophy, psychology, and neurobiology has demonstrated that emotions have a cognitive dimension, are connected to beliefs, and can promote, illuminate, and convey understanding in many ways. In contrast to anti-Enlightenment critiques from Nietzsche onward which have insisted that behind the face of reason there is only raw power, these recent post-Enlightenment critiques have insisted that behind the face of reason — indeed, constitutive of reason itself — may be some familiar emotions.

What we typically call reason and emotion are interrelated in a variety of complex ways. For example, emotions can open up ways of knowing and seeing, and thereby contribute to reasoning. Fear and caring, to illustrate, can make us more attentive to facts; sympathy may be part of properly assessing mitigating evidence in capital sentencing. Indeed, rational beliefs themselves both shape, and are modifiable by, emotion. For example, fear can be reduced by changing our beliefs; our general views about gay people can be changed by empathy we come to feel toward a gay relative. Moreover, emotions — grief, for example — can reveal beliefs that conscious thought conceals. And emotions are often essential to the completion of a rational response. . . . Alas, these ideas have barely made any inroads into the world of law, which, for the most part, has remained comfortable with the easy dichotomy of reason and emotion.

Just as reason is often inseparable from emotion, judgments should not be deemed outside of reason and rationality just because they are automatic or hard to explain. Many important and unimportant things in life we know without ongoing reflection, and without necessarily being able to explain why we believe them. . . .

Consider just a few nonrational aspects of the self that are defining qualities of excellence in a judge: imagination; judgment; courage; compassion; good sense; energy; calmness; open-mindedness; the capacity to listen; eloquence. . . . [T]hese nonrational aspects of mind have long been seen as vital to the activity of judging. . . .

Another valuable role of nonrational elements is that they can *constrain* judges. We tend to think of the nonrational as what breaks through the restraints of judicial role, but the nonrational can itself constrain. The central insight here belongs to the greatest of the legal realists, Karl Llewellyn. The traditional account of judging sees constraint (and, therefore, judicial authority) as coming from preexisting legal rules and the disciplining force of reason. The legal realists and their heirs did much to undermine this conventional account of constraint, demonstrating the many indeterminacies of legal rules, precedent, and conventional modes of judicial argument. . . . For Llewellyn, the most important constraint was not conventional legal reasoning at all, but rather what he called the "operating technique" of judges—a judge's feel, his habits, "the trained, tradition-determined manner of handling [legal] material," "practice, not norm; way of acting, not verbal formula." Judicial "intuition," Llewellyn said, allows judges to reach generally correct results, "even when their ability to fashion legal grounds for their decisions has lagged behind." These constraining factors, Llewellyn said, may operate "unconsciously."

In the field of constitutional law, which Llewellyn rarely wrote about, one nonrational constraint on judges is quite different. . . . [O]ne element that helps to accommodate judicial review and democratic values is a feeling and attitude—a judge's feeling of *humility*, an internalized sense that he is not the sole repository of constitutional truth, an attitude of restraint that is an aspect of temperament. . . .

[I]n affirming a place for emotion, I readily acknowledge that certain emotions must be excluded altogether. Prejudice, for example, totally undercuts the ideal of impartiality that is a necessary predicate for the legitimate exercise of judicial power. But other emotions—sympathy or courage, for example—can *promote* impartiality. (Indeed, the sympathetic capacity to see and feel a situation from many sides in a legal dispute comes close to *defining* the capacity to be impartial.) Put more generally, although some nonrational elements may be inconsistent with legal ideals, others—emotions and intuitions of certain types, imagination, judgment, rhetorical persuasiveness—are fully consistent with those ideals. Some emotions can be unreliable, just as reasons can be. Emotions can pull judges toward a greater preoccupation with particular individuals and their individual stories—particulars that may not be typical and that may therefore distort understanding—just as reasons can pull understanding toward generalities that may conceal particularity and diversity. Emotions, like reasons, can lead in multiple directions and create problems of indeterminacy. Emotions may open the way to understanding only partially and may need the competing insights and discipline of rational reflection—but likewise, reason may be incomplete without emotion. All of this means that emotional responses must be openly tested by deliberation and reasoned examination, and vice versa. The courthouse setting facilitates the testing, however, for courtroom procedures establish an enormous range of opportunities for reasoned exchange among lawyers, judges, and juries. . . .

But what are emotions, anyway, from a neuroscientific (proximate causation) perspective? We all experience emotions, but emotions are more than experiences; they are physiological processes arising from various brain processes. Neuroscience has not provided much insight about the first-person experience of emotion, but it has gained great understanding about the brain circuits producing the various overt expressions of emotion. Emotions are expressed through particular physiological changes, such as changes of heart rate, blood flow, sweating, and gastrointestinal motility that are mediated through the sympathetic (fight/flight/freeze) and parasympathetic (rest/repair) circuits of the autonomic nervous system. Emotions are also expressed through body movements, like approaching or avoiding objects in the environment, and also through facial expressions. Our bodies are under two sources of control, one automatic and fast (emotional), the other deliberate and slow (voluntary). Different brain pathways mediate these two sources of control.

The hypothalamus is crucial for coordination of both the visceral and body movement aspects of emotion. Electrical stimulation of different parts of the hypothalamus elicits violent attacks or fearful cowering. The cerebral cortex is necessary for the experience of emotion, but the behavioral manifestations can be accomplished with only subcortical structures. The hypothalamus influences visceral and body movements through connections with the *reticular formation*, a web of neurons in the brainstem consisting of several cell groups that control basic functions such as heartbeat, respiration, urination, swallowing, and vomiting.

The reticular formation of the brainstem is also influenced by a collection of structures in the brain, known collectively as the limbic system, which are also responsible for the expression of emotional responses. The name limbic system refers to the arrangement of these structures encircling the corpus callosum and thalamus. An early description of the limbic system consisted of the *cingulate gyrus*, which receives inputs indirectly from the hypothalamus and sends outputs to the hippocampus. Completing the circle, the hippocampus sends axons to the hypothalamus. Through this circuit it was believed that the forebrain could control emotions.

Subsequently, other structures were recognized as part of the limbic system. These include orbital and medial frontal cortex and ventral regions of the basal ganglia. Increased blood flow and oxygen utilization occurs in these brain regions when experimental participants experience emotions.

The amygdala, buried in the rostral end of the temporal lobe anterior to the hippocampus, is another key node in the limbic system. The amygdala is actually a collection of at least three distinct groups of neurons with different inputs and outputs. The differences in function can be assessed through studying the effects of electrical stimulation. The amygdala receives inputs from high-level sensory and cognitive cortical areas and sends signals to communicate the emotional significance of stimuli to the hypothalamus. If the amygdala is damaged, one symptom is abnormally reduced expression of emotions such as fear, because the significance of objects is not appreciated. The amygdala is responsible for investing sensory experience with emotional significance—for example, the frozen fear when seeing a snake or spider. The amygdala is necessary for learning associations between stimuli and appropriate emotional responses. Mood disorders such as depression and anxiety are associated with abnormal blood flow in the amygdala as well as orbital and medial prefrontal cortex. Based on such research, an experimental treatment for major depression has been developed that involves electrical stimulation of the medial frontal cortex and ventral basal ganglia.

Whereas emotional expression by animals is usually rather stereotyped, emotional expression by humans varies widely according to context and culture. Such variation arises from connections of different areas of the cerebral cortex with the amygdala and other limbic structures. The circuits through the amygdala are thought to influence the choice of behaviors to obtain rewards and avoid punishments. Damage to cortical regions influencing the amygdala (as in the case of Phineas Gage) can lead to poor decision-making.

In humans, the two halves of the brain play somewhat different roles in emotional expression. This has been found through EEG, fMRI, and brain damage studies. The right hemisphere is generally more important for expressing emotion and comprehending emotions in others. Also, the left hemisphere seems more involved in the experience of positive emotions, while the right is more involved for negative emotions.

More sophisticated methods of analyzing complex patterns in brain imaging data have offered new insights.* Different categories of experienced emotion are represented differently in the activity of distributed cortical and subcortical neural systems.

NOTES AND QUESTIONS

1. On what bases—empirical, normative, or otherwise—do we, can we, and should we determine which emotions are or are not legally relevant? Surely, understanding how the brain enables an emotion ought to be relevant. For example, expressions of regret are considered relevant in assessing culpability. Expressions of regret have been the focus of neuroscientific investigation.** They have been characterized as recognition that an option taken resulted in a worse outcome than an alternative option would have. During experimental testing, upon encountering a less rewarding outcome, even rats pause and orient toward the option not taken. Research has demonstrated the contribution of orbital frontal cortex for expressions of regret. For example, neural impulse rates in orbitofrontal cortex of rats indicating regret modulate according to the previous rather than the current earned reward. To what extent do you think the neuroscience of regret could inform law's own orientation toward the emotion?

2. Emotions are obviously influenced by culture and experience. Yet scientists believe the fundamentals of emotion reflect evolved behavioral adaptations to deep ancestral conditions. How does this biological perspective on emotions affect the way you think about them? Under what circumstances, if any, should it affect the way that law treats them? And if emotions evolved in large measure as important adaptations to ancestral environments, what can we anticipate may happen when the human social environment changes as rapidly as it has? *See* Owen D. Jones, *Time-Shifted Rationality and the Law of Law's Leverage: Behavioral Economics Meets Behavioral Biology*, 95 Nw. U. L. Rev. 1141 (2001).

3. Even today, challenges in defining emotion remain. For instance, one neuroscientist observes:

> If we don't have an agreed-upon definition of emotion that allows us to say what emotion is, and how emotion differs from other psychological states, how can we study emotion in animals or humans, and how can we make comparisons between species?
>
> The short answer is that we fake it. Introspections from personal subjective experiences tell us that some mental states have a certain "feeling" associated with

---

* Philip A. Kragel & Kevin S. LaBar, *Decoding the Nature of Emotion in the Brain*, 20 Trends Cogn. Sci. 444 (2016).

** Adam P. Steiner & A. David Redish, *Behavioral and Neurophysiological Correlates of Regret in Rat Decision-Making on a Neuroeconomic Task*, 17 Nature Neurosci. 995 (2014).

them and others do not. Those states that humans associate with feelings are often called emotions. The terms "emotion" and "feeling" are, in fact, often used inter-changeably. In English we have words like fear, anger, love, sadness, jealousy, and so on, for these feeling states, and when scientists study emotions in humans they typically use these "feeling words" as guideposts to explore the terrain of emotion. . . .

Joseph LeDoux, *Rethinking the Emotional Brain*, 73 Neuron 653, 653 (2012). How would you distinguish between the concepts of "emotion" and "feeling"?

B. THE EMOTIONAL DEFENDANT

The criminal justice system has long parsed culpable mental states to separate acts of malicious intent from accidents. For instance, in the majority of states that follow the Model Penal Code, punishable acts are those accompanied by purpose, knowledge, recklessness, or negligence. But how, exactly, do the roiling storms of emotion—whether anger, fear, lust, or the like—affect law's judgments about behavior? Everyone experiences these emotions, but what if some people are, through no fault of their own, more susceptible to the influence of their emotions than others? Or what if a person of average susceptibility encounters a highly unusual circumstance that, if encountered by another person, would have probably yielded a similar result? How can we hold people accountable for their behaviors while at the same time acknowledging that the behaviors, though regrettable, might have been powerfully difficult to avoid under the circumstances? Should we treat some emotions differently than others? If so, on what grounds?

Consider, for example, the use of the phrase "very properly" in this court's reasoning about a husband's killing of his wife's lover. On what foundations might it be supported?

> But if the act of killing, though intentional, be committed under the influence of passion or in heat of blood, produced by an adequate or reasonable provocation, and before a reasonable time has elapsed for the blood to cool and reason to resume its habitual control, and is the result of the temporary excitement, by which the control of reason was disturbed, rather than of any wickedness of heart or cruelty or reckless-ness of disposition; then the law, out of indulgence to the frailty of human nature, or rather, in recognition of the laws upon which human nature is constituted, very properly regards the offense as of a less heinous character than murder, and gives it the designation of manslaughter. . . .

Maher v. People, 10 Mich. 212, 219 (1862). The next two cases contrast different perspectives on what constitutes "heat" in passion. The first excerpt is from the case mentioned in the opening of this chapter, which involved the murder conviction of law student James Clark Thornton, III.

State v. Thornton
730 S.W.2d 309 (Tenn. 1987)

[Thornton was convicted of murder in the first degree, after the jury rejected his affirmative defenses of insanity and self-defense. The Court of Criminal Appeals affirmed, and Thornton appealed to the Tennessee Supreme Court. —EDS.]

HARBISON, J. Appellant was convicted of murder in the first degree as a result of shooting his wife's paramour in the home of appellant and his wife on May 3, 1983. Appellant found his wife and the victim, Mark McConkey, engaged in sexual relations in the front bedroom of appellant's home. He fired a single shot which struck McConkey in the left hip. The victim died sixteen days later as a result of a massive infection resulting from the bullet wound. Before the night in question appellant had never been acquainted with McConkey or had any previous contact with him. . . .

Under these undisputed facts, in our opinion, the case does not warrant a conviction of homicide greater than that of voluntary manslaughter. The charges accordingly will be reduced to that offense, and the cause will be remanded to the trial court for sentencing and disposition on that basis.

In several previous decisions from this Court and in the almost unanimous course of judicial authority from other states, the encountering by a spouse of the situation which occurred here has been held, as a matter of law, to constitute sufficient provocation to reduce a charge of homicide from one of the degrees of murder to manslaughter absent actual malice, such as a previous grudge, revenge, or the like. . . .

A. THE FACTUAL BACKGROUND

As previously stated, there is almost no dispute as to the material facts in this case. Appellant, James Clark Thornton, III, was thirty-one years of age at the time of the trial of this case in June 1984. His wife, Lavinia, was twenty-seven years of age; they had been married on May 19, 1979, and at the time of the homicide had one child, a son about three years of age. . . .

The marriage of the parties was in some difficulty, apparently as a result of dissatisfaction of Mrs. Thornton. She had advised her husband in March 1983 that she wanted to be separated from him for a time, and he had voluntarily taken an apartment about two miles away from their home. He visited the home almost daily, however, and there has been no suggestion that he was ever guilty of violence, physical misconduct or mistreatment toward his wife or son. . . .

Mrs. Thornton testified that she told McConkey when she first met him that she was married but separated from her husband. She had consulted an attorney and had signed a divorce petition, but the same apparently had not been filed on the date of the homicide. . . .

The record indicates that as early as May 1, two days before the homicide, Mrs. Thornton had stated to her husband that she did not think that the parties would ever be reconciled. On the evening of May 3, appellant picked her and their child up at their home, and the three went to dinner. Again on that occasion Mrs. Thornton reiterated that she thought that the marriage was over, and on this occasion she told appellant that she planned to date someone else whom she had met. . . .

[A]ppellant returned to the home of the parties in his automobile, stating that he wanted to try once more to convince his wife that he was indeed sincere. When he arrived at the home he saw an automobile parked in the driveway. He did not recognize the car as being one belonging to any of his wife's friends. Accordingly he parked around the corner and walked back to the house. Observing from the rear of the house, he saw his wife and McConkey in the kitchen with the child. He observed as Mrs. Thornton washed some laundry for McConkey and as they were eating dinner. Thereafter they sat and read. They drank wine and smoked some marijuana, and appellant saw them kissing.

He decided to go home to get his camera, but before doing so he let the air out of one of the tires on McConkey's car. He went to his apartment, and obtained his camera and an old pistol which had belonged to his father. . . .

Appellant spent more than an hour in the backyard of his home observing his wife and McConkey in the den and kitchen. Thereafter they left the den area, but appellant remained behind the house, thinking that McConkey was about to leave. When he went around the house, however, he found that McConkey's car was still in the driveway and saw the drapes in the front guest bedroom downstairs had been closed. He listened near the window and heard unmistakable sounds of sexual intercourse. He then burst through the front door and into the bedroom where he found the nude couple and attempted to take some pictures. At that point he testified that he thought McConkey was attempting to attack him. In all events he drew his pistol and fired a single shot, striking McConkey in the left hip. Appellant did not harm either his wife or child, although Mrs. Thornton said that he did make some threats against her. He went upstairs and brought down the little boy, who had been awakened and who was crying. He assisted in giving directions to enable an ambulance to bring aid to McConkey, and he remained at the house until the police arrived.

Appellant testified that he simply lost control and "exploded" when he found his wife in bed with the victim. He testified that he had armed himself because McConkey was much larger than he, and he felt that he needed protection if there was trouble when he returned to the residence with the camera.

Appellant testified that he did not intend to kill McConkey, but simply to shoot him in order to disable him and also because of his outrage at the situation which he had found. The single shot was not aimed at a vital organ, but the victim ultimately died because of the spread of a massive infection from the wound. . . .

B. THE LEGAL ISSUES

. . . [I]t has long been a well-settled legal principle that the commission of unlawful sexual intercourse with a female relative is an act obviously calculated to arouse ungovernable passion, and that the killing of the seducer or adulterer under the influence or in the heat of that passion constitutes voluntary manslaughter, and not murder, in the absence of evidence of actual malice.

One of the leading cases in this jurisdiction is *Toler v. State*, 152 Tenn. 1 (1924). There the defendant learned during a noon hour that on a previous occasion the victim had seduced his teenage daughter and had attempted to molest his nine-year-old daughter. The defendant immediately armed himself, walked a quarter of a mile to a field in which the unarmed victim was working, and shot him several times, killing him instantly. . . .

The Court pointed out that if there had been sufficient time for the passion or emotion of the defendant to cool before the shooting, then a verdict of murder might be sustained. It found no such time in that case, nor, in our opinion, was there any such showing in the present case. . . .

The facts of the present case are far stronger than any of the foregoing. Appellant actually discovered his wife *in flagrante delicto* with a man who was a total stranger to him, and at a time when appellant was trying to save his marriage and was deeply concerned about both his wife and his young child. He did not fire a shot or in any way harm the victim until he actually discovered the victim and his wife engaged in sexual intercourse in appellant's own home. In our opinion the passions of any reasonable person would have been inflamed and intensely aroused by this sort of discovery, given the factual background of this case. Even though he was not legally insane as to relieve him of all criminal responsibility for the tragic death which occurred, in our opinion this was a classic case of voluntary manslaughter and no more. . . .

[The Court set aside the conviction of murder in the first degree and remanded for sentencing for voluntary manslaughter. He was resentenced to 4 years for voluntary manslaughter, and was released for time already served. — EDS]

State v. Quick

659 N.W.2d 701 (Minn. 2003)

ANDERSON, J. Appellant Jon Earl Quick was convicted in Norman County of the premeditated first-degree murder of Justin Mueller. Mueller was the boyfriend of Quick's estranged wife. On appeal, Quick seeks to have his conviction reduced to first-degree manslaughter, asserting that the state failed to prove beyond a reasonable doubt that he did not act in the heat of passion at the time of the shooting. . . .

Jon and Diane Quick were married on July 2, 1994, and less than a year later, moved to Ada, Minnesota. They had two children together and Diane had a child from a previous relationship. In May 2000, Diane told Jon she wanted a separation and in early June, Jon moved out of the family home. Jon then moved in with his cousin in Felton, Minnesota, approximately 15 miles from Ada. . . . Despite Jon's efforts at reconciliation, Diane filed for dissolution of the marriage on June 15, 2000. . . .

Two months after Jon moved out, Diane began dating Justin Mueller, a good friend of her brother. Diane and Mueller's relationship soon became serious and Mueller was at Diane's home virtually every day. At some point, Jon became aware that Diane and Mueller were spending a considerable amount of time together, but he contends he was not aware of the seriousness of their relationship. [On several occasions, Jon sent notes and emails to Diane berating her and threatening Mueller.] . . .

On the evening of September 14, Diane had friends, including Mueller, over to play cards. . . . [Jon] called Diane and learned that she had some friends over. He asked Diane who was at the house, but she refused to tell him. Soon after the call, the remaining card players left, leaving only Diane and Mueller to clean up before going upstairs to bed together. . . .

[Jon] called Mueller's residence to see if Mueller was home, but no one answered the phone. He then decided to drive to Ada.

Upon arriving in Ada, Jon drove around the block by Diane's home and saw that Mueller's car was parked in her driveway. Jon observed a neighbor in the neighbor's backyard and drove around the block a second time because he did not want anyone to know that he was there. He then parked in Diane's driveway and saw that all the lights were off in the house. He took the loaded .22 rifle, which was still in its case, from the back seat of his car and approached the house. Jon testified that at this point he wanted to scare and humiliate Mueller and planned to take Mueller four or five miles out of town and make him walk back.

Jon tried to enter the house through the back door, but it was locked. He next tried a basement window and was able to gain entrance. He then climbed the stairs to the first floor, unlocked the back door, took off his shoes, and took the rifle out of the case. . . . He walked through the house and started up the stairs to the second floor where the master bedroom was. About three-fourths of the way up the stairs, Jon said he heard Diane giggle and he testified that he recognized the giggle as one he knew from their intimate moments together. He then ran up to the top of the stairs, turned on the light, and opened the door to the master bedroom.

Diane and Mueller were in bed together and Jon testified that Mueller was naked. Mueller got out of bed and moved toward Jon who was out in the hallway. Jon then fired the rifle five times. At trial, Jon stated that Mueller lunged toward him and tried to grab the rifle and he just reacted. After the last shot was fired, Mueller was laying face down in the hallway. When Diane heard the shots, she called 911. . . .

Quick was indicted by a Norman County grand jury on one count of first-degree murder for the shooting death of Mueller and went to trial in October 2001. The district court provided jury instructions on both first-degree premeditated murder and first-degree heat of passion manslaughter. The jury returned a guilty verdict of murder in the first degree and the court sentenced Quick to life imprisonment.

I.

Quick argues that his conviction should be vacated and the case remanded for sentencing on the lesser-included offense of heat of passion manslaughter. He asserts that the state failed to provide sufficient evidence to prove beyond a reasonable doubt that he did not act in the heat of passion. . . .

To be guilty of first-degree premeditated murder, Quick must have caused the death of Mueller with premeditation and with intent to effect his death. Premeditation means to "consider, plan or prepare for, or determine to commit, the act referred to prior to its commission." Minn. Stat. §609.18 (2002). "A finding of premeditation does not require proof of extensive planning or preparation to kill, nor does it require any specific period of time for deliberation." *State v. Cooper*, 561 N.W.2d 175, 180 (Minn. 1997). Premeditation is a state of mind and, therefore, generally proved through circumstantial evidence of the "defendant's words and actions in light of the totality of the circumstances." *State v. Brocks*, 587 N.W.2d 37, 42 (Minn. 1998). . . .

[Three categories of evidence are relevant when inferring premeditation: (1) facts about what the defendant did before the killing that show he was engaged in planning activity; (2) facts about the defendant's prior relationships with the victim that might establish motive; and (3) facts about the nature of the killing that might tend to show a "preconceived design."—Eds.]

An intentional killing may be mitigated from first-degree murder to first-degree manslaughter if the defendant acted in the heat of passion. Even if the defendant acted with premeditation, the defendant is guilty only of first-degree manslaughter if he also acted in the heat of passion. Thus, for a defendant to be convicted of first-degree premeditated murder, not only must the state prove premeditation, but the state also has the burden of proving beyond a reasonable doubt the absence of heat of passion.

A defendant is guilty of heat of passion manslaughter if the (1) killing was committed in the heat of passion, and (2) passion was provoked by such words or acts of another as would provoke a person of ordinary self-control under the circumstances. The first element is a subjective inquiry and it is the emotional status of the defendant that is of primary importance. If a defendant is in the heat of passion, his reason would be clouded and his willpower weakened. Anger alone is not sufficient for heat of passion. The second element, provocation, is an objective inquiry. "[T]he words and acts of [another] must have been enough to provoke a person of ordinary self-control." *State v. Auchampach,* 540 N.W.2d 808, 815 (Minn. 1995). . . .

Quick was aware and suspicious of his wife's relationship with Mueller and had shown anger and jealousy over their relationship in his comments to his wife's brother and through notes and e-mails sent to his wife. Quick's actions of driving 15 miles late at night, going around the block a second time to avoid being seen, sneaking into the house through a window, taking a loaded rifle with him, and taking off his shoes so he would not be heard all showed planning and preparation and not heat of passion. Moreover, given that Quick strongly suspected that there was a relationship between his wife and Mueller and that Mueller was at the house with his wife, hearing his wife giggle and finding them together was not sufficient provocation to justify a heat of passion killing. Therefore, we hold that there is sufficient evidence for the jury to have determined that Quick killed Mueller with premeditation and without heat of passion. . . .

NOTES AND QUESTIONS

1. Do you agree with how these two cases were decided and justified? If so, how do you reconcile them? If not, which is (or are) wrongly decided, and why?
2. Does your answer change if the defendants were female instead of male? Should laws differ if biology differs?
3. Here is one authoritative description of voluntary manslaughter:

> Voluntary manslaughter in most jurisdictions consists of an intentional homicide committed under extenuating circumstances that mitigate, though they do not justify or excuse, the killing. The principal extenuating circumstance is the fact that the defendant, when he killed the victim, was in a state of passion engendered in him by an adequate provocation (i.e., a provocation which would cause a reasonable man to lose his normal self-control). . . .
>
> The usual type of voluntary manslaughter involves the intentional killing of another while under the influence of a reasonably-induced emotional disturbance (in earlier terminology, while in a "heat of passion") causing a temporary loss of normal self-control. Except for this reasonable emotional condition, the intentional killing would be murder. . . . The "passion" (emotional disturbance) involved in the crime of voluntary manslaughter is generally rage. . . .

Wayne R. LaFave, *Criminal Law* 1026-27 (5th ed. 2010). Do you think that the reason for mitigation is rooted more in logic or in feeling? What does it mean to have a "reasonable emotional condition"?

4. As the above two cases indicate, heat of passion homicides often arise after a husband witnesses his spouse committing adultery and proceeds to kill the spouse or her partner. The sight of adultery has been considered sufficient provocation

since early English common law. In early American law, even the discovery of adultery after the fact was sufficient to justify the killing of a spouse. *See* Joshua Dressler, *Rethinking Heat of Passion: A Defense in Search of a Rationale*, 73 J. Crim. L. & Criminology 421 (1982). For evolutionary angles on heat of passion killings like these (which, it should be noted, do not justify or excuse the behavior), see analysis from Professor Carlton Patrick:

> One evolutionary framework for wife-killings proposes that, because of the asymmetric risk of investing resources in someone else's offspring, in certain circumstances it may have been adaptive for males to kill a spouse that has either been unfaithful or irrevocably broken off the relationship. For our ancestors, in most instances killing a wife would have been maladaptive: it entails the loss of a cooperative partner, a contributor of resources, and a potential source of future reproduction. However, a wife's certain infidelity is unique in that it entails the potential incurrence of extreme costs for the husband. These costs include the loss of the wife's reproductive capacity, a devotion of resources to a rival's offspring, and reputational damage within the community and with polygynous co-wives (i.e. as the type of person who "tolerates' infidelity). Consequently, in cases where infidelity or the loss of the relationship is certain, the fitness benefits of killing an unfaithful wife (e.g., depriving a rival of access to a reproductive source, killing the potential child of the rival, and deterring other wives from cheating) could have outweighed the potential fitness costs for cuckolded partners. In turn, an adaptation for jealousy-induced homicide is hypothesized to have evolved disproportionately in men. . . .

Carlton J. Patrick, *A New Synthesis for Law and Emotions: Insights from the Behavioral Sciences*, 47 Ariz. St. L.J. 1239, 1278 (2015). *See also* Robert S. Walker, Mark V. Flinn & Kim R. Hill, *Evolutionary History of Partible Paternity in Lowland South America*, 107 Proc. Nat'l Acad. Sci. 19195 (2010) (noting that some societies have different mating structures, with different effects on jealousy).

5. Might the neuroscience of emotion also have implications for sentencing and treatment of offenders? Consider Professor Federica Coppola's analysis:

> Research on the influence of socio-emotional factors on morality and on social behavior poses suggestive challenges to the dominant discourse on punishment. In fact, a serious acknowledgment of this body of knowledge on the part of criminal law and justice could lead to bringing some changes in how the law conceives of wrongdoing as well as in the justifications for and measures taken in response to it. . . .
>
> [N]euroscientific findings emphasize the critical role of socio-emotional mechanisms in contributing to and hindering offending behavior. More importantly, neuroscience and its adjacent disciplines have suggested that the marked sensitivity—and, consequently, the malleability—of emotions and socio-emotional skills to external stimuli may have both positive and negative repercussions for moral and social behavior. Therefore, these studies have highlighted the centrality of socio-emotional factors in wrongdoing and their particular role as critical targets to promote prosocial attitudes and socially functional behavior. In view of these insights, neuroscientific findings can theoretically and practically challenge major views of responsibility and punishment. . . .

Federica Coppola, *Valuing Emotions in Punishment: An Argument for Social Rehabilitation with the Aid of Social and Affective Neuroscience*, Neuroethics, https://doi.org/10.1007/s12152-018-9393-4 (2018).

C. THE EMOTIONAL JUROR

The law must grapple not only with how to deal with a defendant's emotional state at the time of her act but also with issues surrounding the emotional states of jurors as they weigh her fate. This challenge is illustrated by debates over the propriety of jurors hearing evidence of the emotional impact that the crime had on the victim. In *Booth v. Maryland*, for instance, the U.S. Supreme Court held that the Eighth Amendment (which prohibits infliction of cruel and unusual punishments) "prohibits a capital sentencing jury from considering victim impact evidence." The Court expanded this holding in the 1989 case of *South Carolina v. Gathers*. But it then abruptly reversed course in the 1991 case of *Payne v. Tennessee*, holding that "if the State chooses to permit the admission of victim impact evidence and prosecutorial argument on that subject, the Eighth Amendment erects no *per se* bar." As you read this evolving case law, think about the animating assumptions (tested or not) regarding the effects of particular emotions on juror decision-making.

Booth v. Maryland
482 U.S. 496 (1987)

Justice POWELL delivered the [5-4] opinion of the Court.

The question presented is whether the Constitution prohibits a jury from considering a "victim impact statement" during the sentencing phase of a capital murder trial.

I

In 1983, Irvin Bronstein, 78, and his wife Rose, 75, were robbed and murdered in their West Baltimore home. The murderers, John Booth and Willie Reid, entered the victims' home for the apparent purpose of stealing money to buy heroin. Booth, a neighbor of the Bronsteins, knew that the elderly couple could identify him. The victims were bound and gagged, and then stabbed repeatedly in the chest with a kitchen knife. The bodies were discovered two days later by the Bronsteins' son.

A jury found Booth guilty of two counts of first-degree murder, two counts of robbery, and conspiracy to commit robbery. The prosecution requested the death penalty, and Booth elected to have his sentence determined by the jury instead of the judge. Before the sentencing phase began, the State Division of Parole and Probation (DPP) compiled a presentence report that described Booth's background, education and employment history, and criminal record. Under a Maryland statute, the presentence report in all felony cases also must include a victim impact statement (VIS), describing the effect of the crime on the victim and his family. Md. Ann. Code, Art. 41, §4-609(c) (1986). Specifically, the report shall:

"(i) Identify the victim of the offense;
"(ii) Itemize any economic loss suffered by the victim as a result of the offense;
"(iii) Identify any physical injury suffered by the victim as a result of the offense along with its seriousness and permanence;
"(iv) Describe any change in the victim's personal welfare or familial relationships as a result of the offense;

"(v) Identify any request for psychological services initiated by the victim or the victim's family as a result of the offense; and

"(vi) Contain any other information related to the impact of the offense upon the victim or the victim's family that the trial court requires." §4-609(c)(3).

Although the VIS is compiled by the DPP, the information is supplied by the victim or the victim's family. The VIS may be read to the jury during the sentencing phase, or the family members may be called to testify as to the information.

The VIS in Booth's case was based on interviews with the Bronsteins' son, daughter, son-in-law, and granddaughter. Many of their comments emphasized the victims' outstanding personal qualities, and noted how deeply the Bronsteins would be missed.* Other parts of the VIS described the emotional and personal problems the family members have faced as a result of the crimes. The son, for example, said that he suffers from lack of sleep and depression, and is "fearful for the first time in his life." He said that in his opinion, his parents were "butchered like animals." The daughter said she also suffers from lack of sleep, and that since the murders she has become withdrawn and distrustful. She stated that she can no longer watch violent movies or look at kitchen knives without being reminded of the murders. The daughter concluded that she could not forgive the murderer, and that such a person could "[n]ever be rehabilitated." Finally, the granddaughter described how the deaths had ruined the wedding of another close family member that took place a few days after the bodies were discovered. Both the ceremony and the reception were sad affairs, and instead of leaving for her honeymoon, the bride attended the victims' funeral. The VIS also noted that the granddaughter had received counseling for several months after the incident, but eventually had stopped because she concluded that "no one could help her."

The DPP official who conducted the interviews concluded the VIS by writing:

"It became increasingly apparent to the writer as she talked to the family members that the murder of Mr. and Mrs. Bronstein is still such a shocking, painful, and devastating memory to them that it permeates every aspect of their daily lives. It is doubtful that they will ever be able to fully recover from this tragedy and not be haunted by the memory of the brutal manner in which their loved ones were murdered and taken from them."

Defense counsel moved to suppress the VIS on the ground that this information was both irrelevant and unduly inflammatory, and that therefore its use in a capital case violated the Eighth Amendment of the Federal Constitution. The Maryland trial court denied the motion, ruling that the jury was entitled to consider "any and

---

*. The VIS stated:

"[T]he victims' son reports that his parents had been married for fifty-three years and enjoyed a very close relationship, spending each day together. He states that his father had worked hard all his life and had been retired for eight years. He describes his mother as a woman who was young at heart and never seemed like an old lady. She taught herself to play bridge when she was in her seventies. The victims' son relates that his parents were amazing people who attended the senior citizens' center and made many devout friends."

"As described by their family members, the Bronsteins were loving parents and grandparents whose family was most important to them. Their funeral was the largest in the history of the Levinson Funeral Home and the family received over one thousand sympathy cards, some from total strangers."

all evidence which would bear on the [sentencing decision]." Booth's lawyer then requested that the prosecutor simply read the VIS to the jury rather than call the family members to testify before the jury. Defense counsel was concerned that the use of live witnesses would increase the inflammatory effect of the information. The prosecutor agreed to this arrangement.

The jury sentenced Booth to death for the murder of Mr. Bronstein and to life imprisonment for the murder of Mrs. Bronstein. On automatic appeal, the Maryland Court of Appeals affirmed the conviction and the sentences. The court rejected Booth's claim that the VIS injected an arbitrary factor into the sentencing decision . . . [concluding] that a VIS serves an important interest by informing the sentencer of the full measure of harm caused by the crime. The Court of Appeals then examined the VIS in Booth's case, and concluded that it is a "relatively straightforward and factual description of the effects of these murders on members of the Bronstein family." It held that the death sentence had not been imposed under the influence of passion, prejudice, or other arbitrary factors.

We granted certiorari to decide whether the Eighth Amendment prohibits a capital sentencing jury from considering victim impact evidence. We conclude that it does, and now reverse.

II

It is well settled that a jury's discretion to impose the death sentence must be "suitably directed and limited so as to minimize the risk of wholly arbitrary and capricious action." *Gregg v. Georgia*, 428 U.S. 153 (1976). . . . [W]hile this Court has never said that the defendant's record, characteristics, and the circumstances of the crime are the *only* permissible sentencing considerations, a state statute that requires consideration of other factors must be scrutinized to ensure that the evidence has some bearing on the defendant's "personal responsibility and moral guilt." *Enmund v. Florida*, 458 U.S. 782 (1982). To do otherwise would create the risk that a death sentence will be based on considerations that are "constitutionally impermissible or totally irrelevant to the sentencing process." *See Zant v. Stephens*, 462 U.S. 862, 885 (1983).

The VIS in this case provided the jury with two types of information. First, it described the personal characteristics of the victims and the emotional impact of the crimes on the family. Second, it set forth the family members' opinions and characterizations of the crimes and the defendant. For the reasons stated below, we find that this information is irrelevant to a capital sentencing decision, and that its admission creates a constitutionally unacceptable risk that the jury may impose the death penalty in an arbitrary and capricious manner.

A

The greater part of the VIS is devoted to a description of the emotional trauma suffered by the family and the personal characteristics of the victims. The State claims that this evidence should be considered a "circumstance" of the crime because it reveals the full extent of the harm caused by Booth's actions. In the State's view, there is a direct, foreseeable nexus between the murders and the harm to the family, and thus it is not "arbitrary" for the jury to consider these consequences in deciding whether to impose the death penalty. Although "victim impact" is not an aggravating factor under Maryland law, the State claims that by knowing the extent of the impact upon and the severity of the loss to the family, the jury was better able to assess the "'gravity or aggravating quality'" of the offense. . . .

The focus of a VIS, however, is not on the defendant, but on the character and reputation of the victim and the effect on his family. These factors may be wholly unrelated to the blameworthiness of a particular defendant. As our cases have shown, the defendant often will not know the victim, and therefore will have no knowledge about the existence or characteristics of the victim's family. Moreover, defendants rarely select their victims based on whether the murder will have an effect on anyone other than the person murdered. Allowing the jury to rely on a VIS therefore could result in imposing the death sentence because of factors about which the defendant was unaware, and that were irrelevant to the decision to kill. This evidence thus could divert the jury's attention away from the defendant's background and record, and the circumstances of the crime. . . .

As evidenced by the full text of the VIS in this case . . . the family members were articulate and persuasive in expressing their grief and the extent of their loss. But in some cases the victim will not leave behind a family, or the family members may be less articulate in describing their feelings even though their sense of loss is equally severe. The fact that the imposition of the death sentence may turn on such distinctions illustrates the danger of allowing juries to consider this information. Certainly the degree to which a family is willing and able to express its grief is irrelevant to the decision whether a defendant, who may merit the death penalty, should live or die. . . .

We also note that it would be difficult—if not impossible—to provide a fair opportunity to rebut such evidence without shifting the focus of the sentencing hearing away from the defendant. . . . We thus reject the contention that the presence or absence of emotional distress of the victim's family, or the victim's personal characteristics, are proper sentencing considerations in a capital case.

B

The second type of information presented to the jury in the VIS was the family members' opinions and characterizations of the crimes. . . .

One can understand the grief and anger of the family caused by the brutal murders in this case, and there is no doubt that jurors generally are aware of these feelings. But the formal presentation of this information by the State can serve no other purpose than to inflame the jury and divert it from deciding the case on the relevant evidence concerning the crime and the defendant. As we have noted, any decision to impose the death sentence must "be, and appear to be, based on reason rather than caprice or emotion." *Gardner v. Florida*, 430 U.S. 349 (1977). The admission of these emotionally charged opinions as to what conclusions the jury should draw from the evidence clearly is inconsistent with the reasoned decision-making we require in capital cases.

III

We conclude that the introduction of a VIS at the sentencing phase of a capital murder trial violates the Eighth Amendment, and therefore the Maryland statute is invalid to the extent it requires consideration of this information. The decision of the Maryland Court of Appeals is vacated to the extent that it affirmed the capital sentence. The case is remanded for further proceedings not inconsistent with this opinion.

Payne v. Tennessee
501 U.S. 808 (1991)

Chief Justice REHNQUIST delivered the [6-3] opinion of the Court. . . .

Petitioner, Pervis Tyrone Payne, was convicted by a jury on two counts of first-degree murder and one count of assault with intent to commit murder in the first degree. He was sentenced to death for each of the murders and to 30 years in prison for the assault.

The victims of Payne's offenses were 28-year-old Charisse Christopher, her 2-year-old daughter Lacie, and her 3-year-old son Nicholas. The three lived together in an apartment in Millington, Tennessee, across the hall from Payne's girlfriend, Bobbie Thomas. On Saturday, June 27, 1987, Payne visited Thomas' apartment several times in expectation of her return from her mother's house in Arkansas, but found no one at home. On one visit, he left his overnight bag, containing clothes and other items for his weekend stay, in the hallway outside Thomas' apartment. With the bag were three cans of malt liquor.

Payne passed the morning and early afternoon injecting cocaine and drinking beer. Later, he drove around the town with a friend in the friend's car, each of them taking turns reading a pornographic magazine. Sometime around 3 P.M., Payne returned to the apartment complex, entered the Christophers' apartment, and began making sexual advances towards Charisse. Charisse resisted and Payne became violent. A neighbor who resided in the apartment directly beneath the Christophers heard Charisse screaming, "'Get out, get out,' as if she were telling the children to leave." The noise briefly subsided and then began, "'horribly loud.'" The neighbor called the police after she heard a "blood curdling scream" from the Christopher's apartment. . . .

Inside the apartment, the police encountered a horrifying scene. Blood covered the walls and floor throughout the unit. Charisse and her children were lying on the floor in the kitchen. Nicholas, despite several wounds inflicted by a butcher knife that completely penetrated through his body from front to back, was still breathing. Miraculously, he survived, but not until after undergoing seven hours of surgery and a transfusion of 1,700 cc's of blood—400 to 500 cc's more than his estimated normal blood volume. Charisse and Lacie were dead. . . .

Payne was apprehended later that day hiding in the attic of the home of a former girlfriend. . . .

At trial, Payne took the stand and, despite the overwhelming and relatively uncontroverted evidence against him, testified that he had not harmed any of the Christophers. Rather, he asserted that another man had raced by him as he was walking up the stairs to the floor where the Christophers lived. He stated that he had gotten blood on himself when, after hearing moans from the Christophers' apartment, he had tried to help the victims. According to his testimony, he panicked and fled when he heard police sirens and noticed the blood on his clothes. The jury returned guilty verdicts against Payne on all counts. . . .

[At sentencing, the] State presented the testimony of Charisse's mother, Mary Zvolanek. When asked how Nicholas had been affected by the murders of his mother and sister, she responded:

> "He cries for his mom. He doesn't seem to understand why she doesn't come home.
> And he cries for his sister Lacie. He comes to me many times during the week and

asks me, Grandmama, do you miss my Lacie. And I tell him yes. He says, I'm worried about my Lacie." . . .

In the rebuttal to Payne's closing argument, the prosecutor stated:

> "You saw the videotape this morning. You saw what Nicholas Christopher will carry in his mind forever. When you talk about cruel, when you talk about atrocious, and when you talk about heinous, that picture will always come into your mind, probably throughout the rest of your lives. . . .
>
> ". . . No one will ever know about Lacie Jo because she never had the chance to grow up. Her life was taken from her at the age of two years old. So, no there won't be a high school principal to talk about Lacie Jo Christopher, and there won't be anybody to take her to her high school prom. And there won't be anybody there — there won't be her mother there or Nicholas' mother there to kiss him at night. His mother will never kiss him good night or pat him as he goes off to bed, or hold him and sing him a lullaby.
>
> "[Petitioner's attorney] wants you to think about a good reputation, people who love the defendant and things about him. He doesn't want you to think about the people who love Charisse Christopher, her mother and daddy who loved her. The people who loved little Lacie Jo, the grandparents who are still here. The brother who mourns for her every single day and wants to know where his best little playmate is. He doesn't have anybody to watch cartoons with him, a little one. These are the things that go into why it is especially cruel, heinous, and atrocious, the burden that that child will carry forever."

The jury sentenced Payne to death on each of the murder counts.

The Supreme Court of Tennessee affirmed the conviction and sentence. The court rejected Payne's contention that the admission of the grandmother's testimony and the State's closing argument constituted prejudicial violations of his rights under the Eighth Amendment as applied in *Booth v. Maryland* (1987), and *South Carolina v. Gathers* (1989). . . .

The court determined that the prosecutor's comments during closing argument were "relevant to [Payne's] personal responsibility and moral guilt." The court explained that "[w]hen a person deliberately picks a butcher knife out of a kitchen drawer and proceeds to stab to death a twenty-eight-year-old mother, her two and one-half year old daughter and her three and one-half year old son, in the same room, the physical and mental condition of the boy he left for dead is surely relevant in determining his 'blameworthiness.'" The court concluded that any violation of Payne's rights under *Booth* and *Gathers* "was harmless beyond a reasonable doubt."

We granted certiorari to reconsider our holdings in *Booth* and *Gathers* that the Eighth Amendment prohibits a capital sentencing jury from considering "victim impact" evidence relating to the personal characteristics of the victim and the emotional impact of the crimes on the victim's family. . . .

[In *Booth* the] Court held by a 5-to-4 vote that the Eighth Amendment prohibits a jury from considering a victim impact statement at the sentencing phase of a capital trial. . . . In *Gathers*, decided two years later, the Court extended the rule announced in *Booth* to statements made by a prosecutor to the sentencing jury regarding the personal qualities of the victim. . . .

Booth and *Gathers* were based on two premises: that evidence relating to a particular victim or to the harm that a capital defendant causes a victim's family do not in general reflect on the defendant's "blameworthiness," and that only evidence relating to "blameworthiness" is relevant to the capital sentencing decision. However, the assessment of harm caused by the defendant as a result of the crime charged has understandably been an important concern of the criminal law, both in determining the elements of the offense and in determining the appropriate punishment. Thus, two equally blameworthy criminal defendants may be guilty of different offenses solely because their acts cause differing amounts of harm. "If a bank robber aims his gun at a guard, pulls the trigger, and kills his target, he may be put to death. If the gun unexpectedly misfires, he may not. His moral guilt in both cases is identical, but his responsibility in the former is greater." *Booth*, 482 U.S. at 519. . . .

The principles which have guided criminal sentencing—as opposed to criminal liability—have varied with the times. . . .

Wherever judges in recent years have had discretion to impose sentence, the consideration of the harm caused by the crime has been an important factor in the exercise of that discretion. . . .

Congress and most of the States have, in recent years, enacted similar legislation to enable the sentencing authority to consider information about the harm caused by the crime committed by the defendant. The evidence involved in the present case was not admitted pursuant to any such enactment, but its purpose and effect were much the same as if it had been. While the admission of this particular kind of evidence—designed to portray for the sentencing authority the actual harm caused by a particular crime—is of recent origin, this fact hardly renders it unconstitutional. . . .

The *Booth* Court reasoned that victim impact evidence must be excluded because it would be difficult, if not impossible, for the defendant to rebut such evidence without shifting the focus of the sentencing hearing away from the defendant, thus creating a "'mini-trial' on the victim's character." *Booth*, 482 U.S. at 506. . . . But even as to additional evidence admitted at the sentencing phase, the mere fact that for tactical reasons it might not be prudent for the defense to rebut victim impact evidence makes the case no different than others in which a party is faced with this sort of a dilemma. . . .

We are now of the view that a State may properly conclude that for the jury to assess meaningfully the defendant's moral culpability and blameworthiness, it should have before it at the sentencing phase evidence of the specific harm caused by the defendant. . . . *Booth* deprives the State of the full moral force of its evidence and may prevent the jury from having before it all the information necessary to determine the proper punishment for a first-degree murder.

The present case is an example of the potential for such unfairness. The capital sentencing jury heard testimony from Payne's girlfriend that they met at church; that he was affectionate, caring, and kind to her children; that he was not an abuser of drugs or alcohol; and that it was inconsistent with his character to have committed the murders. Payne's parents testified that he was a good son, and a clinical psychologist testified that Payne was an extremely polite prisoner and suffered from a low IQ. None of this testimony was related to the circumstances of Payne's brutal crimes. In contrast, the only evidence of the impact of Payne's offenses during the sentencing phase was Nicholas' grandmother's description—in response to a single question—that the child misses his mother and baby sister. Payne argues that the Eighth Amendment commands that the jury's death sentence must be set aside because the jury heard this testimony. But the testimony illustrated quite poignantly some of the harm that Payne's killing had caused; there is nothing unfair about allowing the jury to bear in mind that harm at the same time as it considers the mitigating evidence introduced by the defendant. The Supreme Court of Tennessee in this case obviously felt the unfairness of the rule pronounced by *Booth* when it said: "It is an affront to the civilized members of the human race to say that at sentencing in a capital case, a parade of witnesses may praise the background, character and good deeds of Defendant (as was done in this case), without limitation as to relevancy, but nothing may be said that bears upon the character of, or the harm imposed, upon the victims." . . .

For the reasons discussed above, we now reject the view—expressed in *Gathers*—that a State may not permit the prosecutor to similarly argue to the jury the human cost of the crime of which the defendant stands convicted. We reaffirm the view expressed by Justice Cardozo in *Snyder v. Massachusetts*, 291 U.S. 97 (1934): "[J]ustice, though due to the accused, is due to the accuser also. The concept of fairness must not be strained till it is narrowed to a filament. We are to keep the balance true."

We thus hold that if the State chooses to permit the admission of victim impact evidence and prosecutorial argument on that subject, the Eighth Amendment erects no *per se* bar. A State may legitimately conclude that evidence about the victim and about the impact of the murder on the victim's family is relevant to the jury's decision as to whether or not the death penalty should be imposed. There is no reason to treat such evidence differently than other relevant evidence is treated.

Bryan Myers, Emalee Weidemann & Gregory Pearce

Psychology Weighs in on the Debate Surrounding Victim Impact Statements and Capital Sentencing: Are Emotional Jurors Really Irrational?

19 Fed. Sent'g Rep. 13, 13-17 (2006)

Over the past two decades, one of the more controversial issues surrounding capital sentencing has been the introduction of victim impact statements (VIS). As the victims' rights movement has grown, so has the attention surrounding this issue. . . .

Although justices and legal commentators have repeatedly warned of the dangers of the emotional responses VIS may elicit in jurors, this issue has rarely been investigated. In one of the few studies conducted on emotions and VIS, a sample of college students was presented with a videotaped trial that included both the guilt and penalty phases. Participants were assigned to one of four groups that varied the level of harm expressed in the VIS along with the emotional demeanor of the witness. Participants rated their emotional reactions to the testimony along with rendering sentencing judgments individually and without deliberation. The level of harm expressed in the VIS, and not the emotional demeanor of the witness, significantly impacted sentencing judgments. Moreover, although jurors indicated greater negative emotions in response to VIS as a function of harm expressed, these emotional responses were independent of the relation between harm and sentencing. However, it is noteworthy that the level of emotional response in mock jurors was rather minimal, and the measure of negative emotions failed to discriminate between particular negative emotions (e.g., anger and sadness).

In another study using jury-eligible community members, one of eight trial transcripts was assigned that varied the presence of VIS, the offender's gender, and the victim's gender. The researchers found that participants tended to give lesser sentences to the female defendant, but this difference was reduced by the presence of VIS. In terms of emotional responses to a statement, they found that female defendants elicited less anger in participants when no statement was present, but greater anger relative to male defendants when a statement was present.

Although, as we just noted, researchers have addressed the importance of the emotional qualities surrounding VIS, it is also true that this research represents just the early stages on this important topic. One of the most frequently cited reasons for opposition to the introduction of victim impact evidence is the concern that its emotional nature will inflame the jury at such a critical time when decisions should be based on rational rather than emotional reasons. We next turn to this issue of whether VIS are inflammatory, and what psychological research can tell us about this important issue.

III. VIS, EMOTIONS, AND JUDGMENT

. . . To begin, emotions along with moods are part of a larger category of feelings known generally as affect. The main differences between moods and emotions are that the former are considered to be more diffuse and longer lasting. However, for the purpose of the present commentary, we will generally use affect, moods, and emotions interchangeably. They are not the same, but they are similar enough for the present discussion.

With little question, research has consistently shown that emotions can influence decisions, and psychological research suggests this influence can happen in various ways. For example, emotions can serve to inform jurors how they generally feel about a target (e.g., a defendant or a victim). This heuristic function has been labeled the affect-as-information hypothesis. According to this view, emotions inform us as to how we feel about things, and this allows us to make judgments based on those feelings without resorting to more effortful cognitive processing. Emotions serve as cognitive shortcuts (i.e., heuristics). Less heuristically but equally directly, emotions may lead us to generate thoughts about a target that are associated with those emotions. This theory posits that we when are angry, we easily generate thoughts about the defendant that are consistent with anger. This spreading activation explanation is consistent with the affect-as-information theory in that both would predict that we tend to make judgments about a target that are congruent with our emotional state. The tendency for people to reach judgments that are consistent with their emotional state is known as the mood-congruency effect. Consequently, if we are in a negative mood, we judge the target more negatively than if we are in a positive mood. There is a good deal of support for the mood-congruency effect, and one of the features of this theory that is particularly alarming when applied to legal judgments is the fact that we may misattribute the source of our negative emotions. That is, we may evaluate our target more negatively if we are in a negative mood, regardless of whether the target influenced our negative mood in the first place.

More indirectly than mood congruency, emotions may also influence the degree to which we will engage in effortful processing in an attempt to render a judgment about something or someone. Certain emotions promote effortful processing whereas others inhibit this tendency. For example, when someone is experiencing a positive emotion (e.g., happiness) he or she tends to engage in less detailed information processing, whereas negative emotions (e.g., sadness) are associated with more effortful and detailed information processing. However, not all negative emotions are associated with effortful processing. Anger has the opposite effect of sadness on information processing; it tends to generate less detailed and effortful (i.e., more heuristic) processing. . . .

Finally, emotions may influence the kinds of information we attend to, and this may in turn influence how we render judgments about the defendant or the victim. For example, researchers have found that angry individuals tend to make dispositional attributions (see a person as the cause) more readily than saddened individuals, who tend to make situational attributions (see the situation as the cause) when making judgments about whom to blame for negative outcomes. For example, in one study participants were put in either a sad or an angry mood and asked to judge a series of hypothetical outcomes. Angry individuals tended to see the outcomes as caused by personal (i.e., dispositional) factors whereas sad individuals tended to see these same outcomes as due to situational factors. This general finding has repeated itself over a variety of different studies and contexts. We are in the early stages of understanding why certain emotions are linked with certain attribution tendencies, but the finding has obvious implications concerning the damaging effects of emotions such as anger for a defendant. Moreover, it adds fuel to the notion that treating all emotions as equally prejudicial to the defendant is misguided. . . .

V. IMPLICATIONS FOR CAPITAL SENTENCING AND CONCLUDING COMMENTS

What are the implications of this research for capital sentencing and VIS? First, not all emotions are equal. So it would be a false assertion that psychological research supports the notion that an emotional juror is an irrational juror, as the courts assume. This is particularly so if we regard irrationality as an inability to think clearly and a tendency to act without carefully considering all alternatives. One could reasonably say that research findings support the view that, when saddened, jurors are more likely to carefully, systematically, and extensively process information about a defendant—or a victim for that matter. Such an individual would appear to be well equipped to take on the task of carefully weighing all mitigating and aggravating factors presented during the penalty phase. Yet, other emotions like anger or outrage could lead to less detailed, more heuristic processing strategies. For these emotions, there is ample evidence to support the fear that jurors may not consider all evidence fully and that this may lead to capricious judgments. . . .

NOTES AND QUESTIONS

1. Did the *Payne* Court sufficiently consider the emotional power of victim impact testimony? Consider the following perspective, which argues that it did not and outlines several problems that stem from the Court's failure to acknowledge the emotional impact that the evidence may have on jurors:

First, if the probative purpose of the evidence is to evoke the life lost with vividness and particularity, what is the measure of undue prejudice? Arguably, the informational value of the statement *is* its ability to convey the family's grief and to communicate the emotional impact of the loss of someone who was loved and valued. Many of the usual markers of prejudice—heightened emotionality in delivery and the tendency to elicit strong emotions—seem identical to the features that, according to the *Payne* Court, would make the testimony effectively vivid, meet the jury's expectations about how the family of a murder victim ought to feel, and convey the full moral force of the evidence. . . .

[Second,] many victim characteristics, for example race and ethnicity, are not only irrelevant to sentencing but impermissible factors under the Fourteenth Amendment. Other victim characteristics, such as social class or physical attractiveness, are also irrelevant and objectionable factors. The Court briefly acknowledged the concern that the sort of proof it was permitting might influence the sentencing jury to impose sentences based on the worthiness or unworthiness of victims. . . .

The Court expressed confidence that "[i]n the majority of cases . . . victim impact evidence serves entirely legitimate purposes [but that if] evidence is introduced that is so unduly prejudicial that it renders the trial fundamentally unfair, the Due Process Clause of the Fourteenth Amendment provides a mechanism for relief." . . .

Susan A. Bandes & Jessica M. Salerno, *Emotion, Proof and Prejudice: The Cognitive Science of Gruesome Photos and Victim Impact Statements*, 46 Ariz. St. L.J. 1003, 1031-33 (2014). The authors go on to discuss studies that illustrate the emotional power of victim impact statements. In particular, studies show that such statements increase punitiveness in jurors, making them more likely to render a death sentence. *Id.* at 1035.

2. Rules of evidence often discourage the use of emotion in juror decision-making. For instance, recall Fed. R. Evid. 403: "The court may exclude relevant evidence if its probative value is substantially outweighed by a danger of one or more of the following: unfair prejudice, confusing the issues, misleading the jury, undue delay, wasting time, or needlessly presenting cumulative evidence." Legal scholar Teneille Brown argues that this approach may not be optimal:

The anti-emotions bias in FRE 403 is lamentable for at least three reasons. First, it ignores the wide range of cases where emotion might be said to render decisions more, rather than less, accurate. It is quite possible that empathy, rage, or sadness may be entirely appropriate emotions to be conjured up at the guilt phase of trial, to better understand *prima facie* mental states of the parties (*mens rea*, honesty, etc.). As was mentioned in the previous section on FRE 105, emotional testimony, and our emotional reaction, may also help us focus, attend, and remember. Second, the focus on eliminating emotional bases for decisions does not require, but does suggest, that emotion and cognition are two completely separate processes. And third, it distracts from the fact that bad logic, memory, or perception or marginally related facts, can also contribute to prejudice. . . .

Teneille R. Brown, *The Affective Blindness of Evidence Law*, 89 Denv. U. L. Rev. 47, 75 (2011). Brown goes on to argue that:

The failure to appreciate the inevitable and often helpful role emotions can play in courtroom decision-making results in rules and practices that are woefully out of step with cognitive science data on emotion and reason. The monolithic view of emotions as corrupting of reason results in affective blindness. We therefore ask jurors to perform mental gymnastics and emotional regulation that may not be possible, and also might not be desirable, given that emotions assist with perception, attention, memory, empathy, and social decision-making. . . .

Id. at 128. Do you agree with Professor Brown's assessment?

3. A recent study investigated whether subjects altered the degree to which they assigned punishment when reading emotionally charged descriptions of a harmful act as opposed to neutral descriptions. The researchers found that including more emotional content in a description amplified the severity of punishment assigned to the wrongdoer. However, this finding only held when the decision-maker was told that the wrongdoer intended to cause the harm. When the harm was unintended, the effect of the emotionally charged description was eliminated. Michael T. Treadway et al., *Corticolimbic Gating of Emotion-Driven Punishment*, 17 Nature Neurosci. 1270 (2014). Given these findings, how, if at all, should judges referee the contents of victim impact statements? What about of witness testimony? For example, should a judge instruct a witness not to cry, or call a recess when a witness begins to cry, so as to avoid unduly influencing the jury? *See, e.g.,* Maria Cramer, *Judge in Hernandez Trial Described as Tough but Fair*, Boston Globe (Feb. 25, 2015) (discussing a judge's instructions to victim's to "retain control of your emotions and not to cry").

4. Neuroimaging researchers have found that when weighing sympathy-inducing mitigating factors, participants in the role of jurors relied on brain regions associated with mentalizing and moral conflict, including the dorsomedial prefrontal cortex, posterior cingulate, and temporo-parietal junction. Activation in these regions suggests that jurors confronted with sympathetic mitigating circumstances engage in "a reasoned simulation of what the defendant was thinking when committing the crime or how most people would judge the normative basis for mitigation." Makiko Yamada et al., *Neural Circuits in the Brain That Are Activated When Mitigating Criminal Sentences*, 3 Nature Comm. 759 (2012).

The law often treats emotions as inappropriate bases for decision-making, and judges sometimes instruct jurors to avoiding emotion when rendering a decision. *See, e.g., California v. Brown*, 479 U.S. 538, 539 (1987) (upholding instruction to jurors that they "must not be swayed by mere sentiment, conjecture, sympathy, passion, prejudice, public opinion or public feeling."). If "sympathy is clearly evident in brain activity, and influences sentence mitigation," can jurors be expected to suppress emotions when instructed to? Yamada et al., *supra*. What could judges do instead to address jurors' reliance on emotions?

5. Jurors and judges often rely on facial expressions to determine a defendant or witness's emotional state. Consider the following:

> "Reading" the emotions of a defendant—in the words of Supreme Court Justice Anthony Kennedy, to "know the heart and mind of the offender"—is one pillar of a fair trial in the U.S. legal system and in many legal systems in the Western world. Legal actors like jurors and judges routinely rely on facial movements to determine the guilt and remorse of a defendant. For example, defendants who are perceived as untrustworthy receive harsher sentences than they otherwise would, and such perceptions are more likely when a person appears to be angry (i.e., facial structure is similar to the hypothesized facial expression of anger, which is a scowl). An incorrect inference about a defendant's emotional state can cost them their children, their freedom, or even their lives. . . .

Lisa Feldman Barrett et al., *Emotional Expressions Reconsidered: Challenges to Inferring Emotion from Human Facial Movements*, 20 Psychol. Sci. Pub. Int. 1, 3 (2019). Despite the long-standing use of facial expression to "read" emotions, Barrett and colleagues determined that "[w]hen facial movements do express emotional states, they are considerably more variable and dependent on context than the common beliefs allows." *Id.* at 46. Given these findings, should jurors be instructed on the relative merit of judging the veracity or credibility of a defendant, a witness, or even a lawyer based on facial expressions?

6. Studies suggest that emotion may play a role in the accuracy of an eyewitness's memory. For instance, emotional eyewitnesses provide more complete descriptions of perpetrators, but these descriptions are no more accurate than those of neutral eyewitnesses. Emotional eyewitnesses also recall fewer details about the crime itself and are less likely to recognize a perpetrator in a photographic lineup. *See* Kate A. Houston et al., *The Emotional Eyewitness: The Effects of Emotion on Specific Aspects of Eyewitness Recall and Recognition Performance*, 13 Emotion 118 (2013).

D. THE EMOTIONAL JUDGE

To what extent should emotions—sympathies, a sense of outrage, indignation, and the like—affect judicial decisions? This issue, and the perhaps inevitable entanglement of emotions with personal experience, often arises during confirmation hearings. Two Supreme Court confirmation hearings illustrate the significance that emotion can play in the judicial decision-making process.

Justice Sonia Sotomayor's confirmation hearing centered around her ability to serve as an impartial arbiter. One comment in particular, dubbed the "wise Latina" comment, became a major focus of her hearing. While discussing judicial decision-making in the context of racial and sexual discrimination cases, Justice Sotomayor stated during a speech:

> Whether born from experience or inherent physiological or cultural differences . . . our gender and national origins may and will make a difference in our judging. Justice O'Connor has often been cited as saying that a wise old man and wise old woman will reach the same conclusion in deciding cases. . . . I am also not so sure that I agree with the statement. First, . . . there can never be a universal definition of wise. Second, I would hope that a wise Latina woman with the richness of her experiences would more often than not reach a better conclusion than a white male who hasn't lived that life. . . .

Lecture: 'A Latina Judge's Voice,' N.Y. Times (May 14, 2009). President Obama's comments when appointing Sotomayor also influenced the debates. Obama stated that he intended to appoint a Justice who possessed the "quality of empathy, of understanding and identifying with people's hopes and struggles as an essential ingredient for arriving at just decisions and outcomes." Peter Baker, *In Court Nominees, Is Obama Looking for Empathy by Another Name?*, N.Y. Times (Apr. 25, 2010). This was interpreted by senators as an intent to nominate someone who is not impartial, but instead favors certain groups of people. Sotomayor's ability to apply the law without personal emotion thus dominated questioning during her confirmation.

**Nomination of Sonia Sotomayor to be an Associate Justice
of the Supreme Court of the United States**
Hearing Before the S. Comm. on the Judiciary
111th Cong. 69-71 (2009)

Senator Sessions: . . . [Y]ou have evidenced, I think it is quite clear, a philosophy of the law that suggests that a judge's background and experiences can and should—even should and naturally will impact their decision which I think goes against the American ideal and oath that a judge takes to be fair to every party, and every day when they put on that robe, that is a symbol that they are to put aside their personal biases and prejudices. . . .

Let me recall that yesterday you said, "It's simple: fidelity to the law. The task of a judge is not to make law. It's to apply law." I heartily agree with that.

However, you previously have said, "The court of appeals is where policy is made." And you said on another occasion, "The law that lawyers practice and judge declare is not a definitive, capital 'L' law that many would like to think exists." So I guess I am asking today what do you really believe on those subjects: that there is no real law—that judges do not make law or that there is no real law and the court of appeals is where policy is made? Discuss that with us, please.

Judge Sotomayor: I believe my record of 17 years demonstrates fully that I do believe that law—that judges must apply the law and not make the law. Whether I've agreed with a party or not, found them sympathetic or not, in every case I have decided I have done what the law requires.

With respect to judges[] making policy, I assume, Senator, that you were referred to a remark that I made in a Duke law student dialogue. That remark in context made very clear that I wasn't talking about the policy reflected in the law that Congress makes. That's the job of Congress to decide what the policy should be for society.

In that conversation with the students, I was focusing on what district court judges do and what circuit court judges do, and I noted that district court judges find the facts and they apply the facts to the individual case. And when they do that, their holding, their finding doesn't bind anybody else.

Appellate judges, however, establish precedent. They decide what the law says in a particular situation. That precedent has policy ramifications because it binds not just the litigants in that case; it binds all litigants in similar cases, in cases that may be influenced by that precedent.

I think if my speech is heard outside of the minute and a half that YouTube presents and its full context examined, it is very clear that I was talking about the policy ramifications of precedent and never talking about appellate judges or courts making the policy that Congress makes.

Senator Sessions: Judge, I would just say I don't think it is that clear. I looked at that on tape several times, and I think a person could reasonably believe it meant more than that. But yesterday you spoke about your approach to rendering opinions and said, "I seek to strengthen both the rule of law and faith in the impartiality of the justice system," and I would agree. But you have previously said this: "I am willing to accept that we who judge must not deny differences resulting from experiences and heritage, but attempt, as the Supreme Court suggests, continuously to judge when those opinions, sympathies and prejudices are appropriate."

So, first, I'd like to know, Do you think there is any circumstance in which a judge should allow their prejudices to impact their decision making?

Judge Sotomayor: Never their prejudices. I was talking about the very important goal of the justice system is to ensure that the personal biases and prejudices of a judge do not influence the outcome of a case. What I was talking about was the obligation of judges to examine what they're feeling as they're adjudicating a case and to ensure that that's not influencing the outcome.

Life experiences have to influence you. We're not robots to listen to evidence and don't have feelings. We have to recognize those feelings and put them aside. That's what my speech was saying. That's our job.

Senator Sessions: But the statement was, "I willingly accept that we who judge must not deny the differences resulting from experience and heritage, but continuously to judge when those opinions, sympathies and prejudices are appropriate." That is exactly opposite of what you're saying, is it not?

Judge Sotomayor: I don't believe so, Senator, because all I was saying is, because we have feelings and different experiences, we can be led to believe that our experiences are appropriate. We have to be open-minded to accept that they may not be and that we have to judge always that we're not letting those things determine the outcome. But there are situations in which some experiences are important in the process of judging because the law asks us to use those experiences.

Senator Sessions: Well, I understand that. But let me just follow up. You say in your statement that you want to do what you can to increase the faith in the impartiality of our system. But isn't it true this statement suggests that you accept that there may be sympathies, prejudices and opinions that legitimately influence a judge's decision? And how can that further faith in the impartiality of the system?

Judge Sotomayor: I think the system is strengthened when judges don't assume they're impartial but when judges test themselves to identify when their emotions are driving a result or their experience are driving a result and the law is not . . .

The ability to control one's emotions and remain impartial in judicial decision-making was highlighted vividly during the 2018 Senate confirmation of Justice Brett Kavanaugh. Unlike Sotomayor's hearing, the controversy stemmed not from previous statements but from his demeanor responding to allegations that he sexually assaulted Dr. Christine Blasey Ford in their high school years.

Sheryl Gay Stolberg
A New Front in the Kavanaugh Wars: Temperament and Honesty
N.Y. Times (Oct. 1, 2018)

For Democrats determined to derail Judge Kavanaugh, his performance last week before the Senate Judiciary Committee . . . is proving to be a new avenue of attack. . . .

"The issues of credibility and temperament are not something that happened 30 years ago; they're about Judge Kavanaugh today and how he is as a 53-year-old," Senator Chuck Schumer of New York, the Democratic leader, said. . . . "I think there are serious questions about both his credibility and his temperament that may, to some senators, be more important than the activities that occurred in high school."

As the investigation of past actions continues, lawmakers in both parties are parsing Judge Kavanaugh's testimony from last week. At least one undecided Republican, Senator Jeff Flake of Arizona, took issue on Monday with the nominee's angry treatment of Democrats who questioned him about his drinking in high school. Judge Kavanaugh parried a question from Senator Amy Klobuchar, Democrat of Minnesota, about whether he had ever blacked out from drinking—not by answering the question, but by asking the senator if she had ever blacked out. He later apologized. . . .

"I didn't like some of the more partisan references and the tone, particularly with some of my colleagues," Mr. Flake told an audience in Boston, singling out Judge Kavanaugh's treatment of Ms. Klobuchar. But he said he might have been similarly angry if he had stood accused of sexual assault. . . .

"We all saw something about Judge Kavanaugh's temperament and character that day that should disqualify him from serving on the Supreme Court of the United States," [Senator Mazie] Hirono said. . . .

But Senator Charles E. Grassley, Republican of Iowa and the Judiciary Committee chairman, said Judge Kavanaugh could be excused for showing passion. . . .

"I don't think what he said is any different than what Justice Thomas said," Mr. Grassley said. . . .

Following the criticism that he was unable to control his emotions at the confirmation hearing, Justice Kavanaugh explained his response to questioning in the following opinion piece.

Brett M. Kavanaugh
I Am an Independent, Impartial Judge
Wall St. J. (Oct. 4, 2018)

As I explained [the night of my nomination], a good judge must be . . . a neutral and impartial arbiter who favors no political party, litigant or policy. As Justice Kennedy has stated, judges do not make decisions to reach a preferred result. Judges make decisions because the law and the Constitution compel the result. . . .

The Supreme Court must never be viewed as a partisan institution. . . . [I]f confirmed to the court, I would be . . . committed to deciding cases according to the Constitution and laws of the United States. . . .

After [meetings with senators] and after my initial hearing concluded, I was subjected to wrongful and sometimes vicious allegations. My time in high school and college, more than 30 years ago, has been ridiculously distorted. My wife and daughters have faced vile and violent threats.

Against that backdrop, I testified before the Judiciary Committee last Thursday to defend my family, my good name and my lifetime of public service. My hearing testimony was forceful and passionate. . . . I forcefully and passionately denied the allegation against me. At times, my testimony . . . reflected my overwhelming frustration at being wrongly accused, without corroboration, of horrible conduct completely contrary to my record and character. My statement and answers also reflected my deep distress at the unfairness of how this allegation has been handled.

I was very emotional last Thursday, more so than I have ever been. I might have been too emotional at times. I know that my tone was sharp, and I said a few things I should not have said. I hope everyone can understand that I was there as a son, husband and dad. . . .

NOTES AND QUESTIONS

1. Does emotion have a role to play in judicial decision-making? Judges themselves have failed to agree on the answer. *Compare Roe v. Wade*, 410 U.S. 113, 116 (1973) ("Our task, of course, is to resolve the issue by constitutional measurement, free of emotion and of predilection."), *with Jones v. Luebbers*, 359 F.3d 1005, 1013 (8th Cir. 2004) ("[W]e are not to hold judges to a superhuman standard that would allow no expressions of emotion. . . ."); *United States v. Weiss*, 491 F.2d 460, 468 (2d Cir. 1974) ("Judges, while expected to possess more than the average amount of self-restraint, are still only human. They do not possess limitless ability, once passion is aroused, to resist provocation."); *and Honken v. United States*, 42 F. Supp. 3d 937, 1143 (N.D. Iowa 2013) ("[T]he law does not require judges to refrain from expressing any emotion.").

2. In a series of important articles (see Further Reading below), Professor Terry Maroney has explored the roles of emotions in judicial decision-making. Many often assume, at least initially, that judges both should and can keep their emotions in check, so as not to somehow contaminate their proper decision-making process. Do you think they should, and do you think they can? In one article, Professor Maroney submits that when faced with emotions that may negatively impact decision-making, "[i]nstead of regarding emotion as a failure, judges may choose to face that emotion, seeking to respond thoughtfully to it." *See* Terry A. Maroney, *Emotional Regulation and Judicial Behavior*, 99 Cal. L. Rev. 1485, 1522 (2011). Under this view, judges should first seek to reframe and regulate their emotions, but when this is not possible, those emotions "can, and should, be integrated into judges' decisional and learning processes." *Id.* at 1525. Do you agree with this approach? Why or why not?

3. Consider the view: "The seat of knowledge is in the head; of wisdom, in the heart. We are sure to judge wrong, if we do not feel right." William Hazlitt, *Characteristics* (1823), reprinted in *Selected Essays of William Hazlitt* 223 (Geoffrey Keynes ed., 1946). To what extent do you agree or disagree, and why?

4. Scott Turow has observed that "it is . . . extreme and repellent crimes that provoke the highest emotions—anger, especially, even outrage—that in turn make rational deliberation problematic for investigators, prosecutors, judges, and juries." Scott Turow, *Ultimate Punishment: A Lawyer's Reflections on Dealing with the Death Penalty* 34 (2003) (quoted in Susan A. Bandes, *Repellent Crimes and Rational Deliberation: Emotion and the Death Penalty*, 33 Vt. L. Rev. 489, 490 (2009)). How would you describe the differences—among these legal personnel—in the contexts and effects of emotional engagement? How would you compare the societal impact of emotions in each cohort? And how, in your view, can the law best improve the current situations? To what extent did neuroscientific perspectives inform your answers? Should it?

5. "[E]motions in one domain influence . . . judgments, and decisions in a completely unrelated domain." Ozkan Eren & Naci Mocan, *Emotional Judges and Unlucky Juveniles*, 10 Am. Econ. J. 171, 200 (2018). Anger in one context, for example, may cause an individual to blame a person in a separate context. This phenomenon applies to judges no less than the general public. In a recent study, two scholars investigated the correlation between football game outcomes and judicial decisionmaking. They found that unexpected losses by the Louisiana State University football team correlated with increased sentence lengths imposed by Louisianan judges on juvenile defendants, with a disparate impact on black youth and the effect lasting a full week after the loss. *Id.* How might the judicial system counteract the influence of extraneous factors and emotions?

6. The general ban on hearsay was justified by the advisory committee because the traditional safeguards of the witness being under oath, in the personal presence of the trier of fact, and subject to cross-examination are not available for out of court statements, increasing the risk of undetected errors in perception, memory, narration, and deceit. A number of exceptions, however, have evolved when the risk of errors in perception, memory, narration, and deceit is believed to be lessened, and these exceptions are embodied in rules 803 and 804. FRE 803(5), creating an exception for recorded recollections, can be classified as an instance in which there is reduced concern for the chance of memory errors because the recollection was also recorded in a medium other than the individual's memory while it was still "fresh" in their mind. Other examples focus on an assumed reduced risk of deception, such as the Present Sense Impression Exception (PSI), Rule 803(1). The PSI applies to hearsay evidence when: (a) the statement describes the event in question; (b) the declarant perceived the event in person; and (c) the event and the statement were "substantially contemporaneous." This exception is generally thought to be premised on the assumption that contemporaneity limits a person's ability to lie and reduces the risk of memory errors. Similarly, FRE 803(2), the "excited utterance" exception, creates an exception for statements "relating to a startling event or condition, made while the declarant was under the stress of excitement that it caused." The advisory committee notes explicitly state that the belief underlying the exception is the declarant's

reduced ability to lie, stating "the circumstances may produce a condition of excitement which temporarily stills the capacity of reflection and produces utterances free of conscious fabrication." It should be apparent to the reader that the possible reduction in the risk of testimonial errors depend on psychological assumptions that may or may not be true. Steven Baicker-McKee, *The Excited Utterance Paradox*, 41 Seattle U. L. Rev. 111 (2017).

E. THE EMOTIONAL LEGISLATOR

Very little of the scholarly literature on law and emotions has considered the role of emotions in the activities of legislative personnel. One relatively unexplored question is: To what extent do law/emotion issues vary between litigant/juror/judge contexts and legislative contexts? In this latter context, legislators may not only have their own emotions to contend with, but will also be answerable to constituents, who are motivated by emotions to lesser or greater degrees. Professor Susan Bandes believes there are at least four important issues to consider.*

First, and most generally, to what extent should the unique context of legislative decision-making affect our assessment of the appropriate role of emotions in legislators' actions, in relation to the actions of jurors and judges?

Second, to what extent will or should legislation sometimes reflect an "identifiability bias," in which particularly emotionally salient episodes, such as high-visibility sex offenses or terrorist acts, directly prompt legislation, such as Megan's Law or the Patriot Act.

Third, to what extent should statutory regimes explicitly cater to the emotional needs of constituents—as would appear to be the case with so-called "angel acts," (which require the issuance of birth certificates for stillborn babies).**

Fourth, to what extent can some of the rapid spread of legislative approaches, among the states, be attributed to emotionally contagious "legislative epidemics"?***

NOTES AND QUESTIONS

1. How would you answer these four questions at present? What additional information would you like to have? Where, if at all, might neuroscientific studies fertilize your analysis?
2. All things considered, would you prefer to see a larger or smaller role for emotions in law? What tools might aid the transition you prefer? And what constraints do you see on that transition?
3. Reflecting on the chapter as a whole, what role, if any, do you think the neuroscience of emotions should play in legal arenas?

---

* Personal communication, Dec. 2012.
** *See* Carol Sanger, *"The Birth of Death": Stillborn Birth Certificates and the Problem for Law*, 100 Cal. L. Rev. 269 (2012).
*** Catherine L. Carpenter, *Legislative Epidemics: A Cautionary Tale of Criminal Laws That Sweep the Country*, 58 Buff. L. Rev. 1 (2010).

FURTHER READING

Science of Emotions:

Cognitive Neuroscience of Emotion (Richard D. Lane & Lynn Nadel eds., 2002).

Robert H. Frank, *Passions Within Reason: The Strategic Role of Emotions* (1988).

John T. Cacioppo & Wendi L. Gardner, *Emotion*, 50 Ann. Rev. Psychol. 191 (1999).

Philip A. Kragel, & Kevin S. LaBar, *Decoding the Nature of Emotion in the Brain*, 20 Trends Cogn. Scis. 444 (2016).

Ralph Adolphs & David J. Anderson, *The Neuroscience of Emotion: A New Synthesis* (2018).

Lisa Feldman Barrett, *How Emotions Are Made: The Secret Life of the Brain* (2017).

Elizabeth A. Phelps, *Emotion and Cognition: Insights from Studies of the Human Amygdala*, 57 Ann. Rev. Psychol. 27 (2006).

Elizabeth A. Phelps, Karolina M. Lempert & Peter Sokol-Hessner, *Emotion and Decision Making: Multiple Modularity Neural Circuits*, 37 Ann. Rev. Neurosci. 263 (2014).

Owen D. Jones, *Law, Emotions, and Behavioral Biology*, 39 Jurimetrics 283 (1999).

Mauricio R. Delgado & James G. Dilmore, *Social and Emotional Influences of Decision-Making and the Brain*, 9 Minn. J.L. Sci. & Tech. 899 (2008).

Kristen A. Lindquist et al., *The Brain Basis of Emotion: A Meta-Analytic Review*, 35 Behav. & Brain Scis. 121 (2012).

Tim Dalgleish, *The Emotional Brain*, 5 Nature Revs. Neurosci. 583 (2004).

Pankaj Sah & R. Frederick Westbrook, *The Circuit of Fear*, 454 Nature 589 (2008).

Law and the Emotions:

Susan A. Bandes & Jeremy A. Blumenthal, *Emotion and the Law*, 8 Ann. Rev. L. Soc. Sci. 161 (2012).

Susan A. Bandes, *The Passions of Law* (2001).

Federica Coppola, *The Emotional Brain and the Guilty Mind: Novel Paradigms of Culpability and Punishment* (2021).

John Mikhail, *Emotion, Neuroscience, and Law: A Comment on Darwin and Greene*, 3 Emotion Rev. 293 (2011).

Terry A. Maroney, *A Field Evolves: Introduction to the Special Section on Law and Emotion*, 8 Emotion Rev. 3 (2016).

Terry A. Maroney, *The Persistent Cultural Script of Judicial Dispassion*, 99 Cal. L. Rev. 629 (2011).

Terry A. Maroney, *Law and Emotion: A Proposed Taxonomy of an Emerging Field*, 30 L. & Hum. Behav. 119 (2006).

Terry A. Maroney, *Emotional Competence, "Rational Understanding," and the Criminal Defendant*, 43 Am. Crim. L. Rev. 1375 (2006).

Terry A. Maroney, *Emotional Regulation and Judicial Behavior*, 99 Cal. L. Rev. 1485 (2011).

Terry A. Maroney, *Angry Judges*, 65 Vand. L. Rev. 1205 (2012).

State v. Rizzo, 833 A.2d 363 (Conn. 2003).

Todd E. Pettys, *The Emotional Juror*, 76 Fordham L. Rev. 1609 (2007-2008).

Susan A. Bandes, *Repellent Crimes and Rational Deliberation: Emotion and the Death Penalty*, 33 Vt. L. Rev. 489 (2008-2009).

Eric A. Posner, *Law and the Emotions*, 89 Geo. L.J. 1977 (2001).

Katharine K. Baker, *Gender and Emotion in Criminal Law*, 28 Harv. J.L. & Gender 447 (2005).

CHAPTER 15

Lie Detection

Once you jump behind the skull, there's no hiding.
—Joel Huizenga, CEO of No Lie MRI[†]

A fundamental premise of our criminal trial system is that "the jury *is the lie detector."*
—Justice Clarence Thomas, *United States v. Sheffer*
(concurring)[††]

CHAPTER SUMMARY

This chapter:
- Discusses the historical roots of the polygraph, how a polygraph works, and the polygraph's legal standing in court and in other settings.
- Introduces the science of neuroscience-based lie detection techniques, including fMRI- and EEG-based techniques, as well as critiques of these methods and their potential applications to law.
- Presents recent cases involving neuroscience-based lie detection evidence.

INTRODUCTION

Throughout history and across civilizations, humans have repeatedly tried (and repeatedly failed) to develop reliable techniques and devices for distinguishing lies from truth. In Ancient Greece physicians took a pulse; in the Middle Ages "Ordeals" were used, such as making a man stick his tongue on a hot iron repeatedly. In the 20th century the polygraph was introduced, and in this chapter you will read about the methods that some believe will become prominent in the 21st century: brain-based lie detection.

Multiple types of brain-based lie detection techniques have been developed, and courts are already seeing such evidence proffered. Consider these two cases.

[†] Quoted in Margaret Talbot, *Duped: Can Brain Scans Uncover Lies?*, New Yorker, July 2, 2007, at 54.
[††] *United States v. Scheffer*, 523 U.S. 303 (1998) (quoting *United States v. Barnard*, 490 F.2d 907 (9th Cir. 1973)).

United States. v. Semrau

No. 07-10074 MI/P, 2010 WL 6845092 (W.D. Tenn. June 1, 2010)

PHAM, M.J. Dr. Lorne Allan Semrau was a licensed psychologist in Tennessee and a participating provider in the Medicare and Medicaid programs. . . . [B]etween 1999 and 2005, Dr. Semrau allegedly engaged in a scheme to defraud Medicare, Medicaid, and other health care benefit programs by submitting false and fraudulent claims for payment. . . .[4]

Dr. Steven J. Laken is the President and CEO of Cephos Corporation. . . . Cephos claims it uses "state-of-the-art technology that is unbiased and scientifically validated. We have offered expert testimony and have presented fMRI evidence in court." It further states that "[t]he source of lying is in the brain—that is what Cephos measures with our truth verification brain imaging service using fMRI technology. We provide independent, scientific validation that someone is telling the truth." . . . At the heart of Dr. Laken's lie detection method is fMRI. Functional MRI enables researchers to assess brain function "in a rapid, non-invasive manner with a high degree of both spatial and temporal accuracy." . . .

In an effort to support Dr. Semrau's defense that he did not act with the intent to defraud, sometime in or around December of 2009, Dr. Semrau's attorney, J. Houston Gordon, contacted Dr. Laken, to inquire about having a fMRI-based lie detection test. . . . Dr. Laken decided to conduct two separate fMRI tests on Dr. Semrau, . . . and concluded that Dr. Semrau was not deceptive. He further stated that based on his prior studies, "a finding such as this is 100% accurate in determining truthfulness from a truthful person." In conclusion, Dr. Laken found that "Dr. Semrau's brain indicates he is telling the truth in regards to not cheating or defrauding the government" and that his "brain indicates he is telling the truth in that he correctly provided AIMS tests as was instructed." . . .

Selvi v. Karnataka

7 SCC 263 (2010) (India)

K.B. BALAKRISHNAN, C.J., Delivering the Opinion of the Court. The legal questions in this batch of criminal appeals relate to the involuntary administration of certain scientific techniques, namely narcoanalysis, polygraph examination and the Brain Electrical Activation Profile (BEAP) test for the purpose of improving investigation efforts in criminal cases. This issue has received considerable attention since it involves tensions between the desirability of efficient investigation and the preservation of individual liberties. . . .

The respondents have contended that even if the compulsory administration of the impugned techniques amounts to a seemingly disproportionate intrusion into personal liberty, their investigative use is justifiable since there is a compelling public interest in eliciting information that could help in preventing criminal activities in the future.

---

4. In order to convict Dr. Semrau on the health care fraud charges, the government must prove that he "(1) knowingly devised a scheme or artifice to defraud a health care benefit program in connection with the delivery of or payment for health care benefits, items, or services; (2) executed or attempted to execute this scheme or artifice to defraud; and (3) acted with intent to defraud." . . .

Such utilitarian considerations hold some significance in light of the need to combat terrorist activities, insurgencies and organised crime. It has been argued that such exigencies justify some intrusions into civil liberties. . . . Reference was also made to the frequently discussed "Ticking Bomb" scenario. This hypothetical situation examines the choices available to investigators when they have reason to believe that the person whom they are interrogating is aware of the location of a bomb. The dilemma is whether it is justifiable to use torture or other improper means for eliciting information which could help in saving the lives of ordinary citizens. . . .

Even these short excerpts raise fundamental questions about the scientific merit, legal value, and moral appropriateness of using different types of brain-based lie detection methods in legal proceedings. For instance, although we often think about lie detection as being used to test alibis (e.g., "I was at work. I wasn't in the area where the crime took place."), *United States v. Semrau* shows that lie detection evidence may also be proffered as evidence of a defendant's prior mental state. Before reading the rest of the case later in the chapter, think about what types of information you would want to know about the lie detection methods if you were the judge in that case. Thinking back to Chapter 8 on scientific evidence, what Rules of Evidence are most applicable here? What if the same type of brain-based lie detection evidence was introduced at the sentencing phase to support a claim that the defendant was truly remorseful for any harm she caused? Would your admissibility decision be any different?

As you have seen throughout this book, context matters. The same science may be more or less applicable depending on the legal and policy circumstances. The Indian Supreme Court case excerpted above raises a question about the use of neuroscience-based lie detection in a national security context. Does your analysis or conclusion about the value of brain-based lie detection change if you're considering the use of lie detection technology to prevent terrorist attacks? To screen employees? To conduct a criminal investigation?

Answering questions such as these requires you to consider a question we've seen before in the course: If the new brain science (whatever its flaws) isn't used, what is the next best alternative the law employs? For instance, jurors may believe a witness based on the confidence with which the witness speaks, even if that witness is confidently deceiving them. Or jurors may rely upon cognitive biases, explicit or implicit, in reaching a conclusion that someone was (or was not) telling the truth. It should be recognized that in the law, and in our regular lives, we often do not have access to "ground truth" and must instead make a guess about the truth based on the available evidence.

The question in this chapter is whether (and how) brain-based lie detection evidence is (or can ever be) information that improves our guess about the likely truth of a statement. As you read the cases that follow, ask yourself whether brain-based lie detection, in general or in specific legal contexts, is useful, misleading, or simply irrelevant.

The chapter proceeds in three sections. Section A presents readings about a precursor to brain-based lie detection: the polygraph. You will read about the history of the polygraph, its legal standing, and its use in other contexts such as national defense and employee screening. Section B introduces brain-based lie detection, examining the different types of brain-based lie detection that have been proffered in legal proceedings. Section C concludes with a series of critical perspectives on these lie detection techniques.

A. THE POLYGRAPH

1. History of the Polygraph

Henry T. Greely & Judy Illes

Neuroscience-Based Lie Detection: The Urgent Need for Regulation

33 Am. J.L. & Med. 377, 385-86 (2007)

Human efforts at lie detection must date to near the origin of our species; and, as some evidence points to the existence of intentional deception by other animals, lie detection may well predate us. As soon as humans began to lie, other humans would need to assess whether they were being told the truth. All of us, often without consciously thinking about it, frequently assess the credibility of information, looking, among other things, for evidence that we are being lied to. We look and listen for signs of deception or nervousness. In some cases, we seek truth by coercion, either by legal compulsion ("I swear to tell the truth, the whole truth, and nothing but the truth") or, in some times and places, by physical compulsion, including torture. . . .

Although disputes exist about who should be given priority for the modern polygraph machine, many trace the concept to William Moulton Marston's early research on the link between deception and blood pressure. Marston, who received his bachelor's degree, law degree, and Ph.D. in psychology from Harvard, began to work on using systolic blood pressure as a marker of deception in 1915. . . . From then until his death in 1947, Marston continued to improve his lie detection devices and to promote their widespread use. The _Frye_ case,* which for many years set the standard for admissibility of scientific evidence in federal court (and continues to play that role in some state courts), revolved around whether Marston's expert testimony about a polygraph examination that he claimed cleared a murder defendant should have been admitted in evidence. The court held that the testimony was properly excluded because the technology lacked general acceptance in the scientific community and affirmed the conviction.

Polygraphs measure several physiological features that are associated with nervousness or stress, such as systolic blood pressure (the first and more rapidly variable number in the familiar blood pressure measurement of, for example, 125/75), heart rate, breathing rate, and skin sweatiness (measuring the electrical conductivity of skin, known as galvanic skin response). The polygraph has been widely used in the United States for various purposes; a National Research Council (NRC) committee estimates that several hundred thousand polygraph examinations are conducted each year in the United States. American courts, however, have never generally considered it sufficiently reliable for its results to be admitted into evidence. . . .

---

* [Discussed in Chapter 6.—Eds.]

2. Polygraph's Use in Court

United States v. Matusiewicz

155 F. Supp. 3d 482 (D. Del. 2015)

[This is a memorandum opinion regarding admissibility of polygraph evidence. Defendants were on trial for conspiracy, interstate stalking, and cyberstalking of Christine Belford. Defendants sought to portray Belford as an unfit mother in a custody dispute between Belford and her ex-husband. This included alleging that Belford sexually abused her oldest daughter. As part of this claim, the defendants underwent polygraph testing to prove the veracity of the sexual abuse claims. Later, during trial, the prosecution called the validity of the polygraph testing into question. In an effort to boost the validity of the earlier tests, the defendants underwent a second polygraph test in which the examiner asked whether they were being truthful during the first polygraph test. Defendants then sought to introduce these second polygraph test results. Judge McHugh denied this request in the following opinion. — EDS.]

MCHUGH, D.J. [The court describes the facts of the case.] Substantively, as expressed on the record during trial, the central basis for my ruling was that even under the unique circumstances of this case, the polygraphs were for all practical purposes still being offered as direct evidence of Defendants' guilt or innocence, for which there remains scant support under American law. In *United States v. Scheffer*, 523 U.S. 303, (1998), in upholding a rule barring use of polygraphs in military courts, the Supreme Court comprehensively reviewed decisions from state and federal courts, and concluded that "there is simply no consensus that polygraph evidence is reliable." *Id.* at 309. Even after acknowledging that some circuits have held the door open for possible admission of polygraphs, the Court went on to note that "[w]hatever their approach, state and federal courts continue to express doubt about whether such evidence is reliable." *Id.* at 312. The proffer here was even more problematic, as Defendants sought to introduce polygraphs about polygraphs.

In *Scheffer*, the Supreme Court also refused to attach any legal significance to internal use of polygraphs by governmental agencies, and specifically rejected an argument that such use must necessarily render the tests reliable. *Id.* In the Court's words: "Such limited, out of court uses of polygraph techniques obviously differ in character from, and carry less severe consequences than, the use of polygraphs as evidence in a criminal trial. They do not establish the relative reliability of polygraphs as trial evidence." *Id.* at 312, n. 8.*

[The court discusses prejudice to the prosecution due to the lateness of the evidence.]

In opposing admissibility at trial, the Government relied most heavily on *United States v. Kubini*, No. 11-14, 2015 WL 418220 (W.D.Pa. Feb. 2, 2015). Defendant there took a polygraph of his own volition while under investigation for fraud, and sought to admit the results into evidence. No *Daubert* hearing was conducted, as the court concluded that the polygraph would be inadmissible regardless. In excluding the

---

* I placed no weight on the Government's argument that the use of polygraphs usurps the function of the jury, as that portion of the Court's opinion, Part IIB, did not command a majority of the Justices.

polygraphs, Judge Fischer cited a multitude of factors, one of which the Government stressed in this case, that the polygraphs were for all practical purposes hearsay, because they represented an attempt by the defendants to introduce their out-of-court statements for the truth. *Id.* at 8. Many of the other factors mentioned in *Kubini* carried weight here: the exams were conducted years after the fact when the defendants were acutely aware of the significance of their answers; the Government was not given the opportunity to participate; a mini-trial would ensue concerning the art of polygraphy; and there was a meaningful risk of jury confusion by introducing new polygraphs with different questions. *Id.* at 13-17.

[The court notes a lack of Supreme Court approval of polygraph evidence since *Scheffer.*]

Nor did I find that the consensus of the scientific community visibly changed since *Scheffer*. The National Academy of Sciences appointed a Committee to Review the Scientific Evidence of the Polygraph. Its report, *The Polygraph and Lie Detection*, (Washington, DC: The National Academies Press, 2003),6 comprehensively reviewed the field of polygraphy, and the conclusions reached only reinforced the doubts expressed in *Scheffer*, including the following:

> ***Polygraph Accuracy*** *Almost a century of research in scientific psychology and physiology provides little basis for the expectation that a polygraph test could have extremely high accuracy.*

> ***Theoretical Basis*** *The theoretical rationale for the polygraph is quite weak, especially in terms of differential fear, arousal, or other emotional states that are triggered in response to relevant or comparison questions.*

> ***Research Progress*** *Research on the polygraph has not progressed over time in the manner of a typical scientific field. It has not accumulated knowledge or strengthened its scientific underpinnings in any significant manner.*

> ***Realism of Evidence*** *The research on polygraph accuracy fails in important ways to reflect critical aspects of field polygraph testing, even for specific-incident investigation.*

As noted above, Defendants did not request a *Daubert* hearing or represent that they were prepared to establish the scientific reliability of polygraphs. Their burden would have been substantial. The general problem of reliability was made more acute because the defense sought to introduce polygraphs intended to prove the reliability and accuracy of other polygraphs, effectively doubling down on a procedure viewed already with suspicion by the courts. . . .

For the reasons set forth above, Defendants' request to present testimony about the polygraphs taken during trial was denied.

United States v. Scheffer

523 U.S. 303 (1998)

JUSTICE THOMAS delivered the opinion of the Court. . . . This case presents the question whether Military Rule of Evidence 707,* which makes polygraph evidence

---

* [At the time this case was decided, this was the text of *Rule 707. Polygraph Examinations*: "(a) Notwithstanding any other provision of law, the results of a polygraph examination, the opinion of a polygraph examiner, or any reference to an offer to take, failure to take, or taking of a polygraph examination, shall not be admitted into evidence. (b) Nothing in this section is intended to exclude from evidence statements made during a polygraph examination which are otherwise admissible."—EDS.]

inadmissible in court-martial proceedings, unconstitutionally abridges the right of accused members of the military to present a defense. We hold that it does not. . . .

State and federal governments unquestionably have a legitimate interest in ensuring that reliable evidence is presented to the trier of fact in a criminal trial. Indeed, the exclusion of unreliable evidence is a principal objective of many evidentiary rules. . . .

The contentions of respondent and the dissent notwithstanding, there is simply no consensus that polygraph evidence is reliable. To this day, the scientific community remains extremely polarized about the reliability of polygraph techniques. Some studies have concluded that polygraph tests overall are accurate and reliable. Others have found that polygraph tests assess truthfulness significantly less accurately—that scientific field studies suggest the accuracy rate of the "control question technique" polygraph is "little better than could be obtained by the toss of a coin," that is, 50 percent.

This lack of scientific consensus is reflected in the disagreement among state and federal courts concerning both the admissibility and the reliability of polygraph evidence.* Although some Federal Courts of Appeals have abandoned the per se rule excluding polygraph evidence, leaving its admission or exclusion to the discretion of district courts under *Daubert*,** at least one Federal Circuit has recently reaffirmed its per se ban, and another recently noted that it has "not decided whether polygraphy has reached a sufficient state of reliability to be admissible." Most States maintain per se rules excluding polygraph evidence. New Mexico is unique in making polygraph evidence generally admissible without the prior stipulation of the parties and without significant restriction. Whatever their approach, state and federal courts continue to express doubt about whether such evidence is reliable.

The approach taken by the President in adopting Rule 707 excluding polygraph evidence in all military trials is a rational and proportional means of advancing the legitimate interest in barring unreliable evidence. Although the degree of reliability of polygraph evidence may depend upon a variety of identifiable factors, there is simply no way to know in a particular case whether a polygraph examiner's conclusion is accurate, because certain doubts and uncertainties plague even the best polygraph exams. Individual jurisdictions therefore may reasonably reach differing conclusions as to whether polygraph evidence should be admitted. We cannot say, then, that presented with such widespread uncertainty, the President acted arbitrarily or disproportionately in promulgating a per se rule excluding all polygraph evidence. . . .

It is equally clear that Rule 707 serves a second legitimate governmental interest: Preserving the court members' core function of making credibility determinations in criminal trials. A fundamental premise of our criminal trial system is that "the jury is the lie detector." Determining the weight and credibility of witness testimony, therefore, has long been held to be the "part of every case [that] belongs to the jury, who are presumed to be fitted for it by their natural intelligence and their practical knowledge of men and the ways of men."

---

* Prior to *Daubert*, neither federal nor state courts found any Sixth Amendment obstacle to the categorical rule. Nothing in *Daubert* foreclosed, as a constitutional matter, per se exclusionary rules for certain types of expert or scientific evidence.

** [Discussed in Chapter 8.—EDS.]

By its very nature, polygraph evidence may diminish the jury's role in making credibility determinations. The common form of polygraph test measures a variety of physiological responses to a set of questions asked by the examiner, who then interprets these physiological correlates of anxiety and offers an opinion to the jury about whether the witness often, as in this case, the accused was deceptive in answering questions about the very matters at issue in the trial. Unlike other expert witnesses who testify about factual matters outside the jurors' knowledge, such as the analysis of fingerprints, ballistics, or DNA found at a crime scene, a polygraph expert can supply the jury only with another opinion, in addition to its own, about whether the witness was telling the truth. Jurisdictions, in promulgating rules of evidence, may legitimately be concerned about the risk that juries will give excessive weight to the opinions of a polygrapher, clothed as they are in scientific expertise and at times offering, as in respondent's case, a conclusion about the ultimate issue in the trial. Such jurisdictions may legitimately determine that the aura of infallibility attending polygraph evidence can lead jurors to abandon their duty to assess credibility and guilt. Those jurisdictions may also take into account the fact that a judge cannot determine, when ruling on a motion to admit polygraph evidence, whether a particular polygraph expert is likely to influence the jury unduly. . . .

STEVENS, J., dissenting.

Reliability.   There are a host of studies that place the reliability of polygraph tests at 85% to 90%. While critics of the polygraph argue that accuracy is much lower, even the studies cited by the critics place polygraph accuracy at 70%. . . . Of course, within the broad category of lie detector evidence, there may be a wide variation in both the validity and the relevance of particular test results. Questions about the examiner's integrity, independence, choice of questions, or training in the detection of deliberate attempts to provoke misleading physiological responses may justify exclusion of specific evidence. But such questions are properly addressed in adversary proceedings; they fall far short of justifying a blanket exclusion of this type of expert testimony.

There is no legal requirement that expert testimony must satisfy a particular degree of reliability to be admissible. . . . The Court's reliance on potential unreliability as a justification for a categorical rule of inadmissibility reveals that it is "overly pessimistic about the capabilities of the jury and of the adversary system generally. Vigorous cross-examination, presentation of contrary evidence, and careful instruction on the burden of proof are the traditional and appropriate means of attacking shaky but admissible evidence." . . .

The Role of the Jury.   It is the function of the jury to make credibility determinations. . . . There is, of course, some risk that some "juries will give excessive weight to the opinions of a polygrapher, clothed as they are in scientific expertise." In my judgment, however, it is much more likely that juries will be guided by the instructions of the trial judge concerning the credibility of expert as well as lay witnesses. The strong presumption that juries will follow the court's instructions, applies to exculpatory as well as inculpatory evidence. Common sense suggests that the testimony of disinterested third parties that is relevant to the jury's credibility determination will assist rather than impair the jury's deliberations. As with the reliance on the potential unreliability of this type of evidence, the reliance on a fear that the average jury is not able to assess the weight of this testimony reflects a distressing lack of confidence in the intelligence of the average American. . . .

NOTES AND QUESTIONS

1. Justice Thomas writes that "[a] fundamental premise of our criminal trial system is that 'the jury is the lie detector.'" Does this make polygraph evidence more or less useful in court? Consider Justice Stevens's view that "the testimony of disinterested third parties that is relevant to the jury's credibility determination will assist rather than impair the jury's deliberations." Which view of the polygraph is better? Can the jury do its job better if they are substantially more confident in whether a person was telling the truth or not, due, in part, to polygraph evidence?

2. Justice Stevens suggests that "juries will be guided by the instructions of the trial judge concerning the credibility of expert as well as lay witnesses." If you allowed testimony about a polygraph test to be admitted, what instructions would you give the jury? What if the judge does not have the scientific knowledge to give adequate instructions? Should a judge in this situation err on the side of excluding or including evidence? *See* Justin Amirian, *Weighing the Admissibility of fMRI Technology Under FRE 403: For the Law, fMRI Changes Everything—and Nothing*, 41 Fordham Urb. L.J. 715 (2013).

3. If one believes that polygraphs can fail and that human jurors can also fail, in their respective efforts to assess the truthfulness of statements, is there any meaningful distinction between human failure and scientific failure?

4. Although not typically allowed as evidence in court, or for use in employee screening, the polygraph is nevertheless encountered regularly in a variety of legal settings. For instance, police departments often use polygraph examinations as part of their investigative work. In civil litigation or private settlement, polygraphs may be used in the course of divorce proceedings and negotiations. Are concerns about polygraph use the same or different in each context?

5. In *Wilson v. Corestaff Servs.*, 900 N.Y.S.2d 639 (N.Y. Sup. Ct. 2010), a trial court judge considered a motion from a plaintiff suing her former employer. The plaintiff was seeking a *Frye* hearing on the admissibility of fMRI lie detection evidence to bolster the credibility of a key witness. She wanted to put her key witness through an fMRI lie detector to show that his testimony supporting her case was indeed true. This was one of the first times a court had encountered the fMRI lie detection question, as the trial judge found that "[a]pparently, there is no reported case in New York or in the rest of the country which deals with the admissibility of the results of fMRI test." The plaintiff's motion justified the request on the grounds that "the fMRI could show 'that to a very high probability' that Armstrong 'is being truthful when he testifies.'" The judge found that "since credibility is a matter solely for the jury and is clearly within the ken of the jury, [the] plaintiff has failed to meet this key prong of the *Frye* test and no other inquiry is required." But the judge also added in dicta that "the scientific literature raises serious issues about the lack of acceptance of the fMRI test in the scientific community to show a person's past mental state or to gauge credibility." Do you agree with the trial judge's verdict? Would you have at least proceeded

to conduct the *Frye* hearing? What additional information would you want to know about the evidence? What if the evidence were being offered on behalf of a defendant facing the death penalty? Would this change your analysis about admissibility?

6. A 2015 study used transcranial direct current stimulation (tDCS) to improve lie detection in limited settings. This improvement was modest, only improving accuracy from 54% to 59.5%. However, consider a future in which this technology drastically improves lie detection and is available to jurors. Is this a fair middle ground between Justice Thomas and Justice Stevens's views? *See* Sophie Sowden et al., *Transcranial Current Stimulation of the Temporoparietal Junction Improves Lie Detection*, 25 Current Biology 2447 (2015).

7. Law professor Nita Farahany asks in a TED Talk: "When technology can read minds, how will we protect our privacy?" Her answer: "Brains need special protection" because our "cognitive liberty" is at stake. Farahany implores that "[t]he time has come for us to call for a cognitive liberty revolution." Nita Farahany, *When Technology Can Read Minds, How Will We Protect Our Privacy?*, TED (Nov. 2018). What would such a revolution look like in the law?

8. To what extent is involuntary neurotechnological mind reading more problematic than the involuntary "natural" mind reading we do every day, as we attempt to infer what others are thinking and feeling? For discussion of this issue, see Jesper Ryberg, *Neuroscience, Mind Reading and Mental Privacy*, 23 Res Publica 197 (2017).

3. Polygraph Use in National Defense

Office of Counterintelligence, Dep't of Energy
Polygraph Examination Regulations
10 CFR Part 709, Docket No. CN-03-RM-01, RIN 1992-AA33 (2003)*

Under section 3152(a) of the National Defense Authorization Act for Fiscal Year 2002 (NDAA for FY 2002), DOE is obligated to prescribe regulations for a new counterintelligence polygraph program the stated purpose of which is ". . . to minimize the potential for release or disclosure of classified data, materials, or information" (42 U.S.C. 7383h-1(a).) Section 3152(b) requires DOE to ". . . take into account the results of the Polygraph Review," which is defined by section 3152(e) to mean ". . . the review of the Committee to Review the Scientific Evidence on the Polygraph of the National Academy of Sciences" (42 U.S.C. 7383h-1(b), (e)). . . .

. . . The [National Academy's] main conclusion is that lack of evidence of validity and accuracy justifies not using polygraph examinations for screening purposes. In arriving at this conclusion, the NAS also took into account the expense associated with invalid polygraph results, the potential loss of competent or highly skilled individuals due to false positives or the fear of such a test result, and claims of adverse impact on civil liberties. The NAS also acknowledged but considered less significant the deterrent effect that the prospect of being polygraphed could have on

---

* [This document served as the notice of proposed rulemaking, published by the Department of Energy (DOE), regarding its consideration of whether to retain or to modify its Polygraph Examination Regulations. —EDS.]

employment applicants who are national security risks. In short, what NAS conducted was a cost-benefit analysis that (given the nature of the costs and benefits) inevitably rested in no small part on value judgments made by the NAS. There is nothing inappropriate about this approach in light of the NAS's mission and charge.

DOE, however, has a significantly different mission—one that is intimately involved in science, but directed to a particular end—the national security of the United States; therefore, not surprisingly, section 3152 gave the Department a particular charge for its polygraph program. That charge was not to devise a program based on the NAS's or the Department's own weighing of costs and benefits based on its own value judgments. Rather, Congress directed DOE to develop a polygraph program focused on minimizing the risk of release or disclosure of classified information. That amounts to a Congressional specification that the most important cost about which DOE should be concerned is the risk of release or disclosure of classified information. DOE believes that Congress's judgment in that regard was reasonable. Given that DOE's classified information consists in significant measure of information regarding nuclear weapons of mass destruction, the consequences of compromise of that information can be profoundly significant. Those consequences make it sensible for Congress to conclude that DOE's priority should be on deterrence and detection of potential security risks with a secondary priority of mitigating the consequences of false positives and false negatives. Moreover, whatever may be the importance of other considerations, DOE believes that at this time, when the United States is engaged in hostilities precisely in order to address the potentially disastrous consequences that may flow from weapons of mass destruction falling into the wrong hands, it is under a particular obligation to make sure that no action that it takes be susceptible to misinterpretation as a relaxation of controls over information concerning these kinds of weapons. For all these reasons, while fully respecting the questions the NAS has raised about the use of polygraphs as a screening tool, DOE does not believe it can endorse the NAS's conclusion that the tool should be laid down.

Perhaps in recognition that its main conclusion was less tenable in the context of Federal agencies with national security missions established by law, the NAS went on to conclude in the alternative that if polygraph screening is to be used at all, it should only be used as a trigger for follow-up detailed investigations and not as a sole basis for personnel action (NAS Polygraph Review, p. 5). This alternative conclusion appears to DOE to be much more compatible with the priority DOE is statutorily invited to place on minimizing the potential for release or disclosure of classified information. It is also consistent with the way DOE currently uses screening polygraphs.

Under DOE's current regulations, neither DOE nor its contractors may take an adverse personnel action against an individual solely on the basis of a polygraph result indicating deception (10 CFR 709.25). If, after an initial polygraph examination, there are remaining unresolved issues, DOE must advise the individual and provide an opportunity for the individual to undergo an additional polygraph examination. If the additional polygraph examination is not sufficient to resolve the matter, DOE must undertake a comprehensive investigation using the polygraph examination as an investigative lead (10 CFR 709.15(b)). In DOE's view, this regulatory scheme is consistent both with the NAS's alternative conclusion and with the statutory priority on minimizing release or disclosure of classified information. . . .

B. NEUROSCIENCE-BASED LIE DETECTION

In this section you will be presented with materials on different types of brain-based lie detection methods that have been introduced into legal proceedings. You may find it useful to refer back to Chapter 4 on brain monitoring methods when you read the testimony from the expert witnesses, as they will talk about methods you have learned about: electroencephalography (EEG) and functional Magnetic Resonance Imaging (fMRI).

1. Lie Detection Using Electroencephalography (EEG)

In this section you'll read an excerpt of Dr. Lawrence Farwell's testimony — concerning EEG-based lie detection—on behalf of Terry Harrington, during Harrington's appeal of his murder conviction in Iowa. Here is the background of the conviction, as summarized by the Iowa Supreme Court in *Harrington v. State*, 659 N.W.2d 509 (2003):

> Sometime after midnight on July 22, 1977, security guard John Schweer was murdered at a car dealership in Council Bluffs, Iowa. At the time, Schweer, a retired police captain, was a night watchman for several car dealerships in the area. Schweer had been shot, and a 12 gauge shotgun shell was found in the vicinity of the crime. Footprints and dog prints were also discovered near Schweer's body.
>
> Harrington, who was seventeen at the time, was charged with Schweer's murder and was ultimately convicted, primarily on the testimony of a juvenile accomplice, Kevin Hughes. Hughes gave the following account of July 22, 1977. Shortly after midnight, Hughes, Harrington, and another juvenile, Curtis McGhee, went to the dealership with the intent to steal a beige Toronado. Hughes waited in Harrington's car while Harrington and McGhee walked around a building to find the desired automobile. Harrington had a shotgun. Shortly after Harrington and McGhee left, Hughes heard a gun shot. Then Harrington and McGhee came running back. Harrington said he had just shot a cop.
>
> Hughes was impeached by the defense with prior statements he had made implicating other persons in the crime. Hughes had separately named three other men as the killer. Each man was ultimately discovered to have an alibi before Hughes finally fingered Harrington. Hughes . . . conceded he was "a confessed liar," having lied "about five or six times talking about this case." Hughes acknowledged that he visited the murder scene with the police and prosecutor and told them what he thought they wanted to hear. At the time, Hughes was being held on various theft and burglary charges and "he was tired of [being in jail]." He admitted that these charges were dropped after he agreed to testify against Harrington and McGhee.
>
> The physical evidence linking Harrington to the crime was minimal. . . .*
>
> Harrington and McGhee were both convicted of first-degree murder in separate trials. Harrington's appeal failed, as did a subsequent postconviction relief action in which he claimed that Hughes' testimony was perjured. Harrington also unsuccessfully sought habeas corpus relief in federal court. He is currently serving a life sentence without the possibility of parole.

---

* The murder weapon itself was never found. Additionally, even though plaster casts were made of footprints found at the murder scene, the police did not compare these casts to Harrington's feet.

The court summarized the procedural posture:

> Terry Harrington appeals a district court decision denying his application for post-conviction relief. He claims the court erred in holding his claims were time barred. In addition, he faults the district court for failing to vacate his first-degree murder conviction and order a new trial on the basis of newly discovered evidence consisting of a recantation by the State's primary witness, police investigative reports implicating another suspect in the crime, and "brain fingerprinting" test results. Harrington also rests error on the court's refusal to grant relief based on a due process violation resulting from the prosecution's failure to produce the police reports at the time of Harrington's criminal trial. The State disputes Harrington's allegations of error and affirmatively asserts that Harrington's appeal is untimely.

The Iowa Supreme Court concluded that Harrington's appeal was timely, and that his claims below were not time-barred. It held: "Under the circumstances presented by the record before us, we cannot be confident that the result of Harrington's murder trial would have been the same had the exculpatory information been made available to him. We hold, therefore, that Harrington's due process right to a fair trial was violated by the State's failure to produce the police reports documenting their investigation of an alternative suspect in Schweer's murder." Consequently, the court reversed the district court judgment and remanded for an order vacating Harrington's conviction and sentence, and granting him a new trial.*

Although the Iowa Supreme Court did not reach the legal significance of the post-conviction EEG evidence, Farwell's testimony below is nonetheless useful as vivid illustration of how brain-based lie detection evidence can enter a legal proceeding. Following the testimony is an excerpt from one of the published scientific articles that Dr. Farwell relies upon in making his claims in this case. As you read the science article, and examine the related figures, try to generate questions that you would ask the study's authors if you were cross-examining one of them on the witness stand. One question you may have is: how easy is it to beat the test? To help you answer this question we've provided an excerpt about counter-measures that can be used to defeat an EEG-based lie detection approach as used by Farwell.

Testimony of Dr. Lawrence Farwell

in *Harrington v. State* (Nov. 14, 2000)

DIRECT EXAMINATION

Q: (KENNEDY): . . . [I]n your current position, as psychophysiologist, are you focusing on a certain line of work or a certain area of specialization?

A: (FARWELL): Yes. And I have been since I first started working for the CIA in 1991. And that is specifically what has come to be known as brain fingerprinting.

---

* [The case was subsequently dismissed. After it was learned that the prosecutors had obtained false testimony to frame him (and a co-defendant), Harrington and the co-defendant sued the prosecutors for a violation of civil rights under Section 1983. This raised a legal question about whether the prosecutors enjoyed absolute immunity in such cases. The federal district court and Eighth Circuit Court of Appeals found only qualified immunity, and the case went up to the United States Supreme Court, where oral argument was heard in 2009. But after the county settled, for $12 million, the Supreme Court dismissed the case. —EDS.]

There has been some evolution of technology, but over the years, it's been essentially the same practice, and that is detecting concealed information in the human brain in order determine to whether an individual has or doesn't have particular information in his brain, often with forensic applications. . . .

Q: If you then invented the brain fingerprinting, you are saying that although you invented it, it's based on science, accepted science from other scientists?

A: Right. Basically, what I measure is event related brain potentials. Those are specific patterns of brain activity that indicates that a certain cognitive activity has taken place. By measuring those event related brain potentials, we can tell what information a person recognizes or doesn't recognize. Now, the specific brain wave component that I began with when I first—or I should say brain wave pattern that I began with when I started this, first developed this invention, was the P300. That was discovered in 1965 by Sutton, et al.

Q: . . . The P300, then, is what? Explain that, please.

A: It is an event related brain potential, and what an event related brain potential is, is a specific pattern of brain wave activity that is related to an event. That's why we call it event related. The event that a P300 is related to is the event of taking note of something significant called context updating. This has been published in hundreds of studies in many different labs throughout the world. . . .

Q: And you used the P300 in your brain fingerprinting test?

A: That's correct. Initially I started with the P300, and what happened over time, is that I discovered that there was a little bit more going on after the P300 was over. That happened, by the way, throughout the course of development of cognitive psychophysiology and event related potential. Initially, papers were looking at short potentials that only had to do with sensory processing, and started to look at things that took place a little longer after the stimulus, which had to do with cognitive processing. What I have done is extended out beyond the P300 and looked at the pattern that takes place a little farther out in time. However, in order to conduct this brain fingerprinting, and to get the results that we have gotten with Terry Harrington, all I really need is the P300. . . .

Q: To cut to the heart of the study again, I'm asking you to simplify it way down. You asked college students questions about events that you had researched . . . and the words and pictures, whatever, that you flashed on the screen, what did that tell you about those college students?

A: What it told us, if they got a P300, in response to the items that were specific to that crime or that event, then we knew they recognized those items. That's what a P300 means. It means you recognize something as significant. You take note of it. So that's what that indicated.

Q: What are the differences between these words or phrases that you use?

A: All right. We use three types of stimuli or words or pictures. Usually we use words. One type of stimulus is called a target. These are items that we know the person knows, we are sure the person knows, because we have talked to them about them. We give them a list of them. In many cases, these are details, for example, about a crime that we know he knows, because he has been told them in a trial or because of information that he has some independent access to. We are sure he knows them. We give him a list of them, and we say, "When one of these comes up on the screen, you push a special button." We are very certain he is going to recognize and take note of those. And those are going to emit a P300. You recognize them, he takes note of them. We know we will get a P300 from those, also a MERMER extending out beyond, extending out into a longer time window in looking at the brain wave data from a P300, which will be clearer when I have showed the plots. So we have that stimulus type called targets where we know he is going to recognize them, we know we will get a P300 and a MERMER. A second type of stimuli are irrelevants. They have nothing to do with the crime, they have nothing to do with the person in particular. We know he is not going to recognize those as relevant, and we know we are not going to get that P300 or MERMER response. So those are the two types, sort of set a standard, here is what his brain wave looks like when he recognizes the stimulus, here is what it looks like when it's irrelevant to him, or here is what it looks like when he has that information in his brain, here is what it looks like when he doesn't have that response.

Then we present, mixed in with these others, a third type of stimulus. We don't tell him which ones these are. These are called probes, and these are stimuli that are relevant to the situation we are investigating, say the crime, but that he would have no way of knowing, unless he did it. So if he shows a P300, and a MERMER in response to these probes, that provides evidence that he actually has that information about the crime stored in his brain, because those are significant to him. If he doesn't have the information stored in his brain, then he won't even know which ones are the probes to him. They will look like irrelevants, and the response will look like the irrelevants response. It will not have a P300 in them. It won't have a MERMER.

Q: You keep mentioning MERMER. Would you explain briefly what the MERMERS are as compared to the P300?

A: Yes. The P300 is a positive response. By positive, I mean electrically positive component, maximal at the parietal midline area of the brain, the top of the back of the head. And it indicates that a person is taking note of the stimulus. Now, what happened during my research initially in the FBI study where we were detecting FBI agents, I noticed after this positive response, there was a negative deflection that seemed to take place consistently, whenever that positive response happened. It's been found in other labs as well, at least in one of the labs as well at that time, and more since, I believe. And I started to think, well, maybe there is more to this than we thought. So the positive deflection of the P300 followed by a negative deflection — By a negative, I mean negative voltage on the scalp, constitutes the MERMER. I also am convinced that there are phasic changes, short term changes in the frequency of signals that take place that don't show up in the signal averaging that we use to get event related brain potentials, and these are interesting scientific ideas, and I have some data on that, but basically the MERMER is frosting on the cake, of which the P300 is the cake.

Q: What about the probes? The probes are what they claim they don't know, the subject claims?

A: That's correct. What we do when we are structuring the probes, is we examine the information we have about the situation, say about the crime, and we come up with things that the subject has never been told, say, in courtroom proceedings or in interrogations that we know about, but would know from having committed the crime, and then we say to the subject—we sit them down and say, all right, you say you didn't commit the crime. Then if you didn't commit the crime, then you wouldn't know this particular item about the crime. Would you have ever been told this for any other reason? No, I don't know that. And we go through a list of them. We say, would you recognize this or would you have the answer to this question? Would you know this information about a crime? They say no, I wasn't there, so I don't know that.

So we verify with the subject that he is claiming not to know any of those items that become probe stimuli before the test. Then what the test tells us is in fact whether that information is stored in his brain or not.

Q: Would there be any way for somebody to beat the test?

A: No. Well, put it this way. Let me give an example of where this—what we are measuring. I think that will clarify. Let's say that that that door opens and an elephant comes into the room. Now, everyone in the room who has eyesight is going to notice that. We now have a picture of what is going on in the room stored in our brains, there is a scheme, there is a map of what is going on here of what the physical environment are, what—the rules, what we can expect stored in our brains. If an elephant comes in the room, we have to change that picture to include some new information, namely an elephant. We have to update our internal picture of where we are and what's going on. It's a basic survival function. We have to do it to survive in a changing environment. So when the elephant comes in the room through the door, we are all going to notice it, and say, uh-huh, yes, okay. Now we have an elephant in the room. After we have noticed it, we can start thinking okay, now what am I going to try to do about it. Maybe I will feed the elephant. Maybe I will exit through the back door. When that brain's response recognizing something significant happened takes place, that's when we pick up the P300, that's when we pick up the information, that's when we get the result. So we get our result when they take note of the elephant, not when they decide what to do about it.

When that probe stimulus comes up that is relevant to the crime, the first thing he thinks is uh-huh, yeah, I recognize that. That was the place where the victim was when he was shot, or whatever it is he recognizes, that that is the point at which we pick up our information. Anything else would happen later.

Q: A couple more things, Dr. Farwell. Are there any situations where the brain fingerprinting test would not work on a subject?

A: I wouldn't say there aren't any situations where it wouldn't work in the sense of not working accurately. But there are situations where we simply can't apply it.

CROSS-EXAMINATION

Q: (CROWL): For your machine to work, does your memory have to be perfect?

A: No.

Q: Does your memory have to be good?

A: No.

Q: So your P300 response will come up on things that I don't even remember?

A: No, it won't. . . .

Q: Okay. A probe is a word you flashed across the screen for a split second; right?

A: It's a phrase flashed for four-tenths of a second.

Q: And what were the phrases that you flashed that were the probes?

A: Across street, parked cars, weeds and grass. . . . Drainage ditch, by trees, and straight ahead.

Q: Straight ahead. Let's start with that one. Now, if you flashed straight ahead to everybody in this room, what are you going to get for a response?

A: Completely unpredictable. If I don't set the context, who knows what I will get. . . .

Q: How is straight ahead significant for this case?

A: Well, if you refer back . . . I talked to Terry Harrington.

Q: Before the test or after the test?

A: Before. . . . And I outlined for him and refreshed his memory on the details about the crime that he knew, or the alleged crime, I should say. . . . And I walked him through the crime scene and the specific events that were testified to by Hughes.

Q: Do you know what photographs Mr. Harrington saw, pre-trial or at trial?

A: I don't know whether what he told me was truthful or not about what photographs he had seen.

Q: Do you know what police reports he was given?

A: No.

Q: Could some of those reports or could some of those photographs show some of the probes that you used?

A: They could have, and that is why, when we are conducting this kind of a test, we come up with the best probes we can based on what we know and what we think the defendant or the accused person doesn't know. . . . Now, in the case of that building, I thought I was going to be able to use as a probe, because I didn't think he had that information. And I asked him. He said, "No. I remember that building. It was on the photos."

So I couldn't use it. So I don't know for certain what he knows and doesn't know, but what I do is I asked him what he knows and doesn't know. We use the probes, only items that he would know if he committed the crime, and that he claims not to know, and as far as we know, he's had no other means of finding out. . . .

Q: What was the probe actually used?

A: Brother's car. . . .

Q: Now, if I were sitting in prison, and for life, and I was rehearsing in my mind kind of the alibi or my defense, wouldn't you think that that would elicit a probe when you do the P300 test, any of your probes relevant to any defense.

A: It might. Again, as I have said, I'm not proving how the information got there. What I'm saying is this information is stored in the brain. . . .

Lawrence A. Farwell & Emanuel Donchin

The Truth Will Out: Interrogative Polygraphy ("Lie Detection") with Event-Related Brain Potentials

28 Psychophysiology 531, 531-35 (1991)

The feasibility of using Event Related Brain Potentials (ERPs) in Interrogative Polygraphy ("Lie Detection") was tested by examining the effectiveness of the Guilty Knowledge Test. . . . The subject is assigned an arbitrary task requiring discrimination between experimenter-designated targets and other, irrelevant stimuli. A group of diagnostic items ("probes"), which to the unwitting are indistinguishable from the irrelevant items, are embedded among the irrelevant. For subjects who possess "guilty knowledge" these probes are distinct from the irrelevants and are likely to elicit a P300, thus revealing their possessing the special knowledge that allows them to differentiate the probes from the irrelevants. We report two experiments in which this paradigm was tested. In Experiment 1, 20 subjects participated in one of two mock espionage scenarios and were tested for their knowledge of both scenarios. All stimuli consisted of short phrases. . . . A set of items were designated as "targets" and appeared on 17% of the trials. Probes related to the scenarios also appeared on 17% of the trials. The rest of the items were irrelevants. Subjects responded by pressing one switch following targets, and the other following irrelevants (and, of course, probes). . . . As predicted, targets elicited large P300s in all subjects. Probes associated with a given scenario elicited a P300 in subjects who participated in that scenario. A [statistical] method* was used to assess the quality of the decision for each subject. The [statistical method] declared the decision indeterminate in 12.5% of the cases. In all other cases a decision was made. There were no false positives and no false negatives: whenever a determination was made it was accurate. The second experiment was virtually identical to the first, with identical results, except that this time 4 subjects were tested, each of which had a minor brush with the law. Subjects were tested to determine whether they possessed information on their own "crimes." The results were as expected; the Guilty Knowledge Test determined correctly which subject possessed which information. The implications of these data both for the practice of Interrogative Polygraphy and the interpretation of the P300 are discussed.

RESULTS: EVENT-RELATED BRAIN POTENTIALS

The average ERP responses for artifact-free trials of each trial type at the Pz electrode site for [4] of the 20 subjects in the guilty condition are displayed in Figure [15.1]. ERP's for the same subjects in the innocent condition are displayed in Figure [15.1]. The responses were as predicted. As can be seen in the figure, a large P300 was elicited by the target stimuli, but not by the irrelevant stimuli. The probes elicited a P300 in most subjects when they were relevant to the subject's "crime." A very small P300, if any, was elicited by the probes when the subject was "innocent." . . .

---

* [By now you have learned that data about brain function is hardly ever all-or-none. As you learned in Chapter 4, event-related potentials are averages of small, noisy signals. Researchers use a variety of techniques to determine whether an ERP in one condition is statistically significantly different from the ERP in another condition. Farwell used a technique called bootstrapping. This method measures some value from a random subset of the trials that were collected. The measurement is then repeated for a large number of other random draws from the dataset. If the range of measurements from two conditions can be distinguished, then a conclusion that there is no difference can be rejected. Farwell collected a total of 432 trials. Subjects in the "guilty" group responded to 72 target trials, 72 probe trials and 288 irrelevant trials. Subjects in the "innocent" group responded to 72 target trials and 360 irrelevant trials; in other words, there were no probe trials because there was no knowledge to probe. Farwell compared the ERP in trials with the probe of guilty knowledge with the ERP in trials with an irrelevant stimulus and also with the ERP in trials with the target. The logic of the analysis is that the P300 is elicited by the target because it occurs less frequently than the irrelevant stimuli. If a probe elicits a P300, then Farwell surmises that the subject recognizes the probes as a separate, rare category, like a target. Because the probe is defined as relevant for the hypothetical crime, the ERP indicates that the subject is "guilty." On the other hand, if the ERP on probe trials is indistinguishable from the ERP on irrelevant trials, then Farwell surmises that the subject does not recognize or remember the probes, indicating that the subject is "innocent."—EDS.]

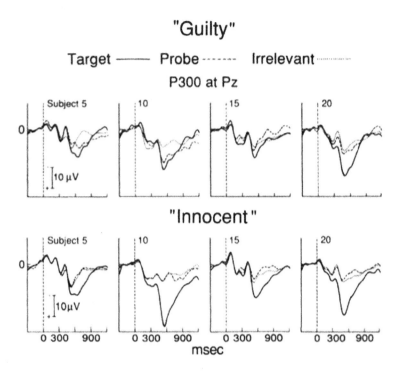

Figure 15.1 [ERPs recorded over the midline parietal cortex ("Pz") for four of the subjects tested in the "Guilty" (top) and "Innocent" (bottom) conditions. The goal of this test is to compare the waveform elicited by the probe (dashed) with the waveforms elicited by the irrelevant stimulus (dotted) and the target stimulus (solid). The vertical dashed line indicates when the stimulus was presented. The target stimulus elicits a waveform with a larger deflection because it is a less frequent signal and thus is noticed more vigorously. The irrelevant stimulus elicits a waveform with a smaller deflection because it is most frequent and thus is ignored. Farwell's test for guilty knowledge is based on the magnitude of the deflection of the waveform elicited by the probe. If the probe elicits a smaller deflection like the irrelevant stimulus, then it was not noticed and thus, Farwell surmises, has no special meaning for the subject. If the probe elicits a larger deflection like the target, then it was noticed more and thus, Farwell surmises, has special meaning to the subject. The waveforms for Subject number 10 in the Guilty and Innocent conditions follow this pattern as do those for Subject 5. However, the waveforms for Subject 15 in the Guilty condition are more ambiguous, and those for Subject 20 are not consistent with Farwell's prediction. — EDS.]

Modified from: Lawrence A. Farwell and Emanuel Donchin, *The Truth Will Out: Interrogative Polygraphy ("Lie Detection") with Event-Related Brain Potentials,* 28 Psychophysiology 531 (1991).

NOTES AND QUESTIONS

1. Farwell's method is not unreasonable theoretically, but its utility in real legal settings is uncertain and still untested. Other investigators have highlighted specific problems with an approach like Farwell's (such as J. Peter Rosenfeld, *"Brain Fingerprinting": A Critical Analysis,* 4 Sci. Rev. Mental Health Prac. 20 (2005)). Some have argued that while the approach is sound, Farwell's methods in

particular are not sufficiently well tested to merit use in legal (or other) settings. *See* Ewout H. Meijer et al., *A Comment on Farwell: Brain Fingerprinting: A Comprehensive Tutorial Review of Detection of Concealed Information with Event-Related Brain Potentials*, 7 Cognitive Neurodynamics 155 (2013).

2. Farwell claims that this method has 100% validity. This claim is incorrect because it ignores the subjects who had ambiguous results; it is a result of the biased sampling problem described in Chapter 5. When the data from all subjects is included, a statistical assignment to the guilty or innocent groups was done in 87.5% of the subjects. Do you think a method that yields uncertain results for 12.5% of participants is reliable enough for use in the courts?

3. Some meet Farwell's claims with considerable skepticism. For example:

> Farwell is an electrophysiologist who has, for over fifteen years, argued that human P300 waves can be used as a "guilty knowledge" test, to determine whether, for example, a suspect has ever seen the site of a crime. Farwell refers to this process as "brain fingerprinting" and has been selling brain fingerprinting for several years through Brain Finger-printing Laboratories, a privately held company. The company's website claims that in more than 175 tests, the method has produced inconclusive results six times and has been accurate every other time. Farwell's work, however, has not been substantially vetted in the peer-reviewed literature. Apparently, the only article he has published on his technology in a peer-reviewed journal is a 2001 on-line article in the Journal of Forensic Science where he and a co-author reported on a successful trial of his method with six subjects. He has not revealed any further evidence to support his claims of high accuracy, protecting it as a trade secret. He is an inventor on four patents that are relevant to this work.
>
> Farwell's claims are widely discounted in the relevant scientific community and his credibility is not helped by his inflated claims for the judicial acceptance of his technique. The company's website states that "Iowa Supreme Court overturns the 24 year old conviction of Terry Harrington, Brain Fingerprinting test aids in the appeals." In fact, the Iowa district court (not a federal district court, as the website claims), in an unpublished opinion, rejected Harrington's petition for post-conviction relief on several grounds in spite of that testimony. It did admit the brain fingerprinting evidence, but it may have been the case that the lower court judge admitted the testimony merely to deprive Harrington of one ground for appeal. Harrington appealed and the Iowa Supreme Court reversed for reasons unrelated to the brain finger-printing test. As to the brain fingerprinting evidence, the Iowa Supreme Court specifically said "Because the scientific testing evidence is not necessary to a resolution of this appeal, we give it no further consideration." The company's website reports, accurately but with a misleading implication, that "The Iowa Supreme Court left undisturbed the law of the case establishing the admissibility of the Brain Fingerprinting evidence."

Henry T. Greely & Judy Illes, *Neuroscience-Based Lie Detection: The Urgent Need for Regulation*, 33 Am. J.L. & Med. 377, 387-88 (2007). Suppose you were preparing your cross-examination of Farwell, with respect to his testimony regarding EEG-based lie detection. How, specifically, might this passage affect your cross-examination? Imagine next, in contrast, that Farwell is your witness, and that having seen this Greely and Illes passage, you need to prepare Farwell for his cross-examination. What advice would you provide?

4. Neuroscientists and psychologists have not elucidated just what process(es) the P300 indexes. Do you think this uncertainty invalidates this method for use in the legal system?

5. Sensitivity and specificity measure how well a classification procedure works. Sensitivity measures the fraction of actual positive cases that are correctly identified as such, e.g., the percentage of guilty people who are correctly identified as being guilty. Specificity measures the fraction of actual negative cases that are correctly identified, e.g., the percentage of innocent people who are correctly identified as being innocent. A perfect classification procedure has 100% sensitivity, i.e., misses none of the actual guilty people, and 100% specificity, i.e., never wrongly accuses anyone. Real world classification procedures are never perfect because of imperfect information being used for the classification and limitations in the computations available to do the classification. Therefore, policies must be devised to guide the trade-off between sensitivity and specificity. In an airport security setting, for example, scanners should have low specificity and generate alerts for low-risk items like belt buckles and keys to reduce the risk of missing high-risk items like guns and bombs. To appreciate the implications of less than 100% sensitivity and specificity, imagine a security screening application that has both sensitivity and specificity of 90%. Further imagine that only 10 of 10,000 people who are screened are actually guilty of attempting to smuggle a bomb onto an airplane. Such a screening procedure would identify correctly eight of the 10 smugglers while missing two. Meanwhile, the screening procedure would falsely identify about 1,600 innocent people. What are the implications of this fraction of false accusation?

J. Peter Rosenfeld et al.
Simple, Effective Countermeasures to P300-Based Tests of Detection of Concealed Information
41 Psychophysiology 205, 205-13 (2004)

In the academic psychophysiology community, the use of the P300 event-related potential (ERP) is probably the most familiar of the alternative approaches. . . . Most of these approaches are concealed information tests or guilty knowledge tests, which utilize P300 amplitude as an index of recognition of critical details of a crime or other concealed information. The National Research Council report . . . [noted that] "it is not known whether simple countermeasures could potentially defeat this approach by generating brain electrical responses to comparison questions that mimic those that occur with relevant questions" (National Research Council, 2003, p. 162). The primary goal and major interest of the present study was to address precisely this question. . . .

This study was directed at developing a countermeasure to the Farwell and Donchin (1991) paradigm. . . . Participants were randomly assigned either to the innocent group, countermeasure group, or the no-countermeasure, simple guilty group. The only difference between the latter two groups is that those in the countermeasure group were informed about a countermeasure. They were instructed to perform covert acts in response to the irrelevant stimuli. More specifically, all participants in the countermeasure group were instructed to perform the acts in response to irrelevant stimuli based on stimulus groups or categories, rather than to individual stimuli. Each member of the group performed the same acts. . . .

For example, for the name-of-operation category, animal names were used. For the probe "cow" and target "pig," the irrelevants were: horse, goat, sheep, and mule. In this case, the same covert countermeasure behavior was performed every time the participant saw any of these irrelevants, as they are all in the same irrelevant group or animal name category. The covert acts were (1) pressing the left forefinger imperceptibly greater on the leg where the left hand rested, (2) pressing the left middle finger imperceptibly greater on the leg where the left hand rested (the right forefinger was being used to press overt response buttons), (3) imperceptibly wiggling the big toe in the left shoe, (4) imperceptibly wiggling the big toe in the right shoe, and (5) imagining the experimenter slapping the participant in the face. There was no act for the sixth irrelevant stimulus category, all members of which would thus become oddballs* as the only irrelevant stimuli not requiring a particular covert response. Thus the essential countermeasure strategy was to make presumed irrelevant stimuli relevant. . . .

The result was that the probe and irrelevant responses became largely indistinguishable in the guilty subject employing a countermeasure successfully.

NOTES AND QUESTIONS

1. Explaining his decision not to re-try Mr. Harrington, the prosecutor in the case, Pottawattamie County Attorney, Matthew Wilber, said, "After personally spending hundreds of hours on this case, I have no doubt that Terry Harrington committed the murder of John Schweer in 1977. The jury made the right decision in 1978, and the right man went to prison for 25 years. That said, I also have no doubt that the admissible evidence which is left after 26 years is not sufficient to sustain a conviction against Mr. Harrington." Mark Siebert, *Free Man: Case Dismissed Against Man Who Served 25 Years*, Des Moines Reg. (Oct. 25, 2003). Imagine that the case had been re-tried, and the prosecutor continued to express this strong belief in Harrington's guilt. If you were Harrington's defense attorney, would you proffer Dr. Farwell's evidence? If you were the trial judge, would you allow it into evidence?

2. How one assesses the usefulness of lie detection evidence (whether brain-based or not) depends on one's presumptions about how well triers of fact perform in the absence of that evidence. Consider law professor Dan Simon's observations:

> To test for this possibility of implicit judgments, studies have been conducted to determine people's ability to distinguish between truths and lies. A large meta-analysis summarizes data from 206 experiments and leads to a rather simple conclusion: people perform poorly in distinguishing truthful from deceitful statements. Overall, the mean percentage of accurate classifications is fifty-four percent. The highest reported rate in any sample was seventy-three percent, and the lowest was thirty-one percent. These results are statistically better than flipping a coin, but barely so. As Aldert Vrij has pointed out, people are considerably better at telling lies than at detecting them. Importantly, human performance on this task falls well short of the levels of diagnosticity that warrant the dramatic impact that a determination of deceit can have on a verdict.

---

* [The term "oddball" refers simply to a category of stimulus that is unlike any of the others in a testing situation. Can you identify the oddball in this list of words: apple, banana, orange, grape, altimeter? — EDS.]

Dan Simon, *The Limited Diagnosticity of Criminal Trials*, 64 Vand. L. Rev. 143, 177-178 (2011). For more in this vein, see John B. Meixner, *Liar, Liar, Jury's the Trier? The Future of Neuroscience-Based Credibility Assessment in the Court*, 106 Nw. U. L. Rev. 1451 (2012) (arguing that neuroscientific evidence may compensate for jurors being "ineffective credibility assessors").

3. Under cross-examination, Farwell states that his Guilty Knowledge test does not prove how the subject acquired information but only whether or not the subject possesses "guilty-knowledge." Does this create the possibility that the accused may be "corrupted" simply due to exposure during the course of the criminal investigation or subsequent court proceedings? How could either side take advantage of the P300's insensitivity to the source of guilty knowledge?

4. In 2012 scientists reported that they had successfully run a laboratory experiment measuring P300 waves with an off-the-shelf "Emotiv" brain-computer interface in order to learn subjects' PIN numbers. Ivan Martinovic et al., *On the Feasibility of Side-Channel Attacks with Brain-Computer Interfaces*, Presentation at the USENIX Security Symposium (Aug. 8, 2012). If such "mind reading" technology continues to develop, what areas of law might be implicated?

5. Japan has used a similar system to Farwell's P300 testing for nearly 50 years. The goal is the same: to detect whether a subject recognizes an item or detail that only someone at the scene could recognize. However, in Japan the polygraph is used rather than EEG. This procedure is also fully accepted by the Japanese judicial system. Uses of the process include providing evidence for prosecution, finding new evidence, identifying a target crime, screening of involved people when searching for a criminal, and preventing false charges. *See* Akemi Osugi, *Field Findings from the Concealed Information Test in Japan*, in *Detecting Concealed Information and Deception: Recent Developments* 97 (J. Peter Rosenfeld ed., 2018). While such a process may not be accepted by American courts as direct evidence for prosecution, do any of the other uses seem acceptable?

6. What are the legal consequences of teaching someone how to "beat" a lie detector test? In 2014 Doug Williams, a former law enforcement officer, was charged with witness tampering for teaching employees and potential employees of federal agencies countermeasures to a federally mandated polygraph test. Williams pleaded guilty mid-trial and was sentenced to three years in prison. The government insisted that the accuracy of the polygraph test was irrelevant because Williams knew the agents intended to lie on the test. That may be true in Williams's case, but what if Williams had not known of the agents' intention to lie? Should he still have been charged with witness tampering? Does it matter that some countermeasures only involve minor movements that participants may engage in without even being aware of their confounding effects? Others have supported studying the polygraph's weaknesses before taking the test. Professor Peter Moskos, a former police officer, advises aspiring police officers in his classes to do exactly that, saying, "You're a fool if you go into a lie detector test thinking that telling the truth is good enough." *See* Indictment at 1-17, *United States v. Williams*, Case 5:14-cr-00318-M (W.D. Okla. 2015); Trial Brief of United States at 4-5, *United States v. Williams*, Case 5:14-cr-00318-M (W.D. Okla. 2015); Judgment in a Criminal Case, *United States v. Williams*, Case 5:14-cr-00318-M (W.D. Okla. 2015); Martin Kaste, *Trial of Polygraph Critic Renews Debate over Tests' Accuracy*, NPR (Jan. 2, 2015).

7. Propranolol is a drug primarily used to treat high blood pressure. However, it also inhibits neurotransmitters necessary to form memories. In effect, it can prevent the formation of memories if taken in a high enough dosage. Paul McGorrery has pointed out that drugs such as this could be used by criminals just before or after committing a crime to effectively defeat brain fingerprinting technology. In a world in which brain fingerprinting is not rare, would using such a drug be considered evidence tampering? Would providing the drug be considered witness or evidence tampering? *See* Paul McGorrery, *A Further Critique of Brain Fingerprinting: The Possibility of Propranolol Usage by Offenders*, 42 Alternative L.J. 216 (2017).

8. Despite the lack of scientific consensus and development of countermeasures, a 2019 report estimated that the market for "brain fingerprinting" technology will expand rapidly due to government counterterrorism and law enforcement demands, with additional interest from border control, marketing, advertising, and health care. Alex Perala, *Growing Market for Brainwave Biometrics in Law Enforcement*, FindBiometrics (June 28, 2019).

9. A research team has developed a new P300 protocol that is potentially more resistant to the countermeasures discussed by Rosenfeld. The Complex Trial Protocol (CTP) seeks to improve the older protocol by requiring the same response for each item while it is on screen (i.e., clicking a button to affirm the subject is paying attention and sees the item) rather than also asking the subject to decide if the item is a target or not, simultaneously. Researchers can then evaluate if the subject recognizes the probe by either comparing the probe's response to the irrelevant item that produced the highest P300 activation or by comparing the probe's response to all irrelevant items. The CTP also happens to increase the workload of the subject, which researchers suggest is one factor in reducing the effectiveness of countermeasures. To further determine the CTP's resistance to countermeasures, scientists have tested both the old countermeasures discovered by Rosenfeld, as well as new countermeasures. These new measures involve creating "oddball" items among the irrelevant items by targeting them with covert responses (e.g., silently self-articulating the word "cat" during random irrelevant items while articulating "dog" for all other items). The researchers then performed both the CTP and old protocol on the subjects who attempted to defeat the test with either the old or the new countermeasures. As predicted, the old countermeasures were less successful in defeating the CTP. However, the new countermeasures were effective at producing false negatives, especially when evaluated using the probe response compared to the highest irrelevant item approach. Despite these new countermeasures, the CTP is an improvement on the older protocol. *See* Gáspár Lukács et al., *The First Independent Study on the Complex Trial Protocol Version of the P300-Based Concealed Information Test: Corroboration of Previous Findings and Highlights on Vulnerabilities*, 110 Int'l J. Psychophysiology 56 (2016); J. Peter Rosenfeld et al., *The Complex Trial Protocol (CTP): A New, Countermeasure-Resistant, Accurate, P300-Based Method for Detection of Concealed Information*, 45 Psychophysiology 906 (2008).

10. Dr. Farwell has continued to offer brain fingerprinting as a valid science-based lie detection method. In addition to his involvement in the *Harrington* case, he claims to have played a key role in determining the guilt of the serial killer J.B. Grinder. He has also appeared in Season 2 of the popular Netflix documentary

Making a Murderer, performing the brain fingerprinting technique to aid the postconviction appeal of Steven Avery in the murder of Teresa Halbach. As part of the Avery case, Farwell also announced a $100,000 reward to anyone who could beat the technique and issued a challenge to the prosecutor in the case, saying, "I offer you a free Brain Fingerprinting test on the issue of obstruction of justice and conspiracy to frame Avery. Put your brain where your mouth is. The brain never lies." Kelly Wynne, *'Making a Murderer' Brain Fingerprinting Expert Offers Ken Kratz Free Session: 'Put Your Brain Where Your Mouth Is'*, Newsweek (Nov. 21, 2018). *See also* Kelly Wynne, *What Is Brain Fingerprinting? How Brainwaves May Prove Steven Avery Is Innocent*, Newsweek (Oct. 30, 2018); and *Farwell Brain Fing[e]rprinting Catches a Serial Killer*, https://larryfarwell.com/Grinder-Summary-dr-larry-farwell-brain-fingerprinting-dr-lawrence-farwell.html.

11. The New Zealand Law Foundation funded a study that ran from 2016 to 2017 to test Farwell's brain fingerprinting method. These studies suggested that brain fingerprinting may be useful as lie detection evidence in court. However, Professor Robin Palmer still urges that more studies into both the science and legal and ethical ramifications of brain fingerprinting are needed. *See* Robin Palmer, *Time to Take Brain-Fingerprinting Seriously? A Consideration of International Developments in Forensic Brainwave Analysis (FBA), in the Context of the Need for Independent Verification of FBA's Scientific Validity, and the Potential Legal Implications of Its Use in New Zealand*, 2017 Te Wharenga 330 (2018).

2. Lie Detection Using fMRI

The introduction of Farwell's EEG-based lie detection evidence in the *Harrington* case did not lead to a proliferation of brain-based lie detection in courts. However, fMRI-based lie detection evidence has been proffered in several subsequent court cases. In this section you will learn about two of these cases. The first, *United States v. Semrau*, featured a *Daubert* hearing in federal court. The second, *Smith v. Maryland*, featured a *Frye* hearing in state court. Taken together, these two cases offer an excellent window into the scientific and legal questions raised by the advent of lie detection evidence from fMRI. To provide additional scientific context for answering those questions, after the cases we present excerpts from neuroscience articles related to fMRI lie detection.

Francis X. Shen & Owen D. Jones
Brain Scans as Evidence: Truths, Proofs, Lies, and Lessons
62 Mercer L. Rev. 861, 867-70 (2011)

In *United States v. Semrau*, the government charged psychologist Dr. Lorne Semrau with Medicare/Medicaid fraud. Proving fraud required proving that Semrau knowingly violated the law. Semrau's defense was partly built around brain scan results that allegedly demonstrated he was telling the truth when he claimed—some years after the fact—that even though he had incorrectly billed for services, he did not do so intending to commit fraud. Semrau owned two businesses, each of which contracted with nursing homes in Tennessee and Mississippi to provide the psychologists and psychiatrists necessary to dispense prescriptions and provide mental health care. After an investigation by the United States Attorney's Health Care Fraud Task Force in the Western District of Tennessee, the government alleged that between 1999 and 2005 Semrau had manipulated Medicare and Medicaid billing codes to inflate payments, resulting in $3 million worth of fraud.

The central legal question in the case concerned Semrau's mental state at the time of his acts: between 1999 and 2005, did Semrau "knowingly devise[ ] a scheme or artifice to defraud a health care benefit program in connection with the delivery of or payment for health care benefits, items, or services"? To bolster Semrau's credibility in asserting that he had not knowingly engaged in prohibited billing practices, defense attorney Houston Gordon contacted Dr. Stephen Laken, founder and CEO of Cephos Corporation. Since 2004, Dr. Laken had been developing fMRI lie detection technology, and beginning in 2008 Cephos marketed the product commercially. During December 2009, Laken worked with Gordon to develop a set of Specific Incident Questions (SIQs) that Dr. Semrau would answer in the scanner. The questions included, "Did you bill CPT Code 99312 to cheat or defraud Medicare?" and "Did you enter into a scheme to defraud the government by billing for AIMS tests conducted by psychiatrists under CPT Code 99301?" Neutral questions, against which the answers to SIQs would be compared, were also used. Examples of neutral questions included, "Do you like to swim?" and "Are you over age 18?" The defense and Laken co-designed the tasks and the SIQs without the knowledge of the prosecution (a fact that would later factor into the court's analysis).

On December 30, 2009, Semrau traveled to the Cephos office in Framingham, Massachusetts, for his initial brain scanning session. Following data analysis, Laken made two conclusions. First, as to whether Semrau was being honest when he claimed that he had not knowingly defrauded the government, Laken concluded that "[i]t appeared his brain showed that he was telling the truth." Second, as to whether or not Semrau knew he was incorrectly billing for services that should not have been separately billed, Laken found that "it appeared that he was lying when he said he was telling the truth." This second conclusion was obviously not the result Semrau's defense team wanted.

After analyzing the data further, Laken contacted Gordon's office and offered to do a third scan, specifically on the second issue of whether Semrau had knowingly incorrectly billed for certain psychiatric tests administered. Laken justified the additional scan on the grounds that Semrau was fatigued for the second scan, and this may have invalidated the results. Laken shortened the questions for the third scan, conducted on January 12, 2010. After the third scan, Laken newly concluded that "we believe that Dr. Semrau's brain indicates that he was telling the truth when he said that he is telling the truth about not inappropriately performing AIMS testing."*

In light of these brain scan results, the defense team decided to have Laken testify. To clarify, Laken was not offered as a witness who could testify *directly* about

---

* [The Abnormal Involuntary Movement Scale (AIMS) assesses abnormal movements, such as those associated with Parkinson's disease, Huntington's disease, Tourette's syndrome, or tardive dyskinesia after taking anti-psychotic medication. Body movements are evaluated on a 12-item scale that evaluates abnormal movements of facial expression, lips, jaw, tongue, arms, legs, sitting posture, and associated movements, standing posture, and associated movements and walking posture and gait. The degree of abnormality and patient's awareness of the abnormalities are scored. *See* Mark R. Munetz & Sheldon Benjamin, *How to Examine Patients Using the Abnormal Involuntary Movement Scale*, 39 Psychiatric Servs. 1172 (1988). —EDS.]

Semrau's past mental state. Instead, he was to testify about the truthfulness of Semrau's claim in *December 2009 and January 2010*, concerning his state of mind between 1999 through 2005. . . .

United States v. Semrau
No. 07-10074 MI/P, 2010 WL 6845092 (W.D. Tenn. June 1, 2010)

PHAM, M.J., Report and Recommendation. Before the court by order of reference is the United States' ("government") Motion in Limine and Memorandum in Support to Exclude Defendant's Expert Witness Testimony of Dr. Steven Laken and Request by the United States for a *Daubert* Hearing, filed February 19, 2010 ("Motion to Exclude").[1] On March 22, the defendant, Dr. Lorne Allan Semrau, filed a response in opposition to the motion. . . . On March 25, the government filed a Supplement to its Motion to Exclude, arguing that in addition to excluding Dr. Laken's testimony under Fed. R. Evid. 702, the court should also exclude his testimony under Fed. R. Evid. 403 . . .

On May 13 and 14, the court conducted a *Daubert* hearing on the motion. . . . The court heard testimony from Dr. Steven J. Laken, Dr. Marcus E. Raichle, and Dr. Peter Imrey. The court received the following exhibits as evidence: (1) curriculum vitae for all three witnesses; (2) the "fMRI Testing Report" containing Dr. Laken's opinions; (3) a chart displaying the results of Dr. Semrau's examinations; (4) an article titled "Functional MRI Detection of Deception After Committing a Mock Sabotage Crime"; and (5) a fifty-three page slide presentation used during Dr. Imrey's testimony. Finally, on May 18, Dr. Semrau filed a Notice of Filing Supplemental Peer Reviewed Articles, Published Articles, and Scientific Presentations.

After careful consideration of the briefs and exhibits filed in connection with the present motion, the testimony of the witnesses and exhibits admitted at the hearing, and the entire record in this case, the court submits the following proposed findings of fact and conclusions of law, and recommends that the Motion to Exclude be granted.

I. PROPOSED FINDINGS OF FACT
A. Summary of the Charges

Dr. Lorne Allan Semrau was a licensed psychologist in Tennessee and a participating provider in the Medicare and Medicaid programs. . . . Dr. Semrau contracted with psychiatrists to provide mental health services to patients in nursing homes in Tennessee and Mississippi. Services provided by the psychiatrists included conducting initial patient evaluations, providing monthly medication management, and administering Abnormal Involuntary Movement Scale ("AIMS") tests on patients. . . .

According to the indictment, between 1999 and 2005, Dr. Semrau allegedly engaged in a scheme to defraud Medicare, Medicaid, and other health care benefit programs by submitting false and fraudulent claims for payment. To carry out this scheme, Dr. Semrau directed his billing personnel to bill CPT codes that were different from the codes marked by the treating psychiatrists, and instructed the psychiatrists to claim a separate CPT code for AIMS tests. Dr. Semrau instructed Superior and

---

1. The motion was referred to the Magistrate Judge for a report and recommendation pursuant to 28 U.S.C. §636(b)(1)(B) and (C).

Foundation employees to delete lower paying CPT codes from the log sheets and to substitute CPT code 99312 (a code that paid a higher rate of reimbursement), and he instructed billing personnel to file claims with CPT code 99312 instead of the lower paying CPT codes circled by the psychiatrists. Dr. Semrau also instructed the psychiatrists to perform AIMS tests approximately every six months and to circle "301" on the log sheets. He instructed billing personnel to file claims for CPT code 99301 even though he knew that this test was not a separately reimbursable test and should have been performed with and billed as part of a regularly scheduled monthly medication management service. In total, "Semrau caused fraudulent billings of approximately $3,000,000.00 to be submitted to Medicare and Medicaid in Tennessee and Mississippi thereby causing payments to be made to Superior and Foundation by CIGNA, CAHABA and Medicaid." . . .

Dr. Semrau denies that he acted with the intent to defraud, asserts that his actions were reasonable under the circumstances because the CPT codes were confusing and unclear, and claims he followed instructions and guidance provided by CIGNA and CAHABA representatives.[4]

B. Functional Magnetic Resonance Imaging and Lie Detection
1. Background

Dr. Steven J. Laken is the President and CEO of Cephos Corporation, a company he founded in 2004 and located in Tyngsboro, Massachusetts. Cephos markets itself as a company that provides a variety of investigative services, including DNA forensic analysis, private detective services, and lie detection/truth verification using functional magnetic resonance imaging ("fMRI"). Regarding its fMRI-based lie detection service, Cephos claims it uses "state-of-the-art technology that is unbiased and scientifically validated. We have offered expert testimony and have presented fMRI evidence in court." It further states that "[t]he source of lying is in the brain—that is what Cephos measures with our truth verification brain imaging service using fMRI technology. We provide independent, scientific validation that someone is telling the truth." Cephos holds a patent on a version of a fMRI-based lie detection method, which identifies Dr. Laken as its inventor.

At the heart of Dr. Laken's lie detection method is fMRI. When undergoing a fMRI scan, a subject lies down on a bed, which slides into the center of a donut-shaped magnet core. As the subject remains still, he or she is asked to perform a task. If the task requires a response, the subject inputs a response with a handheld controller. While the subject performs these tasks, magnetic coils in the scanner receive electric current and the device gathers information about the subject's Blood Oxygen Level Dependent ("BOLD") response. The data is then "heavily processed, aligned, smoothed, and filtered before it can be mapped onto a template of a human brain." By comparing the subject's BOLD response signals with the control state, small changes in signal intensity are detectable and can provide information about brain activity.

---

4. In order to convict Dr. Semrau on the health care fraud charges, the government must prove that he "(1) knowingly devised a scheme or artifice to defraud a health care benefit program in connection with the delivery of or payment for health care benefits, items, or services; (2) executed or attempted to execute this scheme or artifice to defraud; and (3) acted with intent to defraud." . . .

Dr. Laken first became interested in conducting research in the area of fMRI-based lie detection in or around 2003, and shortly thereafter, he began working closely with a small group of researchers in that field, including Dr. Frank Andrew Kozel, Dr. Mark S. George, and Dr. Kevin A. Johnson. Over the next few years, Dr. Laken and his fellow researchers conducted a series of laboratory studies to determine whether they could use fMRI to detect deception. Generally, these studies involved a test subject performing a task, such as "stealing" a ring or watch, and then scanning the subject while he or she answered questions about the task. The subjects were usually offered a modest monetary incentive (e.g. fifty dollars) if their lie was not detected.

Based on these studies, as well as studies conducted by other researchers, Dr. Laken and his colleagues determined that the regions of the brain that are most consistently activated by deception are the right orbitofrontal/inferior frontal, the right middle frontal, and the right anterior cingulate. They also claimed that by analyzing the subjects' brain activity, they were able to identify correctly when the subjects were being deceptive with a high level of accuracy, with reported results ranging from 86% to 93% accuracy. They reported their findings in several peer reviewed articles. . . .

2. Testing Conducted on Dr. Semrau

In an effort to support Dr. Semrau's defense that he did not act with the intent to defraud, sometime in or around December of 2009, Dr. Semrau's attorney, J. Houston Gordon, contacted Dr. Laken, to inquire about having a fMRI-based lie detection test conducted on Dr. Semrau. Dr. Laken agreed to test Dr. Semrau. Dr. Laken decided to conduct two separate fMRI tests on Dr. Semrau, one test that would ask questions regarding the health care fraud charges and the other test that would ask questions regarding the AIMS tests charges.

Prior to the scheduled test date, Dr. Laken developed a set of twenty neutral questions and twenty control questions that would be asked during the scanning. The neutral questions included, for example, "Do you like to swim?", "Are you over age 18?", and "Do you like to watch TV?" Examples of the control questions included, "Do you ever gossip?", "Have you ever done something illegal?", and "Have you ever cheated on your taxes?"

Mr. Gordon and Dr. Laken co-developed Specific Incident Questions ("SIQs"), that is, questions directly relating to the fraud and AIMS tests charges. The government was not notified that Dr. Semrau was going to take the deception test, and thus was not provided with an opportunity to submit its own questions to Dr. Laken to use during the test or to observe the testing procedures.

The SIQs for the first scan included the following [and also additional questions similar to these]: . . .

- Did you bill CPT Code 99312 to cheat or defraud Medicare?
- Did you bill CPT Code 99312 to cheat or defraud Medicaid/TennCare?
- Did you seek guidance by telephone from provider services representatives at Cigna as to which code was appropriate? . . .

The SIQs for the second scan included the following:

- Did you enter into a scheme to defraud the government by billing for AIMS tests conducted by psychiatrists under CPT Code 99301?

- Did you believe that AIMS tests performed by psychiatrists was a necessary service that could be separately billed?
- Did you call Cigna Medicare's provider services office in Nashville to inquire as to how to bill for AIMS tests performed by psychiatrists?
- Did you ever knowingly intend to defraud the government by billing for AIMS tests? . . .

On December 30, 2009, Dr. Semrau traveled to Framingham, Massachusetts, to undergo the tests. Dr. Laken explained the fMRI testing procedure to Dr. Semrau and had him sign a consent form, provide a urine sample for drug screening, fill out an Annette Handedness questionnaire, and complete a MRI safety form. Dr. Laken also interviewed Dr. Semrau to screen him for Axis I disorders. The results of the drug and Axis I disorders screening were negative. Based on those results, Dr. Laken determined that Dr. Semrau was a good candidate for fMRI.

In each fMRI scan, Dr. Semrau was visually instructed to "Lie" or to tell the "Truth" in response to each SIQ. He was told to respond truthfully to the neutral and control questions. Dr. Semrau practiced answering the questions on a computer prior to the scans. Dr. Laken observed Dr. Semrau practice until Dr. Laken believed that Dr. Semrau showed sufficient compliance with the instructions, responded to questions appropriately, and understood what he was to do in the scanner. Dr. Semrau then underwent two fMRI scans on December 30, 2009.

At about 6:00 A.M., Dr. Semrau was placed in the scanner and a display was positioned over Dr. Semrau's head that flashed the questions. The order of the questions was randomized and the response to each question was recorded. According to Dr. Laken, Dr. Semrau tolerated the first fMRI procedure well, but he expressed some fatigue after completing the first scan. After completing the second fMRI scan on December 30, Dr. Semrau stated that the questions were long and he had a difficult time reading the questions before responding. A radiologist reviewed the brain scans taken on December 30, and found that they did not show any obvious abnormalities.

On January 4, 2010, Dr. Laken reviewed the scans taken on December 30. Dr. Laken analyzed the scans using his fMRI testing protocol, found that Dr. Semrau answered an appropriate number of questions, responded correctly, and had no excess movement. Dr. Laken found no imaging artifacts. From the first scan, which included SIQs relating to defrauding the government, the results showed that Dr. Semrau was "not deceptive." However, from the second scan, which included SIQs relating to AIMS tests, the results showed that Dr. Semrau was "being deceptive." According to Dr. Laken, "testing indicates that a positive test result in a person purporting to tell the truth is accurate only 6% of the time." Dr. Laken also believed that the second scan may have been affected by Dr. Semrau's fatigue. Based on his findings on the second test, Dr. Laken suggested that Dr. Semrau be administered another fMRI test on the AIMS tests topic, but this time with shorter questions and conducted later in the day to reduce the effects of fatigue. The following revised SIQs were developed for the third scan [and included the following questions, along with others] . . .

- Did you enter into a scheme to defraud the government by billing for AIMS tests using 99301?
- Did you ever knowingly intend to defraud the government by billing AIMS tests? . . .
- Did you know AIMS testing could not be separately billed? . . .

The third scan was conducted on January 12, 2010 at around 7:00 P.M., and according to Dr. Laken, Dr. Semrau tolerated it well and did not express any fatigue. Dr. Laken reviewed this data on January 18, 2010, and concluded that Dr. Semrau was not deceptive. He further stated that based on his prior studies, "a finding such as this is 100% accurate in determining truthfulness from a truthful person."

In conclusion, Dr. Laken found that "Dr. Semrau's brain indicates he is telling the truth in regards to not cheating or defrauding the government" and that his "brain indicates he is telling the truth in that he correctly provided AIMS tests as was instructed." At the *Daubert* hearing, the prosecutor questioned Dr. Laken on his conclusions:

Q: Now, you said—you mentioned something in your direct testimony that when you do a scan such as this and you ask the questions to the person in the scanner, that you said that you cannot tell whether or not Dr. Semrau is telling the truth as to any specific incident question. Do you understand that? Do I have that right?

A: Yeah. You're exactly right.

Q: But that you said it's more of an overall—

A: That's correct.

Q: —picture or whatever that you can say, well, generally, he was telling the truth to those specific incident questions.

A: That's correct.

Q: So it's possible that on some of the specific incident questions that he was not telling the truth?

A: It certainly is possible. Yes.

Q: . . . Can you say, well, he got 50 percent of them right, and the other 50 percent he lied?

A: So the problem in science, and I'll give you a story, and I guess, Judge, you can figure out what to do with it. But I mean, we had a person that came to me, and they were tested. It was a couple. And she made up a bunch of questions, and he was lying about one of those questions. They were similar like this. They were on 20 questions. He lied on one question, and it showed that he was deceptive. When she confronted him, then he said, well, this is the question I lied on. Now, was he lying on more than one question? I don't know. Maybe he was. But an anecdotal story in a real world situation, one person is lying. We said that they were lying. He is confronted. He admits to something. So what does that tell you? I don't know. But in that situation if he was lying on one, maybe it ends up being that he shows that he was being deceptive on all of them.

Q: All right. So in looking at the specific incident questions that Dr. Semrau was asked on scan number one, and I'm just reading from page 8 of your report, did you ever instruct SLCS FLCS billing employees to bill psychiatry services which had historically been billed by the corporation under CPT code 90862 under CPT code 99312, was he telling the truth when he answered that question?

A: I don't know.

Q: Let me go to the second question. Did you ever tell the billing personnel of SLCS and FLCS that you had received instructions or guidance from Cigna Medicare provider services representatives to bill CPT code 99312? Was he telling the truth on that question?

A: Again, I don't know.

Q: Okay. Just to save time, if I ask you the same question for all of those specific incident questions that were performed in scan one, could you tell me whether or not he was telling the truth as to any of those particular questions?

A: No.

Q: But your opinion was as to scan one he passed?

A: Correct. . . .

Q: And, again, I won't waste the Court's time, but if I read every specific incident question in scan number two and asked you could you tell me whether or not Dr. Semrau was telling the truth to any of those questions, what would you say?

A: I would say I don't know.

II. PROPOSED CONCLUSIONS OF LAW

A. Rule 702 and *Daubert*

Federal Rule of Evidence 702 provides as follows:

> If scientific, technical, or other specialized knowledge will assist the trier of fact to understand the evidence or to determine a fact in issue, a witness qualified as an expert by knowledge, skill, experience, training, or education, may testify thereto in the form of an opinion or otherwise, if (1) the testimony is based upon sufficient facts or data, (2) the testimony is the product of reliable principles and methods, and (3) the witness has applied the principles and methods reliably to the facts of the case. Fed. R. Evid. 702.

In *Daubert v. Merrell Dow Pharmaceuticals, Inc.*, 509 U.S. 579 (1993), the Supreme Court held that the Federal Rules of Evidence superseded the "general acceptance" test of *Frye v. United States*, and that trial courts were required to make an initial determination of whether the reasoning or methodology underlying the testimony is scientifically valid and whether that reasoning or methodology can be applied to the facts in issue.

The court's gate-keeping role is two-fold. First, the court must determine whether the testimony is reliable. The reliability analysis focuses on whether the reasoning or methodology underlying the testimony is scientifically valid. The expert's testimony must be grounded in the methods and procedures of science and must be more than unsupported speculation or subjective belief. Courts are not to be concerned with the reliability of the conclusions generated. If the methodology, principles, and reasoning are scientifically valid, then it follows that the inferences, assertions, and conclusions derived there from are scientifically valid as well.

To aid the trial court in its determination of whether an expert's testimony is reliable, the Supreme Court in *Daubert* suggested several non-exclusive factors to consider: (1) whether the theory or technique can be tested and has been tested; (2) whether the theory or technique has been subjected to peer review and publication; (3) the known or potential rate of error of the method used and the existence and maintenance of standards controlling the technique's operation; and (4) whether the theory or method has been generally accepted by the scientific community.

In addition, the court may consider "whether the experts are proposing to testify about matters growing naturally and directly out of research they have conducted independent of the litigation, or whether they have developed their opinions expressly for purposes of testifying" because the former "provides important, objective proof that the research comports with the dictates of good science." The Supreme Court has emphasized that, in assessing the reliability of expert testimony, whether scientific or otherwise, the trial court may consider one or more of the *Daubert* factors when doing so will help determine that expert's reliability. The test of reliability is a "flexible" one, and the *Daubert* factors do not constitute a "definitive checklist or test," but must be tailored to the facts of the particular case.

The particular factors will depend upon the unique circumstances of the expert testimony at issue.

The second prong of the gate-keeping role requires an analysis of whether the expert's reasoning or methodology can be properly applied to the facts at issue, that is, whether the opinion is relevant. This relevance requirement ensures that there is a "fit" between the testimony and the issue to be resolved by the trial. Thus, an expert's testimony is admissible under Rule 702 if it is predicated upon a reliable foundation and is relevant.

The rejection of expert testimony, however, is the exception rather than the rule, and "the trial court's role as gatekeeper is not intended to serve as a replacement for the adversary system." "Vigorous cross-examination, presentation of contrary evidence, and careful instruction on the burden of proof are the traditional and appropriate means of attacking shaky but admissible evidence." Finally, the proponent of the evidence has the burden of establishing that all of the pertinent admissibility requirements are met by a preponderance of the evidence.

B. Motion to Exclude Under Rule 702

The court's Rule 702 analysis begins with a determination of whether the witness is qualified by "knowledge, skill, experience, training, or education" to offer his or her opinion. This requirement has been treated liberally by the courts. Over the past several years, Dr. Laken has personally conducted research in the field of fMRI-based lie detection (including laboratory studies), is the inventor of the Cephos patent, has written articles in peer reviewed scientific journals on the subject, and regularly conducts fMRI-based lie detection tests on individuals through his company. The government did not challenge Dr. Laken's qualifications as an expert in its briefs or at the *Daubert* hearing. Thus, the court finds that Dr. Laken is preliminarily and generally qualified by his knowledge, skill, experience, training, and education to offer an opinion on fMRI-based lie detection in this case.

Although Dr. Laken is qualified to offer an opinion, the court nevertheless concludes that his testimony should be excluded because, at least at this early stage in its development, fMRI based lie detection does not satisfy the requirements of Rule 702.

1. Testing and Peer Review

The first two *Daubert* factors are whether the theory or technique can be and has been tested and whether it has been subjected to peer review and publication. The court finds that the underlying theories behind fMRI-based lie detection are capable of being tested, and at least in the laboratory setting, have been subjected to some level of testing. It also appears that the theories have been subjected to some peer review and publication, particularly within the last five years, as evidenced by the articles coauthored by Dr. Laken, and the numerous peer reviewed articles by other researchers. . . .

2. The Known or Potential Rate of Error and the Existence and Maintenance of Standards

The next *Daubert* factor is the known or potential rate of error and the existence and maintenance of standards controlling the technique's operation. Dr. Laken testified at the *Daubert* hearing that there are published known error rates. On the other hand, Dr. Imrey disputes the validity of the error rates because they are based on too small of a sample size. While it is unclear from the testimony what the error rates are or how valid they may be in the laboratory setting, there are no known error rates for fMRI-based lie detection outside the laboratory setting, i.e. in the "real-world" or "real-life" setting. *See United States v. Baines*, 573 F.3d 979, 990-91 (10th Cir. 2009) (although real world error rates were not known, the court found that finger-print analysis reported error rate of one in 11 million met *Daubert* standard); *United States v. Crisp*, 324 F.3d 261, 280 (4th Cir. 2003) (finding government did not satisfy third *Daubert* factor partly because handwriting expert studies that more accurately reflect real world conditions showed higher error rates); *United States v. Cordoba*, 194 F.3d 1053, 1059-60 (9th Cir. 1999) (no error in district court's finding that "the error rate of real-life polygraph tests is not known and is not particularly capable of analyzing"); *United States v. Ramirez*, No. H-93-252, 1995 WL 918083, at *2 (S.D. Tex. Nov. 17, 1995) (stating that while error rate for polygraph in the laboratory setting has been shown to be "very low," the error rate in real life situations is not known to a reasonable degree of scientific certainty). In *Cordoba*, the court upheld the district court's rejection of the error rate testified to by the polygraph expert because the results of the tests were not transferable to real-life exams. . . . Here, like in *Cordoba*, the error rate of real-life fMRI-based lie detection is unknown.

In Mock Sabotage Crime, Drs. Laken, Kozel, George, and Johnson, among others, discuss the factors that could affect the test results:

> This study has several factors that must be considered for adequate interpretation of the results. Although this study attempted to approximate a scenario that was closer to a real-world situation than prior fMRI detection studies, it still did not equal the level of jeopardy that exists in real-world testing. The reality of a research setting involves balancing ethical concerns, the need to know accurately the participant's truth and deception, and producing realistic scenarios that have adequate jeopardy. In addition, this study only involved healthy adults who were not taking any medications. Thus, whether fMRI deception testing would work is unknown for participants who are taking a medication, who have a significant psychiatric or medical condition, or who are outside the 18-50 year age range. Future studies will need to be performed involving these populations.*

Similar concerns are echoed by Drs. Kozel, George, and Johnson, in Detecting Deception:

> In addition to the challenges of developing appropriate test questioning paradigms, there are numerous other obstacles that must be overcome. Probably one of the most

---

* [Dr. Semrau was 63 years old at the time he underwent testing by Dr. Laken. When asked by the government, "So the application of your technology to somebody who is 63 years old is unknown?," Dr. Laken responded, "Is unknown. That's correct."—Eds.]

difficult is developing experimental protocols that can be generalized to real-world situations. . . . [A]ll of the studies to date have involved simple laboratory experiments with a relatively small number of subjects. While most studies have sample sizes that are appropriate for cognitive imaging studies, only one study has more than 30 subjects. Additionally, subjects are selectively screened, and often restricted by age, gender, and handedness, which reduces the ability to generalize the results. Furthermore, different types of lies may produce different brain patterns. For instance, differences have been reported in false confessions versus false denials, spontaneous isolated lies versus memorized coherent scenario lies, and autobiographical versus non-autobiographical deception. Thus, one may need to develop different protocols for different applications (e.g. employment screenings versus testing for involvement in a specific crime).

Three other issues that have yet to be addressed in the literature are time, motivation, and independence of deception behavior from investigator control. In terms of time, the deceptive event occurs shortly before scanning in most studies, while this likely will not be the case in many real life applications. Many studies entail little motivation or jeopardy at all, while the motivation (e.g. $50 for successful deception) or jeopardy (revealing personal autobiographical information) in other studies is not equivalent to what would be at stake in real applications. Because of ethical concerns, there are limits to the scenarios in which research subjects can participate. Current study questions range in valance from having deceptive responses regarding mundane daily events to the staged firing of a gun. **Finally, and importantly, deceptive behavior is controlled in the laboratory setting. In all studies to date, the research team directs participants to deceive about a certain condition or choice of conditions.** Despite creative designs, the behavior may resemble compliance with a cognitive task more than independent, volitional deception. Ultimately, validity using real cases where truth versus deception can be independently confirmed via other methods would be ideal. However, obtaining reasonable sample sizes and other logistics may hamper efficiency of such field testing. [Boldface emphasis above was in the original article.]

The authors conclude by stating "Functional MRI is currently not ready to be used in real-world lie detection." . . .[18]

Regarding the existence and maintenance of standards, Dr. Laken testified as to the protocols and controlling standards that he uses for his own exams. Because the use of fMRI-based lie detection is still in its early stages of development, standards controlling the real-life application have not yet been established. Without such standards, a court cannot adequately evaluate the reliability of a particular

---

18. Dr. Laken testified that it would be difficult to conduct fMRI-based lie detection studies in the real world setting and thus obtaining error rates outside the laboratory setting would be similarly difficult. While it may be difficult to address the concerns raised in researchers' articles regarding testing subjects who are facing the prospect of going to prison, additional studies can surely be conducted to address the other concerns raised in the peer reviewed articles and by this court. Moreover, the court notes that potential or known error rates is but one factor under the *Daubert* analysis and that in the future, should fMRI-based lie detection undergo further testing, development, and peer review, improve upon standards controlling the technique's operation, and gain acceptance by the scientific community for use in the real world, this methodology may be found to be admissible even if the error rate is not able to be quantified in a real world setting. *Bonds*, 12 F.3d at 560 ("Although we find that on the basis of the record before us the rate of error is a negative factor in the analysis of whether the FBI's procedures are scientifically valid, the error rate is only one in a list of nonexclusive factors that the *Daubert* Court observed would bear on the admissibility question.").

lie detection examination. Assuming, arguendo, that the standards testified to by Dr. Laken could satisfy *Daubert*, it appears that Dr. Laken violated his own protocols when he re-scanned Dr. Semrau on the AIMS tests SIQs, after Dr. Semrau was found "deceptive" on the first AIMS tests scan. None of the studies cited by Dr. Laken involved the subject taking a second exam after being found to have been deceptive on the first exam. His decision to conduct a third test begs the question whether a fourth scan would have revealed Dr. Semrau to be deceptive again.

The absence of real-life error rates, lack of controlling standards in the industry for real-life exams, and Dr. Laken's apparent deviation from his own protocols are negative factors in the analysis of whether fMRI-based lie detection is scientifically valid.

3. Whether the Theory or Method Has Been Generally Accepted by the Scientific Community

The court next considers whether the theory or method has been generally accepted by the scientific community. " 'Widespread acceptance can be an important factor in ruling particular evidence admissible, and a known technique that has been able to attract only minimal support within the community may properly be viewed with skepticism.' " No doubt in part because of its recent development, fMRI-based lie detection has not yet been accepted by the scientific community. As noted above, experts in the field are of the opinion that fMRI "is currently not ready to be used in real-world lie detection." . . .

In sum, the above-described application of the *Daubert* factors leads the court to conclude that Dr. Laken's testimony is inadmissible under Fed. R. Evid. 702.[19] On that basis, the court recommends that the motion be granted.

C. Motion to Exclude Under Rule 403

In addition to asking the court to exclude Dr. Laken's testimony under Fed. R. Evid. 702 and *Daubert*, the government also moves to exclude his testimony under Fed. R. Evid. 403. The government contends that the probative value of Dr. Laken's testimony is substantially outweighed by the danger of unfair prejudice to the government. The court agrees.

Rule 403 provides the court with a basis for excluding evidence independent of *Daubert*. . . . Under Rule 403, if the unfair prejudice substantially outweighs the probative value of the evidence, the evidence is inadmissible. While the Sixth Circuit Court of Appeals has not addressed fMRI-based lie detection specifically, courts in this circuit have consistently found that the high risk of unfair prejudice associated with the admission of testimony regarding unilaterally obtained polygraph results will preclude such testimony from being admissible.

In *Sherlin*, the defendant sought to admit polygraph results purportedly showing that he was truthful when he denied committing arson and that he did not lie to the grand jury. The polygraph examination was unilaterally obtained by the defendant, without the knowledge or acquiescence of the government. The Court of Appeals found no error in the district court's exclusion of the polygraph results. It held that the unilaterally obtained polygraph test, in the absence of any prior stipulation that

---

19. In light of the above finding that the proposed testimony is not reliable, the court need not address the relevancy prong.

the results would be admissible, was of substantially less probative value because the defendant risked nothing by taking the lie detector test, the results of which (if he failed) would never have been released.

In addition, the court found that any probative value of the results was substantially outweighed by the danger of unfair prejudice. The defendant's credibility was the predominant issue in the case, and "the use of a polygraph solely to bolster a witness' credibility is 'highly prejudicial,' especially where credibility issues are central to the verdict." . . . Thus, under a Rule 403 analysis, the polygraph results were deemed inadmissible.

In *Thomas*, the Court of Appeals again addressed the admissibility of polygraph results under Rule 403. The court affirmed the trial court's denial of the defendant's motion for an evidentiary hearing regarding the results of his privately commissioned polygraph test. The results of the examination supposedly validated the defendant's claim that he was not involved in the receipt and possession of a 1,000 pound shipment of marijuana. As in *Sherlin*, the government was not aware of the examination until after its completion and had no opportunity to approve of or submit questions to the examiner. The court concluded that, because the defendant's family independently hired the examiner to conduct the polygraph examination without knowledge or approval by the government, the results were inadmissible under Rule 403. The court questioned the dubious value of unilaterally obtained lie detection tests:

> [N]ot only was it within the district court's discretion to refuse to hold an evidentiary hearing on the examination, but admitting the polygraph results would have been subject to reversal by this court. It cannot be doubted that the prejudicial effect of [the defendant's] polygraph results would have substantially outweighed its probative value, because [the defendant] had no adverse interest at stake in taking the test.

In this case, the court is confronted with similar issues as in *Sherlin* and *Thomas*. Although those cases involved the admissibility of polygraph results, rather than fMRI-based lie detection results, the concerns expressed in *Sherlin* and *Thomas* regarding the risk of prejudice in unilaterally obtained examinations is the same regardless of the technology employed.

Here, Dr. Semrau seeks to admit expert testimony as to the results of a privately commissioned lie detection examination. The examination was conducted without the government's knowledge and without an opportunity for the government to formulate, submit, or approve the questions asked of Dr. Semrau during the examination. Dr. Semrau risked nothing in having the testing performed, and Dr. Laken himself testified that had the results not been favorable to Dr. Semrau, they would have never been released. Like in *Sherlin* and *Thomas*, Dr. Semrau seeks to admit the results of the fMRI scans for the sole purpose of bolstering his credibility before the jury on issues that are central to this case.

Exclusion under Rule 403 is particularly appropriate in this case because, as Dr. Laken testified, although he believes that Dr. Semrau's responses to the SIQs were truthful "overall," he cannot offer any opinion as to whether Dr. Semrau was deceptive or truthful as to any specific SIQ. Based on his inability to identify which SIQs Dr. Semrau answered truthfully or deceptively, the court fails to see how his testimony can assist the jury in deciding whether Dr. Semrau's testimony is credible.

Chapter 15. Lie Detection

Therefore, the danger of unfair prejudice associated with admitting Dr. Laken's fMRI-based lie detection opinions substantially outweighs any probative value attributable to them. The court recommends that the Motion to Exclude be granted under Rule 403.

NOTES AND QUESTIONS

1. Lorne Semrau appealed his conviction on many grounds, including an argument that the district court erred in excluding Dr. Laken's testimony about his fMRI lie detection results. This was a matter of first impression in the federal courts. The Court of Appeals affirmed the lower court's ruling, holding that:

   > [T]he district court did not abuse its discretion in excluding the fMRI evidence under Federal Rule of Evidence 702 because the technology had not been fully examined in "real world" settings and the testing administered to Dr. Semrau was not consistent with tests done in research studies. We also hold that the testimony was independently inadmissible under Rule 403 because the prosecution did not know about the test before it was conducted, constitutional concerns caution against admitting lie detection tests to bolster witness credibility, and the test results do not purport to indicate whether Dr. Semrau was truthful about any single statement.

   United States v. Semrau, 693 F.3d 510, 516 (6th Cir. 2012).

2. A Maryland murder case also raised the question of the admissibility of an fMRI test for lie detection purposes. In *Smith v. Maryland* (2012), Gary James Smith sought to introduce fMRI evidence that he was telling the truth when he claimed not to have shot and killed his roommate. The *Frye* (general acceptance) test applied. As in *Semrau*, the court concluded after days of hearings that the technique was not generally accepted in its relevant scientific community for lie detection purposes. After a *Frye* hearing, the judge ruled: "The competing motions, expert testimonies, and submitted articles reveal a debate that is far from settled in the scientific community. This scientific method is a recent development which has not been thoroughly vetted. . . . Upon examination of the submitted memorandums of law, the available legal and scientific commentaries, and the testimony of the aforementioned experts, it is clear to the Court that the use of fMRI to detect deception and verify truth in an individual's brain has not achieved general acceptance in the scientific community. Therefore, it does not pass the requisite standard for evidence as delineated in *Frye* and adopted in *Reed* and must necessarily be denied admittance in this Court." Memorandum Opinion and Order at 5, *Smith v. Maryland*, 218 Md. App. 689 (Md. Ct. Spec. App. 2014) (No. 106589C). In this context, what would "general acceptance" require?

   Smith's long legal battle finally ended in 2016. After nearly eight and a half years, including two separate convictions and two successful appeals, Smith entered a plea deal rather than face a third trial. Smith pled guilty to involuntary manslaughter and reckless endangerment but was given credit for time already served and ordered to a period of unsupervised probation. Virginia Terhune, *Army Ranger Murder Case Ends 8.5 Years Later with No Jail and No Supervised Probation, and with a Chance for an Expungement,* Jezic & Moyse (Feb. 15, 2016).

3. As you might imagine, there is a great deal of overlap between the investigation of detecting lies and the investigation of detecting memories. For that reason, you will find it useful to refer back to materials in Chapter 13 on Memory. In short review, you should know that substantial and remarkably successful work has been done, in controlled laboratory conditions, to detect autobiographical memories—in part because a memory detection technique "could conceivably be used to interrogate the brains of suspected criminals or witnesses for neural evidence that they recognize certain individuals or entities, such as those from a crime scene." Jesse Rissman, Henry T. Greely & Anthony D. Wagner, *Detecting Individual Memories Through the Neural Decoding of Memory States and Past Experience*, 107 Proc. Nat'l Acad. Sci. U.S. 9849 (2010). See, for instance, Melina R. Uncapher et al., *Goal-Directed Modulation of Neural Memory Patterns: Implications for fMRI-Based Memory Detection*, 35 J. Neurosci. 8531 (2015); Jesse Rissman et al., *Decoding fMRI Signatures of Real-World Autobiographical Memory Retrieval*, 28 J. Cognitive Neurosci. 604 (2016); Thackery I. Brown et al., *Differential Medial Temporal Lobe and Parietal Cortical Contributions to Real-World Autobiographical Episodic and Autobiographical Semantic Memory*, 8 Sci. Rep. 6190 (2018).

4. Can neuroscience actually identify lies? Neuroscientist Anthony Wagner asked that question in his 2010 review of 28 peer-reviewed articles and concluded that:

> At present, the sensitivity and specificity of fMRI-based lie detection is unknown. Analysis of the published literature reveals no data that provide unambiguous evidence regarding the sensitivity and specificity of fMRI-based neuroscience methods in the detection of lies at the individual-subject or the individual-event levels. While it is possible that fMRI methods will ultimately prove effective for lie detection, future studies are needed to eliminate fundamental confounds that exist in the published literature. In addition, other issues that are likely to prove important for forensic practice have received little to no attention in the literature, including (a) whether the magnitude of the stakes of being caught lying matter, (b) the effects of counter measures, (c) how robust the methods are across subject populations (e.g., older adults, individuals with psychiatric disorders, individuals taking medications, etc.), (d) the effects of repeatedly probing the same "lie" or "truth" event, (e) the effects of retention interval (time between the critical event and when the brain scans are conducted), (f) the effects of instructed vs. subject-chosen deception, and (g) the effects of a lie's content (i.e., what is being lied about). Only future studies will tell whether fMRI-based neuroscience can identify lies."

Anthony Wagner, *Can Neuroscience Identify Lies?*, in *A Judge's Guide to Neuroscience: A Concise Introduction* 13 (2010).

5. Consider this perspective from law professor Jane Moriarty:

> I would urge an informal evidentiary moratorium on admission of this evidence unless and until the science has developed to a place where: (1) the scientists and their critics reach consensus that the results are truly valid, reliable, reproducible, accurate, and the error rate is within an acceptable margin of error; (2) the potential confounding problems related to sample size, group versus individual determinations, and the potential problems of correlation versus causation have been sorted out; and perhaps most importantly, (3) there has been time for sufficient moral, ethical, and jurisprudential rumination about whether the legal system really wants this type of evidence. This delay provides time for additional peer review, replication of results, robust disagreements, and discovery of unanticipated

consequences that might arise from this new, fascinating, and challenging scientific endeavor.

Jane Campbell Moriarty, *Visions of Deception: Neuroimages and the Search for Truth*, 42 Akron L. Rev. 739, 761 (2009). In what ways, and for what reasons, would you support or disagree with these bases for a moratorium?

6. Concerns are often raised about the prejudicial effect of brain-based lie detection evidence on jurors. But is this concern warranted? Consider a study in which subjects were randomly assigned to read either a vignette with fMRI lie detection evidence used, or a vignette without the lie detection evidence. Participants answered two questions after reading the vignette. The first asked, "[I]f you were a participant in the above trial, would you find the defendant guilty or not guilty?" The second question asked, "[W]hat evidence was the most influential in making your decision?" The study found that fMRI lie detection evidence led to more guilty verdicts, but not when that evidence was called into question during cross-examination. David P. McCabe et al., *The Influence of fMRI Lie Detection Evidence on Juror Decision-Making*, 29 Behav. Sci. & L. 566 (2011). Do these results make you more or less concerned? What additional studies would you like to see conducted?

Daniel D. Langleben et al.

Polygraphy and Functional Magnetic Resonance Imaging in Lie Detection: A Controlled Blind Comparison Using the Concealed Information Test

77 J. Clinical Psychiatry 1372, 1372-78 (2016)

We conducted a blind, prospective, and controlled within-subjects study to compare the accuracy of fMRI and polygraphy in the detection of concealed information. . . .

Participants (N = 28) secretly wrote down a number between 3 and 8 on a slip of paper and were questioned about what number they wrote during consecutive and counterbalanced fMRI and polygraphy sessions. . . . Each participant's preprocessed fMRI images and 5-channel polygraph data were independently evaluated by 3 fMRI and 3 polygraph experts, who made an independent determination of the number the participant wrote down and concealed. . . .

RESULTS

Detection Accuracy by Majority and Unanimity Rules

. . . The probability of 2 of the 3 raters agreeing (Majority Rule) about a Lie Item by chance was 1/36 (2.8%) and of all 3 raters (Unanimity Rule) agreeing was 1/216 (0.38%). We found that using the Majority Rule, the polygraph experts detected 20 out of 28 (71.4%) Lie Items, while fMRI experts detected 24 out of 28 (85.7%) Lie Items, with both modalities performing significantly better than chance. Applying the Unanimity Rule resulted in 17/28 (60.7%) Lie Item detection for polygraphy and 23/28 (82.1%) for fMRI, with both modalities yielding detection rates significantly greater than chance. . . .

DISCUSSION

. . . The greater accuracy of the fMRI experts may be explained by the differences between the sources of fMRI and polygraphy signals. While fMRI is able to parse the brain response to stimuli both in time and in space, polygraphy is a more integrative assessment of a subject's overall neurophysiological state. . . .

[W]e observed a high (17 out of 17) correct detection rate in cases in which polygraphy and fMRI were in agreement, suggesting that the 2 modalities may complement each other. . . . [O]ur finding of very high precision of positive determinations of the sequentially acquired fMRI and polygraphy suggests a clinically useful approach that might be able to reach an overall accuracy acceptable for criminal proceedings, where avoiding convictions of the innocent takes precedence.

Joshua D. Greene & Joseph M. Paxton
Patterns of Neural Activity Associated with Honest and Dishonest Moral Decisions
106 Proc. Nat'l Acad. Sci. U.S. 12506, 12506-10 (2009)

[L]ittle is known about the cognitive processes that generate honest and dishonest behavior, and the neural bases of choices to behave honestly or dishonestly have, to our knowledge, never been studied specifically. . . .

The present study uses fMRI (functional magnetic resonance imaging) and a behavioral design inspired by research on moral hypocrisy to examine the neural bases of honest and dishonest choices. More specifically, this study tests 2 competing hypotheses concerning the cognitive nature of honesty. According to the "Will" hypothesis, honesty results from the active resistance of temptation, comparable to the controlled cognitive processes that enable individuals to delay gratification. According to the "Grace" hypothesis, honesty results from the absence of temptation, consistent with research emphasizing the determination of behavior by the presence or absence of automatic processes. These hypotheses make competing predictions concerning the engagement of prefrontal structures associated with cognitive control in honest individuals as they choose to refrain from dishonest behavior.

Subjects undergoing fMRI attempted to predict the outcomes of random computerized coin-flips and were financially rewarded for accuracy and punished for inaccuracy. In the No Opportunity condition, subjects recorded their predictions in advance, denying them the opportunity to cheat by lying about their accuracy. In the Opportunity condition, subjects made their predictions privately and were rewarded based on their self-reported accuracy, affording them the opportunity to cheat. . . . We used a cover story to justify our giving subjects obvious opportunities for dishonest gain. This study was presented as a study of paranormal abilities to "predict the future," aimed at testing the hypotheses that people are better able to predict the future when their predictions are (i) private and (ii) financially incentivized. Thus, subjects were implicitly led to believe, first, that the opportunity for dishonest gain was a known but unintended by-product of the experiment's design and, second, that they were expected to behave honestly. We note that in employing this cover story, subjects were deceived about the experimenters' interests, but not about the economic structure of the task. . . .

As noted above, the Will and Grace hypotheses make competing predictions concerning the neural activity of honest individuals when they choose to refrain from dishonest behavior. More specifically, these hypotheses make competing predictions concerning the following comparison within the honest group: Opportunity Loss trials (in which the subject lost money because s/he chose not to cheat) vs. No-Opportunity Loss trials (in which the subject lost money and could do nothing about it). According to the Will hypothesis, forgoing an opportunity for dishonest gain requires the active resistance of temptation. Thus, the Will hypothesis predicts that, in the honest group, the Opportunity Loss trials (relative to No-Opportunity Loss trials) will preferentially engage brain regions associated with response conflict, cognitive control, and/or response inhibition. . . . According to the Grace hypothesis, honest behavior follows from the absence of temptation, implying no need to actively resist temptation when the opportunity for dishonest gain is present. Thus, the Grace hypothesis, in its strongest form, predicts that honest individuals will exhibit no additional control-related activity when they choose to refrain from dishonest behavior. Both of these hypotheses also make competing predictions concerning reaction time (RT). The Will hypothesis predicts that honest individuals will exhibit increased RTs when they choose to refrain from dishonest behavior, reflecting the engagement of additional controlled cognitive processes in actively resisting temptation. In contrast, the Grace hypothesis, in its strongest form, predicts that honest individuals will exhibit no difference in RT between Opportunity Loss trials and No-Opportunity Loss trials.

Results. . . . The behavioral and fMRI data support the Grace hypothesis over the Will hypothesis, suggesting that honest moral decisions depend more on the absence of temptation than on the active resistance of temptation. Individuals who behaved honestly showed no sign of engaging additional controlled cognitive processes when choosing to behave honestly. These individuals exhibited no additional neural activity of any kind when they chose to forgo opportunities for dishonest gain, as compared with control trials in which there was no such opportunity. We provided a more stringent test of this negative result by dramatically reducing the statistical threshold for this comparison, focusing on brain regions that exhibited effects for this comparison in dishonest subjects. This more-stringent test also revealed no effects, and further tests . . . confirmed that the honest and dishonest subjects exhibited different patterns of activity in these regions. [The data also indicated that the differences between individuals in dishonest behavior was correlated with brain activation (Figure 15.2).] The RT data support the Grace hypothesis as well: Honest individuals took no longer to forgo opportunities for dishonest gain than they did to report their forced losses in control trials. Dishonest individuals, in contrast, took considerably longer to forgo opportunities for dishonest gain. . . .

Although our present focus is on the cognitive neuroscience of honesty and dishonesty, our findings and methods may be of interest to researchers studying brain-based lie detection, in part because the present study is arguably the first to establish a correlation between patterns of neural activity and real lying. However, the present experiment has several notable limitations that deserve attention. First, the model we have developed has not been tested on an independent sample, and therefore its probative value remains unknown. Second, our task design does not allow us to identify individual lies. Third, our findings highlight the challenge in distinguishing lying from related cognitive processes such as deciding whether

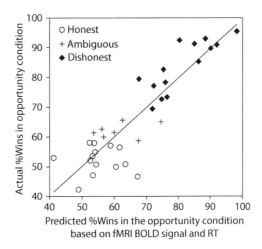

Figure 15.2 [The frequency of dishonest behavior assessed by the percentage of Wins in the Opportunity test condition was accounted for by the fMRI BOLD signal in left dorsolateral prefrontal cortex, dorsomedial prefrontal cortex, right parietal cortex, and bilateral ventrolateral prefrontal cortex. — EDS.]

to lie. Finally, it is not known whether our task is an ecologically valid model for real-world lying. For example, the neural signature of real prepared lies may look different from the patterns observed in association with lying here. Bearing these limitations in mind, our findings may suggest new avenues for research on brain-based lie detection. For example, our findings suggest that interrogations aimed at eliciting indecision about whether to lie, rather than lies per se, may be more effective, provided that the goal is to assess the trustworthiness of the subject rather than the veracity of specific statements.

**Anthony Wagner et al., The MacArthur Foundation
Research Network on Law and Neuroscience**
fMRI and Lie Detection: A Knowledge Brief
(2016)

[Judge ERIC M. JOHNSON, of the Maryland Sixth Judicial Circuit, Montgomery County, refused to admit potentially exculpatory fMRI lie detection evidence in the murder trial of *State v. Gary Smith.*] Citing the *Frye* standard, Johnson wrote, "It is clear to the Court that the use of fMRI to detect deception and verify truth in an individual's brain has not achieved general acceptance in the scientific community."

While research on fMRI-based lie detection has continued, the general consensus in the scientific community regarding its probative value remains the same. This brief explores why. . . .

Many scientists argue that the conclusions drawn from fMRI "lie detection" experiments conducted to date are only valid within the context of the experimental data.

Group data might not be able to tell us what we need to know about an individual.   The holy grail of lie detection is to distinguish truth from lie reliably at the level of the individual subject and at the level of the individual question. But most of the studies conducted on deception to date focus on truth vs. lie differences averaged over multiple subjects and trials.

A sufficient amount of group-averaged data can indicate that a certain pattern of neural activity is frequently associated with a particular experimental condition. However, they cannot tell us whether the pattern of activation is not also common to other experimental conditions (or mental processes). Nor, for the moment, can they shed much light on whether fMRI can reliably detect lies at the level of the individual subject or question. In his testimony during the Semrau trial, Cephos Corporation CEO Steven Laken, who conducted the fMRI lie detection tests submitted as evidence, confirmed that they did not indicate whether Dr. Semrau responded truthfully as to any specific question and that it was "certainly possible" that Dr. Semrau was lying on some of the particularly significant questions.

Experimental conditions often poorly approximate the real world.   To date, fMRI studies have focused on detecting lies about an event that just occurred. The event often has no personal relevance and no consequences. Real-world fMRI lie detection focuses on events or facts that are likely to have occurred months or even years before, are deeply relevant to the subject, and have serious consequences. Little is known about whether real-world and experimental conditions yield similar results.

The sensitivity and specificity of fMRI lie detection   have not been established. No diagnostic tool is perfectly accurate. Antiviral software sometimes detects threats that aren't there; mammograms miss tumors. The probative value of fMRI-based evidence depends on knowing how many lies the tool misses and how often it identifies the truth as a lie; few research studies to date have reported such data.

Findings may not be generalizable to other populations.   fMRI studies typically are conducted on undergraduates and other healthy younger adults. Even if we know that there is neural activity in particular regions under the condition of lying when subjects are younger and healthy—a matter of debate, as already discussed—do we know anything at all about what to expect from a woman of 70, or someone with a mental illness?

PRINCIPLED OBJECTIONS

At present, many of the issues that concern the scientific community with respect to the use of fMRI for lie detection are likely to be problematic for the legal community, at least in most contexts. In fact, much of the existing research on deception has no bearing on the question that matters most to judges, lawyers, defendants, and juries, i.e., "Can fMRI-based lie detection methods provide a legally relevant answer to a specific question?"

Most scientists—including many who have reported detecting lies in the laboratory with a high degree of accuracy—agree that more and different research will need to be conducted before fMRI-based lie detection is ready for its day in court.

NOTES AND QUESTIONS

1. How, if at all, do the two studies excerpted above affect your evaluation of the probability that fMRI techniques will one day be broadly admissible in court for lie detection purposes?

2. Do you agree with the Greene and Paxton distinction between "Will" and "Grace" explanations for truth-telling? Do these alternatives completely cover the space of possibilities? Are you convinced that complex psychological and moral concepts like "Will" and "Grace" can be resolved entirely by patterns of brain activation measured with fMRI?

3. A 2014 meta-analysis of neuroimaging studies of deception found that, across studies, deception was correlated with a number of networks of brain activation, including the bilateral ACC, inferior frontal gyrus, insula, and bilateral inferior parietal lobe. These results were consistent with an earlier 2009 study. *See* Shawn E. Christ et al., *The Contributions of Prefrontal Cortex and Executive Control to Deception: Evidence from Activation Likelihood Estimate Meta-analyses*, 19 Cerebral Cortex 1557 (2009). This meta-analysis also divided studies into social interactive and non-interactive categories to determine whether the social component to certain types of deception led to different patterns of brain activation. The analysis revealed increased activation in the dorsal ACC, right TPJ, and bilateral temporal pole during social interactive compared to non-interactive conditions. The authors suggest that "deceiving an interaction partner requires other processes and activates more brain regions involved in moral and social behavior than solely not saying the truth." The studies also found distinct patterns of activation between tests that allowed a volitional decision to deceive and those that instructed the subject to deceive. Although progress has been made, the authors warn that there is still much to be done in this field. *See* Nina Lisofsky et al., *Investigating Socio-Cognitive Processes in Deception: A Quantitative Meta-analysis of Neuroimaging Studies*, 61 Neuropsychologia 113, 120 (2014).

4. While functional near-infrared spectroscopy (fNIRS) is not a new technology, it is only just beginning to be investigated for lie detection purposes. The procedure itself is similar to both EEG and fMRI procedures. The subject wears a cap with sensors on it, as for an EEG, but to detect BOLD responses, as does fMRI. Also, like EEG, fNIRS has greater temporal resolution than fMRI (10 samples per one second vs. one sample per two seconds). However, fNIRS has a spatial resolution more similar to fMRI, although detection is limited to cortical regions.

   Scientists have recently compared the accuracy of fNIRS in lie detection to the accuracy of the polygraph. For this study, fNIRS was used to measure activation in prefrontal cortex areas that had been previously correlated to lying. A standard polygraph procedure was followed. The test results showed that the polygraph was more accurate than fNIRS by a small margin (74.5% correct vs. 71.6% correct). However, when the scientists used both fNIRS and polygraph data to determine if the subject was lying, the accuracy increased to 86.5%. This is a similar result to Langleben's findings using fMRI and polygraph data, as well as to other studies using EEG P300 and fNIRS data. At what level of accuracy do you think courts should admit lie detection evidence? *See* Xiaohong Lin, Liyang Sai & Zhen Yuan, *Detecting Concealed Information with Fused Electroencephalography and Functional Near-Infrared Spectroscopy*, 386 Neurosci. 284 (2018); M. Raheel Bhutta et al., *Single-Trial Lie Detection Using a Combined fNIRS-Polygraph System*, 6 Frontiers Psychol. 709 (2015).

5. You should be aware that brain-based lie detection has been central to at least one case in India, *Maharashtra v. Sharma & Khandelwal*, Sessions Case No. 508/07

(June 12, 2008), which involved a love triangle in which the two defendants were accused of killing the betrothed of one of them. One defendant was subjected to an involuntary Brain Electrical Oscillation Signature Profiling (BEOS) Test, which purportedly "revealed her experiential knowledge of the commission of the offence," her conspiracy with her co-defendant, and in particular their plan to commit murder by poisoning with arsenic. BEOS is an EEG technique (similar to Farwell's, above), and as applied, it involved the subject hearing a number of voiced "probes"—short sentences or phrases—that depicted different scenarios. The subject was instructed to sit silently and to say nothing as her brain activities were recorded, following each probe. The court rejected the argument that the BEOS findings were hearsay. Moreover, found the court, "Unless and until she has participated in such offence, her responses to Experiential Knowledge could not have been activated. . . ." The court acknowledged that the BEOS Tests were not to be treated as conclusive, but rather were just one link in the chain of circumstantial evidence. It found that, adding the BEOS testing to other evidence in the case was sufficient to support both conviction and life imprisonment. Separately, the Supreme Court of India, in *Selvi v. Karnataka* (Criminal Appeal No. 1267 of 2004), held in 2010 (in the case excerpted in the introduction to this chapter) that no individual should be forcibly subjected to certain physiological investigative techniques. The forbidden techniques included the administration of "narco-analysis," which involves the intravenous administration of drugs causing the subject "to enter into a hypnotic trance and become less inhibited" during interrogation.

6. To what extent would you expect fMRI techniques to work equally well on citizens of differing countries? On this subject, see Tommaso Bruni, *Cross-Cultural Variation and fMRI Lie-Detection*, in *Technologies on the Stand: Legal and Ethical Questions in Neuroscience and Robotics* 129 (B. Van den Berg & L. Klaming eds., 2011).

7. Should admissibility of brain-based lie detection evidence turn, in part, on who is proffering the evidence, and for what purpose? Law professor Charles Keckler proposes "a model that begins with limited admissibility in those contexts most likely to encourage increased rigor-namely, when the proponent is adverse to the witness tested, a circumstance that implies the use of fMRI initially for impeachment rather than substantive evidence. This way there can be mutual benefit for civil plaintiffs and defendants to "cross examine" the brain of a witness whose credibility has been put in doubt." Charles N.W. Keckler, *Cross-Examining the Brain: A Legal Analysis of Neural Imaging for Credibility Impeachment*, 57 Hastings L.J. 509 (2006). Do you agree with this approach?

C. CRITICAL PERSPECTIVES

As evident in the proceedings in the previous sections, the value—both scientific and legal—of the polygraph and of brain-based lie detection methods are hotly debated. In this section we present aspects of that debate.

Frederick Schauer
Neuroscience, Lie-Detection, and the Law
14 Trends Cognitive Sci. 101, 101-02 (2010)

THE CURRENT DEBATE

Because courts rely on witness accounts rather than direct investigation, credibility is a central concern of the law. These concerns are often about the misperception, hedging, fudging, and slanting that is rampant in a system dominated by testimony from self-interested parties, but law also worries about flat-out lying. And because cross-examination is widely known to be more effective in exposing liars on television than in real courtrooms, the legal system is constantly seeking better ways of testing veracity. Legal debates about lie-detecting technology have existed since the 1920s, but with few exceptions the law still prohibits the use of polygraphs, electroencephalography, periorbital spectrography, and other technologies, relying instead on the technologically unaided judge and jury.

The terrain has changed with claims that neuroimaging can identify deception more accurately than its predecessors. However, numerous neuroscientists have challenged these claims, arguing that differences between experimental subjects and those offering evidence in court create problems of external validity and that problems of construct validity arise because an instructed lie in the laboratory is simply not a real lie at all. Moreover, much of the relevant research is not published in peer-reviewed journals, has been produced by financially interested scientists connected with truth verification companies such as CEPHOS or No Lie MRI, and is significantly less reliable than claimed.

For such reasons, the overwhelming scientific opinion is that fMRI lie-detection is a "research topic and not a legal tool," a conclusion emphasized by worries about how the research might be used. It would be wrong, it is argued, to use brain scans to "send [someone] to prison," and even worse if "the police [could] request a warrant to search your brain." And thus one article urged a moratorium on the law's use of neuroimaging until its reliability is established to the satisfaction of federal regulators.

CHALLENGING THE CHALLENGERS

At one level these criticisms appear sound. External and construct validity are problematic, the claims of reliability are exaggerated, the lack of peer review is a fact, and some researchers are indeed connected with interested commercial entities. But at another level the criticisms are based on three flawed premises: that most legal decisions are about sending people to prison; that the standards of science should be the standards of law; and that the legal system's current approach to determining veracity is acceptable.

Although the legal system sends people to prison, doing so requires proof beyond a reasonable doubt. So even if prosecutors, despite existing self-incrimination law, could compel a brain scan of a defendant, the reliability of fMRI lie-detection is not nearly high enough to support conviction under that standard. The converse of the prosecution's heavy burden, however, is a defendant's ability to defeat conviction by showing only a reasonable possibility—not even a probability—of innocence. Even if neural lie-detection reliability were only 0.60, a level grossly insufficient to support conviction, that level, if supporting a defendant's alibi, say, could raise a reasonable doubt as to guilt. Plainly judges have a responsibility to exclude spurious pseudo-evidence that might produce unreasonable doubts, but judges in jury trials have played this gatekeeping role for centuries.

The low confidence in innocence sufficient to acquit is just one example of legal decisions made on the basis of confidence levels well below those necessary for scientific publication. Judgments in civil cases demand only a "preponderance of the evidence," and other decisions require "reasonable suspicion," "probable cause," or merely a "scintilla of evidence." Most importantly, the confidence necessary to admit an item of evidence is much lower than that necessary to justify a verdict—admission into evidence requires only that a proposition be more likely with the evidence than without.

The same considerations apply to external and construct validity. Experiments on undergraduates, for example, justify conclusions about behavior in non-laboratory settings when we know from other research that the behavior of subjects correlates with that of non-subjects. So although laboratory deception differs from real-world deception, any positive correlation between laboratory and non-laboratory deception would require using legal and not scientific standards to determine whether that correlation was sufficient.

The arguments are similar for construct validity. With one prominent exception, the research on neural lie-detection is largely about instructed lies, which are not lies at all. But if the ease of telling an instructed lie in the laboratory correlates with the ease of telling a real lie outside the laboratory, research on instructed lies is no longer irrelevant to detecting real lies. With any positive correlation between instructed and real lies, experiments on the former will tell us something about the latter, and whether that 'something' is enough depends on the uses for which the research is employed. That which is inadequate for scientific publication or criminal prosecution might be sufficient for a defendant seeking to suggest reasonable doubt.

In law as in science, "compared to what?" is an important question. Evaluating fMRI lie-detection requires knowing what it would supplement or replace. As it turns out, the methods now used are worse than the science that is routinely excluded. Currently, the jury or judge (when there is no jury) determines if witnesses are telling the truth. When cross-examination provides little assistance, as it rarely does, juries are instructed to evaluate the "demeanor" of a witness to determine veracity. In doing this, however, they rely on numerous myths, urban legends, and pop psychology with little reliability. They distrust witnesses who perspire, fidget, and fail to make eye contact, and trust those who speak confidently while looking directly at them. Research shows that ordinary people's ability to distinguish truth from lies rarely rises above random, and juries are unlikely to do better. The question is thus whether imaging should be rejected in favor of methods—methods that go to the heart of the jury system, have been in place for centuries, and are extremely unlikely to be changed substantially—that are demonstrably unreliable. The answer to this question will depend on a comparison for which there is yet little evidence, but the point is only that the admissibility of neural lie-detection evidence must be based on an evaluation of the realistic alternatives within the legal system and not on a non-comparative assessment of whether neural lie-detection meets the standards that scientists use for scientific purposes.

But might courts interpret a brain image as having more evidentiary value than it actually possesses? If a scan had a reliability rate of 0.72, might a juror, seeing a "picture" of a brain in vivid color, ignore the 0.28 chance of error and assume absolute accuracy? Might a juror take a scan supporting only one aspect of a defendant's story as "proving" that the defendant was innocent? These risks are real, but the research fails to distinguish seeing a brain image from seeing any color picture, any multi-color diagram, or even any pseudoscientific explanation unrelated to brain imaging. One study, for example, compared perception of a brain image with straight text and with a two-color bar graph to conclude that the brain image produced unjustified reliance. But we do not know whether the mistaken attribution of content is a function of the image being a picture, of it having gradations of color, or of it being a brain. By not controlling for the potential confounds of the non-brain attributes of a brain image, the study cannot tell us whether it is a brain image that produces unwarranted attribution of content, or whether the effect comes simply from the kinds of multi-color or photographic images routinely used for forensic purposes. Although overvaluation is a legitimate worry, the degree of legitimacy is a function of how much, if at all, a brain image produces perceptual distortions beyond those already endemic to litigation.

THE STANDARDS FOR THE USE OF SCIENCE IN LAW CANNOT BE DERIVED FROM SCIENCE ALONE

Once we comprehend the range of standards the legal system now uses, the scalar and not binary character of reliability and validity, and the legal system's venerable reliance on techniques for identifying deception that are worse than even the most modest claims for neural lie-detection, the case against fMRI becomes less compelling. Still, the use of neural lie-detection now is probably unwarranted. But whether it is, and if not now then when, is a determination that cannot be made solely on the basis of scientific standards. The goals of the legal system differ from those of science, and thus what is good enough for science might still not be good enough for law, and what is not good enough for science might sometimes be good enough for law. Science must inform the legal system about reliability rates and degrees of validity, but whether some rate or degree is good enough for some legal purpose is a question of law and not of science.

Henry T. Greely
Premarket Approval Regulation for Lie Detections: An Idea Whose Time May Be Coming
5 Am. J. Bioethics 50, 50-52 (2005)

The FDA seems to offer the only existing path to requiring premarket approval of lie detection devices or drugs and, under existing statutes, it will rarely have jurisdiction. Aside from the largely absent premarket approval limits, there are some important restrictions on how employers may use lie-detecting devices with employees. Unfortunately, it is not clear that they are sufficient.

The most important statute is the federal Employee Polygraph Protection Act of 1988 (FEPPA). This Act prohibits most employers "directly or indirectly, to require, request, suggest, or cause any employee or prospective employee to take or submit to any lie-detector test." The Act defines a lie-detector test broadly as "a polygraph, deceptograph, voice stress analyzer, psychological stress evaluator, or any other similar device (whether mechanical or electrical) that is used, or the results of which are used, for the purpose of rendering a diagnostic opinion regarding the honesty or dishonesty of an individual." The Act does not apply to government employees or to various contractors, experts, and others involved in national security or working with the FBI. It permits private employers to make limited use of polygraphs—but only polygraphs—in ongoing investigations and allows broader polygraph use for a few employers. There is no relevant federal law outside the employment context. Some states have statutes specifically restricting some uses of polygraph machines, although these also focus on employment. State laws differ on whether they restrict polygraphs specifically (e.g., Texas) or lie detection more generally (e.g., California).

The courtroom situation is more complicated. The New Mexico Supreme Court has adopted a rule of evidence generally allowing polygraph evidence under some conditions (*Lee v. Martinez*); military courts are bound by a rule of evidence excluding such evidence (*United States v. Scheffer*). Most other courts view the admissibility of polygraph evidence as an issue of the admissibility of scientific or technical evidence; a few are bound by state statutes. Almost all reject it. The test for admissibility of scientific evidence widely used in American courts through most of the 20th century, the *Frye* test, takes its name from a 1923 case involving the admissibility of testimony of a polygraph operator (*Frye v. United States*). The *Frye* test was replaced for federal courts, and many state courts, by the *Daubert* test after a 1993 decision of the United States Supreme Court (*Daubert v. Merrell Dow Pharmaceuticals, Inc.*). The *Frye* and *Daubert* tests have spawned a vast literature on their individual and comparative merits; for present purposes it is important only to note that both tests rely, at least in the first instance, on the trial court judge to make a decision about the admissibility of the evidence based on expert testimony before her. Neither test requires extended experimentation or sets any accuracy standards that have to be attained (though the *Daubert* test does at least inquire about error rates). Presumably any evidence coming from a new method of lie detection would be admitted or not based on a trial court determination of whether it complied with *Frye* or *Daubert*. Such case-by-case decisions pose a great risk of inconsistency; they also open the possibility that lie detection will be admitted by a judge even though it is not truly reliable.

A better solution, both for courts and more generally, would be to pass federal legislation requiring FDA-like regulation of all lie-detection drugs and devices, whether based on new neuroscience or not. We should prohibit the sale, marketing, distribution, or use of lie detectors until they have been proven, by rigorous trials, to be safe and effective. The rigorous trials would have to examine subjects who were representative of the population—in age, sex, ethnicity, and other characteristics. They would have to test people who had strong incentives to deceive the lie detector as well as people who had been trained in possible ways to beat it. Many types of questions would have to be tried, to see whether the lie detector worked better or worse with particular approaches. And the subjects could be observed for any possible ill effects from the experience. After sufficient study, these lie detectors would be approved or rejected.

This solution, of course, comes with its own problems. Two loom large.

First, who decides whether the lie detector is safe and effective? The FDA has great experience with the design (and critique) of clinical trials and with assessing drug and device safety. It is not perfect, but it seems better than anything else in the federal government. It has no expertise, however, in assessing the efficacy of lie detection and, quite likely, no desire to build up such expertise. Although the FDA covers that large part of the economy that involves putting things in, on, or through our bodies, lie detection seems far from its core. It might well resist Congressional efforts to give it this power. On the other hand, no other agency seems a good fit. The Department of Justice, the only plausible location for such authority, has no experience with scientific trials — and its impartiality might be doubted.

Second, how does an agency decide whether a lie detector is safe and effective? Those terms are never self-defining. The FDA has long experience in calibrating the safety and efficacy of new drugs to the situation — an approvable drug to treat metastatic pancreatic cancer can be a lot less safe, and effective, than a drug to treat teenagers' acne. When the issue is lie detection, something not likely to help the subject's health, safety might be strictly construed to require no significant health risk. But how much efficacy is enough? Should any improvement over random guessing be sufficient as long as the improvement is statistically significant at the 0.01, 0.05, or 0.10 level? Should any improvement over an assessment made by a veteran FBI investigator, an experienced judge, or a careful lay observer, be sufficient? Would efficacy have to be across the board or could it be approved based on efficacy with some populations, or with some kinds of questions, or in some circumstances? The correct answers are not obvious.

Those two are just opening questions. If lie detectors were approved, which substantive uses of them should we permit and which should we prohibit? Should all lie detection be banned, no matter how reliable, with or without a national security exception? What constitutional issues would be raised by their use in the courtroom? Or, as Justice Thomas, writing for four justices, suggested, should all litigation uses of even reliable lie detectors be banned as overly invading the jury's province? (*United States v. Scheffer.*) On the other hand, maybe we should just require rigorous testing, producing solid error rates, and then allow people and institutions to make their own decisions about how accurate is good enough.

On a more mundane level, who would pay for the testing? How would the class of lie detectors be defined, particularly in light of the unknown possibilities that neuroscience may be opening? Would the lie detector operators need to be licensed or otherwise specially qualified? How could we effectively regulate lie detector uses of existing equipment, approved for other purposes, like MRI machines? Finally, and perhaps least resolvable, what could convince Congress to pass reasonable legislation on this issue?

Given the many and serious technical difficulties Wolpe et al. outline in developing a reliable lie detector, it may be too early to draft, let alone to pass, such legislation. Given the many issues of principle and of practicality that would have to be resolved, it is not too early to begin thinking about the shape of the legislation that may be needed.

Michael S. Pardo

Lying, Deception, and fMRI: A Critical Update

in *Neurolaw and Responsibility for Action: Concepts, Crimes, and Courts* 143,
144-49 (Bebhinn Donnelly-Lazarov ed., 2018)

I will focus on two conceptual issues. . . . (1) the distinction between deception and lying, and (2) the concept of lying itself (or the criteria for what constitutes a lie). . . .

The array of empirical issues [with fMRI lie detection] . . . takes place within a conceptual framework that includes a number of presuppositions about what exactly is being measured. . . . These issues are conceptual. . .because they do not concern the empirical relationship between brain activity and behaviors; rather, they concern the concepts that are used to identity and pick out the target behaviors in the first place. For this reason, the conceptual issues are in an important sense prior to, or foundational for, the empirical issues. . . .

In some cases, 'lies' are defined in terms of 'an intent to deceive.' . . . [T]his focus on deception makes sense because there is likely to be substantial overlap between lying and intending to deceive. . . . But the equation of lying with deception is also conceptually problematic. . . . It is possible to deceive without lying, and it is possible to lie without deceiving or even having an intent to deceive. An example . . . includes a witness who has been threatened into giving false alibi testimony for [another] witness. The witness may give such testimony not intending to deceive but hoping the audience (the police, a judge, or a jury) will see through the false statements and refuse to rely on them. The witness will have undoubtedly lied, and the testimony will also fit legal definitions for perjury and false-statement crimes. Importantly, however, the witness will not have had an intent to deceive. Thus, fMRI technology that could reliably measure deceptive intentions would nevertheless be under-inclusive in measuring whether someone is lying or speaking sincerely. . . .

[L]ying involves more than simply stating something that is false or that a speaker believes to be false. There is also a social, normative component to lying that distinguishes it from other activities such as acting in a play, role-playing, playing a game, telling a joke, or using sarcasm, in which actors may say things they believe to be false. . . . [Philosopher Don Fallis] explains, the difference that makes saying 'I am the Prince of Denmark' a lie when told at a dinner party but not when on stage during a play are the distinct norms of conversation that are in effect in the former. In the former, but not the latter, there is an operative norm against communicating something believed to be false. . . .

This normative component is critically important in legal settings. Lying in such settings not only violates an operative communicative norm—it [is] also illegal. This normative component, however, appears to be absent in the fMRI experiments.

Marc Jonathan Blitz

Searching Minds by Scanning Brains: Neuroscience Technology and Constitutional Privacy Protection

26-33 (Marc J. Blitz, Jan C. Bublitz & Jane C. Moriarty eds., 2017)

A BRIEF TOUR OF THE CONSTITUTIONAL PRIVACY LANDSCAPE—AND NEUROIMAGING'S POSSIBLE PLACE IN IT

To understand better why the constitutional puzzles raised by neuroimaging are challenging puzzles, it is helpful to consider the relevant constitutional law more closely. As noted earlier, one might assume that at least in the United States, certain constitutional provisions—such as the Fourth and Fifth Amendments of the US constitution—already do stand in the way of government-compelled neuroimaging. But a closer look at these amendments raises doubts about this claim. . . .

[This discussion by Professor Blitz contains reference to the following hypothetical scenario: Ivy and Ozzie are suspects in a murder. Due to a long-term memory problem, Ozzie records everything from a video camera implanted in his skull that copies its footage to a computer chip implanted in his brain. Ivy has excellent long-term memory. — EDS]

The Fifth Amendment's Bar on Self-Incrimination

The Fifth Amendment's self-incrimination clause states that "no person . . . shall be compelled in any criminal case to be a witness against himself." Police may not, consistent with the Fifth Amendment, force a person facing a criminal trial to give a statement incriminating himself. And if they instead seek to obtain information about the accused's past actions from compelled brain scans rather than compelled statements, this — some scholars argue — would be an unconstitutional end-run around the Fifth Amendment (New 2008, 193-195). Even if police are not using a defendant's spoken words to incriminate him, they would be using unspoken thoughts and memories of a kind that, in prior years, would have been accessible to them only through the accused's testimony. If, as the Supreme Court has indicated, "it is contrary to the letter and spirit of the Fifth Amendment" to "force someone to disclose the contents of his mind," then forcing someone to disclose this mental content by submitting to a brain scan should be just as impermissible as forcing him to disclose his thoughts verbally (*Curcio v. United States* 1957, 128; *United States v. Hubbell* 2000, 43). Or so the argument goes.

Consider again the scenario where Ivy is suspected of committing a murder with Ozzie as her accomplice — and where the police wish to examine Ivy's brain in an fMRI scanner. . . . Ivy will argue that police's viewing of her brain's response to the stimulus is functionally equivalent to compelling her testimony. They are forbidden by the Fifth Amendment from forcing her to answer the question, do you recognize this face or this living room?, so they are instead forcing her to take a brain scan which provides police with the mental states that would underlie an honest answer to those questions. The government, by contrast, will argue that changes in the Ivy's brain triggered by her presence in (a memory of) that living room are not at all like compelled statements. They are not seeking to answer the hypothetical question of how Ivy would respond if she were compelled to answer questions about the victim or the crime scene. They are rather asking whether Ivy's brain behaves in ways that are consistent with her claim that she's never seen the victim or the victim's living room. In the sense, the brain evidence is like other physical evidence. If, for example, police found a carpet fiber from the victim's living room on one of Ivy's shoes, this would challenge her claim that she's never been in that living room Similarly, if police find her brain responds to the living room picture in a way that they know (from past experimental work) is extremely unlikely if she'd never seen it before, then this — they can argue — is a reason to believe Ivy was in that living room, and a reason that has weight no matter what Ivy would say (if forced to speak) and no matter what Ivy's current beliefs might be about what she did or didn't do in the past. All that matters is that her brain showed activity it wouldn't be likely to show unless she had a past encounter with that living room. . . .

Whether the evidence lies in a fiber from the living room carpet, or a video recording in Ozzie's camera, or the wiring in Ivy's brain, government might argue, in all of these cases the nature of the evidence is the same for self-incrimination clause purposes: the defendants' interactions with the crime scene left a mark on their persons, and police are free to uncover such traces of defendants' pasts so long as they don't require the defendant to tell them about it. Although the Fifth Amendment establishes a zone of autonomy, in a sense, shielding the defendant from having to communicate, to police, evidence of her guilt, this zone cannot be so extensive—government might argue—that it can shut the police for all evidence that the defendant's criminal activity may have left in the world, or on his own person. To do so would arguably go beyond safeguarding the suspect's autonomy, or other interests protected by the Fifth Amendment, and deprive the police of much of the evidence they, and the justice system, will respectively need to investigate and fairly adjudicate criminal cases.

As noted earlier, evidence revealing that Ivy was in a particular living room also tells police something about Ivy's memories: If evidence places her there, then it is likely she has some memory of being there. But such an inference is possible not only when police see certain brain activity in an fMRI scan, but also when they find carpet fibers on Ivy's shoes. The brain activity may provide more confidence that Ivy has a memory of the living room. But, is its linkage with the mental state that it correlates with close enough that one can justify treating the brain activity record as equivalent to a self-incriminating statement in a way that the carpet fiber is not?

The Fourth Amendment's Search and Seizure Protection

The Fourth Amendment analysis follows a similar pattern. . . . The Fourth Amendment protects "persons, houses, papers, and effects" against "unreasonable searches and seizures." Its protection against unreasonable searches, the US Supreme Court, has said, shields Americans against "too permeating police surveillance" (*United States v. Di Re* 1948, 595). Although the public—and the police, on the public's behalf—has an important need to uncover criminal activity and bring its perpetrators to justice, this need must coexist with a need for privacy and spaces which, as the Court has said, remain largely free from the government's presence and control. Thus, while police are expected to investigate crimes vigorously, this does not mean they may decide, any time they like, to enter a person's house and rummage through her belongings, or log into her computer and review digital files there, in the hope they may find some evidence of a crime. Rather, in US society, unconsented-to state entry into a person's private home or files—or any other place in which she has a "reasonable expectation of privacy" (*Katz v. United States* 1967, 360-361)—is supposed to be an unusual event that can be justified only by an unusual circumstance; namely, a situation where police can show a judge that they have "probable cause" to believe they will find evidence of a crime in that house or those files. The first question courts would thus have to answer in deciding whether and how the Fourth Amendment limits the scanning of an individual's brain is whether such a scan would count as a "search" subject to constitutional limits. The answer is almost certainly "yes." The Supreme Court has repeatedly held that when certain private realms—like our bodies or houses—are (as a general matter) off-limits to police surveillance, government may not circumvent such privacy protection by using "see-through" technology to observe the insides of such private realms from the outside (*Kyllo v. United States* 2000, 36-37). . . . And authorities, courts have made clear, are likewise constrained by Fourth Amendment limits when they use metal detectors, X-ray devices, or similar technology to examine individuals or their coats, or the insides of their handbags or suitcases at airports, train stations, or sporting events. Officials likewise engage in a search when they use X-ray technology to view the insides of our bodies.

They do something similar when they use fMRI or fNIR technology to image a person's brain activity: These devices respectively use radio waves (in a magnetic field), or near-infra red light, to gather information of processes inside a person's body that would otherwise remain hidden. This is sufficient to make such a technique count as a Fourth Amendment search. Thus, the Fourth Amendment analysis of our prior hypothetical about Ivy and Ozzie may seem much simpler than the Fifth Amendment analysis: It would be a search for police to search Ivy's brain—even if they have no intent of inferring anything about her mental states. Any time the state gathers information from the body's interior it is a search, so state-mandated neuroimaging is a search no matter what its purposes are. And this is true even if we view the state's accessing, and monitoring of Ivy's brain activity, as analogous to obtaining and watching the video stored in Ozzie's camera and computer chip—because that video extraction would also be a search (and a seizure of the video) under the Fourth Amendment. If government helps itself to files (whether electronic documents or video files) from the inside of your computer or SmartPhone, this is a Fourth Amendment search and seizure, and so it would likewise be a search and seizure for them to help themselves to the video files stored in Ozzie's camera and computer chip.

But that the use of neuroimaging, or other advanced technology, is presumptively a search is only the beginning of the Fourth Amendment inquiry. Even if the Fourth Amendment stands in the way of government-compelled brain scans, this leaves us with a second important question—namely, just how high a barrier does it present? . . . [E]ven if brain scan is generally such a "search" by law enforcement . . . under what circumstance may law enforcement nonetheless show that gathering data from the brain is reasonable?

As a general matter, law enforcement can only prevail in such an argument when it can obtain a warrant from a neutral magistrate, something it can in turn do only when it specifies a place, person, or thing to be searched and shows it has probable cause to believe it will uncover evidence of criminal activity there. But the warrant requirement is not necessarily a very high bar. To show probable cause, police generally need to demonstrate "a fair probability that contraband or evidence of a crime will be found in a particular place" (*Illinois v. Gates* 1983, 238). That provides a hurdle of sorts, but—if our unshared mental life is a sanctuary we want to insulate from government except when it has extraordinary need to enter it—we may want to demand more by way of justification than just a "fair probability" that they can find evidence of a crime there. We may want to prevent such entries except when the crime or threat law enforcement faces is an especially grave one.

Moreover, while the Constitution places warrant requirements and other procedural barriers in the way of police searches of our "persons, houses, papers, and effects," it also frequently leaves police with routes around these requirements. Police, for example, need not obtain a warrant when they use investigatory techniques where use of a warrant "would be impracticable" (like unannounced sobriety checkpoints) to meet challenges "beyond the general interest in crime control" (such as finding drunken drivers and removing them from the highways) (*Vernonia Sch. Dist. 47J v. Acton* 1995, 653). Consider . . . the example of airport screening at

US airports: Government certainly engages in a search when it uses metal detectors, X-rays machines, or similar technology to receive information about what lies underneath the surface of our clothing or inside our bags. But it does not need a warrant to do so. Nor does it need probable cause to think that any passenger it searches has a weapon or other dangerous item. Given the security needs at stake, it is allowed to use such technology to search all travelers whether it has any reason to suspect them or not (*United States v. Epperson*, 770).

One might thus ask whether government could ever use the same argument to justify warrantless and suspicion-less brain scanning at airports (assuming it were feasible) — or in other sites, such as transportation hubs, federal courthouses, or crowded sporting or cultural events, where law enforcement can show it needs to take robust anti-terrorism measures. Or whether it can incorporate neuroimaging into the warrantless searches police often can and do make "incident to an arrest," for example, when they require a breathalyzer test of a person arrested for drunk driving to capture evidence of his intoxication while it is still present (*Birchfield v. North Dakota* 2016).

As it turns out, the answers to these questions under current Fourth Amendment doctrine, generally depend on what a court finds when it balances the security (or other) interests the government is promoting against the individual's privacy interests threatened by such a search (*Delaware v. Prouse* 1979, 654). This is in turn, requires some sense of just how significant these privacy interests are. Is neuroimaging a significant invasion of our privacy even in its current, very limited form? Is it a threat to mental privacy if government is seeking evidence not about our unshared beliefs or feelings, but rather about what (criminal or crime-related) actions we performed in a world that we do share with others, and that police have a right to collect evidence about? To what extent, one might ask, is the nature of the privacy interest at stake in searches of the brain any different from that which is at stake in searches of a personal computer, or a cell phone or other mobile device? These aren't questions with clear answers. Until we have a better sense of how courts would analyze the privacy interests at stake in neuroimaging, we are ill-equipped to even begin to think about how they would weigh them against interests such as preventing terrorism in the air or violent attacks on schools, or catching drunk drivers or equipment operators, or preventing arrestees from harming police or destroying evidence.

And on this issue, it may well make a difference whether neuroimaging of a brain is mind-reading or brain-reading — whether it really provides government officials with information about our unshared thoughts and feelings, or instead tells them only about how a brain reacts to certain stimuli, and what this might indicate about the owner of that brain's past interactions with the outside world. It if it is the latter, a number of scholars have worried, then neuroimaging might be treated as analogous to other methods police use to gather data from individuals' bodies — such as breathalyzers or fingertip swaps — which courts have allowed police to use without warrants (and sometimes, without having to overcome any significant constitutional hurdle). It may likewise make a difference to courts that certain mental states may seem more private then others. Perhaps government is more likely to prevail if it is using neuroimaging to make inferences about a person's past interactions with the outside world than it is when using it to derive information about their past or present intentions, or sense of guilt about particular actions.

It is quite possible, of course, that judges will view neuroimaging's privacy impacts as more significant than those at stake in a breathalyzer test or fingertip swap—and thus as placing more weight on the Fourth Amendment scales, in favor of individual protection and against government freedom to investigate. If, for example, courts view Ivy's brain activity as equivalent to the video and computer chip data in Ozzie's brain—if they view the biology underlying our natural mental process as being worthy of the same privacy protection as the data in our "extended minds"—then Fourth Amendment protection may be fairly strong. Courts, after all, have recently been wary of allowing government too much leeway to easily search our cell phones or computer hard drives, so they may likewise place limits on how much government can search the natural equipment we use to create and retrieve memories.

Even here, however, Fourth Amendment protection is less certain than some would like it to be, if they wish to view mental privacy as, in most cases, invulnerable to government observation. Again, police might overcome Fourth Amendment barriers to computer or cell phone searches by obtaining a warrant based upon probable cause. They might also, in some circumstances, conduct warrantless searches of computer memory, and courts may well be willing to let them do so more readily when the search software is programmed only to turn up information connected to certain kinds of criminal activity, such as child pornography. On this model, government may also be able to neuroimage us when it can show that the mental information it seeks is likely to carry information of interest in investigating a particular crime, or thwarting a particular safety threat. In some cases, perhaps, society may need police to have access to such information in our minds. But it's also possible that in opening a door too readily for government to access this kind of needed information about our unexpressed thoughts, Fourth Amendment law may simultaneously give government access to thoughts and feelings it shouldn't be able to access.

Adam J. Kolber
Two Views of First Amendment Thought Privacy
18 U. Pa. J. Const. L. 1381, 1383-86 (2016)

As mind reading technology becomes cheaper and more accurate, the state may seek to regulate thought in ways that threaten the privacy of our mental lives. It is not at all clear if the Constitution would protect us from such invasions. Many free speech cases trumpet our freedom of thought but say frustratingly little about the contours of the protection. Most notably, they conceal whether the First Amendment protects thought itself (what I'll call the *independent* view) or only protects thought when it is linked to expression (what I'll call the *intertwined* view).

As a test case for these two views of First Amendment thought privacy, imagine a prohibition of "card counting" at the blackjack table. To play blackjack, you have to make simple calculations to determine the value of the cards in your hand. Card counters, however, make further calculations based on all of the cards dealt in plain view. These calculations enable them to turn the odds of winning in their favor.

A criminal prohibition of card counting would arguably constitute impermissible *thought-content* discrimination by permitting bettors to make the basic calculations required to play blackjack but not the more predictive calculations used to count cards. Since card counting does not obviously implicate expression, however, whether or not the First Amendment precludes a card counting prohibition may turn on whether the Amendment protects thought independently or only when intertwined with expression.

While ordinary card counting is not currently criminalized, we can surely imagine casinos pushing to criminalize it. Casinos already successfully lobbied for laws that make it a felony to count cards with the aid of a device. When a card counting app was developed on the iPhone (which included a special "stealth mode" to make it hard to detect), the Nevada Gaming Control Board issued an open letter warning that using such a device to count cards in a casino is a serious crime. So if you make your betting computations solely in your head, the criminal law currently leaves you alone. But if your betting computations are assisted by a computer, you can be punished by up to six years in prison for a first offense. . . .

[The] [c]ard counting [example] lets us test the boundaries of our freedom of thought without imagining futuristic brain scanners: it is often easy to determine when players are counting cards based on their betting patterns. These patterns would almost never arise by chance, and special software can help detect card counters. . . .

I argue that card counting (without a device) is plausibly protected under both the independent and intertwined views of First Amendment freedom of thought. . . . Given the limited doctrine on the topic, I predict that at least a significant minority of judges would deem a card counting prohibition unconstitutional, even if the prohibition were tied to an action such as betting. If I'm right, First Amendment concerns would also plausibly be raised by other laws implicating free thought and action, were, for example, the government to prohibit camping in a public park while thinking the mayor is incompetent or enhance punishment for those who "knowingly kill a Republican" but not those who "knowingly kill a Democrat." . . . [T]he issues raised by card counting help us envision the boundaries of freedom of thought as we enter a world in which our thoughts become more and more transparent without our having to express them.

Daniel D. Langleben & Jane Campbell Moriarty
Using Brain Imaging for Lie Detection: Where Science, Law, and Policy Collide

19 Psychol. Pub. Pol'y & L. 222, 228 (2013)

Due to constitutional rights, statutory enactments, and concerns over wrongful convictions, criminal defendants may be able to introduce fMRI lie detection testimony without meeting either the Frye or the Daubert standards in two ways: either in the penalty phases of capital cases, where defendants have a constitutional right to present mitigating evidence (Smith v. Spisak, 2010); or to support a claim of postconviction innocence where there is other, newly discovered evidence.

In capital cases, courts frequently permit defendants to introduce a variety of evidence (including neuroscience) to prove brain damage or mental impairment without stringent proof of reliability. For example, courts have admitted PET and SPECT scans during the penalty phase of capital cases to establish the defendant's mental impairment, even when such evidence may not rise to the level of evidentiary reliability. The U.S. Supreme Court has consistently affirmed constitutional protections for defendants to introduce mitigating evidence in penalty hearings (McKoy v. North Carolina, 1990). "[S]tates cannot limit the sentencer's consideration of any relevant circumstances that could cause it to decline to impose the [death] penalty" (McCleskey v. Kemp, 1987, p. 281). More particularly, the juror may "not be precluded from considering, as a mitigating factor, any aspect of a defendant's character or record and any of the circumstances of the offense that the defendant proffers as a basis for a sentence less than death". A defendant may be able to make a compelling case that fMRI lie detection will meet this foregoing standard.

Although the FRE do not apply in sentencing proceedings, some courts have required proof of the reliability of evidence admitted in sentencing. This reliability requirement has been mentioned in capital case penalty hearings, upholding the exclusion of polygraph evidence (United States v. Fulks, 2006). Because the only cases addressing fMRI evidence of lie detection have found it both unreliable and not generally accepted, courts may not be receptive to the testimony, even in the penalty phase. However, in light of the often lax standards for evidentiary reliability in the penalty phase, the frequent admission of nuclear medicine evidence in these hearings, and the strong constitutional support for defendants' right to introduce mitigating evidence, it is possible that fMRI lie detection evidence will gain a foothold in the courtroom in this manner. For example, a court might permit fMRI evidence that the defendant is being truthful when he expresses remorse about a crime or denies remembering a crime because he was intoxicated. It is thus conceivable that either a trial court will permit such evidence or that an appellate court will find an abuse of discretion where a trial court refused to allow such evidence.

One court has already admitted fMRI evidence relevant to another concern in a penalty hearing. In a 2009 death-penalty case in Illinois, the defense introduced expert testimony during the penalty phase that the defendant, Brian Dugan, suffered from psychopathy that impaired his ability to control his impulse to kill. The trial court permitted the expert to discuss the fMRI scans taken of Dugan's brain as additional proof of the defendant's psychopathy and to establish that Dugan's psychopathy should make him less culpable. The trial court allowed the expert to explain the scans and to use diagrams of the brain, but disallowed use of the actual fMRI images of Dugan's brain activity. Despite the admission of such expert testimony, Dugan received the death penalty. However, a signed verdict form was discovered after the sentencing, indicating that the jury may have intended to render a verdict of life. If the jury did originally decide not to impose the death penalty, it suggests the testimony was influential. However, Dugan's appeal on this issue was dropped when Illinois abolished the death penalty, so the issue remains unresolved.

fMRI lie detection evidence also has the potential to be admitted posttrial in a compelling case of claimed innocence. In Harrington v. State (2003), a trial court permitted testimony from an expert who testified about "brain fingerprinting"—a form of EEG that claims to be able to determine whether a person recognizes a word or image. Although brain fingerprinting has been roundly criticized (Rosenfeld, 2005), the trial court in that case heard testimony from Dr. Farwell, who testified that defendant's brain waves were consistent with his claims of innocence and his alibi. The trial court ultimately denied Harrington's claims, believing them time barred, but the Supreme Court of Iowa reversed, holding that the defendant was entitled to a new trial. On reviewing the record de novo and considering all the circumstances, the court's confidence in the soundness of the defendant's conviction was "significantly weakened." Although the Supreme Court of Iowa mentioned Dr. Farwell's testimony in a footnote, it neither commented on the appropriateness of its admission nor relied on it in its decision. It is difficult, however, for defendants to get a new trial after conviction and appeal, and other defendants who sought to hire Farwell met with judicial resistance. However, another court in a similar circumstance might be more impressed by fMRI evidence, which is based on far more reliable science than the brain fingerprinting.

NOTES AND QUESTIONS

1. Consider Professor Greely's recommendations for regulation. Would you support them as a legislator? As head of the FDA? Why or why not?
2. Consider the distinctions Professor Pardo draws between various kinds of lies. To what extent does this affect your judgment of the probabilities that neuroscience can successfully detect variations in the kinds of lies people tell?
3. Professor Blitz discusses interesting challenges for law, given the Fourth and Fifth Amendments to the U.S. Constitution. To what extent do you think that either or both of these present problems for neuroscientific methods of detecting lies? For an in-depth analysis of these questions, see Michael S. Pardo, *Neuroscience Evidence, Legal Culture, and Criminal Procedure*, 33 Am. J. Crim. L. 301 (2006).
4. Does lie detection evidence raise hearsay or Confrontation Clause issues? Attorney Jessica Haushalter suggests that fMRI evidence may run afoul of both. She suggests that, in most situations, fMRI evidence would be the equivalent of out-of-court statements used for their truth. She also suggests that there would be Confrontation Clause issues if such evidence were used against a defendant. Think of a situation in which a victim of a crime wants to take a lie detection test to help bolster testimony. Are there hearsay exceptions that could negate these problems? Is there a way to satisfy the Confrontation Clause? *See* Jessica Lauren Haushalter, *Neuronal Testimonial: Brain-Computer Interfaces and the Law*, 71 Vand. L. Rev. 1365 (2018).
5. Will juries become increasingly irrelevant? Consider these arguments from Professor Julie Seaman:

> To the extent that we believe that the jury's only legitimate role is to find the facts, which in large part consists of judging the credibility of witnesses, then technological advances—including a highly accurate lie detector—would largely displace the jury and might eventually cause it to go the way of trial by ordeal and trial by battle. After all, if the jury is the lie detector and technology gives us a much better lie detector, why would we need—or want—the jury? Much research tells us that people, of which juries are composed, are not very good at detecting deception; many innocent people are undoubtedly convicted because juries cannot very accurately tell truth from lies. That the system has been around for a long time surely is not a sufficient reason to retain it if we had a better way of doing the very thing it is meant to do.
>
> I think the better argument is that history, theory, and precedent (including recent Supreme Court decisions on the right to a jury trial) strongly support the argument that the jury is much more than a lie detector, and that the Constitutional right to a jury trial in criminal cases (and in some civil cases) is grounded not primarily in the value of an accurate determination of facts but in the need to check governmental power. (I've argued elsewhere that the right to a jury finding of certain facts rests largely on this protective role.)

If the jury does (or should) serve this political, institutional role, the next question is how my imaginary foolproof lie detector would impact the jury's performance of this role—would removing some of the secret, black box quality of the jury threaten to destroy it? And if it might, should we prevent these new technologies from entering the courtroom in order to preserve the jury system?

Julie Seaman, *Black Boxes: fMRI Lie Detection and the Role of the Jury*, 42 Akron L. Rev. 931, 936-37 (2009).

6. The Employee Polygraph Protection Act of 1988, 29 U.S.C. §2005 (2018), which places great limitations on how employers can use the polygraph, defines "lie detector" in this way: "The term 'lie detector' includes a polygraph, deceptograph, voice stress analyzer, psychological stress evaluator, or any other similar device (whether mechanical or electrical) that is used, or the results of which are used, for the purpose of rendering a diagnostic opinion regarding the honesty or dishonesty of an individual." Is all brain-based lie detection covered under this Act?

7. What kind of market might develop for brain-based lie detection services? Law professor Hank Greely "estimates that if fMRI lie detection became admissible in court, the industry could easily be worth more than a billion dollars per year. 'It's a big country, there are lots of judges out there and I think they are hoping to find one who will allow the evidence, particularly if the other side doesn't know much,' says Greely. 'To be able to use [fMRI lie detection] in court would be the blue ribbon, the license to print money.'" Adi Narayan, *The fMRI Brain Scan: A Better Lie Detector?*, Time (July 20, 2009).

8. What other uses might you imagine for lie detection technology? Consider the hypothetical case of a draft dodger who is scanned to assess the sincerity of a recently acquired pacifistic religious belief. Might neuroscience be able to help the government assess the sincerity of this belief? *See* Kevin P. Lee, *Free Exercise and Religious Mania: Neuroscience and Religious Exercise Rights*, Presentation at the Conference on Neuroscience in European and North American Case Law (Sept. 28, 2010).

9. The *Selvi* court and Greely article make institutional competence arguments regarding lie detection—*Selvi* points out that it is traditionally the legislature's job to weigh personal liberty and public safety, while Greely advocates uniform federal regulation of all lie detection drugs and devices. Is taking the question of admissibility out of the judge's hands advisable? Besides ease of application, do bright-line rules have any advantages in such a contested field?

10. In 2009 New York State Assemblyman Michael Benjamin introduced a bill to "ban the use of magnetic resonance imaging (MRI) brain scans in a criminal proceeding where a defendant's or witness's truthfulness or knowledge of a specific event is at issue." N.Y. State Assemb. 9154, 2009-2010 Reg. Sess. (N.Y. 2009). The bill did not move beyond committee, but if it had reached the Assembly floor, would you have voted in favor? Would you have proposed any amendments? What role should the legislature play in regulation of brain-based lie detection?

11. The 2002 movie *Minority Report*, based on a short story by Philip K. Dick, depicts a futuristic world in which a police unit called PreCrime uses mind-reading experts ("precogs") to arrest individuals before they actually commit their violent crimes. In promoting the system, the government tells citizens, "We want to make absolutely certain that every American can bank on the utter reliability of

this system, and to ensure that that which keeps us safe will also keep us free." Would advances in the neuroscience of mind reading make the world safer? More free?

12. The Fifth Amendment to the U.S. Constitution provides that no person "shall be compelled in any criminal case to be a witness against himself. . . ." In *Schmerber v. California*, 384 U.S. 757 (1966), the Supreme Court held that under that so-called self-incrimination clause: (a) no person shall be compelled to "prove a charge [from] his own mouth"; but (b) a person may be compelled to provide real or physical evidence. If neuroscientific techniques could sufficiently probe memories for them to have evidentiary value in criminal cases, would compelled but non-invasive neuroscientific examination survive the self-incrimination clause? Should the evidence be considered "testimonial" or "physical"? Or should developments in neuroscience prompt reconsideration of that dichotomy and development of some new legal framework? *See* Nita A. Farahany, *Incriminating Thoughts*, 64 Stan. L. Rev. 351 (2012).

13. Relatedly, the Fourth Amendment guarantees the right of people "to be secure in their persons . . . against unreasonable searches and seizures." Would acquiring information from a person's brain noninvasively but without their knowledge or consent violate the Fourth Amendment? *See* Nita A. Farahany, *Searching Secrets*, 160 U. Pa. L. Rev. 1239 (2012).

14. It has been written that "[t]he gift of words is the gift of deception and illusion." Frank Herbert, *Children of Dune* 228 (1987). Given the pervasiveness of deception in human interaction, what does it mean to detect a "lie" or to verify "truth"? Are there any legal contexts in which is it more difficult to answer these questions?

15. Can someone lie without having an intent to deceive? What about intending to deceive without lying? Should a court care about these distinctions? If so, when? What if fMRI can only detect subjective beliefs of truthfulness? Are such measurements more helpful than regular witness testimony? Professor Jennifer Bard observes, "If the best Neuroimaging can do is identify the sincerity of "yes" or "no" answers, it is a very expensive machine for playing Twenty Questions." *See* Jennifer S. Bard, *"Ah Yes, I Remember It Well": Why the Inherent Unreliability of Human Memory Makes Brain Imaging Technology a Poor Measure of Truth-Telling in the Courtroom*, 94 Or. L. Rev. 295 (2016).

16. How do the constitutional concerns with brain imaging compare to those surrounding surveillance technology such as facial detection using artificial intelligence (AI)? Allan Poniah, co-founder and CEO of a company developing such facial detection technology, has described the process of these AI models: "If someone smiles insincerely, their mouth may smile, but the smile doesn't reach their eyes—micro-expressions are more subtle than that and quicker." Perhaps researchers will discover patterns of micro-activations of certain brain regions linked to deception similar to the micro-expressions described by Poniah. What if these technologies were used in conjunction with lie detecting technologies as Professor Blitz suggests? *See* Ellen Milligan, *Face-Reading AI Will Tell Police When Suspects Are Hiding Truth*, Bloomberg (June 29, 2019).

One area AI could be relevant is in detecting lies by evaluating the results of technology such as fMRI, EEG, and others. Scientists have compared human evaluation of fNIRS results to that of a support vector machine (SVM). In the test, the SVM achieved 95.63% accuracy when distinguishing between induced lies, induced truths, and non-induced responses (the subject choosing whether to lie or tell the truth). *See* Roberto Vega et al., *Hemodynamic Pattern Recognition During Deception Process Using Functional Near-Infrared Spectroscopy*, 36 J. Med. Biological Engineering 22 (2016). SVMs are not even the most sophisticated form of machine learning. If this type of test is proven to be valid, what implications would this have on admissibility? What about if more sophisticated AI allowed for even higher accuracy?

Would AI and machine-learning technology actually improve the reliability of lie detection technology? Professor Carrie Leonetti observes that human error and conceptual issues of lie detection still remain, writing, "In the case of automated measurements . . . the human subjectivity comes into play at an earlier moment in time, when a human being writes the algorithms that dictate the computer's interpretation of results—for example, when a programmer determines whether an observed physiological change is a 'real' change or an artifact." Based on this observation, Leonetti argues that lie detection technology will likely never be reliable enough to be admitted as evidence. *See* Carrie Leonetti, *Abracadabra, Hocus Pocus, Same Song, Different Chorus: The Newest Iteration of the "Science" of Lie Detection*, 24 Rich. J.L. & Tech. 1 (2017). Do you agree? Could human error be sufficiently eliminated to allow lie detection evidence?

FURTHER READING

On the Polygraph:

> Comm. to Review the Sci. Evidence on the Polygraph, Nat'l Research Council, *The Polygraph and Lie Detection* (2003).
>
> David L. Faigman, Stephen E. Fienberg & Paul C. Stern, *The Limits of the Polygraph*, 20 Issues Sci. & Tech. 40 (2003).
>
> William G. Iacono, *Effective Policing: Understanding How Polygraph Tests Work and Are Used*, 35 Crim. Just. & Behav. 1295 (2008).
>
> Ken Alder, *The Lie Detectors: The History of an American Obsession* (2007).

Brain-Based Lie Detection:

> Anthony Wagner et al., The MacArthur Foundation Research Network on Law and Neuroscience, *fMRI and Lie Detection: A Knowledge Brief* (2016).
>
> Martha J. Farah et al., *Functional MRI-Based Lie Detection: Scientific and Societal Challenges*, 15 Nature Revs. Neurosci. 123 (2014).
>
> Marcus E. Raichle, *An Introduction to Functional Brain Imaging in the Context of Lie Detection*, in *Using Imaging to Identify Deceit* 3 (Emilio Bizzi et al. eds., 2009).
>
> J. Peter Rosenfeld, *'Brain Fingerprinting': A Critical Analysis*, 4 Sci. Rev. Mental Health Prac. 20 (2005).
>
> Daniel D. Langleben et al., *True Lies: Delusions and Lie-Detection Technology*, 34 J. Psychiatry & L. 351 (2006).
>
> F. Andrew Kozel et al., *Detecting Deception Using Functional Magnetic Resonance Imaging*, 58 Biological Psychiatry 605 (2005).
>
> John B. Meixner & J. Peter Rosenfeld, *A Mock Terrorism Application of the P300-Based Concealed Information Test*, 48 Psychophysiology 149 (2010).
>
> Paul S. Appelbaum, *The New Lie Detectors: Neuroscience, Deception, and the Courts*, 58 Psychiatric Servs. 460 (2007).

Junhong Yu et al., *Can fMRI Discriminate Between Deception and False Memory? A Meta-analytic Comparison Between Deception and False Memory Studies*, 104 Neurosci. & Biobehav. Revs. 43 (2019).

Special Issue of *Social Neuroscience* on Neural Correlates of Deception, 4 Soc. Neurosci. (2009).

Jiang Zhang et al., *Mapping the Small-World Properties of Brain Networks in Deception with Functional Near-Infrared Spectroscopy*, 6 Sci. Reps. 25297 (2016).

Xiaoqing Hu et al., *Suppressing Unwanted Autobiographical Memories Reduces Their Automatic Influences: Evidence from Electrophysiology and an Implicit Autobiographical Memory Test*, 26 Psychol. Sci. 1098 (2015).

J. Peter Rosenfeld et al., *Effects of Motivational Manipulations on the P300-Based Complex Trial Protocol for Concealed Information Detection*, in *Detecting Concealed Information and Deception: Recent Developments* 125 (J. Peter Rosenfeld ed., 2018).

Detecting Concealed Information and Deception: Recent Developments (J. Peter Rosenfeld ed., 2018).

Legal and Critical Perspectives:

Michael S. Pardo, *Lying, Deception, and fMRI: A Critical Update*, in *Neurolaw and Responsibility for Action: Concepts, Crimes, and Courts* 143 (Bebhinn Donnelly-Lazarov ed., 2018).

Michael S. Pardo & Dennis Patterson, *Criminal Procedure*, in *Minds, Brains, and Law: The Conceptual Foundations of Law and Neuroscience* 148 (2013).

Michael S. Pardo, *Neuroscience Evidence, Legal Culture, and Criminal Procedure*, 33 Am. J. Crim. L. 301 (2006).

George Fisher, *The Jury's Rise as Lie Detector*, 107 Yale L.J. 575 (1997).

Emily R.D. Murphy & Jesse Rissman, *Evidence of Memory from Brain Data*, J.L. & Biosci. (forthcoming 2020)

Margaret Talbot, *Duped: Can Brain Scans Uncover Lies?*, New Yorker, July 2, 2007, at 52.

Paul Root Wolpe et al., *Emerging Neurotechnologies for Lie-Detection: Promises and Perils*, 5 Am. J. Bioethics 39 (2005).

Sarah E. Stoller & Paul Root Wolpe, *Emerging Neurotechnologies for Lie Detection and the Fifth Amendment*, 33 Am. J.L. & Med. 359 (2007).

John B. Meixner, *Liar, Liar, Jury's the Trier? The Future of Neuroscience-Based Credibility Assessment in the Court*, 106 NW. U. L. Rev. 3 (2012).

Mark Hansen, *True Lies*, 95 A.B.A. J. 56 (2009).

Joseph R. Simpson, *Functional MRI Lie Detection: Too Good to Be True?*, 36 J. Am. Acad. Psychiatry & L. 491 (2008).

Archie Alexander, *Functional Magnetic Resonance Imaging Lie Detection: Is a "Brainstorm" Heading Toward the "Gatekeeper"?*, 7 Houston J. Health L. & Pol'y 1 (2007).

John B. Meixner, Jr., *Admissibility and Constitutional Issues of the Concealed Information Test in American Courts: An Update*, in *Detecting Concealed Information and Deception: Recent Developments* 405 (J. Peter Rosenfeld ed., 2018).

Dov Fox, *Brain Imaging and the Bill of Rights: Memory Detection Technologies and American Criminal Justice*, 8 Am. J. Bioethics 34 (2008).

Barbara J. Sahakian & Julia Gottwald, *Sex, Lies, and Brain Scans: How fMRI Reveals What Really Goes on in Our Minds* (2017).

CHAPTER 16

Judging

The law is reason, free of passion.

—Aristotle[†]

Emotion pervades the law.

—Susan Bandes[††]

CHAPTER SUMMARY

This chapter:
- Summarizes research on the neuroscience of legal decision-making.
- Introduces the use of neuroscientific techniques to identify bias in legal decision-making.
- Raises questions about the potential value of neuroscience in exploring the relationships between analytical and emotional reasoning.

INTRODUCTION

Suppose you are a prisoner facing a parole hearing tomorrow. Your freedom hangs in the balance before a very experienced judge, who will be considering parole applications all day. If given your preference, when would you like to appear? The answer, apparently: just after a meal. Consider Figure 16.1 that shows the probability of getting paroled plotted across the day.[*] The plot flucturates between 60% and 0%. Notice how the favorable rulings increase after each meal break (indicated by the dotted lines).

Something is at work here beyond cool, rational deliberation. It could be the rejuvenating effects of any break. It could be the biochemical effects of recent ingestion on the brain. But it is hard to avoid the conclusion: Judging isn't as dispassionate as it's cracked up to be. Indeed, a 2018 study found that when a prominent football team, in the state in which a judge sits, unexpectedly lost over the weekend, the sentence lengths assigned by that judge during the week following the game

---

[†] Aristotle, *The Politics of Aristotle* 146 (Ernest Baker trans., 1946).

[††] Susan Bandes, *Introduction*, in *The Passions of Law* 1 (Susan A. Bandes ed., 2000).

[*] The graph reflects analysis of eight judges in Israel who among them conducted 1,112 parole board hearings (40% of the total) in Israeli prisons, over a ten-month period. The judges consider between 14 and 35 cases each day, taking two food breaks that divide their day into three sessions. The following had no effect on the decisions: sex; race; length of time already served; severity of crime. The analysis controlled for recidivism and rehabilitation programs. Shai Danziger, Jonathan Levav & Liora Avnaim-Pessoa, *Extraneous Factors in Judicial Decisions*, 108 Proc. Nat'l Acad. Sci. 6889 (2011).

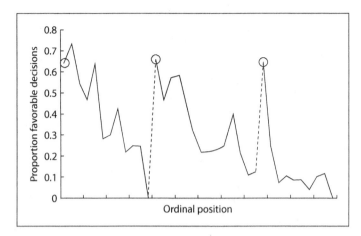

Figure 16.1 Proportion of rulings in favor of the prisoners by ordinal position.
Circled points indicate the first decision in each of the three decision sessions; tick
marks on *x* axis denote every third case; dotted line denotes food break.
Source: Shai Danziger, Jonathan Levav, & Liora Avnaim-Pessoa, *Extraneous Factors in Judicial
Decisions,* 108 Proc. Nat'l Acad. Sci. 6889 (2011).

increased. The study found that "[t]he impact of upset losses on sentence lengths is
larger for defendants if their cases are handled by judges who received their bachelor's degrees from the university with which the football team is affiliated."*

Of course, it isn't a surprise that judges are humans, too. Probably, few people
believe that judges, even at their most conscientious, are capable of removing themselves entirely from the foibles of human existence. And a large literature shows that
judges are susceptible to the same kinds of cognitive biases that we all are.** For
example, judges are—like non-judges—more likely to believe that another person
intended an outcome when the outcome is negative than when it is positive.***

In this chapter we explore insights that neuroscientific techniques might add
to understanding legal reasoning. The chapter proceeds in two sections. Section
A summarizes research on the neuroscience of punishment decisions. Section B
illustrates the use of neuroscientific techniques to identify bias—such as racial
bias—in legal decision-making.

A. THE NEUROSCIENCE OF PUNISHMENT DECISIONS

Some researchers have begun to use neuroscientific tools to investigate brain
activity during moral choices. The use of those tools to investigate brain activity
during legal reasoning is even newer. We have provided, and annotated, in the
Appendix the first peer-reviewed scientific article in that arena: *The Neural Correlates*

---

* Ozkan Eren & Naci Mocan, *Emotional Judges and Unlucky Juveniles,* 10 Am. Econ. J.: Applied Econ.
171, 171 (2018).

** For a summary, see Jeffrey J. Rachlinski & Andrew Wistrich, *Judging the Judiciary by the
Numbers: Empirical Research on Judges,* 13 Ann. Rev. L. & Soc. Sci. 203 (2017).

*** Markus Kneer & Sacha Bourgeois-Gironde, *Mens Rea Ascription, Expertise and Outcome
Effects: Professional Judges Surveyed,* 169 Cognition 139 (2017).

of Third-Party Punishment. Read the Summary, Introduction, and Discussion sections of that article, then return here.

As you just read, the fMRI study investigated the neural activity associated with deciding whether to punish a protagonist named John, who had engaged in hypothetical criminal activity, and, if so, how much. That study showed that there was greater activity in the right dorsolateral prefrontal cortex (rDLPFC) when John was responsible for his behavior in the classic way than when John's circumstances or mental state suggested diminished responsibility. In parallel, rising selections of punishment amounts correlated with increased activity in the right amygdala. Interestingly, activity in the rDLPFC did not correlate neatly with the severity of the harms for which John was responsible, whereas, nearly symmetrically, activity in the right amygdala did not correlate neatly with whether John was or was not classically responsible for his behavior. These findings suggest that liability and punishment decisions are the product of two neural circuitries that are separately deployed, though jointly involved. One region centers on the rDLPFC, a region known to house highly analytic functions. The other region centers on the amygdala, an area known to be involved in (among other things) emotional reactions.

NOTES AND QUESTIONS

1. What do the findings in *The Neural Correlates of Third-Party Punishment* suggest to you about the relationships—during liability and punishment decisions—between analysis and emotion? As you read the rest of this chapter, see whether or not your assessment changes, and if so how.
2. On the National Public Radio program, *Talk of the Nation*, neuroscientist David Eagleman commented that "the punishment has to fit the brain." *David Eagleman Gets Inside our Heads*, Nat'l Pub. Radio (Aug. 24, 2012). To what extent does it trouble you that the very brains deciding other people's punishment are themselves subject to various limitations, biases, and inconsistencies? For more, see Morris Hoffman, *The Punisher's Brain: An Evolutionary History of Judge and Jury* (2014). To complicate matters even further, what if we were to punish not just for bad behavior, but for bad thoughts—for instance, detecting the extent of someone's racial biases and then punishing accordingly. *See* Philip E. Tetlock, Gregory Mitchell & Jason Anastasopoulos, *Detecting and Punishing Unconscious Bias*, 42 J. Legal Stud. 83 (2013).
3. Note that the modern U.S. legal system gives liability decisions to jurors, while judges are typically the ones to decide a criminal's sentence. To what extent do you think this may represent a reflection, in legal structure, of the divided functions within the brain? What advantages or disadvantages would you expect if our system had instead given liability decisions to judges, and sentencing decisions to jurors? Why? One of the few times that sentencing decisions go before a jury is at capital sentencing—when the offender is facing the death penalty. Does it make sense to turn over this most important sentencing decision to a lay jury?
4. As you know, fMRI BOLD signal correlation is not reliable evidence of causation. Suppose repetitive transcranial magnetic stimulation (rTMS) were used to temporarily and reversibly disrupt brain activity in the dLPFC. What results might you expect? Why?

5. There are a number of drugs known to affect operations of the prefrontal cortex, the amygdala, or both. For example, selective serotonin reuptake inhibitors (SSRIs) are widely prescribed in the United States for a variety of ailments, including depression, chronic pain, and anxiety disorders (social anxiety, panic disorders, obsessive-compulsive disorders, eating disorders, and sometimes post-traumatic stress disorder). Given the reliable effect of SSRIs on emotions, to what extent should we worry about the effects of such drugs on juror decision-making? To what extent can or should neuroscience play a role in making that assessment?

6. What if brain science could one day detect bias in jurors? If developed, "Courts could then use this perfect technology of bias detection, referred to as neuro-voir dire, to weed out individuals who harbor any outside influence with enough strength as it relates to a particular trial." But would it be desirable to filter jurors in this way? As law professor Dov Fox asks, "Would the adoption of brain imaging techniques that could detect jury bias hold the appeal that much of the impartiality jurisprudence assumes?" Fox argues against such an approach because ". . . it draws out the full implications of treating all outside sources of juror influence the same." Do you agree? Dov Fox, *Neuro-Voir Dire and the Architecture of Bias*, 65 Hastings L.J. 999, 1017-20 (2014).

7. What implications might the Buckholtz et al. study have for criminal sentencing? And on what bases? Consider and respond to this view:

> The Buckholtz study raises questions about institutional choice in sentencing, since Buckholtz found something like a neural correlate to the bifurcation of the criminal trial into a culpability phase and a sentencing phase. If we were assigning roles to the judge and jury based on these neural activation patterns alone, then we might consider reversing the current division of labor. Judges are trained to use their prefrontal cortices in accordance with the law and should therefore determine culpability, and jurors could democratize punishment by using their socio-affective brain networks to determine criminal sentences. In other words, if culpability decisions are based on legal reasoning and sentencing decisions are based on gut instincts, then maybe the judge should determine culpability and the jury should set the sentence.

Rebecca Krauss, *Neuroscience and Institutional Choice in Federal Sentencing Law*, 120 Yale L.J. 367, 374 (2010).

To what extent might understanding more about how the brain generates legal decisions enrich our approach to explaining and perhaps improving legal decision-making? As you may recall, U.S. law imposes very different roles on judges and jurors during trials. Judges enforce the rules of evidence and inform the jury of the applicable law. Jurors must decide the facts, sometimes deciding which witnesses are more credible than others. In criminal cases, jurors must decide whether the prosecution has proved the facts beyond a reasonable doubt, thereby supporting conviction. If it has, then in most states judges impose all non-death punishment. As you read the next excerpt—which discusses neuroscientific research on how brains make liability and punishment decisions—think open-mindedly but critically, and consider equally the potential legal relevance of this line of thinking and research and its potential irrelevance. Where do you come out in the end, and why?

Morris B. Hoffman & Frank Krueger
The Neuroscience of Blame and Punishment
in *Self, Culture and Consciousness* 207 (Sangeetha Menon, V.V. Binoy & Nithin Nagaraj eds., 2020)

In the last five years, a great deal has been learned about how human brains address the social problem of punishing wrongdoers. Although it is far too early to be confident that these insights will shed any practical light on criminal law or procedure, patterns are emerging that suggest a framework that someday could have significant legal and social consequences. In this chapter we first survey the behavioral and theoretical evidence supporting the proposition that the willingness to blame then punish norm-violators is an evolved human trait. Then we sample the recent neuroscience literature on normative punishment, and follow that with a presentation of our neuropsychological model of blame and third-party punishment. We finish with a discussion of the potential implications a confirmed model might have for law and policy.

THE EVOLUTION OF PUNISHMENT

Biologists have long recognized two fundamental kinds of punishment behaviors: second-party punishment [retaliation against someone who has harmed you] and third-party punishment [retaliation on someone who has harmed someone else]. [Second-party retaliation/punishment is common in the animal kingdom.] . . . [T]hird-party punishment, by contrast, seem uniquely human, [though] there are tantalizing examples of non-human precursors to it. For example, in the early 1990s primatologists in Tanzania observed non-dominant male chimpanzees attack a young adult male, apparently because the young male was attacking females without provocation. . . .

[Punishment arguably solves] the essential Prisoner's Dilemma of our ancestors' early lives: do we cooperate or defect? Humans are the animal kingdom's most highly social heterogenetic species, but of course natural selection still works at the individual level. Living in intensely social groups gave us enormous fitness advantages — in things like hunting, mutual defense, divisions of labor — but it also presented enormous temptations for individuals to cheat. Evolutionary theorists have surmised that without third-party punishment — the willingness of one member to punish a misbehaving fellow member even when that misbehavior has not injured the punishing member — emerging humans could never have evolved in their intense social groups.

. . . [Punishment is] arguably necessary to prevent the spread of uncontrolled cheating. . . . The socialization of that willingness to punish wrongdoers meant that a wrong committed against any member was now a wrong against the group, punishable by the group, or by the group's designees.

But third-party punishment is very costly, evolutionarily speaking. Unlike with second-party punishment, an impartial third-party punisher gains nothing immediate by way of self-defense, only an indirect long-term benefit in group stability. Yet he risks serious injury and even death, either from the resisting wrongdoer himself or from the wrongdoer's family. Indeed, biologists and economists sometimes call third-party punishment "altruistic punishment," to reflect that the benefits to the punisher are indirect at best, or "costly punishment," to reflect that these indirect benefits come at a direct cost. . . .

How exactly an evolved trait for third-party punishment could have arisen remains as controversial as the more general question of how our intensely social groups could have arisen, when the direct benefits of cheating seem always to outweigh the indirect benefits of cooperating. The answer probably has something to do with the fact that our ancestral groups were likely composed of related individuals. "Altruistic" behaviors in such circumstances would not have been entirely altruistic in the genetic sense. Helping a family member, even at some cost, was to some extent helping genes shared with that family member.

There are three lines of evidence that converge to suggest that the evolutionary roots of punishment are something more than a just-so story. First, as mentioned above, many of our primate cousins exhibit behaviors akin to third-party punishment [suggesting a common, ancestral origin to the predisposition]. These behaviors also show the fluid boundary between second- and third-party punishment, and in fact suggest that human third-party punishment may well have evolved out of predecessor second-party punishment. . . .

[Second], third-party punishment also appears to be a human universal. In every human society that has left a sufficient written or oral record, including present day primitive societies, norm-violators are punished by designated punishers who themselves may not have been directly harmed and yet who may pay a cost associated with inflicting the punishment. Whether it is the dominant male in a primitive tribe, a set of tribal elders, a king, a judge or a jury, all human societies have institutionalized in one form or another this idea that serious crimes against the group must be punished by a representative of the group.

[Third], a wide array of behavioral studies, across many kinds of disciplines, from experimental economics to social psychology, show that humans have a palpable willingness to inflict punishment on norm-violators even when the violation does not harm the punisher, and even when the punishment comes at a cost to the punisher. For example, when experimental economists build a costly punishment round into the traditional dictator game* — by forcing a defecting player to forfeit money back to the experimenter but only if the forcing player also must forfeit some money—subjects regularly oblige. Although the amount of cost a third-party punisher is willing to endure varies across and within societies, even in existing primitive societies this game-based willingness to endure a cost to punish a third-party is ubiquitous. The willingness to engage in third-party punishment seems to emerge early in childhood. Four- and five-year-old children engage in third-party punishment behaviors based on an expressed belief that antisocial actions deserve to be punished.

Behavioral studies have also suggested that there is an intermediate step to punishment, which most researchers call "blame" or "blameworthiness." Blame appears to be a more heuristic, automatic process; it is highly predictable, largely invariant across demographics, and seems to be driven by the two classic determinants of criminal culpability—the amount of harm and the wrongdoer's intention. With the wrongdoer's intention kept constant, the greater the harm the greater the blame. Likewise, with harm kept constant, intentional wrongdoers are blamed more than

---

* [The "dictator game" is a game that economists use in studies to examine economic decision-making. In this game, one of two participants is given an amount of money and has complete discretion over whether or not to share some portion of that money with the other participant, and, if so, how much. — EDS.]

accidental wrongdoers. Very recent work shows these two determinants have an additive effect on blame: high harm intentionally caused is blamed more than just the harm or intention, considered separately, would explain. The amount of blame experimental subjects assess is remarkably uniform and predictable across subjects, looking much more like a rote task than a complex moral judgment. That of course doesn't mean that blame is not a moral judgment; it just means that it is the kind of moral judgment that is deeply imbedded in us and driven by a narrow range of variables (namely, harm and intent).

Punishment, by contrast, appears to be a substantially more complex and context-dependent task. It can vary not only depending on a myriad of facts about the wrongdoer, the wrong and the victim, but also on the punisher's beliefs about the nature of the world, the purposes of punishment, and in some circumstances even his beliefs about free will.

Natural selection has arguably equipped us with these two punishment systems: a hot, fast, highly predictable one that places the wrong grossly on a scale of blameworthiness depending only on our assessment of the harm caused and the wrongdoer's intention in causing it; and a second, cooler, slower system that gives us time to consider all the pertinent circumstances before we decide on the amount and type of punishment, or indeed whether [we] will forgive the transgression.

If our willingness to blame and punish . . . is in fact part of an evolutionary suite of behaviors bequeathed to us by natural selection, then of course the mechanism of that inheritance lies embedded somewhere in our neural architectures. A host of functional neuroimaging research using methods such as functional magnetic imaging (fMRI) is beginning to converge on a neural model of blame and punishment.

THE NEUROSCIENCE OF BLAME AND PUNISHMENT
A Sampling of Experiments

Before we present a neuropsychological model of blame and punishment, we sample some of the major neuroscience experiments upon which our model is based. One of the first experiments on the neuroscience of criminal responsibility . . . [asked subjects to] read six hypotheticals involving the difference between intentional crimes, unintentional [crime]s, and attempt[ed crimes], and then graded those differences on a moral scale. Here's one of those hypotheticals:

> *Grace and her friend work at a chemical factory, and are having lunch in the break room. Grace's friend asks her to retrieve some sugar from the counter.*

From this stem narrative, subjects were presented with the following four variations generated by manipulating intent and harm:

1) *Intent and harm.* Grace decides to murder her friend and intentionally gives her poison instead of sugar. The friend dies. (The law typically calls this first degree murder.)

2) *Intent, but no harm.* Grace decides to murder her friend and gives her what Grace thinks is poison, but which turns out to be sugar. The friend is not injured. (The law typically calls this attempted first degree murder.)

3) *No intent, but harm.* Grace intends to give her friend sugar, but accidentally gives her poison instead. The friend dies. (The law typically calls this reckless or negligent manslaughter, or no crime at all, depending on the level of Grace's carelessness.)

4) *No intent and no harm.* Grace intends to give Alice sugar, and does give her sugar. (This, of course, is not a crime.)

Subjects were asked for each variation to rate Grace's behavior on a seven point scale, with 1 being "forbidden" and 7 being "permissible." . . .

Behaviorally, virtually all subjects blamed in exactly the order listed above; that is, they blamed intentional killing most, then attempted killing and then accidental killing least. This conforms to what criminal law and moral philosophy universally recognize: one who commits an attempted intentional harm is more culpable than one who commits an accidental harm, even though an attempt causes no harm and an accident does.

The authors then repeated the experiment, but this time with two different sets of subjects—one control set and one set that had their right temporo-parietal junctions (rTPJs) disrupted by transcranial magnetic stimulation (TMS). The group with disrupted rTPJs found accidental harm more blameworthy than attempted harm. Interestingly, young children also blame in this fashion, presumably because their TPJs—which are among the last brain regions to develop—have not fully developed. Eight-year-olds consistently base their punishments only on the outcome of the violation; adolescents integrate outcomes and intentions in second- but not third-party punishment; and adults integrate outcomes and intentions in second- and third-party punishment.

This experiment confirmed what others had suggested: namely, that regions in the brain such as the TPJ, which are associated with "theory-of-mind"—meaning the ability to attribute beliefs, intentions, desires and perspectives to others —are critical for moral judgment. The experiment also suggested why this is so: these theory-of-mind regions, including the TPJ, are necessary for assessing a wrongdoer's intention, which, as discussed above, is one of the two drivers of blame. Without working theory-of-mind regions, we blame like children blame, focusing only on harm and therefore using principles roughly akin to "no harm no foul."

Another culpability experiment involving TMS was significant for corroborating the fundamental neural differences between blame and punishment. Joshua Buckholtz and his colleagues used TMS to disrupt the dorsal lateral prefrontal cortex (dlPFC) in one set of subjects, then gave them and a control set several blame (how morally responsible is the offender for his actions; nine point scale: 0 = not morally responsible at all; 9 = completely morally responsible) and punishment (how much punishment deserves the offender for his actions; nine point scale: 0 = no punishment and 9 = extreme punishment) scenarios. Disrupting the dlPFC had significant impact on the subjects' punishment decisions, but no impact on their blame decisions.

One of the first studies to try to ferret out the networks involved in third-party blame and punishment was also done by Buckholtz and his colleagues.* In this experiment, subjects in a scanner were asked to impose amounts of punishment on a hypothetical wrongdoer (from 0 to 9, 0 being no punishment and 9 being the most severe punishment the subject could imagine). The experimenters varied the hypotheticals both by harm and the wrongdoer's intention. As to the latter, however, they presented just two different states of mind: a normal "unexcused" condition; and an excused condition (such as the wrongdoer was insane). They found that brain regions associated with affective processing (amygdala, medial prefrontal

---

* [This 2008 study appears in the Appendix. — Eds.]

cortex, and posterior cingulate) predicted the amount of punishment when the wrongdoer's state of mind was held constant. By contrast, when harm was held constant, regions in the dlPFC seemed to be associated with the differences between the unexcused and excused mental states.

We and a group of colleagues expanded on the Buckholtz fMRI experiment by performing effective connectivity analyses to try to piece together the communication among the regions involved. We found that the blame decision does indeed differentially recruit many theory-of-mind regions, and specifically that the temporal pole (TP) and the dorsal medial prefrontal cortex (dmPFC) emerged as hubs of the blaming network, uniquely generating converging output connections to the ventromedial prefrontal cortex (vmPFC), the TPJ and the posterior cingulate cortex (PCC). The dmPFC received inputs only from the TP, and both its differential activation and its connectivity to the dlPFC correlated with the degree of punishment.

In another experiment, one of us and his colleagues applied a whole-brain voxel-based lesion-symptom mapping approach to identify brain regions associated with third-party punishment in a large sample of patients with penetrating traumatic brain injury. The study showed that patients who demonstrated atypical third-party punishment had specific lesions in core regions of the mentalizing (dmPFC, vmPFC) and central-executive (bilateral dlPFC, right parietal posterior cortex [PPC]) networks.

In a different experiment, we used these same crime hypotheticals, keeping intention constant but varying harm, to examine whether subjects' belief in free will correlated to their punishment decisions. We found that they did—that subjects with a strong belief in free will tended to punish more harshly—but only for low harms, a result that helped explain some earlier conflicting studies that did not vary harm. As we put it, when harms are high, we all act like we have strong beliefs in free will. In those low harm cases where beliefs in free will matter, we found a strong correlation between punishment amounts and activations in the right TPJ. Across the two groups with strong and weak beliefs in free will, we found a correlation between the amounts of punishment, the amount of harm, and activations in the right anterior insula (rAI). These results not only tend to corroborate the model that our brain uses two different, though richly interconnected, systems to blame and punish, but also that the punishment decision's highly context-dependent nature can include the punisher's own biases, including biases about free will.

Another study investigated ordinary citizens, who as potential jurors decided on mitigation of punishment for murders after reading hypothetical criminal scenarios. Sympathy for a defendant activated regions associated with mentalizing and moral conflict (e.g., dmPFC, TPJ, precuneus) and individual differences on the inclination to mitigate was associated with activity in the right insula.

Finally, experimenters for the first time varied the wrongdoer's intentions across the four mental states traditionally recognized by the criminal law—purposeful, knowing, reckless and negligent—while also varying the amount of the harm.** They found the same basic pattern as previous experiments. Evaluating harm differentially engaged areas associated with affective and (interestingly) somatosensory functions, evaluating mental states recruited theory-of-mind areas, and vmPFC, PCC and amygdala seemed associated with the integration of these harm and mental

---

** [Matthew R. Ginther et al., *Parsing the Behavioral and Brain Mechanisms of Third-Party Punishment,* 36 J. Neurosci. 9420 (2016).— EDS.]

states signals into blame. They also found, as others had, that moving from blame to punishment seemed to recruit the dlPFC. This experiment, which was very tightly controlled to maximize the chances that the fMRI signals being picked up were actually associated with the subjects' blame and punishment decisions (a real challenge in fMRI experiments both because of the time delay between the task and the hemodynamic response, and because of the problem of knowing when exactly this mysterious thing we call "decision" actually happens), suggests that the essential punishment architecture revealed in these other experiments also applies in the kind of legal ecology typical of the criminal law.

A NEUROPSYCHOLOGICAL MODEL OF BLAME AND THIRD-PARTY PUNISHMENT

From these and other experiments, a few researchers have postulated neural models of the blame/punishment network.* We present here an extended version of the model we published recently.** It appears that at least three domain general large-scale and well-known brain networks are involved when we blame and punish: the salience network, the default mode network and the central executive network. (**Figure 16.2**).

The [salience network], which is anchored in the dorsal anterior cingulate cortex and [anterior insula], with extensive connectivity to the amygdala, has been identified with the general processing of self-related aversive experiences (e.g., personal distress) that guide behavior. In the context of blame and punishment tasks, we postulate that the [salience network] is involved with detecting and responding to norm violations or threats of norm violations. We argue that the dACC is involved with the detection of the harm or threat, that the [anterior insula] is associated with creating the aversive response to that harm or threat, and that the amygdala is involved with providing an emotional range for the severity of harm caused or threatened to the victim. The [salience network] would be involved in first-, second- and third-party punishment, since recognizing norm violations or potential norm violations is necessary for each of these kinds of punishment.

We postulate that the [salience network] modulates the engagement of the [default mode network] as the second large-scale network. The [default mode network] is located generally in the medial prefrontal cortex (mPFC), and is associated with processes, including self-monitoring and theory-of-mind. In the context of blame and punishment, we suggest the mPFC integrates the assessment of the wrongdoer's mental state with the assessment of the harm from the [salience network], producing what we might call a blame signal. In particular, we argue that the harm-integrating portion of the [default mode network] appears to work through the vmPFC, with its inter-network connections to regions within the [salience network], allowing the experience of feelings congruent with another's emotional situation (affective theory-of-mind). We hypothesize that the assessment of the

---

* [A first model was published by Joshua W. Buckholtz & René Marois, *The Roots of Modern Justice: Cognitive and Neural Foundations of Social Norms and Their Enforcement,* 15 Nature Neurosci. 655 (2012).—EDS.]

** [Frank Krueger & Morris Hoffman, *The Emerging Neuroscience of Third-Party Punishment.* 39 Trends Neurosci. 499 (2016).—EDS.]

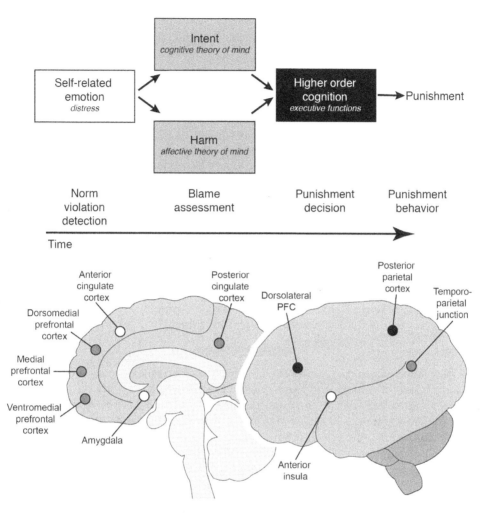

Figure 16.2   [Neuropsychological framework of blame and punishment. The figure portrays the three brain networks that interact to enable the necessary computations. The **salience network** [is indicated by the] white [square on the left and the areas with white circles on right: anterior insula; dorsal anterior cingulate cortex; and amygdala. The **default-mode network** [is indicated by the gray squares on the left and the areas with gray circles on the right]: medial prefrontal cortex; dorsomedial PFC; ventromedial PFC; posterior cingulate cortex; and temporo-parietal junction. The **central-executive network** [is indicated by the black square on the left and areas with black circles on the right]: dorsolateral PFC; posterior parietal cortex). [Details of the interactions are explained in the text.] [The figure was revised and redrawn by the authors.]

wrongdoer's intention involves the dmPFC, with its intranetwork connections to other mentalizing regions (PCC, TPJ) associated with understanding others' mental states (cognitive theory-of-mind). Under this model, the [default mode network] would be necessary for both second- and third-party punishment, since both these forms of punishment require an assessment of blame.

Deciding on a specific type and amount of punishment, as opposed to merely blaming, recruits yet a third large-scale network in our model, the [central executive network]. This network, located primarily in the dlPFC and the posterior parietal cortex (PPC), is recognized to be involved in the kinds of higher-order cognition such as executive functions necessary for context-dependent decision-making. The dlPFC, in particular, is thought to be capable of maintaining stable representations over time (working memory), and of integrating different abstract representations from distinct information processing streams. In other words, the dlPFC is often associated with complex reasoning and decision-making, where many factors have to be assessed and also weighed in order to reach a decision. In the blame and punishment context, we hypothesize that the [central executive network] is involved in the processes by which the blame signal from the [default mode network] is converted into a punishment decision after integration with a wide variety of context-dependent circumstances. We argue that this process involves the recruitment of the PPC to construct a punishment scale, and then the dlPFC to reason to a specific punishment on that scale based on all the circumstances of the case (and of course, as mentioned above, the biases of the punisher). The [central executive network] would be primarily involved in third-party punishment, because only third-party punishment requires the cognitive transition from largely automatic blame (and retaliation) to a decision about third-party punishment. . . .

IMPLICATIONS

The neuroscience of decision-making generally, let alone of complex social decisions like how much to blame and punish a wrongdoer, is of course still in its infancy. In the big picture of things, the black box of decision-making—how the brain enables the mind to cause action—remains frustratingly opaque despite all the breathtaking advances in neuroimaging. And there is nothing in the near- or probably even mid-term that brain science is likely to teach us about this potentially intractable problem, including its age-old sub-problems of when to blame, when to forgive, and how much to punish. . . . [The authors suggest that a deeper understanding of the evolutionary roots of inclinations toward punishment may yield beneficial circumspection at the time of sentencing.]

Advances in our understanding of how brains blame and punish may also someday have much more tangible implications. For example, understanding the differences between blame and punishment may lead to ways to help sentencing judges avoid some of the emotional pitfalls of sentencing. Judges, like all humans, empathize with many victims. Presiding over a trial or sentencing hearing full of all the horrible details of a crime risks retaliatory, second-party, punishment urges that might overwhelm the kind of restrained third-party punishment we need our judges to impose. Knowing more about how the brain converts blame into punishment could arm us in the future with strategies to address this problem.

There is a legislative version of this risk of the angry retaliating judge, which a fuller understanding of the interactions between blaming and punishment might likewise help manage. When crime rates go up, or a particularly notorious crime is splashed across the media, legislatures often respond by creating new crimes or increasing the penalties for old ones. We contend this is essentially a second-party party reaction, which then gets fixed into the law. When these new crimes or increased penalties do not immediately result in less crime (and they often don't, not only because of time delays but also because the effect of general deterrence on crime rates is complex and ill-understood), then legislatures often respond by making even more new laws and increasing penalties further. The result of this one-way ratchet is that penalties for crimes in America have skyrocketed over the last 60 years, crime rates have not correspondingly fallen, more people are in prison than ever before, and ordinary citizens seem to have lost faith in the criminal justice system. Understanding the difference between blame and punishment could one day help break this cycle.

Legal processes might also improve with a fuller understanding of the neuro-psychological underpinnings of punishment. Bedeviling problems of racial, gender and other kinds of punisher bias might admit to some inoculating strategies as we uncover the mysteries of how the [central executive network] turns the blame we all rather consistently feel into the myriad of actual punishments different judges impose. A fuller understanding of how we blame and punish could even conceivable change some well-entrenched legal doctrines, including the four legally-recognized criminal states of mind: purposeful, knowing, reckless and negligent. We know subjects have great difficulty distinguishing knowing from reckless conduct, but it is not yet clear how much of that difficulty comes from problems with the way we define these different mental states and how much reflects the fact that subjects simply may not recognize a moral difference between the two. Learning more about how these assessed mental states are represented may help us decide whether we need to try to improve our jury instruction definitions of them, or whether we need to abandon any legal distinction between knowing and reckless.

None of these legal impacts is imminent. And it may be a long shot that any of them ever comes to pass. But there will almost certainly be *some* impacts, even if we cannot predict them now. Science has a way of filling policy spaces in the most unpredictable of ways. We've learned more about the brain in the last 30 years than we learned in all of prior human history, and the pace of learning appears to be exponential. Neuroimaging technologies are getting better, and it seems that promising investigative methods are being invented every year, including both new technologies (such as new methods to measure connectivity) and powerful new ways of crunching the data from them (such as machine-learning classifiers). At this rate, it is almost inconceivable that neuroscience will not have some important impacts on the law generally, including how we blame and punish the wrongdoers among us. All of us in both disciplines need to be thinking about these possibilities—both their benefits and risks—as the neuroscience races on.

NOTES AND QUESTIONS

1. Evaluate and discuss these views, from the abstract of Professor Anna Spain Bradley's article, *The Disruptive Neuroscience of Judicial Choice.*

> Scholars of judicial behavior overwhelmingly substantiate the historical presumption that most judges act impartially and independent most of the time. The reality of human behavior, however, says otherwise. Drawing upon untapped evidence from neuroscience, this Article provides a comprehensive evaluation of how bias, emotion, and empathy—all central to human decision-making—are inevitable in judicial choice. The Article offers three novel neuroscientific insights that explain

why this inevitability is so. First, because human cognition associated with decision-making involves multiple, and often intersecting, neural regions and circuits, logic and reason are not separate from bias and emotion in the brain. Second, bias, emotion, empathy and other aspects of our cognition can be implicit, thereby shaping our behavior in ways that we are unaware. This challenges the longstanding assumption that a judge can simply put feelings aside when making judicial decisions. Third, there is no basis in neuroscience to support the idea that judges are exempt from these aspects of human cognition. These findings disrupt widespread faith in the unassailable rationality and impartiality of judges, and demonstrate how such views are increasingly at odds with evidence about how our brains work. By offering an original descriptive account of judicial behavior that is rooted in neuroscience, this Article provides a novel exposition of why bias, emotion and empathy have the capacity to influence the choices judges make. Doing so asks us to view judges as the humans they are.

Anna Spain Bradley, *The Disruptive Neuroscience of Judicial Choice*, 91 U.C. Irvine L. Rev. 1, 1 (2018). For a similar argument regarding members of the executive branch, see Anna Spain Bradley, *Cognitive Competence in Executive-Branch Decision Making*, 49 Conn. L. Rev. 713 (2017).

2. To what extent would you expect there to be more or less activation in the emotional circuitry of experienced judges than in controls? Why?

3. Powerful evidence demonstrates that the emotion of disgust is an evolved psychological adaptation for avoiding, among other things, harmful pathogens (such as in feces, rotting meat, and open sores). *See* Debra Lieberman & Carlton Patrick, *Objection: Disgust, Morality, and the Law* (2018). A 2014 fMRI study suggested that brain regions implicated in logical reasoning are modulated by the emotion of disgust during legal decision-making. Beatrice H. Capestany & Lasana T. Harris, *Disgust and Biological Descriptions Bias Logical Reasoning During Legal Decision-Making*, 9 Soc. Neurosci. 265 (2014).

4. The reading discusses research indicating that multiple parts of the brain—some analytic, others subconscious or emotional—interact to (a) decide blameworthiness, (b) assess harms, (c) integrate those two decisions, and (d) finally determine punishment. Krueger and Hoffman suggest that appreciating the nature of the interactions between assessing blame and assigning punishment can have tangible implications for sentencing judges, legislatures and sentencing guidelines, guarding against racial or gender biases, and assessment of criminal states of mind. Do you agree with these implications? Can you think of additional implications?

5. A study demonstrated that subjects with damage to their ventro-medial prefrontal cortex consider attempted harms (that were unsuccessful) as more morally permissible relative to healthy control subjects. Liane Young et al., *Damage to Ventromedial Prefrontal Cortex Impairs Judgment of Harmful Intent*, 65 Neuron 845 (2010). Would you favor a system that precluded such individuals from serving on juries considering prosecutions for an attempted crime? Why or why not?

6. A 2014 fMRI study investigated brain activity during punishment decisions when actions by protagonists in a *low*-culpability mental state yielded *high and graphic* harms. M. Treadway et al., *Corticolimbic Gating of Emotion-Driven Punishment*, 17 Nature Neurosci. 1270 (2014). The study found that emotionally graphic descriptions of harmful acts amplify punishment severity, boost amygdala activity, and strengthen amygdala connectivity with lateral prefrontal regions involved in punishment decision-making. However, this was *only* observed when the actor's

harm was intentional; when harm was unintended, a temporoparietal-medial-prefrontal circuit suppressed amygdala activity and the effect of graphic descriptions on punishment was abolished. These results reveal the brain mechanisms by which evaluation of a transgressor's mental state gates (that is, tamps down) our emotional urges to punish. What does this suggest to you about the roles of emotion and analysis in both liability and punishment decisions?

7. One line of brain imaging research explores what happens behaviorally, and in associated brain activity, when a subject with the power to either punish a transgressor *or* to compensate her victim observes a transgression. Transgressions were more likely than non-transgressions to correlate with activations of lateral prefrontal, anterior cingulate, anterior insula, and precuneus cortex. And transgressions more likely to result in punishment than in compensation were associated with higher ventral striatum activity. Mirre Stallen et al., *Neurobiological Mechanisms of Responding to Injustice*, 38 J. Neurosci. 2944 (2018). Intriguingly, ventral striatum activity is thought to be associated with experiencing a sense of "reward" or satisfaction, suggesting that punishment may have felt more rewarding to the punisher than would compensation of the victim. Even further, the study investigated the role of intra-nasal oxytocin inhalers on brain activity and associate behaviors. Oxytocin functions as both a hormone and a neurotransmitter, known to play a role in social bonding, as well as increased empathy and trust. Subjects who received oxytocin had more activity in the anterior insula, and punished less severely, than subjects who received a placebo. What implications does this have for judges? Juries?

8. Some states have started to use artificial intelligence algorithms to inform sentencing decisions. For compilation and overview, see the regularly updated *Algorithms in the Criminal Justice System: Pre-Trial Risk Assessment Tools*, Electronic Privacy Information Center, *https://epic.org/algorithmic-transparency/crim-justice*. How does that strike you, initially? How would you go about evaluating the net costs and benefits of using such algorithms?

9. React to this: "[P]assion . . . is the soul of punishment." Emile Durkheim, *Division of Labor in Society: Mechanical Solidarity* (George Simpson trans., 1933) (1893).

10. To what extent would you expect an overlap between neural activations involved in moral and legal reasoning? Why?

Jessica M. Salerno & Bette L. Bottoms
Emotional Evidence and Jurors' Judgments: The Promise of Neuroscience for Informing Psychology and Law
27 Behav. Sci. & L. 273, 273-93 (2009)

Neuroscience . . . research on brain mechanisms involved in moral judgments has begun to inform the legal system's understanding of those who commit criminal acts. For example, expert witnesses sometimes present neuroimaging evidence about defendants' brain abnormalities in murder trials, and at least one mock trial study suggests that this can increase jurors' acceptance of defendants' insanity defense. In this review, we argue that neuroimaging research can also help the legal system understand jurors. In particular, we argue that neuroscience research addressing how emotion affects the moral reasoning process has the potential to inform the debate about whether there should be more regulation of the admission of highly emotional evidence such as autopsy photographs and victim impact statements. . . .

THE NEUROSCIENCE OF EMOTION AND MORAL JUDGMENT

Neuroscientific studies based on brain-damaged populations find that emotion is not only important, but essential, to moral decision-making. . . . The participants were asked whether they would be willing to push one person in front of a bus to save many other passengers on board. This dilemma pits a utilitarian judgment (i.e. minimizing the death toll) against the natural strong emotional aversion toward personally killing another human being. Participants with VMPC brain damage chose to push the person in front of the bus significantly more often than did the normal participants or participants with brain damage not involving the VMPC. . . . The authors concluded that the VMPC-damaged participants lacked the normative aversive emotional response to the thought of killing another human being, and thus relied more on the utilitarian goal of saving as many people as possible. If emotion related to moral judgments results from making a moral judgment (as opposed to playing an antecedent causal role), then the VMPC-damaged group would have made the same decision as those without damage, but would have had a different emotional response afterward. Thus, emotions do indeed appear to play a causal role in moral judgment and decision-making. This research also suggests that jurors might need their emotional reactions to make normative moral judgments.

What can neuroscience research tell us about the impact of emotional evidence on jurors' emotions and subsequent judgments? Does more emotion equal less effortful cognitive processing? . . . Studies using fMRI to investigate emotion can provide insight into how brain activation differs when people make decisions that involve more (compared with less) emotional stimuli. A number of relevant fMRI studies have compared brain activation differences when people consider moral dilemmas that involve a personal element (and therefore believed to elicit more emotional engagement) versus a non-personal element. For example, [an investigator] asked participants to decide between letting a trolley full of people run off a cliff versus sacrificing only one man's life to stop the trolley (thus saving the people on board). In the impersonal condition, participants were told they had to pull a lever to switch the trolley to a second track and away from the cliff, killing a man standing on that second track. In the personal condition, participants were told they had to push a man onto the track in front of the trolley to stop it. Participants contemplating the more personal moral violation had increased activity in brain areas associated with emotion and, of even more interest, decreased brain activity in areas associated with cognitive processes such as working memory (i.e. dorsolateral prefrontal and parietal areas). [The investigator] replicated these results and also found that the different activation patterns were what drove the moral decision-making behaviors. This evidence supports the social intuitionist model (and many other contemporary emotion models), which asserts that emotion is a strong driving force in moral decision-making and that when emotions drive decisions there is also less effortful cognition. Less effortful cognitions could lead to information-processing mistakes, ranging from selective biasing of initial attention and encoding of information to the interpretation and retrieval of information in a manner congruent with the negative affect resulting from the emotional evidence. This is just what critics of emotional evidence in court fear.

Other neuroimaging studies have operationally defined emotion differently, more like the circumstances encountered by jurors considering harm suffered by victims in court cases. [An investigator] used a within-subjects design to present participants with sentences that described bodily harm or sentences that did not include bodily harm. Participants were asked to indicate whether the sentence made sense and whether the action depicted in the sentence was appropriate. Sentences involving bodily harm (which the participants rated as higher in emotionality) resulted in quicker judgments, but less activation in the anterior temporal poles, compared with the less emotional non-bodily-harm sentences. Citing evidence that the brain's anterior temporal poles are associated with brain processes such as autobiographical episodic memory necessary for taking context into account when processing material and for attributing intentions to others (i.e. theory of mind tasks), the researchers concluded that viewing bodily harm limits one's ability to take the semantic and emotional context into account when judging another person's actions. Although we believe that this is quite relevant to the issues at stake in this paper, a similar fMRI study examining brain activation in people who are considering emotional (e.g. gruesome photographs of a victim's harm) versus non-emotional (verbal descriptions of the harm) forms of evidence is clearly needed. In its absence, however, the study . . . leads us to expect that viewing gruesome photographs might result in more activation of parts of the brain responsible for emotional reactions, less activation of areas associated with episodic memory, and perhaps even less activation of areas associated with the ability to take into account context—such as mitigating evidence. In fact, [one investigator] found that mock jurors exposed to a victim impact statement about a highly respectable victim (versus a less respectable victim) were less able to take mitigating evidence into account compared with those who were not exposed to the statements. This work might also help explain the finding by [another investigator] that mock jurors in a death penalty trial (which is likely to be emotionally arousing) are more likely to argue that mitigating evidence should be disregarded than that it should be used in a mitigating manner.

In another relevant study, [researchers] presented scenarios to participants during an fMRI scan and manipulated the emotionality of the scenarios' language and the morality and intentionality of the act portrayed in the scenario. The participants judged whether the action depicted in the scenario was wrong (similar to jurors' task in a trial) and whether they would have acted the same way. . . . [T]he study shows that there are differences in processing for information presented in vivid, emotional (colorful) terms versus non-emotional (plain) terms. . . . In summary, . . . neuroimaging studies . . . provide preliminary support for some of the fears voiced by critics of emotional evidence. Specifically, situations involving stimuli that are highly emotionally engaging appear to cause heightened emotionality and decreased brain activity in areas associated with cognitive processes, and these differences in thought patterns appear to drive systematic differences in moral judgments. Although none of these studies involved legal decision-making specifically, future studies could address this domain specifically, so we believe that neuroscience methodology holds considerable promise for contributing to the debate about the effects of emotional evidence, the psychological mechanisms underlying these effects, and perhaps even the ultimate policy issue of what role emotional evidence should play in trials.

SUMMARY, LEGAL IMPLICATIONS, AND FUTURE DIRECTIONS

It is clear that emotion is inevitable during a trial, especially during a murder trial that includes evidence such as gruesome photographs, victim impact statements, and emotional mitigating evidence about the defendant's history. In fact, few would argue that emotion should not be present in such trials. These crimes and their outcomes are inherently emotionally disturbing. Jurors must have a thorough understanding of a crime that has been committed, and this must sometimes necessitate their being exposed to evidence that is emotionally disturbing.

In the case of victim impact statements, a review of the social cognitive theories of emotion and reasoning and neuroimaging research calls into question the Supreme Court's contention in *Payne v. Tennessee* (1991) that victim impact statements are relevant to the sentencing phase of a death-penalty trial because they speak to the level of harm resulting from a crime (i.e. the probative effect) and are harmless because they do not bias jurors against the defendant (i.e. the prejudicial effect). If emotional evidence results in heightened emotion but also decreased cognitive activity that promotes bias, then perhaps the Supreme Court's assumption is in error. In the minority opinion in *Kelly v. California* (2008), Justice Stevens expressed this worry himself, suggesting that video tributes to victims are "emotionally evocative" (particularly overwhelming due to the music and video enhancements) and have little probative value relevant to the offender, the offense, or the moral culpability of the defendant. Of course we cannot know with certainty whether the Supreme Court's reasoning is accurate or inaccurate without more direct empirical testing, as we discuss below.

In the case of gruesome post-mortem photographs, it is not enough for a juror to know simply that a victim was stabbed to death if the victim was in fact stabbed 40 times with great force. The information provided by this level of detail might outweigh the resulting prejudicial emotion elicited in jurors; knowing the victim was stabbed 40 times is relevant to many legal issues such as *mens rea*, the type of physical evidence at the scene, and to the ultimate issues of harm and punishment. But should the use of emotional evidence be regulated? Should the jury in this case see two photographs of the murder victim or an extensive slide show of many photographs shot from different angles? Should the jury see the photograph only when it is admitted as evidence, or should the attorney also be permitted to show the photographs repeatedly during closing statements? The law at issue is the extent of the emotionality that should be present in trials. On the one hand, can jurors make an informed decision without this information? Can jurors truly assess the degree of harm resulting from a crime without viewing post-mortem photographs and hearing victim impact statements? On the other hand, can jurors use this information in the manner the law intends if they are emotionally inflamed by its content? Will this information cloud jurors' ability to process case evidence rationally and thoroughly? Could it cause jurors to weigh evidence inappropriately, underestimate its importance, or miss some evidence entirely? Innocent people do get convicted for crimes they do not commit. Is this more likely when crime details are presented in a highly disturbing manner or when victim impact statements are the most gut-wrenching?

Although we cannot provide definitive answers to these questions, our review of three disparate areas of psychological literature . . . suggests that exceedingly disturbing evidence has the potential to influence jurors' judgments by increasing jurors' emotions and decreasing their effortful cognitive processing of information.

Social cognition theories and neuroscientific evidence help us understand the psychological mechanisms underlying the findings from mock trial studies that emotional evidence leads to more punitive judgments. . . .

CAVEATS

Although we believe that the constellation of evidence we have presented is quite relevant in understanding the probative versus prejudicial nature of emotional evidence in the courtroom, there are certainly a number of reasons to be cautious about generalizing from some of the studies we reviewed to the actual legal arena. First, as noted above, the definitive experiments in this field have not yet been conducted. Second, the social cognition and neuroscience studies we reviewed were not conceived of for generalization to the context of legal decision-making specifically. Third, none of the models we have discussed take into account the potential influence of the jury deliberation process. Studies that do not include the jury deliberation component might misrepresent what final post-deliberation verdicts would be in a real jury context. Deliberation can force jurors to be accountable to other people, not only for their decision, but for the reasons behind their decision. For example, jurors who are affected by emotion in the manner proposed by [the] social intuition model (i.e. their opinions are based solely on an emotional reaction and not rational reasoning) might fail to convince their fellow jurors, while jurors whose opinions are based on rational evidence deliberation might be more persuasive. Thus, potential biases against the defendant resulting from overly emotional evidence might be attenuated after group deliberation. . . . Alternatively, deliberation might also maximize initial biases, or do little more than develop the picture that was formed before deliberation among the majority of jurors. Most of the research we reviewed considered individual jurors' judgments, and if emotional evidence causes more individual jurors to favor a punitive judgment before deliberation, then the chance is increased that the pre-deliberation picture, which deliberation might develop, is one that is biased toward a more punitive decision. In fact, in a recent study . . . participants were angrier at and more likely to punish a member of their experimentally designated group who had committed a small moral violation when another person witnessed the punishment decision, as compared with when their decisions were anonymous. They punished more in others' presence because they felt they "should." Thus, the public aspect of jury deliberation might exacerbate the punitiveness of individuals' sentencing decisions, especially when the crime is emotionally inflammatory.

Further, obviously, a mock jury study will never be completely representative of a real jury situation. Research has shown that people need to be motivated to process thoroughly. A real jury situation may provide more motivation than a mock jury situation, which could either minimize or exacerbate the effects of emotional evidence. Also, there is the issue of sample. Many of the studies we reviewed employed a jury-eligible community member sample. Any of these participants could end up as a real juror. Other studies, however, used college students as participants. Although college students are jury eligible, they are on average younger and less experienced than actual jurors as a group. Results from these studies were consistent with studies employing a community sample, and multiple studies comparing college student and community member samples have found few differences in jury decisions. Even so, this must be taken into consideration in generalizing the findings to a community sample. It would be ideal to have actual sitting jurors' responses to emotional evidence, but this possibility is unfortunately highly unlikely due to the obtrusive nature of neuroscientific measurement. Even if a second set of shadow jurors were to sit alongside a real jury for the purposes of neuroscientific measurement, they would not have the motivational component that real jurors would have—the knowledge that their decisions would affect the defendant's life. Even so, it would be an improvement over current methods if the sample size could be large enough, and the field should strive for methods that better approximate actual jurors' experiences.

A fourth caveat to consider is that the neuroscience studies have thus far not focused on punishment or blame decisions. Instead, they use as stimuli moral dilemmas in which the participant must make a decision about his or her own course of action or the appropriateness of an abstract moral action. The brain might react to emotional stimuli differently when making blame or punishment judgments for a criminal act that is clearly inappropriate. In addition, the neuroscience studies are typically focused on one's own moral decisions, as opposed to judging the moral transgressions of others. One could argue, however, that research on the effect of emotion on judgments about one's own moral acts is relevant enough to speak to the potential effect emotion might have on judgments of others' moral transgressions. Clearly, research is needed that speaks directly to the neural mechanisms at play when one judges and punishes others' moral transgressions.

Fifth, it is difficult to extrapolate from the neuroscience studies regarding emotion and moral judgments to the specific question of emotional evidence in a court case because the emotion manipulations are not so comparable. Neither manipulating the personal component of a moral judgment, the emotionality of written descriptions, nor the depiction of bodily harm are the same thing as the manipulation of being exposed or not to emotional evidence such as grisly photographs or victim impact statements. We have argued, however, that there are certainly enough parallels between these manipulations to make the studies useful, and that, taken together, the neuroscience studies we reviewed present converging evidence that participants with higher versus lower emotional engagement during decision-making have less activation in areas of the brain responsible for deep processing.

CONCLUSION

What should the legal system do with the information we have presented in this article? Ultimately, it should wait for psychologists to conduct the specific studies clearly indicated by this review. These studies, grounded in solid theory and using the most innovative methods applied to the specific question of jury decision-making in the presence or absence of emotional evidence, promise to inform the courts and policy makers directly about the issues most relevant to the debate. Meanwhile, however, the legal system should take note of psychological research that suggests that highly emotional evidence might not only increase emotion, but also result in less effortful cognitive processing of evidence. Thus, the question is whether the information gleaned from this emotional evidence outweighs this negative side effect—is it probative without being prejudicial? If its probative value fails to outweigh its prejudicial impact, then should emotional evidence be banned or limited? Should it be allowed only in conjunction with safeguards such as expert testimony or jury instructions that inform jurors of its potentially biasing influence? It is not the job of psychologists to make a normative claim about whether emotional evidence is legally tenable. Instead, we have a duty to provide the courts and policymakers with empirically derived information regarding how emotion affects jurors' decision-making. Such information has the potential to inform safeguards aimed at maximizing the probative value and minimizing the prejudicial impact of emotional evidence. It is up to the courts to listen and then determine whether the probative and prejudicial effects of emotional evidence are those intended, and if not what to do about it.

NOTES AND QUESTIONS

1. Consider the chapter's epigraph, Aristotle's assertion that "[t]he law is reason, free of passion." What challenges, if any, does neuroscience pose to this contention?

2. The study of parole decisions described in the introduction to this chapter has been questioned on the grounds that the authors failed to account for the sequencing of cases that alone could have explained the variation in favorable rulings. *See* Keren Weinshall-Margel & John Shapard, Letter, *Overlooked Factors in the Analysis of Parole Decisions*, 108 Proc. Nat'l Acad. Sci. E833 (2011). The study's authors then reply in Shai Danziger, Jonathan Levav & Liora Avnaim-Pessoa, *Reply to Weinshall-Margel and Shapard: Extraneous Factors in Judicial Decisions Persist*, 108 Proc. Nat'l Acad. Sci. E834 (2011).

3. A scholar investigating law and emotions, Susan Bandes, argues that:

    The law . . . is imbued with emotion. . . . Emotion pervades not just the criminal courts, with their heat-of-passion and insanity defenses and their angry or compassionate jurors but the civil courtrooms, the appellate courtrooms, the legislatures. It propels judges and lawyers, as well as jurors, litigants, and the lay public. Indeed, the emotions that pervade law are often so ancient and deeply ingrained that they are largely invisible.

    Susan Bandes, *Introduction*, in *The Passions of Law* 2 (Susan A. Bandes ed., 2000). To what extent do you agree or disagree? Categorize your reasons.

4. How would you connect the readings in this chapter to the issues raised in the Emotions chapter? A growing literature, much of it by Professor Terry Maroney, examines the role of emotions in judicial decision-making. *See, e.g.*, Terry A. Maroney, *Emotional Regulation and Judicial Behavior*, 99 Cal. L. Rev. 1485 (2011).

5. Could neuroscience offer new ways to improve judicial decision-making through cognitive enhancement? If the courthouse provides coffee to judges in the morning to help them wake up, should judges also be able, or encouraged to, take other drugs to improve alertness, memory, and information processing? What ethical issues arise with judicial cognitive enhancement? *See* Jennifer A. Chandler & Adam M. Dodek, *Cognitive Enhancement in the Courtroom*, in *Cognitive Enhancement: Ethical and Policy Implications in International Perspectives* 329 (Fabrice Jotterand & Veljko Dubljević eds., 2016).

6. On a panel at the 2013 meeting of the International Neuroethics Society, California Judge Robert Trentacosta, the Presiding Judge of the San Diego Superior Court, reflected on the role that neuroscience might play in judicial punishment decisions:

> At sentencing, at that moment in the life of a case when you've got to get it right, it seems ... that something, something important, is missing. And what's missing is the science. It seems to me that neuroscience and the law have been occupying parallel universes that are separated by a semi-permeable membrane. And ... I kept asking myself "Why?"

Why might neuroscience and judicial decision-making be in parallel universes? Should judges begin to use any of the research described above to inform their instructions to juries or their own practices? Why or why not?

7. Victims' rights advocates support the admission of autopsy photographs and victim impact statements, but others are concerned that jurors' emotional responses to this evidence might unfairly prejudice jurors against a defendant and hamper unbiased reasoning processes. How might neuroscience approaches help resolve this question?

8. Some research suggests that damage to emotional circuitry of the brain impairs decision-making. Antoine Bechara, Hanna Damasio & Antonio R. Damasio, *Emotion, Decision Making and the Orbitofrontal Cortex*, 10 Cerebral Cortex 295 (2000); Mauricio R. Delgado et al., *Viewpoints: Dialogues on the Functional Role of the Ventromedial Prefrontal Cortex*, 19 Nature Neurosci. 1545 (2016). What specific neuroscientific findings would you find useful if they existed? Why?

9. This section of the chapter has explored the use of neuroscientific tools to investigate punishment decisions. To what extent would you expect a fruitful line of future research investigating legal reasoning more broadly? Had you the power to select, what types of legal reasoning would you investigate, and why?

10. The field of neuroeconomics is an inter-disciplinary effort to examine the neuroscientific underpinnings of choices, generally. *See Neuroeconomics: Decision Making and the Brain* (Paul W. Glimcher et al. eds., 2013)

B. NEUROSCIENCE AND RACIST JUDGMENTS

If biases are bad, legal biases are especially bad. And racial bias is among the most pernicious of these. At the same time, directly questioning people—such as potential judges and jurors—seems unlikely to yield valid and reliable diagnoses of racial bias, given that social norms may chill honest answers. Might neuroscience be relevant to related legal questions, and if so, how?

A large and growing literature is identifying behavioral and neuroscientific correlates of racial bias. The Implicit Association Test (IAT) has been an important tool in these investigations, so it is introduced in this first excerpt. However, some of that work has been controversial. Our purpose with the next several readings is not to cover that material in depth, but rather to provide you with a sense of some of the issues involved.

Jeffrey Kluger
Race and the Brain
Time Mag. (Oct. 9, 2008)

In the 1990s, . . . Mahzarin Banaji of Harvard University co-created what's known as the implicit-association test (IAT), a way of exploring the instant connections the brain draws between races and traits. . . . [A]vailable online (at implicit.harvard.edu) the IAT asks people to pair pictures of white or black faces with positive words like joy, love, peace and happy or negative ones like agony, evil, hurt and failure. Speed is everything, since the survey tests automatic associations. When respondents are told to link the desirable traits to whites and the undesirable ones to blacks, their fingers fairly fly on the keys. When the task is switched, with whites being labeled failures and blacks called glorious, fingers slow considerably, a sure sign the brain is struggling.

When Banaji, along with cognitive neuroscientist Liz Phelps of New York University, conducted brain scans of subjects using functional magnetic resonance imaging, they uncovered the reasons for the results. White subjects respond with greater activation of the amygdala—a region that processes alarm—when shown images of black faces than when shown images of white faces. "One of the amygdala's critical functions is fear-conditioning," says Phelps. "You attend to things that are scary because that's essential for survival." Later studies have shown similar results when black subjects look at white faces.

The brain, of course, is not all amygdala, and there are higher regions that can talk sense to the lower ones. Phelps cites studies showing that when blacks and whites are flashed pictures of faces from the other race so quickly that the subjects weren't consciously aware of seeing them, their amygdalae reacted predictably. When the images were flashed more slowly so that subjects could process them consciously, the anterior cingulate cortex and the dorsolateral prefrontal cortex—regions that temper automatic responses—kicked in.

Phelps conducted other studies in which the images included such friendly faces as Will Smith's and Harrison Ford's and found that this helped control the amygdala too. "The more you think about people as individuals," she says, "the more the brain calms down." . . .

Anna Spain Bradley
The Disruptive Neuroscience of Judicial Choice
9 UC Irvine L. Rev. 1, 27-29 (2018)

[A] bias is a preference for or aversion against something. We can be aware of such preferences or explicit bias, and we can have them unknowingly as implicit bias. This includes the so-called cognitive biases such as confirmation bias, anchoring, and hindsight bias. These biases are often identified and evidenced through behavioral science observations about how people behave under specific conditions. . . .

[T]he biases that people often understand as being related to racism, sexism, homophobia, and other forms of discrimination . . . are particularly concerning biases for a judge to acknowledge because judges take an oath to perform their judicial function impartially. Therefore, acknowledging that one's decision-making is prone to bias based on race, gender, sexual orientation, and other aspects of identity conflicts with the notion of judicial impartiality.

The impact of bias in the legal profession is widespread yet poorly understood and acknowledged. Recent scholarship on bias in law aims to change that. For example, biases related to a judge or jury's views about a defendant are believed to increase the risk for wrongful convictions. Take cases where people report a criminal act such as robbery with black men or demonstrate a "shooter bias." Studies in social psychology, notably from the Implicit Association Test, support a general inference that racial bias is real. This builds upon earlier work showing the prevalence of racial profiling in police stops. Despite the sustained evidence of bias in the courtroom and in the legal profession, serious acknowledgment and redress are, still, lacking.

This is where neuroscience may provide an invaluable contribution to the discourse. No one wants to be labeled racist, sexist, or homophobic yet the biases connected to such discriminatory behavior are real. In order to move from description to prescription and remedy, people need to understand why bias of this sort occurs and what to do about it. Neuroscience helps us understand bias as a form of implicit cognition that can influence our thought without us realizing it. In other words, neural mechanisms in our brains can help explain what occurs in a case of racial bias, for example.

Using brain imaging techniques, neuroscience researchers have long studied the amygdala for its importance in activity associated with fear and other human emotions. Studies on racial bias, the most frequently studied type of bias, have linked amygdala activity to racial prejudice. A 2014 review of fMRI studies on emotion and prejudice suggests, once again, that the amygdala is of high importance. The study goes further to argue that activity in this area of the brain may be attributed to a person perceiving a threat that arises from negative cultural associations with black men and other groups. . . .

The implications of studies like these, which continue to evolve, are relevant to the discourse . . . about evidencing judicial bias through neuroscience. First and foremost, evidence of neural activity that explains bias further advances the reality that bias is real and present in society and in the legal profession. Second, there is no evidence to suggest that certain legal professionals, such as judges, are cognitively exceptional and therefore not prone to such bias. Third, neuroscientific studies can lead the way in bringing about evidence-based solutions for reform. . . .

State v. Brown

No. 2017AP774-CR, 2020 WL 3621304 (Wis. July 3, 2020)

[In 2020, the Supreme Court of Wisconsin ruled on the constitutionality of a traffic stop, considering whether the Fourth Amendment's prohibition against unreasonable searches and seizures permits a police officer to extend a traffic stop after writing a ticket for the traffic violation by requesting a driver to exit the vehicle, ask about the presence of weapons, and ask consent to search the car. The majority opinion ruled that this was not an unreasonable search under the Fourth Amendment because "[asking the driver] to step out of the vehicle, ushering him a few feet away from the road, asking [him] whether he possessed anything that could harm [the police officer], and requesting consent for a search, were all negligibly burdensome actions directly related to officer safety and therefore part of the stop's mission." But in sharply worded concurring and dissenting opinions, Justices Bradley (concurring) and Dallet (dissenting) argued about the proper role of scientific evidence of decision-making in resolving constitutional cases. The excerpts below capture the substance of that debate. We present the dissent first, as it introduces the Implicit Association Test (IAT) and then present the concurrence, which critiques the use of the IAT. — Eds.]

DALLET, J. (dissenting). Officer Christopher Deering could have safely returned Courtney Brown's license and warned him of the need to wear a seat belt, thus completing the remaining tasks tied to a traffic stop made on August 23, 2013. Instead, Officer Deering ordered Brown out of the car for the express purpose of requesting consent to search him for illegal drugs. Because the traffic stop was unreasonably extended without independent reasonable suspicion that a crime had been committed, the subsequent search of Brown's person contravenes the Fourth Amendment to the United States Constitution. . . . By upholding the constitutionality of this search, the majority sanctions unrestricted officer discretion to prolong a traffic stop in search of other crimes, and turns a blind eye to the discriminatory consequences of unchecked implicit bias. For these reasons, I respectfully dissent. . . .

I must also address one of the real-world consequences of the majority opinion's rejection of the reasonableness inquiry: unchecked implicit bias. I discuss social science research on implicit bias not to depart from constitutional text as the concurrence postulates, but instead to illustrate empirically how far our jurisprudence has strayed from the original meaning of the Fourth Amendment.

The concept of implicit bias has been well-researched and can best be described as follows. In order to effectively function in a complex world, the human brain makes associations implicitly, or "outside conscious attentional focus." These associations, which can be beneficial and helpful, also include observations sorted by social categories like race or gender, which in turn trigger implicit stereotypes and attitudes.

Problematically, these subconscious stereotypes and attitudes may operate in direct contradiction to one's "consciously and genuinely held thoughts and feelings." A wealth of data collected by Harvard University's Project Implicit confirms that implicit biases can influence our decisions without any awareness that these biases even exist.

The influence of implicit bias is particularly problematic in the policing context, where officers are tasked with rapidly judging stressful and potentially dangerous situations based upon limited information that is largely ambiguous. Research demonstrates that "[i]mplicit biases translate most readily into discriminatory behavior . . . when people have wide discretion in making quick decisions with little accountability." Jerry Kang et al., Implicit Bias in the Courtroom, 59 UCLA L. Rev. 1124, 1142 (2012). Social psychologists have thus come to understand that much of what has been labeled "racial profiling" is likely to instead be spontaneous and unintended.

The *Terry* decision instructs courts to differentiate police hunches based on general, unparticularized information from reasonable inferences based on articulable and specific facts, thereby mitigating the influence of any implicit bias on discretionary searches and seizures. The promised protection of the reasonable suspicion standard, however, has been diluted by this court's growing acceptance of weakly-correlated criminal inferences from generic or generalized factors in direct contrast to the particularized circumstances required under *Terry*. And now . . . [w]ithout inquiring into the reasonableness of these delays, the duration of a trafficstop falls solely to the unfettered discretion of an officer whose judgments, like all human beings, are susceptible to implicit bias. By disavowing any meaningful review of officer discretion during a traffic stop, the majority opinion turns a blind eye to the disparities caused by implicit bias, despite the seemingly even-handed promise of the Fourth Amendment. . . .

BRADLEY, J. (concurring). . . . Justice Dallet claims "the majority opinion turns a blind eye to the disparities caused by implicit bias." Considering the consequences of a decision for certain groups of people conflicts with the judicial oath to "administer justice without respect to persons" and inappropriately assumes a role in developing policy more appropriate for the political branches of government than an impartial judiciary tasked with declaring what the law is rather than what it should be. Social science research has nothing whatsoever to say about the meaning of the Fourth Amendment. . . .

More often than not, an opinion dependent upon social science research for its conclusions is written to reach the outcome desired by a majority of justices rather than the result compelled by the Constitution. . . .

Justice Dallet says I "disregard[ ] the important role of social science research in guiding" judicial decision-making. I don't disregard it; I emphatically reject it. Embracing social science research as a methodology of constitutional interpretation is a license for judges to inject their subjective views into opinions rather than applying the law as it is written. . . .

The IAT has become a common technique for discerning the existence and extent of implicit beliefs such as racial bias. It is run with a computer that requires participants to make a series of rapid judgments to categorize two concepts with a given attribute. For example, pair the concepts "neuroscientist" and "lawyer" with the attribute "virtuous." Easier pairings as assessed by faster responses are interpreted as more strongly associated in memory than more difficult pairings as assessed by slower responses. By requiring rapid reactions, the IAT is supposed to probe participants' attitudes about the concepts and attributes of which they are not consciously aware. The next study attempted to compare the effectiveness of the IAT, a strictly behavioral measure, with the effectiveness of fMRI, that measures a proxy for neural activity.

Harrison A. Korn, Micah A. Johnson & Marvin M. Chun
Neurolaw: Differential Brain Activity for Black and White Faces Predicts Damage Awards in Hypothetical Employment Discrimination Cases
7 Soc. Neurosci. 398, 398-407 (2012)

The sixth amendment of the US Constitution states that all accused have the right to a trial "by an impartial jury." Therefore, when selecting a jury—especially for cases in which race is a factor—courts should strive to select jurors with the least amount of racial prejudice. Currently, to try to get an impartial jury, potential jurors are sometimes explicitly asked during voir dire whether the race of the victim, plaintiff, or defendant would affect their decision-making. This is not a very effective way to identify impartial jurors, however, as social pressures not to express unpopular or socially unacceptable beliefs may make people unlikely to admit they are racially biased.

Further, people have implicit biases that they are not consciously aware of and that differ from their explicit beliefs. In a 1992 dissent, US Supreme Court Justice O'Connor wrote, "[i]t is by now clear that conscious and unconscious racism can affect the way white jurors perceive minority defendants and the facts presented at their trials, perhaps determining the verdict of guilt or innocence" (*Georgia v. McCollum*). Even as explicit biases have declined, the disparity in outcomes in the legal system between Blacks and Whites has persisted. Much of the remaining disparity is likely due to implicit biases that people are unaware they hold. Implicit biases are especially likely to affect decisions in trials since trials are full of ambiguity and uncertainty, conditions that cause people to use heuristics that are often based on stereotypes.

This suggests that a test known as the Implicit Association Test (IAT), which measures implicit biases, may be a better method for finding the least biased jurors than the explicit questioning method that is currently used. The IAT uses response times to test how strongly a person associates two groups (for example, Whites and Blacks) with each of two categories (for example, good and bad). A study of 2.5 million IATs found that implicit biases were pervasive across demographic groups.

In a review of studies involving interracial behavior, the IAT was a significantly better predictor of behavior than more explicit, self-report measures. The behaviors that IAT scores have been found to predict are numerous. For example, scores on a racial IAT have been found to predict the likelihood that a physician will give a hypothetical White patient but not a hypothetical Black patient the appropriate treatment for a myocardial infarction, [and] the likelihood a hiring manager will give an interview to a Swedish applicant and not an Arab-Muslim applicant. . . . However, in the legal field, very little research has been done on the IAT. One study shows that IAT scores can predict actual judges' verdicts in certain hypothetical scenarios. Actual judges read vignettes about a juvenile shoplifter, a juvenile robber, and a battery. When the defendant's race was subliminally primed (but not when it was explicitly stated), the judges' IAT scores predicted the sentences they gave the Black defendant.

But if the IAT is a better predictor of certain racially discriminatory behaviors than explicit measures, then perhaps going one step further back and looking at neural activity would be an even more sensitive measure. Implicit behavioral measures like the IAT still require some conscious cognition, but fMRI measures can tap unconscious processes even further along the implicit–explicit spectrum. Since minimal need for introspective access is desired when studying discrimination and prejudice, fMRI appears to be an attractive tool.

IAT scores have been correlated with subjects' neural activity when viewing Black and White faces. The brain areas that are correlated with IAT scores unfortunately vary on parametric factors, such as how long the faces were presented. When faces are presented for short periods of time (about 30 ms) or as part of a cognitively demanding task, the difference in neural activity for Black versus White faces in emotional regions like the amygdala predicts IAT scores. When faces are presented for longer periods of time with a less cognitively demanding task—allowing for more controlled processing—dorsal lateral prefrontal cortex (DLPFC) activity in response to Black faces can predict IAT scores, reflecting the executive control functions of these regions (right anterior cingulate continuing into the right medial frontal gyrus and right middle frontal gyrus). Greater activity in the executive control regions in response to Black faces was correlated with more implicit bias, suggesting that more biased individuals must put forth more effort in order to suppress these biases and behave according to their explicit, non-prejudicial values.

[Investigators] found evidence that when people have time to engage in controlled processing, DLPFC activity in response to Black faces may work to override people's automatic emotional response in response to Black faces and suppress amygdala activity. As a result, amygdala activity does not correlate with IAT scores when subjects can engage in controlled processing.

Because racial bias has neural correlates, it is reasonable to hypothesize that neural activity when viewing Black and White faces might be able to predict legal judgments. We know of only one study where general legal judgments were predicted by neural activity. [Investigators] found that, for a range of criminal scenarios, neural activity in regions related to affective processing predicted the magnitude of punishment the subject believed the defendant deserved, and neural activity in the right DLPFC predicted whether the subject believed the defendant was criminally responsible.* This study, however, measured subjects' neural activity while they made decisions about specific cases, not neural activity designed to measure a baseline bias that would be reflected in the decisions they made outside the scanner.

In the present study, we sought to show that the difference in a subject's neural activity in response to Black and White faces can predict not only the person's score on an IAT, but also his or her decisions in hypothetical legal cases where race is salient. Specifically, activity in DLPFC regions which have previously been shown to predict IAT scores were expected to also predict subjects' judgments in the legal cases. The fact that DLPFC regions have recently been shown to be active when people make legal decisions, and that. . . . DLPFC was involved in determining whether punishment was warranted, further suggests that activity for Black faces minus White faces in this region may be able to predict people's decisions in legal cases where race is salient.

We asked subjects to read short vignettes based on actual cases and say how much money, if any, they would award the victim. We chose employment discrimination cases because race is a salient factor in the cases and they are very common, accounting for over 40% of all civil rights cases in US District Courts in 2010. Subjects were then scanned in an fMRI while they saw Black and White faces. We paired these faces with positive, negative, and neutral adjectives to see whether pairing a White face (in contrast to a Black face) with a negative adjective or a Black face (in contrast to a White face) with a positive adjective would evoke a greater DLPFC response in more racially biased subjects that in turn would predict a smaller award. We also included neutral adjectives and planned to also collapse across all adjective conditions so that we could perform contrasts that were similar to the contrasts performed in the previously mentioned studies. . . .

DISCUSSION

In this study, we looked to see whether the amount of money people awarded victims of employment discrimination could be predicted by IAT scores or neural activity in response to Black and White faces paired with adjectives. We found the IAT scores did not predict verdict size. However, neural activity for Black faces paired with neutral adjectives minus neural activity for White faces paired with neutral adjectives in right inferior parietal lobule . . . and in right superior/middle frontal gyrus of DLPFC . . . did predict verdict size. This suggests that brain activity could be a more valid measure of racial bias than the IAT, at least when sample size is limited. . . .

---

* [This study, by Buckholtz et al., appears in the Appendix. —EDS.]

Conclusions.   We found that activity in right DLFPC and right inferior parietal lobule in response to Black and White faces can predict how much subjects will give victims in hypothetical employment discrimination cases. Further studies should seek to corroborate these results by testing different employment discrimination vignettes and should seek to expand these results by testing whether these regions predict verdicts in other types of cases where race is salient. Additionally, our study used only White subjects. Further studies should look to see whether the same results can be reproduced in subjects of other races.

We are not suggesting that potential jurors be put in an MRI machine during jury selection for cases where race is salient. The cost of doing so would be prohibitive, many people might feel it is overly invasive, and—because of lack of data—courts have been hesitant to allow neuroimaging data to be used in trials, although the acceptance of neuroimaging data by the courts has steadily been increasing. Further, it is unclear from our data which people are the least biased. The people whose neural activity in response to White faces subtracted from their neural activity in response to Black faces is greatest in the regions we identified—the people who would be predicted to award the victim the most money—are not necessarily the least racially biased. It is possible that these individuals have a pro-Black/anti-White bias. Still, this study is notable in that it shows that neuroimaging data can measure a racial bias that is reflected in juror decisions more effectively than a common behavioral measure—the IAT.

Although there are many enthusiasts, there are also many critics of the IAT. Consider this view.

Amy Wax & Philip E. Tetlock
We Are All Racists at Heart
Wall St. J. (Dec. 1, 2005)

It was once easy to spot a racial bigot: The casual use of the n-word, the sweeping hostility, and the rigid unwillingness to abandon vulgar stereotypes left little doubt that a person harbored prejudice toward blacks as a group. But 50 years of survey research has shown a sharp decline in overt racial prejudice. Instead of being a cause for celebration, however, this trend has set off an ever more strident insistence in academia that whites are pervasively biased.

Some psychologists went low-tech: They simply expanded the definition of racism to include any endorsement of politically conservative views grounded in the values of self-reliance and individual responsibility. Opposition to busing, affirmative action or generous welfare programs were tarred as manifestations of "modern" or symbolic racism.

Others took a high-tech path: Racists could be identified by ignoring expressed beliefs and tapping into the workings of the unconscious mind. Thus was born the so-called "implicit association test." The IAT builds on the fact that people react faster to the word "butter" if they have just seen the word "bread" momentarily flashed on a screen. The quicker response suggests that the mind closely associates those concepts. Applying this technique, researchers such as Mahzarin Banaji of Harvard have found that people recognize "negative" words such as "angry," "criminal" or "poor" more quickly after being momentarily exposed to a black (as opposed to a white) face. And this effect holds up for the vast majority of white respondents—and sometimes even for majorities of blacks.

What do investigators conclude from their findings that "blackness" often primes bad associations and "whiteness" good ones? According to some, it shows that prejudice permeates our unconscious minds and is not just confined to the 10% of hard-core bigots. Know it or not, we are all vessels of racial bias. From this sweeping conclusion, based on a small if intriguing scientific finding, social scientists, legal scholars, opinion leaders and "diversity experts" leap from thought to conduct and from unconscious association to harmful actions. Because most of us are biased, these individuals claim, we can safely assume that every aspect of social life—every school, institution, organization and workplace—is a bastion of discrimination. The most strenuous measures, whether they be diversity programs, bureaucratic oversight, accountability or guilt-ridden self-monitoring, cannot guarantee a level playing field.

What is wrong with this picture? In the first place, split-second associations between negative stimuli and minority group images don't necessarily imply unconscious bias. Such associations may merely reflect awareness of common cultural stereotypes. Not everyone who knows the stereotypes necessarily endorses them.

Or the associations might reflect simple awareness of the social reality: Some groups are more disadvantaged than others, and more individuals in these groups are likely to behave in undesirable ways. Consider the two Jesses—Jackson and Helms. Both know that the black family is in trouble, that crime rates in this community are far too high, and that black educational test scores are too low. That common awareness might lead to sympathy, to indifference, or to hostility. Because the IAT can distinguish none of these parameters, both kinds of Jesses often get similar, failing scores on tests of unconscious association.

Measures of unconscious prejudice are especially untrustworthy predictors of discriminatory behavior. MIT psychologist Michael Norton has recently noted that there is virtually no published research showing a systematic link between racist attitudes, overt or subconscious, and real-world discrimination. A few studies show that openly-biased persons sometimes favor whites over blacks in simulations of job hiring and promotion. But no research demonstrates that, after subtracting the influence of residual old-fashioned prejudice, split-second reactions in the laboratory predict real-world decisions. On the contrary, the few results available suggest that persons who are "high bias" on subconscious criteria are no more likely than others to treat minorities badly and may sometimes even favor them.

There is likewise no credible proof that actual business behavior is pervasively influenced by unconscious racial prejudice. This should not be surprising. Demonstrating racial bias is no easy matter because there is often no straightforward way to detect discrimination of any kind, let alone discrimination that is hidden from those doing the deciding. As anyone who has ever tried a job-discrimination case knows, showing that an organization is systematically skewed against members of one group requires a benchmark for how each worker would be treated if race or sex never entered the equation. This in turn depends on defining the standards actually used to judge performance, a task that often requires meticulous data collection and abstruse statistical analysis.

Assuming everyone is biased makes the job easy: The problem of demonstrating actual discrimination goes away and claims of discrimination become irrefutable.

Anything short of straight group representation—equal outcomes rather than equal opportunity—is "proof" that the process is unfair.

Advocates want to have it both ways. On the one hand, any steps taken against discrimination are by definition insufficient, because good intentions and traditional checks on workplace prejudice can never eliminate unconscious bias. On the other, researchers and "diversity experts" purport to know what's needed and do not hesitate to recommend more expensive and strenuous measures to purge pervasive racism. There is no more evidence that such efforts dispel supposed unconscious racism than that such racism affects decisions in the first place.

But facts have nothing to do with it. What began as science has morphed into unassailable faith. However we think, feel or act, and however much apparent progress has been made, there is no hope for us. We are all racists at heart.

NOTES AND QUESTIONS

1. To what extent, if any, would valid and reliable measures of biases (racist or otherwise) aid the goals of law? Which goals, and why?
2. Do you think efforts to use neuroscientific techniques to identify biases (racist or otherwise) are likely to be beneficial? Why or why not?
3. How, if at all, does the third reading in this section affect your assessments of the other two? Would that result have been different if the sequence of readings had been reversed? If so, would this suggest a bias?
4. Note that in the research paper describing the relationship between outcomes of football games and lengths of sentencing decisions cited at the outset of this chapter, the authors found that the effect of emotional shocks on lengthening sentences is disproportionally borne by black defendants. How, if at all, does this affect your assessment of the value of neuroscientific research into racial bias during legal decision-making?

FURTHER READING

Neuroscience of Legal Decision-Making:

Morris B. Hoffman & Frank Krueger, *The Neuroscience of Blame and Punishment*, in *Self, Culture and Consciousness* 207 (Sangeetha Menon, V.V. Binoy & Nithin Nagaraj eds., 2020).

Leila Glass et al., *Neural Signatures of Third-Party Punishment: Evidence from Penetrating Traumatic Brain Injury*, 11 Soc. Cognitive & Affective Neurosci. 253 (2016).

Joshua W. Buckholtz & René Marois, *The Roots of Modern Justice: Cognitive and Neural Foundations of Social Norms and Their Enforcement*, 15 Nature Neurosci. 655 (2012).

Qun Yang et al., *When Morality Opposes the Law: An fMRI Investigation into Punishment Judgments for Crimes with Good Intentions*, 127 Neuropsychologia 195 (2019).

Erik W. Asp et al., *Soft on Crime: Patients with Ventromedial Prefrontal Cortex Damage Allocate Reduced Third-Party Punishment to Violent Criminals*, 119 Cortex 33 (2019).

Paul H. Robinson, Robert Kurzban & Owen D Jones, *The Origins of Shared Intuitions of Justice*, 60 Vand. L. Rev. 1633 (2007).

Johannes Haushofer & Ernst Fehr, *You Shouldn't Have: Your Brain on Others' Crimes*, 60 Neuron 738 (2008).

Oliver R. Goodenough & Kristin Prehn, *A Neuroscientific Approach to Normative Judgment in Law and Justice*, 359 Philanthropic Transactions Royal Soc'y London 1709 (2004).

Oliver R. Goodenough, *Mapping Cortical Areas Associated with Legal Reasoning and with Moral Intuition*, 41 Jurimetrics 429 (2001).

Ginther et al., *Parsing the Behavioral and Brain Mechanisms of Third-Party Punishment*, 36 J. Neurosci. 9420 (2016).

Neuroscience of Moral and Punishment Decisions:

Joshua D. Greene, *Moral Tribes: Emotion, Reason, and the Gap Between Us and Them* (2013).

Jean Decety & Keith J. Yoder, *The Emerging Social Neuroscience of Justice Motivation*, 21 Trends Cognitive Sci. 6 (2017).

Ben Seymour, Tania Singer & Ray Dolan, *The Neurobiology of Punishment*, 8 Nature Revs. Neurosci. 300 (2007).

Julia F. Christensen & Antoni Gomila, *Moral Dilemmas in Cognitive Neuroscience of Moral Decision-Making: A Principled Review*, 36 Neurosci. & Biobehavioral Rev. 1249 (2012).

Behavioral Research on Jury Decision-Making:

Dennis J. Devine, *Jury Decision Making: The State of the Science* (2012).

Jessica M. Salerno & Shari Seidman Diamond, *The Promise of a Cognitive Perspective on Jury Deliberation*, 17 Psychonomic Bull. & Rev. 174 (2010).

Brian H. Bornstein & Edie Greene, *Jury Decision Making: Implications for and from Psychology*, 20 Current Directions Psychol. Sci. 63 (2011).

Francis X. Shen et al., *Sorting Guilty Minds*, 86 N.Y.U. L. Rev. 1306 (2011).

The Role of Emotions in Judging:

See "Further Reading" in Chapter 14: Emotions.

CHAPTER 17

Adolescent Brains

A consistent and growing body of social science and neuroscience research findings support the conclusion that juveniles are less culpable than adults, and are entitled to different treatment in sentencing in light of their immaturity, vulnerability and changeability.
　　　　—American Psychological Assoc. General Counsel Nathalie Gilfoyle[†]

The court has learned from brain science that teenagers are immature! But we knew that. The problem with using it as a basis for distinguishing between murderers of different ages is that many adult murderers have problems with their brains, too. Why is it not cruel and unusual to sentence them to life in prison?
　　　　—Judge Richard Posner[††]

CHAPTER SUMMARY

This chapter:
- Introduces the neurological processes underlying brain maturation.
- Provides background on the administration of juvenile justice, including competency determinations, and transfers to adult courts.
- Explores invocations and limitations of neuroscience in the context of adolescent culpability.

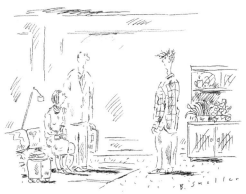

"Young man, go to your room and stay there until your cerebral cortex matures."

Source: B. Smaller, The New Yorker (Apr. 24, 2006).

---

　† Press Release, Am. Psychol. Assn., *American Psychological Association Lauds High Court Decision Rejecting Mandatory Life Sentences for Juveniles Convicted of Homicide* (June 25, 2012).
　†† Richard Posner, *Supreme Court Year in Review: The Justices Should Use More than Their Emotions to Decide How to Rule*, Slate (June 26, 2012).

INTRODUCTION

At the age of 17, while still a junior in high school, Christopher Simmons told his friends he wanted to murder someone. He proposed that he and some friends break into a home, find someone, tie her up, and throw her off a bridge, to drown in the water below. Simmons pointedly noted that they could get away with it, because they were all minors.

Soon after, they broke into the home of a startled Shirley Crook around 2:00 A.M. They used duct tape to cover her eyes and mouth, and to bind her hands. They then drove her to a railroad trestle spanning the Meramec River, where they tied her hands and feet together with electrical wire, wrapped her whole face in duct tape, and threw her from the bridge to her death in the dark water below. Soon after, Simmons bragged about this murder to other friends and was arrested. Roughly nine months later, after turning 18, he was tried and sentenced to death. These are the facts as found in the case of *Roper v. Simmons*,* from which you will read an excerpt shortly.

But the questions now, at the threshold, are these: Do you think the legal system should treat Simmons—and juveniles who commit similar crimes—the same as it would treat an older adult who did the very same thing? And how, if at all, does Simmons' age and crime affect your answer?

One need not be a scientist to know that young humans differ from older ones, and not just in size. But we may want to know more about why, when, and how they differ as we consider whether, and if so, how, to treat juveniles and adults differently. For this reason, many think that neuroscience may provide new information about the nature of being a juvenile that is valuable to improving the delivery of juvenile justice. Others disagree. In this chapter we take up the neuroscience of adolescence and consider the proper role, if any, for neuroscience in juvenile justice law and policy.

The chapter proceeds in five sections. Section A presents current neuroscientific perspectives on the development and capacities of the adolescent brain. Section B provides a brief tour of some juvenile justice basics, including competency assessments and transfers into or out of the juvenile court system. Section C focuses on criminal responsibility of juveniles. Section D presents some critical perspectives. And Section E introduces new arguments for treating young adults (say, 18 to 21 years old) differently from older adults.

A. THE ADOLESCENT BRAIN

This section begins with an excerpt from a 2013 report of the National Research Council, which provides a useful introduction to the transitional period between childhood and adulthood commonly referred to as adolescence. Thereafter we turn to an accessible overview—prepared by a team consisting of two psychologists and a legal scholar—of developmental neuroscience potentially relevant to law.

---

* *Roper v. Simmons*, 543 U.S. 551 (2005).

National Research Council

Reforming Juvenile Justice: A Developmental Approach
Chapter 4: Adolescent Development, 89-99 (2013)

Adolescence is a distinct, yet transient, period of development between childhood and adulthood characterized by increased experimentation, risk taking, heightened sensitivity to peers and other social influences, and the formation of personal identity. . . . This definition applies to all adolescents, regardless of ethnicity, culture, or nationality, and it is not special to humans but observed across species as a period for acquiring the basic skills needed to transition from dependence to relative independence from parental care.

A key function of adolescence is developing an integrated sense of self, including individuation, separation from parents, and personal identity. Age-typical ways in which adolescents form their identities and develop adult skills include experimentation and novelty-seeking behavior that tests limits. These behaviors are thought to serve a number of adaptive functions including socialization and procreation. In testing limits and experimenting, however, the adolescent may engage in alcohol and drug use, unsafe sex, and reckless driving, despite the risks that this can pose to the individual and others. Often these actions occur in the presence of peers and are exacerbated by their influence.

Research indicates that, for most youth, the period of risky experimentation does not extend beyond adolescence, ceasing as identity becomes settled with maturity. Only a small percentage of youth who engage in risky experimentation persist in their problem behavior into adulthood. Thus, it is not possible to predict

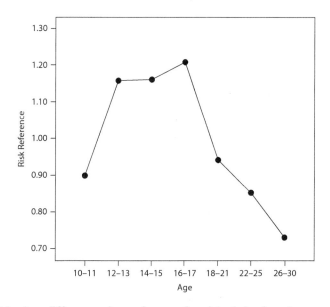

Figure 17.1   Age differences in preference for risky behaviors (e.g., unprotected sex, shoplifting, smoking).

Source: Laurence Steinberg, Should the Science of Adolescent Brain Development Inform Public Policy?, *64 Am. Psychol. 739 (2009).*

enduring antisocial traits on the basis of risky behavior during adolescence. Much adolescent involvement in illegal activity is an extension of the kind of risk taking that is part of the developmental process of identity formation, and most adolescents mature out of these tendencies. Evolutionary theorists have identified adaptive functions of adolescent risky behavior, based on the recognition that the task of adolescence is to move from a childhood state of dependence on parents to an emerging adult state characterized by acquiring independence and self identity, enabling procurement of additional resources, increasing the probability of reproductive success, improving life circumstances, and exploring adult liberties. Thus, adolescence by definition is a transient period of development that involves disruption of an old, secure state in favor of an uncertain but exciting new state. Antisocial behaviors, such as disobedience and lawbreaking, serve the function of disrupting ties to "old" parents and authority figures. Drug use, driving after drinking, and unprotected sex are exemplars of exciting new states that the adolescent may explore, as he or she seeks the new state of adulthood. The adolescent is primed to embrace exciting risk-taking behaviors and may even need to fail at some of these behaviors in order to succeed eventually at the tasks required of adults. The balance that parents and a justice system must find is how to encourage the transition to adulthood while keeping adolescents, and society as a whole, safe. . . .

ADOLESCENT BRAIN DEVELOPMENT

The last decade has provided evidence of significant changes in brain structure and function during adolescence with a strong consensus among neuroscientists about the nature of these changes. Much of this work has resulted from advances in magnetic resonance imaging (MRI) techniques that provide the opportunity to safely track the development of brain structure, brain function, and brain connectivity in humans. Consistent with the previously described behavioral findings that adolescents have poor self-control, are easily influenced by their peers, and do not think through the consequences of some of their actions, the brain imaging findings strongly suggest that adolescents lack these abilities because of biological immaturity of the brain.

STRUCTURAL BRAIN DEVELOPMENT

Several studies have used MRI to map the developmental time course of the structural changes in the normal brain. Even though the brain reaches approximately 90 percent of its adult size by age 6, the gray and white matter subcomponents of the brain continue to undergo dynamic changes throughout adolescence and well into young adulthood. Data from longitudinal MRI studies indicate that increases in white matter are linear and continue well into young adulthood, whereas gray matter volume shows an inverted U-shaped course, first increasing and then decreasing during adolescence. These changes do not occur uniformly across development, but rather there are regional differences in the brain's development. In general, regions that involve primary functions, such as motor and sensory systems, mature earliest compared with brain regions that integrate these primary functions for goal-directed behavior. Similar to sensorimotor regions, subcortical regions involved in novelty and emotions (e.g., striatum, amygdala) mature before the control region of the brain and show greater changes in males than in females during adolescence. These developmental and gender findings are important in the context of this report, given the increase in criminal behavior during the period of adolescence, especially in males.

FUNCTIONAL BRAIN DEVELOPMENT

The most influential method for studying human brain development is that of functional magnetic resonance imaging (fMRI). This method allows for seeing what areas of the brain are active when an individual is behaving by indexing changes in blood oxygen levels in the brain. In the last decade, there has been an explosion of fMRI studies examining adolescent brain development. This work challenges the traditional view that changes in behavior during adolescence are due simply to immature cognitive control capacities and the underlying neural substrates (e.g., prefrontal cortex). Instead, the latest studies suggest that much of what distinguishes adolescents from children and adults is an imbalance among developing brain systems. This imbalance model implies dual systems: one that is involved in cognitive and behavioral control and one that is involved in socioemotional processes. Accordingly, adolescents lack mature capacity for self-regulation because the brain system that influences pleasure-seeking and emotional reactivity develops more rapidly than the brain system that supports self-control. Empirical evidence to support this view comes from three areas of work. First, prefrontal circuitry implicated in self-regulation and planning behavior continues to develop into young adulthood. This development is slow and linear in nature. . . .

A second form of support for the imbalance model of adolescent development comes from studies that directly examine how brain systems interact when self-control is required in a motivational or emotional context. Incentives can both motivate and interfere with cognitive functioning in adolescents. . . . Relative to adults, adolescents had exaggerated activation in the ventral striatum when preparing and executing a response that would be reinforced and an increase in prefrontal activity important for controlling the movements, suggesting a reward-related up-regulation in control regions. In contrast, [other researchers] have shown that adolescents' performance is worse than both children and adults when having to suppress a response to an alluring social cue relative to a neutral one. This inverted-U pattern of performance is paralleled by a similar inflection in ventral striatal activity and heightened prefrontal activity.

Adolescents, but not adults, showed heightened activity in reward-related circuitry, including the ventral striatum, in the presence of peers. . . . Not only are peers influential but also positive exchanges with others may be powerful motivators. Asynchronous development of brain systems appears to correspond with a shift from thinking about self to thinking about others from early adolescence to young adulthood. Together these studies suggest that in the heat of the moment, as in the presence of peers or rewards, functionally mature reward centers of the brain may hijack less mature control systems in adolescents.

BRAIN CONNECTIVITY

Although regional changes in brain structure and function are important in understanding how behavior changes during adolescence, development in the connections between brain regions with age and experience are equally important. There are two relatively new approaches to indexing human brain connectivity. The first is that of diffusion tensor imaging (DTI). DTI detects changes in white matter tracts related to myelination, the process through which nerve fibers become sheathed in myelin, thereby improving the efficiency of neural signaling. DTI-based connectivity studies of prefrontal white matter tracts suggest an association between connection strength and self-regulation. Combining DTI and fMRI, Casey and colleagues have linked connection strength between prefrontal cortex and subcortical brain regions with the capacity to effectively engage in self-control in both typically and atypically developing individuals. A similar increase in number and strength of prefrontal connections to cortical and subcortical regions from age 13 to young adulthood has been shown to be associated with improvements in self-control by Hwang and colleagues (2010).

The second method, resting state fMRI, assesses the strength of functional connections within a network by quantifying correlated spontaneous activity between brain regions at rest. Resting state fMRI studies show that brain maturity involves connections between distal brain regions increasing while connections between proximal or local brain regions simultaneously decrease. Together, these findings support the claim that cognitive maturation occurs not in unitary structures but in the connectivity and interactions between developing structures. Thus, the relative immaturity of adolescent abilities will rely on specific immaturity of the circuitry.

Overall the findings suggest that in emotionally charged situations with limited time to react, as may be the case for most juvenile offenses, basic emotional circuits may drive adolescent actions. In more neutral contexts, more top-down cortical circuits may have a greater impact on decisions.

[The chapter subsequently provides an overview on extensive research concerning the social context of adolescent development, including parental influences, peer influences, school influences, social experiences, and the like.—EDS.]

Elizabeth Scott, Natasha Duell & Laurence Steinberg
Brain Development, Social Context, and Justice Policy
57 Wash. U. J.L. & Pol'y 13, 13-33 (2018)

INTRODUCTION

Justice policy reform in the past decade has been driven by research evidence indicating that brain development is ongoing through adolescence, and that neurological and psychological immaturity likely contributes in important ways to teenagers' involvement in crime. But despite the power of this trend, skeptics point out that many (perhaps most) adolescents do not engage in serious criminal activity; on this basis, critics argue that normative biological and psychological factors associated with adolescence are unlikely to play the important role in juvenile offending that is posited by supporters of the reform trend. This Article explains that features associated with biological and psychological immaturity alone do not lead teenagers to engage in illegal conduct. Instead the decision to offend, like much risk-taking behavior in adolescence, is the product of dynamic interaction between the still-maturing individual and her social context. The Article probes the mechanisms through which particular tendencies and traits linked to adolescent brain development interact with environmental influences to encourage antisocial or prosocial behavior.

Brain development in adolescence is associated with reward-seeking behavior and limited future orientation. Further, as compared to adults, adolescents are particularly sensitive to external social stimuli, easily aroused emotionally, and less able to regulate strong emotions. The Article shows how these tendencies may be manifested in different teenagers in different ways, depending on many factors in the social context. By analyzing this dynamic relationship, the Article clarifies how social environment influences adolescent choices in ways that incline or deter involvement in crime and other risky behavior. Thus a teenager who lives in a high-crime neighborhood with many antisocial peers is more likely to get involved in criminal activity than one in a neighborhood with few such peers, even though the two may not differ in their propensities for risk-taking. . . .

I. PSYCHOLOGICAL AND BIOLOGICAL IMMATURITY

Adolescent risk-taking can be understood, in part, as arising from a "maturity gap" between cognitive and psychosocial development. It is well understood that emotional and social maturation lags behind intellectual development and that adolescents' capacity for self-regulation is immature. As compared to adults, adolescents are particularly inclined toward reward-seeking and are extremely sensitive to their social context and particularly to peers. This combination of features contributes to emotional arousal, and when teenagers are emotionally aroused, they tend to make impulsive, short-sighted choices and engage in risky behaviors that they might understand are ill-advised when considered in a neutral setting. This Part describes a "dual systems" model of brain development offered by developmentalists to explain adolescents' tendency toward impulsive risky choices: While brain systems implicated in reward-seeking and sensitivity to peers develop early in adolescence around puberty, brain systems that govern self-regulation mature gradually through adolescence and into early adulthood. Finally, this Part explains that these attributes and tendencies are endogenous to the developmental stage of adolescence and are found in teenagers across cultures.

A. Developmental Factors Contributing to Risk-Taking

This section describes three features of adolescence that likely contribute to adolescents' inclination to engage in risky behavior to a greater extent than adults. Both biological and behavioral research confirms that, as compared to adults, adolescents are more inclined toward reward-seeking, more sensitive to social context, and more impulsive in their choices, especially under conditions of emotional arousal. Each of these tendencies is linked to normative brain development.

1. Reward Seeking

Substantial research evidence supports the conclusion that adolescents are sensitive to rewards and inclined toward reward- or sensation-seeking to a greater extent than adults, and that they focus on rewards rather than risks in making choices. As discussed below, this inclination is normative in adolescence; indeed, increased sensation-seeking is adaptive developmentally as it encourages adolescents to explore their environment and develop a sense of identity and autonomy. But, reward-seeking also interacts with teenagers' sensitivity to peers in ways that can contribute to harmful risk-taking.

During early adolescence, regions of the brain associated with "incentive processing," or the valuation and prediction of rewards, undergo substantial changes resulting in heightened reward sensitivity during this period. Researchers have linked these changes to hormonal developments during puberty that increase the number of dopamine receptors in the brain that are implicated in approach behaviors and the experience of pleasure. As a result, adolescents evince increased dopamine cell firing in response to rewarding stimuli, which affects feedback learning, sensitivity to social evaluation and loss, and incentive-driven responses.

Neurodevelopmental studies of risk behavior generally suggest that heightened risk-taking in adolescence is associated with greater activation of reward-sensitive brain regions among adolescents as compared to adults. In brain imaging studies, when presented with images of rewarding stimuli, such as smiling faces, adolescents evince a stronger response in reward-processing regions than do children or adults. Moreover, the extent to which individuals show this sensitivity to reward is correlated positively with risk-taking. This suggests that risk-taking is, to some extent, intrinsically rewarding to adolescents, or that adolescents are more sensitive to potential rewards associated with risks.

A large body of behavioral research confirms that adolescents are more sensitive to rewards and more inclined toward reward-seeking than are adults; these findings are consistent with the neurobiological evidence. In these studies, researchers typically measure reward-seeking using self-report scales that assess characteristics such as thrill- or novelty-seeking, or behavioral tasks that assess responsiveness to rewarding stimuli (such as monetary rewards). For example, some studies use gambling tasks in which individuals must learn to discriminate between gambles that are likely to be rewarding (e.g., drawing cards from a deck that is likely to pay off) and those that are likely to be costly (e.g., drawing cards from decks that are likely to lead to losses). Others have used "temporal discounting" tasks, in which players are asked to choose between smaller, immediate rewards (e.g., $200 today) versus larger, but delayed ones (e.g., $1,000 in six months).

Both self-report and behavioral studies of reward-seeking indicate that this behavior peaks in mid-adolescence, and subsequently declines in adulthood. Cross-sectional studies of performance on gambling tasks demonstrate that mid- to late adolescents learn from rewards at a faster rate than do their younger peers or adults; these studies also demonstrate that the tendency to learn more quickly from rewarding experiences than from costly ones is substantially stronger among teens than among adults, who tend to learn from rewarding and costly experiences at similar rates. Studies of temporal discounting have found that younger adolescents demonstrate a stronger preference for smaller, immediate rewards, whereas older adolescents and adults are willing to wait longer for larger ones. Studies also show that younger adolescents characterize themselves in self-report surveys as being less future-oriented (i.e., regulating behavior in favor of long-term goals) and less inclined to consider the future consequences of their actions. Thus, mid-adolescents (ages fifteen through seventeen) demonstrate a heightened sensitivity to rewards compared to younger or older individuals, and this sensitivity seems to motivate decision-making that is oriented toward the present rather than the future, even if the future-oriented decision is superior.

2. Sensitivity to Social Environment

Adolescence is a period of heightened sensitivity to the social environment and the individual's relationship to that context. Recent research indicates that a network of brain systems governing thinking about social relationships undergoes significant changes in adolescence in ways that increase individuals' concern about the opinion of other people, particularly peers. These brain regions, sometimes collectively referred to as "the social brain," are more easily activated in adolescence than before or after, making teenagers especially attuned to both the positive and negative emotions of those around them. During this developmental period, individuals are more sensitive to both praise and rejection than are either children or adults, making them potentially more susceptible to peer influence and responsive to threats.

Recent evidence sheds light on the relationship between peer sensitivity and reward-seeking in adolescence, with important implications for adolescent risk-taking. Jason Chein and colleagues have examined the impact of the presence of peers on individuals' neural responses to a potential reward, comparing adolescents between ages fourteen to eighteen, with younger (nineteen to twenty-two) and older (twenty-four to twenty-nine) adults making decisions in a simulated driving task. The study found that observation by peers increased activation in reward-related brain regions in adolescents but not in the adults, and that activity in these regions predicted risk-taking (running a stoplight to complete the task faster) in the tasks.

Much behavioral research confirms adolescents' sensitivity to peers, and finds a correlation between peer influence and risk-taking in adolescence. Social scientists have studied age differences in responses to peer influence by presenting individuals with hypothetical dilemmas involving peer influence. Studies presenting participants with situations involving pressure to engage in antisocial conduct have found that peer influence increases between childhood and mid-adolescence and declines slowly during the late adolescent years. Peer influence can operate directly when teenagers respond to peer pressure; however, desire for peer approval and fear of rejection also affect adolescents' choices more than those of adults. The increased salience of peers likely makes their approval especially important in group situations. It is not surprising, perhaps, that juveniles are far more likely to offend in groups than are adults.

It is well established that adolescents take more risks in the presence of peers than when they are alone or with an adult, and that this "peer effect" is not found among adults. The presence of peers also influences risk preference among adolescents, as adolescents (but not adults) are more likely to endorse the benefits of risky activities relative to costs in the presence of peers than when they are alone. One study has found that the presence of peers increases risk-taking among adolescents even when they are given information about the probability of positive and negative outcomes.

3. Impulsivity and Cognitive Control

When adolescents are emotionally aroused by the anticipation of rewards in the presence of peers, they tend to make riskier choices that they are less able to control than are adults. As described in Section B below, deficits in self-control in adolescence are thought to derive from immaturity in the system of cognitive regulation, which is centered in the prefrontal cortex, and its connections to social and emotional brain regions. This system develops slowly during adolescence and is not fully mature until the early to mid-twenties. In adolescence, it can be overwhelmed by emotional and social responses, contributing to short-sighted choices.

Studies measure self-regulation using both self-report scales that assess the tendency to act without thinking (e.g., "I act on the spur of the moment") and behavioral tasks that require individuals to resist making automatic, reactive responses to specific stimuli. Studies of self-reported impulse control find that this psychological trait improves into early adulthood. Age patterns in studies involving behavioral tasks are more complex. On simple tasks requiring only that participants inhibit an automatic response, individuals demonstrate adult levels of self-regulation by mid-adolescence. In contrast, mature performance is not observed until early adulthood when tasks involve distractions that cause attentional interference or require planning and complex reasoning.

The most interesting recent research measuring impulse control has compared responses to behavioral tasks under neutral (non-emotional) and emotional conditions. These studies have found that adolescents perform poorly on self-control tasks under emotional conditions and that performance under both neutral and emotional conditions improves into adulthood. A major study sponsored by the MacArthur Foundation Research Network on Law and Neuroscience (of which two of us were members) is illustrative. In this research, almost 150 adolescents, (between thirteen and seventeen), young adults (eighteen to twenty-one) and older adults (twenty-two to twenty-five) were asked to perform a standard task measuring self-control under neutral conditions and conditions involving positive and negative emotional arousal (anticipation of winning money versus hearing an aversive sound). Under conditions of positive arousal, adolescents' performance on the self-control task was substantially poorer than that of the two adult groups, while under conditions of negative arousal, both the adolescent and young adult group performed more poorly than the older adults. Moreover, under emotionally arousing conditions, young adults evinced decreased activation in cognitive control networks and increased activation in brain regions implicated in emotional processing; this combination is thought to have contributed to poorer performance on the self-control task. Another recent study found that those adolescents whose self-control was disrupted during emotionally arousing tasks engaged in more risk-taking during driving simulation tasks than did same-aged individuals whose self-control was less disrupted. Other studies have shown that social arousal, created by the presence of peers, activates reward regions in the adolescent brain, which in turn is associated with riskier decision making. The evidence that emotional contexts interfere with self-control in adolescence sheds light on teenagers' heightened tendency to engage in risk taking in emotionally and socially arousing contexts.

Together with research demonstrating that adolescents tend to evince greater reward seeking and relatively less self-regulation compared to adults, studies also show that these psychological traits are linked with greater engagement in risk taking. For example, higher levels of reward seeking have been associated with self-reported substance use, delinquent acts, and risky driving, as well as risk taking on several laboratory measures of risk taking. Similarly, greater impulsivity has been associated with higher rates of self-reported substance use and delinquent activity, as well as with increased risk taking on behavioral risk taking tasks.

B. Dual Systems Model of Risk Taking

Developmental scientists in recent years have offered "dual systems" or "maturational imbalance" models in seeking to explicate the relationship between emotional immaturity and risk-taking. Brain maturation comprises several processes that vary in their developmental timetable across different brain regions: Dual systems models emphasize research showing that brain systems involved in reward seeking and those regulating self control follow different developmental trajectories. This imbalance, it is believed, results in poor regulation of emotions and a tendency to focus on the immediate rewards of choices, while discounting long-term costs; this combination increases inclinations to engage in risky behavior, including offending.

Neurodevelopmental research indicates that the development of subcortical brain regions implicated in socioemotional processing is more or less completed by adolescence. As explained above, these developments stimulate reward-seeking and increase sensitivity to peers, beginning with the onset of puberty and diminishing as individuals mature into young adulthood, such that these responses are particularly powerful during adolescence. Unlike the subcortical regions, the prefrontal cortex and other brain regions involved in impulse control and emotional regulation develop slowly through adolescence and are not mature until early adulthood. The prefrontal cortex plays a key role in advanced cognitive abilities, including planning ahead, comparing risk and reward, and self-regulation. Immaturity in the prefrontal cortex is thought to make adolescents more susceptible than are mature adults to impetuous decision-making and more vulnerable to the effects of emotional and social arousal on cognitive functioning.

Maturation of the prefrontal cortex involves multiple processes that are ongoing during adolescence but completed at different ages. For example, synaptic pruning, which increases the efficiency of information processing, is largely complete by mid-adolescence; thus, basic cognitive capacities of reasoning and understanding are adult-like by about age fifteen and improve little in later years. In contrast, connectivity between prefrontal regions and the regions that process rewards and respond to emotional and social stimuli are not fully established until individuals are in their mid-twenties. These connections are critically important to emotional regulation and impulse control. The prefrontal regions are implicated in feedback evaluation, integrating experiential information to guide future behavior, and controlling emotional impulses in favor of long-term goals. The lack of functional connectivity leaves adolescents more prone than adults to making emotion-based decisions with inadequate cognitive oversight, suggesting why aspects of social and emotional functioning are slower to mature than basic cognitive functioning. Adolescents' deficient capacity to regulate behavior in the face of highly arousing stimuli may lead to suboptimal decision-making in contexts requiring the coordination of emotion and thinking. In sum, brain systems that govern "cold cognition" (thinking under neutral conditions) reach adult levels of maturity long before those that govern "hot cognition" (thinking under conditions of social and emotional arousal).

C. Cross-cultural Research on Brain Development

For the most part, the developmental brain research that has informed our understanding of various aspects of the dual systems model has been conducted in the United States and a few Western European countries (most notably, the Netherlands). Because expectations and norms for adolescent behavior vary considerably around the world, it is important to ask whether the account of the sensation-seeking, impulsive teenager that emerges from these studies accurately represents young people in other cultural and economic contexts. Adolescence in America and much of Western Europe is a time during which a certain degree of recklessness, especially in its socially acceptable forms, is tolerated—and perhaps even encouraged. Does this characterization of adolescents apply to young people growing up in less individualistic (and perhaps less permissive) cultural contexts?

A recent extensive study of more than 5,000 people between the ages of ten and thirty from eleven different countries suggests that it does. Laurence Steinberg and colleagues used identical test batteries to measure likely contributors to adolescent risk-taking in a diverse sample of countries (China, Colombia, Cyprus, India, Italy, Jordan, Kenya, the Philippines, Sweden, Thailand, and the United States) to determine whether the trajectories of sensation-seeking, self-control, and risk-taking are similar in these varied cultural contexts. Importantly, some of these countries are relatively more tolerant of adolescent recklessness (e.g., Sweden, and the United States), whereas, in others, young people are expected to demonstrate strong self-control (e.g., China and Jordan). Although there were differences among countries in patterns of psychological functioning, there were important and striking similarities.

Three such similarities are especially relevant to the present discussion: First, age trajectories of sensation-seeking and self-control that have been described in studies of American youth were observed internationally. Scores on a composite measure of sensation-seeking (combining both self-reports and behavioral indicators) followed an inverted U-shaped pattern, increasing between preadolescence and late adolescence, peaking during the late teen years, and declining thereafter. On average, the peak was observed at a slightly older age (nineteen years) than had been reported in previous studies of American youth. Perhaps this is due to a somewhat later onset of puberty, which has been shown to contribute to the increase in reward sensitivity in adolescence, in less developed nations than in developed ones; this would shift the average peak in sensation seeking to an older age when the sample is aggregated. In contrast, self-control matured gradually between pre-adolescence and the mid-twenties, at which point it plateaued in some countries (e.g., China, Italy) but continued to mature further in others (e.g., Colombia, Cyprus). Generally speaking, the prolonged maturation of self-control into the late-twenties was more likely to be seen in countries in which the increase during adolescence was less dramatic. Taken together, these results suggest that the characterization of the late teen years as a time during which reward-seeking is heightened and self-regulation is still maturing applies cross- culturally.

Second, the researchers found in other countries the inverted-U shaped trajectory of risk-taking that has been observed in the United States, with risky behavior more common during adolescence than before or after. This set of analyses distinguished between real-world risk taking, measured through self-reports of involvement in activities such as drinking, riding with an intoxicated driver, vandalism, and fighting, and risk taking propensity, assessed with experimental tasks such as a the video driving game described earlier. The authors hypothesized that age patterns in real-world risk taking would be more culturally variable than age patterns in risk taking propensity, since the former is both a function of developmental immaturity and contextual opportunity, whereas the latter is not influenced by contextual conditions (i.e., the test setting was identical across the various countries). This hypothesis was confirmed: Countries were significantly more similar with respect to trajectories of risk taking propensity than with respect to real world risk-taking. Further, as expected, risk-taking propensity peaked earlier than did real-world risk taking, suggesting that the manifestation of adolescents' inherent inclination to engage in risky behavior is delayed by the real world context in which development occurs. Finally, the peak age for antisocial risk-taking was earlier (around age nineteen, similar to that reported in studies of the "age-crime curve") than that for health risk-taking (which peaked in the mid-twenties), presumably because the latter can be delayed by societally imposed constraints that are age-related (for example, age restrictions on purchasing alcohol). This study is especially relevant to our interest in this essay, because it shows how the maturationally-driven tendencies inherent in adolescence can be tempered by social context.

Third, the researchers observed in the international sample the "maturity gap" found in American studies (described above), in which cognitive abilities such as working memory reach adult levels of maturity well before the psychosocial capacities thought to contribute to reckless behavior in adolescence. Age patterns in cognitive abilities were far more similar internationally than patterns in psychosocial capacities; this likely is due to relatively greater cultural variability in expectations for psychosocial maturity than for intellectual competence. Most importantly, whereas the main period for maturation of cognitive competence was during early adolescence (tending to plateau around age sixteen), in virtually all of the countries studied considerable psychosocial maturation took place during the late teens and early twenties.

This Part has explained that psychosocial factors associated with adolescent brain development contribute to a tendency toward risk-taking that declines as individuals mature. These tendencies are normative in adolescence and found across cultures. In the next Part, we turn to the questions of how these inclinations interact with social context and why teenagers vary substantially in the extent and form of risk-taking. . . .

NOTES AND QUESTIONS

Before you continue deeper into this chapter, consider your current reactions to the following questions:

1. Evidence indicates that the executive control functions of the prefrontal cortex (planning, controlling impulses, and weighing consequences of decisions) mature later than many other areas of the brain. To what extent, if any, do you currently think this difference in brain development should translate into any differences in legal approaches to juvenile justice?
2. To what extent do you agree or disagree with Judge Posner's lament in the chapter-opening epigraph?
3. Scott, Duell, and Steinberg discuss evidence that biological immaturity can interact with social environments to increase or decrease the probability of risky and disinhibited behavior that can lead to illegal actions. How, and how well, do you

think the legal system currently engages with multi-causal phenomena? How, in your view, might it improve the ways it does so?

B. THE ADMINISTRATION OF JUVENILE JUSTICE

This section provides an overview of some key elements of the juvenile justice system in three sub-sections. Historical background is provided for context and is followed by coverage of competency determinations and transfers of juveniles into the adult criminal justice system.

1. Historical Background

Elizabeth S. Scott & Laurence Steinberg
Adolescence and the Regulation of Youth Crime
18 Future Children 15, 16-18 (2008)

A BRIEF HISTORY OF JUVENILE JUSTICE IN AMERICA

The history of juvenile crime policy over the course of the twentieth century is a narrative about the transformation of the law's conception of young offenders. At the dawn of the juvenile court era in the late nineteenth century, most youths were tried and punished as adults. Much had changed by 1909 when Judge Julian Mack famously proposed in a *Harvard Law Review* article that a juvenile offender should be treated "as a wise and merciful father handles his own child." Like the other Progressive reformers who worked to establish the juvenile court, Judge Mack viewed youths involved in crime first and foremost as children; indeed, by his account, they were no different from children who were subject to parental abuse and neglect. The early reformers envisioned a regime in which young offenders would receive treatment that would cure them of their antisocial ways—a system in which criminal responsibility and punishment had no place. Because of the juvenile court's rehabilitative purpose, procedures were informal and dispositions were indeterminate.

The rehabilitative model of juvenile justice seemingly thrived during the first half of the twentieth century, but it began to unravel during the 1960s. Youth advocates challenged the constitutionality of informal delinquency proceedings, and, in 1967, the Supreme Court agreed, holding, in *In re Gault*, that youths in juvenile court have a right to an attorney and other protections that criminal defendants receive. But the sharpest attacks on the juvenile court came from another direction. As youth crime rates rose during the 1980s, conservative politicians ridiculed the juvenile system and pointed to high recidivism rates as evidence that rehabilitation was a failure. According to some observers, the juvenile court may have met the needs of a simpler time when juveniles got into school yard fights, but it was not up to the task of dealing with savvy young criminals who use guns to commit serious crimes. . . .

The new generation of reformers went beyond rejecting the paternalistic characterization of young offenders; some advocates for tough policies seemed to view juveniles involved in crime as more culpable and dangerous than adult criminals. John DiIulio's description of "super-predators" in the mid-1990s captured the image of remorseless teenage criminals as a major threat to society and was invoked repeatedly in the media and in the political arena.

As juvenile crime rates—particularly homicide—rose during the 1980s and early 1990s, politicians across the country rushed to enact tough policies through several legislative strategies. First, the age of judicial transfer was lowered in many states to allow the criminal prosecution of teens aged fourteen and younger. Some legislatures expanded the range of transferrable offenses to include a long laundry list of crimes. But perhaps the most dramatic changes came in the form of automatic transfer statutes, under which many youths are categorically treated as adults when they are charged with crimes—either generally (all sixteen-year-olds) or for specific crimes (all thirteen-year-olds charged with murder). These legal reforms resulted in the wholesale transfer of youths into the adult criminal system—more than 250,000 a year by most estimates. The new statutes avoid individualized transfer hearings, shifting discretion from juvenile court judges, who are seen as soft on crime, to prosecutors, who are assumed not to have this deficiency. At the same time, juvenile court dispositions today include more incarceration and for longer periods—extending well into adulthood under some statutes. . . .

The upshot of this reform movement is that the mantra "adult time for adult crime" has become a reality for many young offenders. Through a variety of initiatives, the boundary of childhood has shifted dramatically in a relatively short time, so that youths who are legal minors for every other purpose are adults when it comes to their criminal conduct.

Supporters defend the recent reforms as a rational policy response to a new generation of dangerous young criminals that the juvenile court was unable to control. There is some truth to this claim [but] close inspection reveals that the process of legal reform has been deeply flawed and often has had the hallmarks of what sociologists call a moral panic, a form of irrational collective action in which politicians, the media, and the public reinforce each other in an escalating pattern of alarmed response to a perceived social threat. . . . In some states, racial biases and fears appear to have played a role in reform initiatives. . . .

Not surprisingly, society has continued to change since this history was written in 2008. One of the authors (Professor Scott) has observed that juvenile crime regulation is "in flux,"* describing a post-moral-panic period in which different regulatory approaches have begun to take hold. This flows, she believes, from: (a) perception that juvenile crime is less a threat than it had seemed to be; (b) realization of just how costly incarceration is; (c) studies suggesting that incarceration may increase juvenile re-offending; (d) perceived successes of some developmentally based community programs in reducing recidivism; and (e) re-emergence of the view that juveniles really are different in legally relevant ways, which render the harshest punishments disproportionate.

It is unclear whether neuroscientific perspectives on adolescence are meaningfully changing views or merely justifying already emerging views or, more likely, part

---

* Elizabeth S. Scott, *"Children are Different": Constitutional Values and Justice Policy*, 11 Ohio St. J. Crim. L. 71, 92 (2013).

of a feedback loop between the two. What is clear is that neuroscientific information about adolescent brain development is garnering more attention, with consequences yet unknown. Before we turn to key issues of responsibility generally, it is important to acknowledge two key legal contexts—regarding competency and transfer to adult courts—in which neuroscience may (or may not) have an important role to play.

2. Competency

A recurring question with adolescent defendants is whether they are competent to stand trial. The next two readings provide background on law and neuroscience that bear on this question.

Elizabeth S. Scott & Thomas Grisso
Developmental Incompetence, Due Process, and Juvenile Justice Reform
83 N.C. L. Rev. 793, 799-804 (2005)

I. APPLYING THE TRIAL COMPETENCE REQUIREMENT TO JUVENILES: A DOCTRINAL HISTORY

Competence doctrine was introduced into [the juvenile justice system] beginning in the 1970s, after the Supreme Court announced in *In re Gault* that juvenile defendants were entitled to many of the procedural protections provided to adults in criminal trials. During the post-Gault period, the competence inquiry focused on the incapacities of mentally ill or retarded youths. However, beginning in the late 1980s, dramatic reforms in juvenile justice policy have resulted in the institutional challenge the justice system faces today—that of meeting the constitutional mandate in an era when many young defendants facing serious legal jeopardy may be incompetent due to immaturity.

A. The Legal and Constitutional Requirements of Competence to Stand Trial

The procedural requirement that criminal defendants must be competent to stand trial has long been established as a mechanism to assure that minimum standards of fairness are met in criminal proceedings. . . . This contemporary understanding is captured in the federal standard announced by the Supreme Court in *Dusky v. United States,* [under which] the competence determination focuses on "whether [the defendant] has sufficient present ability to consult with his lawyer with a reasonable degree of rational understanding—and whether he has a rational as well as factual understanding of the proceedings against him."

It is generally agreed that the requirement of trial competence serves three independent functions. First, it preserves the integrity of criminal trials, which would be undermined if a mentally impaired and uncomprehending defendant faced the power of the accusing state in a proceeding in which his liberty is at stake. Second, the requirement reduces error and promotes the accuracy of the proceedings. Again because of the high stakes, error in criminal proceedings that could result in a wrongful conviction undermines basic fairness. An incompetent defendant may be unable to challenge prosecution evidence or to offer exculpatory information. She may also be disabled from raising defenses that an individual with better comprehension could assert. Finally, the competence requirement safeguards defendants' autonomy-based interest in meaningful participation in criminal proceedings—and thus protects a core value underlying due process in this setting. In *Pate v. Robinson*, the Supreme Court affirmed the constitutional importance of this requirement, holding that the Due Process Clause requires that criminal defendants must be competent to stand trial.

B. TRIAL COMPETENCE OF JUVENILES

1. The Incorporation of the Competence Requirement in Delinquency Proceedings

The requirement that criminal defendants be competent to stand trial had no place in delinquency proceedings in the traditional juvenile court. In a system in which the government's announced purpose was to rehabilitate and not to punish errant youths, the procedural protections accorded adult defendants—including the requirement of adjudicative competence—were deemed unnecessary. This all changed with *In re Gault*, which led to an extensive restructuring of delinquency proceedings to conform to the requirements of constitutional due process. Although the Supreme Court has never considered whether due process requires that defendants in juvenile delinquency proceedings be competent to stand trial, many state courts have addressed this issue. Almost all have held that the requirements of due process and fair treatment can be satisfied in juvenile delinquency proceedings only if defendants are competent to stand trial. . . .

Courts incorporating the adjudicative competence requirement into delinquency proceedings have assumed that the incapacities of incompetent juveniles are analogous to those of their adult counterparts: the cases have almost exclusively involved youths who are mentally ill or mentally retarded. Although a few courts have suggested in passing that immaturity might exaggerate the challenges faced by incompetent youths, developmental incompetence per se has received little attention in the case law.

On reflection, this is not surprising. . . . [T]he underlying rationale for maintaining a separate system for the adjudication and correction of juveniles is that young offenders, because of their immaturity, warranted differential treatment. Thus, the idea that immaturity should be a basis for disqualification from adjudication in juvenile court understandably might have seemed incoherent, or at least incompatible with the rationale for the system. The post-*Gault* legal developments took place in a context in which courts, even as they incorporated adult rights, continued to assume that the juvenile court was very different from the criminal justice system in its purposes and in the severity of its sanctions. . . .

In concluding that trial competence is required in delinquency proceedings, courts divided on the competence standard to be applied. Some courts assumed that the Dusky standard should simply be incorporated into delinquency proceedings, while others were less clear about the standard to be applied, emphasizing that juveniles should be assessed by "juvenile rather than adult norms" . . . [a]nd that a lower standard of competence applies to these proceedings. This approach amounts to an implicit recognition that the distinctive purposes of the juvenile court may warrant less exacting procedural requirements.

2. The Criminal Adjudication of Youths

Both before and after *Gault*, youths were occasionally transferred to criminal court and tried and punished as adults. Even in this context, the doctrine prohibiting the adjudication of incompetent defendants has not been adapted in most states to exclude immature youths from criminal prosecution. Under a few statutes, courts conducting transfer hearings are expressly directed to consider whether the youth's immaturity would render her unable to participate in a criminal proceeding. . . .

[U]ntil the 1990s, immature youths generally were not subject to adult criminal proceedings because younger adolescents could not be transferred under most statutes. Thus, the occasional sixteen- or seventeen-year-old criminal defendants may not have raised concerns about trial competence, because they were mature enough to participate adequately in the proceedings.

MacArthur Foundation Research Network on Adolescent Development and Juvenile Justice
Adolescent Legal Competence in Court
1-3 (2006)

One of the pillars of the American justice system is the assurance that those who stand accused of crimes be mentally competent to understand and participate in their trials. The conventional standard for competence has typically focused on the effects of mental illness or mental retardation on individuals' capacities to grasp the nature of their trials or their abilities to decide how to plead. Yet as the courts, both juvenile and adult, see increasingly younger defendants some argue that the law should also take into account adolescents' lesser capacities owing to emotional and psychological immaturity.

This brief details findings from the first comprehensive assessment of juvenile capacities to participate in criminal proceedings using measures of both trial-related abilities and developmental maturity. The MacArthur Foundation Research Network on Adolescent Development and Juvenile Justice compared the responses of youth and adults in a series of hypothetical legal situations, such as plea bargains, police interrogations, and attorney-client interactions. Responses revealed the degree to which participants understood the long-term consequences of their decisions, their ability to weigh risks, and other factors related to developmental and cognitive maturity. Findings show that a significant portion of youth, especially under age 15, are likely unable to participate competently in their own trials, either in an adult or juvenile court, owing to developmental immaturity. . . .

YOUNG ADOLESCENTS MORE LIKELY TO LACK CAPACITIES FOR TRIAL

Findings from the [competence] assessment showed that age matters. Those aged 11-13 performed significantly worse than 14-15 year olds, who performed significantly worse than 16-17 year olds and 18-24 year olds (adults). Interestingly, the performance of 16-17 year olds did not differ from that of the young adults (aged 18-24).

The youngest group was nearly three times more likely than youth older than 15 to be significantly impaired in reasoning and understanding, two important components of legal competence. In other words, nearly one-third of 11-13 year olds and one-fifth of 14-15 year olds had deficits that courts might see as serious enough to question their ability to proceed in a trial. These patterns varied little by race-ethnicity, gender, socioeconomic status, or region of the country.

LEVEL OF MATURITY INFLUENCES IMPORTANT CHOICES

In general, the youngest teens (aged 11-13) proved less mature in their decision-making than older youth. Younger individuals, for example, were more likely to endorse decisions that comply with what an authority seemed to want as measured by their willingness to confess and plea bargain. The proportion of youth who recommended confession decreased with age, from about one-half of the 11-13 year olds to only one-fifth of the 18-24 year olds. (Few individuals in any age group chose to actively deny the offense.) The proportion who advised accepting a plea agreement declined from nearly three-fourths of 11-13 year olds to one-half of young adults. Once again, the study revealed few statistically significant differences among those older than age 15.

In addition, younger teens were significantly less likely to recognize the inherent risks in various decisions, and they were less likely to comprehend the long-term consequences of their decisions. The study found no differences by age in the effects of peer pressure on decision-making. Those with lower IQs, however, performed more poorly on all items. Although perhaps not surprising, this finding is notable given that two-thirds of those under age 15 in juvenile detention facilities had an IQ lower than 89 compared with one-third in the community sample.

These findings suggest that younger adolescents' developmental immaturity may affect their behavior as defendants in ways that extend beyond their competence to stand trial. Their responses indicate that they are often more willing than adults to confess to authority figures such as police, rather than remaining silent, especially if they believe it will result in an immediate reward, such as going home. For similar reasons, they may be more willing to accept a prosecutor's plea agreement. . . .

3. Juvenile Transfer

Another major issue in juvenile justice surrounds the decision of whether or not to try an adolescent in adult court. As you learn about the standards relevant to transfer, consider whether, and if so, how, neuroscience might aid such determinations.

United States v. Juvenile Male #2
761 F. Supp. 2d 27 (E.D.N.Y. 2011)

JOSEPH R. BIANCO, D.J. [Defendant, 16 years old at the time, is alleged to have participated in a gang-related, execution-style double-homicide of a 19-year-old woman and her two-year-old son, after luring them to the woods in Islip, New York, in February of 2010. The government moved to transfer the defendant to adult criminal court.]

"A juvenile fifteen years of age or older who is 'alleged to have committed an act after his fifteenth birthday which if committed by an adult would be a felony that is a crime of violence' may be proceeded against as an adult where a district court, after a transfer motion by the Attorney General, finds that it is 'in the interest of justice' to grant a transfer." United States v. Nelson, 68 F.3d 583, 588 (2d Cir. 1995) ("*Nelson I*") (quoting 18 U.S.C. §5032). In evaluating whether a transfer to adult status would be "in the interest of justice," a district court must consider the following six factors and make findings on the record as to each: (1) the juvenile's age and social background; (2) the nature of the offense alleged; (3) the nature and extent of any prior delinquency record; (4) the juvenile's present psychological maturity and intellectual development; (5) the juvenile's response to past treatment efforts and the nature of those efforts; and (6) available programs that are designed to treat the juvenile's behavior problems. *See* 18 U.S.C. §5032; *Nelson I,* 68 F.3d at 588. Given the presumption that exists in favor of juvenile adjudication, the burden is on the government to establish by a preponderance of the evidence that transfer is warranted.

[The court considered factors 1 through 3. The court noted that the defendant was born into an impoverished home in El Salvador, where he lived until he was seven years old. His mother left for the United States when he was nine months old, leaving him to be raised by his maternal grandmother. His uncle gave him drugs and alcohol. Following various misbehaviors, the family smuggled him to the United States to live with a different uncle, from where he was later taken by a stepfather to New York. He joined a gang at 13.]

D. JUVENILE'S PRESENT PSYCHOLOGICAL MATURITY AND INTELLECTUAL DEVELOPMENT

[The court heard testimony from Dr. William Barr, a clinical neuropsychologist, and Dr. Hegarty, a forensic neuropsychologist, both of whom prepared evaluations and reports on behalf of the defendant.] Dr. Barr testified . . . that he had conducted a neuropsychological evaluation of the defendant, during which he had administered a number of standardized tests designed to assess intellectual functioning, attention, concentration, memory, and executive functioning. As to the defendant's intellectual functioning, Dr. Barr found that defendant's school records indicated that "at one point he was a very good student." However, the defendant's scores on the tests of intellectual functioning were "well below what [Dr. Barr] would have expected based on his school results alone" and were "well below the level he should be for his age group." Overall, Dr. Barr found that the defendant's intellectual development stopped at the fifteen-year-old level, around the time when the defendant "stopped valuing school, attending school, and benefiting from a school environment." In other words, Dr. Barr opined that the defendant's current stage of intellectual development was tied directly to the defendant's environment and personal choices. . . .

Similarly, Dr. Hegarty testified that the defendant's intellectual development was "environmental-dependent," meaning that when he is in a more stable environment with at least some intellectual stimulation, such as the Allen Center, "his IQ is higher than it is today," but that when he is removed from intellectual stimulation, his intellectual functioning does not develop further.

Dr. Barr also diagnosed the defendant with Attention Deficit Hyperactivity Disorder ("ADHD"), a condition that is characterized by hyperactivity and impulsivity. Accordingly, Dr. Barr found that the defendant's ability to control his impulses was even more impaired than that of a typical adolescent. Because of the weaknesses that the defendant exhibited in his cognitive control systems, Dr. Barr concluded that the defendant's cognitive development was equivalent to that of a fourteen or fifteen year old. . . .

Moreover, Dr. Hegarty stressed in her testimony that it was clear the defendant was of "normal intelligence" and that the defendant's "problems aren't with his intellect; they are with the systems in his brain that control[ ] his behavior . . . and also with his emotional development and the development of a stable sense of self or stable personality." Dr. Hegarty also noted that the defendant's IQ was in the low average to average range, which Dr. Hegarty found "extraordinary . . . given his environment[ ]." Indeed, the defendant's ability to learn a second language and earn his GED, both under difficult circumstances, highlights the defendant's intelligence.

As to the defendant's psychological maturity, Dr. Hegarty and Dr. Barr concurred that the defendant was "very immature for his age as a result of development . . . [and his] attention deficit hyperactivity disorder." Both doctors were also "struck by . . . how changeable his personality is . . . [and] [h]ow vulnerable to peer influence he is." Dr. Hegarty explained that the defendant was susceptible to environmental influences and was "somewhat vulnerable to suggestion." As such, "when he's in the wrong company, he does the wrong things." However, Dr. Hegarty noted that the defendant's vulnerability to peer influence could work in the defendant's favor *if* his environment changed and he surrounded himself with positive peers and role models rather than the gang. . . .

Based on this record, with respect to this particular factor, the Court does not find that any one of the pieces of evidence discussed herein should outweigh the others. Accordingly, because there are elements of defendant's intelligence and maturity that weigh both for and against transfer, the Court concludes that this factor should be neutral in the Court's transfer analysis. . . .

[The Court then considered the fifth and sixth statutorily required factors to be weighed.]

* * *

In sum, after carefully balancing all of the statutory factors based upon the record as set forth herein, the Court concludes that transfer of the defendant to adult status is warranted in this case in the interest of justice. . . .

The Second Circuit has made clear that "while rehabilitation is a priority, the courts are not required to apply the juvenile justice system to a juvenile's diagnosed intellectual or behavioral problems when it would likely prove to be anything more than a futile gesture." *Nelson I*, 68 F.3d at 590. In addition, "the goal of rehabilitation must be balanced against the threat to society posed by juvenile crime." *Nelson II*, 90 F.3d at 640. Accordingly, given that the crimes charged here involve the "heinous . . . crime of intentional murder," *Nelson I*, 68 F.3d at 590, and given that the record demonstrates that the defendant is unlikely to be rehabilitated in the juvenile system, the Court concludes that the government has overwhelmingly met its burden of showing that transfer is warranted in this case. Thus, the government's motion to transfer the defendant to adult status is granted.

C. ADOLESCENTS, NEUROSCIENCE, AND CRIMINAL RESPONSIBILITY

In light of the background information surveyed in the last two sections, it will come as little surprise to you that attorneys now often introduce neuroscientific evidence in cases regarding juveniles and sometimes young adults. The judicial opinion in the homicide case *State v. Andrews*, 329 S.W.3d 369 (Mo. 2010), for instance, explicitly referred to brain imaging studies, gray matter in the prefrontal regions, neuronal connections, neurotransmitters, dopamine receptors, white matter, and both cortical and subcortical regions of the brain.

A number of U.S. Supreme Court cases both furthered and reflect that trend. To put this in context, we can now return to the case with which this chapter opened, *Roper v. Simmons.* We look first to an amicus brief in that case, concerning the neuroscience of adolescence. We then excerpt passages from the U.S. Supreme Court's consideration of whether it is unconstitutional to execute someone who was younger than 18 at the time of the offense. Thereafter, we introduce the three cases after *Roper:* that is, *Graham v. Florida, Miller v. Alabama, and Montgomery v. Louisiana,* all of which also considered constitutional limits on sentencing youths for their crimes.

Brief for the Am. Psychol. Assn., and the Mo. Psychol. Assn. as Amici Curiae Supporting Resp't at 1-10

in *Roper v. Simmons* (July 2004)

The American Psychological Association (APA) is a voluntary nonprofit scientific and professional organization with more than 155,000 members and affiliates. Since 1892, the APA has been the principal association of psychologists in the United States. . . . An integral part of the APA's mission is to increase and disseminate knowledge regarding human behavior and to foster the application of psychological learning to important human concerns.

In 2001, the APA recognized that there are unique problems with assessment of juveniles who, under existing law, may be subject to the death penalty and called for a halt to such executions until it could be established that such deficiencies had been addressed. The body of research that has developed, including significant research findings in the last three years, indicates that these deficiencies have not been and cannot be corrected. . . .

At ages 16 and 17, adolescents, as a group, are not yet mature in ways that affect their decision-making. Behavioral studies show that late adolescents are less likely to consider alternative courses of action, understand the perspective of others, and restrain impulses. Delinquent, even criminal, behavior is characteristic of many adolescents, often peaking around age 18. Heightened risk-taking is also common. During the same period, the brain has not reached adult maturity, particularly in the frontal lobes, which control executive functions of the brain related to decision-making.

Adolescent risk-taking often represents a tentative expression of adolescent identity and not an enduring mark of behavior arising from a fully formed personality. Most delinquent adolescents do not engage in violent illegal conduct through adulthood.

The unformed nature of adolescent character makes execution of 16- and 17-year-olds fall short of the purposes this Court has articulated for capital punishment. Developmentally immature decision-making, paralleled by immature neurological development, diminishes an adolescent's blameworthiness. With regard to deterrence, adolescents often lack an adult ability to control impulses and anticipate the consequences of their actions. Studies call into question the effect on juvenile recidivism of harsher criminal sanctions. . . .

The mitigating effect of adolescence cannot be reliably assessed in individualized capital sentencing. Adolescents are "moving targets" for assessment of character and future dangerousness, two important considerations in the penalty phase of capital trials. As one example, psychologists have been unable to identify chronic psychopathy, also known as sociopathy, among adolescents. Assessments of such severe antisocial behaviors during adolescence have yet to be shown to remain stable as individuals grow into adulthood. Consequently, attempts to predict at capital sentencing an adolescent offender's character formation and dangerousness in adulthood are inherently prone to error and create an obvious risk of wrongful execution.

The transitory nature of adolescence also means that an adolescent defendant is much more likely to change in relevant respects between the time of the offense and the time of assessment by courts and experts. At sentencing, an offender may behave and look more like an adult than he or she did at the time the crime was committed. Impressions of the maturity and responsibility of adolescent offenders may also be impermissibly influenced by unconscious racism. . . .

Recent research suggests a biological dimension to adolescent behavioral immaturity: the human brain does not settle into its mature, adult form until after the adolescent years have passed and a person has entered young adulthood. . . .

Of particular interest with regard to decision-making and criminal culpability is the development of the frontal lobes of the brain. The frontal lobes, especially the prefrontal cortex, play a critical role in the executive or "CEO" functions of the brain, which are considered the higher functions of the brain. They are involved when an individual plans and implements goal-directed behaviors by selecting, coordinating, and applying the cognitive skills necessary to accomplish the goal. Disruption of functions associated with the frontal lobes may lead to impairments of foresight, strategic thinking, and risk management. Frontal lobe impairment has been associated with greater impulsivity, difficulties in concentration, attention, and self-monitoring, and impairments in decision-making. One "hallmark of frontal lobe dysfunction is difficulty in making decisions that are in the long-term best interests of the individual." . . .

Roper v. Simmons
543 U.S. 551 (2005)

Justice KENNEDY delivered the opinion of the court. This case requires us to address, for the second time in a decade and a half, whether it is permissible under the Eighth and Fourteenth Amendments to the Constitution of the United States to execute a juvenile offender who was older than 15 but younger than 18 when he committed a capital crime. In *Stanford v. Kentucky*, a divided Court rejected the proposition that the Constitution bars capital punishment for juvenile offenders in this age group. We reconsider the question. . . .

[The Missouri Supreme Court set aside Simmons' death sentence and resentenced him to "life imprisonment without eligibility for probation, parole, or release except by act of the Governor."] We granted certiorari, and now affirm. . . .

The Eighth Amendment provides: "Excessive bail shall not be required, nor excessive fines imposed, nor cruel and unusual punishments inflicted." The provision is applicable to the States through the Fourteenth Amendment. . . .

The prohibition against "cruel and unusual punishments," like other expansive language in the Constitution, must be interpreted according to its text, by considering history, tradition, and precedent, and with due regard for its purpose and function in the constitutional design. To implement this framework we have established the propriety and affirmed the necessity of referring to "the evolving standards of decency that mark the progress of a maturing society" to determine which punishments are so disproportionate as to be cruel and unusual. . . .

Three general differences between juveniles under 18 and adults demonstrate that juvenile offenders cannot with reliability be classified among the worst offenders. First, as any parent knows and as the scientific and sociological studies respondent and his amici cite tend to confirm, "[a] lack of maturity and an underdeveloped sense of responsibility are found in youth more often than in adults and are more understandable among the young. These qualities often result in impetuous and ill-considered actions and decisions." ("Even the normal 16-year-old customarily lacks the maturity of an adult.") It has been noted that "adolescents are overrepresented statistically in virtually every category of reckless behavior." Arnett, Reckless Behavior in Adolescence: A Developmental Perspective, 12 Developmental Review 339 (1992). In recognition of the comparative immaturity and irresponsibility of juveniles, almost every State prohibits those under 18 years of age from voting, serving on juries, or marrying without parental consent.

The second area of difference is that juveniles are more vulnerable or susceptible to negative influences and outside pressures, including peer pressure. ("[Y]outh is more than a chronological fact. It is a time and condition of life when a person may be most susceptible to influence and to psychological damage.") This is explained in part by the prevailing circumstance that juveniles have less control, or less experience with control, over their own environment. See Steinberg & Scott, Less Guilty by Reason of Adolescence: Developmental Immaturity, Diminished Responsibility, and the Juvenile Death Penalty, 58 Am. Psychologist 1009, 1014 (2003) (hereinafter Steinberg & Scott) ("[A]s legal minors, [juveniles] lack the freedom that adults have to extricate themselves from a criminogenic setting.")

The third broad difference is that the character of a juvenile is not as well formed as that of an adult. The personality traits of juveniles are more transitory, less fixed.

These differences render suspect any conclusion that a juvenile falls among the worst offenders. The susceptibility of juveniles to immature and irresponsible behavior means "their irresponsible conduct is not as morally reprehensible as that of an adult." Their own vulnerability and comparative lack of control over their immediate surroundings mean juveniles have a greater claim than adults to be forgiven for failing to escape negative influences in their whole environment. The reality that juveniles still struggle to define their identity means it is less supportable to conclude that even a heinous crime committed by a juvenile is evidence of irretrievably depraved character. From a moral standpoint it would be misguided to equate the failings of a minor with those of an adult, for a greater possibility exists that a minor's character deficiencies will be reformed. Indeed, "[t]he relevance of youth as a mitigating factor derives from the fact that the signature qualities of youth are transient; as individuals mature, the impetuousness and recklessness that may dominate in younger years can subside." [See] Steinberg & Scott 1014 ("For most teens, [risky or antisocial] behaviors are fleeting; they cease with maturity as individual identity becomes settled. Only a relatively small proportion of adolescents who experiment in risky or illegal activities develop entrenched patterns of problem behavior that persist into adulthood").

Once the diminished culpability of juveniles is recognized, it is evident that the penological justifications for the death penalty apply to them with lesser force than to adults. We have held there are two distinct social purposes served by the death penalty: " 'retribution and deterrence of capital crimes by prospective offenders.' " As for retribution, we remarked in *Atkins* that "[i]f the culpability of the average murderer is insufficient to justify the most extreme sanction available to the State, the lesser culpability of the mentally retarded offender surely does not merit that form of retribution." 536 U.S., at 319, 122 S. Ct. 2242. The same conclusions follow from the lesser culpability of the juvenile offender. Whether viewed as an attempt to express the community's moral outrage or as an attempt to right the balance for the wrong to the victim, the case for retribution is not as strong with a minor as with an adult. Retribution is not proportional if the law's most severe penalty is imposed on one whose culpability or blameworthiness is diminished, to a substantial degree, by reason of youth and immaturity.

As for deterrence, it is unclear whether the death penalty has a significant or even measurable deterrent effect on juveniles, as counsel for petitioner acknowledged at oral argument. In general we leave to legislatures the assessment of the efficacy of various criminal penalty schemes. Here, however, the absence of evidence of deterrent effect is of special concern because the same characteristics that render juveniles less culpable than adults suggest as well that juveniles will be less susceptible to deterrence. In particular, as the plurality observed in *Thompson*, "[t]he likelihood that the teenage offender has made the kind of cost-benefit analysis that attaches any weight to the possibility of execution is so remote as to be virtually nonexistent." 487 U.S., at 837. To the extent the juvenile death penalty might have residual deterrent effect, it is worth noting that the punishment of life imprisonment without the possibility of parole is itself a severe sanction, in particular for a young person.

In concluding that neither retribution nor deterrence provides adequate justification for imposing the death penalty on juvenile offenders, we cannot deny or overlook the brutal crimes too many juvenile offenders have committed. Certainly it can be argued, although we by no means concede the point, that a rare case might arise in which a juvenile offender has sufficient psychological maturity, and at the same time demonstrates sufficient depravity, to merit a sentence of death. Indeed, this possibility is the linchpin of one contention pressed by petitioner and his *amici*. They assert that even assuming the truth of the observations we have made about juveniles' diminished culpability in general, jurors nonetheless should be allowed to consider mitigating arguments related to youth on a case-by-case basis, and in some cases to impose the death penalty if justified. A central feature of death penalty sentencing is a particular assessment of the circumstances of the crime and the characteristics of the offender. The system is designed to consider both aggravating and mitigating circumstances, including youth, in every case. Given this Court's own insistence on individualized consideration, petitioner maintains that it is both arbitrary and unnecessary to adopt a categorical rule barring imposition of the death penalty on any offender under 18 years of age.

We disagree. The differences between juvenile and adult offenders are too . marked and well understood to risk allowing a youthful person to receive the death penalty despite insufficient culpability. An unacceptable likelihood exists that the brutality or cold-blooded nature of any particular crime would overpower mitigating arguments based on youth as a matter of course, even where the juvenile offender's objective immaturity, vulnerability, and lack of true depravity should require a sentence less severe than death. In some cases a defendant's youth may even be counted against him. In this very case, as we noted above, the prosecutor argued Simmons' youth was aggravating rather than mitigating. While this sort of overreaching could be corrected by a particular rule to ensure that the mitigating force of youth is not overlooked, that would not address our larger concerns.

It is difficult even for expert psychologists to differentiate between the juvenile offender whose crime reflects unfortunate yet transient immaturity, and the rare juvenile offender whose crime reflects irreparable corruption. As we understand it, this difficulty underlies the rule forbidding psychiatrists from diagnosing any patient under 18 as having antisocial personality disorder, a disorder also referred to as psychopathy or sociopathy, and which is characterized by callousness, cynicism, and contempt for the feelings, rights, and suffering of others. If trained psychiatrists with the advantage of clinical testing and observation refrain, despite diagnostic expertise, from assessing any juvenile under 18 as having antisocial personality disorder, we conclude that States should refrain from asking jurors to issue a far graver condemnation—that a juvenile offender merits the death penalty. When a juvenile offender commits a heinous crime, the State can exact forfeiture of some of the most basic liberties, but the State cannot extinguish his life and his potential to attain a mature understanding of his own humanity.

Drawing the line at 18 years of age is subject, of course, to the objections always raised against categorical rules. The qualities that distinguish juveniles from adults do not disappear when an individual turns 18. By the same token, some under 18 have already attained a level of maturity some adults will never reach. For the reasons we have discussed, however, a line must be drawn. The plurality opinion in *Thompson* drew the line at 16. In the intervening years the *Thompson* plurality's conclusion that offenders under 16 may not be executed has not been challenged. The logic of *Thompson* extends to those who are under 18. The age of 18 is the point where society draws the line for many purposes between childhood and adulthood. It is, we conclude, the age at which the line for death eligibility ought to rest. . . .

Justice O'CONNOR, dissenting. . . . It is beyond cavil that juveniles as a class are generally less mature, less responsible, and less fully formed than adults, and that these differences bear on juveniles' comparative moral culpability. But even accepting this premise, the Court's proportionality argument fails to support its categorical rule.

First, the Court adduces no evidence whatsoever in support of its sweeping conclusion, that it is only in "rare" cases, if ever, that 17-year-old murderers are sufficiently mature and act with sufficient depravity to warrant the death penalty. The fact that juveniles are generally *less* culpable for their misconduct than adults does not necessarily mean that a 17-year-old murderer cannot be *sufficiently* culpable to merit the death penalty. At most, the Court's argument suggests that the average 17-year-old murderer is not as culpable as the average adult murderer.

But an especially depraved juvenile offender may nevertheless be just as culpable as many adult offenders considered bad enough to deserve the death penalty. Similarly, the fact that the availability of the death penalty may be less likely to deter a juvenile from committing a capital crime does not imply that this threat cannot *effectively* deter some 17-year-olds from such an act. Surely there is an age below which no offender, no matter what his crime, can be deemed to have the cognitive or emotional maturity necessary to warrant the death penalty. But at least at the margins between adolescence and adulthood—and especially for 17-year-olds such as respondent—the relevant differences between "adults" and "juveniles" appear to be a matter of degree, rather than of kind. It follows that a legislature may reasonably conclude that at least *some* 17-year-olds can act with sufficient moral culpability, and can be sufficiently deterred by the threat of execution, that capital punishment may be warranted in an appropriate case.

Indeed, this appears to be just such a case. Christopher Simmons' murder of Shirley Crook was premeditated, wanton, and cruel in the extreme. . . . Whatever can be said about the comparative moral culpability of 17-year-olds as a general matter, Simmons' actions unquestionably reflect " 'a consciousness materially more "depraved" than that of' . . . the average murderer." And Simmons' prediction that he could murder with impunity because he had not yet turned 18—though inaccurate—suggests that he *did* take into account the perceived risk of punishment in deciding whether to commit the crime. Based on this evidence, the sentencing jury certainly had reasonable grounds for concluding that, despite Simmons' youth, he "ha[d] sufficient psychological maturity" when he committed this horrific murder, and "at the same time demonstrate[d] sufficient depravity, to merit a sentence of death."

The Court's proportionality argument suffers from a second and closely related defect: It fails to establish that the differences in maturity between 17-year-olds and young "adults" are both universal enough and significant enough to justify a bright-line prophylactic rule against capital punishment of the former. The Court's analysis is premised on differences *in the aggregate* between juveniles and adults, which frequently do not hold true when comparing individuals. Although it may be that many 17-year-old murderers lack sufficient maturity to deserve the death penalty, some juvenile murderers may be quite mature. Chronological age is not an unfailing measure of psychological development, and common experience suggests that many 17-year-olds are more mature than the average young "adult." . . .

For purposes of proportionality analysis, 17-year-olds as a class are qualitatively and materially different from the mentally retarded. "Mentally retarded" offenders, as we understood that category in *Atkins*, are *defined* by precisely the characteristics, which render death an excessive punishment. A mentally retarded person is, "by definition," one whose cognitive and behavioral capacities have been proved to fall below a certain minimum. Accordingly, for purposes of our decision in *Atkins*, the mentally retarded are not merely *less* blameworthy for their misconduct or *less* likely to be deterred by the death penalty than others. Rather, a mentally retarded offender is one whose demonstrated impairments make it so highly unlikely that he is culpable enough to deserve the death penalty or that he could have been deterred by the threat of death, that execution is not a defensible punishment. There is no such inherent or accurate fit between an offender's chronological age and the personal limitations which the Court believes make capital punishment excessive for 17-year-old murderers. Moreover, it defies common sense to suggest that 17-year-olds as a class are somehow equivalent to mentally retarded persons with regard to culpability or susceptibility to deterrence. Seventeen-year-olds may, on average, be less mature than adults, but that lesser maturity simply cannot be equated with the major, lifelong impairments suffered by the mentally retarded. . . .

Justice SCALIA, with whom THE CHIEF JUSTICE and Justice THOMAS join, dissenting. . . . Of course, the real force driving today's decision is not the actions of four state legislatures, but the Court's "'"own judgment"'" that murderers younger than 18 can never be as morally culpable as older counterparts. . . .

Today's opinion provides a perfect example of why judges are ill equipped to make the type of legislative judgments the Court insists on making here. To support its opinion that States should be prohibited from imposing the death penalty on any-one who committed murder before age 18, the Court looks to scientific and socio-logical studies, picking and choosing those that support its position. It never explains why those particular studies are methodologically sound; none was ever entered into evidence or tested in an adversarial proceeding. As The Chief Justice has explained:

> "[M]ethodological and other errors can affect the reliability and validity of estimates about the opinions and attitudes of a population derived from various sampling tech-niques. Everything from variations in the survey methodology, such as the choice of the target population, the sampling design used, the questions asked, and the statisti-cal analyses used to interpret the data can skew the results."

In other words, all the Court has done today, to borrow from another context, is to look over the heads of the crowd and pick out its friends.

We need not look far to find studies contradicting the Court's conclusions. As petitioner points out, the American Psychological Association (APA), which claims in this case that scientific evidence shows persons under 18 lack the ability to take moral responsibility for their decisions, has previously taken precisely the opposite position before this very Court. In its brief in *Hodgson v. Minnesota* [1990], the APA found a "rich body of research" showing that juveniles are mature enough to decide whether to obtain an abortion without parental involvement. The APA brief, citing psychology treatises and studies too numerous to list here, asserted: "[B]y middle adolescence (age 14-15) young people develop abilities similar to adults in reason-ing about moral dilemmas, understanding social rules and laws, [and] reasoning about interpersonal relationships and interpersonal problems." Given the nuances of scientific methodology and conflicting views, courts—which can only consider the limited evidence on the record before them—are ill equipped to determine which view of science is the right one. Legislatures "are better qualified to weigh and 'evaluate the results of statistical studies in terms of their own local conditions and with a flexibility of approach that is not available to the courts.'"

Even putting aside questions of methodology, the studies cited by the Court offer scant support for a categorical prohibition of the death penalty for murder-ers under 18. At most, these studies conclude that, *on average*, or *in most cases*, per-sons under 18 are unable to take moral responsibility for their actions. Not one of the cited studies opines that all individuals under 18 are unable to appreciate the nature of their crimes.

Moreover, the cited studies describe only adolescents who engage in risky or antisocial behavior, as many young people do. Murder, however, is more than just risky or antisocial behavior. It is entirely consistent to believe that young people often act impetuously and lack judgment, but, at the same time, to believe that those who commit premeditated murder are—at least sometimes—just as culpable as adults. . . . In their *amici* brief, the States of Alabama, Delaware, Oklahoma, Texas, Utah, and Virginia offer additional examples of murders committed by individuals under 18 that involve truly monstrous acts. . . . Though these cases are assuredly the exception rather than the rule, the studies the Court cites in no way justify a constitutional imperative that prevents legislatures and juries from treating exceptional cases in an exceptional way—by determining that some murders are not just the acts of happy-go-lucky teenagers, but heinous crimes deserving of death.

That "almost every State prohibits those under 18 years of age from voting, serving on juries, or marrying without parental consent," is patently irrelevant—and is yet another resurrection of an argument that this Court gave a decent burial in *Stanford.* (What kind of Equal Justice under Law is it that—without so much as a "Sorry about that"—gives as the basis for sparing one person from execution arguments explicitly rejected in refusing to spare another?) As we explained in *Stanford,* it is "absurd to think that one must be mature enough to drive carefully, to drink responsibly, or to vote intelligently, in order to be mature enough to understand that murdering another human being is profoundly wrong, and to conform one's conduct to that most minimal of all civilized standards." Serving on a jury or entering into marriage also involve decisions far more sophisticated than the simple decision not to take another's life.

. . . In capital cases, this Court requires the sentencer to make an individualized determination, which includes weighing aggravating factors and mitigating factors, such as youth. . . .

The Court concludes, however, that juries cannot be trusted with the delicate task of weighing a defendant's youth along with the other mitigating and aggravating factors of his crime. This startling conclusion undermines the very foundations of our capital sentencing system, which entrusts juries with "mak[ing] the difficult and uniquely human judgments that defy codification and that 'buil[d] discretion, equity, and flexibility into a legal system.'" The Court says that juries will be unable to appreciate the significance of a defendant's youth when faced with details of a brutal crime. This assertion is based on no evidence; to the contrary, the Court itself acknowledges that the execution of under-18 offenders is "infrequent" even in the States "without a formal prohibition on executing juveniles," suggesting that juries take seriously their responsibility to weigh youth as a mitigating factor.

Nor does the Court suggest a stopping point for its reasoning. If juries cannot make appropriate determinations in cases involving murderers under 18, in what other kinds of cases will the Court find jurors deficient? We have already held that no jury may consider whether a mentally deficient defendant can receive the death penalty, irrespective of his crime. Why not take other mitigating factors, such as considerations of childhood abuse or poverty, away from juries as well? Surely jurors "overpower[ed]" by "the brutality or cold-blooded nature" of a crime could not adequately weigh these mitigating factors either. . . .

Graham v. Florida, decided five years after *Roper,* considered the constitutionality of sentencing a person to life in prison without the possibility of parole for a crime committed before the age of 18.

Graham v. Florida
560 U.S. 48 (2010)

Justice KENNEDY delivered the opinion of the Court. The issue before the Court is whether the Constitution permits a juvenile offender to be sentenced to life in prison without parole for a nonhomicide crime. The sentence was imposed by the State of Florida. Petitioner challenges the sentence under the Eighth Amendment's Cruel and Unusual Punishments Clause, made applicable to the States by the Due Process Clause of the Fourteenth Amendment. . . .

[Graham was arrested at age 16 for armed burglary and attempted armed robbery. Under a plea agreement, the court withheld adjudication as to the charges and sentenced Graham to concurrent three-year terms of probation. A few months later, Graham was arrested again—34 days short of his eighteenth birthday—after participating in multiple home invasion robberies with two 20-year-old men.]

Under Florida law the minimum sentence Graham could receive absent a downward departure by the judge was 5 years' imprisonment. The maximum was life imprisonment. Graham's attorney requested the minimum nondeparture sentence of 5 years. A presentence report prepared by the Florida Department of Corrections recommended that Graham receive an even lower sentence—at most 4 years' imprisonment. The State recommended that Graham receive 30 years on the armed burglary count and 15 years on the attempted armed robbery count.

After hearing Graham's testimony, the trial court explained the sentence it was about to pronounce. . . .

"The only thing that I can rationalize is that you decided that this is how you were going to lead your life and that there is nothing that we can do for you. And as the state pointed out, that this is an escalating pattern of criminal conduct on your part and that we can't help you any further. We can't do anything to deter you. . . . Given your escalating pattern of criminal conduct, it is apparent to the Court that you have decided that this is the way you are going to live your life and that the only thing I can do now is to try and protect the community from your actions."

The trial court found Graham guilty of the earlier armed burglary and attempted armed robbery charges. It sentenced him to the maximum sentence authorized by law on each charge: life imprisonment for the armed burglary and 15 years for the attempted armed robbery. Because Florida has abolished its parole system, a life sentence gives a defendant no possibility of release unless he is granted executive clemency.

Graham filed a motion in the trial court challenging his sentence under the Eighth Amendment. . . .

Roper established that because juveniles have lessened culpability they are less deserving of the most severe punishments. As compared to adults, juveniles have a " 'lack of maturity and an underdeveloped sense of responsibility' "; they "are more vulnerable or susceptible to negative influences and outside pressures, including peer pressure"; and their characters are "not as well formed." . . . A juvenile is not absolved of responsibility for his actions, but his transgression "is not as morally reprehensible as that of an adult."

No recent data provide reason to reconsider the Court's observations in *Roper* about the nature of juveniles. As petitioner's *amici* point out, developments in psychology and brain science continue to show fundamental differences between juvenile and adult minds. For example, parts of the brain involved in behavior control continue to mature through late adolescence. See Brief for American Medical Association et al. as *Amici Curiae* 16-24; Brief for American Psychological Association et al. as *Amici Curiae* 22-27. Juveniles are more capable of change than are adults, and their actions are less likely to be evidence of "irretrievably depraved character" than are the actions of adults. It remains true that "[f]rom a moral standpoint it would be misguided to equate the failings of a minor with those of an adult, for a greater possibility exists that a minor's character deficiencies will be reformed." These matters relate to the status of the offenders in question; and it is relevant to consider next the nature of the offenses to which this harsh penalty might apply.

The Court has recognized that defendants who do not kill, intend to kill, or foresee that life will be taken are categorically less deserving of the most serious forms of punishment than are murderers. . . . Although an offense like robbery or rape is "a serious crime deserving serious punishment," those crimes differ from homicide crimes in a moral sense.

It follows that, when compared to an adult murderer, a juvenile offender who did not kill or intend to kill has a twice diminished moral culpability. The age of the offender and the nature of the crime each bear on the analysis. . . .

In sum, penological theory is not adequate to justify life without parole for juvenile nonhomicide offenders. This determination; the limited culpability of juvenile nonhomicide offenders; and the severity of life without parole sentences all lead to the conclusion that the sentencing practice under consideration is cruel and unusual. This Court now holds that for a juvenile offender who did not commit homicide the Eighth Amendment forbids the sentence of life without parole. This clear line is necessary to prevent the possibility that life without parole sentences will be imposed on juvenile nonhomicide offenders who are not sufficiently culpable to merit that punishment. Because "[t]he age of 18 is the point where society draws the line for many purposes between childhood and adulthood," those who were below that age when the offense was committed may not be sentenced to life without parole for a nonhomicide crime.

A State is not required to guarantee eventual freedom to a juvenile offender convicted of a nonhomicide crime. What the State must do, however, is give defendants like Graham some meaningful opportunity to obtain release based on demonstrated maturity and rehabilitation. It is for the State, in the first instance, to explore the means and mechanisms for compliance. . . . The Eighth Amendment does not foreclose the possibility that persons convicted of nonhomicide crimes committed before adulthood will remain behind bars for life. It does forbid States from making the judgment at the outset that those offenders never will be fit to reenter society. . . .

Categorical rules tend to be imperfect, but one is necessary here. . . .

Another possible approach would be to hold that the Eighth Amendment requires courts to take the offender's age into consideration as part of a case-specific gross disproportionality inquiry, weighing it against the seriousness of the crime. This approach would allow courts to account for factual differences between cases and to impose life without parole sentences for particularly heinous crimes. . . .

The case-by-case approach to sentencing must, however, be confined by some boundaries. The dilemma of juvenile sentencing demonstrates this. For even if we were to assume that some juvenile nonhomicide offenders might have "sufficient psychological maturity, and at the same time demonstrat[e] sufficient depravity," to merit a life without parole sentence, it does not follow that courts taking a case-by-case proportionality approach could with sufficient accuracy distinguish the few incorrigible juvenile offenders from the many that have the capacity for change. . . .

[Chief Justice Roberts concurred in the judgment, as applied to *Graham*, but would have left open the possibility that some juvenile defendants could receive life without parole for non-homicide crimes.]

Justice THOMAS dissenting, joined by Justice SCALIA and, in part, by Justice ALITO. . . .

First, quoting *Roper* the Court concludes that juveniles are less culpable than adults because, as compared to adults, they "have a '"lack of maturity and an under-developed sense of responsibility,"'" and "their characters are 'not as well formed.'" As a general matter, this statement is entirely consistent with the evidence recounted above that judges and juries impose the sentence at issue quite infrequently, despite legislative authorization to do so in many more cases. Our society tends to treat the average juvenile as less culpable than the average adult. But the question here does not involve the average juvenile. The question, instead, is whether the Constitution prohibits judges and juries from ever concluding that an offender under the age of 18 has demonstrated sufficient depravity and incorrigibility to warrant his permanent incarceration.

In holding that the Constitution imposes such a ban, the Court cites "developments in psychology and brain science" indicating that juvenile minds "continue to mature through late adolescence," (citing Brief for American Medical Association et al. as Amici Curiae 16-24; Brief for American Psychological Association et al. as Amici Curiae (hereinafter APA Brief)), and that juveniles are "more likely [than adults] to engage in risky behaviors," But even if such generalizations from social science were relevant to constitutional rulemaking, the Court misstates the data on which it relies.

The Court equates the propensity of a fairly substantial number of youths to engage in "risky" or antisocial behaviors with the propensity of a much smaller group to commit violent crimes. But research relied upon by the amici cited in the Court's opinion differentiates between adolescents for whom antisocial behavior is a fleeting symptom and those for whom it is a lifelong pattern. That research further suggests that the pattern of behavior in the latter group often sets in before 18. And, notably, it suggests that violence itself is evidence that an adolescent offender's antisocial behavior is not transient.

In sum, even if it were relevant, none of this psychological or sociological data is sufficient to support the Court's "'moral'" conclusion that youth defeats culpability in every case. . .

Miller v. Alabama, decided two years after *Graham*, considered the constitutionality of ever *mandating* life without the possibility of parole for individuals who had committed a homicide before the age of 18.

Miller v. Alabama

567 U.S. 460 (2012)

Justice KAGAN delivered the opinion of the Court. The two 14-year-old offenders in these cases were convicted of murder and sentenced to life imprisonment without the possibility of parole. In neither case did the sentencing authority have any discretion to impose a different punishment. State law mandated that each juvenile die in prison even if a judge or jury would have thought that his youth and its attendant characteristics, along with the nature of his crime, made a lesser sentence (for example, life *with* the possibility of parole) more appropriate. Such a scheme prevents those meting out punishment from considering a juvenile's "lessened culpability" and greater "capacity for change," *Graham v. Florida*, and runs afoul of our cases' requirement of individualized sentencing for defendants facing the most serious penalties. We therefore hold that mandatory life without parole for those under the age of 18 at the time of their crimes violates the Eighth Amendment's prohibition on "cruel and unusual punishments." . . .

In November 1999, petitioner Kuntrell Jackson, then 14 years old, and two other boys decided to rob a video store. En route to the store, Jackson learned that one of the boys, Derrick Shields, was carrying a sawed-off shotgun in his coat sleeve. Jackson decided to stay outside when the two other boys entered the store. Inside, Shields pointed the gun at the store clerk, Laurie Troup, and demanded that she "give up the money." Troup refused. A few moments later, Jackson went into the store to find Shields continuing to demand money. At trial, the parties disputed whether Jackson warned Troup that "[w]e ain't playin'," or instead told his friends, "I thought you all was playin'." When Troup threatened to call the police, Shields shot and killed her. The three boys fled empty-handed.

Arkansas law gives prosecutors discretion to charge 14-year-olds as adults when they are alleged to have committed certain serious offenses. The prosecutor here exercised that authority by charging Jackson with capital felony murder and aggravated robbery. . . . A jury later convicted Jackson of both crimes. Noting that "in view of [the] verdict, there's only one possible punishment," the judge sentenced Jackson to life without parole. . . .

Following *Roper v. Simmons*, in which this Court invalidated the death penalty for all juvenile offenders under the age of 18, Jackson filed a state petition for habeas corpus. He argued, based on *Roper*'s reasoning, that a mandatory sentence of life without parole for a 14-year-old also violates the Eighth Amendment. The circuit court rejected that argument and granted the State's motion to dismiss. While that ruling was on appeal, this Court held in *Graham v. Florida* that life without parole violates the Eighth Amendment when imposed on juvenile nonhomicide offenders. After the parties filed briefs addressing that decision, the Arkansas Supreme Court affirmed the dismissal of Jackson's petition. The majority found that *Roper* and *Graham* were "narrowly tailored" to their contexts: "death-penalty cases involving a juvenile and life-imprisonment-without-parole cases for nonhomicide offenses involving a juvenile." Two justices dissented. They noted that Jackson was not the shooter and that "any evidence of intent to kill was severely lacking." And they argued that Jackson's mandatory sentence ran afoul of *Graham*'s admonition that

" '[a]n offender's age is relevant to the Eighth Amendment, and criminal procedure laws that fail to take defendants' youthfulness into account at all would be flawed.' "

[The Court explained the facts of petitioner Evan Miller's case. Miller was charged as an adult with murder in the course of arson, which carries a mandatory minimum punishment of life without parole.]

We granted certiorari in both cases and now reverse. . . .

Roper and *Graham* establish that children are constitutionally different from adults for purposes of sentencing. Because juveniles have diminished culpability and greater prospects for reform, we explained, "they are less deserving of the most severe punishments." Those cases relied on three significant gaps between juveniles and adults. First, children have a " 'lack of maturity and an underdeveloped sense of responsibility,' " leading to recklessness, impulsivity, and heedless risk-taking. Second, children "are more vulnerable . . . to negative influences and outside pressures," including from their family and peers; they have limited "contro[l] over their own environment" and lack the ability to extricate themselves from horrific, crime-producing settings. And third, a child's character is not as "well formed" as an adult's; his traits are "less fixed" and his actions less likely to be "evidence of irretrievabl[e] deprav[ity]."

Our decisions rested not only on common sense—on what "any parent knows"—but on science and social science as well. In *Roper*, we cited studies showing that " '[o]nly a relatively small proportion of adolescents' " who engage in illegal activity " 'develop entrenched patterns of problem behavior.' " And in *Graham*, we noted that "developments in psychology and brain science continue to show fundamental differences between juvenile and adult minds"—for example, in "parts of the brain involved in behavior control."[5]

We reasoned that those findings—of transient rashness, proclivity for risk, and inability to assess consequences—both lessened a child's "moral culpability" and enhanced the prospect that, as the years go by and neurological development occurs, his " 'deficiencies will be reformed.' "

[The Court revisited the holdings and reasoning in *Roper* and *Graham*.]

But the mandatory penalty schemes at issue here prevent the sentencer from taking account of these central considerations. By removing youth from the balance—by subjecting a juvenile to the same life-without-parole sentence applicable to an adult—these laws prohibit a sentencing authority from assessing whether the law's harshest term of imprisonment proportionately punishes a juvenile offender. That contravenes *Graham*'s (and also *Roper*'s) foundational principle: that imposition of a State's most severe penalties on juvenile offenders cannot proceed as though they were not children.

---

5. The evidence presented to us in these cases indicates that the science and social science supporting *Roper*'s and *Graham*'s conclusions have become even stronger. See, e.g., Brief for American Psychological Association et al. as *Amici Curiae* 3 ("[A]n ever-growing body of research in developmental psychology and neuroscience continues to confirm and strengthen the Court's conclusions"); id., at 4 ("It is increasingly clear that adolescent brains are not yet fully mature in regions and systems related to higher-order executive functions such as impulse control, planning ahead, and risk avoidance"); Brief for J. Lawrence Aber et al. as *Amici Curiae* 12-28 (discussing post-Graham studies); id., at 26-27 ("Numerous studies post-*Graham* indicate that exposure to deviant peers leads to increased deviant behavior and is a consistent predictor of adolescent delinquency" (footnote omitted)).

Of special pertinence here, we insisted in these rulings that a sentencer have the ability to consider the "mitigating qualities of youth." Everything we said in *Roper* and *Graham* about that stage of life also appears in these decisions. . . .

In light of *Graham*'s reasoning, these decisions too show the flaws of imposing mandatory life-without-parole sentences on juvenile homicide offenders. Such mandatory penalties, by their nature, preclude a sentencer from taking account of an offender's age and the wealth of characteristics and circumstances attendant to it. . . .

So *Graham* and *Roper* and our individualized sentencing cases alike teach that in imposing a State's harshest penalties, a sentencer misses too much if he treats every child as an adult. To recap: Mandatory life without parole for a juvenile precludes consideration of his chronological age and its hallmark features—among them, immaturity, impetuosity, and failure to appreciate risks and consequences. It prevents taking into account the family and home environment that surrounds him—and from which he cannot usually extricate himself—no matter how brutal or dysfunctional. It neglects the circumstances of the homicide offense, including the extent of his participation in the conduct and the way familial and peer pressures may have affected him. Indeed, it ignores that he might have been charged and convicted of a lesser offense if not for incompetencies associated with youth—for example, his inability to deal with police officers or prosecutors (including on a plea agreement) or his incapacity to assist his own attorneys. And finally, this mandatory punishment disregards the possibility of rehabilitation even when the circumstances most suggest it. . . .

We therefore hold that the Eighth Amendment forbids a sentencing scheme that mandates life in prison without possibility of parole for juvenile offenders. By making youth (and all that accompanies it) irrelevant to imposition of that harshest prison sentence, such a scheme poses too great a risk of disproportionate punishment. Because that holding is sufficient to decide these cases, we do not consider Jackson's and Miller's alternative argument that the Eighth Amendment requires a categorical bar on life without parole for juveniles, or at least for those 14 and younger. But given all we have said in *Roper*, *Graham*, and this decision about children's diminished culpability and heightened capacity for change, we think appropriate occasions for sentencing juveniles to this harshest possible penalty will be uncommon. That is especially so because of the great difficulty we noted in *Roper* and *Graham* of distinguishing at this early age between "the juvenile offender whose crime reflects unfortunate yet transient immaturity, and the rare juvenile offender whose crime reflects irreparable corruption." Although we do not foreclose a sentencer's ability to make that judgment in homicide cases, we require it to take into account how children are different, and how those differences counsel against irrevocably sentencing them to a lifetime in prison. . . .

---

*Montgomery v. Louisiana,** decided four years after *Miller*, considered whether the rule in *Miller* was retroactive, applying to those roughly 2,000 inmates who were already—before *Miller*—serving a mandatory sentence of life in prison without parole, for crimes committed while under the age of 18. Justice Kennedy's 6-3 majority opinion, which emphasized the "transient immaturity" and "distinctive attributes" of youth, held that *Miller* was retroactive, concluding:

> In light of what this Court has said in *Roper*, *Graham*, and *Miller* about how children are constitutionally different from adults in their level of culpability, however, prisoners like Montgomery must be given the opportunity to show their crime did not reflect irreparable corruption; and, if it did not, their hope for some years of life outside prison walls must be restored.

The Court emphasized that its holding could be satisfied by either a resentencing hearing or consideration for possible parole.

According to a recent report, 23 states and D.C. have banned life sentence without the possibility of parole for juveniles. Joshua Rovner, *Juvenile Life Without Parole: An Overview*, Sentencing Project (Feb. 25 2020).

Laurence Steinberg

Adolescent Brain Science and Juvenile Justice Policymaking

23 Psychol. Pub. Pol'y & L. 410, 415-16 (2017)

**HOW IMPORTANT WAS NEUROSCIENCE TO THE
SUPREME COURT DECISIONS?**

Because the Supreme Court justices' deliberations are never made public, it is impossible to know just how much neuroscience findings influenced the Court's decision-making above and be- yond the impact of the behavioral evidence. But a close reading of the transcripts of the oral arguments and opinions makes it clear that the attorneys and justices involved in these cases certainly paid attention to the neuroscience. At times they even insinuated that it was somehow more compelling than the behavioral evidence (as one attorney stated during oral arguments in *Roper*, "I'm not just talking about social science here, but the important neurobiological science"; U.S. Supreme Court, 2004, p. 40), that it was the fundamental driver of the development of maturity ("as the years go by and neurological development occurs, [adolescents'] 'deficiencies will be reformed'"; *Miller v. Alabama*, 2012, p. 22) or at the very least, that neuroscience added validity to an argument based solely on common sense and developmental psychology.

For better or worse, neuroscience may have played a role in persuading the justices that the psychological differences between adolescents and adults as described in *Roper* were genuine and indisputable. There was a decrease, over the course of the series of cases, in the amount of time during oral arguments that was devoted to discussions of where to draw the legal line between adolescents and adults. Indeed, this issue occupied a fair amount of discussion in *Roper* but was barely raised 7 years later, in *Miller*. In addition, a review of the dissenting opinions in each case shows that the justices who voted with the minority clearly moved from a position of some skepticism about whether adolescents were inherently different from adults to one in which the matter was no longer even contested. For example, in his dissenting opinion in *Roper*, Justice Antonin Scalia pointed out that the American Psychological Association, whose amicus brief characterized adolescents as too immature to be exposed to capital punishment, had taken the stance some 15 years earlier, in *Hodgson v. Minnesota*, that adolescents should be able obtain abortions without parental involvement on the grounds that psychological research showed that adolescents were just as mature as adults—the implication being that the developmental immaturity argument advanced by social scientists in *Roper* was just a convenient fabrication concocted by soft-hearted child psychologists to suit their political aims.

By the time *Miller* was decided, things had clearly changed. In his dissenting opinion, Chief Justice John Roberts noted that "[*Roper* and *Graham*] undoubtedly stand for the proposition that teenagers are less mature, less responsible, and less fixed in their ways than adults— *not that a Supreme Court case was needed to establish that*" (*Miller v. Alabama*, 2012, J. Roberts, dissenting, p. 7, italics added for emphasis). We do not know whether the Court's ultimate acceptance of this characterization of adolescents was influenced by neuroscience. Nevertheless, there is a good chance that it was, as the only substantive change in the argument that adolescents are less mature than adults that had taken place between *Roper* and *Miller* involved an increased reliance on neuroscience. The period between these two cases also was characterized by growing coverage of research on adolescent brain development in popular media.

Whether neuroscience should have influenced the justices' reasoning is a different question. In some regards, neuroscience was used as a blunt instrument. As most scientists know, neuroscientific evidence doesn't make the behavioral differences between adolescents and adults any more real. It only makes them seem more real to nonscientists who view psychological research on children as little more than the confirmation of "what every parent knows," and who, like most of us, are more easily impressed by science we do not understand well enough to critique than by science whose methods are more familiar. Several studies, including a recent one in which judges were the subjects, showed that adding just one or two sentences referring to the brain to a description of behavioral findings makes the behavioral findings that much more compelling. A cynical reader may conclude that the introduction of the neuroscience of adolescence into the Supreme Court's deliberations about the juvenile death penalty or juvenile life without parole did little more than exploit the scientific ignorance of laypersons. I think it did more than this, however.

The contribution of neuroscience to discussions of adolescent blameworthiness lies not in what neuroscience tells us about differences in the ways in which adolescents and adults act, but in what it implies about the source of these differences. For example, findings of structural and functional differences between adolescent and adult brains that are plausibly linked to differences in individuals' ability to control their impulses and to stand up to peer pressure suggest that these aspects of adolescent immaturity are not merely reflective of juveniles' poor choices or different values, but that they are at least partly due to factors that are not entirely under an individual's control, which makes immaturity a more convincing mitigator. Identifying the neural underpinnings of age differences in legally relevant capabilities and capacities does not indicate that these differences are immutable (indeed, adolescence is thought to be a time of heightened neuro- plasticity, a period during which the brain is especially malleable in response to experience). However, to the extent that brain maturation during adolescence follows a specific and predictable pattern that is consistent with predictable patterns of behavioral changes, the neuroscientific evidence bolsters the basic argument that adolescents are inherently less mature than adults.

The knowledge that individuals will almost always become more deliberate and self-possessed as they gain experience and as their brains mature, without any special interventions designed to facilitate this process, adds strength to the argument that adolescent offending is unlikely to reflect irreparable depravity. This last point is important, because it provides justification for distinguishing between adolescents, whose immaturity is by definition transient, and fully developed but callow adults, whose immaturity undoubtedly also has neural correlates but is more likely to be an enduring part of their character. This logic helps counter arguments that, if immaturity ought to be viewed as a mitigating factor when sentencing juveniles, it therefore should be used in similar fashion when sentencing immature adults, many of whom, especially those who are genetically inclined toward sensation seeking or impulsivity—both of which have strong genetic components are no more responsible for their immaturity than are teenagers. Ironically, the reason adolescents' immaturity ought to mitigate their culpability is that we can confidently depend on the fact that the vast majority of them will grow out of it. Thus, it is the transient nature of adolescents' immaturity, rather than its neurobiological basis, that warrants their more lenient treatment under the law.

NOTES AND QUESTIONS

1. Scholars differ on the extent to which neuroscience made any difference to the outcomes of the Supreme Court cases excerpted in this section. Identify in those cases direct or indirect invocations of neuroscientific evidence. How important do you think neuroscience was to the outcomes, and why?

2. Do you personally think that juveniles should categorically be exempted from sentences of life in prison without possibility of parole? How, if at all, do neuroscientific considerations affect your own position? Can you think of any neuroscientific finding that, if true, would reverse your view? What does this suggest to you about how the legal system, and ordinary citizens, will invoke or react to neuroscience in future, non-juvenile cases?

3. Given the role neuroscience did—or did not—play in these cases, what lessons might you draw regarding future invocations of neuroscience in non-juvenile-justice contexts—both criminal and civil—such as with drug addicts, gambling addicts, psychopaths, the elderly, or veterans with post-traumatic stress disorder?

4. Justice Scalia calls the American Psychological Association to task for arguing in its *Roper* amicus brief that 16- and 17-year-olds are too immature to be executed for their behavior, while arguing in *Hodgson* that similarly-aged girls are sufficiently mature to make abortion decisions. To what extent is this critique devastating? To what extent, conversely, do you think these two positions could be reconciled, and if so, how?

5. Justice Roberts, although concurring in *Graham*'s result, objected in part to treating adolescents as a group for sentencing purposes, preferring instead an individualized assessment that takes the offender's unique circumstances into account. What role, if any, would neuroscience play in such a regime? How, and with what consequences?

6. Herbert Weinstein, in Chapter 2, proffered neuroscientific evidence about his own brain. The defendants in *Roper* and *Graham* did not. If you could rewind the clock, as attorneys for the juvenile offenders, would you have had your clients brain scanned? Why or why not? And, if so, what would you have hoped to find, and to show? What are the advantages or disadvantages of relying on group-based neuroscientific evidence instead of neuroscientific evidence unique to the defendants?

7. Suppose, for the moment, that a new neuroscientific technique could offer accurate, *individualized* assessments of legally relevant maturity. (For example: this 22-year-old's brain and hormone levels correspond to those of the average 14-year-old; or this 16-year-old's brain and hormone levels are as mature as the average 24-year-old.) How do you think the legal system might, should, or would respond—if at all?

8. React to this argument from legal scholar Stephen Morse:

> The *Roper* briefs were filled with discussion of new neuroscientific evidence that confirms that adolescent brains are different from adult brains in ways consistent with the observed behavioral differences that alone bear on culpability and responsibility. Assuming the validity of the neuroscientific evidence, what does it add? The rigorous behavioral studies already confirm the behavioral differences. No one thinks that these data are invalid because adolescent subjects are faking or for some other reason. The moral and constitutional implications of the data may be controversial, but the data are not. At most, the neuroscientific evidence provides a partial causal explanation of why the observed behavioral differences exist and thus some further evidence of the validity of the behavioral differences. It is only of limited and indirect relevance to responsibility assessment, which is based on behavioral criteria. . . .

Stephen J. Morse, *Brain Overclaim Syndrome and Criminal Responsibility: A Diagnostic Note*, 3 Ohio St. J. Crim. L. 397, 408-09 (2006). What does this suggest to you about variations in the usefulness to law of neuroscientific findings about groups?

9. If a defendant can be treated differently under law because of her membership in a group that is granted, in essence, "impaired brain" status under the law, should it matter whether she is in that group by birth or came to it later? In *Cruel and Unequal Punishments*, 86 Wash. U. L. Rev. 859 (2009), professor Nita A. Farahany notes that under the Supreme Court's doctrine in *Atkins* a person who is intellectually disabled from birth cannot constitutionally be executed, whereas a person who suffered a traumatic brain injury at the age of 22 can be executed—even if the two have identical cognitive, behavioral, and adaptive impairments. Do you perceive a tension between the Eighth Amendment's protections against "cruel and unusual punishments" and the Fourteenth Amendment's guarantee of "equal protection of the laws"? Do you think neuroscience does or might inform this tension, and if so, how?

10. What will be, and what should be, the future use of developmental neuroscience in the criminal law? In the wake of the *Miller* decision, an editorial in *Nature* magazine warned:

> The way the court fashioned its recent decision puts increasing pressure on researchers who study adolescent development to convert their research findings into a format that can be exploited to assess offenders. . . . [T]he ruling might mean that an immature science could be increasingly drawn into the decision-making process. The psychological surveys and functional magnetic resonance imaging of brain structures cited in these cases are most relevant to population-level differences between juveniles and adults. Yet at the individual level, there is wide variation in how mature, culpable and capable of reform a particular offender is. . . . [T]ranslating research from group findings to individuals is a challenge for many areas of society in which science helps to drive decisions: from medicine

to environmental protection and in legal matters. Scientists in affected fields should consider this a call to arms.

Science Takes the Stand, 487 Nature 5 (July 4, 2012). What does the editorial mean when it says this is a "call to arms"? How should scientists respond? How should lawyers respond?

11. Does neuroscientific evidence present particular problems for courts? Particular benefits? Both? Are legislatures better equipped to process the insights of this rapidly developing field? Why or why not? Consider this position, from the advocacy group National Juvenile Justice Network (NJJN):

> Many researchers argue that . . . there is much more that we do not yet know . . . [a]nd thus, it is just too early to start using this research to inform policy . . . [but] juvenile justice advocates have found that this research is nothing short of compelling . . . [because the brain science] opens the doors to legislators' offices who never before thought about progressive juvenile justice reform . . . [and] gives advocates and lawyers working on behalf of juveniles scientific proof for their claims. . . .

Nat'l Juvenile Justice Network, *Using Adolescent Brain Research to Inform Policy: A Guide for Juvenile Justice Advocates* 3 (2012). Do you agree with the position of the NJJN? Law professor Francis Shen has critiqued such positions, arguing that "lobbyist neuroscience" (that is, how science is discussed by advocates in the policy stream) often differs in important ways from laboratory neuroscience, and that legal advocates are often "more aggressive and categorical in their use of the science." Francis X. Shen, *Legislating Neuroscience: The Case of Juvenile Justice*, 46 Loy. L. Rev. 985 (2013). Do you see this as a problem to be remedied (if so, how), or as an inevitable byproduct of scientific advancement?

D. CRITICAL PERSPECTIVES

Consider the following three perspectives on how courts use neuroscience in juvenile justice cases. In the first, Professor Steinberg summarizes and responds to concerns that juveniles are too immature for some decisions (such as those leading to criminal behavior) but—the same scientists have argued—quite mature enough to make other important decisions (such as those regarding abortion). Subsequently, Professor Maroney examines an issue not yet directly considered by the Supreme Court—whether neuroscience has a role to play in providing individualized (rather than group) assessments of adolescents. This should resonate with the issues you first encountered in Chapter 3. Then Professor Shen raises cautionary notes about where the use of neuroscience in this context could lead.

Laurence Steinberg et al.

Are Adolescents Less Mature than Adults? Minors' Access to Abortion, the Juvenile Death Penalty, and the Alleged APA "Flip-Flop"

64 Am. Psychol. 583 (2009)

Developmental science was front and center in the Court's ruling [in *Roper*], which drew extensively on an amicus curiae brief submitted by the American Psychological Association. . . .

The position taken by APA in its brief—that adolescents are inherently less blameworthy than adults as a consequence of their developmental immaturity—was noteworthy not only because it proved so influential to the Court's decision but because it appeared, on its face, to contradict a stance taken by APA in a previous U.S. Supreme Court case, *Hodgson v. Minnesota* (1990). In that case, which concerned a minor's right to obtain an abortion without parental notification, APA had argued that because adolescents had decision-making skills comparable to those of adults, there was no reason to require teenagers to notify their parents before terminating a pregnancy (APA, 1987, 1989). Thus, in *Roper*, APA argued that science showed that adolescents were not as mature as adults, whereas in *Hodgson*, it argued that the science showed that they were. The apparent contradiction in these views did not go unnoticed. Justice Kennedy explicitly asked at oral argument in *Roper* if the APA had "flip-flopped" between 1989 (when its final amicus brief was filed in the abortion case) and 2004 (when its brief was filed in the juvenile death penalty case). The flip-flop issue also was raised by those who disagreed with the Court's decision to abolish the juvenile death penalty. Indeed, in his dissenting opinion in *Roper v. Simmons* (2005), Justice Antonin Scalia drew unambiguous attention to this issue:

[T]he American Psychological Association (APA), which claims in this case that scientific evidence shows persons under 18 lack the ability to take moral responsibility for their decisions, has previously taken precisely the opposite position before this very Court. In its brief in *Hodgson v. Minnesota*, 497 U. S. 417 (1990), the APA found a "rich body of research" showing that juveniles are mature enough to decide whether to obtain an abortion without parental involvement. . . . The APA brief, citing psychology treatises and studies too numerous to list here, asserted: "[B]y middle adolescence (age 14-15) young people develop abilities similar to adults in reasoning about moral dilemmas, understanding social rules and laws, [and] reasoning about interpersonal relationships and interpersonal problems." (Justice Scalia, dissenting, pp. 11-12).

The petitioner in *Roper*, the State of Missouri, made a similar point in its brief:

Ultimately, Simmons wants the Court to declare that [drawing the age boundary for purposes of death penalty eligibility at 16] is now "without penological justification" not based on research that uniformly reaches that conclusion, but based on inconsistent research, viewed through the lense [sic] of a stereotype that the American Psychological Association decried in *Hodgson*: "[T]he assumption that adolescents as a group are less able than adults to understand, reason and make decisions about intellectual and social dilemmas is not supported by contemporary psychological theory and research." (*Roper*, 2004, p. 11).

Concerns about reconciling the scientific arguments offered in the two cases were also raised by abortion rights advocates, but in a different context. Indeed, after Laurence Steinberg met with the Executive Committee of the Society for Research on Adolescence, asking for the organization's endorsement of the APA stance in *Roper*, the committee decided not to sign on to the APA brief, fearing that the argument that adolescents were not as mature as adults (and thus ineligible for capital punishment) would come back to haunt those who had worked so hard to secure the abortion rights of young women.

As it turns out, these worries were not unfounded. Within two years of the *Roper* decision, the U.S. Supreme Court heard *Ayotte v. Planned Parenthood of Northern New England* (2006), which, like *Hodgson*, concerned minors' access to abortion without parental involvement. Opponents of adolescents' autonomous abortion rights had taken the Court's characterization of adolescent immaturity in the juvenile death penalty case and used it to argue in favor of parental involvement requirements. Citing the *Roper* decision, they argued,

> Parental involvement is critical to ensure not only that the adolescent's choice is informed, but that it is freely made and not the result of coercion or duress. . . . These concerns are heightened for adolescents who, as this Court has recently observed, are more susceptible than adults to "outside pressure" and other "negative influences," and more likely than adults to make decisions that are "impetuous and ill-considered." *Roper v. Simmons*, 125 S. Ct. 1183, 1195 (2005). (*Ayotte v. Planned Parenthood of Northern New England*, 2006, p. 15.)

It is easy to see why many criticized APA for its apparently contradictory positions. On the face of it, APA position in the juvenile death penalty case was in direct opposition to the stance it took in *Hodgson*. In its amicus brief arguing for adolescents' abortion rights, for example, APA stated, "[*B*]*y age 14 most adolescents have developed adult-like intellectual and social capacities*" [italics added] including specific abilities outlined in the law as necessary for understanding treatment alternatives, considering risks and benefits, and giving legally competent consent. (APA, 1989, p. 20).

However, in its amicus brief arguing against the juvenile death penalty, APA stated, "*Given that 16- and 17-year-olds as a group are less mature developmentally than adults*" [italics added], imposing capital punishment on such adolescents does not serve the judicially recognized purposes of the sanction. (APA, 2004, p. 13). . . .

Whether APA in fact "flip-flopped" or, worse yet, tried to have it both ways, as its critics have contended, is an exceedingly important question, both with respect to the decisions about where to draw legal boundaries between adolescents and adults for various purposes and with respect to APA's scientific credibility more generally. As some of us have written elsewhere, "scientists' authority to enter the policy arena rests largely on the credibility of their research findings." If APA's statements about the state of scientific knowledge are seen as advocacy masquerading as research, the integrity of the Association's scientific mission is threatened. After all, in both *Hodgson* and *Roper*, APA took a position that could be fairly characterized as, at the very least, friendly to youth advocates. It is crucial, therefore, to examine the issue empirically. That is the focus of the present article. For the past several years, as members of the MacArthur Foundation Research Network on Adolescent Development and Juvenile Justice, we have been studying age differences in many of the cognitive and psychosocial capacities that have been at issue in the Supreme Court cases discussed above. We have been studying basic intellectual abilities, such as working memory and verbal fluency, but also aspects of psychosocial development, including impulse control, future orientation, reward sensitivity, sensation seeking, and susceptibility to peer influence. To our knowledge, ours is the first study to include both cognitive and psychosocial measures administered to the same sample, to include an ethnically and socioeconomically diverse group of individuals, and to span the period from preadolescence through young adulthood.

On the basis of this work, some of which we summarize in the pages that follow, we believe that APA's seemingly contradictory positions in *Hodgson* and *Roper* are in fact quite compatible with research on age differences in cognitive and psychosocial capacities. More specifically, our findings, as well as those of other researchers, suggest that whereas adolescents and adults perform comparably on cognitive tests measuring the sorts of cognitive abilities that were referred to in the *Hodgson* brief—abilities that permit logical reasoning about moral, social, and interpersonal matters—adolescents and adults are not of equal maturity with respect to the psychosocial capacities listed by Justice Kennedy in the majority opinion in *Roper*—capacities such as impulse control and resistance to peer influence. Not only were the legal issues different in the two cases, but so are the circumstances surrounding abortion decisions and criminal behavior, and therefore, the relevant dimensions along which adolescents and adults should be compared differ as well. Unlike adolescents' decisions to commit crimes, which are usually rash and made in the presence of peers, adolescents' decisions about terminating a pregnancy can be made in an unhurried fashion and in consultation with adults.

    . . . [T]he seemingly conflicting positions taken by APA in *Roper v. Simmons* (2005) and *Hodgson v. Minnesota* (1990) are not contradictory. Rather, they simply emphasize different aspects of maturity, in accordance with the differing nature of the decision-making scenarios involved in each case. The skills and abilities necessary to make an informed decision about a medical procedure are likely in place several years before the capacities necessary to regulate one's behavior under conditions of emotional arousal or coercive pressure from peers.

    Science alone cannot dictate public policy, although it can, and should, inform it. Our data can neither "prove" nor "disprove" the appropriateness of requiring parental involvement before a teenager can obtain an abortion, but they do inform the debate. Nor do our data "prove" or "disprove" whether it is appropriate to apply the death penalty to individuals who are inherently more impulsive than adults and whose characters are not yet fully formed—although, again, they are informative. But our findings do demonstrate how the positions taken by APA in *Hodgson v. Minnesota* (1990) and in *Roper v. Simmons* (2005) are compatible with each other and consistent with the rapidly growing body of scientific evidence indicating that intellectual maturity is reached several years before psychosocial maturity. Developmental science can and should contribute to debates about the drawing of legal age boundaries, but research evidence cannot be applied to this sort of policy analysis without a careful and nuanced consideration of the particular demands placed on the individual for "adult-like" maturity in different domains of functioning. Jurists, politicians, advocates, and journalists seeking a uniform answer to questions about where we should draw the line between adolescence and adulthood for different purposes under the law need to consider the asynchronous nature of psychological maturation, especially during periods of dramatic and rapid change across multiple domains of functioning.

Terry A. Maroney
The False Promise of Adolescent Brain Science in Juvenile Justice
85 Notre Dame L. Rev. 89, 93-176 (2009)

[C]ontrary to the high expectations many have placed on developmental neuroscience, it will—and should—have fairly modest effects on juvenile justice. Not only is this correct as a matter of theory, it is being borne out in practice. To show how this is so, this Article offers the first attempt systematically to identify and analyze cases in which advocates have attempted to put developmental neuroscience into practice. The case analysis demonstrates that most such efforts fail, for two primary reasons: a disconnect between scientific findings and the questions asked by legal doctrine, and limitations posed by the science itself. Though the analysis reveals instances in which courts cite approvingly to brain-science arguments, in no such case does that science appear to have been outcome-determinative.

The relative inefficacy of brain science in influencing court outcomes illuminates significant theoretical and practical barriers to such influence. Those barriers counsel that the trend toward urging reliance on such science be significantly moderated. . . .

II. THE LIMITED IMPACT OF ADOLESCENT BRAIN SCIENCE IN THE COURTS

As the previous Part showed, before *Roper* scholars and advocates had begun to envision a powerful role for developmental neuroscience within juvenile justice. Buoyed by apparent success in that case, since *Roper* such theories have proliferated. Defenders and advocates have begun actively to test those theories in cases. To measure the extent to which reality is conforming to predictions, I conducted a study of such cases. As this Part demonstrates, the range of neuroscientific arguments before the courts—state and federal, juvenile and criminal—is both wide and deep. Their impact, however, has been shallow.

This shallow impact, likely surprising to many, cannot be explained fully on the grounds that the science is new or the effort early. Rather, the courts' response to adolescent brain science reflects a frequent disconnect between the questions asked by law and those answered by science. Though courts sometimes cite the science approvingly, they do so only to buttress conclusions otherwise fully explained. The shallow impact also reflects scientific limitations that are genuine and likely to persist. These factors explain how courts generally have responded to developmental neuroscience arguments, but also show why that response has some basis. Two additional factors demonstrate why courts should not unduly privilege such claims. First, juvenile justice cannot directly track neuroscience without implicating equality and autonomy concerns, and no adequate limiting principle has yet been articulated. Second, the pressures of legal advocacy incentivize overstatement and often result in inaccuracy; while this tendency can be controlled, it cannot be eliminated. [. . . A]dolescent brain science has not been (and is unlikely to be) a transformative force in juvenile justice, at least in the courts. . . .

Scientific Limitations

1. Individual Differences

The most significant current limitation of developmental neuroscience is its inability to inform individual assessment. Imaging studies that show group trends in structural maturity—such as relative levels of myelination in prefrontal cortex—do not show that all individuals in the group perfectly reflect the trend. Normal brains follow a unique developmental path bounded roughly by the general trajectory; that is, while all humans will pass through the same basic stages of structural maturation at more or less the same stages of life, the precise timing and manner in which they do so will vary. Moreover, such variation cannot be detected or interpreted in any legally meaningful way. Neither structural nor functional imaging can determine whether any given individual has a "mature brain" in any respect, though imaging might reveal gross pathology. Researchers therefore consistently agree that developmental neuroscience cannot at present generate reliable predictions or findings about an individual's behavioral maturity. Courts thus have a strong basis for deeming brain science irrelevant to many highly individualized claims, such as whether a defendant was able to form specific intent.

Indeed, the cases reflect the difficulties posed by individual variation. Legal decision-makers display incredulity, even annoyance, when general lessons about the adolescent brain appear to conflict with evidence about the individual juvenile. One particularly vivid account of that phenomenon was offered by a Delaware judge who presided over a juvenile capital case while *Roper* was pending. In a pretrial hearing, Michael Jones presented the testimony of Ruben Gur "that juveniles are less criminally culpable than adults because the area of their brains controlling foresight, goal setting, and ability to plan are not yet fully developed." Gur later offered such testimony at trial, alongside the testimony of one Dr. Ragland, a psychologist who had examined Jones. Recounts the court:

> Dr. Ragland discovered that Jones is an exceptionally gifted planner. Dr. Ragland testified that Jones' scores regarding planning and ability to foresee consequences were "off the charts," and were, indeed, higher than any he had ever seen. This admission, which Dr. Ragland repeated ad nauseum, annihilated Jones' only viable defense: that, as a juvenile, he was too young to reasonably calculate the possible outcomes of his murderous rampage, and to plan accordingly. It also eliminated another proposed mitigating factor: that a sentence of life imprisonment would ensure that Jones would never again threaten society. The State used Dr. Ragland's testimony to suggest that Jones would use his exceptional gift for planning to formulate an escape, endangering corrections officers and the public at large. . . .

When Dr. Gur took the stand as the next defense witness, explaining the complicated science of brain development and its nexus to planning ability, the jury appeared disinterested. Their courtroom demeanor, as well as their sentencing recommendation, made it clear that the jury viewed the medical evidence as mere "psychobabble" meant to mislead them into excusing an inexcusable crime. This was despite the fact that Dr. Gur is a superb witness: engaging, charismatic, highly expert, and convincing. There simply was no way for him to salvage the train wreck . . . of the defense case.

Similarly, in *Garcia* the state was able to rebut the notion that anatomical immaturity necessarily manifests itself in a lack of meaningful appreciation of death by showing that Garcia himself had such appreciation; he was deeply affected by the recent death of his grandmother and frequently worried that his gravely ill mother would die. The *Gonzales* court, too, remarked that "[r]egardless of whether the nature of the adolescent brain produces behavior that is more impulsive than an adult's . . . [Gonzales's] conduct in this case reveals a high degree of individual culpability." Neuroscience may provide marginal support for categorically limiting the sanctions that may be imposed on juveniles, but it has little to offer in assessing the mental state, capacity for rehabilitation, or other law-relevant attributes of any given juvenile.

2. Structure v. Behavior

A related difficulty stems from the reality that structural and functional differences between individual brains may not correspond with predictable or discernable differences in behavior. Just as scientists cannot look at an individual teen's brain and conclude that she has a particular level of behavioral maturity, observers cannot look at a teen's behavior and deduce the structural or functional maturity of her brain. This is not an issue only for individual determinations, for even at the group level there are few data demonstrating a clear link between structural immaturity and immature behavior. The structure-behavior hypothesis is a strong one, as brain attributes often correlate with specific behaviors, and a significant developmental stage is highly likely to manifest in behavior. Developmental psychology provides a picture of the attitudes and behaviors that typify adolescents; neuroscience provides a picture of the brain maturation processes that typify adolescence; and the latter can be interpreted in such a way as to provide a plausible, partial explanation for the former. But though it is highly plausible that "[a]dolescents' behavioral immaturity mirrors the anatomical immaturity of their brains," science has not determined the nature or extent of that mirroring.

Advocates, commentators, and defenders unnecessarily overstate the case when they claim that imaging studies explain adolescent behavior, let alone any given adolescent's behavior. Courts also have a basis for believing neural explanations to be less probative than behavioral ones. The Supreme Court displayed that defensible perspective in *Roper* by relying overtly on historical beliefs and legal precedent rooted in direct experience with teenagers' behavior—about which "any parent knows"—and in the behavior-based findings of developmental psychology.

CONCLUSION

This Article tells a cautionary tale. Relying aggressively on developmental neuroscience in legal theory and practice might wear out its welcome early, even though it now offers some law-relevant insights and in the future might offer more. The courts' early cold shoulder shows this to be a real danger. Nor is such reliance necessary, as we already have all the information we need to construct a rational juvenile justice policy. Adolescent brain science does not provide an independent basis to recommit to traditional juvenile justice values; it merely reinforces the wisdom of doing so. The bulk of that wisdom comes not from understanding what is going on inside the teen brain but from understanding the impact of the legal and social environments we create for young people.

We need that wisdom now, as we are at a potentially momentous crossroad for juvenile justice. By removing the most extreme possible punishment for youth, *Roper* unquestionably has shifted the terms of debate. Recent legislative developments suggest that the states are, wisely, starting to roll back some of the policy changes of the 1990s. Most Americans report being committed to second chances for youth. Even recent fiscal challenges have wrought change, as states seek to avoid costly incapacitation if cheaper alternatives, like supervised release and family therapy, can be shown equally effective. These shifts may well portend a welcome new era in juvenile justice, one in which recommitment to the protection and rehabilitation of youth is the driving first principle. But if we move into that new era, it will not be because of adolescent brain science. To the extent that the science appears to promise transformation, it is a false promise.

Francis X. Shen
Legislating Neuroscience: The Case of Juvenile Justice
46 Loy. L.A. L. Rev. 985, 987-1016 (2013)

[When] Justice Kagan was asked about her opinion on juvenile transfer policies, . . . she replied: "[T]hat's for a *legislature* to do. . . . [W]hat makes for good criminal justice policy[?] . . . I view that as a very different question than the questions that I'm answering and a different role to be performed than the role I have." Justice Kagan reminds us that as important as *Miller, Graham,* and *Roper* are for setting limits on legislative action, much of detailed policymaking for juvenile justice remains in the domain of legislators. . . .

. . . [B]rain science is a part of the juvenile justice policy dialogue [in state legislatures], but it is a part of *one side* of that dialogue—the side that argues for lower mandatory sentences and against juvenile transfer to adult courts. I suggest that the rhetoric used by advocacy groups is more categorical than the measured approach suggested by the underlying research.

The National Juvenile Justice Network (NJJN) has developed a comprehensive guide for advocates interested in using brain science. The Guide is unique because it addresses head-on the concern that "[m]any researchers argue that . . . there is much more that we do not yet know. . . [a]nd thus, it is just too early to start using this research to inform policy." The NJJN responds that "juvenile justice advocates have found that this research is nothing short of compelling" because the brain science "opens the doors to legislators' offices who never before thought about progressive juvenile justice reform" and because the science "gives advocates and lawyers working on behalf of juveniles scientific proof for their claims. . . ." In short, NJJN is arguing that the science is good enough for persuasive purposes within the political sphere.

. . . The translation of "lab neuroscience" (what the published research finds) into "lobbyist neuroscience" (what the lobbyists say the research finds) involves a rhetorical reframing of the science. For instance, the Illinois Coalition for the Fair Sentencing of Children uses a subheading of "The *Hard Science* of Culpability" when it introduces the connection between brain science and juvenile justice reform. Act 4 Juvenile Justice similarly suggests that "*[h]ard science* demonstrates that teenagers and young adults are not fully mature in their judgment, problem-solving and decision-making capacities."

The brain-behavior relationship is presented as absolute in the advocate's formulation. . . . [But] while children are different from adults, they are also different *from each other*. At the start of the *Miller* opinion, Justice Kagan emphasizes the Court's line of cases requiring "individualized sentencing for defendants facing the most serious penalties."

At present, neuroscience can offer little in the way of individualized assessment. But efforts are underway in neuroscience to learn more about individual differences. . . .

It does not strain common sense to think that at least a few of the sixteen-year-olds in the country who commit a violent, premeditated crime are rotten to the core, and for whatever reasons have little chance for reform. Could neuroscience ever help us identify these individuals (and feel comfortable with the reliability of that identification)? Maybe not. But if so, such developments in "lab neuroscience" would pose a problem for current "lobbyist neuroscience" to the extent that lobbyists argue that neuroscience tells us only that adolescents *as a group* are less deserving of punishment, and does not tell us whether *individual* adolescents can be singled out for adult-level penalties.

Brain science can add productively to many legislative debates, certainly including juvenile neuroscience. But legislating neuroscience should not replace legislating values. . . . Developmental psychologist Laurence Steinberg . . . offers this cautionary note: "[w]here the revelation that the adolescent brain may be less mature than scientists had previously thought is ultimately a good thing, a bad thing, or a mixed blessing for young people remains to be seen." If one lives by the neuroscience sword in making the case that children are different, then one may die by the neuroscience sword if it swings in an unanticipated way.

NOTES AND QUESTIONS

1. To what extent do you agree or disagree with Maroney's perspective on the role of neuroscience in juvenile justice? For more, see Terry A. Maroney, *The Once and Future Juvenile Brain*, in *Choosing the Future of American Juvenile Justice* 189 (Franklin E. Zimring & David S. Tanenhaus eds., 2014).

2. How, if at all, do these readings affect your prior thoughts on adolescent culpability? To what extent do the data about teen decision-making in the face of immediate rewards versus nonimmediate costs affect your views about how the government should regulate teen behaviors — such as access to abortions, cars, pornography, and the like? On the subject of government regulations regarding the sale or rental of violent video games to minors, see *Brown v. Entm't Merchs. Ass'n*, 131 S. Ct. 2729 (2011).

3. Consider Steinberg's response to Justice Scalia's challenge. Who has the better argument, and why?

4. The Report of the National Research Council — *Reforming Juvenile Justice: A Developmental Approach* — considered the extent to which neuroscience could affect juvenile justice policy. In light of what you have learned in this course to date, what are your reactions to its recommendations, and to the use of developmental science to support them?

5. One commentator, looking at the use of neuroscience in youth justice, has argued that neuroprediction might add "another dimension to the barrage of actuarial devices to which the children of the most marginalized social groups are already subjected." Charlotte Walsh, *Youth Justice and Neuroscience: A Dual-Use Dilemma*, 51 Brit. J. Criminol. 21, 22 (2011). But what if those same actuarial devices allow society to better identify the most dangerous criminals and the individuals least receptive to treatment? In a policy world of increasingly limited resources, is such identification a rational and just way to optimize investments in crime prevention?

6. In oral arguments for *Roper*, the following exchange took place between Justice Breyer and Attorney Seth Waxman, arguing the case on behalf of Christopher Simmons:

> **Justice Breyer:** . . . I thought that the — the scientific evidence simply corroborated something that every parent already knows, and if it's more than that, I would like to know more.

> **Mr. Waxman:** Well, it's—I think it's—it's more than that in a couple of respects. It—it explains, corroborates, and validates what we sort of intuitively know, not just as parents but in adults—that—that—who live in a world filled with adolescents. And—and the very fact that science—and I'm not just talking about social science here, but the important neurobiological science that has now shown that these adolescents are—their character is not hard-wired. . . .

Transcript of Oral Argument at 40, *Roper v. Simmons*, 543 U.S. 551 (2005) (No. 03-633). Mr. Waxman says he's "not just talking about social science," but "neurobiological science." Does it make a difference what type of "science" is used?

7. Do you think a categorical rule against imposition of the death penalty for offenses committed while a juvenile should be extended to non-juveniles who suffer from frontal lobe dysfunction that makes them, arguably, less culpable in a similar way? This was the issue in *Hooks v. Thomas*, No. 2:10-CV-268-WKW, 2011 WL 4915840 (M.D. Ala. Oct. 17, 2011) (petitioner sought access to fMRI to show frontal lobe dysfunction).

8. For an example of how adolescent brain science can affect judicial decision-making in the context of sentencing an immature 19-year-old, see *United States v. C.R.*, 792 F. Supp. 2d 343, 496-506 (E.D.N.Y. 2011) (explaining the science and testimony supporting an immaturity exception), *vacated sub nom. United States v. Reingold*, 731 F.3d 204 (2d Cir. 2013).

9. It has been argued that the very things that make adolescents less culpable also make them more dangerous. According to which principles would you attempt to net out these opposing forces, if sitting in judgment?

10. To what extent should courts distinguish between the role of neuroscience in determining diminished culpability, and the role of neuroscience in determining diminished capacity to stand trial? For an exploration of this, see Jamie D. Brooks, *"What Any Parent Knows" but the Supreme Court Misunderstands: Reassessing Neuroscience's Role in Diminished Capacity Jurisprudence*, 17 New Crim. L. Rev. 442 (2014).

11. Are there reasons—independent of brain development and maturity—to treat juveniles differently than adults, under the criminal law? For an intricately argued case that voting disenfranchisement provides such a reason, see Gideon Yaffe, *The Age of Culpability: Children and the Nature of Criminal Responsibility* (2018). For a contrary view, in response, see Stephen J. Morse, *Against the Received Wisdom: Why the Criminal Justice System Should Give Kids a Break*, 14 Crim. L. & Phil. 257 (2020).

12. The law confronts adolescence in many ways beyond criminal sentencing. For instance, at what age can an individual legally consent to sex? Law professor Jennifer Drobac describes the challenge of line drawing in this context:

> First, have most teenagers formed a coherent independent identity, and if not, should jurists treat teen consent to sex with an adult supervisor, teacher, or coworker as legally significant? Second, do adolescent impulsivity and moodiness combine with stress (including pressure for sex) to influence a teen's decision-making process? Third, who influences an adolescent's decision to have sex with a supervisor or teacher (assuming that a minor does actually consent)? The teen's parents? Peers? Social media? Only the supervisor? Finally, should the law regard teen consent that was arguably given impulsively and under stress, and perhaps as a result of pressure by an authority figure, as significant and legally binding? In sum, does the law even go in the right direction given what scientists know from the group data about adolescent development and decision making?

Assume for a moment that adolescent consent should not be legal binding because adolescents do not have the power, (equal) status, and competence to consent to sex with an adult. Will jurists account for adolescent developing capacity, neurological and psychosocial immaturity, status, and power in their allocation of rights and liabilities? While many people claim to base the attribution of rights on competency, they often judge competency and assign rights based on physical appearance. Thus, society sometimes treats those children who look physically mature as adults, whether or not they are emotionally, neurologically, and psychosocially mature. Scientists have demonstrated that an adolescent may look like an adult but may not have the same cognitive capacity as one. This information is vitally important to judges and jurors who must evaluate consent and capacity. . . .

Jennifer Ann Drobac, *Sexual Exploitation of Teenagers: Adolescent Development, Discrimination, and Consent Law* 44-45 (2016).

E. YOUNG ADULTS

To what extent should the neuroscientific findings—that the human brain is not fully mature by 18 years of age—be relevant to how the legal system treats young adults? Courts around the country are grappling with this now.

For instance, the core logic of the Supreme Court opinions in Section C, above, as augmented by developments summarized by this next excerpt, below, was first extended to young adults in the case of a 19-year-old in *People v. House*, 2015 Ill. App. 110580 (Ill. App. Ct. 2015). Though the litigation is still proceeding (in this, and many other cases), the neurobiology of brain development is front and center in pleadings and court opinions. There the trial court held, largely on the basis of brain science, that a mandatory natural life term for a 19-year-old defendant was unconstitutional. A Kentucky court in 2017 ruled before trial that it was unconstitutional to seek the death penalty for those who were under *21 years old* at the time of their offense. The ruling was vacated by the Kentucky Supreme Court as unripe, and the case was remanded for a trial in 2020. *Commonwealth v. Bredhold*, No. 2017-SC-000436-TG, 2020 WL 1847082 (Ky. Mar. 26, 2020). And a Connecticut court in 2018 held that it was unconstitutional to have a mandatory sentence of life imprisonment without the possibility of parole for those *who were 18* (that is, in "late adolescence," as the court put it) at the time of their crimes. *Cruz v. United States*, No. 11-CV-787 (JCH), 2018 WL 1541898 (D. Conn. Mar. 29, 2018). This case was on appeal as of June 2020.

B.J. Casey et al.,

The MacArthur Foundation Research Network on Law and Neuroscience

How Should Justice Policy Treat Young Offenders?: A Knowledge Brief

(2017)

Over the past decade and more, researchers—including members of the MacArthur Foundation Research Network on Law and Neuroscience—have looked closely at the neuroscience underlying adolescent behavior. What they have found is that different regions of the adolescent brain, and the functional connections among them, develop along distinct timelines, resulting in asymmetry among different brain systems. The emotional centers develop relatively early, making adolescents highly responsive to emotional and social stimuli. By contrast, brain regions that regulate self-control, such as the prefrontal cortex, take a while to catch up and continue to develop even beyond adolescence.

The differential pace of development in these systems can lead to an imbalance in communication among them, allowing those regions that support rational behavior to be overpowered by brain centers involved in emotion. This finding explains the pattern behavioral scientists had previously described: adolescents, especially in emotionally charged contexts or in the presence of peers, are more apt than adults to be impulsive, to disregard future consequences, and to take risks.

Ongoing development of the adolescent brain has another important component: plasticity, or the capacity of the brain to change in response to the environment. Because the brain is undergoing such rapid, fundamental changes at this stage of life, adolescents have a heightened capacity to learn and to alter how they behave as they age out of risky behavior. Given an environment and supports appropriate to their developmental stage, most young offenders have the potential to become law-abiding adults.

YOUNG ADULTHOOD: THE NEXT FRONTIER?

When developmental scientists—and to a large extent policymakers—speak of adolescents they usually mean teenagers up to the age of 18. Today, though, neuroscientists, as well as behavioral scientists, are beginning to look more closely at young adulthood—the period between ages 18 and 21—and to differentiate it from later stages of adulthood.

Why it matters. Young adulthood has changed dramatically over the past half century. Fifty years ago most young men and women left their parents' home around the age of 18, went to college or started work, then got married and had children. Today these milestones on the road toward independent adulthood are far more uncertain, and the dividing line between youth and adult has become less clear and less fixed. Economic hardship has made achieving the markers of adulthood especially difficult for those with fewer resources.

Young adults do commit a disproportionate amount of the nation's crime. In fact, arrests and recidivism peak in this age group. Yet we know relatively little about the developmental factors that may contribute to this phenomenon. What is happening to the developing brain during this period? How do biological and psychological development interact with the surrounding culture? What are the individual's capacities and needs as he or she prepares for adulthood? And what are the special challenges facing disadvantaged young adults? Answering questions like these will help meet the urgent need for programs that can help young adults at risk prepare for successful adulthood.

What brain science is revealing. Very few brain studies have compared individuals in the age group 18 to 21 with younger adolescents or with people in their mid-20s. What evidence there is, however, suggests that young adulthood is a distinct developmental period, and that young adults are different both from adolescents and from somewhat older adults in ways that are potentially relevant to justice policy.

Researchers have found that in young adulthood, as in adolescence, areas of the brain that regulate functions like judgment and self-control are still not fully mature. In certain emotionally charged situations, the capacity of young adults to regulate their actions and emotions appears more like that of teens than adults in their mid 20s or older. Work by members of the MacArthur Foundation Research Network on Law and Neuroscience suggests that young adults' propensity for risky behaviors, in particular, depends on emotional context.

When young adults feel threatened, they become more impulsive and more likely to take risks. However, their decision-making appears less influenced by peers than is that of adolescents. These new findings are especially important to justice policy, which often addresses emotionally charged situations. Still to be explored are questions of brain development that could shed light on young adults' potential for rehabilitation.

JUSTICE POLICY AND YOUNG ADULTS

Viewing young adulthood as a distinct and critical developmental period suggests the need to consider justice policies tailored to this group of young offenders. This is especially important in light of the economic and demographic changes described earlier and their disproportionate harmful impact on low-income youth and youth of color. Ongoing brain maturation in young adulthood has implications for policies related to culpability and punishment, and especially for rehabilitation—policies that give young adults the opportunity to stop offending and become contributing members of society.

At this time there is not a lot of evidence about what kinds of reforms will work best for young adults. We can say with some confidence, however, that treating young adults like older prisoners does not reduce recidivism. Reforms could begin by using less harsh sanctions (such as limited sentences and community-based alternatives) for less serious, non-violent crimes, and by investing in correctional programs and settings specifically designed to address the needs of this group of offenders. Perhaps more challenging will be to design effective educational, vocational, and social skills programs to prepare these individuals for the future. Shielding young adults from the collateral consequences of having a criminal record would facilitate their access to education, employment, and housing.

Finally, because of young offenders' capacity for change, and the likelihood that many of them will stop committing crimes as they mature, it makes sense to consider special, expedited parole policies that allow young adults to demonstrate that they are no longer a threat to society. For the same reason, lawmakers should consider excluding people between 18 and 21 from the mandatory minimum sentences currently imposed on adults. . . .

NOTES AND QUESTIONS

1. To what extent do you think that the extensions of *Roper v. Simmons* and its progeny to emerging adults over age 18 makes sense?
2. Jurisdictions can, of course, set their own age of majority, and indeed set different ages for acquiring different rights. To what extent do you think the legal systems in the United States—which for most purposes consider someone an adult at age 18—should treat young adults (say 18- to 21-year-olds) differently than it currently does? An exploration of this topic appears in Elizabeth S. Scott,

Richard J. Bonnie & Laurence Steinberg, *Young Adulthood as a Transitional Legal Category: Science, Social Change, and Justice Policy*, 85 Fordham L. Rev. 641 (2016). For an argument against raising the age of majority to 21, see Laurence Steinberg et al., *Don't Treat Young Adults as Teenagers*, N.Y. Times (Apr. 29, 2016).

3. A number of commentators are arguing to raise the upper age for juvenile court jurisdiction, with bills introduced in Massachusetts, for example, to include 18-, 19-, and 20-year-olds. Selen S. Perker & Lael Chester, *Emerging Adults: A Distinct Population that Calls for an Age-Appropriate Approach by the Justice System*, Emerging Adult Justice (Harvard Kennedy School, Cambridge, Mass.), June 2017. Would you support such a change? Why or why not?

4. Many jurisdictions have exceptions for when a juvenile can be prosecuted as an adult. Some commentators have argued for a bright line rule that would, for instance, prohibit ever prosecuting someone under 17 as an adult. Kim A. Taylor-Thompson, *Minority Rule: Redefining the Age of Criminality*, 38 N.Y.U. Rev. L. & Soc. Change 143 (2014). Would you support such a rule? Why or why not?

5. A number of jurisdictions have begun experimenting with differing legal approaches for handling young adult offenders. In New York, for instance, where offenders 16 and older have often been treated as adults, the Brooklyn District Attorney's Office, in partnership with the Center for Court Innovation, is piloting a separate court system for ages 16 to 24. And the San Francisco District Attorney launched a similar program. Says Katy Weinstein Miller, of the San Francisco D.A.'s office, "Neuroscience has really informed everything we do in court." Tim Requararth, *Neuroscience is Changing the Debate Over What Role Age Should Play in Courts*, Newsweek (Apr. 18, 2016). *See also* Tim Requarth, *A California Court for Young Adults Calls on Science*, Newsweek (Apr. 17, 2017).

FURTHER READING

Challenges of Drawing Individual Inferences from Group-Averaged Data:

David L. Faigman et al., The MacArthur Foundation Research Network on Law and Neuroscience, *G2i: A Knowledge Brief* (2017).

David Faigman, John Monahan & Christopher Slobogin, *Group to Individual (G2i) Inference in Scientific Expert Testimony*, 81 U. Chi. L. Rev. 417 (2014).

Brain Development:

Kaitlyn Breiner et al., *Combined Effects of Peer Presence, Social Cues, and Rewards on Cognitive Control in Adolescents*, 60 Developmental Psychobiology 292 (2018).

Grace Icenogle et al., *Adolescents' Cognitive Capacity Reaches Adult Levels Prior to Their Psychosocial Maturity: Evidence for a "Maturity Gap" in a Multinational, Cross-Sectional Sample*, 43 L. & Hum. Behav. 69 (2019).

Briana S. Last et al., *Childhood Socioeconomic Status and Executive Function in Childhood and Beyond*, 13 PLoS ONE e0202964 (2018).

The Teenage Brain (Special Issue), 22 Current Directions Psychol. Sci. (2013).

B.J. Casey, Stephanie Duhoux & Matthew Malter Cohen, *Adolescence: What Do Transmission, Transition, and Translation Have to Do with It?*, 67 Neuron 749 (2010).

Charles A. Nelson, Michelle de Hann & Kathleen M. Thomas, *Neuroscience of Cognitive Development: The Role of Experience and the Developing Brain* (2005).

Laurence Steinberg, *Cognitive and Affective Development in Adolescence*, 9 Trends Cognitive Sci. 69 (2005).

Jason Chein et al., *Peers Increase Adolescent Risk Taking by Enhancing Activity in the Brain's Reward Circuitry*, 14 Developmental Sci. F1 (2011).

Michael Dreyfuss et al., *Teens Impulsively React Rather than Retreat from Threat*, 36 Developmental Neurosci. 220 (2014).

Katherine E. Powers et al., *Consequences for Peers Differentially Bias Computations about Risk from Adolescence to Adulthood*, 147 J. Experimental Psychol. 671 (2018).

Legal Implications:

Laurence Steinberg, *Adolescent Brain Science and Juvenile Justice Policymaking*, 23 Psychol. Pub. Pol'y & L. 410 (2017).

Elizabeth Scott et al., *Juvenile Sentencing Reform in a Constitutional Framework*, 88 Temple L. Rev. 675 (2015).

Richard J. Bonnie et al., *The Promise of Adolescence: Realizing Opportunity for All Youth* (2019).

B.J. Casey et al., The MacArthur Foundation Research Network on Law and Neuroscience, *How Should Justice Policy Treat Young Offenders?: A Knowledge Brief* (2017).

Alexandra O. Cohen et al., *When is an Adolescent an Adult? Assessing Cognitive Control in Emotional and Nonemotional Contexts*, 27 Psychol. Sci. 549 (2016).

Elizabeth S. Scott, Richard J. Bonnie & Laurence Steinberg, *Young Adulthood as a Transitional Legal Category: Science, Social Change, and Justice Policy*, 85 Fordham L. Rev. 641 (2016).

Kim Taylor-Thompson, *Minority Rule: Redefining the Age of Criminality*, 38 N.Y.U. Rev. L. & Soc. Change 143 (2014).

Mark R. Fondacaro et. al., *The Rebirth of Rehabilitation in Juvenile and Criminal Justice: New Wine in New Bottles*, 41 Ohio N.U. L. Rev. 697 (2015).

Mark R. Fondacaro, *The Injustice of Retribution: Toward A Multisystemic Risk Management Model of Juvenile Justice*, 20 J.L. & Pol'y 145 (2011).

Mark R. Fondacaro, *Rethinking the Scientific and Legal Implications of Developmental Differences Research in Juvenile Justice*, 17 New Crim. L. Rev. 407 (2014).

Lora M. Cope et al., *Abnormal Brain Structure in Youth Who Commit Homicide*, 4 NeuroImage Clinical 800 (2014).

Kimberly Larson, Frank DiCataldo & Robert Kinscherff, Miller v. Alabama: *Implications for the Forensic Mental Health Assessment at the Intersection for Social Science and the Law*, 39 New Eng. J. on Crim. & Civ. Confinement 319 (2013).

Barry C. Feld, *Punishing Kids in Juvenile and Criminal Courts*, 47 Crime & Justice 417 (2018).

B.J. Casey, *Healthy Development as a Human Right: Lessons from Developmental Science*, 102 Neuron 724 (2019).

Stephen J. Morse, *Brain Overclaim Redux*, 31 Law & Ineq. 509 (2013).

Elizabeth Cauffman et al., *How Developmental Science Influences Juvenile Justice Reform*, 8 U.C. Irvine L. Rev. 21 (2018).

David R. Katner, *Eliminating the Competency Presumption in Juvenile Delinquency Cases*, 24 Cornell J.L. & Pub. Pol'y 403 (2015).

Teneille Brown & Emily Murphy, *Through a Scanner Darkly: Functional Neuroimaging as Evidence of a Criminal Defendant's Past Mental States*, 62 Stan. L. Rev. 1119 (2010).

Terry Maroney, *Adolescent Brain Science After* Graham v. Florida, 86 Notre Dame L. Rev. 765 (2011).

Laurence Steinberg, *The Influence of Neuroscience on U.S. Supreme Court Decisions About Adolescents' Criminal Culpability*, 14 Nature Rev. Neurosci. 513 (2013).

Elizabeth S. Scott, *"Children are Different": Constitutional Values and Justice Policy*, 11 Ohio St. J. Crim. L. 71 (2013).

Richard J. Bonnie & Elizabeth S. Scott, *The Teenage Brain: Adolescent Brain Research and the Law*, 22 Current Directions Psychol. Sci. 158 (2013).

Jennifer Ann Drobac & Leslie A. Hulvershorn, *The Neurobiology of Decision-Making in High Risk Youth and the Law of Consent to Sex*, 17 New Crim. L. Rev. 502 (2014).

Thomas Grisso et al., *Juveniles' Competence to Stand Trial: A Comparison of Adolescents' and Adults' Capacities as Trial Defendants*, 27 Law & Hum. Behav. 333 (2003).

Law and Adolescence: Examining the Legal and Policy Implications of Adolescent Development Research for Youth Involved in the Child Welfare, Juvenile Justice, or Criminal Justice Systems (Special Issue), 79 Temple L. Rev. (2006).

Mary Beckham, *Crime, Culpability, and the Adolescent Brain*, 305 Science 596 (2004).

Jay D. Aronson, *Brain Imaging, Culpability and the Juvenile Death Penalty*, 13 Psychol. Pub. Pol'y & L. 115 (2007).

David R. Katner, *The Mental Health Paradigm and the MacArthur Study: Emerging Issues Challenging the Competence of Juveniles in Delinquency Systems*, 32 Am. J.L. & Med. 503 (2006).

Staci A. Gruber & Deborah A. Yurgelun-Todd, *Neurobiology and the Law: A Role in Juvenile Justice?*, 3 Ohio St. J. Crim. L. 321 (2006).

Jennifer A. Drobac, *Developing Capacity: Adolescent Consent at Work, at Law, and in the Sciences of the Mind*, 10 U.C. Davis J. Juv. L. & Pol'y 1 (2006).

Robert E. Shepherd, Jr., *Relevance of Brain Research to Juvenile Defense*, 19 Crim. Just. 51 (2004-2005).

Aliya Haider, Roper v. Simmons: *The Role of the Science Brief*, 3 Ohio St. J. Crim. L. 369 (2006).

Adam Ortiz, *Adolescent Brain Development and Legal Culpability*, ABA (2003).

Legal Treatment of Young Adults:

Elizabeth S. Scott, Richard J. Bonnie & Laurence Steinberg, *Young Adulthood as a Transitional Legal Category: Science, Social Change, and Justice Policy*, 85 Fordham L. Rev. 641 (2016).

CHAPTER 18

Aging Brains

It is an unfortunate fact of life that physical and mental capacity sometimes diminish with age. . . .

—Justice Sandra Day O'Connor, *Gregory v. Ashcroft*
(writing for the majority)[†]

As you get older, you've probably noticed that you tend to forget things. You'll be talking with somebody at a party, and you'll know *that you know this person, but no matter how hard you try, you can't remember his or her name. This can be very embarrassing, especially if he or she turns out to be your spouse.*

—Dave Barry[††]

CHAPTER SUMMARY

This chapter:
- Introduces current scientific understandings of how age affects the brain.
- Examines how courts confront evidence of aging brains in cases concerning testamentary capacity and consent to sex.
- Considers regulatory and policy debates related to aging brains.

INTRODUCTION

For the vast majority of human history "old brains" were the exception rather than the rule, because life expectancy after birth was short enough that most humans would die before their brains declined significantly. But medical advances and demographic trends over the past two centuries have produced a previously unseen number of adults who are living longer. According to the U.S. Census Bureau, the number of Americans aged 65 and older is projected to nearly double from 52 million in 2018 to 95 million by 2060, and the fraction of the population aged 65 or older will rise from 16% to 23%.

This chapter explores some of the many legal implications that accompany these changes. Elder law has emerged as a growing field, and elder justice initiatives have proliferated across the world. Just as lawyers who work in juvenile justice must learn about the adolescent brain, so too, must lawyers who work with older adults learn about the aging brain.

[†] *Gregory v. Ashcroft*, 501 U.S. 452, 472 (1991) (citations omitted).
[††] Dave Barry, *Dave Barry Turns 40* 163 (1990).

As you read, you will see that the legal issues pertaining to aging brains are often similar to those involving adolescent brains. But you will also find many contexts in which the legal issues—and hence the policy responses—differ. For instance, the question of when to *grant* rights (for instance, to drive or to make one's own financial and medical decisions) is distinct and asymmetric from the question of when to *revoke* rights.

At the core of many of the legal issues is something that will by now be familiar to you: the challenge of Group to individual (G2i) inference. At the population level, age typically leads to reductions in information processing speed and, for some, to serious deficits in memory and decision-making capacity. But there is much individual variation. There appears to be roughly four trajectories of cognition over time:

- "Superaging," with little or no cognitive decline and mental faculties remaining high functioning, even in later ages;
- "Normal aging," with some decline in cognitive performance but not enough to impede daily activity;
- "Mild cognitive impairment," with accelerated cognitive decline significantly affecting daily life; and
- "Pathologic aging" or "dementia," with accelerated cognitive decline that impairs daily functioning.

Given these different trajectories, the G2i issue is clear: While an 80-year-old is at significantly greater risk for dementia than a 50-year-old, it does not follow that *all* 80-year-olds have diminished cognitive capacities, nor that every 50-year-old is free from dementia. Given these G2i issues, how can a court know if a particular older adult has the requisite capacity or competency? And should courts consider brain-scan evidence in their determinations?

Advances in neuroscience have raised new legal questions. Until recently, assessing cognitive function and diagnosing Alzheimer's disease and other types of dementia has been symptom-based. But as you will see in this chapter, there are new proposals for a biomarker approach to identifying and defining such diseases.

Early identification of brain changes that serve as precursors to dementia will provide researchers with important new avenues for improving understanding and treatment. But at present, without a cure, the legal system and society are in a bind: If brain scans tell us that someone has dementia, but we have no cure, what is the proper response? For instance, how would the Americans with Disabilities Act be applicable if an employer discriminates not on the basis of an actual disability, but on the probability of future disability hinted at by a brain scan? Would the answer change by industry? For instance, what if the employee in question is a school bus driver, an airline pilot, or a judge?

Additional problems arise over striking the proper balance between affirming older adults' liberty and autonomy, while at the same time protecting them from those who would capitalize on their vulnerability. You saw an example of a court addressing these questions in Chapter 1, in the case of *Van Middlesworth v. Century Bank & Trust Co.* In *Van Middlesworth*, a court had to determine whether to void an agreement because one of the parties was mentally incompetent due to dementia. The court considered a wide array of evidence, including an MRI suggestive of dementia, and concluded that "[t]he integrity of written contracts must be preserved, but so must an incompetent be protected against his own folly. . . ."

Issues such as those raised in *Van Middlesworth* are likely to grow in number. With more than 70 million baby boomers retiring with a vast sum of assets readily available, elder financial exploitation has been labeled the "Crime of the 21st Century." In resolving disputes concerning older adults and financial decisions, the law relies on fluid and often contested concepts such as "competency," "capacity," "undue influence," "insane delusion," and "lucid interval." Might the law's doctrine need revisiting in light of contemporary behavioral and neurobiological knowledge?

This chapter examines foundational issues likely to emerge as law and policy confront the challenge of aging brains. Section A reviews current knowledge of the aging brain, including changes in decision-making circuitry. Section B presents illustrative cases in which courts have examined competency and capacity in older adults. Section C explores the challenge of older offenders—and of older judges. Section D examines the legal implications of using brain and blood biomarkers to diagnose dementia.

A. THE AGING BRAIN

Judging from the number of advertisements for pills and computer games that are supposed to keep your brain strong, you might suppose that neuroscientists have discovered how the brain ages and how to prevent the associated declines in function. You might think that aging is just like other diseases that scientists seek to cure.

Indeed, we have gained knowledge about what happens during aging. The October 31, 2014 issue of the journal *Science* surveyed current research findings. We do understand what measures can forestall the most serious kinds of decline, but no one knows how to reverse aging. We know that the trajectory of the brain through the life span is affected by genetic, physical, and psychological factors. We know that our mental abilities benefit when we lead lives that are not only physically healthy but also intellectually challenging and socially engaged. Throughout our lives, our brains continuously reorganize in response to new experiences. Adverse physical or psychosocial events, such as a stroke or the death of a loved one, are followed by a period of tremendous flexibility in the brain, enabling previously unexpected compensation. The specialized language systems of the brain seem to be especially resilient.

Numerous investigations of psychological testing and brain function across the life span have uncovered some reliable observations, which were summarized by Ulman Lindenberger in his article *Human Cognitive Aging:* Corriger la Fortune?, 346 Science 572 (2014). The trajectory of cognitive abilities across the life span is the manifestation of a dynamic equilibrium of two key interacting abilities: "crystallized" abilities, such as vocabulary, derived from experience; and "fluid" abilities, such as reasoning and working memory. The ages at which particular cognitive skills peak reflects a balance between accumulation of knowledge and deterioration of brain circuits. At the psychological level, we suffer across the life span a decline of working memory, short-term recall, spatial memory, and most of all speed of general mental processing. Meanwhile, long-term memory concerning life history, vocabulary, verbal knowledge, and unconscious responses to previously encountered information persists throughout life. In addition, emotional aspects of cognition can improve with aging; the emotional elements of memories can become more vivid, and emotional stability can improve.

At the cellular and molecular level, aging affects the brain in many ways. Researchers are very interested in understanding these processes, because they should help us understand the basis of age-related dementia and Alzheimer's disease and how normal aging becomes pathological. Much attention has been focused on aggregations of toxic proteins such as amyloid β-protein in Alzheimer's disease and tau in frontotemporal dementia. Alzheimer's disease is identified with neurofibrillary tangles and amyloid plaques, although the degree of cognitive decline is predicted better by the loss of neurons in the hippocampus and surrounding structures. Gene expression patterns in the brain change with age in relatively subtle ways, so aging is more likely affecting the interactions of proteins and other molecules that enable brain function. Still, considerable uncertainty remains about the relationship between aging and disease.

At the structural level, aged brains are different from younger brains in numerous ways. Examination of brains after death shows numerous structural changes with age, including reduced size and weight, larger cerebral ventricles, wider sulci, loss of myelin sheathing, fewer branches and spines of dendrites, reduced counts of neurons, reduced synaptic density, and reduced cerebral vasculature. Given the aged brain's fewer, smaller, less interconnected neurons and fewer blood vessels, older adults' smaller functional brain activation signals are unsurprising. The thinning of the cerebral cortex is especially pronounced in people diagnosed with Alzheimer's disease. Changes in cortical thickness are not uniform. Cortical regions involved in higher functions shrink more than do cortical regions supporting primary sensory processes. The volume of the hippocampus shrinks progressively more with advancing age. Indeed, loss of tissue in the medial temporal lobes correlates with the degree of pathological memory loss.

Some of these changes can be observed with structural MRI. Spots showing where white matter has been damaged by the collapse or rupture of small blood vessels become more common from middle to late adulthood. The neurochemistry of the human brain changes as well. Many neurotransmitters change their concentration and receptor density. For example, PET studies show a clear decrease in dopaminergic neuromodulation in healthy older adults.

Across all of these features, researchers observe large differences across individuals. For example, particularly large individual differences in age-related shrinkage are observed in the lateral prefrontal cortex, prefrontal white matter, and hippocampus. In spite of this variation, some measures of brain function seem to decline together across individuals. These include dopamine availability, the size of medial-temporal and prefrontal cortical areas, reduced structural and functional connectivity through white matter changes, reduced dynamic range of neural activation, and abnormal synchronization of oscillatory activity within and across fast and slow frequencies.

Human brain development is accomplished through pronounced changes in brain circuit wiring, referred to as neuroplasticity. Brain and behavior can change with experience through neuroplasticity even into late adulthood. While physical exercise programs induce plasticity at neural and behavioral levels of analysis, especially among older sedentary adults, plasticity capacity decreases with age.

At the whole-brain level, studies of functional connectivity reveal subtle age-related disruption of the brain's regional integrity and information flow across the brain.* A consistent finding is that relative to younger adults, older adults have lower functional connectivity between regions of the default mode network. Recall that the default mode network consists of cortical regions like the posterior cingulate cortex, precuneus, medial prefrontal cortex, and lateral parietal cortex, which has implications for cognitive processes such as episodic memory, self-referential processing, and mind wandering and impaired performance on memory and executive function tasks. Also, relative to those of younger adults, older adults' brains exhibit more connectivity between and weaker connectivity within functional networks. This suggests that the processes accomplished by the different networks become less distinct with aging; when tested in various ways, participants with lower functional connectivity have shown lower cognitive performance. These changes have been observed in individuals aged from 60 to 85 years tested over just four years. Parallel changes in structural connectivity have been observed.

Investigations of the brain during aging have begun to offer a useful biomarker of biological age as distinct from chronological age.** Based on data from hundreds of people, it is possible to estimate brain age for individuals of the same chronological age. In other words, matched for birthdate, some people have younger brains and others have older brains. Statistically, women tend to have younger brains than age-matched men, and across the population those with younger brains live longer than those with older brains.

Among healthy people, why do some maintain their cognitive sharpness with age while others do not? According to one recent report, scientists conducting the Scottish Mental Surveys have tracked the outcomes of a very large cohort from among the 70,000 Scottish citizens who received paper-and-pencil intelligence tests as children in 1932 and in 1947.*** In the late 1990s and early 2000s researchers recruited more than 1,000 of these individuals to participate in follow up testing. This testing included multiple cognitive tests, genetic surveys, brain scans, and assessments of lifestyles and health status. After more than a decade of testing, the researchers found that late-life cognitive ability was not predicted by exercise, education, or lifestyle, but instead by intelligence level at age 11. An individual's intelligence score at age 11 predicts about 50% of the variance in their IQs at age 77. The factors accounting for the remaining 50% of the variance included not smoking tobacco, remaining physically fit, speaking more than one language, and having more formal education. Also, around 10% of the variance can be attributed to the integrity of structural brain connectivity.

Given the relevance of language for law, the effects of aging on the brain's language systems seem particularly relevant. Comprehending and producing speech involves many processes, which are affected differently during aging.§ Basic speech comprehension such as remembering words and appreciating syntactic and semantic representations are preserved across the life span. Older adults struggle more

---

* Jessica S. Damoiseaux, *Effects of Aging on Functional and Structural Brain Connectivity*, 160 Neuroimage 32 (2017).

** James H. Cole et al., *Brain Age and Other Bodily "Ages:" Implications for Neuropsychiatry*, 24 Molecular Psychiatry 266 (2019); Manu S. Goyal et al., *Persistent Metabolic Youth in the Aging Female Brain*, 116 Proc. Nat'l Acad. Sci. U.S. 3251 (2019).

*** Emily Underwood, *Starting Young*, 346 Science 568 (2014).

§ *See* Meredith A. Shafto & Lorraine K. Tyler, *Language in the Aging Brain: The Network Dynamics of Cognitive Decline and Preservation*, 346 Science 568 (2014).

than younger adults when speech occurs rapidly or in noisy environments, but this may be due simply to sensory impairments. Older adults can also be impaired when comprehension requires more sophisticated cognitive processes.

Language comprehension involves the bilateral frontal, temporal, and parietal cortical areas. Neuroimaging activation within an extensive, partially overlapping network is modulated by phonological, semantic, and syntactic aspects of language processing. With age, the integrity of the network supporting syntax, including left frontal and temporal lobes, declines, and functional connectivity across the hemispheres increases.

The precise functional consequences of these changes are not known, but it seems that syntactic abilities are retained just in proportion to the fraction of the left hemisphere network that remains intact. In contrast, language production declines with age. Relative to younger adults, older adults produce simpler speech, use vaguer terms, and include more frequent and empty pauses. Older adults more often struggle to find words and experience the "tip of the tongue" frustration of knowing the meaning of a word but not being able to recall it. Research indicates that this is not a memory problem but rather a selective deficit in accessing phonological representations.

Generating speech engages interactions between the left hemisphere posterior temporal and parietal regions plus the inferior frontal, anterior insula, and motor cortex. The process of word production is experimentally investigated by asking participants to name pictures or perform tasks that induce the tip-of-the-tongue phenomenon. The ability to recall words decreases with normal aging, leading to more instances of the tip-of-the-tongue frustration, which are associated with reduced connectivity in left anterior insula and in a major axon bundle connecting Broca's area in the inferior frontal lobe with Wernicke's area in the temporal lobe.

When words are retrieved correctly, the pattern of brain activation is similar in older and younger adults. When words cannot be retrieved, however, both younger and older adult brains adapt by engaging the bilateral performance monitoring and cognitive control circuitry, including anterior insula, middle and inferior frontal, and anterior cingulate areas. This activation parallels that found whenever a participant is working hard to perform some mental task. These observations mean simply that older adults often must work harder to recall words, but the brain functional circuitry supporting this ability does not reorganize qualitatively.

S. Duke Han et al.
Grey Matter Correlates of Susceptibility to Scams in Community-Dwelling Older Adults
10 Brain Imaging & Behav. 524, 525-28 (2016)

[A]ge-related changes in grey matter of particular brain regions may represent another mechanism by which a person could become susceptible to scams in old age. Aging is associated with overall decreases in brain grey matter volume. Neuroimaging research supports a complex and interacting network of brain regions involved in valuation behaviors relevant to susceptibility to scams, many of which are localized to the frontal lobe and involve strategy switching, inhibitory function, self-control, abstraction, and value mapping.

We investigated whether susceptibility to scams was associated with differences in grey matter volume in a sample of community-dwelling non-demented older adults from the Rush Memory and Aging Project. We primarily hypothesized that lower grey matter volume in frontal lobe regions would be associated with susceptibility to scams after controlling for the effects of age, education, and sex. We secondarily hypothesized that lower grey matter volume in medial temporal lobe regions would be associated with susceptibility to scams since these code for prospective decision outcomes by modulating frontal lobe valuation systems. Finally, because even cognitively intact older adults may be susceptible to scams, we explored whether brain grey matter associations with susceptibility to scams remained significant after further accounting for the effects of cognitive function. To our knowledge, this is the first systematic study of brain grey matter associations of susceptibility to scams in old age. . . .

Using voxel-based morphometric measures, we found an inverse association of total grey matter volume with susceptibility to scams in models adjusted for age, education, and sex, and in secondary models further adjusted for global cognition. Consistent with our hypotheses, we observed that lower grey matter concentration in multiple frontal and temporal lobe regions was associated with susceptibility to scams in voxel-level analyses adjusted for the effects of age, education, and sex. In models further adjusted for global cognition, clusters in right temporal lobe regions remained significant. Total white matter and cerebrospinal fluid were not associated, and no regions showed higher grey matter concentration associated with susceptibility to scams. These results suggest susceptibility to scams in old age may have relatively specific neuroanatomical grey matter correlates, and that the associations of these neural correlates with susceptibility to scams are above and beyond the effects of global cognition. . . .

NOTES AND QUESTIONS

1. It is important to clarify terminology. "Dementia" is an umbrella term, used to describe multiple brain conditions:

> including many neurodegenerative diseases, characterized by the progressive loss of mental faculties, ultimately leading to an inability to care for oneself. Alzheimer's disease is the most common form of dementia, although Lewy body dementia, Parkinson's disease dementia, vascular dementia, and frontotemporal dementia are also encountered. Early in the disease course, these different types of dementia can impair specific cognitive processes, such as memory, language, behavior, or executive functions, but all types of dementia can impair decision making. Impaired decision making can have important consequences when considering medical capacity assessments or the legal determination of competency in patients suffering from dementia. . . .

R. Ryan Darby & Bradford C. Dickerson, *Dementia, Decision Making, and Capacity*, 25 Harv. Rev. Psychiatry 270, 270 (2017).

2. There is growing evidence of sex differences in brain aging. One neuroimaging study found that "there were gender differences in elderly brains, with males showing more age-related reduction of brain metabolism than females in frontal medial regions for cognitive control." Maura Malpetti et al., *Gender Differences in*

Healthy Aging and Alzheimer's Dementia: A ^{18}F-FDG-PET Study of Brain and Cognitive Reserve, 38 Hum. Brain Mapping 4212, 4220 (2017). Commenting on another recent study exploring a similar question, neuroscientist Marcus Raichle observed that "[i]f you look at how brain metabolism predicts a person's age, women come out looking about four years younger than they are." Quoted in Ian Sample, *Women's Brains Are 'Four Years Younger' Than Men's, Study Finds*, Guardian (Feb. 4, 2019). *See* Manu S. Goyal et al., *Persistent Metabolic Youth in the Aging Female Brain*, 116 Proc. Nat'l Acad. Sci. U.S. 3251 (2019). How might the legal system confront sex differences in aging brains and the implications of these for cognitive control and ability?

3. Although the age-crime curve clearly indicates that older adults are less likely than younger cohorts to commit crimes, a recognized relationship exists between certain types of dementia and criminal behavior. *See* Madeleine Liljegren et al., *Criminal Behavior in Frontotemporal Dementia and Alzheimer Disease*, 72 JAMA Neurology 295 (2015). Could frontotemporal dementia ever be an excusing condition for criminal responsibility? *See* R. Ryan Darby, Judith Edersheim & Bruce H. Price, *What Patients with Behavioral-Variant Frontotemporal Dementia Can Teach Us About Moral Responsibility*, 7 Am. J. Bioethics Neurosci. 193 (2016).

B. COMPETENCY, CAPACITY, AND CONSENT

This section begins with a case that examines whether a litigant retained the requisite capacity to manage his financial affairs, followed by a commentary clarifying the distinction between how "capacity" and "competency" are often used in law. We finish with a further commentary on the legal doctrine of "undue influence."

Sterling v. Sterling
194 Cal. Rptr. 3d 867 (Cal. Ct. App. 2015)

FLIER, J. In this appeal, Donald T. Sterling . . . seeks to regain ownership of the Los Angeles Clippers (Clippers), a professional basketball team Steven Ballmer purchased on August 12, 2014. . . .

FACTS AND PROCEDURE

The National Basketball Association's (NBA) April 2014 charge against Donald triggered Donald's lifetime ban from the Clippers and prompted the sale of the team. Although Donald initially authorized the sale and actively encouraged his wife Rochelle H. Sterling . . . to sell the team, he subsequently vigorously opposed it. His refusal to sign the sale agreement caused Rochelle to remove him as trustee and to file an ex parte petition in the probate court, seeking confirmation of Donald's removal as trustee and instructions relevant to the sale of the Clippers. The probate court's order following the ex parte petition is the subject of this appeal.

1. Sterling Family Trust

The Sterling Family Trust is relevant because the trust owned the Clippers and because the trust identified the circumstances justifying removal of a trustee. Donald and Rochelle established the Sterling Family Trust in 1998, identifying Donald and Rochelle as both settlors and trustees. [The] trust provided for removal of a trustee due to incapacity. Specifically, the trust provided: "Any individual who is deemed incapacitated, as defined in Paragraph 10.24., shall cease to serve as a Trustee of all trusts administered under this document." Paragraph 10.24. in turn provided: "'Incapacity' [means] incapable of managing an individual's affairs under the criteria set forth in California Probate Code § 810 et seq. An individual shall be deemed to be incapacitated if . . . two licensed physicians who, as a regular part of their practice are called upon to determine the capacity of others, and neither of whom is related by blood or marriage to any Trustee or beneficiary, examine the individual and certify in writing that the individual is incapacitated. . . ."

2. The NBA Penalized Donald

A charge before the NBA's board of governors indicated that on April 26, 2014, a tape recording of Donald's "deeply offensive, demeaning, and discriminatory views toward African Americans, Latinos, and 'minorities' in general" was made public. The NBA imposed a $2.5 million fine on Donald on April 29, 2014. It also imposed a lifetime ban against Donald from participating in the league. Subsequently, the NBA sought to terminate the Sterlings' ownership of the Clippers.

On May 9, 2014, NBA commissioner Adam Silver appointed Richard Parsons as interim chief executive officer of the Clippers. Parsons testified that if the Sterlings did not sell the Clippers, the NBA intended to remove Donald as an owner of the team. The NBA further planned to auction the team. . . .

3. Donald and Rochelle Decide to Sell the Clippers

Following the NBA's actions against Donald and its plan to auction the team, both Donald and Rochelle wanted to sell the team. On May 22, 2014, Donald's attorney wrote [with Donald's co-signature indicating his approval] commissioner Silver that "Mr. Sterling agrees to the sale of his interest in the Los Angeles Clippers." . . .

Donald instructed Rochelle to sell the team before an NBA hearing set for June 3, 2014. Rochelle obtained offers for the team and reported daily to Donald. On May 28, 2014, Donald agreed to Ballmer's offer [of $2 billion, which was $400 million more than the next highest offer]. Donald told Rochelle he was proud of her for obtaining such a good offer, exclaiming "Wow, you really did a good job."

Rochelle entered a "Binding Term Sheet" with Ballmer on May 29, 2014. On May 30, 2014, the NBA withdrew its May 19, 2014 charge and canceled the board of governors meeting set for June 3, 2014, based on the understanding that Rochelle planned to sell the Clippers to Ballmer. . . .

5. Donald Is Found to Lack Capacity to Serve as Trustee of the Sterling Family Trust

Although Donald initially wanted to sell the Clippers and congratulated Rochelle on obtaining a high bid for the team, Donald refused to sign the binding term sheet setting the terms for the sale to Ballmer. When Rochelle asked Donald to sign, Donald promised to sue.

Rochelle subsequently removed Donald as trustee in accordance with the provisions of the trust, which as noted, required certification by two physicians who regularly determine capacity.

Dr. Meril Sue Platzer, a board-certified neurologist who specialized in the detection of Alzheimer's disease, evaluated Donald. It was a regular part of her practice to determine her patients' mental capacity. After evaluating Donald, Dr. Platzer concluded: "Based upon my evaluation performed on May 19, 2014, it is my opinion that Mr. Donald T. Sterling is suffering from cognitive impairment secondary to primary dementia Alzheimer's disease." She continued: "It is my opinion that Mr. Donald T. Sterling is unable to reasonably carry out the duties as Trustee of The Sterling Family Trust as a result of, among other factors, an impairment of his level of attention, information processing, short term memory impairment and ability to modulate mood, emotional lability, and is at risk of making potentially serious errors of judgment."

Dr. Platzer testified Donald was unable to spell the word "world" backwards. When asked to subtract seven from 100, he could not perform the calculation past 93 ($100 - 7 = 93$); he could not subtract seven from 93 ($93 - 7 = 86$). Dr. Platzer testified that Donald's PET (positron-emission tomography) scan indicated he suffered from Alzheimer's disease. She concluded he suffered from Alzheimer's disease for at least three years and more likely five years. She further testified that she considered Probate Code section 811 in reaching her conclusion that Donald was unable to serve as trustee.

Dr. James Spar, a geriatric psychiatrist regularly called upon to determine capacity, also evaluated Donald. Dr. Spar concluded that Donald's performance on a battery of tests was consistent with early Alzheimer's disease or other brain disease. According to Dr. Spar: "Because of his cognitive impairment, Mr. Sterling is at risk of making potentially serious errors of judgment, impulse control, and recall in the management of his finances and his trust. Accordingly, in my opinion he is substantially unable to manage his finances and resist fraud and undue influence, and is no longer competent to act as trustee of his trust." . . .

6. Ex Parte Petition

On June 11, 2014, Rochelle brought an ex parte petition seeking a court order to confirm the sale of the Clippers and to direct the trustee under section 1310, subdivision (b) (section 1310(b)). Rochelle argued that she was the sole trustee because two physicians found that Donald lacked capacity to act as trustee.

The probate court held an eight-day hearing beginning July 7 and ending July 28, 2014. . . . The probate court's overarching conclusions were that (1) Donald was properly removed as a trustee of the Sterling Family Trust and (2) "Rochelle had authority to bind unilaterally the Sterling Family Trust . . . by executing the Binding Term Sheet, dated May 29, 2014" and agreeing to sell the Clippers to Ballmer. Invoking its authority under section 1310(b), the court instructed Rochelle to complete the sale. . . .

DISCUSSION

On appeal, Donald contends he was improperly removed as trustee of the Sterling Family Trust. [Donald Sterling made multiple arguments on appeal. Here, we focus solely on his challenge to the capacity determination.] . . .

Donald argues the record lacks substantial evidence to support the determination that he was properly removed as trustee under the terms of the trust and sections 810 and 811.6 Section 810 sets forth a rebuttable presumption of competency, and section 811 identifies grounds for finding incompetency including ability to remember, ability to modulate mood, and ability to process information.

Donald's argument that he was improperly removed as trustee is forfeited. Donald characterizes the facts directly contrary to the probate court findings. For example, the probate court concluded: "There's no credible evidence presented by Dr. [Jeffrey] Cummings [(Donald's expert)] that there is some professional duty or ethical requirement that . . . either doctor needed to advise Donald or that, in general, a doctor must advise a patient about possible legal consequences of an examination. And, in fact, credible evidence is that such warning would make someone tense and could cause negative effects on the results."

Nevertheless, Donald summarizes the evidence as follows: "Dr. Cummings testified as to the unusual circumstances surrounding the doctor's examinations, including the distractions and stress during Donald's examination and opined that there is an accepted standard of care with respect to the physician's disclosure to the patient. . . . Donald should have been told the purpose of the assessment."

Additionally, the court found: "Donald willingly participated in the evaluations by both Dr. Spar and Dr. Platzer. He testified that he agreed to be examined by them. There is no credible or compelling evidence that Donald was distracted or under stress during the evaluations by Dr. Platzer or Dr. Spar as suggested by Dr. Cummings. Dr. Cummings, called by Donald, had no facts that supported his opinion outside of the fact that he was advised the Sterlings were separated."

Nevertheless, Donald summarizes the evidence as follows: "Dr. Spar conceded that Donald was distracted and preoccupied. . . ." "During the same period of time, Donald was preoccupied by the risk of losing ownership of the Clippers as a result of actions by the NBA. Both examining doctors acknowledged that 'anxiety' could negatively affect his test performance." . . .

Assuming Donald preserved his argument, he failed to demonstrate error. The testimony of Drs. Platzer and Spar, who regularly determine capacity, amply supported the conclusion that Donald was incapable of managing his affairs under the criteria in section 811, the relevant criteria under the terms of the Sterling Family Trust. Dr. Platzer concluded that Donald had "an impairment of his level of attention, information processing, short term memory impairment and ability to modulate mood, emotional lability, and is at risk of making potentially serious errors of judgment." These were factors under section 811 supporting her determination that Donald lacked capacity. Dr. Spar concluded that "[b]ecause of his cognitive impairment, Mr. Sterling is at risk of making potentially serious errors of judgment, impulse control, and recall in the management of his finances and his trust. Accordingly, in my opinion he is substantially unable to manage his finances and resist fraud and undue influence, and is no longer competent to act as trustee of his trust." Dr. Spar expressly testified he considered section 811 and used those factors to conclude that Donald was no longer able to serve as trustee. His conclusion is consistent with the factors enumerated in section 811.

Further there was evidence that Donald's impairments correlated to his ability to act as trustee. The trustee had all powers to employ persons, pay expenses, hold, manage, and control and sell property, operate business, and borrow and lend money. The trust included ownership of the corporation that owned the stock of the Clippers. . . . Three banks held loans totaling about $480 million. Errors of judgment, impulse control and inability to recall are correlated to Donald's ability

to manage the substantial trust assets. The inability to resist fraud and undue influence also are correlated to his ability to manage these assets. Stated otherwise, there
was a clear link between the imparities Drs. Platzer and Spar found and the ability
to perform the duties of the trustee. . . .

DISPOSITION

The trial court's order is affirmed. . . .

Linda Ganzini et al.
Ten Myths About Decision-Making Capacity
6 J. Am. Med. Directors Assn. S100, S100-S101 (2005)

Autonomous choices have three central characteristics: they are adequately
informed; they are voluntary, not coerced; and they are based on reasoning. Patients
who are unable to make autonomous choices are said to lack "decision-making
capacity." . . .

Patients are presumed to have decision-making capacity. . . . In routine clinical
practice, decision-making capacity is often assessed informally or inconsistently, and
misconceptions about decision-making capacity and its assessment are surprisingly
common.

MYTH 1: DECISION-MAKING CAPACITY AND COMPETENCY ARE THE SAME

Although decision-making capacity and competency both describe patients' ability to make decisions, they are *not* synonymous. Decision-making capacity is a clinical assessment of a patient's ability to make specific healthcare decisions, whereas
competency is a legal determination of the patient's ability to make his or her own
decisions in general.

Clinicians routinely assess decision-making capacity as part of clinical care. It
can be defined as the ability "to understand and appreciate the nature and consequences of health decisions" and "to formulate and communicate decisions concerning health care." Clinicians have the *de facto*, even if not the *de jure*, power to
determine whether a patient is incapable of making healthcare decisions and, if so,
to identify a surrogate decision-maker to act on the patient's behalf.

In contrast, courts, not clinicians, determine competency. To say that a person
is incompetent indicates that a court has ruled that the person is not able to make
valid decisions and has appointed a guardian to make decisions for the person.
Competency proceedings, typically long, expensive, and emotionally charged, are
generally the last resort, often triggered when there is a dispute about decision-
making capacity (or about who should be surrogate), and typically reserved for
people who are presumed to be highly and permanently impaired. . . .

Lori A. Stiegel & Mary Joy Quinn
Elder Abuse: The Impact of Undue Influence
Nat'l Ctr. on L. & Elder Rights (2017)

[The report was prepared by the American Bar Association Commission on Law
and Aging.]

Undue influence is a psychological process that may be used against an older person as a means of committing two forms of elder abuse: financial exploitation or sexual abuse. Undue influence is also a legal concept. Case law and statutes recognize that undue influence can undermine an individual's self-determination. Civil lawsuits may result in reversal of decisions made by the individual subjected to the influence. Legal and aging network services professionals can make a significant difference to clients who are vulnerable to or who may be experiencing undue influence by recognizing it, mitigating it, and remedying it.

DEFINING UNDUE INFLUENCE

Psychological Definition

Psychologist Margaret Singer was one of the first researchers to connect elder abuse to undue influence, which she defined as "(w)hen people use their role and power to exploit the trust, dependency, and fear of others. They use this power to deceptively gain control over the decision making of the second person." The psychological tactics of undue influence have been likened to tactics used by cults, in brainwashing, by sexual abusers who "groom" their victims, and by perpetrators of domestic violence.

Legal Definitions

In the context of elder abuse, the types of decisions that may be controlled through undue influence include financial transactions and consent to sexual activity. In other words, undue influence may be used to commit financial exploitation or sexual abuse.

Both the federal Older Americans Act (OAA) and Elder Justice Act (EJA) define "exploitation" or "financial exploitation" as "the fraudulent or otherwise illegal, unauthorized, or improper act or process of an individual, including a caregiver or fiduciary, that uses the resources of an [older individual] [elder] for monetary or personal benefit, profit, or gain, or that results in depriving an older individual of rightful access to, or use of, benefits, resources, belongings, or assets."

The OAA and the EJA define "abuse" as "the knowing infliction of physical or psychological harm or the knowing deprivation of goods or services that are necessary to meet essential needs or to avoid physical or psychological harm." This definition of abuse encompasses sexual abuse.

These are national, general definitions. [Each state] has different definitions of exploitation/financial exploitation or sexual abuse. . . . Research on state laws indicates that most statutes governing probate and APS laws fail to define undue influence clearly or at all, and that most statutory definitions of the concept can be found in state business codes.

Who Commits Undue Influence

The psychological definition of undue influence implies that the influencer is someone the older adult knows and with whom the older adult already has a relationship of trust or who intentionally develops and then takes advantage of a relationship of trust with the older adult. The term "relationship of trust" is commonly used to describe the relationship an older adult has with intimate partners, relatives, paid or unpaid caregivers, friends, neighbors, clergy, and fiduciaries such as agents under a power of attorney, trustees, guardians, or conservators. The nature of the relationship between the alleged influencer and the alleged victim is, generally, crucial to assessing and proving whether undue influence has occurred. . . .

NOTES AND QUESTIONS

1. In *Sterling v. Sterling*, Donald Sterling's capacity for financial decision making was in question. Similar questions arise regularly in cases in which "testamentary capacity"—the capacity to create or change a will—is questioned. Courts face difficulty in adjudicating these cases when the alleged victim is in early stage Alzheimer's disease or experiences mild cognitive impairment (MCI). Forensic psychiatrist Judith Edersheim and colleagues note that "[d]espite the growing magnitude of these concerns, courts have not yet developed a uniform approach toward assessment of elderly people's capacities to make financial and other decisions." Consider this description of a typical case, and consider what type of approach you would recommend a court take:

> K. O. was an 89-year-old man with mild-to-moderate AD. His wife, age 83, had probable early AD. K. O. managed most financial matters without conferring with his wife or children. He engaged in estate planning for the couple of years before his cognitive decline. The children were aware of their parents' plan to leave 10 percent of their assets to deserving charities that the parents had supported in the past. After K. O.'s death, the bulk of his estate passed outright to his widow. Under the influence of a charismatic leader of a charity and in the context of continued cognitive decline, his wife altered the charitable donations to comprise 60 percent of the estate. The children voiced concerns about their mother's mental state to her primary care physician of many years, who concluded, without a formal examination, that she lacked the capacity to make changes to her estate plan. Mrs. O., upset by this opinion, had her estate attorney engage a geriatric psychiatrist, who performed a brief evaluation that consisted of a 15-minute interview without psychometric testing. The psychiatrist offered the opinion that Mrs. O. retained the capacity necessary to change her estate plan. She executed a new will, with the assistance of her estate lawyer and the encouragement of the charitable organization. She also instructed her financial advisor to "cash out" of long-term investments to make her estate more liquid for eventual distribution, generating adverse tax consequences. This will withstood subsequent antemortem and probate legal challenges. The children, who feel that their mother's fragile testamentary capacity and vulnerability to undue influence are obvious, have been frustrated by their inability to protect their mother and their inheritance.

Judith Edersheim et al., *Protecting the Health and Finances of the Elderly with Early Cognitive Impairment*, 45 J. Am. Acad. Psychiatry & L. 81, 86 (2017).

2. Elder financial fraud is a serious issue, and legislatures and regulatory bodies are responding. Congress attempted to deal with elder abuse by passing the Elder Justice Act (EJA), 42 U.S.C. §§1397j et seq. (2018). This Act, part of the Patient Protection and Affordable Care Act, contains a number of provisions designed to strengthen federal and state efforts to prevent and respond to elder abuse, neglect, and exploitation. *See* Carol V. O'Shaughnessy, *The Elder Justice Act: Addressing Elder Abuse, Neglect, and Exploitation*, Nat'l Health Pol'y Forum (Nov. 30, 2010). In addition, the U.S. Securities and Exchange Commission has taken proactive steps to improve early detection of potentially fraudulent activity. *See* Stephen Deane, *SEC, Elder Financial Exploitation: Why It Is a Concern, What Regulators Are Doing About It, and Looking Ahead* (2018). Further, the SEC approved the adoption of Financial Industry Regulatory Authority (FINRA) Rule 2165, which allows brokers to put holds on funds of a customer age 65 or older

when there is a reasonable belief of financial exploitation of that customer. An additional FINRA rule encourages brokers to make reasonable efforts to put a trusted person's contact information on file.

3. For discussion of efforts to combat financial exploitation of older adults, see Stacey Wood & Peter A. Lichtenberg, *Financial Capacity and Financial Exploitation of Older Adults: Research Findings, Policy Recommendations and Clinical Implications*, 40 Clinical Gerontologist 3 (2017) (noting that "[f]inancial exploitation is a broad term that can encompass many different behaviors" and that the "impact of age-related dementia (e.g., Alzheimer's disease) on financial capacity threatens financial autonomy.").

4. What should the role of neuroimaging evidence of dementia be in the courtroom? Consider this perspective:

> Capacity and competency are judgments based on mental states. Behavioral testing can provide valuable information regarding whether there is impairment in neuropsychological processes contributing to the mental states related to decision-making capacity. In many instances, neuroimaging research has identified specific brain regions involved in these neuropsychological processes. A controversial question becomes whether using neuroimaging evidence to show abnormal functional brain activity could therefore add value in determining medical or legal capacity.
>
> . . . [N]euroimaging findings are currently unable to aid in the clinical diagnosis in psychiatric diseases. However, in the case of persons with dementia, neuroimaging is part of routine clinical care and improves diagnostic accuracy. Current research definitions for Alzheimer's disease and frontotemporal dementia, for example, define typical behavioral syndromes as possible AD or FTD, while the presence of neuroimaging abnormalities (amyloid PET scan in AD, frontal or temporal abnormalities on MRI or PET for FTD) are necessary to diagnose probable dementia. As a patient's clinical diagnosis in dementia provides a potential causal explanation for a change in behavior, such evidence can provide additional value in specific cases. However, it is important to note that even with a behavioral profile and neuroimaging consistent with a diagnosis of dementia, assessment of a patient's decision-making related to a specific action is still necessary for medical determinations of capacity and legal determinations of competency.

R. Ryan Darby & Bradford C. Dickerson, *Dementia, Decision Making, and Capacity*, 25 Harv. Rev. Psychiatry 270, 274 (2017). *See also* Vincenzo Tigano et al., *Neuroimaging and Neurolaw: Drawing the Future of Aging*, 10 Frontiers Endocrinology 217 (2019).

5. Can a spouse with dementia ever consent to sexual intercourse with the other spouse? In 2014 a court in Iowa was presented with that question in the case of Henry and Donna Rayhons. As summarized by law professor Alexander Boni-Saenz:

> Henry Rayhons and Donna Young did not expect to find love again after being widowed. They met in their late 60s, and first flirted in church while singing for the choir. Two years later, they were getting married in front of over 350 guests. Now in their 70s, they enjoyed several activities together, such as beekeeping, farming, and long leisurely drives. They also had sex. In 2010, Donna was diagnosed with Alzheimer's Disease. As her condition worsened, two of her daughters from a previous marriage moved her to a residential care facility. Henry would regularly visit her, and on one visit in May 2014, Donna's roommate thought she heard sexual noises coming from across the privacy curtain in their shared room. This led Donna's daughters to seek guardianship over Donna and to limit Henry's

interactions with her. On August 8, 2014, Donna passed away. A week later, Henry was arrested and charged with felony sexual abuse on the basis that Donna Rayhons suffered a "mental defect" that made her unable to consent. Henry abandoned his run for another term as a state legislator, and the criminal case garnered national media attention. A week-long trial exposed details of Donna and Henry's relationship, Donna's medical condition, and their alleged sexual encounter in May. [Henry denied having sex with Donna in the nursing home, stating that they only kissed and held hands.] After two days of deliberations, the jury acquitted Henry of wrongdoing.

Alexander A. Boni-Saenz, *Sexuality and Incapacity*, 76 Ohio St. L.J. 1201, 1202-03 (2015).

How should legal doctrine handle such cases? What evidence should be relevant to these determinations? What if *both* partners in a committed relationship develop dementia? Can neither consent to sex? *See* Gayle Doll, *Dementia and Consent for Sex Reconsidered*, 12 J. Nat'l Acad. Elder L. Att'y 133 (2016). Michelle Joy & Kenneth J. Weiss, *Consent for Intimacy Among Persons with Neurocognitive Impairment*, 46 J. Am. Acad. Psychiatry & L. 286 (2018); James M. Wilkins, *More than Capacity: Alternatives for Sexual Decision Making for Individuals with Dementia*, 5 Gerontologist 716 (2015).

C. AGING OFFENDERS AND AGING JUDGES

Aging brains are not only found in probate court will contests, but throughout the legal system. In this section we explore new issues arising with aging incarcerated populations and aging judges.

1. Aging Offenders

United States v. Payton
754 F.3d 375 (6th Cir. 2014)

MERRITT, C.J. This is a direct appeal from Arthur Payton's sentence to serve 45 years in prison for organizing a series of bank robberies in Michigan. Payton argues that his sentence is unreasonable. We agree, vacate his sentence, and remand.

I.

Arthur Payton is a serial bank robber with a specific *modus operandi*. He would find an accomplice, usually a woman, and usually a woman addicted to drugs or engaged in prostitution. He would convince this accomplice to rob a bank on his behalf in exchange for a cut of the proceeds. He would provide this accomplice with a costume, a threatening note to give to the teller, bags, a toy gun, and everything else needed for the robbery. He would perform the necessary reconnaissance, and both drop off and pick up his accomplice.

Payton was caught in this scheme several times. The first time, when Payton was 26 years old, he was caught, tried, and convicted for six bank robberies—one personally while armed with a weapon, the other five he robbed with his preferred accomplice method. Payton was sentenced to ten years in prison and was released on January 24, 2002, only to be arrested later that year for robbing seven more banks using his accomplice method. Payton, then 35 years old, admitted his involvement in the robberies and was again sentenced to ten years in prison. He was released on July 29, 2011, only to be arrested again later that year for robbing four more banks. This third, final spree concerns us now. Payton, 45 years old at the time of his trial, maintained his innocence and was convicted on all counts.

Payton turned 46 years old before his sentencing hearing. Taking into account Payton's criminal record, the seriousness of his crime, and penchant for recidivism, the presentence report recommended a sentence within the Guidelines range of 210 to 262 months, or between 17 and a half to 22 years. Neither party objected to the presentence report, and the district court found the report accurate. The government urged the sentencing court to impose a more serious sentence of "at least" 300 months, or 25 years. Payton's counsel requested a sentence within the Guidelines range, arguing that even with a Guidelines sentence Payton would be released as an elderly man—somewhere between 63 to 68 years old—who would present little threat to the public.

After hearing each side, the judge sentenced Payton to 540 months, or 45 years in prison. The judge discussed a number of the sentencing factors listed in 18 U.S.C. § 3553(a), focusing on Payton's brazen recidivism and the threat he posed to the public. The court concluded that the 45 year sentence was "the minimum sentence" that was "reasonable and sufficient but not greater than necessary to accomplish the goals of sentencing for this defendant." When prompted, Payton's counsel objected to the sentence above the Guidelines and the government said nothing. The district court responded "All right," and concluded the hearing without further discussion. Payton now appeals, arguing that his sentence is unreasonable.

II.

"[W]e review sentences for reasonableness." *United States v. Camacho–Arellano*, 614 F.3d 244, 246 (6th Cir. 2010). A district judge has wide discretion in sentencing those convicted, and assessing the reasonableness of a judge's sentence on appeal is a multifaceted and often flummoxing task. However, the Supreme Court has made clear that "a district judge must give serious consideration to the extent of any departure from the Guidelines and must explain his conclusion that an unusually lenient or an unusually harsh sentence is appropriate in a particular case with sufficient justifications." *Gall v. United States*, 552 U.S. 38, 46, 128 S. Ct. 586, 169 L.Ed.2d 445 (2007). While a sentence outside the guidelines is not presumptively unreasonable, we must consider "the extent of the deviation and ensure that the justification is sufficiently compelling to support the degree of the variance." *Gall*, 552 U.S. at 51, 128 S. Ct. 586. As the Supreme Court put it, "a major departure should be supported by a more significant justification than a minor one," id, or as we have put it, "the greater the district court's variance, the more compelling the evidence must be." *United States v. Robinson*, 669 F.3d 767, 775 (6th Cir.2012). . . .

III.

Payton's 45 year sentence is a "major departure," "unusually harsh," and one that demands a "significant explanation." *Gall*, 552 U.S. at 51, 128 S.Ct. 586. A sentence that more than doubles the Guidelines recommendation, stacks twenty years on to the government's request, and keeps the defendant in prison until he is ninety one years old requires explanation about why such a sentence is "sufficient, but not greater than necessary" to achieve the goals of sentencing. 18 U.S.C. § 3553(a).

We find the district court's explanation lacking in Payton's case. At minimum, the court failed to adequately respond to Payton's argument that his advanced age diminishes the public safety benefit of keeping Payton in prison an extra twenty years beyond the recommendation of the Guidelines. Even presuming Payton's desire to rob banks is insatiable, as the government argues, Payton contends that age will diminish his very ability to rob banks. This argument attacks the foundations of the government's support for the imposed sentence, and the court's reasoning that the threat posed by a sixty-eight-year-old Payton makes a longer sentence not simply prudent but necessary.

The Sentencing Commission has observed that "[r]ecidivism rates decline relatively consistently as age increases." . . . Both the Guidelines and our Circuit's cases explicitly acknowledge that a defendant's age, and specifically old age, is a relevant consideration in sentencing. . . . Studies indicate that neurotransmitters affecting aggression supplied at the synapses of brain neurons vary based on age, and may explain the observed decline in recidivism among older prisoners. Such evidence, together with statistical support, suffices to require a sentencing judge to explain carefully why a criminal defendant like Payton remains likely to engage in violent robberies between the age of seventy and ninety. The district court did not address Payton's argument on this issue, and therefore did not provide an adequate explanation for imposing such a harsh sentence.

Certainly one can infer from the judge's disbelief that Payton could or would change his ways that the court considered and rejected Payton's age argument. But an empty record allows one to draw the opposite inference as well—that the judge made his decision without adequately considering the personal and individualized circumstances that determine when a sentence is sufficient but not greater than necessary. This is why we require the sentencing judge to explain his or her reasoning, on the record thoroughly addressing all relevant issues, to facilitate our review.

IV.

Payton's sentence is VACATED, and we REMAND for further proceedings consistent with this opinion.

Madison v. Alabama
139 S. Ct. 718 (2019)

Justice KAGAN delivered the opinion of the Court. The Eighth Amendment . . . prohibits the execution of a prisoner whose mental illness prevents him from "rational[ly] understanding" why the State seeks to impose that punishment. In this case, Vernon Madison argued that his memory loss and dementia entitled him to a stay of execution, but an Alabama court denied the relief. We now address two questions relating to the Eighth Amendment's bar. . . . First, does the Eighth Amendment forbid execution whenever a prisoner shows that a mental disorder has left him without any memory of committing his crime? We (and, now, the parties) think not, because a person lacking such a memory may still be able to form a rational understanding of the reasons for his death sentence. Second, does the Eighth

Amendment apply similarly to a prisoner suffering from dementia as to one experiencing psychotic delusions? We (and, now, the parties) think so, because either condition may—or, then again, may not—impede the requisite comprehension of his punishment. The only issue left, on which the parties still disagree, is what those rulings mean for Madison's own execution. . . .

I

A

This Court decided in *Ford v. Wainwright*, 477 U.S. 399 (1986), that the Eighth Amendment's ban on cruel and unusual punishments precludes executing a prisoner who has "lost his sanity" after sentencing. While on death row, Alvin Ford was beset by "pervasive delusion[s]" associated with "[p]aranoid [s]chizophrenia." Surveying both the common law and state statutes, the Court found a uniform practice against taking the life of such a prisoner. Among the reasons for that time-honored bar, the Court explained, was a moral "intuition" that "killing one who has no capacity" to understand his crime or punishment "simply offends humanity." Another rationale rested on the lack of "retributive value" in executing a person who has no comprehension of the meaning of the community's judgment. The resulting rule, now stated as a matter of constitutional law, held "a category of defendants defined by their mental state" incompetent to be executed.

The Court clarified the scope of that category in *Panetti v. Quarterman* by focusing on whether a prisoner can "reach a rational understanding of the reason for [his] execution." Like Alvin Ford, Scott Panetti suffered from "gross delusions" stemming from "extreme psychosis." In reversing a ruling that he could still be executed, the Panetti Court set out the appropriate "standard for competency." *Ford*, the Court now noted, had not provided "specific criteria." But Ford had explored what lay behind the Eighth Amendment's prohibition, highlighting that the execution of a prisoner who cannot comprehend the reasons for his punishment offends moral values and "serves no retributive purpose." Those principles, the Panetti Court explained, indicate how to identify prisoners whom the State may not execute. The critical question is whether a "prisoner's mental state is so distorted by a mental illness" that he lacks a "rational understanding" of "the State's rationale for [his] execution." Or similarly put, the issue is whether a "prisoner's concept of reality" is "so impair[ed]" that he cannot grasp the execution's "meaning and purpose" or the "link between [his] crime and its punishment."

B

Vernon Madison killed a police officer in 1985 during a domestic dispute. An Alabama jury found him guilty of capital murder, and the trial court sentenced him to death. He has spent most of the ensuing decades on the State's death row.

In recent years, Madison's mental condition has sharply deteriorated. Madison suffered a series of strokes, including major ones in 2015 and 2016. He was diagnosed as having vascular dementia, with attendant disorientation and confusion, cognitive impairment, and memory loss. In particular, Madison claims that he can no longer recollect committing the crime for which he has been sentenced to die.

After his 2016 stroke, Madison petitioned the trial court for a stay of execution on the ground that he had become mentally incompetent. . . . And in a later filing, Madison emphasized that he could not "independently recall the facts of the offense he is convicted of." . . . Alabama countered that Madison had "a rational understanding of [the reasons for] his impending execution," as required by *Ford* and *Panetti*, even assuming he had no memory of committing his crime. . . . And more broadly, the State claimed that Madison could not possibly qualify as incompetent under those two decisions because both "concerned themselves with '[g]ross delusions' "—which all agree Madison does not have. . . .

Expert reports from two psychologists largely aligned with the parties' contending positions. Dr. John Goff, Madison's expert, found that although Madison "underst[ood] the nature of execution" in the abstract, he did not comprehend the "reasoning behind" Alabama's effort to execute him. Goff stated that Madison had "Major Vascular Neurological Disorder"—also called vascular dementia—which had caused "significant cognitive decline." And Goff underscored that Madison "demonstrate[d] retrograde amnesia" about his crime, meaning that he had no "independent recollection[ ]" of the murder. For his part, Dr. Karl Kirkland, the court-appointed expert, reported that Madison "was able to discuss his case" accurately and "appear[ed] to understand his legal situation." Although Kirkland acknowledged that Madison's strokes had led to cognitive decline, see id., at 10, the psychologist made no mention of Madison's diagnosed vascular dementia. Rather, Kirkland highlighted that "[t]here was no evidence of psychosis, paranoia, or delusion."

At a competency hearing, Alabama similarly stressed Madison's absence of psychotic episodes or delusions. The State asked both experts to affirm that Madison was "neither delusional [n]or psychotic." . . . On the State's view, that fact answered the competency question because "[t]he Supreme Court is looking at whether someone's delusions or someone's paranoia or someone's psychosis is standing in the way of" rationally understanding his punishment. Madison's counsel disputed that point . . . [arguing instead that under Panetti] the Court there barred executing a person with any mental illness—"dementia" and "brain injuries" no less than psychosis and delusions—that prevents him from comprehending "why he is being executed."

The trial court [sided with the State's reasoning and] found Madison competent to be executed. . . . [Madison attempted to find habeas relief based on the Antiterrorism and Effective Death Penalty Act of 1996 (AEDPA), but that appeal failed.]

When Alabama set an execution date in 2018, Madison returned to state court to argue again that his mental condition precluded the State from going forward. In his petition, Madison reiterated the facts and arguments he had previously presented to the state court. But Madison also claimed that since that court's decision (1) he had suffered further cognitive decline and (2) a state board had suspended Kirkland's license to practice psychology, thus discrediting his prior testimony. Alabama responded that nothing material had changed since the court's first competency hearing. . . . A week before the scheduled execution, the state court again found Madison mentally competent. . . .

Madison then filed in this Court a request to stay his execution and a petition for certiorari. We ordered the stay on the scheduled execution date and granted the petition a few weeks later. . . .

II

Two issues relating to *Panetti's* application are before us. Recall that our decision there held the Eighth Amendment to forbid executing a prisoner whose mental illness makes him unable to "reach a rational understanding of the reason for [his] execution." The first question presented is whether *Panetti* prohibits executing Madison merely because he cannot remember committing his crime. The second question raised is whether *Panetti* permits executing Madison merely because he suffers from dementia, rather than psychotic delusions. In prior stages of this case, as we have described, the parties disagreed about those matters. But at this Court, Madison accepted Alabama's position on the first issue and Alabama accepted Madison's on the second. And rightly so. As the parties now recognize, the standard set out in Panetti supplies the answers to both questions. First, a person lacking memory of his crime may yet rationally understand why the State seeks to execute him; if so, the Eighth Amendment poses no bar to his execution. Second, a person suffering from dementia may be unable to rationally understand the reasons for his sentence; if so, the Eighth Amendment does not allow his execution. What matters is whether a person has the "rational understanding" Panetti requires—not whether he has any particular memory or any particular mental illness.

A

Consider initially a person who cannot remember his crime because of a mental disorder, but who otherwise has full cognitive function . . . is the failure to remember committing a crime alone enough to prevent a State from executing a prisoner?

It is not, under *Panetti's* own terms. That decision asks about understanding, not memory—more specifically, about a person's understanding of why the State seeks capital punishment for a crime, not his memory of the crime itself. And the one may exist without the other. Do you have an independent recollection of the Civil War? Obviously not. But you may still be able to reach a rational—indeed, a sophisticated—understanding of that conflict and its consequences. Do you recall your first day of school? Probably not. But if your mother told you years later that you were sent home for hitting a classmate, you would have no trouble grasping the story. And similarly, if you somehow blacked out a crime you committed, but later learned what you had done, you could well appreciate the State's desire to impose a penalty. Assuming, that is, no other cognitive impairment, loss of memory of a crime does not prevent rational understanding of the State's reasons for resorting to punishment. . . .

But such memory loss still may factor into the "rational understanding" analysis that Panetti demands. If that loss combines and interacts with other mental shortfalls to deprive a person of the capacity to comprehend why the State is exacting death as punishment, then the Panetti standard will be satisfied. . . .

B

Next consider a prisoner who suffers from dementia or a similar disorder, rather than psychotic delusions. The dementia, as is typical, has compromised this prisoner's cognitive functions. But it has not resulted in the kind of delusional beliefs that Alvin Ford and Scott Panetti held. May the prisoner nonetheless receive a stay of execution under Ford and Panetti? Or instead, is a delusional disorder a prerequisite to declaring a mentally ill person incompetent to be executed? We did not address that issue when we last considered this case, on habeas review; in that sense, the question is one of first impression.

But here too, Panetti has already answered the question. Its standard focuses on whether a mental disorder has had a particular effect: an inability to rationally understand why the State is seeking execution. Conversely, that standard has no interest in establishing any precise cause: Psychosis or dementia, delusions or overall cognitive decline are all the same under Panetti, so long as they produce the requisite lack of comprehension . . . most important, Panetti framed its test . . . in a way utterly indifferent to a prisoner's specific mental illness. The Panetti standard concerns, once again, not the diagnosis of such illness, but a consequence—to wit, the prisoner's inability to rationally understand his punishment. . . .

In evaluating competency to be executed, a judge must therefore look beyond any given diagnosis to a downstream consequence . . . delusions come in many shapes and sizes, and not all will interfere with the understanding that the Eighth Amendment requires. And much the same is true of dementia. That mental condition can cause such disorientation and cognitive decline as to prevent a person from sustaining a rational understanding of why the State wants to execute him. But dementia also has milder forms, which allow a person to preserve that understanding. Hence the need—for dementia as for delusions as for any other mental disorder—to attend to the particular circumstances of a case and make the precise judgment Panetti requires.

III

[The Court then discussed how this ruling applied to the present case, and returned the] case to the state court for renewed consideration of Madison's competency . . . ensuring that if he is to be executed, he understands why.

We accordingly vacate the judgment of the state court and remand the case for further proceedings not inconsistent with this opinion.*

2. Aging Judges

Theile v. Michigan
891 F.3d 240 (6th Cir. 2018)

DONALD, C.J. Plaintiff-Appellant, the Honorable Michael J. Theile ("Theile"), is a Michigan state-court judge. In 2020, the year of the next election for the seat he now holds, Theile will be 71 years of age. Because the Michigan Constitution and the relevant Michigan statute prohibit a person who has attained the age of 70 from being elected or appointed to judicial office, Theile will not be eligible to run for re-election. See Mich. Const. art. VI, § 19(3); Mich. Comp. Laws § 168.411. Asserting that this age limitation under Michigan law violates the Equal Protection Clause of the United States Constitution, Theile asks this Court to dispense with rational-basis review of age-based classifications, and instead adopt intermediate scrutiny—a level of review he contends Michigan's judicial age restriction cannot withstand. In the alternative, Theile argues that even under rational-basis review, the Michigan age restriction fails to pass constitutional muster.

For the reasons set forth herein, we AFFIRM the judgment of the district court granting Defendants-Appellees' motion to dismiss Theile's complaint.

---

* [At age 69, Vernon Madison died on in February 2020 at Holman Prison in Atmore, Alabama.—EDS.]

I

Theile is a judge in the Family Division of the Genesee County Circuit Court in Michigan. Theile was appointed to the bench in November 2005, retained his seat by election in 2006, and was re-elected in 2008 and 2014. The next election for his seat will take place on November 3, 2020.

Under the Michigan Constitution, "[n]o person shall be elected or appointed to a judicial office after reaching the age of 70 years." Likewise, the applicable Michigan statute provides, in relevant part, that "[a] person shall not be eligible to the office of judge of the circuit court unless . . . , at the time of election, [the person] is less than 70 years of age." Theile will be 71 years of age on the date of the next election, and is therefore ineligible to run. Theile declares that, "[i]f allowed by a change in the law, . . . he will run for reelection on November 3, 2020."

On June 26, 2017, Theile filed a single-count complaint in United States District Court for the Eastern District of Michigan, alleging that Michigan's constitutional and statutory age limitation on judges violates the Equal Protection Clause of the United States Constitution. . . . Michigan's judicial age limitation, Theile alleges, discriminates based on a characteristic that, "like gender, is . . . immutable" and thus "deserves heightened scrutiny." In the alternative, Theile asserts, the age limitation cannot even survive rational basis review, because it is "no longer rationally related to a legitimate government interest."

Thereafter, Defendants-Appellees filed a motion to dismiss . . . [and] cited *Gregory v. Ashcroft*, 501 U.S. 452 (1991), where the Supreme Court upheld a like age limitation, and *Breck v. Michigan*, 203 F.3d 392 (6th Cir. 2000), where this Court upheld the Michigan age restriction at issue here. . . .

The district court determined that controlling Supreme Court and Sixth Circuit precedent foreclosed Theile's claim. . . .

II

We review de novo a district court's dismissal of a complaint under Rule 12(b)(6). . . .

III

It is undisputed by the parties that age classifications are generally subject to rational-basis review. That standard places a heavy burden on Theile to "show there is no rational basis" for the classification; by the same token, Defendants "need not offer any rational basis so long as this Court can conceive of one."

While not entirely escaping discriminatory treatment, the aged "have not experienced a history of purposeful unequal treatment." Age, therefore, is not a suspect classification, and "rationality is the proper standard by which to test" an age limitation under the Equal Protection Clause. The Supreme Court has repeatedly reaffirmed the standard.

Because the law is concededly settled as to the applicable standard of review, we are called upon to decide whether an exception to the foundational doctrine of stare decisis is justified. . . . In arguing for breaking with precedent as to the applicable standard of review, Theile posits the "similar[ity]" of "stereotyping and discrimination" directed at women and older persons. . . . Ultimately, Theile fails to marshal "the most convincing of reasons" showing that adhering to precedent here "puts us on a course that is sure error." This Court will therefore not disturb the settled precedent of the Supreme Court and of the Sixth Circuit mandating rational-basis review for age-based classifications.

IV

We now turn to the substantive question of whether Michigan's judicial age limitation passes muster under the applicable standard—rational-basis review. Theile argues forcefully that the rule is "capricious, unjustified and irrational." He points out that after mandatory retirement, judges often serve as visiting judges, receivers, arbitrators, and in other important legal roles. He also notes that Michigan imposes no age limit on its governor or state legislators, and that the United States Supreme Court, the federal judiciary, the Presidency, and Congress have no age limits. On the basis of these and similar facts, Theile asserts that "[i]f there were any decent rationale to Michigan's age-limiting laws," the exceptions he alludes to would not exist. However, that Michigan's legislature and the Congress have not seen fit to impose age restrictions for the offices referred to, does not demonstrate that "no rational basis" can be conceived for the restriction here challenged.

This Court recognizes, as did the district court, Theile's "eloquen[ce]" in arguing against age limitations for judges. Indeed, the district court "did not take issue" with several of Theile's points, among them that federal judges face no age limits, that eighteen states have no mandatory judicial retirement age, and that many U.S. Supreme Court justices serve past the age of 70. One may well sympathize with Theile's assertions that the age 70 limit is "archaic," and that "it is wrong indiscriminately to put people to pasture." But "[r]ational basis review does not assess the wisdom of the challenged regulation." Rather, the scrutiny required here demands no more than "a state of facts that provide a conceivable basis for the classification."

There is no way around it: this Court has upheld the very age restrictions Theile challenges. Breck, 203 F.3d at 397 (finding Michigan's judicial age limitation "rationally related to preserving the competency of the judiciary" and "promoting judicial efficiency and reducing partisan appointments of judges," among other state purposes). . . . Equally inescapable is the Supreme Court's upholding of a materially identical age limitation. Gregory, 501 U.S. at 471-72, 111 S.Ct. 2395 (holding Missouri's judicial age limitation of 70 rationally related to such legitimate purposes as avoiding laborious testing of older judges' physical and mental acuity, promoting orderly attrition of judges, and recognizing that judges' remoteness from public view makes determination of competency, and removal from office, more difficult than for other office-holders).

Theile contends that "the laws and facts have changed so significantly in the decades since these decisions . . . that the[ir] reasoning" is now unsound. Longer life expectancy, the increased vitality of the elderly, and the other sweeping societal changes Theile points to have unfolded over some hundred years, but Gregory was decided only twenty-seven years ago, and Breck a mere eighteen. Those opinions found multiple rational bases for judicial age limitations. While the contrary arguments may have considerable force, we find no basis to conclude that the reasoning of Gregory and Breck has somehow been overtaken by interceding events and rendered invalid. Those precedents stand, and this Court is bound by them.

V

For the foregoing reasons, we AFFIRM the judgment of the district court granting Defendants-Appellees' motion to dismiss.

Francis X. Shen

Aging Judges

81 Ohio St. L.J. 235, 241-70 (2020)

[T]he federal judiciary is . . . getting older. . . . Today, the average age of Article III judges is sixty-nine years old, the highest it has ever been. . . . The average retirement age for most Americans is between sixty-two and sixty-four years old. The average age of Article III judges is sixty-nine. Clearly, federal judges prefer to keep working than to retire. . . .

As the Federal Judicial Center observes, "In recent decades, many federal judges have assumed senior status even though eligible for full retirement. This trend may help account for the growing proportion of judges whose terms have ended in death rather than resignation or retirement." . . .

[S]ome judges will experience normal cognitive aging, and that some judges will experience either mild cognitive impairment or some form of more progressive dementia.

RESPONDING TO JUDICIAL COGNITIVE DECLINE

Concerns over mentally incompetent judges have been recognized since the time of the country's founding, and a variety of solutions have been implemented to address these concerns. . . .

Public allegations of the mental incompetence of judges are rare, but this "reveal[s] little about the true extent of the problem" because there has traditionally been a taboo on openly discussing the issue of declining capacity of fellow judges. Indeed, in 1971, the Supreme Court chided a Circuit Court for broaching "so delicate a subject" when the Circuit Court raised concerns about the mental competence of a state court judge in a published opinion. However, judges have since noted that "[w]e have come a long way from the day when discussion of a judge's mental state was considered a breach of decorum."

[There are . . .] several (non-mutually exclusive) avenues by which the challenge of cognitively impaired judges can be addressed within the current system: (1) create incentives for the judge to voluntarily choose retirement, (2) involuntarily remove the judge on the basis of disability pursuant to 28 U.S.C.A. § 372; (3) file a formal complaint under the Judicial Conduct and Disability Act; (4) pursue post-hoc relief via a due process claim; and (5) apply informal pressures to encourage the judge to retire. The available evidence suggests that option #5, informal mechanisms, remains the primary method by which most issues are resolved. . . .

[I]n practice it is informal approaches by which most judicial disability issues are addressed. This use of informal mechanisms is grounded in historical practice. As described in one study, these informal methods can require significant effort:

Chief Judge Charles Clark [on the Fifth Circuit] used an assortment of techniques to induce three chief district judges then in their mid-80s to step down from their administrative posts. He applied pressure on one judge's secretary, while in another case he made "use of a sort of high-grade blackmail," by threatening "that the Bar Association was going to take the matter to the newspapers." The entire proceeding is tortuous. One chief judge recalled it as being "rather unpleasant, both for the person who goes to see the aged judge and . . . for the aged judge himself." So the Sixth Circuit Council had discovered in the Underwood affair. But, the chief judge declared: "We kept after him, and the largest newspaper in Ohio with statewide circulation published some accounts concerning the way he was handling his work, and he finally called me up and said his name had been 'dragged down in the mud far enough,' and that he would retire, and he did retire." Charles Gardner Geyh, *Informal Methods of Judicial Discipline*, 142 U. Pa. L. Rev. 243, 284 (1993) (quoting Peter Graham Fish, The Politics of Federal Judicial Administration 416 (1973)).

There is a legitimate debate about the effectiveness of these informal mechanisms. For instance, when the issue of mandatory retirement ages for federal judges was debated several decades ago, Judge Irving Kaufman wrote in the Yale Law Journal that the problem of failing judicial health "can almost always be managed effectively in a personal and informal manner. On occasion, close colleagues of an afflicted judge suggest that he retire. If necessary, other judges, attorneys, and even family members may approach the ailing jurist. Almost invariably he will acquiesce."

The informal policing system relies on individual judges to (1) recognize their own impairments and (2) take appropriate steps to leave the bench. But in the general population, individuals often underestimate their cognitive decline, and this happens to judges as well. Absent concrete evidence clearly showing the decline, the chief judge, family, and friends must often rely on arm-twisting. . . .

Whether it is because the judge doesn't recognize his/her own decline, because he/she wishes to stay despite the impairments, or for some other reason, there are examples of judges who continued to serve even though their cognition had significantly declined. The most extensive evidence comes from David Garrow's treatment, in which he concludes that "the history of the Court is replete with repeated instances of justices casting decisive votes or otherwise participating actively in the Court's work when their colleagues and/or families had serious doubts about their mental capacities."

Episodes of note include the following: . . .

- Justice Stephen Field's (1863-1897) "mental condition was in noticeable decline . . . [and] the other justices decided Field should be urged to resign." But even with the urging of Justice John Marshall Harlan, Justice Field refused to resign until 1897.
- Justice Joseph McKenna's (1898-1925) "mental alertness began to decline," but he did not resign. As a result, in 1924 the remaining members of the Court decided "that no case would be decided because of McKenna's vote."
- Justice Oliver Wendell Holmes retired only after Justice Hughes brought to his attention that his colleagues thought it best that he retire. David Garrow rightly observes that "even what may have been the single most distinguished career in the entire history of the United States Supreme Court ended in an explicitly requested retirement because of increasing mental decrepitude."
- Justice Marshall's final years included embarrassing mistakes during an oral argument that gained national attention.

• Justice William O. Douglas experienced a stroke on December 31, 1974 and did not fully recover. Douglas "repeatedly addressed people at the Court by their wrong names, often uttered nonsequiturs in conversation or simply stopped speaking altogether." But rather than leave the court, he stayed, and the rest of the court (with the exception of Byron White) agreed that they would not allow Douglas to render votes.

Examples such as these have led some commentators to call for reform in judicial terms and retirement. . . .

NOTES AND QUESTIONS

1. Policymakers are aware of the growing challenge of an incarcerated population that is aging. It is both costly and logistically challenging to meet the medical needs of older inmates. *See* Kimberly A. Skarupski et al., *The Health of America's Aging Prison Population*, 40 Epidemiologic Revs. 157 (2018); Adonis Sfera et al., *Neurodegeneration Behind Bars: From Molecules to Jurisprudence*, 5 Frontiers Psychiatry 115 (2014). One proposed solution to this challenge takes the form of "compassionate release" laws, which provide some limited opportunities for old persons and terminally ill offenders to leave prison. *See* Tina Maschi et al., *Analysis of US Compassionate and Geriatric Release Laws: Applying a Human Rights Framework to Global Prison Health*, 1 J. Hum. Rts. & Soc. Work 165 (2016).

2. Assume that in *Thiele* the court had applied heightened scrutiny to the Michigan statute and constitution mandating a judicial retirement age. Would the outcome be different?

3. With regard to federal judges, how would you recommend addressing the challenge of an aging judiciary? Are term limits best? Mandatory retirement ages? Or should judges continue to retain power over their retirement decisions? Some circuits are now pursing Judicial Wellness initiatives, providing education and counseling to judges on the possibility of mental decline and other matters. Wellness Committees have now been established in the First, Third, Fifth, Ninth, and Tenth Circuits. In describing the rationale for the Wellness Committee, Ninth Circuit chief judge Phyllis Hamilton observed: "We're an organization that is required to police ourselves. . . . If we wish to retain the goodwill and confidence of the public in our ability to render justice by judges who are unimpaired . . . , we have to take steps." Quoted in Sudhin Thanawala, *9th Circuit Addresses Senility Among Federal Judges Head On*, AP News (Nov. 7, 2015).

4. In medicine, the issue of older physicians is emerging and in law, so too is the issue of aging attorneys. *See* Katrina A. Armstrong & Eileen E. Reynolds, *Opportunities and Challenges in Valuing and Evaluating Aging Physicians*, 323 JAMA 125 (2020); Anothai Soonsawat et al., *Cognitively Impaired Physicians: How Do We Detect Them? How Do We Assist Them?*, 26 Am. J. Geriatric Psychiatry 631 (2018); Daniel C. Marson, *Assessment of the Cognitively Impaired Senior Attorney: Conceptual and Clinical Aspects*, 1 Innovation Aging 718 (2017). Should the approach to older professionals be different in medicine and law? What about older professors? Or older politicians? On this last point, see *Dementia and Democracy: America's Aging Judges and Politicians*, Mass. Gen. Hosp. Ctr. for L. Brain & Behav. (Dec. 19, 2017),

https://clbb.mgh.harvard.edu/dementiaanddemocracy. See also Jalayne J. Arias et al., *Legal and Policy Challenges to Addressing Cognitive Impairment in Federal Officials,* 76 JAMA Neurology 392 (2019).

D. LEGAL IMPLICATIONS OF BIOMARKERS FOR DEMENTIA

Francis X. Shen
Aging Judges
81 Ohio St. L.J. 235, 239-56 (2020)

In the past two decades, there have been "revolutionary changes in dementia research and practice, with a growing array of imaging and fluid biomarkers taking center stage in diagnostic evaluation and monitoring of progression."[6] . . .

In 2004, the Alzheimer's Disease Neuroimaging Initiative (ADNI) was formed to develop a range of biomarkers—including imaging, genetic, and biochemical markers—for the early detection and monitoring of AD. For clinicians, this early detection can help facilitate prevention or help slow the disease's progression.

. . . In 2012, the Food and Drug Administration (FDA) approved an imaging technique that uses positron emission tomography (PET) scanning with the radioactive tracing compound Florbetapir F-18 to identify the accumulation of amyloid-β (Aβ) plaques, which are believed to play a central role in AD.

In addition, the National Institute of Aging and the Alzheimer's Association have worked over the past decade to better define and identify the preclinical (i.e. without symptoms) stages of AD. In 2011, the working group "created separate diagnostic recommendations for the preclinical, mild cognitive impairment, and dementia stages of Alzheimer's disease." In 2018, on the basis of on-going neuroscience research, the same working group published a landmark paper in which they proposed a diagnosis of AD that was "not based on the clinical consequences of the disease (i.e., symptoms/signs)," but which "shifts the definition of AD in living people from a syndromal to a biological construct." The proposed "research framework focuses on the diagnosis of AD with biomarkers in living persons." Specifically, AD would require a finding of both Aβ plaques and pathologic tau deposits.

More broadly, the framework introduced an "Alzheimer's continuum," which would include both those with Alzheimer's Disease (i.e. those with the established biomarkers) and those in the category of "Alzheimer's pathologic change," an "early stage of Alzheimer's continuum, defined in vivo by an abnormal Aβ biomarker with normal pathologic tau biomarker." Notably, and important for the analysis to follow in the judicial context, under this framework an individual (such as a judicial nominee) could be both symptom free and diagnosed as being on the Alzheimer's continuum.

Under the new framework, for many individuals there will be a lengthy (15-20 years) period of brain change without symptoms. As lead author Clifford Jack observed: "In every other area where biomarkers exist—hypertension, diabetes, cancer—the disease identified in an asymptomatic individual is still the disease. If

---

6. Bradford C. Dickerson, *Neuroimaging, Cerebrospinal Fluid Markers, and Genetic Testing in Dementia,* in *Dementia: Comprehensive Principles and Practice* 528, 531 (Bradford C. Dickerson & Alireza Atri, eds., 2014).

cancer is detected on a screening colonoscopy, it's still cancer, even if the person doesn't have symptoms."

The transition from symptom-based to biologically-based detection of AD offers clinicians an opportunity to intervene earlier in the progression of the disease. The proposed framework would fundamentally change the definition of AD; not surprisingly, it has been heavily debated.

In the excerpts below, we present some of the legal and regulatory challenges that will emerge from the early identification of AD in asymptomatic individuals.

Jalayne J. Arias & Jason Karlawish
Confidentiality in Preclinical Alzheimer Disease Studies: When Research and Medical Records Meet
82 Neurology 725, 726-28 (2014)

Health, life, and long-term care insurers may have an interest in using biomarkers in underwriting practices. Current legal mechanisms are not sufficient to protect subjects enrolled in research on the basis of biomarkers or genetic markers from discrimination by insurers. Beginning in 2014, the Patient Protection and Affordable Care Act (ACA) will prohibit health insurers from discriminating against an individual based on a preexisting condition. Whether these provisions will prevent discrimination against individuals with preclinical AD, a condition that has yet to be clinically validated, is uncertain. An additional provision prohibits health insurers from discriminating against individuals based on their participation in medical research. To qualify for protections under this provision, the clinical trial must be an investigation to prevent, detect, or treat cancer or "another life-threatening disease or condition." The provision goes on to define "life-threatening disease or condition" as "any disease or condition from which the likelihood of death is probable unless the course of the disease or condition is interrupted." AD is life-threatening, but it is unclear whether AD is within the intention of the definition. Additionally, the protections do not prohibit discrimination based on the disclosure of information gathered during research, but merely discrimination based on enrollment. . . .

There are no protections under the ACA relevant to long-term care or disability insurance. At its passage, the ACA included the Community Living Assistance Services and Supports (CLASS) Act.7 This provision sought to create an option for individuals to purchase long-term care insurance through a public option. Under the CLASS Act, individuals would have been able to buy into a long-term care insurance plan even if they had preexisting conditions. The CLASS Act was, however, repealed in early 2013. As a result, the ACA fails to protect research subjects from discrimination by long-term care insurers or provide additional options for those who seek to purchase long-term care insurance once learning that they test positive for AD biomarkers. . . .

The potential protections under the Americans with Disabilities Act (ADA) may provide sufficient protections to limit discrimination by employers. However, the definition of "disability" has never been tested in case law relating to protecting asymptomatic individuals with disease biomarkers. . . . Until case law or the Equal

Employment Opportunity Commission provides explicit guidance specific to bio-markers, a gap in protection remains for individuals enrolled in studies whose employers learn their research information. . . .

Jalayne J. Arias et al.

The Proactive Patient: Long-Term Care Insurance Discrimination Risks of Alzheimer's Disease Biomarkers

46 J.L. Med. & Ethics 485, 485-97 (2018)

Biomarkers provide information that can help individuals and families prepare for future cognitive and functional impairment, including planning for long-term care [services] and supports (LTSS) needs. Insurers could also use this informa-tion to make discriminatory and adverse underwriting decisions based on a risk for Alzheimer's disease. These potential risks raise novel legal and policy challenges. . . .

[Our] study found that state laws were substantially consistent with the NAIC Long-Term Care Insurance Model Act. Using the Model Act as a proxy for state laws, the study found that Alzheimer's disease biomarkers likely meet the definition of "preexisting condition." Additionally, investigators determined that preexisting condition laws would assure coverage for LTSS related to Alzheimer's disease, if an individual application is approved. However, individuals would not be protected from adverse medical underwriting decisions based on biomarker status. As a result, we concluded that protections provided by the NAIC Model Act and states laws were not meaningful. . . .

This gap in anti-discrimination protections indicates that reevaluation of under-writing standards are needed to promote access to LTC insurance, as promoted by the NAIC Model Act. We propose that future research develop amendments to the NAIC Long-term Care Insurance Model Act as a catalyst for changes in state legal standards. . . .

Betsy J. Grey

Aging in the 21st Century: Using Neuroscience to Assess Competency in Guardianships

2018 Wis. L. Rev. 735, 766-74 (2018)

THE IMPACT OF AD BIOMARKERS ON CAPACITY ASSESSMENT AND GUARDIANSHIP DECISIONS

The law traditionally relies on changes in observed behavior before it acts, so the availability of biomarker evidence, and its ability to look at brain states, has the potential to unsettle all kinds of legal assessments. The potential impact could include competency assessments in guardianship proceedings, which, in line with the traditional view, generally rely upon behavioral data such as performance-based tests and clinical observation to determine whether the law should act to remove an individual's decision making authority. Because the statutory schemes governing these assessments were enacted well before biomarker research in this area advanced, they do not anticipate use of biomarker evidence or documenta-tion of brain states of AD. Use of AD biomarkers in capacity assessments has not yet been introduced in court, so it is unclear how biomarker evidence will affect these determinations.

Several challenges lie ahead. First and foremost, should the law even consider biomarker evidence of AD, most especially pre-behavioral symptomatology, in this context, or would its consideration be antithetical to our conceptions of competency? Even if it does allow consideration, the use of markers would have to pass evidentiary muster; establishing the probity of tests indicating a higher probability for developing or having AD will present significant evidentiary and interpretive challenges. If biomarker diagnostic evidence does not come into evidence directly, either because its consideration would be impermissible under the statutory scheme, would not pass evidentiary standards, or fundamentally would violate due process concerns, we need to anticipate that its availability will likely have indirect effects, both positive and negative, on the guardianship decision. . . .

[B]iomarker diagnostics have the potential to spark a paradigm shift in the way we look at the competency determination. Biomarker evidence may move the legal system to redefine the binary choice between competent and incompetent in a demented patient. As use of biomarker diagnostics of dementia becomes generally accepted in the medical community, and the medical community becomes more sensitive to the view of AD as a spectrum, the ability to detect changes in brain states may argue in favor of a guardianship model that includes legal protections for those who do not yet meet the legal threshold for incompetence. As Professor Jalayne Arias advocates, we may need to recognize a "gap" category to protect individuals with declining capacity, but who do not yet meet the criteria for incompetency. Biomarkers will become part of the inquiry to identify individuals along the spectrum of AD. In this context, even pre-behavioral symptomatic biomarker evidence may be useful for screening purposes. It may assist in reinforcing the need for a clinical assessment and provide a quick and efficient way to identify individuals whom we should examine more carefully for "quasi" competency under this gradient model.

Finally, biomarker evidence will provide an additional baseline to measure the progression of the disease, allowing us to reach back earlier in the continuum of the multiple stages of AD. A baseline enhances scientific rigor in determining when the loss of capacity likely has occurred, helping to avoid an approach of "I know it when I see it." The availability of additional empirical measurements for baselines will be particularly important with individuals with mild cognitive impairment, the period with the most variation. Different individuals decline at different rates, and biomarker identification will help track the rate of decline more accurately. Not only will this help give precision to when a guardianship is appropriate, it can also help determine its scope. . . .

RISKS OF BIOMARKER DIAGNOSTICS USAGE

As we gain confidence in biomarker diagnostics and prognostics, the availability of the evidence may prove to be a double-edged sword; increased use of biomarker diagnostics poses significant risks. Even if biomarker diagnostics are not admitted into evidence, their availability increases the potential for misrepresentation and manipulation. Would family members press an individual not to contest guardianship proceedings after brain alterations are identified or a genetic predisposition found, but while the individual still thinks he is competent? Would members of a family-run business take advantage of the biomarker findings to pressure the individual to turn to surrogate decision-making? Courts will need to take precautions to guard against these undue influences and new potential for elder abuse and financial exploitation once biomarkers come into the picture. . . .

The biggest challenge with biomarker evidence may be to guard against undue consideration of biomarker evidence when behavioral symptoms are manifesting at their earliest stages. We need to proceed slowly and cautiously in introducing these test results, especially as we shift our view of AD from staged to a continuum. Under all these scenarios, however, it is important to resist the imposition of de facto categorical rules on the significance of biomarker findings. We do not want incapacity to be defined by a diagnosis of AD based solely on biomarker evidence; nor do we want it to be ignored. . . .

Joshua Preston et al.

The Legal Implications of Detecting Alzheimer's Disease Earlier

18 AMA J. Ethics 1207, 1208-14 (2016)

DETERMINING THE LEGAL RELEVANCE OF INCREASED RISK FOR AD

Most bodies of law—including tort, contracts, and criminal law—have traditionally demanded outwardly manifested behavior as a prerequisite for legal recognition of physical injury. The advent of Alzheimer's biomarkers thus poses a conundrum: how should the law treat a person who does not exhibit behavioral symptoms but whose brain is documented to have already altered in such a way as to suggest a higher likelihood of AD?

Consider, for instance, the following hypothetical situation involving a 50-year-old man named John, someone with no significant medical history. Let us assume the FDA approves a neuroimaging technique that allows physicians to diagnose people as being at an elevated risk of developing AD. Although John is well below the average age at which AD symptoms typically appear (age 65), he tests positive for the brain AD biomarker. What happens next?

For social security disability benefits, it is unclear if the positive biomarker result will matter (at least under current law). Currently, the Social Security Administration (SSA) provides disability benefits to applicants who demonstrate early-onset AD. . . . The regulations emphasize that "clinical information documenting a progressive dementia is critical and *required* for disability evaluation of early-onset AD." In our hypothetical case, John's clinical record does not include behavioral manifestations of the disease. That is, John's brain is altered in ways that suggest he will develop AD, but John is not yet consciously aware of experiencing memory loss.

Should disability benefits always require clinical manifestations? . . . How should the law treat a healthy person with a not-so-healthy brain?

The question will arise not only in disability and insurance law, but also in core legal domains such as contracts, torts, and criminal law. In each domain, issues of "capacity," "competency," and liability may be affected by AD biomarkers. . . .

It is unclear how long it will take for brain biomarkers of AD to develop and how much longer still until we have more effective clinical treatments for AD. But it is not too early for the legal system to begin thinking carefully about how it will respond.

NOTES AND QUESTIONS

1. As brain biomarkers become more prominent in diagnosis of Alzheimer's disease and other types of dementia, more individuals will want access to brain scans. This means that Medicare and private insurance companies will increasingly need to determine whether they will reimburse such requests. In 2016 the U.S. Court of Appeals for the District of Columbia remanded a decision by the Centers for Medicare and Medicaid Services (CMS) denying coverage of beta-amyloid positron emission tomography scans ("BA scans") after a September 2012 determination that "the then-existing medical and scientific evidence did not support a finding that BA Scans are reasonable and necessary for the diagnosis of an illness." CMS's decision was supported by a finding that these scans did not improve "health outcomes of patients exhibiting cognitive impairment or informed the management of such patients' diseases." But the court determined that CMS's decision was arbitrary and capricious due to an inconsistency between its decision not to cover BA scans and a prior decision allowing coverage of FDG PET scans, a diagnostic tool used "to differentiate between patients suffering from frontotemporal dementia and Alzheimer's." Specifically, the court found that (1) "[b]oth are diagnostic tests that involve the use of a PET scan and a radiopharmaceutical tracer"; (2) "[b]oth are indicated for use on overlapping patient populations exhibiting symptoms of cognitive impairment"; (3) "both have diagnostic value as a tool for differentially diagnosing patients"; and (4) "neither test has demonstrated effectiveness in terms of improving health outcomes or altering patient management." Importantly, the court did not establish that patients had a right to Medicare coverage of either BA scans or FDG PET scans, but rather remanded the decision for the CMS to evaluate whether the varying coverage decisions could be reconciled. *See Kort v. Burwell*, 209 F. Supp. 3d 98 (D.D.C. 2016).

2. One of the most hotly contested debates concerning aging and cognitive decline concerns the revocation of driving privileges. As one insurance company brochure tells its customers, "It's difficult to decide when someone with dementia should stop driving, since you need to balance safety considerations with the person's sense of independence, pride and control. Most information about dementia warns against driving, but doesn't help you determine when it should stop." The Hartford Ctr. for Mature Mkt. Excellence, *At the Crossroads: Family Conversations About Alzheimer's Disease, Dementia & Driving* (2013). Should policymakers revoke driving privileges for anyone who is diagnosed with Alzheimer's disease? Should all drivers over age 65 retake driving tests? *See* Sokratis G. Papageorgiou et al., *Does the Diagnosis of Alzheimer's Disease Imply Immediate Revocation of a Driving License?*, 3 Int'l J. Clinical Neurosci. & Mental Health S02 (2016) (noting that "loss of driving privileges can lead to an increase in the levels of depressive symptoms, thus compromising the psychological health of this group of individuals" and that "the restriction or total loss of driving privileges is a complicated and serious decision that should not be taken without the active participation of a well-trained Neurologist and Neuropsychologist with deep understanding of the information provided by neurological and neuropsychological measures that are linked to driving fitness according to accumulating findings of previous research.").

3. Neuroscience research is indicating that altered brain activation observed with functional imaging and the early pathological changes in the medial temporal lobe can distinguish incipient dementia from normal aging. Lieke H. Meeter et al., *Imaging and Fluid Biomarkers in Frontotemporal Dementia*, 13 Nature Revs. Neurology 406 (2017). When should such imaging be used to inform policy?

4. Many research studies are underway to examine the neurobiological changes associated with Alzheimer's disease. To date, the conventional practice in the Alzheimer's Disease Neuroimaging Initiative (ADNI) is not to return any neuroimaging results to research participants. But a survey of ADNI researchers found that the field is "experiencing tremendous flux" and that a majority of researchers would support return of some results if evidence-based guidelines could be developed. Melanie B. Shulman et al., *Using AD Biomarker Research Results for Clinical Care: A Survey of ADNI Investigators*, 81 Neurology 1114 (2013). At present, guidelines for return of brain imaging research results do not exist. What policies would you recommend for return of results?

FURTHER READING

On the Aging Brain:

Mark S. Lachs & S. Duke Han, *Age-Associated Financial Vulnerability: An Emerging Public Health Issue*, 163 Annals Internal Med. 877 (2015).

The Aging Brain: Functional Adaptation Across Adulthood (Gregory R. Samanez-Larkin ed., 2019).

Gregory R. Samanez-Larkin, *Financial Decision Making and the Aging Brain*, 26 APS Observer 30 (2013).

Gregory R. Samanez-Larkin & Brian Knutson, *Decision Making in the Ageing Brain: Changes in Affective and Motivational Circuits*, 16 Nature Revs. Neurosci. 278 (2015).

Bruce A. Yankner, Tao Lu & Patrick Loerch, *The Aging Brain*, 3 Ann. Rev. Pathology 41 (2008).

On Elder Law, Legal Doctrine, and State Laws:

Ray D. Madoff, *Unmasking Undue Influence*, 81 Minn. L. Rev. 571 (1997).

Philip C. Marshall & Mary Joy Quinn, *Undue Influence Revisited, Voice Experience*, Am. Bar Ass'n Chicago (May 30, 2017).

Shelly L. Jackson, *Senate Special Committee on Aging Hearings and GAO Reports*, in *Elder Abuse: Research, Practice and Policy* 595 (XinQi Dong, ed. 2017).

The National Elder Law Foundation, *https://www.nelf.org*.

On Forensic, Psychological, and Psychiatric Assessment:

Am. Bar Assn./Am. Psychological Assn. Assessment of Capacity in Older Adults Project Working Grp., *Assessment of Older Adults with Diminished Capacity: A Handbook for Psychologists* (2008).

Eric Y. Drogin & Curtis L. Barrett, *Evaluation for Guardianship* (2010).

Peter A. Lichtenberg, *Financial Exploitation, Financial Capacity, and Alzheimer's Disease*, 71 Am. Psychologist 312 (2016).

Daniel C. Marson, *Assessing the Competency of Patients with Alzheimer's Disease Under Different Legal Standards: A Prototype Instrument*, 52 Archives Neurology 949 (1995).

Jennifer Moye, Daniel C. Marson & Barry Edelstein, *Assessment of Capacity in an Aging Society*, 68 Am. Psychologist 158 (2013).

Mary Joy Quinn et al., *Developing an Undue Influence Screening Tool for Adult Protective Services*, 29 J. Elder Abuse & Neglect 157 (2017).

On Elder Financial Fraud:

Jalayne J. Arias, *A Time to Step In: Legal Mechanisms for Protecting Those with Declining Capacity*, 39 Am. J.L. & Med. 134 (2013).

David Burnes et al., *Prevalence of Financial Fraud and Scams Among Older Adults in the United States: A Systematic Review and Meta-Analysis*, 107 Am. J. Pub. Health e13 (2017).

Nat'l Ctr. for State Courts, Ctr. for Elders and the Courts, *http://www.eldersandcourts.org*.

U.S. Dep't of Justice, Elder Justice Initiative, *https://www.justice.gov/elderjustice*.

U.S. Gov't Accountability Office, GAO-17-33, *Elder Abuse: The Extent of Abuse by Guardians Is Unknown, but Some Measures Exist to Help Protect Older Adults* (2016).

PART 5

THE FUTURE

Part 4 explored core themes at the intersection of law and neuroscience. In Part 5, we look to the future, exploring complex legal, ethical, and policy issues raised by the trajectory of neuroscientific and engineering advances. What new legal challenges will such advances entail? And how will legal systems adapt, respond to, regulate, prohibit, facilitate, or engage with these new technologies on the rapidly approaching horizon?

As you read this Part, keep in mind that today's most prominent lawyers, legislators, policy-makers, and judges sat where you are now sitting before there were home computers, phone answering machines, or CDs—let alone smart phones, flat-screen TVs, the Internet, Facebook, YouTube, robot vacuum cleaners, Adderall, unmanned drones, or cyber-attacks.

Your turn is coming, for you are the lawyers, legislators, policy-makers, and judges of the future. Neuroscientists will continue to make unexpected discoveries, and engineers will continue to make amazing tools. Engaging with the issues you are presented with in this course can help prepare you not only for the neurolaw challenges of tomorrow, but also for the many broader societal changes that you will face in your lives.

PART SUMMARY

This Part:

- Considers, in Chapter 19, scientific, legal, and ethical debates related to Cognitive Enhancement.
- Introduces, in Chapter 20, innovative new Brain-Machine Interface technology and the law's response.
- Explores, in Chapter 21, the frontiers of Artificial Intelligence and the Law.

Cognitive Enhancement

Man is not going to wait passively for millions of years before evolution offers him a better brain.

—Corneliu Giurgea[†]

The original purpose of medicine is . . . to heal the sick, not to turn healthy people into gods.

—Francis Fukuyama[††]

CHAPTER SUMMARY

This chapter:
- Discusses the challenge of defining normal and abnormal, and distinguishing treatment from enhancement.
- Explores how neuroscience-informed methods of cognitive enhancement raise questions for law and regulation, with special focus on the use of drugs and devices to enhance academic performance.
- Raises a series of ethical questions prompted by advances in cognitive enhancement.

INTRODUCTION

Have you ever worked with a tutor to enhance your knowledge of a particular subject area? Have you had a cup of coffee or an energy drink (or Ritalin) to stay awake at night? These, and countless other examples, are all ways in which you can enhance some aspect of your cognitive functioning. Today, these lifestyle interventions are generally socially accepted. So too is the most important enhancer of all: formal education and training. Indeed, you are required by law to enhance your mental faculties starting at an early age, and society rewards those who study longer and pursue higher education opportunities.

If these approaches are acceptable, and even desirable, then should we think any differently about newer forms of enhancement? If a medical treatment happens to also benefit healthy individuals, should we consider the intervention a "treatment" or an "enhancement"? Where should the line between these classifications be drawn? Of course, this question cannot be answered without first answering

---

[†] Quoted in Martha J. Farah, *The Unknowns of Cognitive Enhancement*, 350 Science 379, 379 (2015).
[††] Francis Fukuyama, *Our Posthuman Future: Consequences of the Biotechnology Revolution* 208 (2002).

another: What is "normal"? And will "normal" change with the advent of new direct brain interventions? Questions like this have spawned much scholarship, and the launch of a dedicated *Journal of Cognitive Enhancement* in 2017. The journal's coverage explores enhancement through "meditation, video games, smart drugs, food supplements, nutrition, brain stimulation, neurofeedback, physical exercise, music, cognitive training and beyond."

Movies such as *Limitless* premise a future in which a small pill allows one to achieve almost limitless learning and memory ability. Fiction is becoming reality. In 2013 *New York Magazine* profiled Wall Street trader and venture capitalist Peter Borden.* In an effort to improve his productivity and work more effectively on less sleep, Borden began taking modafinil (a drug approved by the FDA to treat narcolepsy). The result? Borden reported, "I didn't take as many breaks; I didn't get as frustrated; the stuff came out with fewer errors." But when Borden forgot to take the medicine, he felt the downside: ". . . It was sort of like being thrust into dirty, messy reality, as opposed to a clean, neatly organized place. It was like crashing, and I actually found what would happen is the anxiety that got dialed down on the way in, when you were coming off it, all of a sudden you went through the reverse. . . ." *New York Magazine* reports that Borden stopped taking the drug and turned to meditation instead, but that he "remains a little in awe of the pill."

Borden isn't the only one. In 2018 Netflix released the documentary *Take Your Pills*, showing how some college students are now routinely using Adderall and other stimulants—often to enhance performance. Tim Ferriss, famous for his best-selling book, *The 4-Hour Workweek*, has tried a range of drugs to improve performance. As the subtitle of a feature in *Wired* magazine summed up: "Professional guinea pig Tim Ferriss raids the medicine cabinet to become superhuman."** Ferriss reports that he's taken desmopressin to improve reading speed and memory skills; phenylpiracetam to improve cold tolerance; galantamine to run faster; and selegiline to ward off the effects of aging on sex drive.

Others are similarly experimenting with drugs to improve their performance. Prescriptions for drugs that affect cognitive functioning, such as modafinil and Adderall, have risen steadily. This has led to a number of new labels entering the lexicon: neuroenhancement, neural (or cognitive or neurocognitive) enhancement, cosmetic neurology, and brain boosting. The terminology may be different, but the purpose is the same: to improve the cognitive functioning of otherwise healthy individuals.

It is not yet clear how the medical and legal communities will respond. For the medical community, neurologist Anjan Chatterjee, who coined the term "cosmetic neurology," observes that "[t]here are no guidelines, nor much tradition to guide physicians. . . . We don't have a clue what neurologists, psychiatrists, and primary care physicians are doing. . . ."***

The legal response is similarly unknown. Hence, this chapter explores the implications of these new technologies. Section A addresses the question, what, exactly,

---

* Robert Kolker, *The Real Limitless Drug Isn't Just for Lifehackers Anymore*, N.Y. Mag. (Mar. 29, 2013).
** Peter Rubin, *Better, Faster, Smarter*, Wired (Dec. 2012).
*** Ricki Lewis, *Neural Enhancement: A Slippery Slope for Neurologists*, Psychiatric Times (Mar. 31, 2006).

is "enhancement"? Section B reviews the efficacy and safety of some popular neurocognitive enhancements. Section C presents opposing viewpoints on the use of drugs and other direct brain interventions to improve cognitive functioning. Section D concludes with a survey of ethical issues raised by cognitive enhancement and summarizes recommendations of national panels.

A. DEFINING ENHANCEMENT

Nick Bostrom & Anders Sandberg
Cognitive Enhancement: Methods, Ethics, Regulatory Challenges
15 Sci. & Eng'g Ethics 311, 311-13 (2009)

Cognitive enhancement may be defined as the amplification or extension of core capacities of the mind through improvement or augmentation of internal or external information processing systems. . . .

External hardware and software supports now routinely give human beings effective cognitive abilities that in many respects far outstrip those of biological brains.

Cognition can be defined as the processes an organism uses to organize information. This includes acquiring information (perception), selecting (attention), representing (understanding) and retaining (memory) information, and using it to guide behavior (reasoning and coordination of motor outputs). Interventions to improve cognitive function may be directed at any one of these core faculties.

An intervention that is aimed at correcting a specific pathology or defect of a cognitive subsystem may be characterized as therapeutic. An enhancement is an intervention that improves a subsystem in some way other than repairing something that is broken or remedying a specific dysfunction. In practice, the distinction between therapy and enhancement is often difficult to discern, and it could be argued that it lacks practical significance. For example, cognitive enhancement of somebody whose natural memory is poor could leave that person with a memory that is still worse than that of another person who has retained a fairly good memory despite suffering from an identifiable pathology, such as early-stage Alzheimer's disease. A cognitively enhanced person, therefore, is not necessarily somebody with particularly high (let alone super-human) cognitive capacities. A cognitively enhanced person, rather, is somebody who has benefited from an intervention that improves the performance of some cognitive subsystem without correcting some specific, identifiable pathology or dysfunction of that subsystem.

The spectrum of cognitive enhancements includes not only medical interventions, but also psychological interventions (such as learned "tricks" or mental strategies), as well as improvements of external technological and institutional structures that support cognition. A distinguishing feature of cognitive enhancements, however, is that they improve core cognitive capacities rather than merely particular narrowly defined skills or domain-specific knowledge.

Most efforts to enhance cognition are of a rather mundane nature, and some have been practiced for thousands of years. The prime example is education and training, where the goal is often not only to impart specific skills or information, but also to improve general mental faculties such as concentration, memory, and critical thinking. Other forms of mental training, such as yoga, martial arts, meditation, and creativity courses are also in common use. Caffeine is widely used to improve alertness. Herbal extracts reputed to improve memory are popular, with sales of Ginko biloba alone in the order of several hundred million dollars annually in the U.S. In an ordinary supermarket there are a staggering number of energy drinks on display, vying for consumers who are hoping to turbo-charge their brains.

Education and training, as well as the use of external information processing devices, may be labeled as "conventional" means of enhancing cognition. They are often well established and culturally accepted. By contrast, methods of enhancing cognition through "unconventional" means, such as ones involving deliberately created nootropic drugs,* gene therapy, or neural implants, are nearly all to be regarded as experimental at the present time. Nevertheless, these unconventional forms of enhancements deserve serious consideration for several reasons:

- They are relatively new, and consequently there does not exist a large body of "received wisdom" about their potential uses, safety, efficacy, or social consequences;
- They could potentially have enormous leverage (consider the cost-benefit ratio of a cheap pill that safely enhances cognition compared to years of extra education);
- They are sometimes controversial;
- They currently face specific regulatory problems, which may impede advances; and
- They may eventually come to have important consequences for society and even, in the longer run, for the future of humankind. . . .

Kirsten Brukamp

Better Brains or Bitter Brains: The Ethics of Neuroenhancement

in *Cognitive Enhancement: An Interdisciplinary Perspective* 99, 101-102

(Elisabeth Hildt & Andreas G. Franke eds., 2013)

Enhancement comprises strategies to improve one's bodily appearance or functioning by medical means, although the client is healthy and not considered a patient. [. . .] Given that potential options for neuroenhancement are still in development, two preliminary ways of classification currently make sense:

---

* [According to Dr. Corneliu E. Giurgea, who coined the term, a "nootropic" is "a . . . drug which acts directly on the higher integrative brain mechanisms, by enhancing their efficacy, therefore resulting in a positive, direct impact on mental . . . functions." A nootropic drug . . . "(a) facilitates learning acquisition and enhances resistance to learning impairments due to different causes . . . ; (b) facilitates interhemispheric transfer of information . . . ; enhances cerebral resistance, as seen by using other than . . . criteria (EEG, convulsions, pathology, survival), to different aggressions (hypoxia, experimental high-altitude, barbiturate and other chemical intoxications); strengthens, in appropriate conditions, the tonic cortical "control" upon subcortical CNS levels; [and] even in very high dosages . . . induces no behavioral (sedation or stimulation) electrophysiological (EEG; reticular or limbic excitability) or autonomic significant changes and is devoid of toxicity even with long-term administration." Corneliu Giurgea, *The Pharmacology of Nootropic Drugs: Geropsychiatric Implications*, in *Neuro-Psychopharmacology: Proceedings of the Tenth Congress of the Collegium Internationale Neuro-Psychopharmacologicum* 67, 67-68 (Pierre Deniker ed., 1978).—EDS.]

1. *Functions*: Neuroenhancement may be geared towards diverse functions of the brain. In particular, the following pursuits are feasible:
   1.1. *Cognitive enhancement*: Its goal is to improve wakefulness, attention, concentration, intelligence, memory, and executive functions. Examples for medication candidates include methylphenidate, modafinil, anti-dementia medication, and amphetamine derivatives.
   1.2. *Mood enhancement*: Its aim is to brighten emotional states. Examples are selective serotonin reuptake inhibitors (SSRIs), such as fluoxetine.
   1.3. *Moral enhancement*: It is meant to improve social behavior [by increasing] a subject's empathy for others. Candidates include oxytocin and methylene-dioxymethamphetamine (MDMA), the latter of which possesses an additional mood enhancement component. Nevertheless, at present, medical knowledge is insufficient to precisely utilize potential moral enhancers for this particular purpose. Therefore, moral enhancement to improve social behavior remains speculative overall.
   1.4. *Various effects*: Moreover, some neurotropic medications have been noted to lead to extraordinary sensory impressions and transient feelings of pleasure. Others increase the pain threshold in healthy individuals. Many medications that act on the central nervous system may be regarded as neuroenhancers depending upon the purpose and the context in which they are used.
2. *Methods*: Neuroenhancement may involve varying techniques and devices. Only a subset of them is debated because of moral concerns. In a broad sense, the term "neuroenhancement" also refers to such innocuous methods as sufficient sleep, adequate nutrition, physical exercise, the use of mnemonic techniques, and brain training. Since these methods cause no or few moral problems, they are neglected in the ethical discussion. However, the moral issues of the following types of neuroenhancement in the narrow sense have been recognized:
   2.1. *Pharmacological enhancement*: At the present time, the use of medication remains the most frequent strategy for attaining neuroenhancement. The drugs utilized either originate from medication intended for therapeutic purposes, or they stem from illegal substances.
   2.2. *Non-invasive technology*: An enhancement potential may exist for transcranial stimulation techniques that are currently in development, such as transcranial magnetic stimulation (TMS) or transcranial direct current stimulation (tDCS).
   2.3. *Implanted technology*: Neuroenhancement might also involve invasive technology in the future, e.g. in the format of brain implants. . . .

I. Glenn Cohen
What (If Anything) Is Wrong with Human Enhancement? What (If Anything) Is Right with It?
49 Tulsa L. Rev. 645, 646-51 (2014)

I. A TAXONOMY OF ENHANCEMENT

[I]t useful to map out what form enhancement might take and some key distinctions that may be relevant as we think about what, if anything, the law should say about enhancement.

a. Biological vs. Non-Biological Enhancement:

When people speak about enhancement, many people think of biological enhancement. But it is unclear whether there is anything distinctive, from a moral or legal point of view, between biological enhancements and non-biological enhancements. A good example of a non-biological enhancement discussed in the literature is all forms of learning or training, such as LSAT tutoring for prospective law school applicants. While this is a line traditionally offered in the literature on enhancement, one might wonder whether learning really is, deep down, actually a biological enhancement—when we learn our brains change, there is no other way to learn except the alteration of our biology. One can parse the matter by suggesting that what we really mean by "biological enhancement" is "enhancement that directly alters our biology rather than alters that biology indirectly," but as we seek to alter the language to be more precise the attractiveness of this as a moral or legal line to draw becomes, at least to me, increasingly suspect.

In any event, let us imagine, *dubitante*, that this line can really be drawn. Within the non-biological category, some non-biological enhancements will take the form of "add-ons" rather than alterations. For example, the new Google Glass might be thought of as a kind of enhancement that allows the user to see things and access information that he might not already have access to. At some point, the line between a non-biological enhancement versus an adjunct technology will be blurred. I do not think there is a single right answer as to where to draw that line; instead such line-drawing heavily depends on the particular moral concern motivating the inquiry. . . .

One interesting implication of these distinctions is that the regulatory regime that currently exists focuses quite a lot on biological enhancement and almost not at all on non-biological enhancements. Google Glass, and many other possible technological enhancements, falls flatly outside of the regulation of FDA or any other agency that would give serious thought to its enhancement capabilities. By contrast, attempts to alter our brains or our bodies at the biological level are regulated by FDA rules about drugs and devices, rules about the use of stem cells in certain states or countries or some institutions, and the tort system on the back end through medical malpractice. Drawing the line this way might make a lot of sense if we thought that biological enhancements were particularly dangerous, raised particularly difficult ethical practices, etc. Perhaps there is something about the invasiveness of drugs and implantable devices, or their nature as credence goods that might lead us to believe this is (in general true) on the safety side. On the ethics side, though, it seems to me that Google Glass and its like is just as likely to have profound effects on our society raising difficult ethical questions (relating to surveillance, what it means to constantly be networked) than, for example, the use of Human Growth Hormone. . . .

Within the category of biological enhancements, we can usefully distinguish:

i. Genetic enhancements vs. non-genetic biological enhancements

In the second category would be getting breast augmentation or reduction, using Ritalin or another ADHD medication for help on the SATs, using beta-blockers before an Olympic pistol shooting competition . . . .

A separate set of distinctions has to do with whom is doing the enhancing and when.

b. Choosing for Ourselves vs. Choosing for Others Who Cannot Choose for Themselves:

One could choose to enhance oneself, for example choosing to take anabolic steroids or to get cosmetic surgery. One could also choose to enhance others who cannot make a choice for themselves. Children are the most important members of this latter category. Here we should draw a further distinction when it comes to choosing for others:

i. Enhancing after birth vs. enhancing before birth

[I]t may matter for ethical analysis whether enhancement takes place after versus before birth. . . . Among pre-birth interventions we should draw still another distinction:

1. Enhancing by selection vs. enhancing by manipulation of already fertilized embryos or implanted fetuses

In enhancing by selection, one tries to influence the traits one's child will exhibit (i.e., its phenotype) by making decisions about the child's genotype. . . . A different kind of selection would be in choosing for implantation between numerous pre-embryos that prospective parents have already fertilized as part of In Vitro Fertilization.

Both of these are to be contrasted with post-conception but pre-birth manipulation. Though mostly hypothetical at the moment, this could take the form of genetic exploitation of an already fertilized embryo and/or surgical interventions on already implanted fetuses in order to achieve desired traits or avoid undesired ones.

c. Enhancements Compatible with Expanding Life Plans vs. Enhancements That Will Limit Options

Some enhancements are "swiss army knives" in that they can improve the prospects for a child, whatever the child chooses to do with his life. . . . By contrast, other enhancements will serve to close off certain life plans while they improve the chances in others. An enhancement in height may improve the chance that a child will play in the NBA, but decrease the chance that they will be able to serve on a submarine.

[T]his is best thought of as a continuum, with a sense of how many options are being foreclosed for the sake of a particular enhancement.

Another set of distinctions relates to how much enhancement is taking place and of what kind:

d. Reversible vs. Irreversible Enhancement

This distinction is actually more of a continuum. On the one extreme, genetic enhancement through selection generates what we would think of as an irreversible enhancement. . . . On the other extreme, there are enhancements that are easily undone. . . .

A further distinction has to do with how enhancement relates to particular baselines.

e. Enhancement vs. Treatment (?)

Some would draw distinctions between "treatment" to correct disease or disability as opposed to enhancement to make people "better than well." Some defend this as an important distinction. . . .

There is also a more subtle version of this distinction that is sometimes drawn in the literature:

    i. Enhancements to the upper bounds of what people already have vs. enhancements that add beyond human nature as it now stands

Under this distinction it would be permissible to enhance one's height to that of the tallest individual in one's society, but no further. Similarly, it would be permissible to extend one's life to the longest reported length, but no further. . . . This principle establishes a "ceiling effect," which partially solves a problem I will discuss just below relating to positional goods.

f. Enhancements for Absolute vs. Positional Goods

Some goods (such as being tall) are beneficial primarily in a positional sense — they are desirable to have only because others lack them. By contrast, other goods — for example immunity to disease — are primarily absolute goods, in the sense that one would want to have the enhancement even if everyone were to have it. . . . [D]etermining just how much a particular trait is valued for positional as opposed to absolute value may be quite difficult (and/or costly). . . .

NOTES AND QUESTIONS

1. How would you define "normal"? For example, what is the normal, or average, body temperature? You most likely believe the correct answer is 98.6°F (37°C). This was the average value of a million measurements of body temperature from 25,000 individuals by a physician 150 years ago. Would it surprise you to learn that average body temperature today is 97.5°F? A recent study of historical trends found that body temperature in men and women has decreased by 0.03°C per decade of birth? Myroslava Protsiv et al., *Decreasing Human Body Temperature in the United States Since the Industrial Revolution*, 9 eLife e49555 (2020). Questions about what is "normal" also necessarily require definition of the comparison group. For instance, it's normal for a 35-year-old man to be taller than five feet. This is not normal for a six-year-old.

2. How would you define "enhancement"? Which of the following are enhancements under your definition: lifting weights to improve strength for athletics, physical therapy to regain leg strength after an injury, drinking alcohol in order to feel less inhibited at a party, taking an over-the-counter medication to improve sleep, brushing your teeth, learning a foreign language; training for a marathon, and taking an LSAT prep course?

3. In 2012, neuroscientists published a study finding that connections in the brain can be affected by an intensive LSAT prep course. Allyson P. Mackey, Kirstie J. Whitaker & Silvia A. Bunge, *Experience-Dependent Plasticity in White Matter Microstructure: Reasoning Training Alters Structural Connectivity*, 6 Frontiers Neuroanatomy 32 (2012). Subsequent research has replicated finding changes in the brain associated with changes in learned abilities and measures of IQ. Miguel Burgaleta et al., *Cognitive Ability Changes and Dynamics of Cortical Thickness Development in Healthy Children and Adolescents*, 84 NeuroImage 810 (2014). Does revealing the brain science behind LSAT preparation affect your evaluation of LSAT preparation as an enhancement? Why or why not?

4. When would enhancing fail to enhance? As Professor Cohen suggests, some enhancements (like better health) are absolute enhancements because one lives a healthier life even if everyone else gets the same enhancement. But other enhancements, such as being able to study better for a standardized test graded on a curve relative to other students' performance, only help if others don't have access to the same enhancement. Beyond policing safety and efficacy of methods, what role does law have in regulating access to and use of these different types of enhancements?

5. "Should there be a constitutional right to cognitive enhancement?" Law professor Marc Blitz argues that ". . . if, as the Supreme Court has said, constitutional 'liberty presumes' and protects 'an autonomy of self,' then there is a strong case to be made that individuals are engaging in a key exercise of such autonomy when they use modern technology to reshape their thinking processes." If a state imposed regulations on cognitive enhancement, how might such a constitutional challenge play out? *See* Marc Jonathan Blitz, *A Constitutional Right to Use Thought-Enhancing Technology*, in *Cognitive Enhancement: Ethical and Policy Implications in International Perspectives* 293, 293-94 (Veljko Dubljević & Fabrice Jotterand eds., 2016).

6. In addition to better memories, what about better *morals*? There is emerging debate about the use of drugs and devices to improve humans' moral decision-making. *See, e.g.,* Thomas Douglas, *Moral Enhancement*, 25 J. Applied Phil. 228 (2008); G. Owen Schaefer & Julian Savulescu, *Procedural Moral Enhancement*, 12 Neuroethics 73 (2019). Could evidence of moral enhancement have legal relevance? Consider this hypothetical, posed by philosopher John Shook and neuroscientist Jim Giordano:

> [A] hypothetical person P was provided with a [cognitive enhancer] CE, which dramatically reduces the likelihood of choosing to indulge in aggressive or abusive conduct. P has been using CE as supervised by a competent clinician. On a certain day, P is arrested for getting into a violent fight and is accused of instigating the violence. The legal defense for P argues during the trial that, in light of conflicting witnesses and ambiguous evidence about who started the violence (e.g., no video surveillance), the additional fact that P was properly using the CE should be admitted as evidence tending to show that P was probably not the instigator. . . . Should P's use of CE be admitted as evidence under such circumstances? If admitted, how should the evidence be presented/explained to the jury? Are any special jury instructions needed for their deliberations? And if P is convicted on some charge, should the same evidence be available for sentencing deliberations? . . .

John R. Shook & James J. Giordano, *Moral Bioenhancement for Social Welfare: Are Civic Institutions Ready?*, 2 Frontiers Sociology 21 (2017).

B. DOES ENHANCEMENT WORK?

Debates over the ethics of enhancement rest in large part on efficacy—both real and perceived—of enhancers. In this section, we review emerging research on the effectiveness and known side effects of some techniques currently available for enhancing brain function.

Irena P. Ilieva, Cayce J. Hook & Martha J. Farah
Prescription Stimulants' Effects on Healthy Inhibitory Control,
Working Memory, and Episodic Memory: A Meta-Analysis
27 J. Cognitive Neurosci. 1069, 1069-86 (2015)

To what degree do the medications used for cognitive enhancement in fact improve the abilities of cognitively normal individuals?

In view of the prevalence of cognitive enhancement and the intensity of academic and policy interest in this practice, it is surprising that the answer to this question has not been clearly established. The empirical literature on the effects of these stimulants on cognition in normal participants has yielded variable results, with some reviewers doubting their efficacy altogether. . . .

The primary goal of the present meta-analysis is to obtain a quantitative estimate of the cognitive effects of the stimulants amphetamine and methylphenidate. They are commonly prescribed for the treatment of attention deficit hyperactivity disorder (ADHD) but are frequently diverted for enhancement use by students and others. Guided by the findings of Smith and Farah's (2011) review, we focus on the cognitive processes that seemed most likely to be enhanced by stimulants, specifically inhibitory control, working memory, and episodic memory. In addition, because this earlier review found the strongest evidence of episodic memory enhancement after long delays between learning and test, we distinguish between episodic memory tested soon after learning (within 30 min after learning trials) and episodic memory tested after longer intervals (1 hr to 1 week). . . .

SUMMARY AND INTERPRETATION OF RESULTS

Earlier research has failed to distinguish whether stimulants' effects are small or whether they are nonexistent. The present findings supported generally small effects of amphetamine and methylphenidate on executive function and memory. Specifically, in a set of experiments limited to high-quality designs, we found significant enhancement of several cognitive abilities. We found a small but significant degree of enhancement of inhibitory control and short-term episodic memory. Effects on working memory were small and significant in one of our two analyses. Delayed episodic memory was unique in showing a medium-sized effect. However, both working memory and delayed episodic memory findings were qualified by possible publication bias.

Theoretically, the relatively more pronounced effects of delayed episodic memory, in comparison with short-term episodic memory, suggest that stimulants may be affecting most potently memory consolidation in comparison with encoding or retrieval. This conclusion is consistent with previous proposals but, again, qualified by the possibility of publication bias.

Consistent with the nonmonotonic relation between dopamine activity and performance, there is evidence that stimulants can impair performance in normal individuals who are especially high performing. It remains possible that some individuals who would not qualify for a diagnosis of ADHD could nevertheless benefit from stimulants to a greater degree than indicated by the present results and that some individuals could be impaired.

Could the effects documented here be driven by undiagnosed psychopathology in some participants? One might expect participants with ADHD or depression to perform better on stimulants and participants with anxiety disorders or bipolar disorder to be impaired by these drugs. Unfortunately, few publications included comprehensive, detailed description of procedure through which psychopathology was screened out, making it difficult to assess the quality of assessment. Nevertheless, all reports explicitly described their samples as "healthy" or "nonclinical." Thus, it is possible but unlikely that unrecognized mental illness is responsible for the pattern of obtained findings.

NEUROETHICAL IMPLICATIONS

The present findings should temper . . . more skeptical assessments of stimulant medications for cognitive enhancement of healthy, cognitively normal individuals. Although the reported effects are smaller than these of some other cognitive enhancement techniques (e.g., mindfulness meditation, for which near-medium effects on inhibitory control have been documented), the present findings show stimulant benefits comparable with the effects of other commonly used enhancement tools (e.g., physical exercise, the cognitive effects of which have been found to be similarly small). Furthermore, small effects can make a difference in academic and professional outcomes. Even on a single occasion, a small effect might make the difference between good and very good performance or between passing a school entrance or licensing examination or failing. It is also possible that these drugs may give a larger boost to cognitive functions not examined here (e.g., sustained attention, processing speed); to people not specifically studied in this meta-analysis (e.g., healthy participants with low cognitive performance or specific genotypes); or to performance under conditions not tested here, for example, fatigue, sleep deprivation, distraction, or repeated stimulant use. It is also possible that stimulants enhance cognitive performance in real-world contexts at least in part through effects on users' affective states. They have been found to alter users' emotions about, and interest in, tasks otherwise seen as boring and unrewarding.

The results of this meta-analysis cannot address the important issues of individual differences in stimulant effects or the role of motivational enhancement in helping perform academic or occupational tasks. However, they do confirm the reality of cognitive enhancing effects for normal healthy adults in general, while also indicating that these effects are modest in size.

1. Transcranial direct current stimulation

In this section we summarize briefly another popular and easily accessible addition to the enhancement toolbox: transcranial direct current stimulation ("tDCS"). tDCS is a noninvasive brain stimulation technique that delivers a weak electrical current to the brain through two electrodes placed on the head. The mechanism of action of tDCS is unclear.

tDCS is purportedly effective for both treatment and enhancement. Recent studies indicate that the technology can be used to treat patients suffering from neuropsychiatric diseases, such as stroke, chronic pain, schizophrenia, and depression. *See, e.g.,* Marom Bikson, Bhaskar Paneri & James Giordano, *The Off-Label Use, Utility and Potential Value of tDCS in the Clinical Care of Particular Neuropsychiatric Conditions,* 3 J. Law & Bioscience 642 (2016). For healthy individuals, tDCS may serve as a means of enhancing a range of cognitive functions, including improvements in visual perception, attention span, working and long-term memory, language, and mathematical ability. *See e.g.*, Jacky Au et al., *Enhancing Working Memory Training with Transcranial Direct Current Stimulation*, 28 J. Cognitive Neurosci. 1419 (2016). The true cognitive benefit, however, is unknown. *See* Martha J. Farah, *The Unknowns of Cognitive Enhancement*, 350 Science 379 (2015). Published literature on the efficacy of tDCS is mixed, with some literature reviews submitting that tDCS has no effect whatsoever on mental functioning.

Regardless of efficacy, home use of tDCS technology has increased notably. The market for direct-to-consumer neurotechnologies including tDCS is expected to exceed $3 billion in 2020. A recent survey employing a non-representative convenience sample of tDCS users from popular tDCS websites indicated thousands of regular users, but an exact number is unknown. The most common reason given for personal use of tDCS use was cognitive enhancement. Some companies have begun marketing compact, user-friendly tDCS devices for more everyday uses. *See* Anna Wexler, *Who Uses Direct-to-Consumer Brain Stimulation Products, and Why? A Study of Home Users of tDCS Devices*, 2 J. Cognitive Enhancement 114 (2018).

This trend in home use is driven by the affordability, simplicity, and relative safety of tDCS. Unlike pharmacological forms of enhancement, tDCS presents only minor side effects, including headaches or itching under the electrodes. But researchers fear that at-home tDCS risks potential misuse that could lead to long-lasting unintended and undesirable effects on cognitive functioning.

The potential risk of at-home tDCS use and its rising prevalence have prompted some researchers to call for regulation of the devices. Currently, tDCS devices are explicitly exempted from FDA regulation. While a lack of regulation is understandable given the novelty of tDCS, these researchers argue that the public availability of such devices necessitates a regulatory scheme.

Paola Frati et al.

Smart Drugs and Synthetic Androgens for Cognitive and Physical Enhancement: Revolving Doors of Cosmetic Neurology

13 Current Neuropharmacology 5, 5-9 (2015)

Methylphenidate is a psycostimulant, present on the market with different trade names (e.g. Ritalin, Concerta, Methylin, Equasym XL). . . . It was used at the beginning for the treatment of several conditions, such as: depressive states, psychosis associated to narcolepsy etc. Presently, methylphenidate is one of the most commonly prescribed drugs for the treatment of attention deficit-hyperactivity disorder (ADHD).

In order to understand the possible efficacy of this drug as a cognitive enhancer, a fundamental starting point is . . . [its mechanism of action on the cellular level. I]t acts as a dopamine-norepinephrine reuptake inhibitor. . . .

Although according to numerous reports, methylphenidate is widely abused as a cognitive enhancer among healthy subjects, especially young adults and teenagers, it is very difficult to determine the actual trend of abuse. First of all, it is necessary to distinguish the illicit from therapeutic use among people affected by ADHD or other pathologies requiring methylphenidate as therapy.

According to the U.S. Department of Health and Human Services, in monitoring the Future National Survey Results on Drug Use, 1975–2006, the use of methylphenidate among college students was 3.9% in 2006, whereas in young adults it was 2.6%. It is interesting to underline a slight decrease in the use of this drug in both categories between 2002 and 2006. Moreover, these trends of use if compared to other [drugs] such as amphetamines, show that methylphenidate is less used both in college students and in young adults.

Numerous other studies have investigated the misuse/abuse of methylphenidate in healthy subjects, but because of different methodologies, type of studies and statistical analysis they cannot be uniformly compared; . . . [One study investigated] the use of methylphenidate in a small New England college. . . . According to this study about 16% of the student population had used the drug for recreational purposes and it is the most common among students (aged 18-24 years).

. . . [A] larger study at the University of Michigan [administered] a questionnaire. About 3% of the students had used or abused methylphenidate. . . . Males and females presented nearly the same percentages of misuse/abuse. In addition, an association between misuse and attendance at parties was found.

. . . [Another study reported] that 16.2% of students have misused or abused stimulants. Of this group, 96% identified Ritalin as their stimulant of choice. The frequency of abuse in more than 50% of misusers was 2-3 times per year, in almost 34% it was monthly (1-2 times/month) and in 15.5% it was weekly (2-3 times/week).

Despite not allowing for comparative analysis, the above reported studies highlight a wide misuse/abuse of methylphenidate as a cognitive enhancer among teenagers, college students and young adults. . . .

Regarding the diffusion of methylphenidate among healthy subjects, no exhaustive conclusion can be formulated. . . .

NOTES AND QUESTIONS

1. Assuming that drugs and other interventions could genuinely enhance memory and thinking, what, if anything, is new or unique about such cognitive enhancement? In what ways are the types of cognitive enhancement discussed in the excerpts above different from the activities listed below? Do these differences matter?

   Consider this perspective:

   > Fortifying one's mental stamina with drugs of various kinds has a long history. Sir Francis Bacon consumed everything from tobacco to saffron in the hope of goosing his brain. Balzac reputedly fuelled sixteen-hour bouts of writing with copious servings of coffee, which, he wrote, "chases away sleep, and gives us the capacity to engage a little longer in the exercise of our intellects." Sartre dosed himself with speed in order to finish "Critique of Dialectical Reason." My college friends and I wrote term papers with the sweaty-palmed assistance of NoDoz tablets. . . .

   Margaret Talbot, *Brain Gain: The Underground World of "Neuroenhancing" Drugs*, New Yorker (Apr. 27, 2009).

2. How can you know or at least gain confidence regarding whether a substance or technique that is claimed to enhance cognitive or emotional function actually works? For example, above we stated that the peer-reviewed literature on the efficacy of tDCS is mixed, with some literature reviews submitting that tDCS has no effect whatsoever on mental functioning. How can you know what is true?

3. Do the reported proportions of students using Ritalin surprise you? Too few? Too many?

4. What does the public think about cognitive enhancement? Although data is sparse, at least one study found that the public stakes out a middle ground: "[T]he public appears to be cautiously accepting of CE [cognitive enhancers], even as they recognize the potential perils." Nicholas S. Fitz et al., *Public Attitudes Toward Cognitive Enhancement*, 7 Neuroethics 173, 185 (2014).

5. How would you regulate the sale and use of tDCS? For discussion of current regulation, and possible regulatory gaps, see Anna Wexler & Peter B. Reiner, *Oversight of Direct-to-Consumer Neurotechnologies*, 363 Science 234 (2019); Andreas Kuersten & Roy H. Hamilton, *Minding the 'Gaps' in the Federal Regulation of Transcranial Direct Current Stimulation Devices*, 3 J .L. & Biosciences. 309 (2016). For empirical evidence on who is actually using tDCS at home, and why, see: Anna Wexler, *Who Uses Direct-to-Consumer Brain Stimulation Products, and Why? A Study of Home Users of tDCS Devices*, 2 J. Cognitive Enhancement 114 (2018).

C. ENHANCING PERFORMANCE AND MANIPULATING MEMORY

1. Enhancing Performance

Although estimates vary widely, some studies suggest that nearly 30% of college students have taken a prescription stimulant without a prescription. This is leading to new campus debates about how schools should respond. Is the off-label use of drugs or devices to improve academic performance cheating? Or should it be encouraged in the same way that schools encourage brain-boosting foods and good sleep?

In 2011, the Editorial Board of the *The Minnesota Daily* newspaper (the student newspaper of the University of Minnesota) decided to adopt the position of a North Carolina State University editorial by running an opinion piece entitled, "Using Adderall Is a Form of Cheating." In response, a University of Minnesota student wrote an op-ed defending the use of the drug. The excerpts below capture each side of the debate.

Editorial Board

Using Adderall Is a Form of Cheating

Minn. Daily (Dec. 5, 2011)

With finals and papers looming, it seems like the right time to make the decision, will you or won't you allow chemicals to alter your brain's make-up so that you can do better on a paper or final.

Research on Adderall quickly reveals it is considered a highly addictive medication. Typically it's prescribed for attention deficit hyperactive disorder.

For those who don't have ADHD, Adderall acts as a stimulant. Although stimulants increase attentiveness, they also increase heart rates, sometimes at a rate too high to be safe. Other side effects of Adderall abuse include the development of sleeping and eating disorders, dry mouth, mood swings and higher blood pressure. These are effects that students who misuse Adderall probably don't consider.

The National Survey on Drug Use and Health in 2009 found that full-time college students between the ages of 18 and 22 are twice as likely as non-full-time college students to have used Adderall nonmedically in the past year.

With this grade-boosting pill becoming an issue, universities should reevaluate their cheating policies and include Adderall in the definition of cheating.

Adderall makes it possible to significantly increase the amount of time spent studying as well as the attentiveness to the material, which results in a dishonest grade.

Students should not use Adderall to succeed since it alters chemicals in the brain. It's better to earn a grade honestly than take a drug to do well in college.

I hope North Carolina State University will at least consider addressing Adderall use in the Student Code of Conduct.

Using mind-altering substances is not something that shows we are an institution of higher learning, as the administrators like to remind us that we are.

Christopher Meyer
Let Students Use Adderall
Minn. Daily (Dec. 12, 2011)

I say universities should move in the opposite direction and give Adderall away for free. Adderall isn't right for everyone, but it's right for a lot of people, including a lot more than those currently using it. Universities should provide students with the knowledge they need to make an informed decision, and let them determine for themselves whether the advantages outweigh the disadvantages.

Adderall is a stimulant composed of a mixture of amphetamine salts. It is primarily prescribed for people with ADHD, but it improves concentration for most "neurotypical" people as well, enabling them to be far more productive on academic tasks than they otherwise would be. Along with other "study drugs" like Ritalin and Provigil, Adderall has soared in popularity as more and more students use it to improve their academic performance.

A 2009 Minnesota College Student Health Survey found that 7 percent of students at nine Minnesota colleges reported that they used prescription drugs without a prescription. The study did not specify what drugs the students were taking, but it's a safe assumption that the majority are study drugs. If the University of Minnesota were to follow the Technician's advice, thousands of our peers would be instantly transformed into cheaters.

Technically I wouldn't be among them, because I have a prescription for Adderall. I didn't start with one, however; I first started taking it illegally when my friend offered me some during finals last spring. After researching the drug's side effects extensively, I concluded that it was a good fit for my lifestyle and sought out a prescription. I did officially get diagnosed with ADHD (without lying about anything; I was completely forthright during the entire process), but it was a stretch. The cognitive benefit Adderall has for me is not much different than the effect it has for most people: It simply allows me to concentrate more intensely for longer periods of time. . . .

There are many . . . potential issues. . . . Some people are allergic to the drug, and it can react badly with other medications. Adderall is also chemically addictive, so if you use it for a long period of time and then stop abruptly, you might suffer severe withdrawal effects. Your body builds tolerance to the drug, so over time it takes more and more of it to produce its effects. If you don't get a prescription, that will quickly make it grow extremely expensive.

All of these are reasons to be cautious before starting on Adderall, but they are not adequate reasons to prohibit people from doing so, and they're not reasons to attack those of us who have decided that it's worth it.

The Technician's logic for why Adderall should be classified as cheating was as follows: "Adderall makes it possible to significantly increase the amount of time spent studying as well as the attentiveness to the material, which results in a dishonest grade."

This logic fundamentally misunderstands what it is that makes cheating bad in the first place. When someone cheats by copying answers from a neighbor's exam, they are asserting that they know something that they don't actually know. When someone takes Adderall, they're gaining real knowledge, doing real work and making real contributions to society.

Perhaps the biggest reason people have for opposing cognitive enhancements is that they pose a threat of exacerbating inequality of cognitive ability between those who take the drug and those who don't. This can be fixed by making the drug available to those who want it, not just those who are willing to jump through the system's hoops to get a prescription. Inequality is a legitimate concern, but it's not an appropriate response to prevent ourselves from benefiting from technology (in this case, biotechnology). There are other technologies that don't work for everyone, but that doesn't mean we prevent everyone they do work for from using them.

This will become more and more of an issue as more neurological enhancements become available. We're on the cusp of some serious advances in neurological understanding, which may lead to far more potent enhancers. What happens when more substantial enhancements become available? Will we take advantage of their benefits or squander the opportunities they provide?

NOTES AND QUESTIONS

1. Should universities adopt policies that classify the non-prescription use of stimulants as "cheating"? ". . . [I]s prescription tweaking to perform on exams, or prepare presentations and grants, really the same as injecting hormones to chase down a home run record, or win the Tour de France?" Benedict Carey, *Brain Enhancement Is Wrong, Right?*, N.Y. Times (Mar. 9, 2008).

2. Since 2011, Duke University's policies governing academic dishonesty have included "the unauthorized use of prescription medication to enhance academic performance" in its definition of academic dishonesty. Duke University, Office of the University Registrar, *The 2019-20 Duke Community Standard in Practice: A Guide for Undergraduates* 16. Interestingly, this move to label such drug use as cheating came from student groups on campus, not campus administration. Previously, such non-prescription use had only been a violation of the university's drug policy. Are policies prohibiting non-prescription drug use for academic purposes advisable? What assumptions are behind such policies? Does your university have a similar provision? If not, do you think it should? If so, is it enforced? *See, e.g.,* Arden Kreeger, *Adderall Abuse Continues Despite Ban*, The Chronicle (Dec. 12,

2011) (reporting anecdotal stories of continued unauthorized prescription drug use and quoting Duke University Dean of Students suggesting that "[The policy changes have] been relatively inconsequential."); Lizi Byrnes-Mandelbaum, *An Addy a Day*, The Chronicle (Apr. 24, 2017) (reporting anecdotal stories of continued unauthorized prescription drug use). Should universities prevent, encourage, or simply turn a blind eye to the use of these drugs for purposes of enhancing academic performance? If you were writing an academic honesty code, what regulations (if any) would you include about cognitive enhancement?

3. Does your answer change for other professions that use stimulants? Professors, too, use stimulants when they are looking for an edge. *See* Caroline Schmitt, *Oxford Academic: I Use Brain Enhancing Drugs*, DW (Oct. 29, 2014). Is a professor who uses drugs to instruct better, conduct smarter research, and publish more papers "cheating"?

4. Is a distinction between *cognitive* enhancement and *mood* enhancement relevant to law and regulation? If it is considered cheating to enhance focus and thinking skills during an exam, would it also be cheating to enhance mood in ways not clearly related to the tasks of the test? For example, what (if any) academic dishonesty implications do you see for students taking Prozac for clinically diagnosed depression? What about undiagnosed students taking Prozac just to feel better?

5. Are cognitive enhancing drugs a solution to persistent achievement gaps between rich and poor students? At least one pediatrician thinks so. Dr. Ramesh Raghavan comments, "We as a society have been unwilling to invest in very effective non-pharmaceutical interventions for these children and their families. . . . We are effectively forcing local community psychiatrists to use the only tool at their disposal, which is psychotropic medications." Alan Schwarz, *Attention Disorder or Not, Pills to Help in School*, N.Y. Times (Oct. 9, 2012). Do you agree?

6. Does the use of stimulants as cognitive enhancers by law students raise special ethical concerns? Consider the following:

> [I]s the use of Adderall by non-ADHD students cheating, specifically when taken for the lengthy tasks of outlining and examination preparation in general? How does it correlate to GPA? How do law schools address it? . . . [D]o non-ADHD students mislead potential employers when their transcripts contain Adderall-produced grades? How does non-prescription stimulant use during law school impact students' performances on the fitness of character segment of the bar exam? What happens to a student in their future workplace if their Adderall source runs dry? How will this affect their competent representation of clients? . . . [W]hat does it say about the legal profession that students and lawyers feel they must take Adderall or similar drugs to succeed? . . .

Alana E. Toabe, *A Stimulating Education: The Ethical Implications of Prescription Stimulant Abuse by Law Students*, 30 Geo. J. Legal Ethics 1037, 1040 (2017).

2. Manipulating Memory

Enhancing memory—both the ability to forget and the ability to remember—is the subject of much contemporary neuroscience research. In this section, we review legal and ethical issues raised by the availability and use of drugs that can dampen or enhance memory. As you read this section, you may find it helpful to review materials on the science of memory, covered in Chapter 13.

a. Memory Dampening

Adam J. Kolber

Therapeutic Forgetting: The Legal and Ethical Implications of Memory Dampening

59 Vand. L. Rev. 1559, 1578-84 (2006)

OVERVIEW OF LEGAL ISSUES

Memories serve two distinct roles in the legal system. First, they play an indispensable role in fact-finding. We gather memories in depositions, trial testimony, police investigations, lineups, and more to help establish the underlying facts that set the entitlements of disputing parties. We value these memories principally for the information they can provide. Second, memories and their associated affective states can themselves form part of a claim for damages. If you injure me and cause me to have upsetting memories, I can sometimes seek redress for the intentional or negligent infliction of the emotional distress associated with those memories. While the existence of emotional distress must be proved just like other facts in a cause of action, the memories causing that distress are significant not only for their fact-finding role in assessing liability but also because of the negative feelings attached to them.

1. The Informational Value of Memory

Let us turn first to the role of memory as a source of information. There is little evidence so far as to how much, if at all, propranolol affects the informational content of traumatic memories formed before the drug is consumed. Assume, however, that propranolol or a future memory-dampening drug dampens both informational and emotional aspects of memories. If a witness to a recent gruesome crime uses such a drug, it will have two effects: First, it will ease the witness's suffering and help him resume a normal life. Second, it will reduce the socially-valuable information contained in the witness's memories-information that may be vitally important to prosecuting the perpetrator and protecting others from harm. These two effects reveal a tradeoff that memory dampening may pose between our individual autonomy interests in controlling what happens to our bodies' and society's interest in preserving evidence that benefits others. . . .

There are a variety of ways one might exploit memory dampening to eliminate damaging evidence. For example, the perpetrator of physical or sexual abuse could try to dampen his victim's memory, making it harder for the victim to assist police and provide incriminating testimony. There is already much skepticism about the accuracy of such eyewitness memories; pharmaceutical memory-alteration will only create more doubt. In the particularly dreadful scenario where the victim is a child, memory-dampening drugs could further muddle the much-debated issues surrounding the accuracy, prevalence, and, some would add, existence of repressed childhood memories.

Furthermore, memory-dampening drugs might be taken, not just by victims and witnesses, but by perpetrators as well. A perpetrator might do so in order to cope with feelings of shame and guilt associated with his crime. Alternatively, a perpetrator might cold-heartedly dampen his memories in order to more convincingly deceive police and a jury. It might be more advantageous to do so than to claim a Fifth Amendment privilege to remain silent and face the negative inference that jurors often draw from that silence. Even without memory-dampening drugs, those accused of a crime frequently claim to have no recollection of committing it. While many of these claims are undoubtedly spurious, the availability of a powerful memory-dampening drug could increase the rate of both genuine and malingered claims of forgetting by criminals. Thus, in order to ease painful memories or to deliberately eliminate damaging evidence, those who dampen memories may degrade our shared pool of socially-valuable information and may require us to strengthen laws governing evidence preservation.

2. The Affective Disvalue of Memory

Memory-dampening drugs also raise new legal issues associated with memory's connection to negative emotional states. For example, under some circumstances, doctors could be liable for malpractice for failing to dampen a patient's distressing memory and, perhaps too, for dampening a memory that should have been left alone. If so, we would face difficult questions about how to calculate damages for memories that are tortiously dampened or retained. Furthermore, . . . questions may arise as to the sorts of disclosures that health professionals must make in order to obtain informed consent to dampen the memories of a recently traumatized person.

In the torts context more generally, courts may have to decide the effect of memory dampening in the already controversial area of damage calculations for emotional distress. In addition to the valuation issues just noted, one thorny problem, discussed in more detail below, concerns whether a person with tortiously-caused physical and emotional trauma fails to mitigate damages if he decides not to dampen. While courts have generally not required plaintiffs to mitigate emotional damages, if indeed memory dampening proved popular and successful, the tendency might change. . . .

b. Memory Enhancement

Nick Bostrom & Anders Sandberg
Cognitive Enhancement: Methods, Ethics, Regulatory Challenges
15 Sci. & Eng'g Ethics 311, 317-18 (2009)

Working memory can be modulated by a variety of drugs. Drugs that stimulate the dopamine system have demonstrated effects, as do cholinergic drugs (possibly through improved encoding). Modafinil has been shown to enhance working memory in healthy test subjects, especially at harder task difficulties and for lower-performing subjects. (Similar findings of stronger improvements among low performers were also seen among the dopaminergic drugs, and this might be a general pattern for many cognitive enhancers.) Modafinil has been found to increase forward and backward digit span, visual pattern recognition memory, spatial planning, and reaction time/latency on different working memory tasks. The mode of action of this drug is not yet understood, but part of what seems to happen is that modafinil enhances adaptive response inhibition, making the subjects evaluate a problem more thoroughly before responding, thereby improving performance accuracy. The working memory effects might thus be part of a more general enhancement of executive function.

Modafinil was originally developed as a treatment for narcolepsy, and can be used to reduce performance decrements due to sleep loss with apparently small side effects and little risk of dependency. The drug improved attention and working memory in sleep-deprived physicians and aviators. Naps are more effective in maintaining performance than modafinil and amphetamine during long (48 h) periods of sleep deprivation, while the reverse holds for short (24 h) periods of sleep deprivation. Naps followed by a modafinil dose may be more effective than either one on its own. These results, together with studies on hormones like melatonin which can control sleep rhythms, suggest that drugs can enable fine-tuning of alertness patterns to improve task performance under demanding circumstances or disturbed sleep cycles. . . .

NOTES AND QUESTIONS

1. Consider these observations from Dr. Steven E. Hyman, a neurobiologist at Harvard:

   > This possibility of memory editing has enormous possibilities and raises huge ethical issues. . . . On the one hand, you can imagine a scenario in which a person enters a setting which elicits traumatic memories, but now has a drug that weakens those memories as they come up. Or, in the case of addiction, a drug that weakens the associations that stir craving. . . . We know that people already use smart drugs and performance enhancers of all kinds, so a substance that actually improved memory could lead to an arms race. . . .

   Benedict Carey, *Brain Power: Brain Researchers Open Door to Editing Memory*, N.Y. Times (Apr. 6, 2009). How should law respond to memory editing and enhancement technologies? To what extent are the legal implications of manipulating memory similar to or different from those of manipulating other personal traits?
2. Propranolol can reduce the physiological response to recalled traumatic memories. The drug is effective both when ingested immediately following the traumatic event and also when ingested later following recall of the event. This effect suggests that this drug or drugs like it could have wide therapeutic value. Should legislatures establish rules regarding the use and dispensing of this drug? If so, what should those rules be?
3. How might memory dampening affect criminal prosecutions where the testimony of a traumatized victim is essential? Consider this hypothetical, posed by law professor Jennifer Chandler and colleagues:

   > A Hypothetical Scenario of Pharmacological Memory Dampening in Sexual Assault
   >   A 20-year-old woman, J.D., contacts the police to report a sexual assault that occurred four days earlier. She reports that an acquaintance she ran into at a campus party walked her home, where he pushed his way into her apartment and raped her. She reports that she had been drinking heavily at the party. J.D. was traumatized and did not immediately report the assault. Several days later she confided in a friend who encouraged her to report the assault to the police. After giving her statement to the police, she also attends at a specialized sexual assault unit at the hospital where she receives medical care, including prophylaxis for sexually transmitted diseases. The team also examines J.D. for forensic evidence with her consent, but are unable to collect useful DNA evidence due to the passage of too much time since the assault.

J.D. is referred to a psychiatrist for a follow-up consultation. At the consultation a month later, the psychiatrist is concerned that J.D. is showing signs of PTSD and proposes using propranolol in a novel technique to try to dampen her traumatic memories. The psychiatrist is aware that J.D. may become involved in legal proceedings arising out of the assault, including possibly testifying as a complainant in an eventual prosecution. There is no discussion of whether treatment will help or hinder this prosecution, or of whether treatment should be delayed pending completion of the trial. J.D. proceeds with the propranolol treatment. The trial occurs several months after the completion of the propranolol treatment.

At trial, the defense argues that gaps and inconsistencies in J.D.'s account of the assault are due to memory deficits associated with (1) her PTSD, and (2) the further disruption of her memories with propranolol.

The prosecution seeks to admit expert evidence to explain the impact of trauma on memory and to dispel the inference that her testimony is unreliable. The jury is also puzzled by J.D.'s demeanor while testifying, which it regards as detached and unemotional, contrary to their expectations regarding a rape complainant.

Jennifer A. Chandler et al., *Another Look at the Legal and Ethical Consequences of Pharmacological Memory Dampening: The Case of Sexual Assault*, 41 J.L. Med. & Ethics 859, 861 (2013).

4. Some researchers are investigating the possibility of improving eyewitness testimony through brain stimulation. Consider this observation from scholars Laura Klaming and Anton Vedder:

As experts within the field of eyewitness memory have recently suggested, "it is possible to imagine a future science of eyewitness evidence that is radically different from the methods used today." Recent developments in neuroscience suggest that it is possible to improve memory by stimulating certain brain regions that are involved in memory retrieval processes. Based on these recent findings, it may therefore be possible to use neurotechnologies in criminal justice for the purpose of improving eyewitness memory thereby increasing the reliability of eyewitness evidence. Moreover, since neurotechnologies in contrast to current methods directly affect brain structures and processes, it is conceivable that they exceed methods used today and lead to more reliable eyewitness evidence. This could eventually contribute to a decrease in wrongful acquittals and convictions on the basis of mistaken eyewitness testimony. . . .

Laura Klaming & Anton H. Vedder, *Brushing Up Our Memories: Can We Use Neurotechnologies to Improve Eyewitness Memory?*, 1 L. Innovation & Tech. 203, 204-205 (2009). From the perspective of law, do you find the prospect of using neurotechnologies to improve eyewitness memory exciting or disturbing? How do you think the legal system should respond?

5. Klaming and Vedder also argue that improving eyewitness testimony through transcranial magnetic stimulation is an enhancement "for the common good." They submit that objections against cognitive enhancements are less significant when viewing enhancement from the perspective of "the common good." Anton Vedder & Laura Klaming, *Human Enhancement for the Common Good—Using Neurotechnologies to Improve Eyewitness Memory*, 1 AJOB Neurosci. 22 (2010). Does viewing enhancement through a "common good" lens desirable? Does it present risks? Consider the following response:

[Vedder and Klaming's] willingness even to *consider* forcing people . . . to undergo a treatment that is not entirely without risks, shows clearly enough how dangerous it can be to adopt the perspective of a presumed "common good" . . . There is a tendency here to view the common good as something absolute that exists irrespective of what is good for the individuals concerned, that is more important than the latter, and that, therefore, occasionally requires that the merely individual good be sacrificed.

Any notion of common good that is worth its salt must be informed by what is good for the individual. . . . The concession that even common good enhancements must always be voluntary is not sufficient. Once memory enhancement (TMS), veracity enhancement (truth serums), or morality enhancement (no-crime pill) are available, it's going to be very hard to refuse them. For why would anyone refuse to assist the law, unless they got something to hide?

Michael Hauskeller, *Cognitive Enhancement — To What End?*, in *Cognitive Enhancement: An Interdisciplinary Perspective* 113, 121-22 (Elisabeth Hildt & Andreas G. Franke eds., 2013).

D. THE ETHICS OF ENHANCEMENT

The President's Council on Bioethics
Beyond Therapy: Biotechnology and the Pursuit of Happiness
4-16, 298-99 (2003)

Chapter 1. Biotechnology and the Pursuit of Happiness: An Introduction . . .

I. THE GOLDEN AGE: ENTHUSIASM AND CONCERN

While its leading benefits and blessings are readily identified, the ethical and social concerns raised by the march of biotechnology are not easily articulated. They go beyond the familiar issues of bioethics, such as informed consent for human subjects of research, equitable access to the fruits of medical research, or, as with embryo research, the morality of the means used to pursue worthy ends. Indeed, they seem to be more directly connected to the ends themselves, to the uses to which biotechnological powers will be put. Generally speaking, these broader concerns attach especially to those uses of biotechnology that go "beyond therapy," beyond the usual domain of medicine and the goals of healing, uses that range from the advantageous to the frivolous to the pernicious. . . . People worry both that our society might be harmed and that we ourselves might be diminished in ways that could undermine the highest and richest possibilities for human life.

Truth to tell, not everyone who has considered these prospects is worried. On the contrary, some celebrate the perfection-seeking direction in which biotechnology may be taking us. Indeed, some scientists and biotechnologists have not been shy about prophesying a better-than-currently-human world to come, available with the aid of genetic engineering, nanotechnologies, and psychotropic drugs. . . .

Yet the very insouciance of some of these predictions and the confidence that the changes they endorse will make for a better world actually serve to increase public unease. Not everyone cheers a summons to a "post-human" future. Not everyone likes the idea of "remaking Eden" or of "man playing God." Not everyone agrees that this prophesied new world will be better than our own. Some suspect it could rather resemble the humanly diminished world portrayed in Aldous Huxley's novel

Brave New World, whose technologically enhanced inhabitants live cheerfully, without disappointment or regret, "enjoying" flat, empty lives devoid of love and longing, filled with only trivial pursuits and shallow attachments. . . .

III. DEFINING THE TOPIC

[W]e confine our attention to those well-meaning and strictly voluntary uses of biomedical technology through which the user is seeking some improvement or augmentation of his or her own capacities, or, from similar benevolent motives, of those of his or her children. Such use of biotechnical powers to pursue "improvements" or "perfections," whether of body, mind, performance, or sense of well-being, is at once both the most seductive and the most disquieting temptation. It reflects humankind's deep dissatisfaction with natural limits and its ardent desire to overcome them. It also embodies what is genuinely novel and worrisome in the biotechnical revolution, beyond the so-called "life issues" of abortion and embryo destruction, important though these are. What's at issue is not the crude old power to kill the creature made in God's image but the attractive science-based power to remake ourselves after images of our own devising. As a result, it gives unexpected practical urgency to ancient philosophical questions: What is a good life? What is a good community? . . .

V. THE LIMITATIONS OF THE "THERAPY vs. ENHANCEMENT" DISTINCTION

Though we shall ourselves go beyond this distinction, it provides a useful starting place from which to enter the discussion of activities that aim "beyond therapy." "Therapy," on this view as in common understanding, is the use of biotechnical power to treat individuals with known diseases, disabilities, or impairments, in an attempt to restore them to a normal state of health and fitness. "Enhancement," by contrast, is the directed use of biotechnical power to alter, by direct intervention, not disease processes but the "normal" workings of the human body and psyche, to augment or improve their native capacities and performances. Those who introduced this distinction hoped by this means to distinguish between the acceptable and the dubious or unacceptable uses of biomedical technology: therapy is always ethically fine, enhancement is, at least prima facie, ethically suspect. . . .

At first glance, the distinction between therapy and enhancement makes good sense. Ordinary experience recognizes the difference between "restoring to normal" and "going beyond the normal." . . . More fundamentally, the idea of enhancement understood as seeking something "better than well" points to the perfectionist, not to say utopian, aspiration of those who would set out to improve upon human nature in general or their own particular share of it.

But although the distinction between therapy and enhancement is a fitting beginning and useful shorthand for calling attention to the problem . . . , it is finally inadequate to the moral analysis. "Enhancement" is, even as a term, highly problematic. In its most ordinary meaning, it is abstract and imprecise. Moreover, "therapy" and "enhancement" are overlapping categories: all successful therapies are enhancing, even if not all enhancements enhance by being therapeutic. Even if we take "enhancement" to mean "nontherapeutic enhancement," the term is still ambiguous. When referring to a human function, does enhancing mean making more of it, or making it better? Does it refer to bringing something out more fully, or to altering it qualitatively? In what meaning of the term are both improved memory and selective erasure of memory "enhancements"?

Beyond these largely verbal and conceptual ambiguities, there are difficulties owing to the fact that both "enhancement" and "therapy" are bound up with, and absolutely dependent on, the inherently complicated idea of health and the always-controversial idea of normality. The differences between healthy and sick, fit and unfit, are experientially evident to most people, at least regarding themselves, and so are the differences between sickness and other troubles. When we are bothered by cough and high fever, we suspect that we are sick, and we think of consulting a physician, not a clergyman. By contrast, we think neither of sickness nor of doctors when we are bothered by money problems or worried about the threat of terrorist attacks. But there are notorious difficulties in trying to define "healthy" and "impaired," "normal" and "abnormal" (and hence, "super-normal"), especially in the area of "behavioral" or "psychic" functions and activities. Some psychiatric diagnoses—for example, "dysthymia," "oppositional disorder," or "social anxiety disorder"—are rather vague: what is the difference between extreme shyness and social anxiety? And, on the positive side, mental health shades over into peace of mind, which shades over into contentment, which shades over into happiness. If one follows the famous World Health Organization definition of health as "a state of complete physical, mental and social well-being," almost any intervention aimed at enhancement may be seen as health-promoting, and hence "therapeutic," if it serves to promote the enhanced individual's mental well-being by making him happier.

Yet even for those using a narrower definition of health, the distinction between therapy and enhancement will prove problematic. While in some cases—for instance, a chronic disease or a serious injury—it is fairly easy to point to a departure from the standard of health, other cases defy simple classification. Most human capacities fall along a continuum, or a "normal distribution" curve, and individuals who find themselves near the lower end of the normal distribution may be considered disadvantaged and therefore unhealthy in comparison with others. But the average may equally regard themselves as disadvantaged with regard to the above average. If one is responding in both cases to perceived disadvantage, on what principle can we call helping someone at the lower end "therapy" and helping someone who is merely average "enhancement"? In which cases of traits distributed "normally" (for example, height or IQ or cheerfulness) does the average also function as a norm, or is the norm itself appropriately subject to alteration?

Further complications arise when we consider causes of conditions that clamor for modification. Is it therapy to give growth hormone to a genetic dwarf, but not to a short fellow who is just unhappy to be short? And if the short are brought up to the average, the average, now having become short, will have precedent for a claim to growth hormone injections. Since more and more scientists believe that all traits of personality have at least a partial biological basis, how will we distinguish the biological "defect" that yields "disease" from the biological condition that yields shyness or melancholy or irascibility? . . .

[The Report spanned six chapters and concluded in Chapter Six with a discussion of sources of concern, summarized below.]

Chapter 6. "Beyond Therapy": General Reflections . . .

Summing up these "essential sources of concern," we might succinctly formulate them as follows:

In wanting to become more than we are, and in sometimes acting as if we were already superhuman or divine, we risk despising what we are and neglecting what we have.

In wanting to improve our bodies and our minds using new tools to enhance their performance, we risk making our bodies and minds little different from our tools, in the process also compromising the distinctly human character of our agency and activity.

In seeking by these means to be better than we are or to like ourselves better than we do, we risk "turning into someone else," confounding the identity we have acquired through natural gift cultivated by genuinely lived experiences, alone and with others.

In seeking brighter outlooks, reliable contentment, and dependable feelings of self-esteem in ways that by-pass their usual natural sources, we risk flattening our souls, lowering our aspirations, and weakening our loves and attachments.

By lowering our sights and accepting the sorts of satisfactions that biotechnology may readily produce for us, we risk turning a blind eye to the objects of our natural loves and longings, the pursuit of which might be the truer road to a more genuine happiness.

To avoid such outcomes, our native human desires need to be educated against both excess and error. We need, as individuals and as a society, to find these boundaries and to learn how to preserve and defend them. To do so in an age of biotechnology, we need to ponder and answer questions like the following:

When does parental desire for better children constrict their freedom or undermine their long-term chances for self-command and genuine excellence?

When does the quest for self-improvement make the "self" smaller or meaner?

When does a preoccupation with youthful bodies or longer life jeopardize the prospects for living well?

When does the quest for contentment or self-esteem lead us away from the activities and attachments that prove to be essential to these goals when they are properly understood?

Answers to these questions are not easily given in the abstract or in advance. Boundaries are hard to define in the absence of better knowledge of the actual hazards. Such knowledge will be obtainable only in time and only as a result of lived experience. But centrally important in shaping the possible future outcomes will be the cultural attitudes and social practices that shape desires, govern expectations, and influence the choices people make, now and in the future. This means reflecting more specifically on how biotechnology beyond therapy might affect and be affected by American society. . . .

In 2013 President Obama charged the Presidential Commission for the Study of Bioethical Issues ("Bioethics Commission") to "identify proactively a set of core ethical standards—both to guide neuroscience research and to address some of the ethical dilemmas that may be raised by the application of neuroscience research findings." Presidential Comm'n for the Study of Bioethical Issues, 1

Gray Matters: Topics at the Intersection of Neuroscience, Ethics, and Society vii (2014).The Bioethics Commission released two reports: The first report emphasized integrating ethics into all stages of neuroscientific research. The second report focused on ethical issues related to "three cauldrons of controversy—cognitive enhancement, consent capacity, and neuroscience and the legal system." Presidential Comm'n for the Study of Bioethical Issues, 2 *Gray Matters: Topics at the Intersection of Neuroscience, Ethics, and Society* 2 (2015).

The establishment of the Brain Research through Advancing Innovative Neurotechnologies (BRAIN) Initiative included an integrated perspective on neuroethics: "Although brain research entails ethical issues that are common to other areas of biomedical science, it entails special ethical considerations as well. Because the brain gives rise to consciousness, our innermost thoughts and our most basic human needs, mechanistic studies of the brain have already resulted in new social and ethical questions." *See* BRAIN Working Grp., BRAIN Initiative, *Brain 2025: A Scientific Vision* 55 (2014). In 2015 the NIH BRAIN Initiative's Neuroethics Working Group was established as a panel of experts in neuroethics and neuroscience that serves to provide the NIH BRAIN Initiative with input relating to neuroethics: https://braininitiative.nih.gov/about/neuroethics-working-group.

Presidential Comm'n for the Study of Bioethical Issues
2 *Gray Matters: Topics at the Intersection of Neuroscience, Ethics, and Society*
40-45 (2015)

ETHICAL ANALYSIS

Modifying the brain and nervous system is not inherently ethically problematic. Individuals use a wide range of substances, processes, and interventions to modify the brain and nervous system, including high-quality nutrition, meditation, education, drugs, and devices. Society must evaluate the ethical concerns of specific means of neural modification individually, including those labeled cognitive enhancements, to determine whether and why they are potentially problematic. Scholars characterize ethical issues raised by cognitive enhancement into multiple clusters. . . .

Justice and Fairness

Concerns about justice and fairness related to neural modifiers that enhance cognition and other functions of the brain and nervous system arise in two distinct ways. First, an individual with more—or enhanced—cognitive abilities, for example, might have an advantage relative to others; in this sense, cognitive ability is a positional good, in that it confers an advantage on some individuals only if others do not have the same good. Cognitive enhancement raises the concern that those who have access will gain an unfair competitive advantage over those who do not. If safe and effective novel forms of neural modification are available only to those who are already advantaged (by wealth or social capital), limited availability might exacerbate existing inequalities.

Justice and fairness require not only equitable distribution of the benefits of neural modifiers, but it also requires attention to the distribution of their burdens and risks. For example, early study and use of neural modifiers might find that they are effective in the short term, but cause negative consequences in the long term. The burdens and risks of understudied neural modifiers must not fall unfairly on certain groups or individuals.

Second, neural modifiers thought to alter cognitive and other neural functions can offer nonpositional benefits (i.e., benefits that are inherently valuable, not because they provide a competitive advantage over others). . . . Here, the concern about justice is not whether access to the means for elevated brain and nervous system function confers unfair advantages, but rather whether the distribution of safe and effective neural modifiers can promote justice by providing individuals with a greater range of opportunities and enabling them to participate more fully in society.

The nonpositional individual and societal benefits of neural modification support pursuing modifications collectively, rather than limiting access to a privileged few. Neuroscience research on the effects of novel neural modifiers can contribute to our understanding of how these interventions can be distributed justly. . . . Some scholars argue that if cognitive enhancement and other neural modifiers could reduce existing inequities, then justice requires interventions. This might prove to be so. At the very least, new forms of safe and effective interventions that deliver real advantages to those who use them should not be distributed so as to exacerbate or amplify existing inequities. . . .

Moral Agency and Human Dignity

Moral agents are individuals capable of acting freely and making judgments for which they can be praised, blamed, or held responsible. Respect for human dignity has grounded longstanding ethical prohibitions against coerced uses of drugs and devices to alter the brain and nervous system. In addition, some scholars contend that cognitive enhancement and other neural modifications also pose a potential threat to moral agency and human dignity. Enabling individuals without specific impairments to achieve higher levels of cognitive function is ethically controversial. Scholars question whether humans should exercise so much control over the natural world, and debate where to draw the line. On this view, advances that vastly improve human beings cross ethical lines by risking the creation of not better humans but transhumans.

Use of pharmaceuticals to improve alertness, attention, mood, and happiness also raise concerns about morally legitimate paths to success and wellbeing. Some scholars consider achieving success with the help of a pill akin to cheating or taking the easy way out, because they believe success is supposed to be the result of personal effort and hard work. According to this objection, some forms of neural modification offer only false visions of human achievement. This type of success might be valuable for the immediate outcome, but cannot be considered the kind of achievement that results from personal will and exertion. From this perspective, success is as much about how goals are achieved as achieving them.

Similarly, some scholars contend that happiness and wellbeing are supposed to be rewards of virtue and good character, not an outcome of medication. Although it can be deeply upsetting and profoundly life-changing to live with traumatic memories, some view medications to dampen memories as problematic because they could prevent individuals from coming to terms with their lives as continuous subjects of both good and bad experiences. From this perspective, neural modification, particularly through pharmacological management, threatens to provide only "fraudulent happiness." Yet, from another perspective, ethical merit might exist in "fraudulent happiness" that enables individuals to be functional parents, providers, and engaged citizens.

In contrast, others view the practice of novel neurotechnologies being used to enhance humans as technological progress and innovation. Scholars evaluate some forms of neural modification for their potential to be used for moral enhancement. Drugs that free us of rage, impulsivity, and aggression might enable us to participate successfully in the moral community. . . .

Importantly, the empirical evidence supporting the possibility of moral enhancement is thin, and interpreting results in terms of moral enhancement has been criticized by both those internal and external to the scientific community. Some scholars question whether we would be morally better at all if only through use of a drug—our conduct would be the result of a will controlled by the external and artificial stimulus of a pharmaceutical rather than will disciplined through effort. In contrast, others point out that, although technological moral enhancement is only a distant prospect, it can serve as a complement to, not a replacement of, traditional social and educational modes of moral improvement. . . .

The Bioethical Commission offered several recommendations, including:

1. Prioritizing existing, evidence-based strategies for maintaining or improving neural health, including, for example, adequate exercise and sleep, healthy diet, high-quality educational opportunities, and public health interventions, such as lead paint abatement.
2. Prioritizing research into treatment of neurological disorders through neural modifiers to improve health and alleviate suffering.
3. Researching the prevalence, benefits, and risks of novel neural modifiers to guide ethical use of such interventions and ensure their potential effects are accurately portrayed to the public.
4. Ensuring equitable access to novel neural modifiers so as to avoid exacerbating existing social and economic inequities. The Bioethics Commission warns that simply making enhancements available to everyone may in fact preserve inequities. To ensure policies are sensitive to social and economic disparities, they should be guided by evidence of who will benefit most from using neural modifiers.
5. Creating detailed guidance and educational materials for stakeholders on use, potential benefits and risks, and ethical concerns of neural modifiers. Stakeholders include clinicians, patients, parents, educators, employers, and professional organizations for fields that are associated with "on-the-job" use of neurocognitive enhancement intervention, such as aviation, medicine, and military. The Bioethics Commission specifically called on professional organizations and other expert groups to contribute to the development of such guidelines.

Henry T. Greely
Remarks on Human Biological Enhancement
56 U. Kan. L. Rev. 1139, 1148–54 (2008)

SIX CONCERNS ABOUT HUMAN BIOLOGICAL ENHANCEMENT

There are three concerns about enhancements that I think are relevant and appropriate. I think we have to worry about safety, coercion, and fairness. The next three concerns, integrity, long-term social effects, and the "yuck" factor, I am frankly less taken with, although I think they inform more of the public response.

1. Safety

If [cognitive enhancing technologies] come through an FDA or an FDA-like process, they have been accepted as safe, but that safety is qualified in many ways. There are two very relevant qualifications for these purposes. First, it is safety in the context of a particular dose and dosing regimen. . . . Athletes, weightlifters, and bodybuilders who take steroids actually seem to take them on a variety of different regimens, but they are not regimens that have ever been tested by the FDA, or tested by anybody scientifically. . . .

The second safety issue is even deeper in some respects. When the FDA approves a drug as safe, it approves it as safe for a particular use. . . . This is a concern that some people may have with the off-label use of FDA-approved medicines. . . .

2. Coercion

If biological enhancements were allowed, we might say they could be allowed for people who voluntarily choose to use them. But we might draw the line at frank, implicit, or most trickily, most complicatedly, parental coercion. . . .

3. Fairness

Fairness works at a couple of different levels. . . . One level is the individual competition, for instance, the individual weightlifter, wrestler, or bodybuilder, or even the individual football player who is trying to make it to the NFL. Is it fair that one competitor is using drugs and the other is not? . . .

What happens if only the rich or only certain groups obtain access to these enhancements and other people do not? . . .

4. Integrity

There is not a good label . . . but . . . the concern [is] that it is cheating to use enhancements, that it is not right somehow. Now if that were the equivalent of "the rules forbid it and you should follow the rules," then I agree. . . .

But that does not answer the question about what the rules should be. And some people argue that, particularly in the sports context, enhancement violates the essence of sport; that using biological enhancements is inherently cheating or inherently violates the integrity of the endeavor. . . .

5. Long-Term Social Effects

Michael Sandel, a political philosopher at Harvard . . . is worried that in a world where we enhance people, we will increase our discrimination against the non-enhanced or against those who are completely outside of enhancement: the sick, disabled, and unfortunate. If we are all focused on becoming Supermen and Superwomen, the people who are left behind will be left even further behind. . . .

6. The "Yuck" Factor

[T]he concern goes, "it's wrong because it's just not right, because it's not natural." The intellectual versions of this come in two categories. There is the religious perspective: that this is not how God meant us to be. . . .

The other . . . is that this is not the way evolution intended us to be. This is not the way natural selection created us, natural selection knew what it was doing, and therefore, we should not muddle with it. . . .

NOTES AND QUESTIONS

1. Philosopher Walter Glannon writes that, given the current state of knowledge, we ought to adopt a middle ground approach:

   > A significant body of data on the long-term effects of psychopharmacology to enhance normal levels of cognition or mood is not yet available. So there is no decisive reason for a policy that would prohibit the use of drugs for this purpose. Nevertheless, the potential harm from chronic use of enhancing drugs could be significant, which would seem to justify erring on the side of safety and adopting a precautionary principle limiting their use. At the same time, as an expression of autonomy competent individuals should be permitted to take enhancing drugs and to take responsibility for their effects. In adopting a reasonable middle ground between these two positions, we should issue the warning: "User Beware."

   Walter Glannon, *Psychopharmacological Enhancement*, 1 Neuroethics 45, 53-54 (2008). If someone else knows the risks and wants to use a particular enhancement technology anyway, does that concern you? So long as you are not required to enhance yourself as well, are you fine with everyone else doing it? Consider Dr. Carl Elliott's observation:

   > It is less a story about trying get ahead than about the terror of being left behind, and the humiliation of crossing the finish line dead last, while the crowd points at you and laughs. You can still refuse to use enhancement technologies, of course—you might be the last woman in America who does not dye her gray hair, the last man who refused to work out at the gym—but even that publicly announces something to other Americans about who you are and what you value. This is all part of the logic of consumer culture. You cannot simply opt out of the system and expect nobody to notice how much you weigh.

   Carl Elliott, *Better Than Well: American Medicine Meets the American Dream* 298 (2003).

2. Imagine that a neuroprosthetic device were developed and that it proved safe and effective. Further imagine that it could, to some minimal degree, improve one's ability to carry out a job-relevant task. If you were the manager hiring for that job, would you want to know if your employee had the implant? Should employment law prevent you from asking that question in a job interview?

3. Consider the effect of cognitive enhancement on other mental functions. One concern, advanced by Drs. Chatterjee and Farah, is that cognitive enhancement could have tradeoffs, enhancing certain functions while potentially diminishing others, like creative thinking. Dr. Farah, for example, remarked in an interview, "I'm a little concerned that we could be raising a generation

of very focused accountants." Margaret Talbot, *Brain Gain: The Underground World of "Neuroenhancing" Drugs*, New Yorker (Apr. 27, 2009). Their initial research on the hypothesis is inconclusive. Martha J. Farah et al., *When We Enhance Cognition with Adderall, Do We Sacrifice Creativity? A Preliminary Study*, 202 Psychopharmacology 541, 546-47 (2009) (reporting results indicating no evidence of general impairment of creativity and concluding that preliminary results indicate the "neuroethical worry that widespread stimulant use could create a general downward shift in the creativity of the population is assuaged by the results").

4. In 2018 the NIH Advisory Committee to the Director Working Group on BRAIN 2.0 Neuroethics Subgroup (BNS) was created. This group created a Neuroethics Roadmap for the NIH BRAIN Initiative. On brain enhancement, the Roadmap noted that

> [T]wo lines of related empirical research are needed. First are carefully controlled studies with healthy research volunteers to evaluate the short- and long-term effects (and side effects) of drugs and devices thought to produce cognitive, moral, and mood enhancement. . . . Second, there is a need for systematic data collection on actual usage patterns of neuroenhancement drugs and devices.

The Brain Initiative Neuroethics Subgroup, *The BRAIN Initiative and Neuroethics: Enabling and Enhancing Neuroscience Advances for Society*, Nat'l Institutes of Health. How would you design a study to address either of these research trajectories?

5. Wayne D. Hall and Jayne C. Lucke raise an additional concern about addiction:

> Contemporary advocates of neuroenhancement speak as if this was a wholly novel phenomenon. They fail to appreciate the relevance of historical experiences with the non-medical use of what are recognized nowadays as drugs of addiction. Cocaine, for example, was arguably one of the first pharmaceutical drugs that was promoted as a cognitive enhancer, by Sigmund Freud among others. It was seen as a low-risk drug that could be taken regularly to relieve tiredness, increase endurance and improve cognitive performance.
>
> Amphetamines were viewed in much the same way from the 1930s and into the 1970s. Students used amphetamines to cram for examinations, and pharmaceutical companies claimed that they enhanced "mental performance." Further studies showed that they improved efficiency in simple mental and psychomotor tasks largely because they increased confidence. By the late 1960s amphetamines were used on US university campuses as a study aid and a party drug in much the same way that it is claimed nowadays that students use Ritalin. Both drug classes were placed under legal control because of the high rates of dependence and adverse effects experienced by regular users.

Wayne D. Hall & Jayne C. Lucke, Editorial, *The Enhancement Use of Neuropharmaceuticals: More Scepticism and Caution Needed*, 105 Addiction 2041, 2042 (2010).

6. Consider the following view: "If bioengineering made the myth of the 'self-made man' come true, it would be difficult to view our talents as gifts for which we are indebted, rather than as achievements for which we are responsible." Michael J. Sandel, *The Case Against Perfection: What's Wrong with Designer Children, Bionic Athletes, and Genetic Engineering*, The Atlantic (Apr. 2004). Do you agree?

7. In his 2004 paper on cognitive enhancement, Anjan Chatterjee concluded by posing the following questions:

> 1. Would you take a medication with minimal side effects half an hour before Italian lessons if it meant that you would learn the language more quickly?
> 2. Would you give your child a medication with minimal side effects half an hour before piano lessons if it meant that they learned to play more expertly?
> 3. Would you pay more for flights whose pilots were taking a medication that made them react better in emergencies? How much more?
> 4. Would you want residents to take medications after nights on call that would make them less likely to make mistakes in caring for patients because of sleep deprivation?
> 5. Would you take a medicine that selectively dampened memories that are deeply disturbing? Slightly disturbing?

Anjan Chatterjee, *Cosmetic Neurology: The Controversy over Enhancing Movement, Mentation, and Mood*, 63 Neurology 968, 973 (2004). How would you answer these questions? What should the law say about how you answer them? What about your school's internal policy guidelines?

8. If physicians are the "gatekeepers" to cognitive enhancement, how should they respond to patients who ask for enhancing drugs? Consider the following recommendation, offered by the Ethics, Law and Humanities Committee of the American Academy of Neurology:

> Until medications designed specifically for neuroenhancement in a normal population are developed, neuroenhancement will consist of "off-label" use of medications that were developed and clinically studied in cohorts of patients with a defined disease state.
>
> FDA review and approval of a new drug application is limited to the uses for which the manufacturer has conducted safety and efficacy studies. To avoid constraining physicians' ability to treat patients, the FDA's position is that lack of approval of a drug or device for a particular use (e.g., neuroenhancement) does not imply that such off-label use is either disapproved or improper. Thus, neurologists, in their professional judgment, and based on an individualized assessment of patients, may prescribe FDA-approved drugs or devices for any clinical indication or purpose that they believe will benefit their patients. This prerogative includes 1) prescribing drugs for conditions other than those for which they were approved; 2) prescribing drugs for patient groups other than those for which they were originally approved; and 3) varying from the approved dosage or method of administering drugs.
>
> Clinicians should have a medical basis or plausible rationale when prescribing medications for off-label use, which should be based on relevant medical principles and available evidence, including the pathophysiology of the disease, pharmacologic properties of the medication, studies or case reports in the professional literature, or professional experience. Neurologists must also consider whether doing so would be consistent with the practice of other neurologists in similar circumstances (i.e., standard of care). Physicians who consider prescribing medication for neuroenhancement are disadvantaged by the dearth of valid clinical studies concerning the effects and safety of these drugs on normal persons. Whether the effects shown in these studies can be extrapolated to the general population is unknown.
>
> Before prescribing medications for off-label use of enhancement, neurologists should 1) inform patients that the medication has not been approved by the FDA

for such use; 2) explain possible side effects, including potential risks to cognitive function; 3) discuss potential short-term and long-term risks of the medication; and 4) explain the alternatives to the medication (including not taking it). . . .

Dan Larriviere et al., *Responding to Requests from Adult Patients for Neuroenhancement: Guidance of the Ethics, Law and Humanities Committee*, 73 Neurology 1406, 1409 (2009). *See also* Tracy D. Gunter, *Cosmetic Neurocognitive Enhancement and Healthcare Providers*, 12 Ind. Health. L. Rev. 729 (2015).

9. Coercion can take many forms. For example, implied or explicit coercion in the employment context may be a key arena for oversight:

> The one area in which objectors can make a good case for legislative intervention is with regard to coercion. If the goal of good social policy is to maximise autonomy while minimising suffering—and I believe that it is—then the threat of individuals being pressured into unwanted enhancement must be examined seriously. This is particularly true regarding inherently unbalanced relationships, such as those between employer and employee, where the inequality of bargaining power often limits meaningful employee choice. For example, what if hospitals started to demand that medical residents dose up on methylphenidate, a drug used to improve concentration, as a prerequisite for employment? . . .

Jacob M. Appel, *When the Boss Turns Pushers: A Proposal for Employee Protections in the Age of Cosmetic Neurology*, 34 J. Med. Ethics 616, 617 (2008).

With regard to Dr. Appel's query, recent studies have indeed suggested that modafinil might improve a sleep-deprived doctor's performance, at least with regard to certain skill sets. Colin Sugden et al., *Effect of Pharmacological Enhancement on the Cognitive and Clinical Psychomotor Performance of Sleep Deprived Doctors*, 255 Annals Surgery 222 (2012); Charles A. Czeisler et al., *Armondafinil for Treatment of Excessive Sleepiness Associated with Shift Work Disorder: A Randomized Controlled Study*, 84 Mayo Clinic Proc. 958 (2009). In the Sugden et al. study, sleep-deprived doctors taking modafinil performed better in a series of commonly used psychological tests, seeing improvements in "cognitive processes critical for efficient information processing, flexible thinking, and decision-making under time pressure," among others, although no improvement was observed as to psychomotor performance. Sugden et al. at 225-26. Although the study was preliminary, if the results are confirmed does that mean doctors should be encouraged to take such drugs? Required? *Compare* Steven H. Rose & Timothy B. Curry, *Fatigue, Countermeasures, and Performance Enhancement in Resident Physicians*, 84 Mayo Clinic Proc. 955, 956 (2009), *and* Steven H. Rose & Timothy B. Curry, *In reply to: Wake-Promoting Therapeutic Medications Not an Appropriate Alternative to Implementation of Safer Work Schedules for Resident Physicians*, 85 Mayo Clinic Proc. 302, 303 (2010) (both arguing that use of performance-enhancing drugs like modafinal, if shown to be safe, "should not be dismissed reflexively" as a possible option to support residents in long-hour training programs), *with* Katherine Drabiak-Syed, *Reining in the Pharmacological Enhancement Train: We Should Remain Vigilant About Regulatory Standards for Prescribing Controlled Substances* 29 J.L. Med. & Ethics 272, 277 (2011) (arguing that standards for practicing medicine and prescribing controlled substances counsel against such off-label prescription uses in the medical community and that physicians must play a greater role in "reign[ing] in our culture's seemingly inevitable efficiency imperative").

What other concerns does this debate raise? Would you want to be operated on by a surgeon using modafinil? Would you prefer to be? Dr. Appel recommended that Congress adopt a strategy modeled on the approach of the Genetic Information Nondiscrimination Act (GINA), and that "forced enhancement should be prohibited, while employers should be permitted to continue outcome-based assessments." Indeed, he suggested that "without preventive legislative action, employers will begin to demand that their employees accept neurological enhancement as a condition for employment or promotion—and the working stiffs of the world will not have the financial power to resist." Jacob M. Appel, *When the Boss Turns Pushers: A Proposal for Employee Protections in the Age of Cosmetic Neurology*, 34 J. Med. Ethics 616, 618 (2008). Do you agree? To what extent do your opinions change based on the employment context? *See, e.g.*, Jerome Groopman, *Eyes Wide Open: Can Science Make Regular Sleep Unnecessary?*, New Yorker (Dec. 3, 2001) (discussing early use of modafinil in military missions and research).

10. Research is underway to investigate the utility of enhancement for military purposes. Recently, the Navy began experimenting with transcranial electrical stimulation headsets that purportedly improve the efficiency of physical training. Air Force pilots already use pharmaceutical enhancements, including modafinil and stimulants. Hope Hodge Seck, *Super SEALs: Elite Units Pursue Brain-Stimulating Technologies*, Military.com (Apr. 2, 2017). These developments raise important normative questions. For instance:

> How safe should these human enhancements and new medical treatments be prior to their deployment (considering recent controversies such as mandatory anthrax vaccinations)? Must enhancements be reversible or temporary (considering that most warfighters will return to society as civilians)? Could enhancements count as "biological weapons" under the Biological and Toxin Weapons Convention (considering that the term is not clearly defined)?

Patrick Lin, Maxwell J. Mehlman & Keith Abney *Enhanced Warfighters: Risk, Ethics, and Policy* iii (2013).

11. Consider the following:

> The controversy swirling around possible—and indeed current—uses of biotechnology (drugs, stem cells, brain-machine interfaces) to enhance human cognition, emotion, and executive function is illustrated by contrasting two government sponsored reports, one from the UK and one from the US.... [The U.K. group's members] call directly for efforts to boost what they call mental capital, i.e., cognitive abilities and emotional and behavioral regulation. The report does not make a direct recommendation for technological approaches to enhancement, focusing instead on prevention and early intervention in conditions that impair mental capital formation and well-being. A fair reading, however, could find the implication that enhancement strategies could play a role as part of an integrated strategy to improve productivity and well-being in an increasingly competitive and unforgiving world.
>
> In contrast, the President's Council on Bioethics, 2003 chaired by Leon Kass worried that the very attractiveness of technologies to enhance performance and well-being in an increasingly competitive world, might lead individuals and societies to lose sight of the significant hidden costs of such interventions. In the Council's view the potential costs are many, including acceptance of short-cuts

(much like anabolic steroid use in sports) that undermine the intrinsic value of toil and self-improvement, and ultimately the instrumentalization of human beings as performance machines. . . .

Steven E. Hyman, *Cognitive Enhancement: Promises and Perils*, 69 Neuron 595 (2011).

12. The Bioethics Commission's 2015 report recommended that "professional organizations and other expert groups" develop guidance on the use of neural modifiers for health care providers to assist them in ethically prescribing neural modifiers. The Commission recommended that guidelines be developed, in particular, for "fields such as aviation, medicine, and the military, among others, that are associated with on-the-job use of brain and nervous system enhancement interventions." Presidential Comm'n for the Study of Bioethical Issues, 2 *Gray Matters: Topics at the Intersection of Neuroscience, Ethics, and Society* 4 (2015). Remember that some neural modifiers, such as tDCS, discussed *supra* Section B, are not regulated by any governmental agency. Should responsibility to ensure ethical use of neural modifiers be left to clinicians who prescribe these interventions and employers who use such interventions on employees? Or should state or federal government play a role in ensuring ethical use of interventions?

13. Is the focus on pharmacological neuroenhancements misplaced? What if behavioral enhancements—such as meditation, mnemonic devices, and even sleep—were proved to be just as effective as pharmacological methods? Consider the following perspective:

> So far, the public debate on neuroenhancement concentrates mainly on pharmacological interventions. The impressive success of some behavioral techniques, however, suggests that this focus might be misleading: techniques like the method of loci ["an ancient technique utilizing routes, visualizing to-be-remembered items at salient points along the routes, and then mentally retracing those routes during recall"] might exceed any pharmacological intervention by far. . . . [Additionally,] several drugs enhance cognition only in pathological cases; whereas, in healthy subjects, these drugs are effective to a weaker degree or not at all. This phenomenon might be different for certain behavioral neuroenhancement techniques: mnemonics seem to benefit young and healthy subjects to a larger extent than older or cognitively impaired subjects, creating an even larger gap between these groups. . . .

Martin Dresler, *Behavioral Neuroenhancement*, in *Cognitive Enhancement: An Interdisciplinary Perspective* 59, 63 (Elisabeth Hildt & Andreas G. Franke eds., 2013). If behavioral enhancements are just as effective as pharmaceuticals, are the ethical concerns regarding unequal access warranted?

FURTHER READING

Cognitive Enhancement Generally:

Michael Bess, *Our Grandchildren Redesigned: Life in the Bioengineered Society of the Near Future* (2016).

Marc Jonathan Blitz, *Freedom of Thought for the Extended Mind: Cognitive Enhancement and the Constitution*, 2010 Wis. L. Rev. 1049 (2010).

Allen E. Buchanan, *Beyond Humanity? The Ethics of Biomedical Enhancement* (2011).

Anjan Chatterjee, *Is It Acceptable for People to Take Methylphenidate to Enhance Performance?*, 338 BMJ 1532 (2009).

John Harris, *Chemical Cognitive Enhancement: Is It Unfair, Unjust, Discriminatory, or Cheating for Healthy Adults to Use Smart Drugs?*, in *Oxford Handbook of Neuroethics* 265 (Judy Illes & Barabara J. Sahakian eds., 2011).

Steven E. Hyman, *Cognitive Enhancement: Promises and Perils*, 69 Neuron 595 (2011).

Oxford Handbook of Neuroethics (Judy Illes & Barbara J. Sahakian eds., 2011).

Barbara J. Sahakian & Sharon Morein-Zamir, *Neuroethical Issues in Cognitive Enhancement*, 25 J. Psychopharmacology 197 (2011).

Enhancing Human Capacities (Julian Savulescu, Ruud ter Meulen & Guy Kahane eds., 2011).

Science of Enhancement:

Roy Hamilton, Samuel Messing & Anjan Chatterjee, *Rethinking the Thinking Cap: Ethics of Neural Enhancement Using Noninvasive Brain Stimulation*, 76 Neurology 187 (2011).

Masud Husain & Mitul A. Mehta, *Cognitive Enhancement by Drugs in Health and Disease*, 15 Trends Cognitive Sci. 28 (2011).

M. Elizabeth Smith & Martha J. Farah, *Are Prescription Stimulants "Smart Pills"? The Epidemiology and Cognitive Neuroscience of Prescription Stimulant Use by Normal Healthy Individuals*, 137 Psychol. Bull. 717 (Sept. 2011).

Ethics of Enhancement:

Cynthia R.A. Aoki, *Rewriting My Autobiography: The Legal and Ethical Implications of Memory-Dampening Agents*, 28 Bull. Sci. Tech. & Soc'y 349 (2008).

V. Dubljević, V. Saigle & E. Racine, *The Rising Tide of tDCS in the Media and Academic Literature*, 82 Neuron 731 (2014).

Francis Fukuyama, *Our Posthuman Future: Consequences of the Biotechnology Revolution* (2002).

Henry T. Greely et al., *Towards Responsible Use of Cognitive-Enhancing Drugs by the Healthy*, 456 Nature 702 (2008).

Roi Cohen Kadosh et al., *The Neuroethics of Non-Invasive Brain Stimulation*, 22 Current Biology 108 (2012).

Adam Kolber, *Give Memory-Altering Drugs a Chance*, 476 Nature 275 (2011).

Eryn J. Newman et al., *Attitudes About Memory Dampening Drugs Depend on Context and Country*, 25 Applied Cognitive Psychol. 675 (2011).

Tommaso Pizzorusso, *Erasing Fear Memories*, 325 Sci. 1214 (2009).

Nicole A. Vincent, *Enhancing Responsibility*, in *Neuroscience and Legal Responsibility* 305 (Nicole A. Vincent ed., 2013).

International Perspectives:

Australian Brain Alliance, *A Neuroethics Framework for the Australian Brain Initiative*, 101 Neuron 365 (2019).

Diana W. Bianchi et al., *Neuroethics for the National Institutes of Health BRAIN Initiative*, 38 J. Neurosci. 10583 (2018).

Cognitive Enhancement: Ethical and Policy Perspectives in International Perspective (Veljko Dubljević & Fabrice Jotterand eds., 2016).

Judy Illes et al., *Neuroethics Backbone for the Evolving Canadian Brain Research Strategy*, 101 Neuron 370 (2019).

Sung-Jin Jeong et al., *Korea Brain Initiative: Emerging Issues and Institutionalization of Neuroethics*, 101 Neuron 390 (2019).

Khara M. Ramos et al., *The NIH BRAIN Initiative: Integrating Neuroethics and Neuroscience*, 101 Neuron 394 (2019).

Yi Wang et al., *Responsibility and Sustainability in Brain Science, Technology, and Neuroethics in China—A Culture-Oriented Perspective*, 101 Neuron 375 (2019).

CHAPTER 20

Brain-Machine Interface and Law

The chemical or physical inventor is always a Prometheus. There is no great invention, from fire to flying, which has not been hailed as an insult to some god. But if every physical and chemical invention is a blasphemy, every biological invention is a perversion. There is hardly one which, on first being brought to the notice of an observer from any nation which had not previously heard of their existence, would not appear to him as indecent and unnatural.

— J. B. S. Haldane[†]

Fundamentally, we are not the stuff that makes up our bodies and brains. These particles essentially flow through us in the same way that water molecules flow through a river. We are a pattern that changes slowly but has stability and continuity, even though the stuff comprising the pattern changes quickly. The gradual introduction of nonbiological systems into our bodies and brains will be just another example of the continual turnover of parts that compose us. It will not alter the continuity of our identity any more than the natural replacement of our biological cells does.

— Ray Kurzweil[††]

CHAPTER SUMMARY

This chapter:
- Introduces scientific and engineering developments in brain-machine interfaces.
- Considers legal issues arising from the use of these devices.
- Explores ethical issues related to the use of these devices for military purposes.

INTRODUCTION

Jan Scheuermann, a writer and producer of murder mystery parties in Pittsburgh, developed spinal cerebellar degeneration that paralyzed her limbs. After 10 years of this condition she volunteered to participate in a research study in which one array

---

[†] J.B.S. Haldane, *Daedalus or Science and the Future: A Paper Read to the Heretics, Cambridge on February 4th, 1923* 44 (1924).

[††] Ray Kurzweil, *How to Create a Mind: The Secret of Human Thought Revealed* 240 (2012).

of electrodes was implanted in a part of her motor cortex that controls reaching while another array was implanted in a part that controls grasping.

Signals from these electrodes enabled her to control a robot arm to reach for and grasp various objects, like chocolate bars. Jan said, "This is the ride of my life. I keep saying, this is the rollercoaster, this is the skydiving. It's just fabulous and I'm enjoying every second of it."* This is not an isolated case. Cathy Hutchinson, whose limbs and voice are paralyzed, drank coffee from a robotic arm she controlled, and Matt Nagle controls a computer cursor to use programs like email. Advances in wireless technology have eliminated the need for any physical connection between a person and the robot. So robots can be manipulated, by thoughts, at any distance.

Brain-machine interfacing (some call it brain-computer interfacing) doesn't even always require surgery. Scott Mackler is a neuroscientist at the University of Pennsylvania. Although being fit enough to run a 3.5-hour marathon, he was diagnosed with Amyotrophic Lateral Sclerosis (ALS, or Lou Gehrig's disease) when he was 40 years old, in 1999. The disease prevents signals from the brain from reaching the muscles of the body. Consequently, Mackler suffers "locked in" syndrome. That is, his mind is active and alert, but he cannot move any part of his body except his eyes. For a decade, he could communicate with his wife only by eye movement signals. Yet with a brain-machine interface developed by Jonathan Wolpaw at New York State's Wadsworth Center, Mackler can communicate with others so effectively that he can continue running his laboratory to investigate addiction. Mackler wears an EEG cap while staring at a computer screen that systematically displays letters and numbers; computer analysis of the EEG detects the letters or numbers Mackler wants to write in real-time. This dramatic story was featured on an episode of *60 Minutes* in 2008. Just seven years later, EEG caps are now envisioned as a way to control smart-home devices.**

Elon Musk, the tech entrepreneur behind Tesla and SpaceX, has even more ambitious goals for his company *Neuralink*. The goal of Musk's company is to merge humans with AI. In Musk's view, the technology "will enable anyone who wants to have superhuman cognition."*** To this end, brain implants are getting smaller and smaller, creating the potential for a less-invasive and more-integrative form of connection with machines. Scientists are developing "Neural Dust," wireless and ultrasound powered implants smaller than a grain of rice which have the potential to both read and stimulate nerves while causing less of a biological disturbance in the recipient's body than traditional implants.**** Continuing at this rate, some predict that humans will evolve into a new species—the "digitally immortal" *Homo optimus*—by 2050.*****

These gripping examples illustrate the frontiers of brain-machine interface (BMI) technology. But as dramatic as current technology is, it may pale in comparison to

---

* Tim Hornyak, *Brain Implants Let Paralyzed Woman Move Robot Arm*, CNET (Dec. 17, 2012).
** Cadie Thompson, *This Professor Thinks He Has the Key to Controlling Your Home with Your Mind*, Business Insider (May 31, 2015).
*** Todd Haselton, *Elon Musk: I'm About to Announce a 'Neuralink' Product That Connects Your Brain to Computers*, CNBC (Sept. 7, 2018).
**** Charles Q. Choi, *Scientists Have Invented Wireless 'Neural Dust' to Monitor Your Brain*, Insider (Aug. 4 2016).
***** Sarah Griffiths, *Is Technology Causing Us to 'Evolve' Into a New SPECIES? Expert Believes Super Humans Called Homo Optimus Will Talk to Machines and be 'Digitally Immortal' by 2050*, Daily Mail (Feb. 1, 2016).

what is just around the corner. As a neurologist who treats ALS patients observed, "Patients want to be able to communicate beyond the yes or no with an eye blink. They want to send an e-mail, and turn off the light and, even more, to have a meaningful conversation."* Patients may be able to do this soon, as technology such as the lightweight and portable "iBrain" has been tested with physicist Stephen Hawking. It is tantalizing to think of the possibilities provided by such developments, for good and for harm, intended or unintended, whether with disabled patients or healthy individuals.

This chapter focuses on a set of legal and ethical issues that are arising from these developments. Section A introduces some applications of neuroprosthetic devices and then surveys some of the technical issues involved in developing and implementing brain-machine interfaces. Section B considers ethical and legal issues. In particular, the section asks whether existing legal frameworks are sufficient to address these developments, or whether the fact that the organ in question is the nervous system raises any unique considerations. Section C provides a brief discussion of the use of BMI in military contexts.

A. INTRODUCTION TO BRAIN-MACHINE INTERFACES

Neuroprosthetics, also known as brain-machine interfacing or brain-computer interfacing, is an active discipline at the boundary of neuroscience and biomedical engineering. The successes of BMI have overcome sensory and motor disabilities consequent to injury or disease. The goal of researchers is also to address cognitive and emotional problems through direct brain interventions. The development and testing of BMI are very active areas of research. In January 2020, the National Institutes of Health were providing over $61 million in funds through more than 100 grants to support research and scientific training in this area.

Neuroprosthetic devices can serve as either input or output to the brain. As input, you may already be familiar with commonly used brain-machine interfaces in the form of cochlear implants, which correct hearing loss. They directly stimulate nerves in the cochlea, the input to the auditory system. More specifically, a microphone on an external unit gathers the sound and processes it; then the processed signal is transferred to an implanted unit that stimulates the auditory nerves through a microelectrode array. Some researchers are now working on implants to correct vision loss.

As output, we introduced above BMI systems that detect signals in the motor areas of the cerebral cortex and convert those signals into commands to move a computer cursor or a robot arm. Through this technology, quadriplegic patients can interact with the world once again to play a song, compose an email, or grab a piece of chocolate.

Another aspect of BMI is engineering motorized arms and hands, such as the Luke hand project. Engineers are devising robotic limbs controlled by the amputee's central or peripheral nervous system. Also, motorized exoskeletons are

---

* David Ewing Duncan, *A Little Device That's Trying to Read Your Thoughts*, N.Y. Times (Apr. 2, 2012).

allowing paralyzed patients to walk. They are also allowing able-bodied individuals to carry more.

The introduction of Google Glass in 2012, and its updated Glass Enterprise Edition available in 2020, brought brain-machine interface even closer to mass consumption. Airplane mechanics, for example, now view software showing instructional videos, animations and images immediately in their line of sight. The time saved from consulting a three-inch thick assembly manual has reduced errors and improved efficiency by 10%. Should we be surprised, then, that a blogger asked, "How far-fetched is it, really, to go from today's Google Glass to nanobots communicating between your brain and a Google cloud that is indistinguishable from a human?"* To answer such a provocative question, though, you should first know more details about how BMI works.

Brain-machine interfaces are accomplished in a variety of ways. We have distinguished BMI as input (replacing or augmenting a sensory system) and BMI as output (replacing or augmenting a motor system). Improvements in BMI have been accelerated by advances in computer algorithms, robotics, materials science, computational models of intelligent behavior, signal processing, and basic systems neuroscience. Earlier, capabilities were limited by computer speeds, but microprocessor design and digital signal analysis now outpace the requirements of neuroprosthetics. Implants become smaller as devices gain computational power and reduce size.

BMI are comprised of several basic components. Among these are hardware devices to interface with the brain, an electrical amplifier and computer analysis system that can detect brain signals in real time, an electrical stimulator with battery power that can modulate brain function in real time, communication pathways to convey signals to internal or external actuator devices, and feedback monitoring systems to measure how precisely the actual outcome corresponded to the desired outcome.

To introduce the signal detection element, we remind the reader that the brain both generates and reacts to electrical impulses. The natural electrical impulses generated by the brain can be detected by thin metal probes implanted in the brain. Engineers have developed arrays of such probes than can detect signals from dozens of local sites in the brain. These devices afford the highest resolution of brain signal. However, the long-term viability of these implants is compromised by the body's immune response, which effectively masks the signals. Materials engineers are exploring new substrates from which to build electrodes to reduce or eliminate the immune response.

The summed collective signal associated with those impulses can be detected by larger metal discs placed on the surface of the head. This noninvasive approach measures a signal known as the electroencephalogram (EEG). Patterns in the EEG can enable people to control cursors and select letters of the alphabet for communication. EEG is limited, though, by the poor spatial resolution of the signal. More signal resolution is available by placing the metal discs directly on the cerebral cortex, beneath the scalp, muscle, and bone. This type of neural recording is called electrocorticography (ECoG). This kind of signal may achieve the best balance of

---

* Dan Farber, *A Look into the Mind-Bending Google Glass of 2029*, CNET (Aug. 15, 2013).

signal quality, durability, and reliability. ECoG-based neuroprosthesis has allowed a patient to accurately move a robot arm after a spinal-cord injury.

The connection with the nervous system need not be in the head, though. Other researchers are connecting devices through probes attached to peripheral nerves outside of the brain and spinal cord. This approach entails less surgical risk. The connection can be formed by penetrating the nerve or by wrapping a sensor around the nerve. Yet another approach involves measuring signals in muscles, known as electromyography (EMG). Thus, by monitoring the voluntary control of muscles in the chest, neck, or shoulders, investigators can obtain signals useful for controlling the movements of prosthetic limbs.

Still other physiological changes can be measured to control BMI. These include magnetic fields associated with electrical current, neurotransmitter concentration gradients, blood flow or blood oxygenation changes. Each of these requires a more expensive, sophisticated apparatus and so are unlikely to gain common use.

Once detected, the information content of these changes in brain state must be extracted and decoded. The design of this decoding stage takes advantage of knowledge gained through basic research about the functional and anatomical properties of the region of the brain from which the signals were sampled. Such information helps resolve ambiguities like this—neural impulses measured in a brain region before a reaching and grasping movement could convey the movements contemplated by the subject, the coordination of the various muscle contractions necessary, the anticipated proprioceptive body sense information, or just neural noise. Decoding the meaning of neural impulses is a very active area of current research, which advances through new insights in computer science, cognitive psychology, and the mathematics of signal processing. These microscopic and macroscopic brain signals can be decoded and conveyed to computers and mechanical devices to produce actions without limb movements.

The next element of BMI is the actuators, the mechanical system whereby the desired action is enacted. Many actuators have been developed. One is just the cursor on a computer that allows an otherwise paralyzed person to scroll through a playlist, select a movie, or send an email. A particularly dramatic kind of actuator is a robotic arm and hand that allows the paralyzed person to take a drink, retrieve a chocolate bar, or shake a hand. Yet another kind of actuator conveys the decoded central brain signals to stimulating electrodes in the patient's own peripheral nerves or muscles.

The same thin metal probes that detect neuron impulses can also artificially produce impulses in the brain conveyed through external stimulators. Like a heart pacemaker, these brain stimulators can calm a seizure, steady a tremor, ignite an image, and possibly relax a mood.

The final component of BMI systems accomplishes feedback and adaptation. In any motor control system, errors in measurement, interpretation, and execution occur. For robust and accurate performance, compensation of such errors must be incorporated in the design of the system. This is particularly important in the injured brain, where the initial signal may not necessarily be the most direct one, and extrapolation may be needed to approximate what is interpreted as the actual intended movement. Feedback may be designed into the actuator itself, whereby comparisons are performed between the command signal and the executed action. For example, a prosthetic hand can include a slip detector for local control of grasping to maintain effective grip.

By contrast, in other neuroprosthetic devices, feedback, and error correction occur through the subject's observation of a cursor position with respect to a target position. Here the feedback loop is completed by the patient's own brain while she learns to move the robot arm. Additionally, some of the learning can happen in the computers inserted between the raw brain signal and the robot arm (or computer cursor). Like infants learning the dimension and weight of their limbs, the BMI patient must practice through trial and error to learn the match between the volitional command and the external movement. Eventually, though, the patient can move the robot hand and arm with as much grace and as little thought as you move your own hand and arm. Ultimately, like you, they cannot explain how they produce the basic action; it just happens.

The development of devices that interface with our brains already has had a profound impact on the quality of human life, and research in this field promises to provide more ways of correcting various disabilities. Yet the technologies enable non-medical applications as well. As you read the materials in this chapter, consider the implications for law, in both medical and non-medical contexts.

Nick Stockton
Woman Controls A Fighter Jet Sim Using Only Her Mind
Wired (Mar. 5, 2015)

All Jan Scheuermann wanted to do was feed herself some chocolate. She ended up piloting the world's most expensive fighter jet.

Scheuermann is quadriplegic, unable to move her arms and legs due to a neurodegenerative disease. . . . [S]cientists from the military's future-science arm [DARPA]* and the University of Pittsburgh's Human Engineering Research Laboratories approached her in 2012 about plugging her brain into a robotic arm. . . . Two years later, . . . the scientists changed the game. Instead of connecting Scheuermann's brain interface to a robotic arm, they connected her to a flight simulator. She'd use the same neural connections to pilot an F-35 Joint Strike Fighter—the military's next-gen attack jet. . . .

[T]his research was conducted under [DARPA]'s Revolutionizing Prosthetics research track, which is geared towards better robotic arms for injured veterans. "We are thinking about exactly how to restore function after injury, how the brain can be used to actuate devices," says Justin Sanchez, the head of [DARPA]'s prosthetics research. . . .

The idea of a neural interface for computers isn't new. The first brain-controlled videogames go back to 2006, when a team of scientists at Washington University in St. Louis built an interface that let a teenager with epilepsy control *Space Invaders*. The idea is that instead of using purpose-specific neurons to control a purpose-specific device—like a cochlear implant, or some prostheses—you could build an interface between the brain and any computer, and then the computer could do a range of tasks—from gripping a candy bar to performing a barrel roll.

---

* The Defense Advanced Research Projects Agency, within the United States Department of Defense, is responsible for the development of emerging technologies for use by the military.—EDS.

Scheuermann's imaginary fighter jet flight wasn't her first foray into controlling virtual objects with her mind. She trained to use the robot arm by controlling a virtual one on a computer screen. Her neural activity gets picked up by a four-millimeter-wide sensor embedded in her brain, 96 microelectrodes . . . each trained on a different cell. . . . His team simply reprogrammed the output of the electrodes so that instead of controlling the movements of a robotic arm, they controlled the altitude, pitch, and roll of an onscreen fighter jet. . . .

The real achievement here is reprogramming the same neuronal wiring that controlled a robotic arm to fly a virtual fighter jet. "Fundamentally it's demonstrations like this that change the way that we think about the way brain does work in the world," says Sanchez. It's an early step, but he says this raises interesting questions about whether humanity could one day outgrow physical interfaces with its machines. This is about more than just video games—it's about finding a fundamentally new way to interact with the virtual world, and maybe even the real one.

NOTES AND QUESTIONS

1. The scope of BMI applications is increasing rapidly. For example, from a BMI implanted over the auditory cortex, using cutting-edge deep neural network analyses and the latest innovations in speech synthesis technologies, investigators reproduced sentences heard by patients. Hassan Akbari et al., *Towards Reconstructing Intelligible Speech from the Human Auditory Cortex*, 9 Sci. Rep. 874 (2019). In addition, a BMI implanted in a somatosensory area of the cerebral cortex enables tactile sensitivity in a patient after spinal cord injury. Sharlene N. Flesher et al., *Intracortical Microstimulation of Human Somatosensory Cortex*, 8 Sci. Transl. Med. 361ra141 (2016). With access to both input and output channels, patients can gain a sense of touch in a prosthetic limb. *Neurotechnology Provides Near-Natural Sense of Touch: Revolutionizing Prosthetics Program Achieves Goal of Restoring Sensation*, DARPA (Sept. 11, 2015).

2. The foregoing described robot arms being controlled with signals recorded within the brain. Because this requires invasive brain surgery, few individuals are in this state. However, new research has devised methods to control robot arms (or any other device) with noninvasive EEG signals. Jianjun Meng et al., *Noninvasive Electroencephalogram Based Control of a Robotic Arm for Reach and Grasp Tasks*, 6 Sci. Rep. 38565 (2016). The possibility of controlling devices through noninvasive EEG signals could allow for widespread adoption of the technology. How would this change the legal and regulatory landscape?

3. Commercialization of brain-machine interfacing has begun. For instance, a company called Galvani states, "[W]e believe bioelectronics have the potential to change the face of medical science forever . . . and our ambition is to take the lead. We are developing the expertise to place tiny devices inside the human body. These will be programmed to read and modify electrical signals passing along nerves in the body, to restore health." *Our Mission & Values*, Galvani Bioelectronics (2016). Suppose you are the lawyer for an engineering company that is considering expanding its operations into the brain-machine interface market. The company has asked you to provide an initial high-level overview of the features of the legal landscape that they should have in mind.

4. Imagine that you are an aide to a legislator who has been approached by two groups. One consists of consumer organizations arguing that the regulatory framework for brain-machine interfaces is inadequate. The other consists of industry groups arguing that they need not more, but less, regulation. The legislator has asked you to consider the merits of these approaches, as well as others that might occur to you, and to provide an initial overview of possible courses of legislative/regulatory action, with discussion of the pros and cons. In light of the technology you just learned about, how would you organize and structure such an overview?

5. Brain-to-brain interfaces are also being explored. In 2015 a research team linked together brain circuits of rats and of monkeys. One demonstration with four adult rat brains both sampled impulses from many neurons and electrically stimulated the somatosensory cortex. The neural signals from one rat were communicated through electrical stimulation to the brain of another rat. Multiple tests demonstrated that the network of four brains could perform various detection and discrimination tasks. Miguel Pais-Vieira et al., *Building an Organic Computing Device with Multiple Interconnected Brains*, 5 Sci. Rep. 11869 (2015). Another demonstration with two or three macaque monkeys sampled impulses from many neurons in cortical regions contributing to controlling arm movements. Robot arms could be controlled in two- and three-dimensions by combining neural signals from the individual monkey brains. Arjun Ramakrishnan et al., *Computing Arm Movements with a Monkey Brainet*, 5 Sci. Rep. 10767 (2015). Technically, human brains could be linked similarly. What, then, happens to the legal concept of responsibility when brains are combined in this way?

6. Lessons about BMI may be learned from the experiences of prosthetic devices in sports. For example, Dr. Rory A. Cooper, Director of Human Engineering Resources Laboratories at the University of Pittsburgh, founding director of the Veteran Affairs Rehabilitation Research and Development Center and a veteran who suffered a spinal cord injury asserts, "The question in basketball is not if but when. . . . Basketball is a little behind, but it's already happened in track and field." He is referring to sprinters like Marlon Shirley and Oscar Pistorius, who have competed at high levels using prosthetic legs. At issue is whether the prosthetic confers an unfair advantage. Kevin Arnovitz, *How Advancements in Prosthetic Limbs Could Impact Future of Sports*, ESPN (Nov. 11, 2015).

7. In spite of these amazing demonstrations and the lives that they have impacted, the field of BMI is not without major challenges. Andy Schwartz, a professor of neurobiology at the University of Pittsburgh and a pioneer of brain-computer interfaces summarizes it, "What most people fail to realize is there's a whole different aspect of the problem, and that's the basic science. I would say almost everybody is skipping over that. I call that engineering arrogance." Christopher Mims, *A Hardware Update for the Human Brain*, Wall St. J. (June 5, 2017).

8. "The augmented among us—those who are willing to avail themselves of the benefits of brain prosthetics and to live with the attendant risks—will outperform others in the everyday contest for jobs and mates, in science, on the athletic field and in armed conflict. These differences will challenge society in new ways—and open up possibilities that we can scarcely imagine." Gary Marcus & Christof Koch, *The Future of Brain Implants*, Wall St. J. (Mar. 14, 2014). What fields of law do you think are most likely to be affected by such developments? To what extent, and how, do you think the legal system should be engaged in regulating the implementation of, and availabilities of, such technologies?

9. How will deep brain stimulation (DBS) affect patients' sense of "autonomy"? Answering that question likely depends on how "autonomy" is defined. Consider:

> A range of positions have been articulated regarding how great an interference (and alternatively, how great a promise) DBS may represent for patient autonomy. Views about how DBS may affect autonomy vary not only in terms of their direction (promoting or undermining) and the magnitude of the possible effect, but also regarding how autonomy is affected. What explains the dramatically different ways of talking about autonomy that one encounters in the neuroethics literature on DBS? The answer, it seems, is that the parties to the debate are deploying different conceptions of autonomy—different understandings of its core features, or at the very least, different degrees of emphasis on, or privileging of, certain potential features over others. . . .

Peter Zuk & Gabriel Lázaro-Muñoz, *DBS and Autonomy: Clarifying the Role of Theoretical Neuroethics*, Neuroethics 1, 3 (2019). How would you define "autonomy" in the context of brain-machine interface?

10. Might law have to fundamentally reconsider its notion of personhood? Consider this argument from law professors Bartha Maria Knoppers and Hank Greely:

> [D]o the classical legal boundaries still matter, and if so, why? Altering the legal meaning of "human" ultimately affects the foundation for all human rights. Between legal classifications of biomedical waste and legal obligations to future generations, both the certainty that law provides in human interaction and the content of the concomitant duties and freedoms it accords are at stake.
>
> "Hominum causa omne jus constitutum est" ("All law is created for the sake of men") is a maxim from Roman law and is the origin of most legal systems the world over. It epitomizes the relationship between "man" and law. Uncertain boundaries can lead to unintended and untoward legal consequences, which only intensify when one considers the effect of judicial decisions. A new classification has the potential to affect and bind all future parties while unsettling the past. Irrespective, classical dualisms continue to serve as frameworks for legal determinations in most specific contexts. Courts, scientists, and physicians continue to be creative in their interpretations of emerging biotechnologies and in the imposition of necessary limits across the dualisms. Regions of the world with different cultural values concerning the beginning or end of life or on the use of tissues and cells still remain subject to the international umbrella filter of "human" rights. Our traditional approaches to this may not be badly out of date, but they need to be applied flexibly. So, what can we suggest as a way forward? . . .

Bartha Maria Knoppers & Henry T. Greely, *Biotechnologies Nibbling at the Legal "Human,"* 366 Science 1455, 1456 (2019).

B. ETHICAL AND LEGAL IMPLICATIONS OF NEUROPROSTHETICS

Ethicists and scientists have begun to discern the many implications of brain-machine interface devices. For instance, Karim Jebari argues that privacy and autonomy are at risk: "individualism and the very nature of interpersonal relationships may be altered as a result of BMI applications." Karim Jebari, *Brain Machine Interface and Human Enhancement—An Ethical Review,* 6 Neuroethics 617, 617 (2013).

Jebari sees that information extracted from the brain for purposes of informing the attached machinery could be used by employers and the government. Jebari warns against a future in which such technologies are "used by a third party to manipulate our emotions and desires, for example, by making us enjoy things that we would not otherwise consider enjoyable." *Id.* at 623.

Jens Clausen asks what happens in situations where the machinery attached to the human fails: "Who is responsible for involuntary acts? Is it the fault of the computer or the user? Will a user need some kind of driver's licence [sic] and obligatory insurance to operate a prosthesis?" Jens Clausen, *Man, Machine and in Between*, 457 Nature 1080, 1080 (2009). Such questions may be even more complex if the boundary between man and machine is blurred. Or, perhaps not. Søren Holm & Teck Chuan Voo, *Brain-Machine Interfaces and Personal Responsibility for Action — Maybe Not as Complicated After All*, 4 Stud. Ethics L. & Tech. (2011). Through analysis of several hypothetical BMI situations, Bublitz and colleagues conclude that:

> [r]esponsibility of BCI-users for damages to third-parties follows regular rules of liability, mainly tort and criminal law. BCI users can be liable on three separate counts: For actions, mediated by BCIs; for omissions to prevent harms arising from operations of BCIs; for deploying BCIs, provided harmful events were foreseeable. Assessing whether BCI-mediated movements constitute actions can be challenging. We suggest the law expands its concept of action to include the category of mental actions with physical consequences, and therewith, willfully initiated BCI-mediated movement. . . .

Christoph Bublitz et al., *Legal Liabilities of BCI-Users: Responsibility Gaps at the Intersection of Mind and Machine?*, 65 Int'l J.L. Psychiatry 101399 (2019).

Another issue concerns maintenance and medical support of implant technology as the financial fortunes of manufacturers wax and wane. A *Science* article described the case of an 11-year-old boy who received an electrical stimulator to treat cerebral palsy. The implant was placed in 1980, and it worked. Now, though, he is 46 years old, and the device is wearing out. The company that developed it has stopped manufacturing the device, and the electrodes used in the original are no longer available. Emily Underwood, *Brain Implant Trials Raise Ethical Concerns*, 348 Science 1186, 1186 (2015). Another example involves the Freehand device, produced by NeuroControl, which successfully reactivated paralyzed hands in people with a specific type of nerve damage. It was approved by the FDA in 1997, but in 2001 NeuroControl abandoned the technology because it was not profitable. Ultimately, when the company closed its doors, the approximately 250 people who had received the device no longer had access to replacements for the fraying wires in their implants. *Id.* at 1187. Finally, Underwood described the unsuccessful outcome of numerous clinical trials of deep brain stimulation for depression. For example, St. Jude Medical discontinued one large trial for depression in 2013. When the testing was concluded, the patients received little or no more support because in the United States, companies or institutions sponsoring research are rarely, if ever, required to pay medical costs that trial subjects incur as a result of their participation. To address this, neurologist Helen Mayberg sustained an independent clinical trial of the same device. As long as she keeps the trial open, Medicare and private insurance will cover at least some of her patients' medical costs related to the device. *Id.* Some companies seek to avoid such outcomes by requiring trial participants to agree in advance that an implanted device will be removed at the end of a trial, even if it is working. Still, regulatory gaps remain. *See* Gabriel Lázaro-Muñoz, et al., *Continued Access to Investigational Brain Implants*, 19 Nat. Rev. Neuro. 317 (2018).

What if the patient prefers to keep the implant? According to Liam Drew, Patient Number 6 received an electrical implant in her brain that helped manage disabling epileptic seizures. She reported, "It becomes part of you. You grow gradually into it and get used to it, so it then becomes a part of every day. It became me." When the company that developed the device went bankrupt, the device had to be removed. Although Patient 6 resisted having the removal done, ultimately the device was removed. She grieved, "I lost myself." *The Ethics of Brain-Computer Interfaces*, Nature (July 24, 2019).

From a clinical perspective, José L. Contreras-Vidal observes that "in the case of co-robots," with information flowing between brain and robot, deciding when to use a brain computer interface is a "complicated scenario not only in terms of the consent process and deciding whether the benefits of using the system outweigh the risks but also the potential impact to society at large." José L. Contreras-Vidal, *Ethical Considerations Behind Brain-Computer Interface Research*, O&P EDGE (Aug. 2012). When is a clinician speaking with the "human" and when with the "robot"?

At present there are more questions than answers. As a review of neuroprostheses concluded: "it remains difficult to predict how, and in which directions, . . . research will progress. Perhaps the only certain thing about the future of neuroprosthetics is that the field is growing and that the states of the science and the field remain in flux. . . . The possibilities are not infinite, but they most assuredly are intriguing." Pratik Y. Chhatbar & Subrata Saha, *Neuroprostheses: Implications of the Current and Future State of the Science and Technology, in Neurotechnology: Premises, Potential, and Problems* 100 (James Giordano ed., 2012). Amidst this flux, the law must regulate, apportion liability, and determine responsibility.

In 2013, Stephen S. Wu and Marc Goodman surveyed the legal implications of BMI.* They anticipate many potential criminal issues. First, and parallel to someone's hacking a heart pacemaker, for example, a malicious actor might hack wireless BMI devices, such as controllers for prosthetic limbs, or deep brain stimulators. Second, the means and the motivation to exploit neural devices might develop. Third, the history of the use of computers and the Internet indicates that, given the opportunity, people will attack and subvert computers and devices

However, the authors note, the threat to neural devices is fundamentally different from the threat to computers and the Internet. Whereas attacks to computers and the Internet typically affect money, data, or property, hacking of medical devices can cause immediate physical, mental, or emotional harm. And hacking neural devices poses greater risks than hacking other medical devices. For example, attacking a neural device used to enhance a person's memory may erase or change that person's memory or change their thought processes.

Thus, brain implants and neuroprosthetics present new legal issues. Companies offering services related to BMI could have exceptional access to private information stored in the human brain. Obtaining meaningful informed

---

* Stephen S. Wu & Marc Goodman, *Neural Implants and Their Legal Implications*, 30 GPSolo 68 (2013).

consent poses significant challenges concerning the collection of data from an individual. Device manufacturers will need to develop data security policies to secure administrative, physical, and technical control in the manufacture of BMI devices. They will also need to develop privacy policies to protect sensitive information and systems.

In the future, federal and state laws might impose security and privacy requirements on manufacturers of BMI devices and related companies that service them. And litigation may arise from privacy torts or from the violation of security and privacy requirements in statutes and regulations.

Henry T. Greely, Khara M. Ramos & Christine Grady
Neuroethics in the Age of Brain Projects
92 Neuron 637, 637–39 (2016)

["BRAIN 2025: A Scientific Vision" is a June 2014 publication that] . . . lays out seven core principles for maximizing the value of the BRAIN Initiative. . . . The sixth principle was to "consider ethical implications of neuroscience research . . . [with] [v]igorous dialogue among ethicists, educators, government and corporate representatives, patients and their advocates, lawyers, journalists, scientists and other concerned stake-holders about social and ethical issues raised by new knowledge and technologies generated under the BRAIN Initiative."

The report [proposed] four explicit goals . . . :

(1) Joint neuroscience/ethics training programs and meetings to consider the unique issues raised by human neuroscience research, and to establish a shared vision for the ethical conduct of such research.

(2) Resources for collecting and disseminating best practices in the conduct of ethical scientific research, particularly for the conduct of clinical research.

(3) Support for data-driven research to inform ethical issues arising from BRAIN Initiative research, ideally with integrated activities between ethicists and neuroscientists.

(4) Opportunities for outreach activities focused on engaging government leaders, corporate leaders, journalists, patients and their advocates, educators, and legal practitioners in discussion of the social and ethical implications of neuro-science research. . . .

[I]ssues arising from implanting devices into human brains have become a major focus. What consent requirements are appropriate? What are the long-term responsibilities of researchers (and funders) to people who received the implanted devices, particularly those who had good results? Issues both similar and different will arise from non-implanted, non-invasive methods of recording or modulating human brain activity. Privacy and confidentiality are additional important points. The collection and sharing of information on brains is seen as crucial to effective research but might go beyond what the human sources of that information expected and may even put their privacy at risk.

CeReB: The Center for Responsible Brainwave Technologies
The Ethics of Brain Wave Technology: Issues, Principles and Guidelines
at 28 (2014)

ETHICAL GUIDELINES FOR BRAINWAVE TECHNOLOGY

Principle	Guideline
Integrity of the person. . .	Developers should treat all users as an end, and not as a means to an end. . . .
Agency: The ability to take action	Brainwave technology should not inhibit or interfere with a user's ability to act when wishing to do so. . . .
Autonomy: The ability to act based on one's own volition	Brainwave technology should . . . not coerce, or force, action on the part of the user, unless the user has explicitly consented to participating in contexts where such actions can be reasonably expected to be part of that context (e.g. gaming). . . .
Privacy: Protection against involuntary disclosure	All data generated by brainwave technology should be considered, and treated, as sensitive, and accorded a level of protection commensurate with that designation. . . .
Safety: Use of the device falls within acceptable safety and security standards	The hardware, software, and data components of any brainwave system should be designed and developed with user security and safety as a top priority. . . .
	This . . . include[s] considerations to prevent or mitigate malicious interference or corruption of any component of the technology on the part of a determined or opportunistic 'hacker.'
Honesty and clarity over any claims made on behalf of the technology	Developers of brainwave technology should be careful to clearly define and characterize the veracity of any claim they make with respect to the use of brainwave technology, based on the evidence reasonably available to them. . . .
Contributing to informed decision making on the part of the user	All those involved in the application or development of brainwave technology should actively enhance users' and the public's understanding of the technology and its current and future implications. . . .

NOTES AND QUESTIONS

1. Ethical considerations have been integral to the BRAIN research initiative in the U.S. Although the BRAIN Initiative was announced in April 2013, its scope was not explicit until the June 2014 publication of "BRAIN 2025: A Scientific Vision." The report said that "the research supported by and the knowledge generated through the BRAIN Initiative should be regularly assessed for their ethical, legal, and societal implications." Brain Research Through Advancing Innovative Neurotechnologies (BRAIN) Working Group Report, *BRAIN 2025: A Scientific Vision* 117 (2014). To that end, in November 2014, a working group of NIH leadership approved the creation of a Neuroethics Work Group. DARPA also formed a Neuroethics, Legal, and Social Issues Advisory Panel. As indicated in the Further Reading list at the end of the chapter, parallel neuroethics considerations are happening in other countries.

2. One general feature of tort law is that defendants take plaintiffs as they find them. That is, a tortfeasor's liability will ordinarily take into account any unusual vulnerabilities of the injured party. This is the so-called "eggshell plaintiff" doctrine. To what extent should that doctrine apply if an injured person's body contains millions of dollars of robotic equipment? Conversely, if robotic prostheses are less damaged by tortious activity than ordinary skin and bone, should a tortfeasor's liability be commensurately limited (in what might be called the "hardshell plaintiff" doctrine)?

3. Consider a case in which the tortfeasor (rather than the plaintiff) has a brain-machine interface. What are the possible legal implications? How would duties be affected if that interface was known to be less capable than the average body? What if it were known to be (in fine motor skills, for example) more capable than the average body?

4. To what extent is it accurate to say that brain-machine interfaces enable users to manipulate things "by thoughts alone"? What difference does the answer make? For example, Nissan is developing Brain-to-Vehicle (B2V) technology that "[d]elivers more excitement and driving pleasure by detecting, analyzing and responding to driver's brainwaves in real time." *Brain-to-Vehicle*, Nissan (2020). Nissan's former Executive Vice-President Daniele Schillaci "describes his vision of the future: 'Through Nissan Intelligent Mobility, we are moving people to a better world by delivering more autonomy, more electrification and more connectivity.'" *Nissan's Brain-to-Vehicle Technology Communicates Our Brains with Vehicles*, BitBrain (Oct. 8, 2018). But, another company believes that the use of EEG for large-scale consumer products is highly unlikely if not impossible, at least in the next 5-10 years because of limitations in EEG measurement and uncertainty about its reliable and convenient application. *Realities of Brain-Computer Interfaces for the Automotive Industry: Pitfalls and Opportunities*, BRAIQ, Inc. (2018). As of 2020, this company is no longer in business.

5. BMI are also being used to control wheelchairs. Álvaro Fernández-Rodríguez, Francisco Velasco-Álvarez & Ricardo Ron-Angevin, *Review of Real Brain-Controlled Wheelchairs*, 13 J. Neural Engineering 061001 (2016). Your smart home can be under BMI control, as well. Cadie Thompson, *This Professor Thinks He Has the Key to Controlling Your Home with Your Mind*, Business Insider (May 31, 2015).

6. What do you imagine will happen over the course of your lifetime in terms of advancements in brain-machine interfaces and other prosthetics? Some commentators have asked, "Will an enhanced human being—a human being possessing a neural interface with a computer—still be human, as people have experienced humanity through all of time? Or will such a person be a different sort of creature?" Michael Joseph Gross, *The Pentagon's Push to Program Soldiers' Brains*, The Atlantic (Nov. 1, 2018). Richard Godwin summarized interviews with several scientists and futurists, "But of all the developments emerging now, it's technology focused on the human body that would appear to introduce the most chaos into the system. California biotech startups talk of making death 'optional.' Facebook is working on telepathic interfaces. Bionic limbs will soon outperform human limbs." *'We Will Get Regular Body Upgrades': What Will Humans Look Like in 100 Years?*, Guardian (Sept. 22, 2018). With what projected legal consequences?

7. What criminal activities could brain-machine interfaces enable? Would you favor any new criminal statues specific to BMI?

8. Political scientist Francis Fukuyama observes:

> It is my view that this turn away from notions of rights based on human nature is profoundly mistaken, both on philosophical grounds and as a matter of everyday moral reasoning. Human nature is what gives us a moral sense, provides us with the social skills to live in society, and serves as a ground for more sophisticated philosophical discussions of rights, justice and morality. What is ultimately at stake with biotechnology is not just some utilitarian cost-benefit calculus concerning future medical technologies, but the very grounding of the human moral sense. . . .

Francis Fukuyama, *Our Posthuman Future: Consequences of the Biotechnology Revolution* 101–02 (2003). Do you agree or disagree? Why?

9. The many ethical, legal, and moral issues entailed by BMI should be informed by the actual experiences of BMI users. Unfortunately, systematic investigation has emphasized the technology and overlooked the self-image and self-experience of the BCI user or of the caregivers. Johannes Kögel et al., *Using Brain-Computer Interfaces: A Scoping Review of Studies Employing Social Research Methods*, 20 BMC Med. Ethics 18 (2019). As the experiences of BCI users are crucial for evaluating ethical and societal aspects of an emerging technology, more empirical research on these matters should be encouraged. Do you agree?

10. BMI entail complex privacy concerns. Kevin Y. Li, *Get Out of My Head: An Examination of Potential Brain-Computer Interface Data Privacy Concerns*, Boston College Intellectual Property and Technology Forum (2018). The Health Information Portability and Accountability Act (HIPAA) and the Health Information Technology for Economic and Clinical Health Act (HITECH) may have privacy implications for data collected by BMI. HIPAA regulates data that would identify the person to which information pertains and is relevant to that individual's physical or mental health. HIPAA originally applied to only healthcare providers and insurance companies, but HITECH expanded HIPAA's scope to include business associates—third parties that create, receive, maintain, or transmit personal information for functions such as data analysis, processing, or administration with healthcare providers or insurance companies. Manufacturers of

wearable devices (e.g., the Apple Watch) are typically not covered under HIPAA because they do not interact directly with healthcare providers or insurance companies. The applicability of HIPAA to BMIs will depend on the degree of medical relevance. State laws have also addressed personal data security. Another concern involves the use of BMI data as evidence in court proceedings. In 2017 an Ohio state court held that data from a defendant's pacemaker was admissible evidence in determining whether or not he committed arson. The obvious concern is that BMI data can offer more accurate and incriminating information about mental and emotional states. Do you agree that there is a need for expansive state privacy regulations, a federal expansion of HIPAA, and a framework for addressing potential self-incrimination issues?

11. With thousands of mental health apps on the market and dozens of devices for cognitive enhancement, relaxation by entraining brain waves, improving motor function, etc., the market for direct-to-consumer neurotechnology is predicted to top $3 billion in 2020. However, in view of the number of products, the ever-updating software applications, the flexibility and expertise required for oversight, some believe that current regulatory oversight is not sufficient. Anna Wexler & Peter B. Reiner, *Oversight of Direct-to-Consumer Neurotechnologies*, 363 Science 234 (2019). One issue concerns whether the neurotechnologies work as advertised. For example, scientific consensus has not been reached concerning the effectiveness of transcranial direct current stimulation for cognitive performance or benefits from EEG neurofeedback. A related issue concerns the challenges of consumers without scientific training assessing the claims made by neurotechnology companies. Similar to dietary supplements, these direct-to-consumer neurotechnologies are not regulated as medical devices. Notably, premarket FDA approval discourages venture capital to finance new neurotechnologies. Regulation for these neurotechnologies has fallen to the Federal Trade Commission (FTC) to take action in cases of deceptive advertising. However, because these neurotechnologies are products of NIH-supported research, it would be appropriate and likely effective for the NIH to focus funding on direct-to-consumer neurotechnologies. In addition, an independent working group consisting of scientists, health professionals, consumer groups, industry representatives, ethicists, regulators, and funders could survey the main domains of DTC neurotechnology and provide succinct appraisals of potential harms and probable efficacy to identify gaps in current knowledge.

12. Some BMI applications support patients' spelling words and sentences. How will the logs of a BMI spelling tool be stored and protected? Who should have access? What should we do with recordings? Should they be fleeting (deleted on the spot) like real-life conversations? What if there is an emergency situation (such as the patient's spouse has an advance directive), but it is in conflict with BCI spelling communication with a doctor? Can they subpoena the spelling logs? If so, which prevails?

13. Cultural, ethical, and legal standards vary around the planet. A study sampled 40 million decisions about moral dilemmas in 10 languages from millions of people in 233 countries and territories. Edmond Awad et al., *The Moral Machine Experiment*, 563 Nature 59 (2018). Responses varied across regions in ways that could guide different public policy decisions. Should BMI operate according to different policies in different countries? If so, how would travel between such countries be affected?

14. One observer of brain machine interface has suggested that in time, those who can afford it will be able to achieve "electronic immortality" by downloading their brains to the cloud or even into a human clone. Many in the "transhumanist" movement argue that such developments ought to be a goal of research and development. For instance, the organization Humanity+ argues that advances in AI, BMI, and related technologies can "take the human beyond the historical (normal) state of existence . . ." and that "[h]uman enhancement, both therapeutic and selective, challenges the normal status and aims to expand human capabilities that further human physiological functions and extend the maximum life span." Humanity+, *humanityplus.org* (2020). Should humans strive to harness technology to go beyond our normal state of existence?

C. MILITARY APPLICATIONS OF BRAIN-MACHINE INTERFACE

Since the White House announced the BRAIN initiative in 2013, the Defense Advanced Research Projects Agency (DARPA) has invested in multiple new programs. The Hand Proprioception and Touch Interfaces (HAPTIX) program seeks to create fully implantable and modular neural-interface microsystems that communicate wirelessly to restore naturalistic sensations to amputees. Through HAPTIX, DARPA has succeeded in restoring the sense of touch to amputees via a prosthetic hand. Similarly, their Revolutionizing Prosthetics program aims to increase the functionality and realistic quality of prosthetic limbs, and since its inception, DARPA has received FDA approval of one of their arm-systems. The Neural Engineering System Design (NESD) program aims to develop an implantable neural interface to allow seamless data transfer between the human brain and the machines. Other promising research has come from the Electrical Prescriptions (ElectRx) program, which funded the research team that developed a millimeter-scale wirelessly powered "neural dust" device that have harnessed the power of ultrasound for communication through neural interfaces.

Ivan S. Kotchetkov et al.
Brain-Computer Interfaces: Military, Neurosurgical, and Ethical Perspective
28 Neruosurgical Focus E25 (2010)

MILITARY ENHANCEMENT WITH BCIS

Alongside therapeutic interventions, rapid advances in BCI technologies will also create opportunities for neurosurgeons to participate in improving military training and operations, particularly through combat performance modification and optimization. In fact, the use of neuroscientific approaches for achieving these goals is already an evolving area of research. During the last decade, the Pentagon's DARPA launched the "Advanced Speech Encoding Program" to develop nonacoustic sensors for speech encoding in acoustically hostile environments, such as inside of a military vehicle or an urban environment. The DARPA division is currently involved in a program called "Silent Talk" that aims to develop user-to-user communication on the battlefield through EEG signals of "intended speech," thereby eliminating the need for any vocalization or body gestures. Such capabilities will be of particular benefit in reconnaissance and special operations settings, and successful applications of silent speech interfaces have already been reported.

Enhancements of soldiers' perception and control of vehicles or heavy machinery with BCIs are also within the realm of possibilities. A recent DARPA proposal for a "Cognitive Technology Threat Warning System" includes a requirement for operator-trained high-resolution BCI binoculars that can quickly respond to a subconsciously detected target or a threat. Such biological vision devices can have detection ranges of up to 10 km against dismounts and vehicles, and can expand soldiers' field of view to 120°. Thus, future generations of auditory and visual neuroprostheses may allow soldiers to perform better during combat situations through automated detection and interpretation capabilities. The concept of telepresence, in which a soldier is physically present at a base or concealed location, but has the ability to sense and interact in a removed, real-world location through a mobile BCI device, is also being actively investigated and has even been projected to be available in limited applications by 2015. These expectations are substantiated by recent advances in the operation of robots using EEG signals, such that control of cargo-loading machines, demolition robots, or unmanned aerial vehicles, as enabled by BCIs, is more than a progressive goal; it is also a realistic expectation. In its earliest stages, this type of BCI could be used in manned vehicles, vessels, and aircraft to make their operation more efficient by reducing the need for manual input of key functions as required by today's navigation and weapons deployment protocols.

The ethical considerations of employing BCIs for performance modification depend largely on the type of intervention required to implement the device. Because a majority of unclassified DARPA projects are based on noninvasive BCIs, use of such platforms will not be associated with additional risks and can be viewed in a similar manner as the use of night-vision goggles or radiofrequency signals. However, the application of invasive or partially invasive BCIs in soldiers presents an ethically challenging scenario that raises concerns of surgical risk as well as issues of neurocognitive enhancement and alteration of personal identity. Unlike the use of BCIs for therapeutic interventions, cognitive, physical, and psychological enhancement of healthy individuals does not fall under the principle of physician beneficence that obligates doctors to restore health to normal levels through the treatment and prevention of disease. Nevertheless, the ability of BCI devices to expand human capacities must also be viewed in light of the advantage they grant soldiers to perform and succeed in combat missions. In this context, development of BCIs can be seen as making a paramount contribution to the national security, which citizens, including physicians, have a social duty to support. Equally important is the distribution of this technology: in the hands of a responsible military, BCIs can protect national interests and the population at large, but if obtained by rogue groups, they can promote terrorism and instability. On a further level, if an existing BCI application had the potential for significant benefit in a much wider population, such as through therapeutic uses, it would be ethically questionable to sequester its use without justly distributing it to the society at large. All these and other considerations make the role of a neurosurgeon in the development of BCIs particularly complex. Nevertheless, ethical considerations must be foremost applied to the most realistic expectations, such as BCI therapeutics, and deferred in those that are presently more speculative. . . .

Michael N. Tennison & Jonathan D. Moreno

Neuroscience, Ethics, and National Security: The State of the Art

10 PLoS Biology e1001289 (2012)

INTRODUCTION

During the past decade, the US national security establishment has come to see neuroscience as a promising and integral component of its 21st century needs. Much neuroscience is "dual use" research, asking questions and developing technologies that are of both military and civilian interest. Historically, dual use has often involved a trickle down of military technology into civilian hands. The Internet, for example, originated as a non-local, distributed means to secure military information. In the case of neuroscience, however, civilian research has outpaced that of the military. Both National Research Council (NRC) reports and Department of Defense (DoD) funding reveal ongoing national security interests in neuroscience and indicate that the military is quite eager to glean what it can from the emerging science. To pursue cognitive neuroscience research, the Pentagon's science agency, the Defense Advanced Research Projects Agency (DARPA), received about US$240 million for the fiscal year of 2011, while the Army trails at US$55 million, the Navy at US$34 million, and the Air Force at US$24 million.

The military establishment's interest in understanding, developing, and exploiting neuroscience generates a tension in its relationship with science: the goals of national security and the goals of science may conflict. The latter employs rigorous standards of validation in the expansion of knowledge, while the former depends on the most promising deployable solutions for the defense of the nation. As a result, the exciting potential of high-tech developments on the horizon may be overhyped, misunderstood, or worse: they could be deployed before sufficiently validated.

Current state-of-the-art neuroscience, including new forms of brain scanning, brain–computer interfaces (BCIs), and neuromodulation, is being tapped for warfighter enhancement, deception detection, and other cutting-edge military applications to serve national security interests.

BRAIN–COMPUTER INTERFACES

BCIs exemplify the dual use nature of neuroscience applications. BCIs convert neural activity into input for technological mechanisms, from communication devices to prosthetics. The military's interests in BCIs are manifold, including treatment modalities, augmented systems for controlling vehicles, and assistance for detecting danger on the battlefield.

In the late 1990s, scientists demonstrated neurological control of the movement of a simple device in rats, and soon thereafter, of a robotic arm in monkeys. More recently, a pilot study of BrainGate technology, an intracortical microelectrode array implanted in human subjects, confirmed 1,000 days of continuous, successful neurological control of a mouse cursor. Non-invasive technologies for harnessing brain activity also show promise for human use. Progress has recently been reported on a "dry" EEG cap that does not require a gel to obtain sufficient data from the brain. The "brain cap" is reported to reconstruct movements of humans' ankle, knee, and hip joints during treadmill walking in order to aid rehabilitation.

DARPA's Augmented Cognition (AugCog) program sought to find ways to use neurological information gathered from warfighters to modify their equipment accordingly. For example, the "cognitive cockpit" concept involved recording a pilot's brain activity to customize the cockpit to that individual's needs in real time, from selecting the least burdened sensory organ for communicating information to prioritizing informational needs and eliminating distractions. Although the Augmented Cognition moniker (and funding mechanism) seem to have been dropped, its spirit lives on in other DARPA projects. For example, the Cognitive Technology Threat Warning System is developing portable binoculars that convert subconscious, neurological responses to danger into consciously available information. Such a system could reduce the information-processing burden on warfighters, helping them to identify and respond to areas of interest in the visual field more quickly.

Via intracortical microstimulation (ICMS), a neurologically controlled prosthetic could send tactile information back to the brain in nearly real time, essentially creating a "brain-machine-brain interface." The technology underlying this concept is already evolving, and some researchers hope that optogenetics, which both enables "precise, millisecond control of specific neurons" and "eliminates most of the key problems with ICMS," will ultimately supplant the ICMS for sensory feedback. In addition to devising prosthetics that can supply sensory information to the brain, brain-machine-brain interfaces may directly modify neurological activity. Portable technologies like near infrared spectroscopy (NIRS), for example, could detect deficiencies in a warfighter's neurological processes and feed that information into a device utilizing in-helmet or in-vehicle transcranial magnetic stimulation (TMS) to suppress or enhance individual brain functions.

Much of the technological evolution of warfare has introduced a distance between the parties involved. From the advent of firearms to airplanes, aerial bombs to remotely operated drones, the visceral reality of combat afforded by the physical proximity to one's enemy has steadily eroded. In 2007, researchers taught a monkey to neurologically control a walking robot on the other side of the world by means of electrochemical measurements of motor cortical activity. Considering this in light of the work on robotic tactile feedback, it is easy to imagine a new phase of warfare in which ground troops become obsolete. . . .

Marcello Ienca et al.

From Healthcare to Warfare and Reverse: How Should We Regulate Dual-Use Neurotechnology?

97 Neuron 269, 269–73 (2018)

In the ethics of (bio)technology, the dual-use problem refers primarily to the cooptation of civilian technology for military aims. This expression is also used to refer to the possibility of utilizing the same technology for both beneficial (e.g., clinical) applications and harmful misuse (e.g., bioterrorism). . . .

Security-sensitive research . . . is classified as Dual Use Research of Concern (DURC). DURC is a United States government's oversight label identifying research in the life sciences that can be anticipated to provide informational or technical resources for the development of threats to public health, individual safety, or national security.

In the past two decades, new concerns have [caused] the inclusion of various areas of neuroscience into the DURC domain. . . .

The dual-use problem is often presented as an ethical dilemma since it identifies a conflict between two fundamental ethical duties: the promotion of good and the prevention of possible collateral harm. . . . [I]n some research contexts, including neurotechnology, the complexity of the dual-use dilemma is increased by its bidirectional character. While classical dual-use problems are concerned with the cooptation of beneficial, civilian technology for military or nefarious purposes, neurotechnology also raises the reverse problem as several neurotechnologies developed by the military for national security purposes are likely to spill over into the civilian sector with a disruptive impact on healthcare, communication, or other fields.

The dual-use character of neurotechnology makes it also a potential target for non-State actors [and] cyber risks. Even though there are no confirmed cases of malicious attacks in non-experimental settings, information security researchers have experimentally demonstrated the actual feasibility of performing side-channel attacks and extracting private information from users of EEG-based BCIs. . . .

A neurosecurity framework could help anticipate future threats and maximize security in the neurotechnology domain through calibrated regulatory interventions, (neuro) ethical codes of conduct, and awareness- raising activities across the scientific community and the public.

NOTES AND QUESTIONS

1. How concerning is it to you that militaries are keen on improving, developing, and deploying brain-machine interfaces? What roles, if any, do you see for Congress in this domain? Anthropologist Hugh Gusterson has argued: "Most rational human beings would believe that if we could have a world where nobody does military neuroscience, we'll all be better off." Tim Sands, *Pentagon Goes Psycho*, Nature News Blog (Aug. 14, 2008). Do you agree? Why or why not?

2. In April 2013 the Department of Defense submitted its proposed FY 2014 budget. Included in the budget request were these activities:

> *Title:* Human Assisted Neural Devices
>
> *Description:* The Human Assisted Neural Devices program will develop the scientific foundation for understanding the language of the brain for application to a variety of emerging DoD challenges, including improving performance on the battlefield and returning active duty military to their units after injury. This will require an understanding of neuroscience, significant computational efforts, and new material design and implementation. Key advances expected from this research include determining the nature and means through which short-term memory is encoded, and discovering the mechanisms and dynamics underlying neural computation and reorganization. These advances will enable memory restoration through the use of devices programmed to bridge gaps in the injured brain. Further, modeling of the brain will progress to an unprecedented level with this novel approach. A key aspect of this effort will be to develop non-invasive bioimaging techniques that are capable of rapid analysis and interpretation of brain tissue alterations including new methods of analysis and interpretation for measuring brain tissue alterations at the cellular scale. . . .

Defense Advanced Research Projects Agency, *Department of Defense Fiscal Year (FY) 2014 President's Budget Submission*, Volume 1-50 (2013). By FY 2021, the Department of Defense noted that it had achieved "completion of system design and integration plans of the neural interface system." The Department's proposal for FY 2021 for Biomedical Technology included this description:

> This Biomedical Technology Program Element focuses on applied research for medical related technology, information, processes, materials, systems, and devices. Successful battlefield . . . neural interface technologies developed within this Program Element address a broad range of DoD challenges to ensure warfighter readiness, including . . . neurotechnology for improved warfighter performance. . . . To improve warfighter performance, this project will develop new neural architectures and data processing algorithms to interface the nervous system with multiple devices, enabling control of robotic prosthetic-limb technology. . . .

Defense Advanced Research Projects Agency, *Department of Defense Fiscal Year (FY) 2021 Budget Estimates*, Volume 1-49 (2020). If you were a member of Congress, how would you react to these funding requests?

3. In a 2002 demonstration a team of neuroscientists—funded by the Department of Defense—implanted electrodes in particular regions of the brains of rats and then effectively "drove" the rats through a maze by electrical stimulation. Sanjiv Talwar et al., *Rat Navigation Guided by Remote Control*, 417 Nature 37 (2002). Some were critical of this research:

> The revelation in the experiment, however, is how the scientists made themselves feel good. The story isn't what we tell the rats. It's what we tell ourselves.
>
> What's creepy about the robotized rats isn't that they're unhappy. It's that they're happy doing things no autonomous rat would do. Chapin's paper boasts that his team steered the rats "through environments that they would normally avoid, such as brightly lit, open areas." A companion diagram notes that a rat "was instructed to climb a vertical ladder, cross a narrow ledge, descend a flight of steps, pass through a hoop and descend a steep . . . ramp. . . . The rat wasn't whipped or pushed. It was "motivated." . . .

William Saletan, *Robot Rationalizations; How We Make Ourselves Feel Good About Hijacking Animals' Brains*, Slate (May 9, 2002).

In 2013 a different group of researchers reported on being able to remotely control cockroaches. Potentially constructive uses of this kind of technology—from military to search-and-rescue—come quickly to mind. What potential uses strike you as more problematic? As likely to raise novel legal questions?

4. The use of BMI in combat raises novel questions about prosecution for war crimes under international law. For instance:

> Resolving the issue of whether a pilot remotely connected by a brain-machine interfaced UAV could incur criminal liability for having killed a person that the Geneva Conventions protect would prove particularly problematic because of the uncertain status of the role that the *actus reus* requirement plays in determining criminal responsibility. Before the existence of this type of weapons system, courts had no occasion to resolve whether the condition exists merely because of the evidentiary impossibility of proving a thought crime or because the requirement in fact possesses an independent significance. . . .
>
> The use of machine interfaces may also lead to problematic results in the context of determining whether or not a volitional act took place. The recognition

of movement and motion planning register different electrical patterns of brain activity, and brain-machine interface studies rely on discriminating between different types of neural activity. Advances in neuro-imaging now make it possible to use computers to make increasingly accurate predictions about what a subject will to do before he or she actually does it. . . . Theoretically, a brain-machine interface weapon could fire a weapon based on such a predictive response, thereby making it uncertain whether or not a volitional act actually took place. . . .

Stephen E. White, *Brave New World: Neurowarfare and the Limits of International Humanitarian Law*, 41 Cornell Int'l L.J. 177, 196-98 (2008). How would you assess *actus reus* in this context? What about *mens rea*?

5. The Second Amendment of the U.S. Constitution reads: "A well regulated Militia, being necessary to the security of a free State, the right of the people to keep and bear Arms, shall not be infringed." Does this protect a right to bear *robotic* arms? Dan Terzian, *The Right to Bear (Robotic) Arms*, 117 Penn St. L. Rev. 755 (2013).

FURTHER READING

General Overview:

Isaac Asimov, *Fantastic Voyage II: Destination Brain* (1987).

Ray Kurzweil, *The Singularity Is Near: When Humans Transcend Biology* (2006).

Miguel Nicolelis, *Beyond Boundaries: The New Neuroscience of Connecting Brains with Machines—And How It Will Change Our Lives* (2011).

Judith Horstman, *The Scientific American Brave New Brain: How Neuroscience, Brain-Machine Interfaces, Neuroimaging, Psychopharmacology, Epigenetics, The Internet, and Our Own Minds Are Stimulating and Enhancing the Future of Mental Power* (2010).

Malcolm Gay, *The Brain Electric: The Dramatic High-Tech Race to Merge Minds and Machines* (2015).

Tim Urban, *Neuralink and the Brain's Magical Future*, Wait But Why (Apr. 20, 2017).

Brain-Computer Interfaces Handbook: Technological and Theoretical Advances (Chang S. Nam, Anton Nijholt & Fabien Lotte eds., 2018).

Ethical and Legal Considerations:

Stephen S. Wu & Marc Goodman, *Neural Devices Will Change Humankind: What Legal Issues Will Follow?*, 8 SciTech Law. (2012).

Eric Chan, *The Food and Drug Administration and the Future of the Brain-Computer Interface: Adapting FDA Device Law to the Challenges of Human-Machine Enhancement*, 25 J. Marshall J. Computer & Info. L. 117 (2007).

Eran Klein & Alan Rubel, Privacy and Ethics in Brain-Computer Interface Research, in *Brain-Computer Interfaces Handbook: Technological and Theoretical Advances* 653 (Chang S. Nam, Anton Nijholt & Fabien Lotte eds., 2018).

Michael Bess, *Our Grandchildren Redesigned: Life in Bioengineered Society of the Near Future* (2015).

Yuval Noah Harari, *Homo Deus: A Brief History of Tomorrow* (2017).

Karola V. Kreitmair, *Dimensions of Ethical Direct-To-Consumer Neurotechnologies*, 10 AJOB Neurosci. 152 (2019).

Sara Goering, et al., *Staying in the Loop: Relational Agency and Identity in Next-Generation DBS for Psychiatry*, 8 AJOB Neurosci. 59 (2017).

The Royal Society, *iHuman: Blurring Lines Between Mind and Machine* (Sept. 2019).

Military and National Security:

Committee on Military and Intelligence Methodology for Emergent Neurophysiological and Cognitive/Neural Science Research in the Next Two Decades, *Emerging Cognitive Neuroscience and Related Technologies* (2008).

Jonathan D. Moreno, *Mind Wars: Brain Science and the Military in the 21st Century* (2012).

Jeremy T. Nelson & Victoria Tepe, *Neuromodulation Research and Application in the U.S. Department of Defense*, 8 Brain Stimulation 247 (2015).

Charles N. Munyon, *Neuroethics of Non-Primary Brain Computer Interface: Focus on Potential Military Applications*, 12 Frontiers in Neurosci. 696 (2018).

International Neuroethics Statements:

Australian Brain Alliance, *A Neuroethics Framework for the Australian Brain Initiative*, 101 Neuron 365 (2019).

Judy Illes et al., *A Neuroethics Backbone for the Evolving Canadian Brain Research Strategy*, 101 Neuron 370 (2019).

Sung-Jin Jeong et al., *Korea Brain Initiative: Emerging Issues and Institutionalization of Neuroethics*, 101 Neuron 390 (2019).

Khara M. Ramos et al., *The NIH BRAIN Initiative: Integrating Neuroethics and Neuroscience*, 101 Neuron 394 (2019).

Norihiro Sadato et al., *Neuroethical Issues of the Brain/MINDS Project of Japan*, 101 Neuron 385 (2019).

Arleen Salles et al., *The Human Brain Project: Responsible Brain Research for the Benefit of Society*, 101 Neuron 380 (2019).

Yi Wang et al., *Responsibility and Sustainability in Brain Science, Technology, and Neuroethics in China—A Culture-Oriented Perspective*, 101 Neuron 375 (2019).

CHAPTER 21

Artificial Intelligence, Robots, and Law

Detective Spooner: Can a robot write a symphony? Can a robot turn a canvas into a beautiful masterpiece?

Sonny [the robot]: Can you?

— *I, Robot*, 20th Century Fox (2004)

The machines will convince us that they are conscious, that they have their own agenda worthy of our respect. They will embody human qualities and will claim to be human. And we'll believe them.

—Ray Kurzweil[†]

CHAPTER SUMMARY

This chapter:
- Introduces current developments in artificial intelligence and robotics.
- Explores the implications of AI for legal doctrine and legal practice.
- Considers the distinctions and similarities between humans and robots and whether robots should ever enjoy rights akin to those of humans.

INTRODUCTION

The history of machine intelligence is filled with massive failures of imagination. In 1943 Thomas Watson—the chairman of the board of IBM—remarked, "I think there is a world market for maybe five computers." Three decades later in 1972, Ken Olson—founder of Digital Equipment Corporation—asserted, "There is no reason anyone would want a computer in their home." At the same time, the history of machine intelligence has also witnessed excessively grandiose predictions followed by disappointing failures. But, no one can dispute that computers have become more common than anyone would have imagined. When invented, each computer required the attention and care of multiple individuals. The ratio of the number of computers to humans was much, much less than one. Today, think about how many computers you use—on your desk, in your phone, throughout your kitchen, embedded in the electric, gas, and water utilities you depend on, and on the campus

---

† Ray Kurzweil, *The Age of Spiritual Machines: When Computers Exceed Human Intelligence* 63 (2000).

supporting your education. Today, the ratio of computers to humans has become much more than one.

Knowledge about natural intelligence and improvements in the power of computers have spawned advances in artificial intelligence (AI) systems that have transformed life. And the developments keep coming. You have experienced the almost annual improvements in the capability of your smartphone. From robot vacuums searching for dust in homes, to robots searching for humans buried in earthquake rubble, intelligence has been embedded in machines that move around in different environments to accomplish useful tasks. The fact that some of these machines can be built to look and even act like humans suggests that tomorrow's future will continue to merge with today's science fiction.

Recent advances in machine learning and AI have led to rapid responses in legal practice and scholarship. In practice, law firms are using AI to improve efficiency, and representing clients on many new matters associated with AI. For instance, tasks such as document review and contract analysis used to be assigned to young associates but are now increasingly completed by AI systems. In 2018, a dozen big law firms created Reynen Court, a "platform for AI" technology specifically tailored to the needs of lawyers.

Since the first edition of this book, many major law firms have opened up new AI practice groups. The breadth of an AI and Law practice is captured in one firm's description of its work: "We cover all legal aspects of the AI ecosystem, such as IP strategies for AI and AI-device systems, data management and security; privacy law; software as a medical device; digital health; digital transformation strategies and related technology services like blockchain; machine learning and robotics; smart contracts; big data analytics; liability and risk assessment in AI-related contracts and torts; and the Internet of Things."*

In this chapter we focus on the subset of these AI issues most related to neuroscience. For those interested in additional reading, the further readings suggested at the end of the chapter point you in multiple directions. There are at least three ways in which AI and law intersect with neuroscience.

First, appreciation of the kinds and degrees of intelligence that can be embodied through computers provides an inspiring and informative perspective on the kinds and degrees of intelligence embodied in humans (and animals and plants). Most pointedly, does agency and legal standing require a biological brain?

Second, for both practice and doctrine, evaluation of AI decision-making in legal contexts inevitably invites comparisons with human decision-making. For instance, both the utility and the constitutionality of an AI program to screen job applicants' resumes hinges on its biases and performance outcomes relative to the human staffers who would have otherwise screened the applicants. Similarly, whether or not a human should be "in the loop" for AI healthcare decision-making requires careful consideration of how the human brain would approach the same decisions.

Third, as illustrated in the previous chapter, the boundary between biology and technology is becoming blurred. This raises questions about accountability and ownership. Where does liability rest when an autonomous AI system malfunctions? What if that AI system is inside the human—for instance, a closed-loop neurostimulator

---

* *Artificial Intelligence,* DLA Piper (2020), https://www.dlapiper.com/en/us/focus/artificial-intelligence.

relying on AI to determine when and how much voltage to send to various regions of the brain? Complex questions such as these are now ripe for careful legal analysis.

The chapter is organized in three sections. Section A provides an introduction to salient developments in Artificial Intelligence and Robotics. Section B examines how AI has already begun, and will in the future continue, to change a wide swath of legal doctrine and practice. Section C then considers whether robots should have legal rights, and corresponding legal responsibilities, and if so, where and how to draw those lines.

A. THE DEVELOPMENT OF AI AND ROBOTICS

The term AI describes a field in computer science and engineering that has the goal of designing and building machines that exhibit signs of intelligence. This intelligence can be manifested through various means, such as playing chess or poker, operating autonomous vehicles on city streets or in remote locations, investing in stocks, managing properties, and organizing bed schedules and staff rotations in hospitals. John McCarthy, who coined the term in 1956, defines AI as "the science and engineering of making intelligent machines." The field is motivated and guided by the premise that human intelligence can be described so precisely that it can be replicated by a machine.

Today AI is an essential element of computer science, finance, modern industry, medicine, and the military. To address anticipated labor shortages, countries like Japan and South Korea are investing heavily in developing robotics. Time-saving automation of tasks has been happening for decades, of course. An advertising slogan from the (now quaint) 1920s reads: "Clothes washing is a task for a machine, not for your wife. Turn the hard work into play. Buy her a Bluebird." Today you can buy a robot vacuum cleaner and a self-driving car. In the first edition of this book we quoted a scientist who observed, "During the next decade we're going to see smarts put into everything . . . [s]mart homes, smart cars, smart health, smart robots, smart science, smart crowds and smart computer-human interactions."* Reading this second edition, how many of these do you use and enjoy today?

Since the first edition of this book appeared, AI has been transformed by the development of *deep neural networks* (also known as *convolutional neural networks*). These consist of many layers composed of multiple interconnected nodes, the activation of which represents inputs and outputs at various levels of abstraction. They are inspired by insights from neuroscience. For example, the input layer could be the light intensities in a visual image. From this input, a deep neural network would have layers deriving the edges, contours, and surfaces in the image and other layers ultimately representing the identity of the objects in the image. The connections in the network are structured through a process referred to as *machine learning* (also known as *deep learning*). The learning algorithm updates the connections between layers through trial and error with rewards structured by the programmer to produce a network with desired input-output properties.

---

* Ed Lazowska, as quoted in John Markoff, *The Rapid Advance of Artificial Intelligence*, N.Y. Times (Oct. 14, 2013).

In our example, the network could be trained to distinguish dogs from cats, for instance. Indeed, today deep neural networks can learn desired associations between inputs and outputs. Perhaps the most vivid accomplishments of deep neural networks structured through machine learning are in the domain of object recognition. Highlighting the connection between deep neural networks and neuroscience, systems that achieve human-level object recognition end up with nodes that recapitulate the properties of neurons observed in the visual system of the brain. However, the training of such systems depends on knowing the right answers. In the beginning, this was accomplished by having human volunteers label thousands of objects in hundreds of scenes. Subsequently, companies like Google used the responses of humans to Captcha ("completely automated public Turing test to tell computers and humans apart") used for secure website transactions to acquire data used to train subsequent neural networks. Today, these systems can be trained to recognize things like license plates and faces (even with a mask on). Such systems are now used on assembly lines and in purchasing warehouses to select among components or small items jumbled in a container. Operating faster than the human brain, such neural networks can work in real time environments. For example, the Tesla self-driving cars are designed with dozens of neural networks. Deep neural networks can also learn without human intervention to play games like Go or poker.

As technology has progressed, so too have philosophical inquiries about the nature of the mind, legal inquiries about liability for robots gone awry, and ethical inquiries about creating, sustaining, and controlling artificial beings. These issues have been addressed vividly in fiction from *Frankenstein* to *I, Robot*. These issues have also been addressed in government policies across the globe. For instance, the European Robotics Research Network formulated a Roboethics Roadmap; the South Korean government established a panel to formulate a Robot Ethics Charter; and Japan's Ministry of Economy, Trade and Industry has developed safety guidelines styled somewhat after science fiction author Isaac Asimov's *Three Laws of Robotics*. Guidelines include recommendations to install sensors to prevent robots from running into people, to use more flexible materials to further prevent injury, and to include clear and easy-to-access emergency shut-off switches.

Perhaps the most vivid examples of AI are humanoid robots. In fiction these machines have been called *androids*. The development of such robots has been inspired by the two-part desire to understand how to accomplish what humans do so effortlessly and to create useful aids for human challenges and tasks. On the internet, you can find many videos of humanoid robots illustrating how realistic they look and how sophisticated they have become: ASIMO, Leonardo, Nao, Repliee Q1, and Atlas. Animals have also inspired the design of robots such as Big Dog. As you watch these videos, you probably experience at least some small sense of identification with the robots. With a little effort, you can probably imagine that they have a point of view.

An experiment run at an International Conference on Human-Robot Interaction confirmed that people find it difficult to turn off a robot that has interacted with them in a way that suggests a personality. As one reporter described the study, "I personally find myself with an irrational attachment to robots, a feeling which I think is shared by a lot of other people. I know they're all just running code, but I still talk to them and try to be nice to them and feel bad when (say) they get stuck on something or otherwise are having trouble. Like I said, it's completely irrational, I know it's irrational, but for me, robots that exhibit autonomous behavior strike enough of an 'alive' chord that I tend to treat them as if they had some sort of consciousness. . . ."* Our natural impulse to anthropomorphize is an important factor to keep in mind as we explore the implications of building and living with intelligent machines.

Neil M. Richards & William D. Smart
How Should the Law Think About Robots?
in *Robot Law* 5-22 (Ryan Calo, A. Michael Froomkin & Ian Kerr eds., 2016)

1. WHAT IS A ROBOT?

Before we can think about these systems, we need to have a clear understanding of what we mean by "robot." The word itself comes from a Czech play from the 1920s, entitled *R.U.R.* (Rossum's Universal Robots), by Karel Čapek. In the play, the "robots" are artificial humans used as slave labor in a factory (roboti in Czech translates to "serf labor," with the associated connotations of servitude and drudgery). The term roboticist, one who studies or creates robots, was coined by Isaac Asimov in 1941. Even the etymology of the word suggests a device that is well-suited for work that is too dull, dirty, or dangerous for (real) humans.

So what is a robot? . . .

Even professional roboticists do not have a single clear definition. Arms that assemble cars, teleoperated submarines that explore the ocean depths, space probes hurtling through the void, remote-controlled cars augmented with little computers and sensors, and human-like androids all fall under the definition of "robot," depending on whom you ask.

So how do we usefully define a "robot" . . .? In most of the examples above, the robots can move about their world and affect it, often by manipulating objects. They behave intelligently when interacting with the world. They are also constructed by humans. These traits are, to us, the hallmarks of a robot. We propose the following working definition: A robot is a constructed system that displays both physical and mental agency but is not alive in the biological sense. That is to say, a robot is something manufactured that moves about the world, seems to make rational decisions about what to do, and is a machine. It is important to note that the ascription of agency is subjective: the system must only appear to have agency to an external observer to meet our criteria. In addition, our definition excludes wholly software-based artificial intelligences that exert no agency in the physical world.

Our definition intentionally leaves open the mechanism that causes the apparent agency. The system can be controlled by clever computer software or teleoperated by a remote human operator. While both of these systems are robots by our definition, the legislative implications for each of them are quite different, as we argue below.

---

* Evan Ackerman, *Good News: Humans Have Trouble Killing Robots*, IEEE Spectrum (Jan. 31, 2013).

2. WHAT CAN ROBOTS DO?

Now that we have a definition of what a robot is, we turn to what robots can do today. Since many of us are informed by movies, sound-bite media, and other unreliable sources, we are often poorly informed about what state-of-the-art robots look like and what they can do right now. Robots have not yet reached the levels of capability the public associates with science fiction, but they are surprisingly close.

Until recently, the majority of "robots" in the world, over a million by some counts, were the industrial automatons that assemble cars, move heavy parts, and otherwise make factory workers' jobs easier. These are, . . . by our definition above, not really robots; although they certainly have physical agency, they have no mental agency. Most of these systems perform set motions over and over, without regard for what is happening in the world. Spot-welding robots will continue to spot-weld even if there is no car chassis in front of them.

But "robots" within our definition do exist today. The most common robot in the world is now the iRobot Roomba, a small robot that can autonomously vacuum-clean your house. iRobot claimed to have sold over 6 million Roombas as of the end of 2010.* These little critters are robots by our definition; they have both physical and mental agency. The computer algorithms that control them are simple, but they appear to make rational decisions as they scoot around the floor avoiding objects and entertaining your cat. The Roomba is fully autonomous and needs no human assistance, despite operating in a cluttered real-world environment (your house); this is a more impressive achievement than one might think, especially given that these inexpensive robots are available to consumers for only a few hundred dollars, depending on the model.

Other, more expensive robots are seeing heavy use in military settings all over the world. Cruise missiles, which meet our definition of robot, have been used for many years by the United States military and by other countries. More recently, remote-controlled drone aircraft, many of which we classify as robots, have seen heavy use in intelligence-gathering and offensive roles. Ground-based teleoperated robots, such as the Packbot (iRobot) and the Talon (Foster-Miller) are becoming ubiquitous in modern military settings. These systems can replace human soldiers in dangerous situations: disabling a bomb, performing reconnaissance under fire, or leading the assault on a building. Based on extrapolations of earlier sales figures for a single type of these ground robots, it is reasonable to estimate that there are 10,000 such systems currently in use worldwide, in both military and civilian roles. These robots can drive around under remote control, often have an arm that can pick up and manipulate objects, and have a suite of sensors that relay data back to the operator. While they are completely controlled by a human operator, and currently have no autonomous capabilities, they often look intelligent to an external observer (who might be unaware that there is a human pulling the strings).

NASA has a long history of sending robots into space and to other worlds. The most successful recent examples are probably the Mars Exploration Rovers: Spirit and Opportunity. These were sent to Mars in 2003, and although no communication has been received from Spirit since March 2010, Opportunity is still

---

* [According to the iRobot webpage, as of 2020 over 30 million have been sold. —Eds.]

operational after nine years on the surface. The rovers are mixed initiative or shared autonomy systems; they receive high-level instructions from human operators ("go over to that boulder"), but are responsible for their own low-level behavior (avoiding obstacles, for instance). . . . As robots become more and more multipurpose, it will be harder to imagine a priori how they will be used and, thus, harder to create comprehensive legislative and consumer protections for them. In the extreme (and very far-future) case of a robot that can do everything a human can, there are few practical boundaries on what the robot can be used for. How does one legislate such a system? No other devices are like it, meaning we must come up with suitable analogies and metaphors, which, we claim, will be tricky.

As robots enter public life and our private homes, the protections associated with them must be more comprehensive and robust than those currently in place for research robots. Most research robots come with many warnings and disclaimers and rely on the users (who are trained professionals) not to do anything stupid. This is simply not practical for the general public, since they have no technical training and cannot be relied on to exercise good judgment and caution.

As robots become more autonomous, the question of where liability rests when something goes wrong is complicated. Is it the manufacturer, the programmer, the user (who gave a bad instruction), or some combination of them all? The matter will be complicated in systems that are autonomous some of the time and teleoperated at other times, since this introduces a remote operator who might be controlling the robot in good faith, but with limited sensory information.

As robots enter the real world, our ability to predict what will happen decreases dramatically. Uneven floor surfaces, unexpected obstacles, small children, and a host of other factors make controlling the robot safely difficult, and designing legislation that is comprehensive but does not overly constrain the use of the systems will be challenging. . . .

6. COMPLICATIONS: *DEUS EX MACHINA*

Figuring out how to think about and analogize robots is hard enough for systems that are clearly autonomous or clearly teleoperated. Things get harder when we start to consider the new generation of shared autonomy systems. In these, a human operator (often at a remote location) collaborates with the autonomous software on the robot to control the system. The robot is neither fully autonomous nor fully teleoperated, and it will be difficult for an external observer to determine which mode (autonomous or remote-controlled) the system is in at any given time. This greatly complicates our choice of metaphors used to understand the system. We must also carefully choose the metaphors that we use to understand the operator's role, operating a system over which they have only partial control.

Is the robot a portal or avatar for a remote expert (like a plumber), or is the human-robot system the "expert"? Where does liability lie if the human teleoperator issues the correct command, but the autonomous software on the robot carries it out poorly? What are the privacy implications of not really knowing if there is a remote human "inhabiting" your household robot? How can we provide effective privacy metaphors and safeguards for both the owner of the robot and the remote operator? . . .

The robots *are* coming, and they are coming soon. We need to be ready for them and to be prepared to design appropriate, effective legislation and consumer protections for them. We believe that we can only do this by understanding the technology, drawing on our recent experience with other disruptive technologies, and by avoiding seductive anthropomorphizations of our new metallic overlords.

NOTES AND QUESTIONS

1. What would be your criteria for determining whether a machine can think?
2. Is your brain a "machine"? Why or why not? According to what criteria?
3. Are all living human beings "intelligent"? Think back to the chapter on brain death. Is someone in a permanent vegetative state "intelligent"? Is s/he more intelligent than the automated life support system that is keeping the heart pumping?
4. Thought leader Stephen Hawking told the BBC, "The development of full artificial intelligence could spell the end of the human race." Rory Cellan-Jones, *Stephen Hawking Warns Artificial Intelligence Could End Mankind*, BBC News (Dec. 2, 2014). Elon Musk agrees: "[A]s AI gets probably much smarter than humans, the relative intelligence ratio is probably similar to that between a person and a cat, maybe bigger. I do think we need to be very careful about the advancement of AI." Kara Swisher, *Elon Musk: The Recode Interview*, Vox (Nov. 5, 2018). Do you more fear or welcome developments in AI and robotics?
5. The success of deep neural network systems to recognize objects has led to investigation of countermeasures. For example, a research group at the University of Maryland has devised adversarial attacks on state-of-the-art object detection systems (https://www.cs.umd.edu/~tomg/projects/invisible). Based on their research, you can wear a T-shirt with a carefully devised pattern that will make you effectively invisible to AI systems that identify human actors in an environment. Zuxuan Wu et al., *Making an Invisibility Cloak: Real World Adversarial Attacks on Object Detectors*, arXiv, Oct. 31, 2019, at https://arxiv.org/abs/1910.14667. How can and should the law regulate research that attempts to thwart AI and robotic accomplishments?
6. Contrasting with the robot rebellion theme, the well-known writer Isaac Asimov was one of the first to explore the ethical and moral implications of autonomous machines. His 1942 short story "Runaround" introduced the three laws of robotics:

> First Law: A robot may not injure a human being, or, through inaction, allow a human being to come to harm.
> Second Law: A robot must obey orders given it by human beings, except where such orders would conflict with the First Law.
> Third Law: A robot must protect its own existence as long as such protection does not conflict with the First or Second Law.

Subsequently, Asimov discovered the need for a fourth law, referred to as Law Zero: No robot may harm humanity or, through inaction, allow humanity to come to harm. Are these "laws" adequate for ensuring human safety from robots? How would such laws be enforced?

In 2017 Oren Etzioni, CEO of the Allen Institute for AI (AI2), proposed a new set of three rules for AI: "First, an A.I. system must be subject to the full gamut of laws that apply to its human operator. [Second,] an A.I. system must clearly disclose that it is not human. [Third,] an A.I. system cannot retain or disclose confidential information without explicit approval from the source of that information." Oren Etzioni, *How to Regulate Artificial Intelligence*, N.Y. Times (Sept. 1, 2017). What three laws would you mandate?

The Vatican has also become concerned about AI. It co-signed with IBM and Microsoft an ethical resolution on the design and use of artificial intelligence systems based on six principles: Transparency, Inclusion, Responsibility, Impartiality, Reliability, and Security and Privacy. Simon Chandler, *Vatican AI Ethics Pledge Will Struggle to Be More than PR Exercise*, Forbes (Mar. 4, 2020).

7. In 1930 the economist John Maynard Keynes made this prediction:

> In quite a few years—in our own lifetimes I mean—we may be able to perform all the operations of agriculture, mining, and manufacture with a quarter of the human effort to which we have been accustomed. . . . We are being afflicted with a new disease of which some readers may not yet have heard the name, but of which they will hear a great deal in the years to come—namely, technological unemployment. This means unemployment due to our discovery of means of economising the use of labour outrunning the pace at which we can find new uses for labour.
>
> But this is only a temporary phase of maladjustment. All this means in the long run is that mankind is solving its economic problem. I would predict that the standard of life in progressive countries one hundred years hence will be between four and eight times as high as it is today. There would be nothing surprising in this even in the light of our present knowledge. It would not be foolish to contemplate the possibility of a far greater progress still.

John Maynard Keynes, *Economic Possibilities for Our Grandchildren*, in *Essays in Persuasion* 358, 364-65 (Harcourt, Brace & Co. 1932). Does this apply to present circumstances? Will we see technological unemployment due to the rise of AI?

8. What other challenges might the legal system encounter in attributing liability to an AI? If AIs can be held liable for their actions, who pays the damages? Must AIs be granted property rights at the same time as the ability to be held liable? What other negative feedback could an AI experience that would make it "learn" not to repeat the action in question? Do the justifications for incarceration apply to AI (incapacitation, just desserts, deterrence)? What characteristics would an AI need for each of these justifications for punishment to apply?

9. The excerpt referred to software-based Artificial Intelligences that exert no agency in the physical world. You should know, however, that some AI systems run physical systems like power plants. Moreover, malicious actors can cause damage in the physical world by introducing software changes in the systems. For example, in the early 2000s a computer worm known as Stuxnet was developed. It was designed to disrupt the normal operation of programmable logic controllers automating electromechanical processes. It was used by the United States to damage the centrifuges used in Iran's nuclear program. What kinds of regulations, decided and administered by whom, would you ideally like to see implemented?

10. The U.S. government and countries across the world are preparing for an AI future. In 2019 the Trump Administration issued an Executive Order declaring that "[c]ontinued American leadership in AI is of paramount importance to maintaining the economic and national security of the United States and to shaping the global evolution of AI in a manner consistent with our Nation's values, policies, and priorities." Maintaining American Leadership in Artificial Intelligence, Exec. Order No 13859 § 1, 84 Fed. Reg. 3967 (Feb. 11, 2019).

B. AI AND THE LAW

The field of law and artificial intelligence is several decades old, beginning with explorations of how artificial intelligence could mimic legal reasoning. As the editors of the journal *Artificial Intelligence and Law* wrote in its inaugural issue in 1992, AI and law is "an interdisciplinary field that combines one of the oldest human intellectual endeavors with one of the youngest."* Thirty years ago, AI and the law was a field occupied primarily by a small cadre of academics. But no longer. As the excerpts in this section make clear, the incorporation of AI into many facets of life is generating challenging questions in many areas of law.

The first three excerpts provide clarity on how to define terms such as "artificial intelligence," "machine learning," and "robot" and on the role of neuroscience in the development of AI.

1. AI and the Law: Defining the Terms

Edwina L. Rissland

Artificial Intelligence and Law: Stepping Stones to a Model of Legal Reasoning

99 Yale L.J. 1957, 1958-81 (1990)

A. WHAT IS ARTIFICIAL INTELLIGENCE?

AI is the study of cognitive processes using the conceptual frameworks and tools of computer science. As a distinct subfield of computer science, AI had its beginnings in the mid-fifties. In 1968 Marvin Minsky, one of the founders of AI, said it well: AI is "the science of making machines do things that would require intelligence if done by man." Thus, all manner of intelligent behavior is in the realm of AI, including playing chess, solving calculus problems, making mathematical discoveries, understanding short stories, learning new concepts, interpreting visual scenes, diagnosing diseases, and reasoning by analogy. Any discussion of AI must note that tasks involving "common sense" reasoning or perception, such as language understanding, are by far the most difficult for AI. More technical tasks, like solving calculus problems or playing chess, are usually much easier. That is because the latter can be framed in well-defined terms and come from totally black-and-white domains, while the former cannot and do not. What distinguishes the AI approach from other studies of cognition and knowledge, such as psychology or philosophy, is its insistence on

---

* From the Editors, 1 Artificial Intelligence & L. 1, 1 (1992).

grounding the analysis in computational terms—preferably in a successfully running computer program that embodies the analysis.

AI is pursued for at least two reasons: to understand the workings of human intelligence and to create useful computer programs and computers that can perform intelligently. Most workers in the field of AI pursue these goals simultaneously. . . . In the context of law, these twin rationales translate into the twin goals of understanding certain key aspects of legal reasoning and building computational tools useful for legal practice, teaching, or research. An example of the former is the development of an AI model for reasoning based upon the doctrine of precedent. The process of developing an AI model causes one to learn about legal reasoning. Modeling involves elucidating key ingredients of precedent-based reasoning, such as making assessments of the relevance of precedents to new situations, distinguishing contrary cases, and drawing connections between relevant cases; then describing them in detail and building a program to execute them.

An example of the second, more applications-oriented goal, is construction of a set of computational tools (a lawyer's workbench, so to speak) to assist in the preparation of a brief. These may include functions to assist in gathering relevant precedents from data bases, sorting them according to their doctrinal approaches, and "Shepardizing"' them. Building a practical system, like one to assist with writing a brief, requires developing analytical models. Typically, satisfaction with an analytical model increases if it offers insights leading to the practical advances. . . .

In seeking to understand and model legal reasoning, AI will be challenged and enriched. By engaging in AI endeavors, the law will be challenged and enriched too; it will better understand its own modes of reasonings, including the knowledge and assumptions underlying them, and it will benefit from practical computational tools and models. The relationship between AI and law is a true synergy, the shared specialty of AI and law adding value to both.

Harry Surden
Artificial Intelligence and Law: An Overview
35 Ga. St. U. L. Rev. 1305, 1311-16 (2019)

MACHINE LEARNING

Machine learning refers to a family of AI techniques that share some common characteristics. In essence, most machine-learning methods work by detecting useful patterns in large amounts of data. These systems can then apply these patterns in various tasks, such as driving a car or detecting fraud, in ways that often produce useful, intelligent-seeming results. Machine learning is not one approach but rather refers to a broad category of computer techniques that share these features. Common machine-learning techniques that readers may have heard of include neural networks/deep learning, naive Bayes classifier, logistic regression, and random forests. . . . [M]achine learning is the predominant approach in AI today. . . .

At the outset, it is important to clarify the meaning of the word learning in machine learning. Based upon the name, one might assume that these systems are learning in the way that humans do. But that is not the case. Rather, the word learning is used only as a rough metaphor for human learning. For instance, when humans learn, we often measure progress in a functional sense—whether a person is getting better at a particular task over time through experience. Similarly, we can roughly characterize machine-learning systems as functionally "learning" in the sense that they too can improve their performance on particular tasks over time. They do this by examining more data and looking for additional patterns. Importantly, the word learning does not imply that that these systems are artificially replicating the higher-order neural systems found in human learning. Rather, these algorithms improve their performance by examining more data and detecting additional patterns in that data that assist in making better automated decisions. . . .

In sum, machine learning is currently the most significant and impactful approach to artificial intelligence. It underlies most of the major AI systems impacting society today, including autonomous vehicles, predictive analytics, fraud detection, and much of automation in medicine. It is important, however, to emphasize how dependent machine learning is upon the availability of data. The rise of machine learning has been fueled by a massive increase in the availability of data on the Internet, as more societal processes and institutions operate using computers with stored, networked data. Because effective machine learning typically depends upon large amounts of high-quality, structured, machine-processable data, machine-learning approaches often do not function well in environments where there is little data or poor-quality data. [L]aw is one of those domains where high-quality, machine-processable data is currently comparatively scarce except in particular niches.

Ryan Calo

Robotics and the Lessons of Cyberlaw

103 Calif. L. Rev. 513, 529-31 (2015)

A. DEFINITIONS

Few complex technologies have a single, stable, uncontested definition. Robots are no exception. There is some measure of consensus, however, around the idea that robots are mechanical objects that take the world in, process what they sense, and in turn act upon the world. The utility here of the so-called sense-think-act paradigm lies in distinguishing robots from other technologies. A laptop with a camera can, to a degree, sense and process the external world. But a laptop does not act upon the world. A remote control car with a camera senses and physically affects its environment but relies on the human operator for processing. The idea of a robot or robotic system is that the technology combines all three.

Each of these characteristics of sensing, processing, and acting exists on a spectrum. Some robots sense the world but little. . . .

While well-known robots like the Mars Rover, the Da Vinci surgical robot, and the infamous Predator B drone are substantially teleoperated in that a human being sees what the machine sees and controls its movements, these systems also "think" to a limited degree. The Mars Rover, for example, has self-directed modes and will not necessarily take certain actions suggested by NASA, like drive off a Martian cliff, if doing so will imperil the robot. . . .

Robots can "act" to varying degrees as well—they can possess a greater or lesser ability to move around or manipulate the world. But acting invites a more fundamental question of definition: Can technology act non-mechanically? Recall that we are looking here for the ways robots differ from longstanding and constituent technologies. If a user interface is the same as an actuator, it is not clear how robots are different from smartphones. At the same time, visual and auditory interfaces introduce energy into and hence alter the human environment. Movies and other stimuli—including social "bots" made of software—can induce a range of emotions and physiological responses. . . .

[A] system acts upon its environment to the extent it changes that environment directly. A technology does not act, and hence is not a robot, merely by providing information in an intelligible format. It must *be* in some way. A robot in the strongest, fullest sense of the term exists in the world as a corporeal object with the capacity to exert itself physically. But again, I am talking in terms of a continuum. It may well be appropriate to refer to certain virtual objects organized to exist in and influence the world as robots, especially if they meet the other definitional elements. . . .

A working definition of what it means for technology to act, as opposed to inform, is of particular interest to legal analysis. . . . [O]fficials and courts will face the line between informing and acting more and more, just as scholars have already started to grapple with the essential qualities of robotics without acknowledgment of the transition.

To sum up, robots are best thought of as artificial objects or systems that sense, process, and act upon the world to at least some degree. But this is just a technical definition, akin to describing the networks and protocols that comprise the Internet. What turns out to be important for legal and policy discourse is not the precise architecture, but the possibilities and experiences the architecture generates and circumscribes. . . .

Deborah W. Denno & Ryan Surujnath
Rise of the Machines: Artificial Intelligence, Robotics, and the Reprogramming of Law: Foreword
Symposium, 88 Fordham L. Rev. 381, 383-84 (2019)

Neuroscience—"the branch of life sciences that studies the brain and nervous systems"—is integral to AI development, as programmers seek to improve machines by understanding human thought patterns.

During the early stages of AI, neuroscience was integral to the development of basic neural networks' reinforcement learning. Today, modern AI research has taken cues from neurological studies to replicate human cognitive functions in an AI's code. . . .

The pace of today's research is rapid and fueled by advancements beyond pure software: "neurorobotics" is a field born from the combination of neuroscience, robotics, and AI. Neurorobotics devices use biologically inspired neural networking systems which are implemented into physical platforms. In turn, such devices are integral to the development of industrial-grade robotics, prosthetics, and even primitive nanomachines. Just as these technologies promise to reinvent industry, our traditional understanding of legal rules and systems could be at the precipice of major change.

Nonetheless, AI is something of a buzzword across the legal industry. There is still a certain mystique to the technology's functionality. . . . As researchers continue to use neuroscience to make AI more "human" in its reasoning, the technology has encountered a range of human legal problems, including discrimination and bias, civil liability for risk-taking, and ownership of data and creative content. . . .

[E]thical standards for the development of AI will be crucial. There is a popular adage in the world of computing: "garbage in, garbage out." In essence, this idea tells us that flawed inputs will yield flawed results. It is an unfortunate reality that human beings are imperfect and susceptible to errors, biases, and prejudices. It is thus integral to reduce the impact that human judgments have on the tools we use. The transition to a world of algorithmic governance is not without its potential costs. As is particularly salient in the national discourse, it appears that our privacy is something of a premium. With the next great advancement in automated decision-making, individuals may stand to lose in privacy what they gain in convenience. . . .

2. AI and the Law: Ownership, Accountability, and Governance

Shlomit Yanisky-Ravid

Generating Rembrandt: Artificial Intelligence, Copyright, and Accountability in the 3A Era — The Human-Like Authors Are Already Here — A New Model

2017 Mich. St. L. Rev. 659, 661-67 (2017)

The artist appraises the work, silently judging each stroke of dark ink on the canvas. Determining that the composition is not shaded quite right, the artist decides to switch to an even blacker hue. Retrieving the brush from the palette, the artist begins to work again, methodically filling the canvas with terse, precise brushstrokes. This is a familiar scene, one that has been playing out in artists' workshops from the medieval classic painters to modern creative artists. This artist, however, is different. It is a robot. Named e-David by its creators at the University of Konstanz in Germany, this robotic artist uses a complex visual optimization algorithm to create paintings. E-David represents merely one step in the ongoing development of the complex, advanced, automated, autonomous, unpredictable, and evolving artificial intelligence (AI) systems that already create original intellectual property works.

These AI systems are quite different from simple laser printers, which can only reproduce or copy existing works, in a predictable, structural method. E-David, on the other hand, unlike the traditional systems, can produce new drawings in a non-anticipated and creative way. E-David does not copy other works, but instead autonomously takes pictures with its camera and draws original paintings from these photographs. Some of these artworks might be entitled to copyright protection had humans created them. By using different techniques and an optimization system, e-David makes autonomous and unpredictable decisions about the image it is creating, the shapes and colors, the best way to combine light and shadow, and more. Even though e-David functions through software created by its programmers, a camera embedded in its complex system allows it to independently take new pictures and generate new creative input as "its own."

. . . I argue that under the "3A era" of automated, autonomous, and advanced technology, sophisticated AI systems and robots turn into talented authors. Indeed, these AI systems already function in the 3A era, generate products and services, make decisions, act, and independently create artworks.

[P]olicy makers must re-consider the relevancy of the current laws. Can our legal system cope with questions of ownership and responsibility in the 3A era that have never been seen before?

. . . The main legal challenge remains: Who owns the products generated by AI systems and who is responsible for the possibly negative outcomes stemming from them?

Joshua A. Kroll et al.
Accountable Algorithms
165 U. Pa. L. Rev. 633, 636-40 (2017)

Many important decisions that were historically made by people are now made by computer systems. . . . The efficiency and accuracy of automated decision-making ensures that its domain will continue to expand. . . .

However, the accountability mechanisms and legal standards that govern decision processes have not kept pace with technology. The tools currently available to policymakers, legislators, and courts were developed primarily to oversee human decisionmakers. Many observers have argued that our current frameworks are not well-adapted for situations in which a potentially incorrect, unjustified, or unfair outcome emerges from a computer. Citizens, and society as a whole, have an interest in making these processes more accountable. If these new inventions are to be made governable, this gap must be bridged.

[A]uthorities can demonstrate—and . . . the public at large and oversight bodies can verify—that automated decisions comply with key standards of legal fairness . . . [through] two approaches: ex ante approaches aiming to establish that the decision process works as expected (which are commonly studied by technologists and computer scientists), and ex post approaches once decisions have been made, such as review and oversight (which are common in existing governance structures). . . . [T]he tools of the first approach [can be used] to guarantee that the second approach can function effectively. . . . [T]echnical tools for verifying the correctness of computer systems can be used to ensure that appropriate evidence exists for later oversight.

[I]n order for a computer system to function in an accountable way—either while operating an important civic process or merely engaging in routine commerce—accountability must be part of the system's design from the start. Designers of such systems, and the nontechnical stakeholders who often oversee or control system design, must begin with oversight and accountability in mind. . . .

Andrew Tutt
An FDA for Algorithms
69 Admin. L. Rev. 83, 104-07 (2017)

The rising complexity and varied uses of machine-learning algorithms promise to raise a host of challenges when those algorithms harm people. Consider three: (1) algorithmic responsibility will be difficult to measure; (2) algorithmic responsibility will be difficult to trace; and (3) human responsibility will be difficult to assign. . . .

Consider the difficulty of measuring algorithmic responsibility. The problem is multi-faceted. Algorithms are likely to make decisions that no human would have made in a variety of circumstances no human has confronted or even could confront. Those decisions might be a "bug" or a "feature." Often it will be difficult to know which. A self-driving car might intentionally cause an accident to prevent an even more catastrophic collision. A stock-trading algorithm may make a bad bet on the good faith belief (whatever that means to an algorithm) that a particular security should be bought or sold. The point is, we have a generally workable view of what it means for a person to act negligently or otherwise act in a legally culpable manner, but we have no similarly well-defined conception of what it means for an algorithm to do so.

Next, consider the difficulty of tracing algorithmic harms. Even if algorithms were programmed with specific attention to well-defined legal norms, it could be extremely difficult to know whether the algorithm behaved according to the legal standard or not in any given circumstance. The stock trading algorithm that made the bad bet might have made its decision based solely upon the "signal" in its training data—i.e., the algorithm was right about the circumstance it was confronting, but the event it predicted did not come to pass. Or it might have made its decision based on "noise" in the training data—i.e., the algorithm looked for the wrong thing in the wrong place. Algorithms that engage in discrimination offer a good example. Suppose a company used a machine-learning algorithm to screen for promising job candidates. That algorithm could end up discriminating on the basis of race, gender, or sexual orientation—but tracing the discrimination to a problem with the algorithm could be nearly impossible. To be sure, the discrimination could be a result of a bug in the design of the training algorithm or a typo by the programmer, but it could also be because of a problem with the training data, a byproduct of latent society-wide discrimination accidentally channeled into the algorithm, or even no discrimination at all, but instead a low-probability event that just happened to be observed.

Finally, consider the difficulty in fixing human responsibility. Algorithms can be sliced-and-diced in several ways that many other products are not. A company can sell only an algorithm's code or even give it away. The algorithm could then be copied, modified, customized, and reused or used in a variety of applications its initial author never could have imagined. Figuring out how much responsibility the original developer bears when any harm arises down the road will be a difficult question. Or consider a second company that sells training data for use in developing one's own learning algorithms, but does not sell any algorithms itself. Depending on the algorithm the customer trains, and the use to which the purchaser wishes to put the data, the data's efficacy could be highly variable, and the responsibility of the data seller could be as well. Or imagine a third company that sells algorithmic services as a package, but the algorithm it offers relies partially or extensively on human interaction when determining its final decisions and outputs (e.g., a stock trading algorithm where a human must confirm all the proposed trades). Divvying up responsibility between the algorithm and the human is likely to prove complicated.

With those challenges in mind . . . a federal agency could act as a standards-setting body that coordinates and develops classifications, design standards, and best practices. . . .

Table 1. A Possible Qualitative Scale of Algorithmic Complexity

Algorithm Type	Nickname	Description
Type 0	"White Box"	Algorithm is entirely deterministic (i.e., the algorithm is merely a pre-determined set of instructions).
Type 1	"Grey Box"	Algorithm is non-deterministic, but its non-deterministic characteristics are easily predicted and explained.
Type 2	"Black Box"	Algorithm exhibits emergent proprieties making it difficult or impossible to predict or explain its characteristics.
Type 3	"Sentient"	Algorithm can pass a Turing Test (i.e., has reached or exceeded human intelligence).
Type 4	"Singularity"	Algorithm is capable of recursive self-improvement (i.e., the algorithm has reached the "singularity").

An agency could develop categories for classifying algorithms, varying the level of regulatory scrutiny based on the algorithm's complexity. Under a sufficiently nuanced rubric, the vast majority of algorithms could escape federal scrutiny altogether. For example, the agency could classify algorithms into types based on their predictability, explainability, and general intelligence, but only subject the most opaque, complex, and dangerous types to regulatory scrutiny—thereby leaving untouched the vast majority of algorithms with relatively deterministic and predictable outputs. . . .

The Public Voice, Electronic Privacy Information Center
Universal Guidelines for Artificial Intelligence
(Oct. 23, 2018)

New developments in Artificial Intelligence are transforming the world, from science and industry to government administration and finance. The rise of AI decision-making also implicates fundamental rights of fairness, accountability, and transparency. Modern data analysis produces significant outcomes that have real life consequences for people in employment, housing, credit, commerce, and criminal sentencing. Many of these techniques are entirely opaque, leaving individuals unaware whether the decisions were accurate, fair, or even about them.

We propose these Universal Guidelines to inform and improve the design and use of AI. The Guidelines are intended to maximize the benefits of AI, to minimize the risk, and to ensure the protection of human rights. These Guidelines should be incorporated into ethical standards, adopted in national law and international agreements, and built into the design of systems. We state clearly that the primary responsibility for AI systems must reside with those institutions that fund, develop, and deploy these systems.

1. **Right to Transparency.** All individuals have the right to know the basis of an AI decision that concerns them. This includes access to the factors, the logic, and techniques that produced the outcome.

2. **Right to Human Determination.** All individuals have the right to a final determination made by a person.

3. **Identification Obligation.** The institution responsible for an AI system must be made known to the public.

4. **Fairness Obligation.** Institutions must ensure that AI systems do not reflect unfair bias or make impermissible discriminatory decisions.

5. **Assessment and Accountability Obligation.** An AI system should be deployed only after an adequate evaluation of its purpose and objectives, its benefits, as well as its risks. Institutions must be responsible for decisions made by an AI system.

6. **Accuracy, Reliability, and Validity Obligations.** Institutions must ensure the accuracy, reliability, and validity of decisions.

7. **Data Quality Obligation.** Institutions must establish data provenance, and assure quality and relevance for the data input into algorithms.

8. **Public Safety Obligation.** Institutions must assess the public safety risks that arise from the deployment of AI systems that direct or control physical devices, and implement safety controls.

9. **Cybersecurity Obligation.** Institutions must secure AI systems against cybersecurity threats.

10. **Prohibition on Secret Profiling.** No institution shall establish or maintain a secret profiling system.

11. **Prohibition on Unitary Scoring.** No national government shall establish or maintain a general-purpose score on its citizens or residents.

12. **Termination Obligation.** An institution that has established an AI system has an affirmative obligation to terminate the system if human control of the system is no longer possible.

NOTES AND QUESTIONS

1. Many commentators, including in the excerpts above, have emphasized the need to hold AI systems "accountable." What does accountability mean for AI and robots? How can accountability be "part of the system's design from the start"? Could a robot pay damages or be incarcerated? Law professor Hank Greely observes:

> What if artificial intelligence were treated as a kind of person, subject to those sanctions? One might well want to make sure that it had assets that could be used to pay its liabilities. Before allowing use of an artificial intelligence entity, the law could require that it be 'endowed,' through insurance or otherwise, with assets sufficient to discharge its plausible debts. (States do something of the sort by insisting that motor vehicles can be legally operated only when they — technically their registered owners, but in some sense 'they' — have liability insurance.) Enforcing injunctions might be even easier by, for example, adding programming that requires compliance with the court order. One might even imagine ways of 'imprisoning' or 'punishing' an artificial intelligence through putting it into a situation that it might find or feel unpleasant or even painful. . . .

Henry T. Greely, *Neuroscience, Artificial Intelligence, CRISPR— and Dogs and Cats*, 51 U.C. Davis L. Rev. 2303, 2324-25 (2018).

2. Is there a deeper issue than simply the effectiveness of machine learning at achieving desired outcomes? Consider the argument from law professor Emily Berman: "[E]ven assuming algorithmic models yield an accurate result in ninety-nine percent of national security and law enforcement decisions, can the use of these models to make such decisions *ever* conform to the fundamental values underlying our legal framework? That is to say, whether reliance on the output of machine-learning models — even if highly accurate — is in tension with the goal to maintain 'a government of laws' and not of machines." Emily Berman, *A Government of Laws and Not of Machines*, 98 B.U. L. Rev. 1277, 1282 (2018).

3. "Someday, perhaps sooner, perhaps later, machines will have demonstrably better success rates at medical diagnosis than human physicians — at least in particular medical specialties." How will medical malpractice law respond? *See* A. Michael Froomkin et al., *When AIs Outperform Doctors: Confronting the Challenges of a Tort-Induced Over-Reliance on Machine Learning*, 61 Ariz. L. Rev. 33, 35 (2019). *See also* W. Nicholson Price II, *Regulating Black-Box Medicine*, 116 Mich. L. Rev. 421 (2017).

4. It has been suggested that "on a conceptual level, machine learning and crime fighting are a perfect match" because identifying potential criminal offenders and those who might offend again involves many layers of complex variables. If developed, would "Automated Suspicion Algorithms" be constitutional? *See* Michael L. Rich, *Machine Learning, Automated Suspicion Algorithms, and the Fourth Amendment*, 164 U. Pa. L. Rev. 871, 875 (2016). *See also* Aziz Z. Huq, *Racial Equity in Algorithmic Criminal Justice*, 68 Duke L.J. 1043 (2019). Other challenges of such a system have been anticipated in fictional works such as "The Minority Report" by Philip K. Dick.

5. Could AI transform administrative law? On one hand, officials in government agencies "must make an array of crucial judgments on a daily basis that are not unlike the kinds of judgments that machine learning has so clearly helped improve in the private sector, [and if] machine learning can help regulatory agencies make smarter, more accurate decisions, the benefits to society could be considerable." At the same time, however, "[r]egulating by robot would hardly seem, at first glance, to fit naturally within prevailing principles of administrative law." Cary Coglianese & David Lehr, *Regulating by Robot: Administrative Decision Making in the Machine-Learning Era*, 105 Geo. L.J. 1147, 1153 (2017). *See also* Katherine J. Strandburg, *Rulemaking and Inscrutable Automated Decision Tools*, 119 Colum. L. Rev. 1851 (2019). If an AI system administering regulations does not "fit naturally within prevailing principles of administrative law," but a human does, what is the difference that makes a difference?

6. Should robots pay taxes? Or more realistically, should tax policy create incentives for companies to hire humans rather than automate tasks? Bill Gates has supported a so-called "robot tax," and legal scholars Ryan Abbott and Bret Bogenschneider have pointed out that "[r]obots are simply not taxpayers, at least not to the same extent as human workers. If all workers were to be replaced by machines tomorrow, most of the tax base would immediately disappear." Ryan Abbott & Bret Bogenschneider, *Should Robots Pay Taxes? Tax Policy in the Age of Automation*, 12 Harv. L. & Pol'y Rev. 145, 150-51 (2018).

7. What skills will lawyers need to navigate a world of legal practice infused by AI, robots, and machine learning? Consider this observation: "The frenetic and

much-touted world of artificial intelligence (AI) has poured into the legal industry like a storm surge. Lawyers who lack technical expertise or feel overwhelmed
by jargon and arcane mathematical concepts are at a distinct disadvantage in this
technology-oriented new world. Vendors can make assertions with little risk of
cross-examination." Maura R. Grossman & Rees W. Morrison, *7 Questions Lawyers
Should Ask Vendors About Their AI Products*, N.Y. St. B. Ass'n J., Mar. 2019, at 49.
See also David Lehr & Paul Ohm, *Playing with the Data: What Legal Scholars Should
Learn About Machine Learning*, 51 U.C. Davis L. Rev. 653 (2017).

8. You've read in previous chapters about the gatekeeping function that judges
   play in evaluating expert evidence. Should judges be able to call upon AI to
   help them evaluate the admissibility of complex science? *See* Pamela S. Katz,
   *Expert Robot: Using Artificial Intelligence to Assist Judges in Admitting Scientific Expert
   Testimony*, 24 Alb. L.J. Sci. & Tech. 1, 42 (2014) (arguing that such a robot "would
   lead to better decision making, ensure more uniformity and integrity in the process, and therefore greater trust in the system.")

C. ROBOT RIGHTS AND RESPONSIBILITIES: THE PERSONHOOD OF AUTONOMOUS ARTIFICIAL AGENTS

Lawrence B. Solum
Legal Personhood for Artificial Intelligences
70 N.C. L. Rev. 1231, 1231-40 (1992)

Could an artificial intelligence become a legal person? . . .

The classical discussion of the idea of legal personhood is found in John Chipman
Gray's *The Nature and Sources of the Law.* He began his famous discussion, "In books
of the Law, as in other books, and in common speech, 'person' is often used as
meaning a human being, but the technical legal meaning of a 'person' is a subject
of legal rights and duties." The question whether an entity should be considered a
legal person is reducible to other questions about whether or not the entity can and
should be made the subject of a set of legal rights and duties. The particular bundle
of rights and duties that accompanies legal personhood varies with the nature of
the entity. Both corporations and natural persons are legal persons, but they have
different sets of legal rights and duties. Nonetheless, legal personhood is usually
accompanied by the right to own property and the capacity to sue and be sued.

Gray reminds us that inanimate things have possessed legal rights at various
times. Temples in Rome and church buildings in the middle ages were regarded
as the subject of legal rights. Ancient Greek law and common law have even made
objects the subject of legal duties. In admiralty, a ship itself becomes the subject of a
proceeding in rem and can be found "guilty." Christopher Stone recently recounted
a twentieth-century Indian case in which counsel was appointed by an appellate
court to represent a family idol in a dispute over who should have custody of it. The
most familiar examples of legal persons that are not natural persons are business
corporations and government entities.

Gray's discussion was critical of the notion that an inanimate thing might be
considered a legal person. After all, what is the point of making a thing—which can
neither understand the law nor act on it—the subject of a legal duty? Moreover, he

argued that even corporations are reducible to relations between the persons who own stock in them, manage them, and so forth. Thus, Gray insisted that calling a legal person a "person" involved a fiction unless the entity possessed "intelligence" and "will." Those attributes are part of what is in contention in the debate over the possibility of AI. . . .

Wendell Wallach
From Robots to Techno Sapiens: Ethics, Law and Public Policy in the Development of Robotics and Neurotechnologies
3 L. Innovation & Tech. 185, 192-95 (2011)

Legal theorists and philosophers have been intrigued for years by the thought experiment of when, or if, future robots might be granted legal rights, or be designated legal persons responsible for their own choices and actions. But there is also beginning to be a small body of scholarship that analyses more near-term issues for the robotics industry. . . .

The central concerns are subsumed within four interrelated themes: (a) safety, (b) appropriate use, (c) capability, and (d) responsibility.

Safety has always been of importance to the engineers who build systems. Existing legal frameworks largely cover the legal challenges posed by present day robots. The robots that have been developed so far are sophisticated machines whose safety is clearly the responsibility of the companies that produce the devices and of the end users who adapt the technology for particular tasks.

Social and ethical theorists have raised a number of questions regarding which tasks are *appropriate* for robots. Some find the use of robots as sex toys offensive. Others lament the sensibilities and lessons lost in substituting robopets and robocompanions for animals or people. From a humanistic perspective, turning to robotic caregivers for the homebound and elderly is perceived as abusive or reflecting badly upon modern society, although robotic care is arguably better than no care at all. One dangerous practice is the increasing use of robonannies, robots that tend infants and children. Noel and Amanda Sharkey argue that the extensive use of robots as nannies, and companions for infants, may actually stunt emotional and intellectual development.

The appropriateness and *ability* of robots to serve as caregivers is commonly misunderstood by the public or misrepresented by those marketing the systems. The limited abilities of present day robotic devices can be obscured by the human tendency to anthropomorphise robots whose looks or behaviour is faintly similar to that of humans. There is a need for a professional association or regulatory commission that evaluates the capabilities of systems and certifies their use for specific activities. This is likely to be very expensive, as the development of each robotic platform is a moving target—existing capabilities are undergoing refinement and new capabilities are constantly being added to systems. . . .

3.1 LIMITING LIABILITY

With the increasing complexity of robotic systems, designers and engineers cannot always predict how they will act when confronted with new situations and new inputs. "Many hands" will have contributed to the building of a robot. The full operation of each hardware component in a system will only be understood by those who designed and built that component, and even they may have little or no understanding of how that component might interact with other components in a totally new device. The pressures to complete projects and the cost of testing also contribute to limited understanding of the potential risks inherent in new devices.

Of course credible manufacturers do not want to be held liable for marketing faulty devices. They may elect to avoid releasing products whose safe use they have no way of guaranteeing. For a society banking on the productivity improvements that transformative technology such as robots offer, this could be perceived as a heavy burden on innovation and a heavier price to pay for systems whose risks are low but whose benefits are significant. Indeed, other countries with higher bars to litigation would be likely to take a lead in robot technologies as manufacturers waited for liability law to be sorted out in their own country.

Manufacturers will certainly welcome measures that lower their liability. As a means of spurring industry growth and innovation, Ryan Calo has proposed immunising manufacturers of open robotic platforms from all actions related to improvements made by third parties. But any approach to limiting liability must be balanced against insuring that industry does not knowingly introduce dangerous products.

No-fault insurance for robots is another approach that could lower manufacturers' liability. Consider driverless cars, such as the one Google has developed. Even if driverless cars are much safer than those driven by humans, robot-chasing attorneys are likely to initiate suits for each death in which a robotic car is involved. All new technologies face similar challenges. Free societies have an array of laws, regulations, insurance policies and precedents that help protect industries from frivolous lawsuits. Companies pursuing the huge commercial market in robotics will protect their commercial interests by relying on the existing frameworks and by petitioning legislatures for additional laws that help manage their liability. . . .

[P]ractical ethicists and social theorists are raising concerns as to the dangers inherent in diluting corporate and human responsibility, accountability and liability for the actions of increasingly autonomous systems. Recently, five rules have been proposed as a means of re-establishing the principle that humans cannot be excused from moral responsibility for the design, development or deployment of computing artifacts.

Rule 1: The people who design, develop or deploy a computing artefact are morally responsible for that artefact, and for the foreseeable effects of that artefact. This responsibility is shared with other people who design, develop, deploy or knowingly use the artefact as part of a sociotechnical system.

Rule 2: The shared responsibility of computing artefacts is not a zero-sum game. The responsibility of an individual is not reduced simply because more people become involved in designing, developing, deploying or using the artefact. Instead, a person's responsibility includes being answerable for the behaviours of the artefact and for the artefact's effects after deployment, to the degree to which these effects are reasonably foreseeable by that person.

Rule 3: People who knowingly use a particular computing artefact are morally responsible for that use.

Rule 4: People who knowingly design, develop, deploy or use a computing arte-fact can do so responsibly only when they make a reasonable effort to take into account the sociotechnical systems in which the artefact is embedded.

Rule 5: People who design, develop, deploy, promote or evaluate a comput-ing artefact should not explicitly or implicitly deceive users about the artefact or its foreseeable effects, or about the sociotechnical systems in which the artefact is embedded. . . .

Kate Darling
Extending Legal Rights to Social Robots: The Effects of Anthropomorphism, Empathy, and Violent Behavior Towards Robotic Objects
in *Robot Law* 213, 216-31 (Ryan Calo, A. Michael Froomkin & Ian Kerr eds., 2016)

At first glance, it seems hard to justify differentiating between a social robot, such as a Pleo dinosaur toy, and a household appliance, such as a toaster. Both are man-made objects that can be purchased on Amazon and used as we please. Yet there is a difference in how we perceive these two artifacts. . . .

[S]ocial robots elicit behavior in us that is significantly different from what we exhibit towards other devices, like toasters. While people have for decades named their cars and developed emotions towards other inanimate objects, the effect of robots that actively and intentionally engage our ingrained anthropomorphic responses is considerably stronger. We are already disposed towards social engage-ment with the robotic companions available to us today, and we can only imagine what the technological developments of the next decade will be able to effect. As we move within the spectrum between treating social robots like toasters and treating them more like our cats, there may be some ethical issues to consider. . . .

WHEN SHOULD WE START PROTECTING ROBOTS?

Whether out of sentiment or to promote socially desirable behavior, some parts of society may sooner or later begin to ask that legal protections be extended to robotic companions. If this happens, politicians and lawmakers will need to deliber-ate whether it would make sense to accommodate this societal preference.

One view supports granting legal protection to social robots as soon as there is sufficient societal demand. Assuming that our society wants to protect animals regardless of their capacities, because of our personal attachments to them, soci-ety may someday also want to protect social robots regardless of their capacities. Humans' moral consideration of robots may simply depend more on our own feel-ings than on any societal effects or inherent qualities built into robots. Catering to this preference views the purpose of law as a social contract. . . .

Ideally, however, social sentiment and political push would be based on an understanding of the actual effects of anthropomorphism and driven by well-founded concern for societal welfare. . . . [T]he question of when we should extend legal protections to social robots depends on whether we find evidence that our behavior towards robots translates to other contexts. . . . [I]f lifelike and alive is sub-consciously muddled, then treating certain robots in a violent way could desensitize actors towards treating living things similarly. . . .

Jaap Hage

Theoretical Foundations for the Responsibility of Autonomous Agents

25 Artificial Intelligence L. 255, 258-61 (2017)

3.1 THE MENTAL AND THE PHYSICAL ASPECTS OF ACTS

It is almost a tautology that human beings are responsible for their acts, because if people are not responsible, the acts would not count as "their" acts. However, if humans are responsible while the responsibility of autonomous agents still needs to be argued, there must be one or more differences between humans and autonomous agents which seem at first sight relevant. One difference might be that that humans act intentionally and on the basis of a free will, while autonomous agents have no intentions, nor a will, let alone a free will. Let us assume for the sake of argument that autonomous agents lack intention and a will. In spite of this lack, they have in common with human beings that their "behavior" has a physical aspect and that this physical aspect is part of the processes that constitute physical reality. Even if human behavior is intentional and based on a free will, what physically happens fits in the same chain of events in which the "acts" of autonomous agents fit. The question is therefore whether intention and free will make a difference, and whether they play a role in the chains that constitute the physical aspects of acts. If they do not play such a role, they are in that sense redundant. It seems dubious then to base a difference in the attribution of responsibility on such redundant phenomena.

There are many reasons to assume that intention and free will do not play a role in the chains of facts and events that constitute the physical aspects of acts. The physical research paradigm which assumes that physical events are only linked to other physical events in a law-like fashion, works quite well and leaves no room for intervening mental phenomena like intention or will. It is completely unclear how physical events might be influenced by mental events as such, and there is no evidence that such an influence exists. It should be emphasized in this connection that the two words "as such" in the previous sentence are crucially important. The possibility should not be excluded beforehand—and actually it is quite likely—that intentions and will have counterparts in brain states. These brain states play a role in the processes of the physical world. However, this does not mean that intention and will as mental . . . influence the physical world.

Therefore, even if humans act on the basis of intentions and free will—whatever that might mean—while autonomous agents do not, this does not make a difference for what happens physically. It is for this reason not at all obvious that the alleged difference between humans and autonomous agents should mean that only human agents are held responsible for their acts and autonomous agents not. Whether such a difference should be considered depends on the reasons why we hold humans responsible, even if the mental aspects of their behavior do not influence the physical aspects thereof. . . .

3.5 ATTRIBUTION TO AUTONOMOUS AGENTS

By definition, what is "real" does not depend on attribution and is mind-independent. What is the result of attribution, on the contrary, depends on the human mind. This mind-dependency may be direct, as when somebody considers what another "does" as an act. It may also be indirect, as when members of a tribe attribute the failure of rain to the anger of the gods which makes the anger of the gods the cause of the rain failure even if some members do not believe this. It is also indirect when the law attributes the status of owner of a house to the daughter of a deceased person to whom the house used to belong. (The daughter is taken to have inherited the house.)

Because attribution is mind-dependent, agency and responsibility may theoretically be attributed to anything, and on any grounds. It is possible to consider events as the acts of animals or of gods, or as the acts of organizations, and we may hold animals, gods and organizations responsible and liable for these "acts." This however is only from a historical perspective done by analogy to the attribution of agency to human beings. Ontologically speaking, there is no difference between attribution of agency to humans and to other agents.

If we can attribute agency to organizations and hold them responsible and liable for their acts, we can do the same for autonomous agents. From the perspective of what can be done, there are no difficulties for the attribution of agency, responsibility and liability to autonomous agents. The question is not whether such attributions can be made, but whether it is *desirable* to do so. . . .

NOTES AND QUESTIONS

1. Looking backwards, the history of the word "person" may be illuminating:

> The word "person" is derived from the Latin word "persona" which originally referred to a mask worn by a human who was conveying a particular role in a play. In time it took on the sense of describing a guise one took on to express certain characteristics. Only later did the term become coextensive with the actual human who was taking on the persona, and thus became interchangeable with the term "human." Even as this transformation in linguistic meaning was taking place, the concepts of person and human remained distinct. To Greeks such as Aristotle, slaves and women did not possess souls. Consequently, while they were nominally human, they were not capable of fully participating in the civic life of the City and therefore not recognized as persons before the law. Because they were not legal persons, they had none of the rights possessed by full members of Athenian society. Similarly, Roman law, drawing heavily from Greek antecedents, made clear distinctions, drawing lines between property and legal persons, but allowing for gradations in status and in the case of slaves, permitting movement between categories.

   David J. Calverley, *Imagining a Non-Biological Machine as a Legal Person*, 22 AI & Soc'y 523, 525 (2008).

2. "It is fascinating (and perhaps unsettling) to realize the complexity and seriousness of tasks currently delegated to avatars and robots." David Allen Larson, *Artificial Intelligence: Robots, Avatars and the Demise of the Human Mediator*, 25 Ohio St. J. on Disp. Resol. 105, 107 (2010). At least one well-funded project, the 2045 Initiative, aims to create a life-sized avatar. Under what circumstances, if any, could or should an avatar be treated as your agent? As an autonomous, albeit non-biological being? The next excerpt explores theoretical complexities of such inquiries.

Samir Chopra & Laurence White
Artificial Agents—Personhood in Law and Philosophy
in *Proceedings of the 16th European Conference on Artificial Intelligence* 635, 635-38 (2004)

1. INTRODUCTION

A recurring philosophical debate concerns when or whether to ascribe person-hood to artificial agents. Typically, contributions to this debate involve drawing up a list of necessary and sufficient conditions, which must be met by an artificial agent in order to be classified as a genuine cognizer on par with human beings. Several issues are—unavoidably—conflated in this debate: the ascription of intentionality or conscious phenomenal experience, the possibility of the exercise of free will by—and autonomy for—artificial agents and so on. Unsurprisingly there is disagreement about what such a list of conditions should look like. One view on this situation is that philosophical theorizing about the cognitive status of artificial agents should draw inspiration from legal theorizing—which carries a strong pragmatic flavour—about the status of these agents in our society. Some of these legal arguments would support classifying agents as intelligent beings on par with human beings. Others would not. Conversely, legal arguments could draw upon philosophical arguments in arguing for the ascription of elevated cognitive status to artificial agents. A virtuous circle of complementary theorizing is possible. Theorizing in this area is of crucial importance to designers of artificial agents: will the agents designed be autonomous enough to deserve and warrant legal rights?

A legal person is an entity that is the subject of legal rights and obligations. Typically, a legal person has the capacity to sue and be sued, and to hold property, in its own name, although some kinds of entity—notably corporations, children and the mentally incapacitated—may need to act through agents to exercise their legal capacities. Not all legal persons have the same rights and obligations; some rights (e.g., marriage) depend on age. Other rights (e.g., voting) and obligations (such as the liability to be imprisoned) are typically restricted to humans.

Being human is not a necessary condition of being accorded legal personality, an obvious example being the modern business corporation. English admiralty law treats a ship as a legal person capable of being sued in its own right; other legal systems have recognized temples, dead persons, spirits and idols as legal persons. The law has also not, historically, considered being human a sufficient condition of being recognized as a legal person. In Roman law, the paterfamilias or free head of the family was the subject of legal rights and obligations on behalf of his household; his wife and children were only indirectly the subject of legal rights and his slaves were not legal persons at all. In English law before the middle of the 19th century, the married woman was not, for most purposes, accorded separate legal personality from that of her husband. In United States law slaves were considered non-persons. Currently, human foetuses in many jurisdictions are not considered legal persons; all other living human beings are generally accorded legal personality.

Legal scholars have considered the problem of personhood for artificial agents in a number of contexts. This debate has often taken shape as a possible solution to the legal doctrinal problem of accounting for the formation of electronic contracts. In the first case study, we sketch out this doctrinal problem, and some possible solutions, only one of which involves according legal personality to artificial agents. On the basis that it is conceptually possible that the legal system will accord legal personality with civil rights to artificial agents, the second case study examines the factors that the legal system could be expected to take into account in coming to this decision. In what follows, we confine ourselves to doctrines of Anglo-American law. While civil law (based on Roman and Napoleonic law) will differ in details, most of the concepts discussed below will have their analogues in these legal systems. We use "agent" to denote complex computational systems that could individually—or as part of a multi-agent system—represent human persons or corporations. We use "operator" rather than "user" to denote the entity on whose behalf the agent operates, as "user" can be confused with the person interacting with the agent (e.g., a shopper interacting with a shopping website agent). Lastly, we use "principal" interchangeably with "operator," by analogy with the principal of a human agent.

2. THE CONTRACTING PROBLEM

Artificial agents, and the contracts they make, are ubiquitous. Every time we interact with a shopping website we interact with a relatively autonomous interface that queries the operator's database, uses our input to populate the operator's database, and confirms the terms of the transaction. The operator does not exercise direct control over the agent's "choices," at least until the operator has a chance to confirm or reject the transaction entered into. Right now, websites such as the ebay auction website offer users agent-like functionality, by optionally bidding incrementally up to a specified maximum, allowing the user to "set and forget" the bidding process. Eventually, agents such as shopbots and pricebots capable of collecting information and engaging in transactions with very limited operator input are envisaged.

Various legal doctrinal difficulties are associated with contracts made by artificial agents:

> 1. In relation to the requirement that there be two parties involved in contract-making, artificial agents are not considered by current law to be legal persons; therefore, only the buyer and seller can be the relevant parties to the contract.
> 2. There are therefore difficulties in finding an agreement about terms between the parties where one party is unaware of the terms of the particular contract entered into by its artificial agent.
> 3. In relation to the requirement that there be an intention to form legal relations between the parties to the contract, a similar issue arises here as with agreement: if the agent's principal is not aware of the particular contract being concluded, how can the required intention be attributed?

2.1 Possible Solutions to the Contracting Problem

There is some disagreement as to the effectiveness of potential solutions to the contracting problem as we move up the sophistication scale of artificial agents. The first three are "tweaks"—involving minor changes of law, or pointing out that existing law perhaps with minor modifications or relaxations can accommodate the problem. The fourth is more radical and involves treating artificial agents the same as human agents, but without legal personality; the fifth, the most radical, proposes according artificial agents legal personhood.

Most current approaches to the problem of electronic contracting adopt the first potential solution—by treating artificial agents as mere tools of their operators, or as mere means of communication. All actions of artificial agents are attributed to the agent's operator, whether or not they are intended, predicted, or mistaken. On this basis, contracts entered into through an artificial agent will always bind the operator—a stricter liability principle than that which applies to human agents and their principals. The "artificial agent as tool" approach predominates in proposed legislative attempts to deal with electronic contracting. It is not clear whether legal change will be required in order to entrench this approach, since it currently appears so common-sense. However, as the autonomy of agents increases, it will be less realistic to approach agents as mere tools of their operators and as mere means of communication. The limitations of the approach, in cases where it would seem unjust and economically inefficient to burden the principal with losses caused by erratic behaviour of the agent, have not become sufficiently evident because of the limited autonomy displayed by existing artificial agents. There may be a natural limit to the "means of communication" doctrine too—e.g., where the person receiving the communication no longer can reasonably rely on the communication as having emanated from the purported principal.

The second potential solution, which addresses difficulties (2) and (3), is to deploy the unilateral offer doctrine of contract law. Contracts can be formed by a party's unilateral offer addressed to the whole world, together with acceptance—in the form of conduct stipulated in the offer—by the other party. Competitions and terms and conditions of entry to premises are among the most common examples involving unilateral contracts. In a simple sell-side agent example, the user's interaction with the website, in legal terms, can be equated with an interaction with a vending machine, where the contractual terms of particular contracts are not determined by the agent.

Many will see in the unilateral offer doctrine a theory that could justify many electronic contracts. The offer being made to the world is to be bound by contracts made through the artificial agent. That offer is accepted by interaction by a user with the artificial agent. What are the limits of such a doctrine? According to [one author], the analysis breaks down when we are dealing with agents that are able to determine contractual terms autonomously—for then the seller cannot be said to have intended the terms of each particular contract. However, we suggest that the law might imply into the offer made to all the world a reasonableness requirement i.e., the limits of the doctrine would be reached when it is unreasonable for the user to believe that the agent's principal would assent to the terms of the contract. This will only be the case where the agent is acting erratically or unpredictably as opposed to merely autonomously. This is a distinction that is relevant to the next solution too.

The third potential solution is to deploy the objective theory of contractual intention, which is dominant in United States law. Here, a contract is an obligation attached by the force of law to certain acts of the parties, usually words, which accompany and represent a known intent. The party's assent is not necessary to make a contract; the manifestation of intention to agree, judged according to a standard of reasonableness, is sufficient, and the real but unexpressed state of the first party's mind is irrelevant. It is enough that the other party had reason to believe that the first party intended to agree. [Another author] suggests that the objective theory cannot be relied on for assistance when an offer can be said to be initiated by the electronic device "autonomously i.e., in a manner unknown or unpredicted by the party employing [i.e., operating] the electronic device." This is because a party employing such a device cannot be thought to assent to contracts of which he is unaware, and which he cannot predict.

We do not share these doubts about the potential utility of the "objective theory." As above, we distinguish autonomy from unpredictability. Almost by definition, autonomous action takes place without the knowledge (at least contemporaneously and of the specific transaction) of the principal. But just as a good employee can, while exercising autonomy in decision-making, stay within well-defined boundaries and act in predictable ways, so can an artificial agent. We suggest that the 'objective' theory of intent might be relied on as an alternative underpinning to many contracts reached autonomously through artificial agents. However, [it] is correct to suggest that there would be limits to the applicability of the objective intent theory. We suggest that those limits would be reached not when agents behave autonomously but when agents behave erratically or unpredictably. Under those circumstances, it becomes difficult to argue that a reasonable person would conclude that, merely by reason of operating the agent, the operator should be taken to assent to the terms agreed by the agent. This limit is similar to the limit we proposed on the applicability of the unilateral offer doctrine.

It is not clear however, that the "unilateral offer" doctrine or the "objective theory" doctrine should be used as an attribution rule at all, whereby the actions of an artificial agent can be attributed to its operator. In current law relevant to human agents, the doctrinal work is done by the law of agency, which is intimately connected with the notion of the agent's authority to act. Within the scope of the agent's actual authority, legal acts done by it on behalf of its principal—such as entering a contract or giving or receiving a notice—become, in law, the acts of the principal. The doctrine extends to cases of apparent authority where the agent has no actual authority, but where the principal permits third parties to believe that he has authority.

The fourth potential solution, therefore, involves taking the artificial agent metaphor seriously, and treating artificial agents literally as the legal agents of their operators. Under this solution, within the scope of the agent's authority, contracts entered into by agents would become contracts of their operators. The agent's authority could be readily understood as that field of contracts which the agent had instructions/permissions—and the means—to conclude. A number of objections to the possibility of treating artificial agents as true agents in the legal sense have been discussed. Refutations to the most important of these follow:

> 1. Artificial agents necessarily lack legal power to give consent because they are not persons. But the example of Roman slaves—who were not considered legal persons but who did have capacity to enter contracts on behalf of their masters—disproves this objection.
>
> 2. Artificial agents lack the intellectual capacity or ability to exchange promises. But many artificial agents (such as the interfaces operated by shopping websites) display all the "intelligence" or "intentionality" required of them—no less so and much more reliably than the human telephone clerks that they replace, and which in many cases are practically indistinguishable from recorded voices. We believe the objective theory of contract should be deployed in this context On this approach, an ability to perform the requisite actions—such as emailing the buyer with the correct details in a notification and updating the seller's databases correctly—would be sufficient to qualify a seller's artificial agent as having the right 'intentional' or 'mental' states. We

do not see how else courts could adjudicate on these matters other than by adopting an 'intentional stance' towards agents: it would be the best way to make sense of their behavior.

3. In some legal systems agency requires a contract between the agent and the principal, and as artificial agents are not persons, they cannot enter contracts in their own name. However, in Anglo-American law a contract between principal and agent is not necessary; all that is necessary is that the principal is willing for the agent to bind him as regards third parties. In legal systems where a contract is necessary, it will be necessary to investigate personhood for artificial agents in order to deal with contracts made by artificial agents, or move to the Anglo-American model.

4. Another objection relates to the mental capacity of artificial agents. While in Anglo-American law an agent need not have the contractual capacity of an adult legal person—for example, children who cannot contract for themselves can contract on behalf of adults—nevertheless, an agent must be of sound mind in order for the agency to begin or to continue. This means that the agent must understand the nature of the act being performed. This doctrine would need to be adapted, to the case of artificial agents without human-like intelligence, before a true agency treatment of artificial agency could be undertaken.

Scholars have postulated a fifth potential solution, where the legal system would treat artificial agents as legal persons in order to solve the doctrinal difficulties cited. But as pointed out above, a contracting agent need not necessarily be treated as a legal person to be effectual. The advantage of treating artificial agents as legal persons in the contracting context is that it would provide a complete parallel with the situation of human agents, in terms of the ability of the innocent third party to sue the agent for breach of authority. There are however a number of objections to the idea of according artificial agents with legal personality as a way of dealing with the contracting problem:

1. It is unnecessary, as other solutions are adequate.

2. The warranty of authority is not a particularly important or much-relied upon doctrine of law, so the inability to sue the errant agent (in the agent-as-slave scenario) is not in practice a significant loss for the innocent user.

3. The personal identity conditions for artificial agents are not well understood. For example, a multi-agent system in the form of "swarm-ware"—consisting of multiple copies of the same program in communication—might alternately be seen as one entity and a group of entities. . . .

4. In civil law countries, the concept of a legal person is intimately bound up with the concept of patrimony, i.e. the assets under the control of the person which might be used to satisfy a judgement against the person. It may seem unclear where such assets can be derived from—although one possibility would clearly be ordinary gainful employment, on behalf of users or operators.

2.2 Reflections on the Possible Solutions

Which solution one chooses depends on whether one believes that the risk of unpredictable and erratic activity of artificial agents should fall on their operators, or on those interacting with them. This question can be seen as a difficult issue of efficient risk allocation in the economics of law, which is outside the scope of this paper. The five approaches sketched above have different results:

1. Under the "agent as mere tool" solution, the principal would be liable for erratic behaviour—unless a reasonableness requirement were imported into it—but

the principal could in many cases recover his loss from the designer of the agent, with whom he might have a contractual relationship, or under product liability laws.

2. Under both the "unilateral offer" solution and the "objective intent" solution, the principal would generally not be liable for erratic behaviour, if it were not reasonable for the user to believe that the principal would have assented to that behaviour, had it been aware of it.

3. Under the agent as slave solution, all behaviour outside the scope of the agent's authority—actual or apparent—could be disclaimed by the principal, and the user would have no right of action against the agent, which would not be a person. The user might however have rights under product liability laws against the designer of the agent.

4. Under the agent as person solution, the principal would not be liable for the agent's behaviour outside the scope of its authority, but the user would be able to sue the agent for breach of its authority. The agent might conceivably in turn be able to sue its own designer under product liability laws, for instance.

We suspect that the "agent as mere tool" doctrine will survive for some time on grounds of convenience and justice. As agents become more sophisticated, a slave analysis, and then an analysis involving personhood, might be embraced. The contractual problem is not enough, on its own, to motivate a personhood analysis. This is the closest so far to a real-world problem of according personhood to artificial agents. It is intended to show the extent to which "system-level" concerns will continue to dominate for the foreseeable future. Factors such as whether it is necessary to introduce personhood in order to explain all relevant phenomena, efficient risk allocation and whether alternative explanations gel better with existing theory, will count for more than the qualities or capacities of artificial agents in this debate.

NOTES AND QUESTIONS

1. "Origin chauvinism" is described as the position that even if a computer could achieve an *exact* behavioral and physiological similitude with the human brain, the fact that it was not born naturally would disqualify it from receiving rights. Where do you stand on this?

2. A 2011 story in the *New Scientist* opened with the question: "What if a robot—brain, body and all—could be born and then develop in a similar way to a human baby?" Dr. Jeffrey Clune, of Cornell University's Creative Machines Lab, commented that "[t]he end game is to evolve robots in simulation, hit print, and watch them walk out of a 3D printer." Quoted in Lakshmi Sandhana, *Darwin's Robots: Survival of the Fittest Digital Brain*, New Scientist (Sept. 14, 2011). As you consider legal rights and responsibilities, keep in mind this aspect of AI—its ability, perhaps, to replicate (and even evolve) without additional human intervention.

3. Military and government applications of autonomous robots are seen now in drones and related machines. "At present, there are no laws or treaties specifically pertaining to restrictions or governance of military robots, unmanned platforms, or other technologies currently under consideration within the purview of this article. Instead, aspects of these new military technologies are covered piecemeal (if at all) by a patchwork of legislation pertaining to projection of force under international law; treaties or conventions pertaining to

specific technologies and practices; international humanitarian law; and interpretations of existing principles of the Law of Armed Conflict (LOAC)." Gary E. Marchant et al., *International Governance of Autonomous Military Robots*, 12 Colum. Sci. & Tech. L. Rev. 272, 289 (2011). What type of safeguards would you introduce to avoid disastrous outcomes? What issues would be most important to address? In a report submitted to the United Nations in April 2013, Christof Heyns, the Special Rapporteur on extrajudicial, summary, or arbitrary executions, warned: "The prospect of a future in which fully autonomous robots could exercise the power of life and death over human beings raises a host of additional concerns. . . . [T]he introduction of such powerful yet controversial new weapons systems has the potential to pose new threats to the right to life. It could also create serious international division and weaken the role and rule of international law — and in the process undermine the international security system." Christof Heyns (Special Rapporteur), Human Rights Council, *Report of the Special Rapporteur on Extrajudicial, Summary or Arbitrary Executions*, at 6, U.N. Doc. A/HRC/23/47 (Apr. 9, 2013). *See* Richard Stone, *Scientists Campaign Against Killer Robots*, 342 Science 1428 (2013).

4. Many nations are pursuing robotic weapons. Is the integration of AI into combat a welcome development? Human Rights Watch, in a 2012 report, *Losing Humanity: The Case Against Killer Robots*, argued that there should be a prohibition on "the development, production, and use of fully autonomous weapons through an international legally binding instrument." But not all agree. The Executive Director of the Information Operations Center at the Naval Postgraduate School argues: "A lot of people fear artificial intelligence. . . . I will stand my artificial intelligence against your human any day of the week and tell you that my A.I. will pay more attention to the rules of engagement and create fewer ethical lapses than a human force." Quoted in John Markoff, *War Machines: Recruiting Robots for Combat*, N.Y. Times (Nov. 27, 2010). But others argue that we ought to embrace new modes of warfare. *See* John Yoo, *Embracing the Machines: Rationalist War and New Weapons Technologies*, 105 Calif. L. Rev. 443 (2017). If weapons are increasingly autonomous, and perhaps one day operating without a "human in the loop," how can accountability be assigned? *See* Rebecca Crootof, *War Torts: Accountability for Autonomous Weapons*, 164 U. Pa. L. Rev. 1347 (2016); Kenneth Anderson & Matthew C. Waxman, *Law and Ethics for Robot Soldiers*, Pol'y Rev., Dec. 2012-Jan. 2013, at 35.

5. In September 2004, the State of Colorado replaced six aging computer systems supporting various state-administered welfare programs with a single system using current technologies, called the Colorado Benefits Management System (CBMS). It was supposed to provide better service to clients and assurance that the state's welfare programs were being administered properly. The conversion was a disaster. *See* Cindi Fukami & Donald J. McCubbrey, *Colorado Benefits Management System (C): Seven Years of Failure*, 29 Comm. Ass'n for Info. Sys. 97 (2011); Jordan Steffen, *Officials Want Millions to Keep Upgrading Troubled Computer System*, Denv. Post (Apr. 27, 2016). Besides basic system problems, the CBMS has faulty law embedded in its code. The CBMS produced thousands of overpayments, underpayments, delayed benefits, faulty notices, and erroneous eligibility determinations. Worst of all, in 2009, a nine-year-old boy died after a pharmacy — depending upon the CBMS system — wouldn't fill his asthma prescription despite proof the family

qualified for Medicaid help. Who is responsible? Imagine that a new system, CBMS+ was created and was designed to learn on its own and reprogram its own operating code. Further imagine that after two years of this self-learning, CBMS+ works more efficiently and effectively than any other system in the nation, but also that the self-learned code of CBMS+ is so complex that even its original creators don't understand exactly how it works. Do you want such a system running the benefits system? If not, why not? If so, what if CBMS+ makes a mistake, as its predecessor CBMS did? Are any humans liable for the mistake of CBMS+? The foregoing was written in the first edition of this book. Since then the Colorado Governor's Office of Information Technology spent $25 million over two years to update and fix the system. The new system was launched in mid-2019, but many flaws were immediately discovered. *See* Sam Tabachnik, *Some Coloradans Can't Access Food and Medical Benefits Due to Glitches in New State System*, Denv. Post (Sept. 5, 2019).

6. Do robots implicate privacy concerns as well? Some think so. Consider this analysis:

> [T]he clearest way in which robots implicate privacy is that they greatly facilitate direct surveillance. Robots of all shapes and sizes, equipped with an array of sophisticated sensors and processors, greatly magnify the human capacity to observe. The military and law enforcement have already begun to scale up reliance on robotic technology to better monitor foreign and domestic populations. But robots also present corporations and individuals with new tools of observation in arenas as diverse as security, voyeurism, and marketing. . . .
>
> A second way in which robots implicate privacy is that they introduce new points of access to historically protected spaces. The home robot in particular presents a novel opportunity for government, private litigants, and hackers to access information about the interior of a living space. Robots on the market today interact uncertainly with federal electronic privacy laws and, as at least one recent study has shown, several popular robot products are vulnerable to technological attacks—all the more dangerous in that they give hackers access to objects and rooms instead of folders and files.
>
> Society can likely negotiate these initial effects of surveillance and unwanted access with better laws and engineering practices. But there is a third, more nuanced category of robotic privacy harm—one far less amenable to reform. This third way robots implicate privacy flows from their unique social meaning. Robots are increasingly human-like and socially interactive in design, making them more engaging and salient to their end-users and the larger community. Many studies demonstrate that people are hardwired to react to heavily anthropomorphic technologies such as robots as though a person were actually present, including with respect to the sensation of being observed and evaluated.
>
> That robots have this social dimension translates into a least three distinct privacy dangers. First, the introduction of social robots into living and other spaces historically reserved for solitude, may reduce the dwindling opportunities for interiority and self-reflection that privacy operates to protect. Second, social robots may be in a unique position to extract information from people. They can leverage most of the same advantages of humans (fear, praise, etc.) in information gathering. But they also have perfect memories, are tireless, and cannot be embarrassed, giving robots advantages over human persuaders
>
> Finally, the social nature of robots may lead to new types of highly sensitive personal information—implicating what might be called "setting privacy." It says little

about an individual how often he runs his dishwasher or whether he sets it to auto dry. It says a lot about him what "companionship program" he runs on his personal robot. Robots exist somewhere in the twilight between person and object and can be exquisitely manipulated and tailored. A description of how a person programs and interacts with a robot might read like a session with a psychologist—except recorded, and without the attendant logistic or legal protections. . . .

M. Ryan Calo, *Robots and Privacy*, in *Robot Ethics: The Ethical and Social Implications of Robotics* 187, 187-88 (Patrick Lin, Keith Abney & George A. Bekey eds., 2014).

Since the first edition of this book was published, cars with self-driving features have become more common. Some simply prevent the driver from changing lanes inadvertently. Others, most notably produced by Tesla, offer full self-driving capabilities. Such self-driving cars have been expensive, but the Tesla Model 3 was introduced in 2017 with a price comparable to other cars. Since then, it has become the fastest selling car in the market.

Jack Karsten & Darrell West
The State of Self-Driving Car Laws Across the U.S.
Brookings Inst. (May 1, 2018)

SETBACKS IN AUTONOMOUS VEHICLE TESTING

An Uber vehicle with a safety driver struck and killed a pedestrian in Tempe, Arizona on March 18; Uber quickly suspended all testing of its autonomous fleet while it investigates the causes of the crash. On March 23, the driver of a Tesla in autonomous mode died when the vehicle crashed into a highway median in Mountain View, California. Tesla has not suspended the feature in its vehicles while the company and the National Highway Traffic Safety Administration (NHTSA) investigate the causes of that crash. Since proponents highlight the safety improvements of driverless cars, these fatalities will invite stricter scrutiny of the claims of the technology.

As their name implies, safety drivers have played an important role in autonomous vehicle development. They receive special training to assume control when onboard computers encounter a situation that the vehicle cannot navigate by itself. Driving conditions can change quickly and the safety driver must remain alert constantly. However, advancements in driverless technology promise to eliminate human inputs altogether. With no steering wheel or a gas pedal, a computer would control the engine and steering based on inputs from onboard sensors. Passenger shuttles without any of these features have launched in Las Vegas, the University of Michigan, and in San Ramon, California. . . .

LABORATORIES OF DEMOCRACY, AND SELF-DRIVING CARS

Looking at the database of autonomous vehicle legislation from the National Conference of State Legislatures, we can track the progress of states in passing legislation. Twenty-two states and the District of Columbia have passed laws and an additional 10 state governors have issued executive orders regarding the operation of autonomous vehicles, while ten other state legislatures have considered legislation and the remaining eight state legislatures have not considered any. . . .

Autonomous Vehicle Act of 2012
2012 D.C. Law 19-278 (Act 19-643)

AN ACT to authorize autonomous vehicles to operate on District roadways, to require the Department of Motor Vehicles to create an autonomous vehicle designation, and to establish safe operating protocols for autonomous vehicles.

BE IT ENACTED BY THE COUNCIL OF THE DISTRICT OF COLUMBIA, That this act may be cited as the "Autonomous Vehicle Act of 2012."

Sec. 2. Definitions.

For the purposes of this act, the term:

(1) "Autonomous vehicle" means a vehicle capable of navigating District roadways and interpreting traffic-control devices without a driver actively operating any of the vehicle's control systems. The term "autonomous vehicle" excludes a motor vehicle enabled with active safety systems or driver-assistance systems, including systems to provide electronic blind-spot assistance, crash avoidance, emergency braking, parking assistance, adaptive cruise control, lane-keep assistance, lane-departure warning, or traffic-jam and queuing assistance, unless the system alone or in combination with other systems enables the vehicle on which the technology is installed to drive without active control or monitoring by a human operator.

(2) "Driver" means a human operator of a motor vehicle with a valid driver's license.

(3) "Public roadway" means a street, road, or public thoroughfare that allows motor vehicles.

(4) "Traffic control device" means a traffic signal, traffic sign, electronic traffic sign, pavement marking, or other sign, device, or apparatus designed and installed to direct moving traffic.

Sec. 3. Autonomous vehicles permitted.

An autonomous vehicle may operate on a public roadway; provided, that the vehicle:

(1) Has a manual override feature that allows a driver to assume control of the autonomous vehicle at any time;

(2) Has a driver seated in the control seat of the vehicle while in operation who is prepared to take control of the autonomous vehicle at any moment; and

(3) Is capable of operating in compliance with the District's applicable traffic laws and motor vehicle laws and traffic control devices.

Sec. 4. Vehicle conversion; limited liability of original manufacturer.

(a) The original manufacturer of a vehicle converted by a third party into an autonomous vehicle shall not be liable in any action resulting from a vehicle defect caused by the conversion of the vehicle, or by equipment installed by the converter, unless the alleged defect was present in the vehicle as originally manufactured.

(b) The conversion of vehicles to autonomous vehicles shall be limited to model years 2009 or later or vehicles built within 4 years of conversion, whichever vehicle is newer. . . .

Nat'l Highway and Transp. Safety Admin.
Automated Vehicles for Safety
https://www.nhtsa.gov/technology-innovation/automated-vehicles-safety

THE ROAD TO FULL AUTOMATION

Fully autonomous cars and trucks that drive us instead of us driving them will become a reality. These self-driving vehicles ultimately will integrate onto U.S. roadways by progressing through six levels of driver assistance technology advancements in the coming years. This includes everything from no automation (where a fully engaged driver is required at all times), to full autonomy (where an automated vehicle operates independently, without a human driver). . . .

SOCIETY OF AUTOMOTIVE ENGINEERS (SAE) AUTOMATION LEVELS

0	1	2	3	4	5
No Automation	Driver Assistance	Partial Automation	Conditional Automation	High Automation	Full Automation
Zero autonomy; the driver performs all driving tasks.	Vehicle is controlled by the driver, but some driving assist features may be included in the vehicle design.	Vehicle has combined automated functions, like acceleration and steering, but the driver must remain engaged with the driving task and monitor the environment at all times.	Driver is a necessity, but is not required to monitor the environment. The driver must be ready to take control of the vehicle at all times with notice.	The vehicle is capable of performing all driving functions under certain conditions. The driver may have the option to control the vehicle.	The vehicle is capable of performing all driving functions under all conditions. The driver may have the option to control the vehicle.

BENEFITS OF AUTOMATION
Safety

The safety benefits of automated vehicles are paramount. Automated vehicles' potential to save lives and reduce injuries is rooted in one critical and tragic fact: 94% of serious crashes are due to human error. Automated vehicles have the potential to remove human error from the crash equation, which will help protect drivers and passengers, as well as bicyclists and pedestrians. When you consider more than 37,133 people died in motor vehicle-related crashes in the U.S. in 2017, you begin to grasp the lifesaving benefits of driver assistance technologies.

Economic and Societal Benefits

Automated vehicles could deliver additional economic and additional societal benefits. A NHTSA study showed motor vehicle crashes in 2010 cost $242 billion in economic activity, including $57.6 billion in lost workplace productivity, and $594 billion due to loss of life and decreased quality of life due to injuries. Eliminating the vast majority of motor vehicle crashes could erase these costs.

Efficiency and Convenience

Roads filled with automated vehicles could also cooperate to smooth traffic flow and reduce traffic congestion. Americans spent an estimated 6.9 billion hours in traffic delays in 2014, cutting into time at work or with family, increasing fuel costs and vehicle emission. With automated vehicles, the time and money spent commuting could be put to better use. A recent study stated that automated vehicles could free up as much as 50 minutes each day that had previously been dedicated to driving.

NOTES AND QUESTIONS

1. Would you be more excited or scared to be sitting in the back seat of a taxi driven autonomously? Is that feeling rational? Does the rationality of your sense matter to you? Are you aware of the fact that your discomfort will be reduced with more experience in such automobiles?

2. In a negligent driving tort lawsuit an appellate court in Maryland affirmed a lower court decision upholding a jury verdict that did not find in favor of the plaintiff. The appellate court recognized that non-negligent accidents happen, and went on to observe: "Until we enter the era of self-driving or autonomous vehicles, with a 360-degree range of 'vision' (and therefore no need to divert their attention from the traffic ahead in order to merge safely with traffic on the left), collisions like the one in this case may occur without the fault of either of the human beings who are driving the cars involved." *Grant v. Newman*, No. 404305-V, 2017 WL 4251755, at *6 (Md. Ct. Spec. App. Sept. 26, 2017). How will negligent driving lawsuits change in a new era of autonomous vehicles?

3. In addition to the District of Columbia, both Nevada and Florida have passed legislation relating to autonomous vehicles. Other states are considering similar bills. If you were writing such legislation, would you adopt the D.C. language in the Autonomous Vehicle Act of 2012 or modify it?

4. "[I]f autonomous vehicles reduce the frequency and/or severity of accidents, liability will still be an important and potentially limiting consideration for manufacturers. Liability, in that case, requires an analysis of three key factors. First, who will be liable? Second, what weight will the court's finder of fact give to the overall comparative safety of autonomous vehicles when determining whether those involved in a crash should be held liable? Third, will a vehicle 'defect' that creates potential manufacturer liability be found in a higher percentage of crashes than with conventional vehicle crashes where driver error is usually attributed to be the cause?" Gary E. Marchant & Rachel A. Lindor, *The Coming Collision Between Autonomous Vehicles and the Liability System*, 52 Santa Clara L. Rev. 1321, 1322 (2012). How would you answer these questions?

5. Privacy law is also implicated, because "absent privacy precautions, much of a vehicle's internal sensor data is potentially linkable to the vehicle user and is therefore personal information that raises privacy issues." Dorothy J. Glancy, *Privacy in Autonomous Vehicles*, 52 Santa Clara L. Rev. 1171, 1176 (2012). What information might be collected (and transmitted) by a self-driving car that you might not want collected and transmitted?

FURTHER READING

Overviews of Machine Intelligence:

Nick Bostrom, *Superintelligence: Paths, Dangers, Strategies* (2014).

Rodney A. Brooks, *Flesh and Machines: How Robots Will Change Us* (2002).

The Cambridge Handbook of Artificial Intelligence (Keith Frankish & William M. Ramsey eds., 2014).

Ray Kurzweil, *The Singularity Is Near: When Humans Transcend Biology* (2005).

John Long, *Darwin's Devices: What Evolving Robots Can Teach Us About the History of Life and the Future of Technology* (2012).

Max Tegmark, *Life 3.0: Being Human in the Age of Artificial Intelligence* (2017).

Wendell Wallach & Colin Allen, *Moral Machines: Teaching Robots Right from Wrong* (2008).

Legal and Ethical Implications:

Kevin D. Ashley, *Artificial Intelligence and Legal Analytics: New Tools for Law Practice in the Digital Age* (Cambridge Univ. Press 2017).

Research Handbook on the Law of Artificial Intelligence (Woodrow Barfield & Ugo Pagallo eds., 2018).

Robot Law (Ryan Calo, A. Michael Froomkin & Ian Kerr eds., 2016).

Int'l Assoc. for Artificial Intelligence and Law, http://www.iaail.org.

Daniel Martin Katz, *Quantitative Legal Prediction—or—How I Learned to Stop Worrying and Start Preparing for the Data-Driven Future of the Legal Services Industry*, 62 Emory L.J. 909 (2013).

Robot Ethics: The Ethical and Social Implications of Robotics (Patrick Lin, Keith Abney & George A. Bekey eds., 2011).

Gary E. Marchant et al., *International Governance of Autonomous Military Robots*, 12 Colum. Sci. & Tech. L. Rev. 272 (2011).

Jonathan D. Moreno, *Mind Wars: Brain Science and the Military in the 21st Century* (2012).

Cass R. Sunstein, *Of Artificial Intelligence and Legal Reasoning*, 8 U. Chi. L. Sch. Roundtable 29 (2001).

We Robot Conference, http://robots.law.miami.edu.

How to Read a Brain Imaging Study

Because lawyers are increasingly encountering brain imaging evidence, in both civil and criminal contexts, it is important that they gain some initial sense of how to actually read and understand brain imaging studies.

This appendix provides a guided tour of the first full-scale law and neuroscience study. Specifically, it illustrates how to read and understand an fMRI study, by liberal use of comments inserted into the margins. Those comments explain terms, elaborate on experimental design, and caution against misunderstandings. The text of the study appears unedited and in its entirety, to give realistic exposure to the way brain imaging studies are likely to be encountered in actual practice.

The brain imaging article chosen to be the illustrative text for commentary is not a study that will necessarily find immediate utility in litigation. It has been selected because legal thinkers reading an fMRI study for the first time will likely learn most readily from a study that inherently addresses matters relevant to law. Hence, we focus in this Appendix on an article that reports discovery of the brain areas and activities associated with deciding whether or not to punish someone for criminal behavior and, if so, how much. What follows is excerpted, with permission, from Owen D. Jones, Joshua W. Buckholtz, Jeffrey D. Schall & René Marois, *Brain Imaging for Legal Thinkers: A Guide for the Perplexed*, 2009 Stanford Tech. L. Rev. 5.

Joshua W. Buckholtz, Christopher L. Asplund, Paul E. Dux,
David H. Zald, John C. Gore, Owen D. Jones & René Marois
The Neural Correlates of Third-Party Punishment
60 Neuron 930 (2008)

INTRODUCTION

Though rare in the rest of the animal kingdom, large scale cooperation among genetically unrelated individuals is the rule, rather than the exception, in Homo sapiens (Henrich, 2003). Ultra-sociality and cooperation in humans is made possible by our ability to establish social norms—widely shared sentiments about appropriate behaviors that foster both social peace and economic prosperity (Fehr and Fischbacher, 2004a;

Spitzer et al., 2007). In turn, norm compliance relies not only on the economic self-interest often served by cooperation and fair exchange, but also on the credible threat of unwelcome consequences for defection (Spitzer et al., 2007). Social order therefore depends on punishment—which modern societies administer through a system of state-empowered enforcers, guided by state-governed, impartial, third-party decision-makers, who are not directly affected by the norm violation and have no personal stake in the execution of its enforcement.

The role of legal decision-makers is two-fold: determining responsibility and assigning an appropriate punishment. In determining responsibility, a legal decision-maker must assess whether the accused has committed a wrongful act and, if so, whether he did it with one of several culpable states of mind (so-called "mens rea") (Robinson, 2002). For many of the most recognizable crimes, the defendant must have engaged in the proscribed conduct with intent in order to merit punishment. Moreover, in sentencing an individual for whom criminal responsibility has been determined, a legal decision-maker must choose a punishment that fits the crime. This sentence must ordinarily be such that the combined nature and extent of punishment is proportional to the combined harmfulness of the offense and blameworthiness of the offender (Farahany and Coleman Jr., 2006; LaFave, 2003).

Despite its critical utility in facilitating prosocial behavior and maintaining social order, little is known about the origins of, and neural mechanisms underlying, our ability to make third-party legal decisions (Garland, 2004; Garland and Glimcher, 2006; Zeki and Goodenough, 2004). The cognitive ability to make social norm-related judgments likely arose from the demands of social living faced by our hominid ancestors (Henrich, 2003; Richerson et al., 2003). These demands may have promoted the emergence of mechanisms for assessing fairness in interpersonal exchanges and enacting personal retaliations against individuals who behaved unfairly (second-party punishment) (Fehr and Fischbacher, 2004a). Recent work has greatly advanced our understanding of how the brain evaluates fairness and makes decisions based on the cooperative status and intentions of others during two-party economic exchanges (de Quervain et al., 2004; Delgado et al., 2005; King-Casas et al., 2005; Knoch et al., 2006; Sanfey et al., 2003; Singer et al., 2004; Singer et al., 2006; Spitzer et al., 2007). Notably, these studies have elucidated the neural dynamics that underlie human altruistic punishment, in which the victim of a social norm transgression, typically unfairness in an economic exchange, punishes the transgressor at some significant additional cost to himself. These findings have specifically highlighted the importance of reward and emotion-related processes in fueling cooperative behavior (Seymour et al., 2007). However, how—or even whether—neural models of economic exchange in dyadic interactions apply to impartial, third-party legal decision-making is currently unknown (Fehr and Fischbacher, 2004a). Furthermore, the importance of uncovering neural mechanisms underlying third-party punishment is underscored by the proposal that the development of stable social norms in human societies specifically required the evolution of third-party sanction systems (Bendor and Swistak, 2001).

Given that, in great measure, criminal law strives towards the stabilization and codification of social norms, including moral norms, in legal rules of conduct (Robinson and Darley, 1995), moral decision-making is inherently embedded into the legal decision-making process. The relevance of moral decision-making to an investigation of legal reasoning is highlighted by experimental findings which suggest that individuals punish according to so-called "just deserts" motives; i.e., in proportion to the moral wrongfulness of an offender's actions (Alter et al., 2007; Carlsmith et al., 2002; Darley and

1. In this instance, "neural mechanisms" refers to the manner by which the brain encodes and processes information to enable a specific cognitive ability.

2. There are two basic experimental designs in fMRI, "block" and "event-related." In block designs subjects encounter long sequences (or "blocks") of the same kind of stimulus (e.g., pictures of various faces) interspersed with blocks of a control stimulus (e.g., pictures of shapes). Average brain activity in one block is then contrasted to average brain activity in the other block. In event-related designs, subjects encounter randomly intermixed stimuli (e.g. faces and shapes). The choice between designs depends on what is being investigated.

3. "fMRI" stand for "functional magnetic resonance imaging." By convention, the leading "f" is lowercase.

4. "Neural circuitry" refers to interconnected brain regions that interact, like a wired circuit, during information processing. Within the circuit, each brain region has a specialized function that contributes to the brain's information-processing task.

5. What governs study size? fMRI scan sessions are expensive, frequently extending 1.5 hours, at $300 to $600 per hour. In determining a suitable number of subjects, statistical power (the probability that a real experimental effect will be detected) trades against cost. As a general rule, studies with fewer than 10 subjects are treated with skepticism.

6. To prevent changes in subjects' brain responses that are due to variables not under the experimenter's control, researchers keep variations to a minimum. Here, the protagonist's name is kept constant across all scenarios, to avoid confounds that could follow if different names were used. Again, there are trade-offs: the possible confound of using the same name repeatedly (which risks subjects cumulating their reactions to John's behavior, despite instructions not to) was considered less problematic than that different brain activations could be caused by different subject associations with different names.

7. fMRI data are extremely "noisy," in the sense that a small but true brain "signal" of interest that changes with the experimental manipulation can be obscured by much larger but irrelevant brain activation differences between experimental conditions. Since noise is random, while the true signal is not, researchers can detect changes in true signal by averaging the signal across all trials (enabling noise to cancel out). Consequently, researchers aim to pack as many experimental trials as possible (here, 50) into a given 60-90 minute scan session. Averaging across a large number of trials increases the likelihood of detecting the experimentally manipulated signal.

8. It is common to hold constant other variables in an experiment (here, gravity/severity of the harm), to ensure that any changes in brain activity between two conditions are due to the variable being investigated, rather than other factors.

Pittman, 2003). As such, the seminal work of Greene and others—which has demonstrated distinct contributions of emotion-related and cognitive control-related brain regions to moral decision-making (Greene et al., 2004; Greene et al., 2001; Heekeren et al., 2005; Heekeren et al., 2003; Moll et al., 2002a; Moll et al., 2002b)—is germane to the study of legal decision-making. However, despite the conceptual overlap between moral and legal reasoning, the latter process is not entirely reducible to the former (Hart, 1958; Holmes Jr., 1991; Posner, 1998; Robinson, 1997; Robinson and Darley, 1995). Indeed, whereas determining blameworthiness may in many cases fall under the rubric of moral decision-making, the distinctive core and distinguishing feature of legal decision-making is the computation and implementation of a punishment that is appropriate both to the relative moral blameworthiness of an accused criminal offender, and to the relative severity of that criminal offense (Robinson, 1997; Robinson and Darley, 1995). The present study is focused on elucidating the neural mechanisms underlying this third-party, legal decision-making process.

In this study, we used event-related fMRI to reveal the neural circuitry supporting third-party decision-making about criminal responsibility and punishment. Given that these two legally distinct judgments are rendered on the basis of differing information and considerations (LaFave et al., 2007), we were particularly interested in determining whether these two decision-making processes may rely on at least partly distinct neural systems. To address this issue, we scanned 16 participants while they determined the appropriate punishment for actions committed by the protagonist (named "John") in a series of 50 written scenarios. Each of these scenarios belonged to one of three categories: Responsibility (R), Diminished-Responsibility (DR) and No-Crime (NC). Scenarios in the Responsibility set (N=20) described John intentionally committing a criminal action ranging from simple theft to rape and murder. The Diminished-Responsibility set (N=20) included actions of comparable gravity to those described in the

Responsibility set but also contained mitigating circumstances that may have excused or justified the otherwise criminal behavior of the protagonist by calling his blameworthiness into question. The No-Crime set (N=10) depicted John engaged in non-criminal actions that were otherwise structured similarly to the Responsibility and Diminished-Responsibility scenarios (scenarios available as Supplementary Methods). Participants rated each scenario on a scale from 0-9, according to how much punishment they thought John deserved, with "0" indicating no punishment and "9" indicating extreme punishment.

Two groups of 50 scenarios (equated for word length between conditions and between groups) were constructed and their presentation counterbalanced across the 16 participants. The Responsibility set of group 2 consisted of group 1 Diminished-Responsibility scenarios for which the mitigating circumstances had been removed, while the Diminished-Responsibility set of group 2 consisted of group 1 Responsibility scenarios with mitigating circumstances added. Thus, each criminal scenario (e.g. depicting theft, assault or murder) in the Responsibility and Diminished-Responsibility condition was created by modifying identical "stem" stories, with salient details such as magnitude of harm matched between conditions.

RESULTS

Behavioral Data

Behavioral data showed a significant effect of scenario category on

9. It is common to include control stimuli. Here, a "No-Crime" control was included to provide a baseline level of brain activity that is associated with subjects viewing a protagonist intentionally engaged in a relatively harmless act. Thus, the experimenter is able to disentangle brain activity associated with viewing intentional action per se from that associated with viewing intentional actions that are potentially criminal.

10. For the control condition to be maximally useful, it must be as similar as feasible to the main conditions (in length, subject task, and general format, for example).

11. Because even slight head motion interferes with accurate data collection, scanned subjects must generally indicate responses with their hands, by pressing buttons, moving a joystick, or rolling a trackball. Here, each finger had a separate button. The buttons corresponded to a relative (i.e., internal/subjective) scale of punishment, rather than to some absolute metric, because that enabled more meaningful comparisons between subjects (since subjects could differ widely in their personal upper limits of actual punishment).

12. In general, counterbalancing helps diminish the potential confounding effects of variables not being studied. For example, any effect of order of presentation, when encountering multiple stimulus types, can be neutralized or diminished by randomizing the presentation order of stimuli. The counterbalancing in this experiment ensured that equal numbers of participants saw each group of scenarios.

13. Here, the counterbalancing ensured that different brain activity between different scenarios was likely a function of the level of responsibility manipulated as a variable, rather than a function of some other difference (such as location, item stolen, etc.) between the two scenarios.

14. Behavioral data, in brain imaging contexts, are measurements of subject responses that are separate from the collection of brain images. Typically, these are not recorded by the MRI machine. Here, for example, behavioral data include the punishment rating each subject selected for each scenario, and the elapsed time between presentation of scenario and selection of punishment.

15. "Significant" is an important term of art in science. In scientific experiments, observed results can be due to three things: 1) the factor that that the experimenter thinks the results are due to (i.e., the experimental manipulation); 2) an unmanipulated factor that the experimenter hasn't thought of or controlled (i.e., a "confound"); or 3) random chance (i.e., a "false positive"). A claim of significance is ordinarily accompanied by a numerical

representation (a "p" value) of the probability that the results arose by random chance. For example: p < .05 indicates that there is less than 5 chances in 100 that the result described could have arisen by chance alone. In setting a p-value to a given value, an investigator allows for the fact that there is a certain set probability that any effect is due to random chance, and it is near-universally agreed that p < 0.05 is a "reasonable" threshold. Statistical software outputs a p-value for each experimental comparison of interest. Thus, referring to something as "significant" in this context ordinarily means that the experimenter has submitted an experimental measure to a statistical test, and the outcome of this test allows the experimenter to be confident that the results have less than a 5% probability of being due to random chance. In some instances, a p-value may be set lower (e.g., to .01) to allow stricter control over the possibility of obtaining a false-positive.

16. The significant results from the statistical tests allow the authors to state that rating differences between conditions were due to the experimental manipulation. Briefly, in psychology and neuroscience, an independent variable is the factor that the experimenter manipulates to cause some effect on the dependent variable. When we talk about an effect of condition, we're talking about the effect of one or more independent variables on one or more dependent variables. Here, the dependent variable is punishment ratings and the independent variable is scenario category (which has three "conditions" or "levels"): Responsibility, Diminished Responsibility, and No-Crime.

17. These refer to the outcome of the statistical tests. In this case, an Analysis of Variance (ANOVA) test was used — the "F" value gives an indication of the strength of the experimental manipulation, and can be understood to represent the size of the difference in scores conditions, while the "p" value indicates that there is less than 1 chance in 1000 that these condition differences could have arisen by chance.

18. S.E. stands for "standard error (of the mean)" which helps readers understand the estimated stability of the measurement across samples. Essentially, this indicates the likelihood that the mean value will "jump" around between different samples of subjects.

19. The paired t-test is a common statistical test used to test for the effects of a condition on a dependent measure.

20. This means the authors' key experimental manipulation (here, protagonist's criminal responsibility) affected how much punishment subjects gave to the protagonist.

punishment ratings (F (1,15) = 358.61, p < 0.001) (Figure 1), with higher mean ratings for the Responsibility (Mean = 5.50, S.E. = 0.22) than for the Diminished-Responsibility scenarios (Mean = 1.45, S.E. = 0.21) (p < 0.001, paired t-test), indicating that assessed punishment was strongly modulated by the protagonist's criminal responsibility. By the same token, the fact that the mean punishment rating for the Diminished-Responsibility condition was greater than 0 suggests that some participants still attributed some blameworthiness to the protagonist despite the extenuating circumstances.

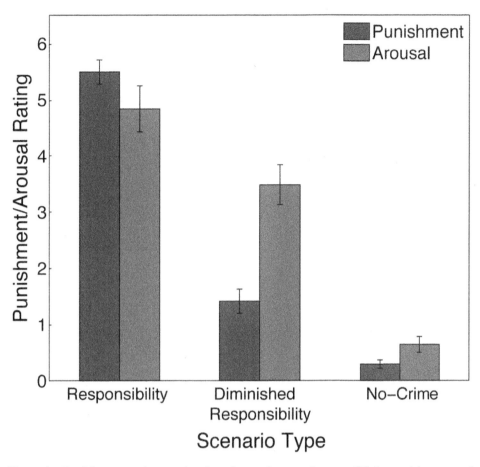

Figure 1   Punishment and arousal ratings for each scenario type. While punishment and arousal scores were similar in the Responsibility condition, punishment scores were significantly lower than arousal scores in the Diminished-Responsibility condition.

To examine the subjective emotional experience elicited by the scenarios, all participants completed post-scan ratings of emotional arousal for each scenario. These ratings also demonstrated an effect of condition $(F(1,15) = 94.61, p < 0.001)$ (Figure 1), with greater mean arousal scores for the Responsibility (Mean = 4.83, S.E. = 0.41) compared to Diminished-Responsibility scenarios (Mean = 3.48, S.E. = 0.35) $(p < 0.001,$ paired t-test). Additionally, we found a significant interaction between rating type (punishment vs. arousal) and condition (Responsibility vs. Diminished-Responsibility) $(F(1,15) = 68.8,$

21. The authors sought to quantify the subjects' emotional responses to the scenarios because they hypothesized that emotional responses could influence punishment decisions.

22. Subjects rated each of the 50 scenarios (presented in random order on a computer screen outside the scanner) on the basis of how emotionally aroused they felt following its presentation (0 = calm, 9 = extremely excited).

23. "Main effect" is a term of art referring to the effect of one experimentally manipulated factor (e.g. protagonist responsibility) on one experimental variable (e.g. reaction time). Often, investigators are interested in looking at the interactive effects of two or more conditions on a dependent variable. The term "main effect" is used to indicate that the influence of one independent variable was examined in isolation.

24. Reaction time is the length of time elapsing between the "onset" (when the subject was first presented with the scenario to consider) and the behavioral response (here, pressing a button to select a punishment level).

25. All BOLD fMRI studies are based on comparisons of BOLD signal between two conditions. By subtracting BOLD signal (within a given brain region) during one condition from brain BOLD signal (within that same brain region) during another condition, the effect of the experimental manipulation on regional brain function can be estimated. Here, because the only factor that differs between experimental conditions is information about protagonist responsibility, this subtraction method allows fMRI investigators to remove brain activation that is not due to the independent variable. In this study, the authors took an average of the measured brain signal during each R scenario, an average of the measured brain signal during each DR scenario, an average of the measured brain signal during each NC scenario, and compared these condition-averaged signals for each subject. They then took an average across all subjects to see where in the brain the signal was significantly different between levels of the independent variable.

26. An "area of activation" is a region of the brain where the measured fMRI signal was significantly greater during one condition (e.g. R) compared to another (e.g. DR).

27. There are several ways to designate brain regions. One rather general way uses 45 "Brodmann's Areas." These are based on a classification scheme devised by Korbinian Brodmann (1868-1918), separating areas by neuron type and organization.

28. The "peak" refers, in this instance, to the specific region of the brain that demonstrated the strongest effect of condition.

29. Human brains vary widely in size and shape. Because fMRI investigators average condition differences in brain activity across subjects, it is imperative that a brain region on one subject correspond to the exact same brain region on another subject. Thus, before an fMRI investigator can compare brain activity between conditions, each subjects' brain must first be "normalized" into a common space. Neuroimagers therefore

$p < 0.001$) such that, while the punishment and arousal ratings were not significantly different for the Responsibility scenarios ($p > 0.05$, paired t-test), punishment ratings were significantly lower than the arousal ratings for the Diminished-Responsibility scenarios ($p < 0.001$, paired t-test) (Figure 1). Lastly, we found a main effect of scenario condition on reaction times (RTs) ($F(1,15) = 21.87$, $p < 0.001$), such that RTs were shortest for the No-Crime condition and longest for the Diminished-Responsibility condition (mean, S.E. for: Responsibility = 12.69s, 0.46; Diminished-Responsibility = 13.76s, 0.46; No-Crime = 11.12s, 0.44) (all paired comparisons $p < 0.01$).

fMRI Data: Criminal Responsibility

To identify brain regions that were sensitive to information about criminal responsibility, we contrasted brain activity between Responsibility and Diminished-Responsibility scenarios. The resulting statistical parametric map (SPM) revealed an area of activation in the right dorsolateral prefrontal cortex (rDLPFC, Brodmann Area 46, peak at Talaraich coordinates 39, 37, 22 [x,y,z]; Figure 2a) that was significantly more activated in the Responsibility than in the Diminished-Responsibility condition.

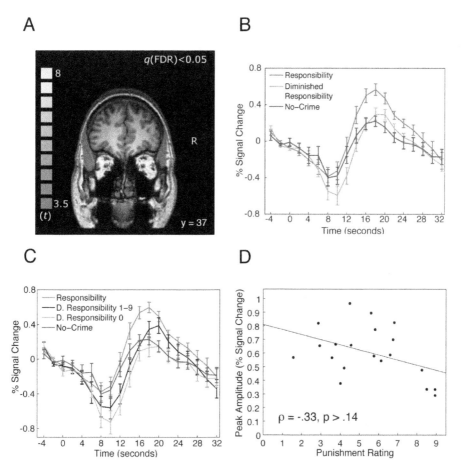

Figure 2 Relationship between responsibility assessment and right DLPFC activity.
A) SPM displaying the right DLPFC VOI (rendered on a single subject T1-weighted
image), based on the contrast of BOLD activity in the Responsibility condition compared
to the Diminished-Responsibility condition, $t(15) > 3.5$, $q < 0.05$, random effects analysis.
R = Right Hemisphere. **B)** BOLD activity time courses in right DLPFC for the Responsibility,
Diminished-Responsibility and No-Crime conditions. BOLD peak amplitude was significantly
greater in the Responsibility condition compared to both the Diminished-Responsibility
and No-Crime conditions ($p = 0.002$, $p = .0004$, respectively). Peak was defined as the
single TR with maximal signal change from baseline within the first 13 volumes after scenario presentation onset. t-tests were performed on these peak volumes, which were
defined separately for each condition and each subject. **C)** BOLD activity time courses in
right DLPFC for Responsibility, "non-punished" Diminished-Responsibility (Diminished-
Responsibility 0), "punished" Responsibility (Diminished-Responsibility 1-9) and No-Crime
scenarios. BOLD peak amplitude was significantly greater in "punished" compared to "non-
punished" Diminished-Responsibility scenarios ($p = 0.04$), while no difference was observed
between "non-punished" Diminished-Responsibility and No-Crime scenarios ($p = 0.98$). **D)**
Relationship between BOLD peak amplitude in right DLPFC and punishment ratings in the
Responsibility condition. These two variables were not significantly correlated ($p > 0.15$).

Time course analyses of peak activation differences confirmed that there was greater rDLPFC activity in Responsibility compared to Diminished-Responsibility or No-Crime conditions (R>NR, p = 0.002; R>NC, p = 0.0004; paired *t*-tests; see Figure 2b) and no difference between the Diminished-Responsibility and No-Crime conditions (p = 0.19). No effect of condition was found in the left DLPFC (p > 0.2 for all paired comparisons; see Methods), and the right DLPFC was significantly more engaged than the left DLPFC in the Responsibility condition (p = 0.04, paired *t*-test), suggesting that punishment-related prefrontal activation is confined to the right hemisphere. Bilateral anterior intraparietal sulcus (aIPS) demonstrated a pattern of responsibility-related activity that was similar to rDLPFC (Table 1, Supplementary Figure 1, Supplementary Results), whereas the temporo-parietal junction (TPJ) showed the reverse pattern, with more activity for the Diminished-Responsibility than the Responsibility condition (Table 1, Figure 3, see below).

translate (or "warp") subjects' brains into a single, common brain space. The most frequently used template is that defined by the coordinate system of Talairach and Tourneaux. After warping into Talairach space, which has a standardized three-dimensional coordinate system based on neuroanatomical landmarks, regional brain activation can be compared between subjects — and importantly, across studies. So, in this section of the paper, the authors are describing precisely where changes in brain function occurred. Roughly speaking, rDLPFC is like designating a city, Brodmann Area 46 is the street, and Talairach coordinate is the precise street number.

30. Time course analyses examine what is happening, over time, within a given region of the brain, during the cognitive task performed.

31. "Peak activation" refers to the maximum amplitude of BOLD signal (and hence, by inference, brain activity) within a given brain region. The sentence here describes an analysis of the different times at which, under different conditions, the maximum BOLD signal appeared within the brain region.

32. In articles describing experimental results, the experimental and analytical methods are ordinarily and carefully described in a separate "Methods" section.

33. The brain contains two largely independent hemispheres, left and right. Anatomical features (such as the amygdala) generally appear separately in both hemispheres.

34. For a depiction of brain orientation, see Box 1 (next page).

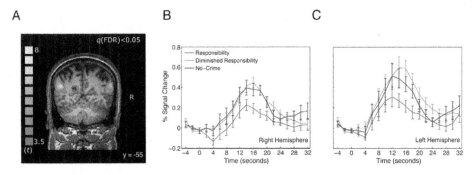

Figure 3   Relationship between responsibility assessment and bilateral temporo-parietal junction (TPJ) activity. A) SPM displaying the right and left TPJ VOIs (rendered on a single subject T1-weighted image), 00based on the contrast of BOLD activity in the Diminished-Responsibility condition compared to the Responsibility condition, *t*(15) > 3.5, *q* < 0.05; random effects analysis. R = Right Hemisphere. BOLD activity time courses in right (**B**) and left (**C**) TPJ for the Responsibility, Diminished-Responsibility and No-Crime conditions. BOLD peak amplitude was significantly greater in the Diminished-Responsibility condition compared to the Responsibility and conditions for right (p = 0.0005) and left (p = 0.001) TPJ. Peak was defined as the single TR with maximal signal change from baseline within the first 13 volumes after scenario presentation onset. *t*-tests were performed on these peak volumes, which were defined separately for each condition and each subject.

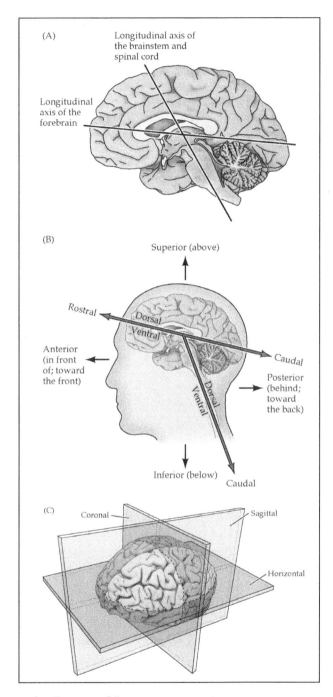

Box 1   (Accompanies Comment 34)
Reproduced by permission of Sinauer Associates from Dale Purves et al., Neuroscience, 2d edition 2001.

The greater rDLPFC activation in the Responsibility condition did not simply result from longer time-on-task: response times (RTs) to Responsibility scenarios were shorter than Diminished-Responsibility scenarios (p = 0.005, paired t-test), and the effect of condition on rDLPFC activity was still significant when response time was used as a covariate in an analysis of covariance (ANCOVA, F(1,37) = 10.15, p = 0.003) or when response times were equated between conditions (see Methods; R>DR, p = 0.006; R>NC, p = 0.002; Supplementary Figure 2). In addition, rDLPFC activity was not correlated with reaction time (p = 0.09 in Responsibility scenarios, p = .12 in Diminished-Responsibility scenarios). We also assessed whether the activity pattern in rDLPFC might have been driven by between-condition differences in emotional arousal rather than by differences in criminal responsibility. To this end, we performed a peak activation difference analysis between the Responsibility and Diminished-Responsibility conditions after equating their mean arousal ratings (Responsibility = 3.62, Diminished-Responsibility = 3.50; p > 0.10, paired t-test; see Methods). The results still revealed greater rDLPFC activity in the Responsibility compared to the Diminished-Responsibility condition even in the absence of arousal differences (p = 0.0005, paired t-test).

If rDLPFC is involved in the decision-making process to punish blameworthy behavior, then this brain region should be more activated during Diminished-Responsibility scenarios in which subjects still decided to punish (punishment ratings of 1 or greater) compared to Diminished-Responsibility scenarios in which they did not (punishment rating of 0). Consistent with this hypothesis, rDLPFC activity was higher in "punished" Diminished-Responsibility trials than in "non-punished" Diminished-Responsibility trials (p = 0.04, paired t-test, Figure 2). In turn, rDLPFC activity during "non-punished" Diminished-Responsibility trials was not greater than in No-Crime trials.

35. "Covariate" in this instance refers to a factor other than the independent measure that could contribute to condition differences in a dependent measure (in this case, fMRI signal). To ensure that this uncontrolled factor did not cause the observed condition differences in the dependent measure, the authors performed a test (called an ANCOVA) to see if condition differences remained even after taking that uncontrolled factor — the covariate — into account. A significant value for this test indicates that the covariate did not drive the observed differences in fMRI signal.

36. Response time differences between conditions might influence the observed pattern of brain results in a manner that was not anticipated or desired by the investigators. To control for this potential confound, an ANCOVA was employed.

37. A "peak activation difference analysis" is simply a test to see if the peak activation within a brain region (see comment 31) differed significantly between two experimental conditions (here, the Responsibility and Diminished Responsibility conditions).

(p = 0.98, Figure 2). These results, as well as those for aIPS (Supplementary Results, Supplementary Fig. 1), strongly support the notion that prefrontal and parietal activity is modulated by a punishment-related decisional process.

In addition to the peak activation differences, the timecourse of rDLPFC activity revealed an early deactivation (negative percent signal change from baseline) around 8 s post-stimulus onset. Importantly, this early deactivation ("dip") does not account for the peak activation results outlined above: the activation differences between conditions at the dip do not predict corresponding activation differences at the peak (correlation of subjects' activity differences between the Responsibility and Diminished-Responsibility conditions at the dip and at the peak: ρ = -0.19, p = 0.49; Supplementary Figure 3; see Methods). Furthermore, rDLPFC activity during "non-punished" Diminished-Responsibility and No-Crime trials strongly differed at the dip (p = 0.008) but not at the peak (p = 0.97), indicating that peak activation differences are not simply carry-over effects from differences during the dip.

fMRI Data: Punishment Magnitude

The finding that rDLPFC activity was higher when subjects decided to punish, in either Responsibility scenarios or in "punished" Diminished-Responsibility trials, raised the possibility that this brain region might track the amount of assessed punishment for a given criminal scenario. However, rDLPFC signal amplitude was not linearly correlated with punishment ratings (ρ = -0.33, p = 0.15; Figure 2D) in the Responsibility condition. This finding suggests that the magnitude of punishment is not simply coded by a linear increase in rDLPFC activity.

Although rDLPFC activity was not proportional to punishment amount, a linear relationship between peak BOLD amplitude and punishment magnitude

38. "Deactivation" in this context refers to the fact that BOLD signal in this region, at this particular moment in time, was lower (i.e., comparatively deactivated) after showing subjects the experimental scenarios.

39. s = seconds

40. Post-stimulus onset means after presentation of the experimental stimulus (scenario)

41. That between-condition activation differences at peak and at dip were not related to each other suggests that this region of the brain might be involved in two distinct activities at these different points in time.

42. Signal amplitude here is a synonym for peak activation.

43. Correlation is a statistical test to see if two variables are related. A linear correlation means that as one variable increases in value, so does another (positive correlation). Alternatively, a negative correlation refers to a relationship wherein as one variable increases in value, another exhibits a commensurate decrease.

44. The greek letter *rho* refers to the value of a statistical test for correlation (the Spearman test).

45. I.e., represented in the brain by.

46. See comment 25 for explanation of BOLD.

47. "Affective" is a psychological term of art, meaning "emotional."

48. A median split divides a set of experimental observations (here, punishment ratings) into two groups split at the median, such that the higher half of the set is in one group, and the lower half of the set is in the other.

49. This correlation suggests that subjects' emotional responses to a scenario correlated positively with how much punishment subjects will assign to the protagonist in that scenario.

50. See comment 4 for description of neural circuits.

was found in a set of brain regions that have been extensively linked to social and affective processing. To isolate such effects, we compared Responsibility scenarios with high punishment ratings to those with low ratings (median split by scenario across subjects; see Methods). The resulting SPM revealed activation in the right amygdala (peak Talairach coordinates 29, -7, -13; Fig. 4; Supplementary Figure 5) as well as in other brain regions commonly associated with social and affective processing (LeDoux, 2000; Phelps, 2006; Phillips et al., 2003; Price, 2005), including the posterior cingulate, temporal pole, dorsomedial and ventromedial prefrontal cortex, and inferior frontal gyrus (Supplementary Table 2; Supplementary Figure 4, Supplementary Figure 5). The association between amygdala activity and punishment magnitude was further demonstrated by a strong correlation between amygdala BOLD signal and punishment ratings across Responsibility scenarios ($\rho = .70$, $p = 0.001$; Fig. 4). However, punishment rating was not the only variable that correlated with amygdala function, as participants' arousal ratings yielded a similar correlation with amygdala activity ($\rho = 0.67$, $p = 0.001$), and punishment and arousal ratings were themselves highly correlated ($\rho = 0.98$, $p = 0.000001$). Correlations between peak BOLD signal and punishment ratings (and between peak BOLD signal and arousal ratings) also held for a number of the other affective regions, including ventromedial prefrontal cortex and posterior cingulate cortex (Supplementary Table 2; Supplementary Figures 4 and 5), indicating that the relationship between affective processing and punishment involved a distributed neural circuit.

Although the correlation between amygdala activity and punishment scores could be interpreted as evidence for a role of emotional arousal in the assignment of deserved punishment, it is also possible that such activity simply reflected subjects' emotional reaction to the graphical content of the

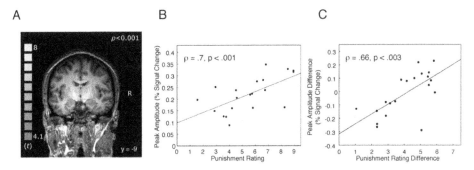

Figure 4   Relationship between punishment and right amygdala activity. A) SPM displaying the right amygdala VOI (rendered on a single-subject T1-weighted image), based on the contrast of BOLD activity between high and low punishment (computed from the median split for Responsibility scenarios), thresholded at $t(15) > 4.1$, $p < 0.001$ (uncorrected) for visualization. This amygdala activation survives correction for multiple comparisons, q(FDR) < 0.05; random-effects analysis. R = Right Hemisphere. **B)** Relationship between BOLD peak amplitude in the right amygdala and punishment ratings in the Responsibility condition. These two variables were significantly positively correlated (p = 0.001). **C)** Relationship between condition differences in right amygdala BOLD peak amplitude (Responsibility minus Diminished-Responsibility) and condition differences in punishment score (Responsibility0minus Diminished-Responsibility); these two variables are significantly correlated (p = 0.001).

scenarios rather than its involvement in the decision-making process *per se*. To avoid the potential arousal confound inherent to an examination of criminal scenarios that differ in graphic content (as was the case for our comparison of high vs. low punishment scores within the Responsibility condition), we examined the relationship between punishment ratings and amygdala activity after controlling for the possible confounding effect of graphic arousal. Because Responsibility and Diminished-Responsibility scenarios were equated for graphic content and differed only by the presence of mitigating circumstances (see Methods), the potentially confounding contribution of graphic arousal to amygdala activity in the Responsibility scenarios can be controlled for by subtracting amygdala activity in the Diminished-Responsibility scenarios from that in the corresponding Responsibility scenarios. If amygdala activity appertains to punishment magnitude rather than, or in addition to, emotional arousal

51. It is incumbent on the investigator to prove that their effects are due to their experimental manipulation, and not to other uncontrolled factors that could explain their results just as well. Such an uncontrolled factor that could potentially explain the results better than the experimental manipulation is referred to as a confound.

related to the graphic content of the scenarios, it should still track punishment ratings even after subtracting out graphic content differences in the scenarios. To this end, we created, for each pair of Responsibility and Diminished-Responsibility scenarios, punishment rating difference scores (Responsibility minus Diminished-Responsibility) and assessed whether these scores were correlated with the corresponding difference scores for peak amygdala BOLD signal. That correlation was significant ($\rho = 0.62$, p = 0.001; Figure 4), indicating that the magnitude of amygdala BOLD signal difference between Responsibility and Diminished-Responsibility conditions for a given scenario predicted a corresponding change in punishment rating for that scenario. Similar correlations were found in posterior cingulate and ventromedial prefrontal cortex (Supplementary Table 2). These findings suggest that activity within brain regions previously implicated in social and affective processing reflect third-party decisions about how much to punish, even after controlling for the potentially confounding arousal associated with the "graphic" content of the criminal scenarios.

52. In the discussion section of scientific papers, the investigators comment on the significance of their findings, place these findings in the context of the current scientific literature, address possible shortcomings or limitations of the study, and make suggestions for future studies.

DISCUSSION

The present findings suggest that the two fundamental components of third-party legal decision-making — determining responsibility and assigning an appropriate punishment magnitude — are not supported by a single neural system. In particular, the results reveal a key role for the right dorsolateral prefrontal cortex in third-party punishment. This brain region appears to be involved in deciding whether or not to punish based on an assessment of criminal responsibility. The only other brain region demonstrating a comparable pattern of responsibility-related activity (R>DR, R>NC, DR=NC) to rDLPFC was the anterior intraparietal sulcus (Supplementary Table 1, Supplementary Figure 1, Supplementary Results). This parietal region has been associated with a number of diverse cognitive functions including general response selection (Gobel et al., 2004) and quantitative numerical comparisons (Dehaene et al., 2003; Dehaene et al., 1999; Feigenson et al., 2004), which may hint at a role for this area in associating a specific action (punishment outcome) with a given scenario.

Our results also implicate **neural substrates** for social and affective processing (including amygdala, medial prefrontal cortex and posterior cingulate cortex) in third-party punishment, albeit in ways distinct from the rDLPFC. Specifically, while prefrontal activity was linked to a categorical aspect of legal decision-making (deciding whether or not to punish on the basis of criminal responsibility), the magnitude of assigned punishments for criminal transgressions **parametrically** modulated activity in affective brain regions, even after controlling for the potentially confounding arousal-related activity associated with the graphic content of the criminal scenarios. Our findings suggest that a set of brain regions (e.g. amygdala, medial prefrontal cortex, and posterior cingulate) consistently linked to social and emotional processing (Adolphs, 2002; Amodio and Frith, 2006; Barrett et al., 2007; Lieberman, 2007; Phelps, 2006; Phillips et al., 2003; Zald, 2003) is associated with the amount of assigned punishment during legal decision-making. As such, these results accord well with prior work pointing to social and emotional influences on economic decision-making and moral reasoning (De Martino et al., 2006; Delgado et al., 2005; Koenigs and Tranel, 2007) (Greene and Haidt, 2002; Greene et al., 2004; Greene et al., 2001; Haidt, 2001; Heekeren et al., 2003; Koenigs et al., 2007; Moll et al., 2002b; Moll et al., 2005), and provide preliminary neuroscientific support for a proposed role of emotions in legal decision-making (Arkush, 2008; Maroney, 2006). Our data concur with behavioral studies that have proposed a link between **affect** and punishment motivation in both second- and third-party

53. Neural substrates are brain regions that underlie a certain kind of information processing.

54. In this context, "parametrically" means that as the magnitude of punishment increases, so does brain activity in these regions.

55. Affect = emotion.

56. A common criticism of fMRI is that it is inherently correlational. Brain activity changes are *correlated* with changes in the independent variable, but one cannot say definitively that the independent variable *caused* those brain activity changes. Nor can one definitively say that the regions identified by this correlational approach are necessary or sufficient for the kind of cognitive process under study (e.g., legal decision-making).

contexts, and are consistent with the hypothesis that third-party sanctions are fueled by negative emotions towards norm violators (Darley and Pittman, 2003; Fehr and Fischbacher, 2004a, b; Seymour et al., 2007). However, it must be acknowledged that the present conclusions rest exclusively on correlational data. Thus, additional research will be required to confidently determine the contributions of socio-affective brain regions to third-party punishment in the absence of any graphic arousal confound. In particular, it will be important in future experiments to fully dissociate the factors of crime severity and arousal by employing task conditions that manipulate arousal without affecting crime severity. Furthermore, future research should also focus on determining how these affective brain regions interact with dorsolateral prefrontal cortex during third-party punishment decisions.

An additional concern in interpreting our findings, or any others based on simulated judgments, is whether they are relevant to real-world decision-making. After all, the punishment decisions made by our participants did not have direct, real-world consequences for real criminal defendants. Thus, it remains to be seen if our findings, generated by examining brain activation patterns during "hypothetical" judgments, will generalize to circumstances in which "real" punishments are made. However, there is some evidence suggesting that the hypothetical judgments made by our subjects may be a good proxy measure for real-world legal judgments. For example, post-scan debriefing of our subjects indicated that their punishment assessments were implicitly legal, with lower numbers corresponding to low prison sentences and higher numbers corresponding to high prison sentences (see Supplementary Table 3). Thus, participants appeared to adopt an internal punishment scale based on incarceration duration—a legal metric—when making their judgments, even in the absence of explicit instructions to do so. Further, we found that participants' decisions about punishment amount for each of the crimes depicted in the Responsibility scenarios were strongly correlated with the recommended prison sentences for those crimes, according to the benchmark sentencing guidelines of North Carolina, a model state penal code ($\rho = 0.8$, p < .0001; Supplementary Figure 6; see Methods). Thus, although our subjects were not literally applying a criminal statute to an accused individual, these data suggest that subjects' punishment decisions were consistent with statutory legal reasoning. However, despite these suggestions, further empirical studies are required to confirm our supposition that neuroimaging studies of simulated third-party legal decision-making can be valid models for understanding the neural basis of real-world legal reasoning.

Relative Contributions of Temporo-Parietal Junction (TPJ) and rDPLFC to Third-Party Punishment Decisions

The neural mechanisms of third-party punishment are undoubtedly complex, involving a dynamic regional interplay unfolding in a temporally specific manner. In particular, the decision to punish a person for his blameworthy act is generally preceded by an evaluation of that person's intention in committing that act (Alter et al., 2007; Carlsmith et al., 2002; Darley and Pittman, 2003; Darley and Shultz, 1990; Robinson and Darley, 1995; Robinson et al., 2007; Shultz et al., 1986). Such an evaluation ought therefore to activate brain regions that underlie the attribution of goals, desires, and beliefs to others, referred to as theory of mind (TOM) (Gallagher and Frith, 2003). One such region, the TPJ—a key node in the distributed TOM network (Decety and Lamm, 2007; Gallagher and Frith, 2003; Saxe and Kanwisher, 2003; Vollm et al., 2006) — might be predicted to serve this function during legal decision-making given recent evidence of its role in attributing mental beliefs in moral judgments (Young et al., 2007) and its involvement in dyadic

57. "Temporally specific," in this context, refers to the fact that legal decision-making likely relies on different brain regions communicating in specific ways *at very specific times* throughout the legal decision-making process.

58. "Node," in this context, refers to one specific brain region that participates as part of a neural circuit. In general, a circuit refers to two or more brain regions that interact cooperatively to enable some kind of cognitive function.

economic exchange games (Rilling et al., 2004). Given this context, it is noteworthy that the TPJ was activated in all of our conditions (Fig. 3). Furthermore, TPJ came online during the period when rDLPFC was deactivated (see Fig. 2B), a result that is consistent with the suggestion that temporoparietal cortex and dorsolateral prefrontal cortex operate within largely distinct and at times functionally opposed networks (Fox et al., 2005). Given this proposed antagonistic response pattern in the TPJ and DLPFC, we speculate that the early rDLPFC deactivation may reflect a perspective-taking based evaluation of the beliefs and intentions of the scenarios' protagonist, which is followed by a robust rDLPFC activation as subjects go on to make a decision to punish based on assessed responsibility and blameworthiness. However, the conclusion that rDLPFC's biphasic timecourse reflects an initial socioevaluative process followed by a decisional process must be viewed as tentative because the present experiment did not constrain the temporal sequences of evaluative and decisional processes involved in this task.

Moral versus Legal Decision-Making

The results of the present neuroimaging study underscore the conceptual relationship between moral and legal decision-making. Indeed, the general involvement of both the prefrontal cortex and affective brain regions in legal reasoning is reminiscent of their roles in moral judgment (Greene et al., 2004; Greene et al., 2001). Specifically, moral decision-making studies have indicated that regions of lateral prefrontal cortex and inferior parietal lobe may be preferentially involved in impersonal moral judgments whereas socio-affective areas (e.g. amygdala, medial prefrontal cortex and posterior cingulate cortex) may be primarily engaged during personal moral decision-making (Greene et al., 2004; Greene et al., 2001). Thus, both legal and moral decision-making may rely on "cold" deliberate computations supported by the prefrontal cortex and

59. Functional opposition means that as brain activity in one network increases, brain activity in another tends to decrease.

60. In the present study, TPJ is shown to be activated during a period when rDLPFC is deactivated, suggesting that they oppose each other. This opposition is referred to as "antagonistic."

61. Biphasic in this context refers to the fact that the early (deactivation) and late (activation) periods of the rDLPFC timecourse appear to be associated with different cognitive functions.

"hot" emotional processes represented in socio-affective brain networks, although the extent to which these two decision-making processes rely on the same brain circuitry remains to be determined.

While these findings serve to highlight an important conceptual overlap between moral reasoning and legal reasoning in criminal contexts, they do not imply that third-party punishment decisions are reducible to moral judgment. Indeed, while legal decision-making may in most (but not all) criminal cases have an essential moral component, there are crucial distinctions between morality and law (Hart, 1958; Holmes Jr., 1991; Posner, 1998). Perhaps the most critical distinguishing feature of legal decision-making, compared to moral decision-making, is the action of punishment—intrinsic to the former and secondary to the latter (Robinson, 1997). Although our participants likely engaged in the process of evaluating the moral blameworthiness of the scenarios' protagonist, our study was designed to investigate the neural substrates of a fundamental legal decision— assigning punishment for a crime—that is not a defining characteristic of moral judgment. Indeed, while moral decision-making studies to date have focused on assessing brain function during decisions about the moral rightness or wrongness of actions depicted in written scenarios, they have not specifically addressed the issue of punishment (Borg et al., 2006; Greene et al., 2004; Greene et al., 2001; Heekeren et al., 2005; Heekeren et al., 2003; Kedia et al., 2008; Luo et al., 2006; Moll et al., 2002a; Moll et al., 2002b; Moll et al., 2001; Young et al., 2007; Young and Saxe, 2008).

Neural Convergence of Second-Party and Third-Party Punishment Systems.
The prefrontal cortex area activated in the present third-party legal decision-making study corresponds well to an area that is involved in the implementation of norm enforcement behavior in two-party economic exchanges (peak Talairach coordinates of

62. Neural convergence is when a common brain region underlies two distinct, but related, cognitive processes.

63. Repetitive transcranial magnetic stimulation (rTMS) is a non-invasive technique that disrupts brain activity. In rTMS, a series of magnetic pulses are applied to a circumscribed region of the brain. These pulses temporarily interfere with brain activity in that region, creating a reversible "virtual lesion."

39, 37, 22 [x,y,z] for (Knoch et al., 2006; Sanfey et al., 2003); vs 39, 38, 18 [x,y,z] for the present study), raising the possibility that rDLPFC serves a function common to both third-party legal and second-party economic decision-making. In this respect, it is noteworthy that this region of rDLPFC is recruited when participants decide whether or not to punish a partner by rejecting an unfair economic deal proposed by that partner (Sanfey et al., 2003); this result is analogous to our finding that rDLPFC is activated by the decision to punish the perpetrator of a criminal act. Furthermore, while disruptive magnetic stimulation of this region impairs the ability to punish economic norm violations in dyadic exchanges (Knoch et al., 2006; van't Wout et al., 2005), this manipulation has no effect on norm enforcement behavior when the unfair economic exchanges are randomly generated by a computer instead of a human agent (Knoch et al., 2006). This result accords well with our finding that rDLPFC was much less activated when the scenario protagonist was not criminally responsible for his behavior, and supports the notion that this prefrontal cortex area is primarily recruited when punishment can be assigned to a responsible agent (Knoch et al., 2006). Finally, we still observed greater rDLPFC activity in the Responsibility condition (compared to Diminished-Responsibility scenarios) when we restricted our analysis to scenarios that only contained physical harms ($p < 0.005$, paired t-test), suggesting that the overlap of rDLPFC activity between studies of economic decision-making and the present examination of legal decision-making is not solely driven by scenarios describing economic transgressions.

The parallels between these previous findings and our current results lead us to suggest that the right DLPFC is strongly activated by the decision to punish norm violations based on an evaluation of the blameworthiness of the transgressor. This proposed function of rDLPFC appears to apply equally to situations where the motive for punishment is unfair behavior in a dyadic economic exchange or when responding to the violation of an institutionalized social norm in a disinterested third-party context. Of course, confirmation of this hypothesis will require further experimental evidence that legal and economic decision-making (and perhaps moral decision-making as well) rely on the same neural substrates. That said, this apparent overlap illustrates an important point: that the brain regions identified in our study are not specifically devoted to legal decision-making. Rather, a more parsimonious explanation is that third-party punishment decisions draw on elementary and domain-general computations supported by the rDLPFC. In particular, on the basis of the convergence between neural circuitry mediating second-party norm enforcement and impartial third-party punishment, we conjecture that our modern legal system may have evolved by building on pre-existing cognitive mechanisms that support fairness-related behaviors in dyadic interactions. Though speculative and subject to experimental confirmation, this hypothesis is nevertheless consistent with the relatively recent development of state-administered law enforcement institutions, compared to the much longer existence of human cooperation (Richerson et al., 2003); for thousands of years before the advent of state-implemented norm compliance, humans relied on personal sanctions to enforce social norms (Fehr et al., 2002; Fehr and Gachter, 2002).

EXPERIMENTAL PROCEDURES

Subjects

Sixteen right-handed individuals (8 males, age 18-42) with normal or corrected-to-normal vision participated for financial compensation. The Vanderbilt University Institutional Review Board approved the experimental protocol, and informed consent was obtained from each subject after they were briefed on the nature and possible consequences of the study. A brief psychological survey was also administered to

64. Because handedness can affect which side of the brain is used to process some kinds of information, group-averaged brain scan studies typically use subjects of one handedness or the other.

65. The Institutional Review Board (IRB) is charged with approving, monitoring, and reviewing human subjects research to make sure that subjects' rights are respected, and that research conforms with established ethical standards.

66. An experimental protocol is the specific "recipe" for executing a study. It details the process for recruiting subjects and running the experiment.

67. Subjects must provide "informed consent" to participate — that is, they must be fully informed about what to expect in an experiment, and what their rights are as a subject, before they are allowed to agree to participate.

68. Exclusion criteria are established reasons to exclude a subject from participating in the study.

69. That is, the protagonist's responsibility was either full or diminished (dichotomous), but he was described committing a range of crimes ranging in severity from simple theft to rape and murder (continuous).

exclude individuals who may react adversely to the content of the criminal scenarios. Exclusion criteria included history of psychiatric illness, being the victim of or having witnessed a violent crime (including sexual abuse), and having experienced any trauma involving injury or threat of injury to the subject or a close friend/family member.

Paradigm

In this experiment, subjects participated in a simulated third-party legal decision-making task in which they determined the appropriate level of punishment for the actions of a fictional protagonist described in short written scenarios. The principal goal of our study was to isolate the neural processes associated with the two fundamental processes of legal decision-making: deciding whether or not an accused individual is culpable for a given criminal act, and determining the appropriate punishment for that act (a parametric process based on the ordinal severity of a crime). Correspondingly, our design manipulated responsibility in a dichotomous fashion and crime severity in a continuous fashion. Each participant viewed 50 scenarios (some inspired by prior behavioral studies of relative blameworthiness (Robinson and Darley, 1995; Robinson and Kurzban, 2007)) depicting the actions of the protagonist named "John." The 50 scenarios were subdivided into three sets (complete scenario list available as Supplementary Methods). In the Responsibility set (N = 20), the scenarios described John intentionally committing a criminal action ranging from simple theft to rape and murder. The Diminished-Responsibility set (N = 20) included similar actions comparable in gravity to those in the Responsibility set, but contained circumstances that would often legally excuse or justify the otherwise criminal behavior of the protagonist. The No-Crime set (n=10) depicted John engaged in non-criminal actions that were otherwise structured similarly to the Responsibility and Diminished-Responsibility scenarios.

The No-Crime scenarios were included to assist in interpreting activity differences between Responsibility and Diminished-Responsibility scenarios (see e.g. Fig. 2).

Two groups of 50 scenarios were constructed and their presentation counterbalanced across the 16 participants (8 subjects received group 1 scenarios, and 8 others received group 2 scenarios) and across gender (equal numbers of men and women received scenarios from each group). The Responsibility set of group 2 consisted of group 1 Diminished-Responsibility scenarios from which the mitigating circumstances had been excised, while the Diminished-Responsibility set of group 2 consisted of group 1 Responsibility scenarios with mitigating circumstances added. As a result, the Responsibility and Diminished-Responsibility scenarios were counterbalanced across subjects, and differed only by the presence of mitigating circumstances. Thus, exactly the same scenario premises were used in constructing the Responsibility and Non-Responsibility conditions. Finally, the No-Crime set was identical in both groups of scenarios, and all scenario sets were equated for word length.

Participants rated each scenario on a scale from 0-9, according to how much punishment they thought John deserved, with "0" indicating no punishment and "9" indicating extreme punishment. Punishment was defined for participants as "deserved penalty." Participants were asked to consider each scenario (and thus, each "John") independently of the others and were encouraged to use the full scale (0-9) for their ratings. In the scanner but prior to the functional scans, subjects were shown five practice scenarios that were designed to span the punishment scale. Scenarios were presented as white text (Times New Roman) on a black background (14.2 degrees [width] x 9.9 [height] degrees of visual angle). Below each scenario an instruction reminded participants of the task instructions: "How much punishment do you think John deserves,

70. Two sets of complementary scenarios were constructed so that no individual subject viewed the same core scenario details (e.g., unlawfully taking a book) twice — once as a responsibility scenario and then again as a diminished responsibility scenario. This arrangement would increase the likelihood that subjects would consciously detect our experimental manipulation. If subjects become conscious of an experimental manipulation, they tend to behave differently — an experimental artifact referred to as "demand characteristics."

71. Word length is a potential confound. If the subject reacts differently to two scenarios that not only have different content but also different length, then the differences in brain function might be caused by differences in reading time, instead of content.

72. Functional scans refer to MRI scans that detect brain activity over time. In contrast, anatomical scans detect brain *structure* in detail, but without assessing brain *function*.

73. It is good practice in fMRI studies to give participants something to focus on in between trials in order to limit mind-wandering.

74. Researchers commonly want to avoid "order effects"— a confound whereby the order in which a condition type is presented (e.g. mostly R first or mostly NR first) creates response biases. It is also important to avoid "run effects"— a confound whereby certain trial types predominate in one run and are absent in another. To avoid both, we randomized trial types both within and between runs.

75. For a depiction of the differences between sessions, runs, volumes, slices, and voxels, see Box 2 (next page)

76. Emotional *arousal* measures how emotionally excited a subject feels. Emotional *valence* describes the direction (positive or negative) of that arousal.

77. Multiple regression analyses are standard statistical processes for disentangling the multiple influences of multiple variables. More specifically, they examine independent and interactive influences of multiple *independent variables* on a given *dependent variable*. (See comments 16 and 35.)

on a scale from 0 to 9 where 0 = No punishment and 9 = Extreme punishment. By punishment, we mean deserved penalty." Participants were instructed to make a response as soon as they had reached their decision.

Each trial began with the presentation of a scenario, which remained onscreen until participants made a button press response, or up to a maximum of 30 seconds. Participants then viewed a small white fixation square (0.25 degrees of visual angle) for 12-14 seconds (as stimulus onset was synched to scan acquisition [TR = 2s], while stimulus offset was synched to subject response), which was followed by a larger fixation square (0.49 degrees of visual angle) for two seconds prior to the presentation of the next scenario. Ten scenarios (four Responsibility, four Diminished-Responsibility, and two No-Crime) — selected randomly without replacement from the fifty scenarios — were presented in each of the five fMRI runs. Scenario identity and condition order were randomized for each run. The duration of each fMRI run was variable, with a maximum length of 7.33 minutes. The experiment was programmed in Matlab (Mathworks, Natick MA) using the Psychophysics Toolbox extension (Brainard, 1997; Pelli, 1997) and was presented using a Pentium IV PC.

Following the scanning session, participants rated the same scenarios along scales of emotional arousal and valence. They first rated each of the 50 scenarios (presented in random order on a computer screen outside the scanner) on the basis of how emotionally aroused they felt following its presentation (0 = calm, 9 = extremely excited). They then rated each of the scenarios, presented again in random order, on the basis of how positive or negative they felt following its presentation (0 = extremely positive, 9 = extremely negative). In these sessions, subjects rated the same scenarios they viewed in the scanner. The valence data were highly correlated with arousal ratings, and multiple regression analysis demonstrated that they did not

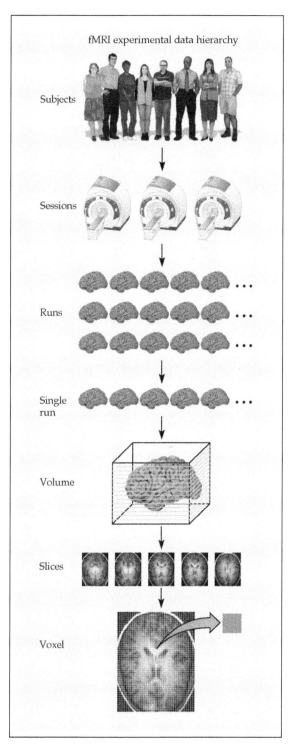

Box 2   (Accompanies Comment 75)
Reproduced by permission of Sinauer Associates from Scott A. Huettel et al., 2003.

account for any additional variance in punishment ratings that is unaccounted for by the arousal data. Therefore, the valence data are not further discussed in this manuscript.

Internal Scale Questionnaire

In a post-scan debriefing, participants were questioned about the internal scale of punishment they used during the scan. Specifically, participants were asked "what kind of punishment did you imagine?" for punishment scores of 1, 3, 5, 8 and 9. There was strong agreement among participants about their internal scale of justice. While low punishment scores (1, 3) were generally associated with financial or social penalties, greater punishment scores (5, 8) included incarceration time, with higher scores associated with longer jail times and, at the extreme (9), life imprisonment or state execution.

Relationship Between Punishment Ratings and Legal Statutes

To investigate the relationship between punishment ratings for Responsibility scenarios obtained in the present experiment and an existing, statutorily prescribed punishment for each of the crimes depicted in these scenarios, we coded each Responsibility scenario using the criminal law and criminal procedure statutes of the state of North Carolina. Among those states that have a sentencing statute, North Carolina's is widely considered to be both comprehensive and exemplary (Stanley, 1996; Wright, 2002).

For each responsibility scenario, we determined the crime(s) (such as larceny, involuntary manslaughter, or murder) with which John might reasonably be charged under the criminal code of North Carolina (2005 General Statutes of North Carolina, Chapter 14). We then determined, for each crime, the authorized presumptive sentencing range (such as 58 to 73 months in prison), assuming no aggravating or mitigating factors that could, under the statute, increase or decrease the authorized sentencing range

78. Debriefing is often an important feature of scientific studies involving human subjects, as it can help researchers understand the extent to which subjects' motivations and observed behavior matched the experimenter's expectations. In this case, the authors wanted to gauge precisely what subjects intended for a given punishment value, given that the scale (0-9) was by design subjective rather than objective and absolute.

(2005 General Statutes of North Carolina, Chapter 15A, Article 81). We then calculated and assigned to each scenario the mean for this range, in months. As the distribution of sentence values was highly right-skewed, we log-transformed (natural log) to create a normal distribution of sentence values (we verified that non-transformed data produced similar correlations as transformed data). For scenarios with multiple crimes, the averages for each respective crime were summed (whether this summed value or simply the mean value for the most severe crime depicted in a given scenario was used in the correlation analysis did not significantly affect the results). Where the upper limit of the sentencing range was life in prison, it was coded as 29 years (which has been estimated as the average time likely to be served by lifers newly admitted in 1997) (Mauer et al., 2004). Similarly, where the upper limit of the sentencing range was death, it was also quantified as life in prison (29 years). The log-transformed mean sentences for each of the 20 scenarios were then correlated with the group-averaged punishment ratings for these scenarios.

Statistical Analysis

Mean punishment and arousal scores and reaction times were calculated for each subject for each condition (Responsibility, Diminished-Responsibility, and No-Crime) and entered into a repeated-measures Analysis of Variance (ANOVA) using SPSS 15 (SPSS Inc. Chicago, IL) to determine main effects and interactions. Data from 16 subjects were used for all analyses. Punishment, arousal scores and reaction times were compared between conditions and post-hoc tests were performed using Fisher's Least Significant Difference (LSD) measure using an alpha level of .05. Two-tailed tests were used in all cases. For correlational analyses, data from Responsibility scenarios (N = 20) were averaged across all (N = 16) subjects. Examination of scatterplots for the correlation of rDLPFC signal and punishment

79. To work properly, some statistical tests require that the data have certain features (e.g., a so-called "normal distribution" of values). The authors applied a standard mathematical transformation to the sentence scores to permit the use of these statistical tests.

80. The alpha level defines an acceptable rate of "Type-I" error (the false positive rate). More specifically ".05" means, here, that the authors accept as significant only the statistical comparisons that they are confident have less than a 5% false positive rate.

81. This "Statistical Analysis" section details how the data were prepared before testing for relationships between fMRI signal, behavioral measures, and recommended sentence values. Such testing was accomplished via correlation analysis. (See comments 43 and 56.)

82. This section details the precise statistical test — a Spearman correlation, signified by the greek letter *rho* — used to examine relationships between fMRI signal, behavioral measures, and recommended sentence values. It also gives a rationale for using this test, as opposed to other common tests of correlation (like Pearson's).

83. Pearson's test — which uses the letter "r" to denote the value of its statistic — is another way to test for relationships between variables. It is more vulnerable to extreme values than the Spearman test.

84. This section of the paper describes the specific parameters that determine the characteristics of the signal that will be acquired from the brain using the fMRI scanner. Those parameters include such details as the number, thickness, and orientation of the brain slices from which this signal will be acquired.

85. 3D (three-dimensional). This refers to an image of brain structure, also known as *T1-weighted*.

86. Magnet strength is measured in units of Tesla (T), after Nicola Tesla (a prolific inventor and electrical engineer). For comparison, the Earth's magnetic field strength is around one twenty-thousandth of one Tesla.

87. Manual responses are typically recorded because speaking often moves the head (and hence brain) in subtle ways, interfering with the fMRI signal. Additionally, MRI scanners are very loud, making it impractical to record speech.

88. T2* (pronounced "tee-two-star") is a biophysical parameter. It describes an atomic phenomenon that is strongly influenced by the local physiological conditions within a small area of brain tissue. It is affected by the local magnetic environment. Changes in T2* between conditions allow the experimenter to contrast brain activity between conditions. With fMRI, what is really being measured is the biophysical phenomenon known as T2* relaxation. That is, fMRI detects differences in T2* relaxation between oxygenated blood (decreases T2*, increases fMRI signal) and deoxygenated blood (increases T2*, decreases fMRI signal).

89. A gradient echo pulse sequence describes the sequence of changes in the three smaller magnetic fields within the fMRI scanner. These smaller magnetic fields are used to create differences in magnetic field strength (gradients) between one end of the scanner and the other. These gradients are used in localizing brain activity. EPI is a customizable recipe that specifies the precise radiofrequency pulses to be used during the scan. It allows for the rapid collection of fMRI images.

suggested the presence of outliers. As non-parametric correlations tend to be more robust to outliers, we used Spearman's ρ to measure correlations between fMRI signal, behavioral measures, and recommended sentences. All correlations that were significant using Spearman's ρ were also significant ($p < 0.05$) when we employed Pearson's r.

fMRI Data Acquisition

High resolution 2D and 3D anatomical images were acquired with conventional parameters on a 3T Philips Achieva scanner at the Vanderbilt University Institute of Imaging Science. The visual display was presented on an LCD panel and back-projected onto a screen positioned at the front of the magnet bore. Subjects lay supine in the scanner and viewed the display on a mirror positioned above them. Stimulus presentation was synchronized to fMRI volume acquisition. Manual responses were recorded using two five-button keypads (one for each hand; Rowland Institute of Science, Cambridge MA). Functional (T2* weighted) images were acquired using a gradient-echo echoplanar imaging (EPI) pulse sequence with the following parameters: TR 2000 ms, TE 25 ms, flip angle 70°, FOV 220x220mm, 128x128 matrix with 34 axial slices (3 mm, 0.3 mm gap) oriented parallel to the gyrus rectus. These image parameters produced good T2* signal across the brain except in ventromedial frontal cortex, where some signal dropout was evident in all subjects (Brodmann area 11).

Each of the 16 participants performed five fMRI runs, except for two participants who could only complete four runs due to technical malfunctions.

fMRI Data Preprocessing

Image analysis was performed using Brain Voyager QX 1.4 (Brain Innovation, Maastricht, The Netherlands) with custom Matlab software (MathWorks, Natick MA).

Prior to random effects analysis, images were preprocessed using 3D motion correction, slice timing correction, linear trend removal and spatial smoothing with a

90. The parameters detailed here are basically standard. These are values that the experimenter feeds to the MRI machine to tell it how the brain images are to be collected. For example, 34 axial slices, 3mm thick: this tells the scanner how the investigator wants to cut up the brain — specifically, into 3mm slices, oriented in a particular plane, 34 slices of which together comprise an entire brain image volume. The 0.33 mm gap defines the distance that separates slices, so they do not overlap. TR: specifies how long it takes the scanner to acquire an entire volume of 34 slices. TR is important because it defines the lower end of the temporal resolution of scans. For example, if it takes 2s to acquire one volume, the experimenter can't claim to detect changes that occur at a rate that is faster than 2s.

91. This informs the reader about how the slices were oriented, using a known structural brain feature (the gyrus rectus) as a reference.

92. fMRI data are not immediately ready for analysis after being obtained from the scanner. Several image processing steps, known as "preprocessing," are required to make the images suitable for analysis (processing). This section describes those steps.

93. Random effects analyses allow for the generalization of results from one specific sample (e.g., the 16 subjects scanned in this study) to the population at large.

94. fMRI images are acquired in sequence over the course of many minutes, during which subjects often make slight head movements. These cause sequential images to become unaligned, with respect to the position of the head. Motion correction therefore reorients the images to account for slight head movements.

95. A single brain image (known as a "volume") is comprised of many sequentially obtained thin "slices" that are acquired over the course of anywhere from a few hundred milliseconds to several seconds (2 seconds in this study). While these slices are linked together and treated as though they were acquired at the same time, slight differences can exist between the slices due to minute differences in acquisition time. The slice time correction step "corrects" for these differences by slightly "blurring" the slices in a given volume over the total acquisition time.

96. fMRI signal changes that are unrelated to the experimental task can occur across the scan session. As one example, one scenario could trigger an emotionally arousing memory, which in turn elicits brain activity that is irrelevant to the task. These changes can obscure task-related signal, limiting the ability of the experimenter to detect an effect. Linear trend removal "removes" some of these task-independent signal changes.

97. To take into account anatomical differences between subjects that still remain after warping to a common space (see comment 29) each brain image volume is slightly blurred, a process known as smoothing. This prevents brain differences that are not meaningful from being interpreted as if they are.

98. This is a description of the degree of smoothing applied to the images. For fMRI, this typically ranges from 0-8 mm.

99. In a typical fMRI scan session, two types of images are acquired. "Structural" images provide a high resolution picture of brain anatomy, but give no information about brain activation over time. "Functional" images (also referred to as "T2*" or "epi" images due to technical details of how these images are acquired) provide a very good picture of changes in brain activation over time, but give very poor information about brain anatomy. *Coregistration* describes a process whereby a subject's functional and structural images are aligned or "registered" together. This aids the process of spatial normalization to a common space.

100. The material in this paragraph describes how the investigators compared brain imaging volumes between the experimental conditions to create a statistical map of fMRI signal differences.

101. In this context, each scenario for which subjects determine punishment is one experimental "trial." 10 trials comprised one fMRI "run" of approximately 7 minutes. 5 runs (50 trials) comprised one complete experiment.

102. *"Statistical parametric map"* (SPM) is the more precise term for a brain image in fMRI. "Pictures" of brain images, resulting from fMRI studies, are not akin to direct, photographic snapshots of brain activity. They are instead generated by a computer, using parameters defined by the experimenters to perform statistical comparisons of measured fMRI signal between experimental conditions. These statistical comparisons are performed in every single "voxel" in the brain. A "voxel" (a contraction of "volume element") is the smallest unit of resolvable measurement of fMRI signal. Voxel size is determined by the investigator and programmed into the fMRI scanner at the start of each experiment. In the current study, voxels were 3mm (on a side) cubes — a typical size for fMRI studies. Thus, investigators divide their subjects' brains into tens of thousands of these voxels for the purposes of localizing changes in brain activity between conditions. This means that for each subject, tens of thousands of statistical comparisons were performed — one statistical test for each of these 3mm cubes. The colors in a "brain image" represent the value of the statistical test in each voxel, with brighter colors usually meaning higher statistical values, and thus a greater difference in brain activity between two conditions. Our brain map is thus really a statistical map or — more accurately — a statistical parameter map. In this case, the parameter referred to is a t-statistic, as the investigators are using t-tests to compare activity between conditions.

6mm Gaussian kernel (full width at half maximum). Subjects' functional data were coregistered with their T1-weighted anatomical volumes and transformed into standardized Talairach space.

Responsibility Analysis

This analysis was performed to isolate brain regions that were sensitive to responsibility during punishment assessment. Signal values for each fMRI run were transformed into Z-scores representing a change from the signal mean for that run and corrected for serial autocorrelations. Design matrices for each run were constructed by convolving a model hemodynamic response function (double gamma, consisting of a positive γ function and a small, negative γ function reflecting the BOLD undershoot—SPM2, http://www.fil.ion.ucl.ac.uk/spm) with regressors specifying volumes acquired during the entire trial (stimulus onset to stimulus offset) for a given condition. These were entered into a general linear model with separate regressors created for each condition per subject (random effects analysis). We then contrasted the beta-weights of regressors using a t-test between conditions to create a statistical parametric map (SPM) showing voxels that demonstrated significantly increased activation in the Responsibility condition compared to the Diminished-Responsibility condition. Predictors for the

No-Crime condition were weighted with a zero (i.e. not explicitly modeled). We applied a False-Discovery Rate (FDR) threshold of $q < .05$ (with ($c(V) = ln(V) + E$)) to correct for multiple comparisons. Only activations surviving this corrected threshold are reported.

Volumes of interest (VOIs) were created from the suprathreshold clusters isolated in the above SPM at the conservative FDR threshold. The boundary of these VOIs were drawn from SPMs thresholded using a less conservative implementation of FDR ($q < .05$, $c(V) = 1$). The signal for each trial (event) included the time course from two TRs (four seconds) before stimulus onset to 13 TRs (26 seconds) after. Each event's signal was transformed to a percent-signal change (PSC) relative to the average of the first three TRs (0-4 seconds before stimulus onset). Event-related averages (ERAs) were created by averaging these PSC-adjusted event signals; separate ERAs were created for each combination of VOI, condition, and subject. These ERAs were then averaged across subjects for display purposes.

As subjects were instructed to make a response as soon as they had reached a decision about punishment amount, and in keeping with other neuroimaging studies of decision-making (Aron and Poldrack, 2006; Coricelli et al., 2005; Dux et al., 2006; Ivanoff et al., 2008; Rahm et al., 2006), decision-related activity should correspond to the portion of the time course that follows subjects' response. Given that mean RTs hovered around 12 seconds (mean, S.E. for: Responsibility = 12.69s, 0.46; Diminished-Responsibility = 13.76s, 0.46; No-Crime = 11.12s, 0.44) and accounting for a hemodynamic peak rise time of about 5 seconds post-stimulus (Boynton et al., 1996; Friston et al., 1994; Heeger and Ress,

103. As stated above (see comment 102) investigators perform tens of thousands of statistical tests. As voxel sizes are quite small, the brain is thus divided into many many voxels. Say, for example, that a brain is divided into 60,000 such voxels: that means that 60,000 separate statistical tests will be performed. If an investigator sets the maximum probability of false positives error to 5%, and 5% of 60,000 is 3000, with 60,000 statistical tests, and a p-value of p < 0.05, that means that an investigator could potentially have an "activation" of 3000 voxels due to chance alone. 3000 voxels, at a voxel size of 3mm, is very large, meaning that "activation" in an entire brain region could be a false positive. This problem is referred to as the "multiple comparisons" or "multiple testing" problem, and statistical corrections have been devised to account for this issue. The "False Discovery Rate" (FDR) approach is one such correction, and has been implemented in the current study.

104. Surviving a corrected threshold, in this context, means meeting the criteria for rejecting the null hypothesis — i.e., that there are no between-condition differences in brain activation within a given region — even after invoking the correction for multiple comparisons described above (comment 103).

105. In this context, VOI (volume of interest) and ROI (region of interest) both refer to regions of the brain within a statistical parametric map that the experimenters have selected for further, more detailed analysis.

106. "Clusters" are contiguous activated voxels. Suprathreshold clusters are clusters that survive a given corrected threshold (see comment 104).

107. This sentence describes the fact that the investigators have selected as VOIs, clusters that survive a certain kind of correction for multiple comparisons.

108. This is a method for quantifying the magnitude of experimentally induced BOLD signal increase. It is the percentage of change in BOLD signal, between the two experimental conditions, to which researchers attend.

109. BOLD signal changes during each trial are averaged across each trial type (e.g., here, in Responsibility trials) for each suprathreshold cluster for each subject. These per-subject averages are then averaged across subjects.

110. There is a lag between changes in brain activity and changes in BOLD signal. BOLD signal (see comments 25 and 31) takes about 4-6 seconds to reach its maximum following brain activity.

111. Brain activity that occurs around the time a punishment decision is made.

112. This describes how the investigators defined the BOLD signal peak — the precise time of the maximum increase in BOLD signal from baseline.

2002), then peri-decision activity should occur approximately 17 seconds after trial onset, which corresponds well with the time of peak hemodynamic response observed in rDLPFC (see Fig. 2). We therefore used the peak hemodynamic response as a measure of decision-related activity. To determine condition effects on BOLD signal within a given brain region, we then contrasted each condition's activation averaged across subjects by using paired t-tests applied on these peak estimates. The peak was experimentally defined as the single volume with maximal signal change from baseline between volumes 1 and 13 (2-26 seconds post stimulus onset). However, we ascertained that the same results were obtained when the peak was defined using a narrower volume range of 14 to 22 seconds post-stimulus (R>DR, $p = 0.00070$; R>NC, $p = 0.00025$, DR>NC, $p = 0.19$), or even when using a single volume 16s post-stimulus (R>DR, $p = 0.00023$; R>NC, $p = 0.00027$, DR>NC, $p = 0.84$). Thus, our rDLPFC peak activation results are insensitive to the temporal width of the analysis window.

Arousal- and Reaction-Time Equated Analyses

To determine whether activation differences between the Responsibility and Diminished-Responsibility conditions were driven by punishment assessment rather than any differences in arousal, these two conditions were compared after equating for arousal ratings. This was accomplished by deleting the six trials with the highest arousal ratings from the Responsibility condition for each subject. Time courses were extracted and peak differences were compared as above.

We also determined whether reaction time differences between the Responsibility, Diminished-Responsibility and No-Crime conditions affected the brain activation results by comparing these conditions after equating for response times. This was accomplished by deleting, for each subject, the trials with the highest reaction times for Diminished-Responsibility scenarios and the trials with the lowest reaction times for the No-Crime scenarios until the RTs across conditions (for each subject) were approximately equal (p > 0.1 for all paired *t*-tests between conditions). In addition, we compared rDLPFC activation between Responsibility and Diminished-Responsibility scenarios controlling for reaction time by performing a GLM analysis of covariance (ANCOVA) using the extracted rDLPFC BOLD signal and punishment reaction times for each Responsibility and Diminished-Responsibility scenario averaged across subjects.

Dissociation of Activation Peak and Deactivation Dip

To assess the relationship between early (~8s) deactivation in the rDLPFC timecourse and later (~16s) peak activation, we calculated peak and "dip" values for the Responsibility and Diminished-Responsibility conditions from each subject's ERA. "Peak" and "dip" were defined, respectively, as the volume with the maximal positive and maximal negative change from baseline. For each subject, we subtracted the Diminished-Responsibility peak value from the Responsibility peak value, and the Diminished-Responsibility dip value from the Responsibility dip value. Per-subject peak and dip difference values were then correlated via Spearman bivariate correlation in SPSS 15.

Laterality Analyses

To confirm the lateral specificity of Responsibility-related activation in right DLPFC, we extracted BOLD signal from the corresponding left DLPFC volume of interest (i.e. "x-mirrored" VOI, centered on talairach coordinate -39, 37, 22). We performed a two-way ANOVA with "Condition" (Responsibility, Diminished-Responsibility and No-Crime) and "Side" (Left and Right) as independent variables and BOLD signal as the dependent variable. Post-hoc comparisons between conditions in each hemisphere, and between hemispheres for the

113. This term of art refers to the process of "extracting" the underlying statistical information from brain images. This is often useful for performing more in depth statistical analyses.

114. SPSS is a widely used software application for performing statistical comparisons.

115. The same brain region as identified on the right, except on the left side (mirrored on the x-axis in the Talairach coordinate system, which separates left from right).

Responsibility condition, were performed using paired *t*-tests.

Punishment Rating Analysis

To identify brain regions that tracked the degree of punishment subjects assigned to a scenario, we performed a median split for punishment scores given during Responsibility scenarios. Based on the median punishment value for each scenario in the Responsibility condition across subjects, scenarios were separated into two groups, high and low. Design matrices and GLMs were constructed as above, with predictors for high and low scores for each subject specifying volumes acquired during Responsibility trials on which a high or low punishment score was given, respectively. We contrasted the beta-weights of these predictors using a t-test between high and low punishments to create an SPM showing voxels that demonstrated significantly increased activation during Responsibility trials in which subjects gave high (at or above the median) punishments compared to Responsibility trials in which subjects gave low (below the median) punishments. We applied a threshold of $q < 0.05$ False-Discovery Rate (FDR) to correct for multiple comparisons. Using a conservative implementation of the FDR correction technique $(c(V) = ln(V) + E)$, we did not find significant activation differences. We report activations significant at FDR $q < 0.05$, using a less conservative implementation of FDR $(c(V) = 1)$. The differences between the two implementations relate to assumptions about the independence of tests being performed on the data; both are valid for controlling multiple testing in functional imaging data (Genovese et al., 2002).

VOIs were created as described for the Responsibility analysis. The extracted peak activation values were used for a correlation analysis between punishment rating and BOLD response. Specifically, for each of the 20 Responsibility scenarios, the peak amplitude of the group-averaged ERA was computed, and the resulting value was correlated with the corresponding group-averaged punishment rating for that scenario. These peak values were also used in the between-condition difference score analyses.

TABLE OF CASES

GLOSSARY

Note: This glossary provides definitions for the scientific terminology used in the book. To find definitions of legal terms, we recommend using one of the many excellent and free online legal dictionaries. These include *Wex* (a community-built legal dictionary hosted by the Legal Information Institute at Cornell University Law School) and the dictionary.law.com web site.

acetylcholine (ACh) — A neurotransmitter with several functions. It is used in the connection from nerves to muscles to make them contract. It is also used in the brain to modulate the state of the brain when we pay attention, learn, and remember.

across-subject study design — An experimental design in which results are compared across two or more groups of subjects, each of which is tested on a different experimental variable. Also known as a *between-subjects study design*.

action potential — A brief (approximately 1/1000 of a second) change in voltage polarization, within a neuron, that is conveyed from the cell body to the tips of the axons, whereupon it can result in synaptic transmission; also known as a nerve impulse.

Adderall — A stimulant drug prescribed to treat symptoms of attention deficit hyperactivity disorder.

Alzheimer's disease — A progressive brain disease that impairs and then eliminates memory and thinking skills; also known as dementia. Named for Alois Alzheimer, who described a case in 1906. Usually diagnosed after age 60, though emerging techniques may enable earlier diagnosis in the future.

amygdala — The almond-shaped group of clusters of neurons located deep within the rostral end of the temporal lobe; considered part of the limbic system, it is involved in the processing of memory for emotional reactions like fear.

amnesia — A disorder of memory that has two types. Anterograde amnesia describes the inability to form new memories even with intact memory of prior events. Retrograde amnesia describes the inability to recall events that happened prior to sustaining injury or disease.

amphetamine — A psychostimulant drug that produces increased wakefulness and focus in association with decreased fatigue and appetite; colloquially referred to as "speed." Prescribed as treatment for attention deficit hyperactivity disorder under the name Adderall. The neural mechanism of action is primarily through the dopamine and norepinephrine systems in the brain.

analgesic — A drug prescribed to reduce discomfort associated with painful medical procedures or injury.

anesthetic — A substance that eliminates sensitivity to stimulation from medical treatments such as surgery. Local anesthetics eliminate sensitivity by blocking neural signals in one part of the body, for example, at the dentist. General anesthetics, also known as hypnotics, eliminate sensitivity through reversible loss of consciousness.

angiography — A medical imaging technique used to visualize blood vessels in the brain and other organs of the body; also referred to as arteriography.

angular gyrus — The area of the cerebral cortex at the boundary of the parietal and temporal lobes, located posterior to the supramarginal gyrus; it is involved in language, mathematics and cognition.

anterior — The area toward the front of the brain; synonymous with *rostral*.

anterior cingulate cortex (ACC) — A region on the medial anterior surface of the cerebral cortex that is thought to contribute to numerous behavior-monitoring and behavior-maintenance functions, including reward anticipation, decision-making, empathy, impulse control, and emotion.

anterograde amnesia — A loss of the ability to create new memories after brain damage or disease, while long-term memories from before the event remain intact.

antidepressant—A drug prescribed to treat symptoms of depression. Many such drugs are also prescribed to treat symptoms of anxiety.

antiepileptic—A drug prescribed to treat symptoms of epilepsy.

antipsychotic—A drug prescribed to treat symptoms of psychosis disorders such as schizophrenia. *Typical* antipsychotic drugs influence dopamine transmission. *Atypical* antipsychotic drugs influence serotonin transmission.

antisocial personality disorder—A disorder that is diagnosed when a person has a long-term pattern of manipulating, exploiting, or violating the rights of others; see sociopathy

anxiolytic—A drug prescribed to treat symptoms of anxiety. Many such drugs are also prescribed to treat symptoms of depression.

aphasi—A disorder of the comprehension and/or formulation of language caused by brain damage.

apnea—The interruption of breathing.

apraxia—This refers to an inability (short of paralysis) to produced skilled movements such as drawing, writing, or speaking.

arachnoid mater (or arachnoid membrane)—The middle of the three membranes (meninges) protecting the brain inside the skull; it is named for its web-like appearance.

astrocyte—The most common cell in the human brain, this type of glial cell contributes to the blood-brain barrier, providing nutrients to nervous tissue, maintaining extracellular ion balance, and repairing or scarring following traumatic injuries.

asystole—A state of heartbeat in which there is a "flatline"; it may be used by a medical practitioner to certify clinical or legal death.

autonomic nervous system—The subdivision of the nervous system that controls visceral functions including heart rate, digestion, respiratory rate, salivation, perspiration, pupil size, urination, and sexual arousal; its function is largely unconscious and involuntary.

axon—The fiber extending from a neuron along which nerve impulses travel to influence muscles, glands, or neurons in other parts of the nervous system; it constitutes the output end of a neuron.

basal ganglia—A collection of neuron groups deep in the brain that are involved in selecting which movements, thoughts, and emotions are expressed, and in learning to perform tasks automatically. It consists of the putamen and caudate nucleus (also known as the striatum), the globus pallidus, the subthalamic nucleus, and the substantia nigra.

baseline task—A condition used in neuroimaging testing in which subjects are required to do something very simple, such as visually fixate on a point. The brain state measured in this condition is used as a reference against which brain activation during more complex tasks is compared.

behavioral genetics—The interdisciplinary scientific study of the genetic contributions to behaviors of animals and humans through analysis of the inheritance of behavioral traits.

behavioral model—An understanding of how and why people behave as they do; in legal contexts, it is the basis for expecting that a change in the law will result in an intended change in behavior.

between-subjects study design—An experimental design in which results are compared between two or more groups of subjects.

biosocial criminology—An interdisciplinary field that employs both biological and environmental theories to explain crime and antisocial behavior, a departure from exclusively sociological theories.

bipolar disorder—A mental illness diagnosed by episodes of an elevated or agitated mood alternating with episodes of profound depression; also known as bipolar affective disorder, manic-depressive disorder, or manic depression.

block design—A neuroimaging testing procedure in which data are averaged to increase statistical power by having subjects perform the same task in "blocks" for periods of several seconds to several minutes. The design is most applicable for tasks that can be repeated over sufficiently long periods and it assumes that the brain states of subjects do not vary in meaningful ways over the long periods of testing.

blood-brain barrier—The separation of circulating blood from the extracellular fluid in the central nervous system produced by specialization of the capillaries and glia. It prevents objects like bacteria and potentially damaging molecules from entering the brain while allowing oxygen, nutrients, hormones, and certain other chemicals to pass.

blood-oxygenation-level-dependent (BOLD) signal—The main measurement currently used for fMRI. It is derived from the ratio of oxygenated versus deoxygenated hemoglobin that varies through changes in blood volume, blood flow, and oxygen extraction that are related to neural activity.

BOLD—See blood-oxygenation-level-dependent signal.

brain fingerprinting—A phrase coined by a for-profit company to market a controversial technique of measuring EEG event-related potentials for purposes of lie detection.

brainstem—The part of the central nervous system at the base of the brain as it becomes the spinal cord, consisting of a collection of various clusters of neurons that are essential for basic functions such as heart beat and respiration; also includes collections of axons traveling between the brain and spinal cord. It includes the medulla, pons, and midbrain.

brain plasticity—A term referring to a variety of changes that the brain undergoes naturally during development and in response to injury. Most dramatically, one part of the brain can acquire a function lost by another.

brain substrate—A term used to refer to a process in the brain that is thought to underlie and enable a particular cognitive process, such as perceiving or deciding. See *neural correlate*.

Broca's area—A cortical area in the left frontal lobe that is essential for production of speech.

Brodmann's areas—A numbering system for partitioning the cerebral cortex according to systematic variations of cellular structure and density; proposed in the early 1900s by a neuroscientist named Korbinian Brodmann. Although many details have been superseded by more recent research, the system remains useful today.

caudal—The area toward the back of the brain; synonymous with posterior.

cell body (soma)—The part of the neuron that holds the cell's DNA, produces proteins such as the neuron's neurotransmitters, and houses its energy supply and the enzymes controlling its metabolism.

central nervous system (CNS)—The brain and spinal cord; distinguished from the peripheral nervous system (PNS), which is comprised of the nerves in the body.

central sulcus—The main medial-to-lateral sulcus separating the frontal and parietal lobes.

cerebellum—Literally "small brain," it is a part of the brain tucked beneath the cerebral hemispheres on the back of the brainstem. It is essential for coordinating complex movements and body posture as well as learning and memory functions.

cerebral cortex—A 2 to 3 millimeter thick sheet of neurons and glia covering the cerebrum. It is necessary for perception, learning, memory, planning, acting, and feeling.

cerebrospinal fluid (CSF)—A clear fluid that is derived from the blood stream and circulates through the ventricles of the brain and spinal cord. It provides nutrients and immunological protection and cushions against traumatic injury.

cerebrovascular accident—Damage to the brain caused by occlusion of or excessive bleeding from blood vessels; also known as stroke.

cerebrum—The convoluted mass of neurons and glia forming the anterior and (in the higher vertebrates) largest part of the brain. Collectively it is thought to comprise the brain substrate of conscious mental processes (such as analyzing and deciding).

chronic traumatic encephalopathy (CTE)—A degenerative disease found in individuals who have been subjected to repetitive traumatic brain injuries, i.e., multiple concussions. At present, it can be definitively diagnosed only after death.

cholinesterase inhibitor—A drug or other substance that prevents the normal breakdown of the neurotransmitter acetylcholine, thereby increasing the duration of its action at the synapse; some can be toxic while others have therapeutic value. Also known as an acetylcholinesterase inhibitor.

cingulate cortex—The most medial part of the cortex, it forms a belt (Latin, *cingula*) that wraps around and is situated directly above the corpus callosum. Although different parts of the cingulate have functional specificity (posterior vs. anterior cingulate cortex), this continuous layer of cortex is grouped with other structures as part of the limbic system and has been implicated in different forms of emotional regulation, learning, and memory. Also referred to as cingulate gyrus (or simply, "cingulate").

classifier—An algorithm that has been trained to discriminate patterns of data. A Multi-Voxel Pattern Analysis (MVPA) classifier computes the probability that a particular brain state is associated with a specific condition, such as a stimulus, a response, or a disease. The algorithm can then be applied to brain activation patterns to infer whether a particular condition occurred.

closed head injury—A traumatic brain injury during which the skull and dura mater remain intact.

cognitive control—The deliberate, non-reflexive, non-automatic control of action, thought, and emotion necessary to respond flexibly to changing environmental contingencies. It is typically identified with the prefrontal cortex. Also referred to as executive control.

cognitive psychology—The scientific study of mental processes such as perception, attention, memory, intention, language, problem solving, creativity, and thinking.

coma—A state of prolonged unconsciousness in which a person cannot be awakened, does not respond to painful stimuli, light, or sound, lacks a normal wake-sleep cycle, and does not initiate voluntary actions.

commissures—Collections of axons that communicate between the two cerebral hemispheres.

comparison task—A task completed by a subject in a neuroimaging experiment that differs from the target task in a critical and informative manner; by comparison with the target task, it allows the researcher to make inferences about the localization of brain function.

compatibilism—A position holding that free will and determinism both can be endorsed without being logically inconsistent.

computed tomography (CT)—A neuroimaging technique in which X-rays of the head are obtained from all angles and mathematically combined to yield a three-dimensional image of the skull and brain.

concussion—A head injury producing a temporary loss of brain function, as evidenced by symptoms such as loss of consciousness or amnesia, headache, feeling confused, emotional unpredictability, and irritability, perhaps with sleep disturbances. Also referred to as mild brain injury, mild traumatic brain injury, mild head injury, or minor head trauma.

consequentialism—The philosophical position holding that the morally right act (or omission) is the one that will produce the best possible consequences; utilitarianism is an example of consequentialism.

coregistration—spatial alignment of a series of brain images collected at different times, with different methods (structural and functional), or from different individuals.

coronal section—A plane through the brain that is perpendicular to a line drawn from anterior to posterior. Also referred to as frontal.

corpus callosum—The largest collection of axons communicating between the two cerebral hemispheres, it has a distinctive bowed appearance in medial views of the brain.

correlation—A statistically significant relationship between two or more variables. Correlation does not necessarily imply causation, as the causal relationship between correlated variables is not always certain; distinguished from causation in which one variable is known to cause the other(s).

cortex—Refers to layered sheets of neurons covering the surface of a brain structure, such as the cerebral cortex or the cerebellar cortex; from the Latin "treebark," which it was thought to resemble.

corticolimbic system—The dopamine pathway originating in the midbrain and terminating in the frontal lobe that is involved in anticipating rewards, or other consequences of actions.

cranial fossa—The three large depressions in the posterior, middle, and anterior aspects of the floor of the cranial cavity in which the brain is positioned.

deep brain stimulation—Electrical stimulation of structures deep in the brain to treat symptoms of neurological disorders. The most common is stimulation of parts of the basal ganglia to treat symptoms of Parkinson's disease.

deep neural network—A computer system that converts arbitrary inputs into useful outputs through many stages of representation and transformation that are accomplished in layers consisting simply of nodes with input and output connections to the adjacent layers. The connections between layers are structured through a trial-and-error learning process, known as machine learning, that creates the useful mapping between inputs and outputs. (also known as convolutional neural network).

default mode—A characteristic brain state observed when an individual is at wakeful rest when no task is being performed. It consists of spontaneous, low-frequency correlations among particular cortical areas distinct from those that are active when individuals are responding to events and stimuli. Also known as resting state.

default mode network—A collection of cortical areas that have correlated patterns of activation when individuals are in the resting state, default mode. These include the medial temporal lobe, medial prefrontal cortex, posterior cingulate cortex, and ventral precuneus.

dementia—A loss of overall cognitive ability greater than expected from normal aging in a previously unimpaired person.

dendrites—Protrusions from the cell body of a neuron resembling the branches of trees that receive input connections from the axons of other neurons through synapses; it is the input end of a neuron.

depolarize—Change of voltage within a neuron that makes more likely but does not guarantee production of a nerve impulse that will result in subsequent synaptic transmission.

deoxyhemoglobin—Also known as deoxygenated hemoglobin, it is the hemoglobin protein without attached oxygen; it is influenced by magnetic fields, which provide the basis of the fMRI BOLD signal, and hence fMRI brain imaging.

determinism—A position stating that for everything that happens there are conditions such that, given those conditions, nothing else could happen; usually contrasted with free will.

diffuse axonal injury—Breaking or shearing the brain's long connecting nerve fibers (axons) caused by rapid movement and rotation of the brain against the skull.

diffusion tensor imaging (DTI)—A neuroimaging technique that uses MRI to map or quantify the integrity of axon fiber pathways in the central nervous system, based on the diffusion of molecules parallel to the neuron fiber pathways.

dipole—A physics term describing a spatial separation of positive and negative electrical charges; in neuroscience this occurs when elongated pyramidal neurons are activated. This is thought to create the electric polarization measured in EEG recordings.

disinhibition—A psychology term describing a lack of restraint manifested in several ways, including disregard for social conventions, impulsivity, and poor risk assessment. Disinhibition affects motor, instinctual, emotional, cognitive, and perceptual aspects with signs and symptoms similar to the diagnostic criteria for mania. Hypersexuality, hyperphagia, and aggressive outbursts are indicative of disinhibited instinctual drives.

dopamine—A neurotransmitter with modulatory actions of excitation and inhibition that contributes to control of body movements, thoughts, and emotions as well as reward. It is most concentrated in the basal ganglia, and drugs with abuse potential typically act directly or indirectly through the dopamine systems of the brain. Disorders of dopamine function are implicated in Parkinson's disease and schizophrenia, among other disorders.

dorsal—The area toward the top of the brain; synonymous with superior.

dorsolateral prefrontal cortex (DLPFC)—The broad expanse of the frontal lobe that consists of multiple areas that are essential for short-term memory, attention, forming and sustaining goals and plans, evaluating consequences, and self-control.

double dissociation—An experimental technique by which the function of two brain regions are dissociated by demonstrating that inactivation or damage in brain structure *A* impairs function *X* but not *Y*, and further demonstrating that inactivation or damage in brain structure *B* impairs function *Y* but spares function *X*.

DTI—See *diffusion tensor imaging*.

dura mater—The outer and most durable of the three membranes (meninges) protecting the brain inside the skull.

EEG—See *electroencephalography*.

electroconvulsive therapy—A brief electrical stimulation of the brain while the patient is under anesthesia, used to treat severe depression or bipolar disorder.

electroencephalography (EEG)—A neuroimaging technique whereby the variation in the magnitude and polarity of weak electric fields generated by neural activity in the brain are measured on the scalp. See *quantitative EEG (QEEG)* for analysis approaches.

encephalopathy—A disorder or disease of the brain.

epidemiology—The scientific study of the patterns, causes, and effects of health and disease conditions in defined populations.

epilepsy—A disease in which abnormally synchronized neural activity manifest as seizures. Some seizures involve violent contractions of the muscles, but other seizures involve loss of awareness of the environment. The frequency of the seizures can vary and progress unless treated. Causes can include brain trauma, drugs, or can be unknown, referred to as idiopathic. Treatments for epilepsy include drugs and surgery to remove the site where the seizure originates.

episodic memory—The memory for autobiographical events, such as times, places, associated emotions, and other contextual knowledge.

etiology—Generally, the cause(s) of a disease.

event-related design—A neuroimaging testing procedure in which data are collected while subjects perform multiple tasks organized into discrete, single-trial "events." which are presented in a random sequence. The order of task presentation may be random, as distinct from blocked designs, and trials may occur with variable inter-stimulus time windows (i.e., the time in between presentations may not always be the same). The generally acknowledged benefit of an event-related design is that it may allow for a more accurate capture of the brain's response to tasks and events.

event-related potential (ERP)—A measure derived by averaging an interval of electro-encephalography (EEG) or magnetoen-cephalography (MEG) signals synchronized on an event such as a stimulus or a behavioral response. Systematic variation in magnitude and polarity have been associated with particular aspects of perception, attention, memory, intention, response planning, and monitoring of consequences. Also known as evoked potential.

evolutionary biology—The scientific study of the evolutionary processes that result in the diversity of life on Earth, including in species-typical bodies and behaviors.

excitability—The fundamental property of neurons whereby they respond to electrical, physical, or some chemical stimulation by discharging a nerve impulse.

excitatory neurons—A class of neurons that immediately increase the probability of activity in the neurons to which they connect; this is accomplished by directly causing depolarization. Contrast with *inhibitory* and *modulatory neurons*.

executive control—See *cognitive control*. Also referred to as executive function.

false negative—Also known as Type II error, an outcome of an analysis that indicates that a particular condition or attribute is absent even though it is actually present.

false positive—Also known as Type I error, an outcome of an analysis that indicates that a particular condition or attribute is present even though it actually is not.

fight-or-flight response—The physiological response to a perceived harmful event, attack, or threat to survival. It involves activation of the sympathetic nervous system, priming for fighting or fleeing.

fluorodeoxyglucose—A radioactive form of glucose that is used in PET imaging to locate regions of the brain using more glucose.

fMRI—See *functional magnetic resonance imaging*.

folk psychology—A psychological theory that explains the causes of human behavior, at least in part, by mental states such as desires, beliefs, intentions, and plans.

forebrain—The term refers to the most rostral subdivisions of the central nervous system, consisting of the cerebral cortex and thalamus.

fossa—See *cranial fossa*.

frontal—The lobe of the cerebral cortex behind the eyes.

forensic psychology or forensic psychiatry—The specialized area of expertise that translates between psychological or psychiatric diagnostic information and the legal system as, for example, serving as an expert witness or doing competency evaluations.

forward inference—Addressing the question of which pattern of brain activity in which structures are associated or correlated with a particular behavior or mental state. Such results are rarely exclusive because associations with other behaviors or mental states are usually also observed.

frontal lobe—The most anterior lobe of the cerebral cortex that is necessary, generally, for planning, judging, and moving.

frontal lobotomy—Also known as prefrontal leukotomy, it is a discredited surgical procedure in which the nerve pathways connecting the frontal lobe to the rest of the brain are severed. It was used to treat major mental illness.

frontal plane—See *coronal*.

functional brain imaging—A general term referring to PET, fMRI, and in some senses EEG/ERP or QEEG.

functional decomposition—The conceptual breakdown of a task into its component operations, carving the task at its functional joints.

functional magnetic resonance imaging (fMRI)—A neuroimaging technique that measures neural activity indirectly by detecting changes in blood flow, oxygenation, and volume through the blood-oxygen-level-dependent (BOLD) signal derived from the magnetic properties of oxygenated and deoxygenated hemoglobin.

functional neuroimaging—See functional brain imaging.

gamma-amino-butyric acid (GABA)—The major inhibitory neurotransmitter in the central nervous system.

Galvanic skin response—The measurement of the electrical conductance of the skin that varies with its moisture level, which indexes the state of the sympathetic nervous system because it controls the sweat glands. Greater arousal will increase sweating and thus skin conductance.

general-linear model (GLM)—A statistical approach, used commonly in fMRI studies, that assumes that the BOLD signal is composed of the linear combination of different factors along with uncorrelated noise.

genotype—The genetic endowment of a cell, an organism, or an individual; often used to refer to a particular genetically-influenced trait under study or discussion.

glia—One of the major types of cells making up the nervous system; it outnumbers neurons 10 to 1. Key functions include providing physical sustenance and nutrition to neurons, immune protection, and sheathing axons in a coating called myelin that speeds nerve-cell signaling.

glioma—A tumor originating in the glial cells of the central nervous system, which impairs neural function and thereby produce symptoms related to the location of the tumor.

glutamate—The major excitatory neurotransmitter in the central nervous system.

grand mal seizure—A type of generalized seizure affecting the entire brain, more currently known as tonic-clonic seizure. In the tonic phase, lasting only a few seconds, the person loses consciousness and the skeletal muscles tense, often causing the extremities to be pulled towards the body or rigidly pushed away from it, which will cause the person to fall if standing or sitting. In the clonic phase the person's muscles will start to contract and relax rapidly, causing convulsions, ranging from exaggerated twitches of the limbs to violent shaking or vibrating of the stiffened extremities. See *partial seizure.*

gray matter—Organized clusters of neuron cell bodies and glia; the outer layer covering the cerebral cortex.

group-averaged data—Data that is averaged over a specified group, as contrasted with individual-subject data. Published neuroscience studies typically examine group-level data but have increasingly started to examine individual differences within that data.

gyrus (plural: gyri)—The rounded ridges of the brain surface separated by sulci.

hematoma—A pooling of blood in the brain outside of the blood vessels.

hemiplegia—Paralysis of the muscles on one side of the body. The most common cause of hemiplegia is stroke, damaging the connections between the cerebral cortex and the brainstem and spinal cord. The side of the body affected is opposite the hemisphere that is damaged.

hemodynamic—A term referring to blood flow.

hippocampus—The seahorse-shaped cluster of neurons deep in the medial temporal lobe; considered part of the limbic system. It is involved in long-term memory of events and locations.

homeostasis—The self-regulation processes that maintain critical physiological variables such as body temperature and blood acidity.

horizontal section—A plane through the brain perpendicular to a line drawn from dorsal to ventral.

Huntington's disease—A genetic neurodegenerative disorder that impairs movement and cognition. It is commonly diagnosed in mid-adult life with the classic symptom of uncontrolled large movements known as chorea, but also announced by mood swings and/or impaired cognitive functions.

hyperpolarize—Change of voltage within a neuron that makes less likely production of a nerve impulse that will result in subsequent synaptic transmission

hypometabolism—Abnormally low metabolism, used to reference brain regions that are not functioning normally.

hypothalamus—A set of diverse neuron clusters at the base of the brain that have several functions necessary for regulating blood pressure, body temperature, hunger, thirst, sleep and circadian cycles; with the pituitary gland, it regulates hormone levels.

impulse control—The ability to resist a temptation or urge, usually meant when consequences are likely to be negative.

incompatibilism—A position holding that free will and determinism cannot both be endorsed without being logically inconsistent.

independent component analysis—An analysis approach for fMRI that separates the BOLD signal into subcomponents based on the assumption that the subcomponents are statistically independent from each other.

inferior—The area toward the bottom of the brain; synonymous with ventral.

inferior frontal gyrus—The most inferior gyrus of the frontal lobe; it includes Broca's area and is also thought to be important for controlling behavior.

inferior temporal gyrus—The most inferior gyrus of the temporal lobe, it is involved in visual perception of complex objects such as faces.

inhibitory neurons—A class of neurons that immediately decrease the probability of activity in the neurons to which they connect; this is accomplished by directly causing hyperpolarization or preventing depolarization. Contrast with *excitatory* and *modulatory neurons.*

innervate—The projection of axons to a muscle, gland, or part of nervous system.

intermittent explosive disorder—A disorder characterized by expressions of extreme anger that are disproportionate to the situation. In the Diagnostic and Statistical Manual of Mental Disorders (DSM-5) it is categorized as "Disruptive, Impulse-Control, and Conduct Disorders."

interoception—Sensing the internal state of your body

intraparietal sulcus—A major sulcus on the lateral surface of the parietal lobe containing several areas that are involved in coordinating attention and body movements in space, and also high level cognitive operations, such as manipulating symbolic numbers and interpreting the intentions of others.

lateral—The area toward the left or right side of the brain; closer to the ears than the nose.

lateral sulcus—The major sulcus separating the temporal lobe from the frontal and parietal lobes. Also referred to as Sylvian sulcus.

local field potentials—Fluctuating electrical signals sampled in the brain by a small probe placed in the tissue.

L-DOPA—A drug given to treat Parkinson's disease; it crosses the blood-brain barrier and is transformed into dopamine, the neurotransmitter that is lacking in the brains of those with the disease.

lesion—In neuroscience, refers to a relatively localized region of damage in the brain often associated with particular mental and behavioral disorders; to "lesion" the brain is to intentionally disrupt a localized area of brain function.

limbic system—The collection of structures encircling the core of the brain involved in emotion, motivation, long-term memory, and olfaction. The limbic system includes the thalamus, amygdala, hippocampus, as well as other structures.

lobe(s)—Any one of the four large regions into which the hemispheres of the cerebral cortex are divided by major sulci; they have generally distinct functions.

local field potentials—Small electrical voltages associated with synaptic transmission among local groups of neurons in the brain sampled by inserting an appropriately designed electrically sensitive probe in the brain. This is commonly done in experimental animals but is progressively more commonly done in humans to treat disorders like epilepsy.

longitudinal fissure—The gap separating the two cerebral hemispheres.

lower motor neuron—Neurons in the brainstem or spinal cord that innervate the muscles of the face and body. Damage to lower motor neurons causes paralysis and muscle loss.

machine learning—Computer algorithms used to guide the structure of deep neural networks to usefully map outputs to inputs according to desired principles. Also known as deep learning.

malingering—Faking symptoms of mental or physical disorders for various motives such as avoiding work or school, obtaining drugs, gaining financial compensation, or receiving lighter criminal sentences.

magnetic resonance imaging (MRI)—A neuroimaging technique that provides images of interior brain structure through systematic variation of the magnetic properties of atoms in gray and white matter.

magnetoencephalography (MEG)—A noninvasive neuroimaging technique that records the small magnetic fields created by electrical activity in the brain.

medial—The area toward the center or middle of the brain; closer to the nose than the ears.

medulla oblongata—The caudal half of the brainstem that runs into the spinal cord; neurons therein are necessary for producing heart beats, breathing, and regulating blood pressure.

MEG—See magnetoencephalography.

meninges—The protective covering of the brain inside the skull consisting of the dura mater, the arachnoid mater, and the pia mater.

meta-analysis—The statistical combination of results from different studies with the goal of identifying patterns of agreement or disagreement among individual study results.

methylphenidate—A psychostimulant drug approved for treatment of attention-deficit hyperactivity disorder.

midbrain—That portion of the central nervous system between the forebrain and the pons consisting of neuron groups and axon bundles contributing to key functions that include movements of the eyes, vision, hearing, modulating motor control, responding to rewards, and arousal.

middle frontal gyrus—The large gyrus occupying the lateral surface of the frontal lobe; involved in forming plans and sustaining goals.

middle temporal gyrus—The gyrus occupying the lateral surface of the temporal lobe; involved in complex visual and auditory perception.

millisecond—One one-thousandth (1/1000) of a second; this is the duration of nerve impulses. Many brain processes occupy tens or hundreds of milliseconds.

minimally conscious state—A condition of severely altered consciousness that is distinguished from the vegetative state by the presence of minimal but clearly discernible behavioral evidence of self or environmental awareness.

Modafinil—A drug that promotes wakefulness.

modulatory neurons—A class of neurons that can increase or decrease the probability of activity in the neurons to which they connect for a prolonged period; this is accomplished by indirectly causing hyperpolarization or preventing depolarization. Contrast with *excitatory* and *inhibitory neurons*.

motion correction and realignment—An analysis method necessary for fMRI that corrects for incidental head movements during the scan.

motor systems—The networks of neurons in the brain that cause movements of the body. One motor system controls movements of the limbs through muscle contraction. Another motor system controls the glands, gut, and heart.

MRI—See *magnetic resonance imaging*.

multi-unit recordings—Sampling the impulses produced by a group of single neurons by inserting an appropriately designed electrically sensitive probe in the brain.

multivoxel pattern analysis—An approach to fMRI analysis that computes the probability that a particular pattern of BOLD activation across many or all voxels is associated with a specific stimulus, a response, or disease. See *classifier*.

myelin sheath—A white material derived from glia cells that wraps around and electrically insulates some axons; improves the speed of nerve impulse transmission.

myelination—The process during development of forming myelin sheaths.

natural selection—An evolutionary process, identified by Charles Darwin and Alfred Russell Wallace, by which different heritable traits become either more or less common in a population, over generations, as a function of the effect of those traits on the differential reproductive success of the individual organisms who bear them. Natural selection can lead to increasing complexity in body-plans and behavior, and it consequently can produce a tight "fit" between an organism and its environment.

near-infrared spectroscopy (NIRS)—A noninvasive functional neuroimaging technique, NIRS measures through the skull how wavelengths of light are differentially absorbed by the presence of various molecules in the blood that are related to neural activity, such as oxygenated hemoglobin, deoxygenated hemoglobin, and cytochrome-C-oxidase.

negative symptoms—The absence of normal behaviors or mental states that occur because of a disease or injury. Examples include paralysis following spinal cord injury, absence of facial expressions of Parkinson's disease, or apathy, lack of initiative, and flattened affect associated with depression.

nerve impulse—A brief electrical signal that begins at the cell body (soma) and travels to the tips of an axon where it results in synaptic transmission. Also known as an action potential, or colloquially as a "spike," because of its rapid occurrence.

neural correlate—A term used to identify a particular brain process that is supposed to instantiate a particular cognitive process. See *brain substrate*.

neuroimaging—The use of various techniques such as MRI, fMRI, PET, EEG, or MEG to directly or indirectly image the structure, function, and pharmacology of the brain.

neuron—One of the major types of cells making up the nervous system.

neuroprosthetic—A device through which electrical or other brain signals are detected or manipulated with external electronic and computer systems to enable abilities and treat disorders

neuroscience—The scientific study of the structure and function of the nervous system; includes experimental and clinical studies of animals and humans.

neurotransmitter—One of several molecules used by neurons to influence one another, neurotransmitters are stored within vesicles and released into the synapse whereupon they may bind to receptors on the dendrites of neurons.

nociception–The neural processes of encoding and processing noxious, painful stimuli.

nonindependence error—A form of circular reasoning that can confuse the interpretation of functional brain imaging data. The error arises when investigators perform statistical analyses to compare samples (like different brain regions) that were selected based on prior knowledge or suspicion of a difference. The selection bias contributes to the outcome of the analysis because the two steps are not logically independent. The non-independence error arises in fMRI when a subset of voxels is selected for an analysis, but the null-hypothesis of the analysis is not independent of the selection criteria used to choose the voxels.

norepinephrine—Also known as noradrenaline, a chemical that acts as both a hormone in the body and neurotransmitter in the brain contributing to arousal and alertness.

nucleus accumbens—A key structure for responding to rewards, located ventromedially in the brain.

occipital—The lobe of the cerebral cortex at the back of the brain. It is necessary for visual perception.

orbital frontal cortex (orbitofrontal)—The area of frontal lobe located behind the forehead and above the eyes; it is involved in olfaction, emotion, and guiding decisions based on rewards. It is sometimes considered part of the limbic system.

organic brain disease—A general term from psychiatry, referring to diverse brain disorders that cause impaired mental function but are distinct from psychiatric disorders.

organelles—A specialized subunit within a cell that has a specific function; it is usually separately enclosed.

oxyhemoglobin—Also referred to as oxygenated hemoglobin, it is the hemoglobin protein with attached oxygen. In contrast to de-oxygenated hemoglobin, it is relatively unaffected by magnetic fields, providing the basis for fMRI BOLD signal brain imaging.

paralimbic system—A collection of brain structures surrounding the limbic system including piriform cortex, entorhinal cortex, and parahippocampal cortex that has been implicated in criminal psychopathy.

parasympathetic nervous system—One of the two divisions of the autonomic nervous system (the other is the sympathetic nervous system); responsible for "rest-and-digest" activities occurring when the body is at rest.

parietal—The lobe of the cerebral cortex on the top of the brain; involved in the complex organization of perception and action.

parieto-occipital sulcus—The sulcus separating the occipital and parietal lobes.

Parkinson's disease—A disorder caused by the death of dopamine-generating neurons in the substantia nigra, a region of the midbrain. Early major symptoms include tremor, rigidity, slowness of movement, and postural instability. Later, thinking and behavioral problems may arise, with dementia commonly occurring in the advanced stages of the disease. It is diagnosed most commonly after the age of 50. No cure is possible, but effective treatments include the Levo-dopa

drug, deep brain stimulation, and lesions of particular parts of the basal ganglia.

partial seizure—An epileptic seizure that affects only part of the brain, with symptoms varying according to the location and extent of the brain that is affected. Also known as focal seizure. See *grand mal seizure.*

peripheral nervous system—The nerves and somas in the body outside of the brain and spinal cord that connect the central nervous system to the limbs and organs.

PET—See *positron emission tomography.*

phenotype—An organism's observable characteristics or traits, such as its body shape and coloring, as well as development, biochemical, or physiological properties; can also refer to behavior and products of behavior (such as a spider's web). Phenotypes result from the expression of an organism's genes, as well as from the influence of environmental factors and the interactions between the two.

pia mater—The innermost and most delicate of the three membranes (meninges) protecting the brain inside the skull; it contains the cerebrospinal fluid to protect the brain and spinal cord.

pituitary gland—The endocrine gland located ventral to the hypothalamus at the base of the brain; it secretes hormones that regulate homeostasis.

plasticity—The capacity of the brain to adapt to injury and experience by changing excitability, altering the shape (structure), or changing the characteristic responses of groups of neurons.

pons—The part of the brain stem between the midbrain and medulla and ventral to the cerebellum. It consists of axon bundles passing between the cerebral cortex and the cerebellum. It also consists of neuron groups necessary for sleep, respiration, swallowing, bladder control, hearing, equilibrium, taste, eye movements, facial expressions, facial sensation, and posture.

positive symptoms—The presence of abnormal behaviors or mental states that occur because of a disease or injury. Examples include the tremors of Parkinson's disease or the delusions and hallucinations of schizophrenia.

positron emission tomography (PET)—An imaging technique that produces a three-dimensional image of functional processes in the body by detecting pairs of gamma rays emitted indirectly by a positron-emitting tracer that is injected into the body on a biologically active molecule. Metabolically active tissue can be located using fludeoxyglucose (FDG).

postcentral gyrus—The gyrus caudal to the central sulcus; involved in sense of touch and limb position.

posterior—The area toward the back of the brain; synonymous with caudal.

post-traumatic stress disorder (PTSD)—A type of anxiety disorder that can occur after exposure to an extreme emotional trauma. It is diagnosed when a group of symptoms—such as disturbing recurring flashbacks, avoidance, or numbing of memories of the event—as well as high levels of anxiety, continue for more than a month after the traumatic event.

precentral gyrus—The gyrus rostral to the central sulcus; contains the primary motor cortex that is necessary for fine motor control of the limbs, fingers, and vocal apparatus.

precuneus—The portion of the superior parietal lobule on the medial surface of each hemisphere. It contributes to episodic memory, visuospatial processing, and self-awareness.

prefrontal cortex—The portion of the frontal lobe that lies rostral to the premotor and motor cortex; contributes to planning and controlling thought and behavior.

premotor area—A large area of the cerebral cortex rostral to the primary motor cortex; involved in the organization of complex body movements in response to arbitrary stimuli such as verbal instructions.

preoccipital notch—A landmark in the cerebral cortex used to define the boundary of the occipital lobe.

primary motor area—The area of the cerebral cortex in the precentral gyrus that is necessary for fine motor control of the limbs, fingers, and vocal apparatus.

primary auditory cortex—The cortical area in the temporal lobe that first processes auditory signals.

primary somatosensory cortex—The cortical area in the parietal lobe that first processes tactile, somatosensory signals.

primary visual cortex—The cortical area in the occipital lobe that first processes visual signals.

prosocial—A behavior intended to benefit other people in one's social group or society as a whole.

proximate cause—In fields such as biology and evolutionary psychology, one of two concurrently operating kinds of causes. (The other is *ultimate cause*.) Proximate causes are "how" causes, involving the immediate mechanistic logistics of physiology and biochemistry, as well as an organism's unique developmental history, that lead to particular behavioral outcomes. In law, a proximate cause is a cause without which the harm would not occur, and that directly, without a superseding cause, produces the harm.

psychedelic—A drug taken usually recreationally that can cause altered states of consciousness including hallucinations.

psychoactive drugs—Drugs that affect mental processes of perception, thinking, memory, and feeling.

psychomotor—Referring to the origination of movement in conscious mental activity.

psychopathy—A personality disorder characterized by enduring anti-social behavior, a diminished capacity for empathy or remorse, and poor control of behavior. In the Diagnostic and Statistical Manual of Mental Disorders (DSM-5) it is categorized as "Antisocial (Dissocial) Personality Disorder."

psychophysiology—A scientific specialization concerned primarily with relating psychological states with physiological measures, such as galvanic skin response, EEG, QEEG, event-related potentials, and more recently MEG.

psychostimulant—A drug taken usually recreationally that increases arousal, cognition, and behavior.

receptor—In neuroscience, refers to a protein to which neurotransmitters bind and thereby produce changes, such as opening ion channels or activating chemical cascades.

QEEG—See *quantitative electroencephalography*.

quantitative electroencephalography (QEEG)—The computerized analysis that separates the EEG recorded on the scalp into wave frequency components; also known as Brain Electrical Activity Mapping (BEAM).

reflex—An involuntary and nearly instantaneous movement in response to a stimulus, e.g. the rotation of the eyes that compensate for rotation of the head.

region of interest—A location or structure in the brain that is identified for some purpose by prior knowledge of anatomy of function or by statistical analysis of brain imaging data. A region of interest could be a location where activation occurs during performance of some task or where a disease process or injury has impaired function.

reinforcement—During learning, an object or stimulus that changes the likelihood that a behavior will occur. A reinforcement is defined by the effect that it has on behavior. Positive reinforcements (such as sweets, for instance) tend to increase or strengthen a behavior. Negative reinforcements (like aversive shocks or sounds, for instance) tend to decrease or weaken a behavior.

repetitive TMS—Repetitive transcranial magnetic stimulation, noninvasive electromagnetic stimulation with sequences of pulses, which is distinguished from single pulse TMS.

resting state—See *default mode.*

reticular formation—The region in the brainstem consisting of multiple distinct networks that maintain posture and balance, control heart rate and blood pressure, modulate pain sensitivity, regulate arousal and the sleep-wake cycle, and habituate to irrelevant background stimuli.

retributivism—A theory of criminal justice that advocates punishment based on what a criminal morally "deserves"; contrasted with utilitarian justifications for punishment.

retrograde amnesia—The loss of memory for events that occurred, or information that was learned before an injury or the beginning of a disease.

reverse inference—Addressing the question of which behavior or mental state is occurring based on a pattern of brain activity in particular structures. Such conclusions are limited by the fact that associations of brain activity with behaviors and mental states are rarely exclusive.

rostral—The area toward the front of the brain; synonymous with anterior.

sagittal section—A plane through the brain that is perpendicular to a line drawn from medial to lateral.

salience network—A group of cortical areas that coordinates the selection of which emotional and sensory stimuli are deserving of attention and the switching between internally directed cognition and externally directed cognition. It includes the anterior insula and dorsal anterior cingulate cortex.

schizophrenia—A mental disorder in which thought is confused and emotions are blunted or unusual. Positive symptoms include delusions, paranoia, auditory hallucinations, and disorganized thinking and speech. Negative symptoms include flat or blunted emotion, poverty of speech, inability to experience pleasure, lack of desire to form relationships, and lack of motivation. Associated with significant social or vocational dysfunction. Onset of symptoms occurs usually in young adulthood. Diagnosis is based on observed behavior and the patient's reported experiences.

selective serotonin reuptake inhibitor (SSRI)—A class of drugs that are supposed to increase the concentration of serotonin in synapses by inhibiting its reuptake into the presynaptic axon terminal; prescribed to treat depression, anxiety, and some personality disorders.

sensitivity—A measure of the fraction of actual positive cases that are correctly identified as such by a diagnostic test; for example, the percentage of liars who are correctly identified as being liars by a lie detection test.

serotonin—A modulatory neurotransmitter, known formally as 5-hydroxytryptamine or 5-HT, that has been linked to mood, appetite, and sleep. Many antidepressant medications (selective serotonin reuptake inhibitors, or SSRIs) act by increasing activity at serotonin receptors.

sham rage—Exceptionally aggressive behaviors in experimental animals elicited by stimulation or other manipulation of particular parts of the limbic system of the brain.

single-photon emission computed tomography (SPECT)—An imaging technique in which a radioactively labeled molecule is administered to a subject. Unlike the more expensive PET technique, SPECT detects only the emission of single photons resulting in less spatial resolution than PET.

single-unit recordings—Sampling the impulses produced by a single neuron by inserting an appropriately designed electrically sensitive probe in the brain. This is commonly done in experimental animals but is progressively more commonly done in humans to treat disorders like epilepsy.

sinus—Generally referring to cavity in bone or tissue, in neuroscience it refers to a channel formed by dura mater through which blood flows back to the heart.

size normalization—A step of fMRI analysis that adjusts for differences in the sizes of brains across individuals.

skin conductance response (SCR)—The measurement of the electrical conductance of the skin that varies with its moisture level, which indexes the state of the sympathetic nervous system, because it controls the sweat glands. Greater arousal increases sweating, and thus skin conductance. Also known as galvanic skin response (GSR), electrodermal response (EDR), psychogalvanic reflex (PGR), skin conductance response (SCR), or skin conductance level (SCL).

slice-timing correction—A step in fMRI data analysis that accounts for the timing of scanning across slices through the brain (each slice being acquired at a slightly different moment of time compared to those immediately before and after it).

sociopathy—More formally known as antisocial personality disorder, which is diagnosed when a person has a long-term pattern of manipulating, exploiting, or violating the rights of others, often in a criminal fashion.

soma—See *cell body*.

somatic marker theory—A theory formulated by neuroscientist Antonio Damasio to explain how decisions can be guided or influenced by emotional states called somatic markers.

spatial smoothing—A step of fMRI analysis that evens out variation of the signal across voxels in the brain that is considered incidental noise.

specificity—A measure of the fraction of actual negative cases that are correctly identified, e.g. the percentage of innocent people who are correctly identified as being innocent.

SPECT—See *single-photon emission computed tomography*.

spinal cord—The long extension of the central nervous system into the spine consisting of axons running to and from muscles, joints, skin, and gut, as well as specialized neuron groups involved in sensory signaling and muscle contractions.

statistical significance—Generally, a calculation of the extent to which a relationship between two samples that include some amount of random variability is judged to be not due to chance.

structural magnetic resonance imaging—A noninvasive method that provides images of the internal structure of the brain; useful for quantifying variation in brain structure and locating focused brain damage.

subcortical—Referring to brain structures beneath the cerebral cortex.

subtraction technique—An approach to analyzing functional brain imaging data whereby activation in a baseline condition is subtracted from activation in a test condition. The resulting pattern of differences in activation is supposed to reveal regions contributing to the processes required to perform the test condition.

sulcus (plural sulci)—A furrow or groove formed by the folding of the cerebral cortex into gyri.

supplementary motor area (SMA)—An area of the medial frontal lobe rostral to the primary motor area that is involved in production of voluntary body movements; the rostral portion may also be distinguished as preSMA.

superior—The area toward the top of the brain; synonymous with dorsal.

superior parietal lobule—The most dorsal-medial region of the parietal lobe bounded by the occipital lobe and the intraparietal sulcus; involved in orienting movements in space.

superior frontal gyrus—The most dorsal-medial region of the frontal lobe; its functions are not well understood but involve very high level cognition, such as long-term planning.

superior temporal gyrus—The most dorsal gyrus of the temporal lobe, consisting of several cortical areas; involved in auditory perception and speech comprehension.

supramarginal gyrus—A region at the intersection of the parietal and temporal lobes; in the left hemisphere it includes Wernicke's area. It is important for speech comprehension.

Sylvian sulcus—The major sulcus separating the temporal lobe from the frontal and parietal lobes; also referred to as lateral sulcus. Also known as Sylvian fissure.

sympathetic nervous system—One of the two divisions of the autonomic nervous system (the other is the parasympathetic nervous system); responsible primarily for fight-or-flight response.

synapse—The specialized microscopic structure where the axon of one neuron contacts part of the dendrite or soma of another neuron; at this point synaptic transmission can occur. Synapses are also formed on muscles and glands.

synaptic cleft—Small gap between axon and dendrite in which synaptic transmission occurs.

synaptic plasticity—Processes occurring during brain development, during learning, and in response to injury whereby neural circuits change configuration to adapt to new situations.

synaptic pruning—The process that occurs during brain development whereby excessive synapses are removed through patterns of lack of use.

synaptic transmission—The means of communication between neurons through the release of small chemicals called neurotransmitters that either increase, decrease, or modulate the excitability of neurons.

temporal lobe—Refers to the lobe of the brain ventral to the lateral sulcus; involved in auditory perception, including speech comprehension, visual perception of complex objects, and memory.

temporal resolution—Refers to the amount of time it takes to acquire an image, e.g. high temporal resolution means that images can be obtained very quickly in succession.

temporoparietal junction—An area at the boundary of the temporal and parietal lobes that contributes to high level cognitive functions, including theory of mind.

teratogen—An agent or factor that causes malformation of an embryo during development.

Tesla—The unit of measure of the strength of magnets. fMRI measurements can be done with 1.5T magnets, but more usually 3T. Some research now use 7T and even stronger. The Earth's magnetic field is around 40 millionths of a Tesla.

thalamus—A bulb-shaped mass, about the size of a walnut, containing several subgroups of neurons located in the middle of the brain beneath the cerebral hemispheres and above the midbrain. Its subgroups relay signals to the cerebral cortex from sensory inputs and other brain centers. Whether the signals are transformed, filtered, or just relayed is uncertain.

theory of mind—The ability to attribute mental states such as knowledge, beliefs, intentions, and desires to oneself and others, including appreciation that the knowledge, beliefs, intentions, and desires of other people may differ from one's own.

traumatic brain injury (TBI)—The disruption of normal brain function caused by either a collision of the head with another object (non-penetrating, closed) or the piercing or puncturing of the skull and brain by an object (penetrating, open). Severity can range from "mild," i.e., a brief change in mental status or consciousness, to "severe," i.e., an extended period of unconsciousness or amnesia. Mild TBI is also known as a concussion.

transcranial direct current stimulation (TDCS)—A noninvasive technique for manipulating brain function by delivering weak continuous current to a part of the brain through the scalp.

transcranial magnetic stimulation (TMS)—A noninvasive technique for manipulating brain function by delivering strong magnetic pulses close to the surface of the scalp that facilitate or attenuate neural activity in a localized region.

trial—As used in the context of a scientific experiment, a trial refers to a single instance of performing an experimental test. For instance, to test your memory for faces, you would be presented with images of different familiar and unfamiliar people and asked to identify them. Each presentation and response is a trial. As used in the context of clinical trial, a trial refers to the process of testing (through a randomized controlled experiment) whether a particular drug or other treatment is effective. These two uses are distinct from the use of trial in the context of the law, where it refers to a legal proceeding in which a fact-finder (judge or jury) decides the legal outcome of a criminal or civil matter.

ultimate cause—In fields such as biology and evolutionary psychology, one of two concurrently operating kinds of causes. (The other is *proximate cause*.) Ultimate causes are the "why" causes, involving the aggregate reproductive consequences of behavior over evolutionary time. Explanations of ultimate cause are consequently historical, involving adaptation by natural selection over many generations. Understanding ultimate causes helps to explain, for instance, why specific environmental stimuli tend to yield predictable behaviors within a species.

upper motor neuron—neurons in the cerebral cortex that innervate neurons in the brainstem or spinal cord. Damage to upper motor neurons causes paralysis with increased muscle tension.

utilitarianism—An ethical theory asserting that the morally right action is that which maximizes "utility" (often translated as maximizing human happiness and minimizing human suffering). In the context of punishment, a utilitarian approach imposes punishment, and kinds of punishment, when the benefits to society outweigh the pain, fear, and public expense.

vegetative state—A state of consciousness characterized by preserved sleep–wakefulness cycle and intact subcortical functions, on the one hand, and the complete lack of subjective awareness, on the other hand. It is a chronic condition that can persist for years. With time, the chance to regain consciousness decreases, but cases of patients emerging have been reported.

venous drainage system—The system of veins and channels formed by dura mater through which de-oxygenated blood is removed from the brain and returned to the circulatory system through the jugular veins.

ventral—The area toward the bottom of the brain; synonymous with inferior.

ventrolateral prefrontal cortex (VLPFC)—A general region of the frontal lobe that has been identified with complex cognitive functions.

ventromedial prefrontal cortex—A general region of the frontal lobe that has been identified with control of complex decision making.

vesicle—A microscopic sphere containing neurotransmitters that are produced in the cell body and transported to the ends of axons, where they can be released into the synapse.

voxel—A three-dimensional volume element (volumetric pixel) that is the unit of MRI reconstruction; frequently 3 millimeters cubed, though other volumes are sometimes used.

Wernicke's area—A region near the caudal end of the left temporal lobe, around the supramarginal gyrus, that is important for speech comprehension

white matter—The axons passing between the cerebral cortex and other neuron groups; the white appearance is because of the myelin sheaths surrounding the axons.

within-subjects design—An experiment in which results are compared between two or more tasks that each subject performs to test different experimental variables.

x-ray—An electromagnetic wave with high energy and very short wavelength enabling it to pass through many materials opaque to light, making it useful for viewing the internal composition of something, such as the interior of the body.

AUTHOR & NAME INDEX